INTEGRATIVE MEDICINE

INTEGRATIVE MEDICINE

Principles for Practice

BENJAMIN KLIGLER, MD, MPH

Assistant Professor of Family Medicine
Albert Einstein College of Medicine
Bronx, New York
Research Director and Co-Director
Integrative Medicine Fellowship
Center for Health & Healing
Beth Israel Medical Center
New York, New York

and

ROBERTA LEE, MD

Medical Director and Co-Director
Integrative Medicine Fellowship
Center for Health & Healing
Beth Israel Medical Center
New York, New York
Diplomate, Program in Integrative Medicine
University of Arizona
Tucson, Arizona

McGraw-Hill
MEDICAL PUBLISHING DIVISION

New York   Chicago   San Francisco   Lisbon   London   Madrid   Mexico City
Milan   New Delhi   San Juan   Seoul   Singapore   Sydney   Toronto

The **McGraw·Hill** Companies

Integrative Medicine: Principles for Practice

1234567890   DOC DOC 0987654

ISBN 0-07-140239-X

This book was set in Garamond Light by Atlis Graphics
The editors were Andrea Seils and Karen Davis.
The production supervisor was Catherine H. Saggese.
The cover designer was Aimée Nordin.
The index was prepared by Marilyn Rowland.
RR Donnelley was printer and binder.

This book is printed on acid-free paper.

Library of Congress Cataloging-in-Publication Data

Integrative medicine / edited by Benjamin Kligler, Roberta A. Lee.—1st ed.
     p. ; cm.
   Includes bibliographical references and index.
   ISBN 0-07-140239-X
     1. Alternative medicine.   2. Integrated delivery of health care.
 I. Kligler, Benjamin.   II. Lee, Roberta A.
   [DNLM: 1. Delivery of Health Care, Integrated.   2. Complementary
Therapies. W 84.1
 I6048 2004]
 R733.15756 2004
 615.5—dc21
                                                   2003052719

Contents

PART I

Basic Principles / 1

PART II

Therapeutic Modalities / 103

PART III

Integrative Approaches to Specific Conditions / 369

PART IV

Integrative Approaches Through the Life Cycle / 695

PART V

Legal and Ethical Issues / 845

PART VI

Selected Cases in Integrative Medicine / 875

Contributing Editors

WOODSON MERRELL, MD

Assistant Clinical Professor of Medicine
Columbia University College of Physicians
  & Surgeons
Executive Director
Center for Health & Healing
Beth Israel Medical Center
New York, New York

DAVID RILEY, MD

Clinical Associate Professor of Medicine
University of New Mexico Medical School
Albuquerque, New Mexico
Founder and Medical Director
Integrative Medicine Institute
Santa Fe, New Mexico

VICTORIA MAIZES, MD

Assistant Professor of Clinical Medicine
College of Medicine
University of Arizona Health Sciences
Executive Director
Program in Integrative Medicine
University of Arizona
Tucson, Arizona

VICTOR SIERPINA, MD

WD & Laura Nell Nicholson Professor
  in Integrative Medicine
Associate Professor and Clinical Medical Director
Department of Family Medicine
University of Texas Medical Branch
Galveston, Texas

Contributors

G. SRINIVASA ARCHARYA, MD (AYURVED)

Padma Ayurveda Clinic
Ambalpady, Udupitaluk, Karnataka
India

JOHN A. ASTIN, PHD

Research Scientist
California Pacific Medical Center
Research Institute
San Francisco, California

MARYBETH AUGUSTINE, RD, CDN

Registered Dietician
NYS Certified Dietician/Nutritionist
Integrative Medicine Nutritionist
Center for Health & Healing
Beth Israel Medical Center
New York, New York

MARK BLUMENTHAL, BA

Adjunct Associate Professor of Medicinal Chemistry
College of Pharmacy
University of Texas at Austin
Austin, Texas
Founder and Executive Director
American Botanical Council
Austin, Texas

RAYMOND CHANG, MD, FACP

Clinical Assistant Professor of Medicine
Weill Medical College
Cornell University
President
Institute of East-West Medicine
Medical Director
Meridian Medical Group
New York, New York

JAMES N. DILLARD, MD, DC, LAC

Assistant Clinical Professor
College of Physicians & Surgeons
Columbia University
New York, New York

ALAN DUMOFF, JD, MSW

Dumoff & Associates
President
Life Tree Consulting
Rockville, Maryland

DAGMAR EHLING, MAC, LAC, DOM

Oriental Health Source, Inc.
Durham, North Carolina

KAREN ERICKSON, DC

Senior Chiropractor
Center for Health & Healing
Beth Israel Medical Center
New York, New York

KELLY FORYS, MA

Doctoral Candidate
Clinical Psychology/Behavioral Medicine
Department of Psychology
University of Maryland
Baltimore, Maryland

LEO GALLAND, MD

Director
Foundation for Integrated Medicine
New York, New York

SUSAN GERIK, MD

Assistant Professor of Pediatrics
Department of Family Medicine Research Office
University of Texas Medical Branch at Galveston
Galveston, Texas

ANDREA GIRMAN, MD, MPH

Diplomate, Fellowship in Integrative Medicine
Beth Israel Medical Center
New York, New York

SEZELLE GEREAU HADDON, MD

Assistant Professor
Otolaryngology, Head and Neck Surgery
Columbia University Medical Center
Attending Otolaryngologist
Center for Health & Healing
Beth Israel Medical Center
New York, New York
Associate Fellow, Program
   in Integrative Medicine
University of Arizona
Tucson, Arizona

xiii

SUSAN HADLEY, MD

Faculty
Middlesex Family Practice Residency Program
Middletown, Connecticut
Assistant Professor
University of Connecticut, School of Medicine
Farmington, Connecticut

RICHARD HAMMERSCHLAG, PhD

Research Director
Oregon College of Oriental Medicine
Adjunct Professor of Neurology
Oregon Health & Science University
Portland, Oregon

MARSHA J. HANDEL, MLS

Education & Information Co-ordinator
Center for Health & Healing
Beth Israel Medical Center
New York, New York

RANDY J. HOROWITZ, MD, PhD

Medical Director
Program in Integrative Medicine
Clinical Assistant Professor of Medicine
University of Arizona College of Medicine
Tucson, Arizona

STEVEN F. HOROWITZ, MD

Clinical Professor of Medicine and Nuclear Medicine
Albert Einstein College of Medicine
Bronx, New York
Chief, Department of Cardiology
Stamford Hospital
Stamford, Connecticut

JAMAL ISLAM, MD, MS

Assistant Professor
Department of Family Medicine Research Office
University of Texas Medical Branch at Galveston
Galveston, Texas

GEORGE KESSLER, DO

Clinical Instructor of Medicine
Albert Einstein College of Medicine
Bronx, New York
Adjunct Assistant Professor
New York College of Osteopathic Medicine
New York, New York

BENJAMIN KLIGLER, MD, MPH

Assistant Professor of Family Medicine
Albert Einstein College of Medicine
Bronx, New York
Research Director and Co-Director
Integrative Medicine Fellowship
Center for Health & Healing
Beth Israel Medical Center
New York, New York

ROBERTA LEE, MD

Medical Director and Co-Director
Integrative Medicine Fellowship
Center for Health & Healing
Beth Israel Medical Center
New York, New York
Diplomate, Program in Integrative Medicine
University of Arizona
Tucson, Arizona

ROBERT Y. LIN, MD

Professor of Medicine
New York Medical College
Valhalla, New York
Chief
Allergy/Immunology Section
Department of Medicine
St. Vincent's Hospital
New York, New York

SUZANNE LITTLE, PhD

Coordinator, Mind Body Program
Supervising Psychologist
Center for Health & Healing
Beth Israel Medical Center
New York, New York
Assistant Professor of Psychiatry
Albert Einstein College of Medicine
Bronx, New York

JAY LOMBARD, DO

Assistant Clinical Professor of Neurology
Weill Medical College
Cornell University
New York, New York

TIERAONA LOW DOG, MD

Clinical Lecturer
Department of Medicine
University of Arizona
Tucson, Arizona
Clinical Assistant Professor, Family Medicine
University of New Mexico
Albuquerque, New Mexico

ROBERT B. LUTZ, MD, MPH

Research Assistant Professor
University of Arizona College of Medicine
Assistant Professor of Nutritional Sciences
Mel & Enid Zuckerman College of Public Health
University of Arizona
Tucson, Arizona

VICTORIA MAIZES, MD

Assistant Professor of Clinical Medicine
College of Medicine
University of Arizona Health Sciences
Executive Director
Program in Integrative Medicine
University of Arizona
Tucson, Arizona

LEWIS MEHL-MADRONA, MD, PhD

Coordinator for Integrative Psychiatry and
  System Medicine
Program in Integrative Medicine
University of Arizona College of Medicine
Director
Practitioner Core Center for Frontier Medicine
  in Biofield Science
Tucson, Arizona

KENNETH MERCER, MD, MPH

Research Fellow
The Richard and Hinda Rosenthal Center
  for Complementary and Alternative Medicine
Columbia University
New York, New York

WOODSON MERRELL, MD

Assistant Clinical Professor of Medicine
Columbia University College of Physicians
  & Surgeons
Executive Director
Center for Health & Healing,
Beth Israel Medical Center
New York, New York

DANIEL MULLER, MD, PhD

Associate Professor
Departments of Medicine (Rheumatology)
  and Medical Microbiology & Immunology
Institute on Aging, Mind Body Center
University of Wisconsin–Madison
Madison, Wisconsin

SANFORD NEWMARK, MD

Associate Faculty Member
Department of Pediatrics
University of Arizona College of Medicine
Faculty
Program in Integrative Medicine
University of Arizona
Director
Center of Pediatric Integrative Medicine
Tucson, Arizona

ARYA NIELSEN, MA, MS, LAc, FNAAOM

Faculty, Master Acupuncturist
Center for Health & Healing
Beth Israel Medical Center
Practitioner and Professor of East Asian Medicine
Senior Faculty
Tristate College of Acupuncture
New York, New York
Guest Faculty
Anglo-Dutch Institute on Oriental Medicine
Netherlands

AURORA OCAMPO, MA, RN, CS

Adjunct Faculty
School of Nursing
Long Island University
Brooklyn, New York
Education Nurse Manager
Nurse Specialist
Center for Health & Healing
Beth Israel Medical Center
New York, New York

SUNIL PAI, MD

President and Medical Director
Sanjerani LLC
Santa Fe, New Mexico
Diplomate, Associate Fellow,
  Program in Integrative Medicine
University of Arizona
Tucson, Arizona

FRANCINE RAINONE, DO, PhD, MS

Assistant Professor of Family and Social Medicine
Albert Einstein College of Medicine
Bronx, New York
Director of Community Palliative Care
Clinical Director of Inpatient Palliative Care
Department of Family Medicine
Montefiore Medical Center
Bronx, New York

DAVID RAKEL, MD

Director
University of Wisconsin Integrative Medicine Program
Assistant Professor
Department of Family Medicine
University of Wisconsin Medical School
Madison, Wisconsin

DAVID RILEY, MD

Clinical Associate Professor of Medicine
University of New Mexico Medical School
Albuquerque, New Mexico
Founder and Medical Director
Integrative Medicine Institute
Santa Fe, New Mexico

AVIVA ROMM, AHG, CPM

Integrative Midwifery
Carton, Georgia

ANTHONY ROSNER, PhD

Foundation for Chiropractic Education and Research
Arlington, Virginia

KENNETH SANCIER, PhD

Qigong Institute
Menlo Park, California

Foreword

A Harvard study recently reported that almost half of the American population is interested in using some form of complementary and alternative medicine (CAM) for the improvement of health.[1] Without proper guidance from knowledgeable healthcare practitioners, however, the public's enthusiastic embracing of CAM can be counterproductive. Patients need comprehensive treatment plans and guidance in selecting therapies and therapists in order to increase the chance of good therapeutic outcomes. This book illustrates the principles that physicians and other healthcare professionals can use in order to practice CAM in combination with mainstream medicine in a thoughtful manner. If it were simply a collection of protocols for the management of common conditions, it would be valuable, but it is more than that. Its content embodies the philosophy of the emerging field of integrative medicine.

Integrative medicine is not synonymous with CAM. Above all, it seeks to work with the body's natural potential to heal. It recognizes that the body has innate mechanisms to maintain health and promote healing. The aim of integrative treatment is to activate those mechanisms and to address the patient's emotional and spiritual well-being in addition to physical health. All aspects of lifestyle are evaluated in an integrative health assessment, and recommendations are made—about diet, exercise, and stress management, for example—that aim to foster healing. Great emphasis is placed on the therapeutic relationship that forms between practitioner and patient.

When I founded the Program in Integrative Medicine at the University of Arizona in 1997, many who were skeptical about this approach viewed it as unscientific or even antiscientific. But much of this concern seemed rooted in a lack of awareness of the scientific evidence that existed for the safety and efficacy of many CAM treatments. Now, seven years later that body of evidence has increased exponentially. Today, 22 medical institutions have joined the Consortium of Academic Health Centers for Integrative Medicine for the specific purpose of changing medical education, research, and practice in this direction. The deans and chancellors of these institutions recognize that medical education must include the principles of integrative medicine and specific information on CAM. This represents a profound paradigmatic shift within the medical profession and society at large.

Modern medicine has overlooked the body's natural potential to heal. Conventional medical education emphasizes invasive procedures and the use of powerful medications that often produce significant adverse effects. Although the conventional system is able to treat many problems successfully, we must reconsider more carefully its potential for harm. In reality, the evidence base for many allopathic treatments is not as solid as is generally thought. Furthermore, most medical decision-making takes place in an arena where there is much scientific uncertainty. In the absence of a clear therapeutic path, physicians and patients should be partners in making decisions, using both knowledge and intuition.

Some years ago, I had a patient with metastatic breast cancer. Her oncologist persuaded her to opt for a bone marrow transplant, a very

[1] Eisenberg DM, Davis RB, Ettner SL, et al. Trends in alternative medicine use in the United States, 1990–1997: results of a follow-up national survey. *JAMA* 1998;280:1569–1575.

invasive and potentially lethal procedure that is now understood to be worthless. Did the oncologist really employ the strictest standard of evidence possible for a treatment that could jeopardize his patient's life? Did the patient demand adequate evidence from her physician for the efficacy and safety of this procedure?

Thankfully this situation is changing. I meet many medical educators and clinicians who realize that medicine, like all professions, must acknowledge that it is in a state of constant reevaluation in order to move forward. These are people open to change, and they are aware that they must be prepared to meet the needs of patients who desire more natural, less harmful ways of treating disease and supporting health.

This text is a valuable source of information for those interested in meeting this challenge. Many of the authors are graduates of the Program in Integrative (PIM) at the University of Arizona. Others are graduates of the relatively new Integrative Medicine Fellowship at Beth Israel Medical Center–a program co-directed by one of my first students at PIM. I am pleased to see that it provides a base of scientific evidence where possible but also preserves the perspective of many of the alternative practitioners who have extensive experience in their respective disciplines.

It is a pleasure to introduce this book to what I hope will be a broad readership, interested in obtaining greater insight into the process of healing and how it can be maximized in the clinical setting.

Andrew T. Weil, MD
Clinical Professor of Medicine
Director, Program in Integrative Medicine
University of Arizona
Tucson, Arizona

Preface

Integrative medicine is renewing the soul of medicine by combining the advances of science and technology in Western medical training with the whole person approach of traditional healing systems. While the practices and philosophy of complementary and alternative medicine (CAM) comprise an important component of the integrative approach, this new discipline is not synonymous with CAM. Integrative medicine seeks to blend the best of allopathic medicine with the best of CAM in its effort to assist medicine in returning to its original mission: preventing disease in a relationship-centered approach that emphasizes the holistic nature of patient care and utilizes lifestyle components to improve health along with mental and spiritual well-being. These are fundamental values reflected in every ancient and traditional medical system. Although some feel that conventional medical approaches adequately embody these principles, many medical educators, physicians and patients today do not agree.

It is now estimated that as many as 30 to 40 percent of Americans seek some form of alternative therapies to support their conventional care. Although both conventional and CAM approaches can provide much clinical insight and effective tools for healing illness, their views of health and illness can be quite divergent, often leaving both types of practitioners wondering how they can effectively work together. This text seeks to strengthen the bridge between these rapidly converging worlds, augmenting the understanding of each in such a way as to improve the care of our patients. We hope that medical and CAM practitioners alike will find the information in this book a useful reference for effective integrative patient care.

A major challenge in editing this textbook has been to address the dual purpose of an integrative medicine reference: to be comprehensive in describing the spectrum of current clinical practice while being firmly anchored in scientifically based clinical research. At times these two goals are at odds, as much of the clinical practice of integrative medicine is not adequately supported by scientific evidence. For some therapies, scientific evidence may exist but has been produced in a less rigorous manner than we would like to see. Integration requires an open mindedness and willingness to explore the validity of alternative paradigms for health and illness, despite the lack of evidence from clinical trials. Therefore, although we have sought to maintain a perspective rooted in biomedical science, we have decided that a certain amount of material should be included which extends beyond what would be normally accepted in a referenced text.

We used several criteria for deciding which healing traditions and modalities to include, given the paucity of quality clinical research on many of these therapies. Questions of what constitutes legitimate evidence, and the context of how knowledge is evaluated and judged within the medical profession form an important part of this discussion. We decided that additional criteria for inclusion of traditions or modalities within the text should include

- longevity of use within a complex medical system (e.g., Chinese and Ayurvedic medicine);
- a plausible mechanism for effectiveness in treating a given condition, even in the absence of clinical trials; and

- expert opinion and clinical experience, particularly given the standing of many of our authors as leading clinicians in this field.

Understanding of a given condition from the perspective of a traditional medical system often will challenge the current pathophysiologic paradigms of conventional biomedical training. Our view is that this should be a welcome challenge that could open the door to potentially helpful new approaches.

A second challenge facing us as editors is seeking a balance between the systems-oriented, disease-focused approach to organizing information typically used in medical texts, and the whole person, wellness-oriented perspective that captures more accurately the philosophy of the integrative medicine approach. Thus, we begin the book by looking at wellness from the perspectives of physicians as well as practitioners of other healing arts. In subsequent chapters we examine the integrative approach to the treatment of specific conditions. Throughout the text we encouraged the authors to address how principles of healing and homeostasis can be applied in clinical practice. It is clear from these contributions that a whole-person, wellness-oriented approach can be applied even when discussing the treatment of a specific disease or condition. It is this commitment to simultaneously embracing both wellness-oriented and disease-oriented perspectives that is the heart of integrative medicine.

Our experience at the Beth Israel Center for Health & Healing in New York over the past three years has provided the inspiration for approaching integration in this manner. The Center is a group of sixteen practitioners of diverse healing arts ranging from acupuncture to conventional medicine to homeopathy and chiropractic who are deeply committed to the development of this new paradigm. A great deal of effort has been required to forge a common language amongst ourselves to create effective communication and allow space for a diversity of opinions regarding the origins of human health, illness and wellness. Our work with this group of practitioners—many of whom are authors in this text—over the past three years, and with our integrative medicine fellows over the past two years, has provided the intellectual framework for the outline of this new approach that we offer in this textbook. The text is divided into six sections.

- Part I, "Basic Principles," outlines some of the distinctions between the conventional medical approach and the integrative approach, both in terms of principles and in terms of patient approach. The relevance of mind–body–spirit connections and of family, community, and social influences on health and illness are discussed in depth, with reference to specific patient case studies to illustration these basic principles.
- Part II of the text, "Therapeutic Modalities," discusses in depth the major therapeutic approaches which, in addition to allopathic medicine, constitute the "toolbox" of the integrative practitioner. East Asian medicine, manipulative approaches, nutritional therapeutics, homeopathy, Ayurvedic medicine, movement therapies, botanical medicine, exercise, and spirituality are covered in this section. Each chapter is written by a practitioner of the discipline who was charged with balancing the "medical" perspective with that of the practitioners of the various healing arts. These chapters include a discussion of the history and philosophy of the modality, and a current review of the research literature regarding the impact of that particular approach on specific health outcomes. This commitment to find a balance between these two perspectives and a bridge between different healing paradigms is a central part of the philosophy of integrative medicine. It requires from all involved a commitment to appreciate the potential validity of a wide variety of paradigms in health, thus serving the equally

important mission to facilitate cross-cultural awareness. Informatics, which has become an indispensable tool for all health care practitioners, is also covered in this section with a specific emphasis on how to access reliable integrative medicine resources.

- In Part III, "Integrative Approaches to Specific Conditions," we revisit the systems-oriented, disease-focused approach familiar to physicians and medical educators. These chapters, which cover a range of specialties and diagnoses focus on applications of the integrative approach to treatment of specific conditions. These chapters are all written by physicians and emphasize an evidence-based approach. In some areas where clinical research is not very extensive, we encouraged the authors of this section to include guidance for readers regarding some approaches which, although not yet adequately studied, are safe and potentially useful in clinical practice. This section of the text, written by physicians in active clinical practice of integrative medicine, should serve as an easy reference for practitioners looking for reliable information on how to help a patient with a specific illness or health condition using the integrative approach.

- Part IV of the text, "Integrative Approaches through the Life Cycle," discusses the unique discusses the unique dimensions of the integrative medicine approach to the care of children, women (including pregnancy), and the elderly. This section takes a less "disease-oriented" perspective than Part III, and in particular emphasizes aspects of well-person care such as nutrition, exercise, and mind–body–spirit health which are often omitted from the conventional primary care approach to the care of healthy patients. The emphasis on preventive approaches and health-promotion which informs this section are central to the overall philosophy of integrative medicine.

- Part V, entitled "Legal and Ethical Issues," covers a topic with which we feel every physician moving into the realm of integrative medicine should be familiar. This chapter provides illustrations of specific situations which may arise in the practice of integrative medicine and strategies which can help address the legal and ethical concerns which often emerge from those situations. In our teaching we find concerns regarding liability and ethics are often high on the list for physician audiences; this chapter offers concrete recommendations for physicians practicing in a new and unconventional approach.

- Part VI, "Selected Cases in Integrative Medicine" provides three case studies from the Fellowship Program in Integrative Medicine at Beth Israel Medical Center. These case discussions—one of a child with recurrent otitis and respiratory problems, one of a woman with fatigue and hormonal imbalance, and one of an elderly woman with heart disease and chronic pain—emerge from the weekly case conference we hold at the Center for Health and Healing as part of our postresidency clinical fellowship program. In these conferences, the fellows present cases from their practice to a rotating panel of faculty comprised of physicians, acupuncturists, nutritionists, psychotherapist and mind–body practitioners, homeo-paths, and representatives of various other healing arts. The cases in this chapter are offered as illustrations of how the diverse voices of the varied healing arts can come together to form a coherent treatment plan for many challenging problems.

The worlds of alternative practitioners and physicians continue to converge as scientific knowledge advances and the demands of health care evolve. Some of the newest discoveries in genetics and molecular biology hold the promise of potentially reversing disease at the most fundamental level. However, in far too many cases, all physicians can do is quell the symptoms of disease. In addition, physicians now have less time with patients—a brief ten minutes on average. Dissatisfaction by physicians and patients, for different reasons, has forced the re-examination of medicine's purpose. As its central theme, integrative medicine advocates the treatment of both the patient and the disease while seeking to redraft the definition of healing. Toward that end, our hope is that this text can add to the reshaping of current practices into a more humanistic, scientifically rooted body of medicine.

Benjamin Kligler
Roberta Lee

Acknowledgments

▶ **FROM B.K.**

I would like to thank the many friends and colleagues who have inspired me over my own personal and professional healing journey, including Jeanne Anselmo, John Falencki, Barbara Glickstein, Al Kuperman, Dorothy Larkin, Betsy Macgregor, Mark Miller, Red Schiller, Sir Abdulla Smith Ford, Charles Terry, and Gil Tunnel. My gratitude also to my patients and their families, who have taught me most of what I know.

My thanks to my mother, Deborah Krasnow and to my stepfather, Herbert Krasnow, for their love and support, and to my father, the late Dr. David Kligler, for my inspiration to become a physician.

Finally, my deepest thanks and appreciation to my wife, Susan, and to my children, Sophie, Michaela and Zachary, who bring joy and inspiration into my life every day and who are all very glad this project is completed!

▶ **FROM R.L.**

There are a lot of people to whom I would like to express my gratitude. First, thanks to my former colleagues (Fellows and Associate Fellows) at the Program in Integrative Medicine at the University of Arizona for helping to shape some of the many ideas that are expressed in this book. Thanks to Wendy, Russ, Karen, Opher and Craig Schneider for your support throughout the years. Thanks to Victoria Maizes, Dave Rakel, Randy Horowitz, Sunil Pai, Sezelle Gireau-Haddon and Bob Lutz for contributing to the book. Having mentors is always a gift; I am greatly appreciative of the ongoing support and guidance of Andrew Weil, who has always been a great inspiration to me.

I would like to acknowledge those who have been my teachers. Thank you to Dan Shapiro, Marty Hewlett, Tracy Gaudet, John Tarrant, Garchen Rinpoche, Steve Gurgevich, Sue Fleishman, Fredi Kronenberg, Harriet Beinfield, Efrem Korngold, Jon Kabat-Zinn, Saki Santorelli, Kate Worden, Rausa Clark, Jim Dalen, Joseph Alpert and Victor Yano.

A special thanks to my companion, Michael Balick, for his sense of humor, his advice and wisdom as a writer and editor. Thanks to my family for their eternal support especially my parents, Curtis, Millie and Cynthia, my sister Sabrina, brother Chris, as well as Tammy and Daniel Balick.

▶ **FROM B.K. AND R.L.**

We are greatly appreciative of the time, effort, and expertise of all our contributing editors and authors; thank you for spending so much of your "extra time" to write on this project.

Also a big thank you to our wonderful editors at McGraw-Hill, Andrea Seils and Karen Davis, for their patience and guidance through this project, and to our editorial assistant, Margaret Price.

Lastly, there is one individual for whom any words we could think of to express our gratitude would not be enough: Mrs. Dorothy Mills. We are profoundly thankful for her support.

PART I

Basic Principles

CHAPTER 1

Integrative Medicine: Basic Principles

ROBERTA LEE, BENJAMIN KLIGLER, AND SAMUEL SHIFLETT

The doctor of the future will give no medicine, but will interest his patient in the care of the human frame, in diet, and in the cause and prevention of disease.

THOMAS EDISON

▶ THE EVOLUTION OF MEDICINE

The physician's goal has always been to alleviate suffering. This legacy, as passed from one generation of physicians to another, is encapsulated in the Hippocratic Oath taken by all medical students when they complete their medical training (see Figure 1–1).

Although the goal has remained constant, the means by which to achieve this goal have changed and evolved over time. In part, this change in the methodology of medicine has been shaped by a more complete understanding of anatomy and physiology, by the modern approach to treatment of infectious disease, and by the emergence of new areas in science such as genetics and molecular biology. In the twentieth century, rapid acquisition of knowledge in these areas has created a new paradigm for how disease can be influenced and treated.

During the time that the Hippocratic Oath was written, around 300 B.C.,[1] the philosophy of medicine reflected an emphasis on observation of all aspects of the individual, from diet to the nature and content of dreams, as a means of understanding the malady suffered by that individual. Hippocratic physicians were strongly encouraged to resist classifying diseases solely according to the organs affected. Each patient was seen as an individual rather than as a "disease entity." The notion of an individual as a combination of both material and spiritual properties was an accepted medical paradigm. In this era, explanations for ill health were ascribed to the imbalance of the four humors: phlegm, blood, yellow bile, and black bile. A constant thread throughout the writings of this time was a reliance on nature, and the main objective of treatment was to help patients achieve harmony so that the natural

A Modern Hippocratic Oath by Dr. Louis Lasagna

I swear to fulfill, to the best of my ability and judgment, this covenant:

I will respect the hard-won scientific gains of those physicians in whose steps I walk, and gladly share such knowledge as is mine with those who are to follow;

I will apply, for the benefit of the sick, all measures which are required, avoiding those twin traps of overtreatment and therapeutic nihilism.

I will remember that there is art to medicine as well as science, and that warmth, sympathy and understanding may outweigh the surgeon's knife or the chemist's drug.

I will not be ashamed to say "I know not," nor will I fail to call in my colleagues when the skills of another are needed for a patient's recovery.

I will respect the privacy of my patients, for their problems are not disclosed to me that the world may know. Most especially must I tread with care in matters of life and death. If it is given me to save a life, all thanks. But it may also be within my power to take a life; this awesome responsibility must be faced with great humbleness and awareness of my own frailty. Above all, I must not play at God.

I will remember that I do not treat a fever chart, a cancerous growth, but a sick human being, whose illness may affect the person's family and economic stability. My responsibility includes these related problems, if I am to care adequately for the sick.

I will prevent disease whenever I can, for prevention is preferable to cure.

I will remember that I remain a member of society, with special obligations to all my fellow human beings, those sound of mind and body, as well as the infirm.

If I do not violate this oath, may I enjoy life and art, respected while I live and remembered with affection hereafter. May I always act so as to preserve the finest traditions of my calling and may I long experience the joy of healing those who seek my help.

The Oath of Maimonides

The eternal providence has appointed me to watch over the life and health of Thy creatures. May the love for my art actuate me at all time[s]; may neither avarice nor miserliness, nor thirst for glory or for a great reputation engage my mind; for the enemies of truth and philanthropy could easily deceive me and make me forgetful of my lofty aim of doing good to Thy children.

May I never see in the patient anything but a fellow creature in pain.

Grant me the strength, time and opportunity always to correct what I have acquired, always to extend its domain; for knowledge is immense and the spirit of man can extend indefinitely to enrich itself daily with new requirements.

Today he can discover his errors of yesterday and tomorrow he can obtain a new light on what he thinks himself sure of today. Oh, God, Thou has appointed me to watch over the life and death of Thy creatures; here am I ready for my vocation and now I turn unto my calling.

Figure 1-1. Modern Hippocratic Oath by Dr. Louis Lasagna (1923–2003). The Oath of Maimonides (1135–1204).

forces in the body (humors) could return to a state of balance. Relief of suffering from illness was primarily achieved by alterations in lifestyle, in diet, and in the life of the spirit. However, interventions such as botanical substances were sometimes incorporated in treatment as well. Even the writings of this time pertaining to surgery had the focus of restoration in balancing the "humors." The mind and the body were seen as inseparable parts contained within each person, each person a combination of physical and spiritual properties.[2]

In the seventeenth century, René Descartes (1596–1650), a philosopher/scientist/mathematician, wrote a treatise on the relationship of the mind and the body—proposing that each was distinct from the other. This philosophy led to the mind–body duality or what is known as the "Cartesian split,"[3] discussed in detail in Chapter 2 by John A. Astin. Descartes thought that the science of his time did not provide the proper tools or perspective for the study of mind and spirit. Descartes proposed that as science moved forward in its study of the physical body, the study of mind and spirit should be in the domain of the church. He believed that the application of empirical, scientific observation—as it was defined at the time—to the study of mind and spirit, would lead to an incorrect and inappropriate reductionism in the view of these central aspects of the human experience.

The notions of what was contained in the domain of science were influenced by other philosophers after Descartes. John Locke (1632–1704) and David Hume (1711–1776) philosopher/scientists of the seventeenth and eighteenth centuries produced influential writings that promoted reductionism[1] and the use of "rational analysis" as the process of inquiry in science. During this time, great discoveries in physics by Sir Isaac Newton (1642–1727) and others in different areas of science enabled humans to gain mastery in explaining, predicting, and controlling many things in their environment—moving the world further and further into using this process of scientific inquiry

to evaluate any phenomena in nature that needed investigation.

Reductionists viewed the world from a mechanistic perspective, believing that all natural phenomena could be reduced to smaller, simpler pieces and the whole could be understood by studying the sum of its parts. According to this form of thought, in the equation $A = B + C$, A is defined as an identical state equal to the parts summated by $B + C$. But is this really a true representation for A? More recent thinking, as represented, for example, in quantum physics, holds that in more complex systems, although A is whole, $B + C$ does *not entirely equal* A. Rather, it is a *close approximation* of A. Therefore, the equal sign is somewhat of a misnomer. What is significant is that in the reductionistic thinking process, the *whole is regarded* only *as the sum of its parts*, whereas in the more modern model the whole can actually be *more* than the sum of those parts. In the eighteenth and nineteenth centuries, the subtlety of this distinction was lost because the reductionistic model was so effective in explaining many puzzling phenomena of nature.

Another analogy for understanding the distinction between reductionistic and "holistic" ways of understanding systems would be the process of baking a cake. The reductionistic view would assume that by studying the elements of a recipe comprising a cake (flour, water, eggs, and baking soda), we can understand what a cake is. However, this approach overlooks the process that actually transforms a collection of ingredients into a single entity.

▶ EARLY AMERICAN MEDICAL PRACTICE: THE FLEXNER REPORT AND THE TRANSFORMATION OF MEDICAL EDUCATION (1800–1920)

In the early 1800s, "conventional" physicians, known as Heroic medical practitioners, included the use of purging, bleeding, large doses of calomel (mercury chloride), and opiates as therapeutic interventions. In opposition to these practices were a substantial number of other medical professionals who believed these interventions to be toxic. On the basis of this conviction, many of these practitioners turned to systems of natural healing such as osteopathy, homeopathy, and naturopathy—all of which became popular in the United States during the nineteenth century. By the late 1800s, 20% of all practitioners in medicine in the United States were "alternative physicians."[5]

Meanwhile, during this period, conventional physicians organized and lobbied to preserve economic and political dominance by setting up state medical societies to license physicians. "Irregular practitioners" not schooled and approved by orthodox institutions were aggressively pursued with the intent of depriving them of their ability to practice. Battle lines became drawn between the physicians and the alternative practitioners based on philosophical, political, and socioeconomic differences.[6] The criteria for what constituted proper medical treatment and the content of medical education in the early years of this transformation became a heated topic of academic and political debate. At one point, the alternative practitioners, tired of the aggressive moves of the Heroic practitioners, lobbied to repeal all licensing laws that had been implemented, and won. This was known as the Popular Health Movement. By the end of the 1840s, almost all licensing laws had been repealed—creating great ire in the conventional medical community.[7]

Partially in response to this movement, in 1847, the American Medical Association (AMA) was founded to erect a barrier between orthodox medicine and "irregular practitioners."[8] By 1900, the AMA lobbied for state medical licensing laws to reclaim power from "irregular practitioners," and eventually laws regulating practice were enacted in all the states. In 1910, Abraham Flexner, a medical educator, was employed by the Carnegie Foundation to evaluate the state of education in medical and healing schools across North America. The report was initiated to help the leading philanthropists of the day decide where to focus their support. It evaluated most institutions very negatively. A major criticism cited was the weak entrance criteria for most schools; in some schools all that was required for admission was a "common school education." In addition, Flexner dismissed homeopaths, osteopaths, and naturopaths as "unconscionable quacks."[9]

The repercussions of the Flexner report resulted in the closing of more than half of the medical schools and many of the alternative medical schools in the United States. Only medical schools that were grounded in science survived the purge. Medical school curricula became steeped in biomedicine and science. As scientific thinking became more rigorous the toxic treatments of the past were discontinued and more efficacious drugs were used, increasing the public's faith in the biomedical model and the power of science in taming disease. The Flexner report not only influenced allopathic schools to restructure their training but significantly challenged alternative practices to reevaluate their methods and educational curricula as well.[10]

▶ AMERICAN MEDICINE IN THE TWENTIETH CENTURY

In the first half of the twentieth century, three advances produced a dramatic shift in methods of treatment: the discovery of microorganisms as a cause of disease, the development of antibiotics to combat those organisms, and the development of effective anesthesia.[11] Other breakthroughs in the applied sciences created equally dramatic transformations in medicine. Advances in biochemistry, biophysics, physical chemistry, and immunology enabled escape from devastation by the scourges of smallpox, cholera, polio, and diphtheria, first through improved public hygiene and then through the development of vaccines. Henry Dale, the 1936 Nobel laureate in medicine, wrote this description of the therapeutic advances in medicine that had occurred by mid-century:

> Our successors, viewing the times in which we live from the longer perspective of history are likely to recognize the first half of the twentieth century as the period in which civilization first began to feel, for good or ill, the first impact of progress in the natural sciences.[12]

The explosion of the scientific and medical information of this time provided a much different understanding of the pathophysiologic basis of disease and the tools required to combat it. The birth of subspecialization in medical care evolved to accommodate this expansion of knowledge and technology. The focus in training and practice in medicine continued to shift physicians toward a disease-oriented model, as it was so effective in taming disease with the new tools of technology and discoveries in science. This trend continues today in medical education as well as in the clinical arena. As David Rakel and Andrew Weil suggest, physicians have become a body of practitioners who "focus on pieces"[13] of medical care, and our society one that believes in the power of medical technology to conquer all medical ills.[14]

At the beginning of the twentieth century, the life expectancy in the United States was approximately 50 years of age. It has risen steadily since that time and now stands at 76.9 years.[15] The rise in life expectancy has increased the prevalence of chronic disease. And although the life expectancy has continued to rise, the ability of technological medical advances to keep pace in their ability to alleviate suffering from these chronic diseases has been limited in comparison to the impact of the advances on more acute illness.[16] The basis for this gap in success between the treatment of acute and chronic conditions using conventional methods lies in the current approach to both diagnostics and therapeutics. Conventional approaches focus on specific diseases, repairing only a part without addressing the underlying causes.[17]

This method ignores the interconnectedness of all organ systems and the role of mind and spirit in the restoration of health. Although temporary relief may be attained from this organ-specific approach, it may also impart a "sense of false security."[18] For example, cyclooxygenase-2 (COX-2) inhibitors may provide adequate relief from pain for a runner with chronic lower extremity pain from an overuse injury. However, this relief may merely allow the runner to further damage his joints because he has relief from his pain—yet his lifestyle and the reasons for the development of the pain have not been addressed.

▶ TECHNOLOGY AND THE HEALTH CARE CRISIS

The triumphs of medical science have carried with them a great financial burden for our society. Medical advances during and after World War II were primarily in pharmaceuticals, which were relatively inexpensive. After 1960, advances in medical treatment increasingly involved new and complex equipment or procedures that, in contrast, were quite expensive. This created a tremendous rise in medical expenditures. From 1965 to 1975, the share of national health care expenditures paid by the federal government jumped from 26% to 37%[19] and the $10 billion spent by the government in 1965 became $27.8 billion by 1970.[20] In 1999, national health care expenditures as a percentage of gross domestic product was 13%, and in 2000 the overall cost of health care was $1.29 trillion.[21]

By 1969, the awareness of growing health care expenditures was labeled as a "crisis in health care,"[22] even though costs had been steadily rising at that point for almost a decade. Analysis revealed that the crisis was derived from more than just the cost of delivering new technology and procedures; in fact, the system of health care had built-in incentives encouraging use for those providing services. If more procedures were done for the treatment of a disease, financial rewards increased for the physician and/or hospital involved.[23] Furthermore, the system encouraged patients to believe that these tools were the answer to their ill health. In the 1980s, managed care and capitation began to emerge as cost-control strategies. These models of health care, however, had their own costs, as they reduced some excessive expenditures but created more erosion in the patient–provider relationship. As physicians became enmeshed in this system, they acquired new demands on their professional time unrelated to patient care, and began spending less time with their patients as a consequence. A great dissatisfaction developed in both patients and doctors; patients have mourned the loss of medical attention and felt unheard and poorly served, and physicians have experienced a loss of autonomy. Moreover, physicians have lost much of the satisfaction that comes from establishing a genuine connection with the patient.

This situation continues in American medical care to this day. The complexity of achieving successful treatment in chronic illness remains a challenge for both doctor and patient because it must be addressed in an existing medical system that sustains a narrow focus. The "healing tools" of time, touch, and rapport that constituted a major part of how physicians traditionally cared for chronically ill patients remain undervalued and uncompensated in our current system. Meanwhile a growing number of people who are acutely aware of their unmet medical needs have turned to other medical systems—alternative health care and older traditional health systems—for relief from suffering in chronic illness.

► PUBLIC DEMAND AND THE RESURGENCE OF TRADITIONAL MEDICAL SYSTEMS

The 1960s were a pivotal time in American culture, and the ideas that were introduced in American society created a new subculture of people whose values embraced ethnic diversity, environmental awareness, and a reexamination of traditional family and professional roles. Paul Ray, a sociologist, and Sherry Ruth Anderson, a clinical psychologist, have identified these people as "Cultural Creatives." After surveying over 100,000 Americans during a 13-year period, they estimated that there may be as many as 50 million people who have intentionally chosen a style of life that reflects personal authenticity. The authors define authenticity as follows:

> . . . that your actions are consistent with what you believe and what you say. The people in this subculture prefer to learn new information and to get involved in ways that feel most authentic to them. Almost always it involves direct personal experience in addition to intellectual ways of knowing.[24]

One example of this shift toward a different awareness and its effect is in attitudes toward environmentalism: "When Rachel Carson's *Silent Spring* appeared in 1962, the environment was a serious concern for no more than 20% of Americans. Now at least 85% of Americans are concerned about it."[25]

What is the relevance of these facts to medical professionals? These Cultural Creatives seek a more holistic form of health care, including an interest in traditional medical systems such as Chinese medicine and Ayurveda, as well as other modalities that focus on the importance of mind–body awareness. These more holistic approaches, it seems, address more directly the need of this population for a more authentic form of health care.

Much of this shift toward healing arts other than conventional medicine went undetected by the medical community until a landmark publication by David Eisenberg and colleagues, in 1993, revealed that the public was spending $13 billion dollars out of pocket for complementary and alternative care medicine (CAM).[26] A subsequent study, published 5 years later showed a similar trend, with an even higher percentage (42%) of Americans using CAM in

1997, and out-of-pocket expenditures for CAM increasing by 27% over the earlier study.[27] Astin, in 1998, was able to document that this interest was not entirely a result of dissatisfaction with the current medical milieu. His research revealed that the most powerful motivator for patients in choosing therapies other than conventional medicine was the desire for an approach to health and illness more closely aligned with "their own values, beliefs, and philosophical orientations toward health and life."[28] These values, as they are often expressed in healing arts other than medicine, include a commitment to a healing-oriented approach to health; an attempt to choose natural remedies when possible; an emphasis on therapeutic interventions using diet and lifestyle rather than aggressive medical procedures; and an understanding of the centrality of the mind–body connection in the healing process. These are all values very consistent with those of the Cultural Creatives as defined by Ray and Anderson.

▶ THE DEVELOPMENT OF THE NATIONAL CENTER FOR COMPLEMENTARY AND ALTERNATIVE MEDICINE

The public demand for CAM therapies created a need for research in these areas. Physicians largely unfamiliar with these practices were limited in their ability to answer questions that patients might ask about CAM. Huge information gaps were evident in the scientific literature concerning safety and efficacy. In 1993, in answer to this need, an Office of Alternative Medicine was started within the National Institutes of Health (NIH), with an initial budget of $2 million. The office later was expanded and renamed the National Center for Complementary and Alternative Medicine (NCCAM); its budget has been greatly expanded, and, as of 2002, it was $104.6 million per year.[29] The continued expansion of this office has allowed important research in areas that were previously studied either not at all or only with very small groups of patients.

As research in this area has matured, however, it has become clear that the clinical practice of integrative medicine, relying as it typically does on multiple therapeutic interventions applied in an individualized treatment plan for a given patient, poses a great challenge for conventional research methodology. Our "gold standard"—the reductionistic, randomized, controlled, double-blind study—may not be the most effective tool for studying individualized treatments or complicated remedies that act in combination and are not amenable to reduction. The phenomenon of synergy, in which the whole is actually equal to more than the sum of the individual parts, is felt by many integrative medicine practitioners to play a critical role in this model. Randomized controlled trials (RCTs) and the reductionistic model in general—at least as they are widely used today—are not entirely applicable tools for measuring or describing the phenomenon of synergy.

Equally challenging to conventional science is the question of what constitutes sufficient evidence as a source of knowledge. We have been entrained by our scientific education to value the randomized, controlled, double-blind study as the highest process by which to study and evaluate efficacy in medicine and in science at large. However, at the root of its development as an evaluative process, this method approaches whatever is studied by dissection of the component parts while ignoring the concept that the whole has some value beyond the summation of these components.[30] In a realm where personal perception, belief, cultural influence, or even the community has significant influence, this reductionistic perspective may be too narrow to be of value as an evaluative tool. That is not to say that it is not useful: we have gained and will continue to gain great insight from studies using this methodology. But the complexity of converging systems, some with distinctly less material aspects, should be acknowledged and accommodated as we pursue a greater understanding of how and why things work. More specific issues, challenges, and new developments pertaining to research are discussed later in this chapter in the section "General Research Issues."

▶ WHAT IS INTEGRATIVE MEDICINE?

According to Rakel and Weil,

> Integrative medicine is about changing the focus in medicine to one of healing rather than disease. This involves an understanding of the influences of mind, spirit, and community as well as of the body. It entails developing insight into the patient's culture, beliefs, and lifestyle that will help the provider understand how best to trigger the necessary changes in behavior that will result in improved health. This cannot be done without a sound commitment to the doctor–patient relationship.[31]

Integrative medicine is a medical practice that is healing-oriented. It is a practice that is oriented toward prevention of illness and toward the active pursuit of an optimum state of health. It is the marriage of conventional biomedicine, other healing modalities, and traditional medical systems (Chinese medicine, Ayurveda, homeopathy, and Western herbalism, among others.). An integrative practice neither rejects conventional medicine nor uncritically embraces alternative practices.[32] It is an approach that belongs to no specific specialty and describes a state of dynamic health. Therapeutic choices in integrative medicine are prioritized according to the level of benefit, risk, potential toxicity, and cost. The relationship between the physician and patient is central to the practice of integrative medicine, and involves the *art* of relationship as much as it does the *knowledge* of science. Finally, the integrative approach is a perspective that acknowledges the full spectrum of being in health in all realms: the mind, the body, and the spirit. A major objective is a life that is *lived* from a stance of enjoyment as wellness is maintained rather than a focus on regimens that make up an obligatory "checklist" of health prescriptions to extend longevity. Community and environment are seen as integral components to wellness. Implicit in this process is the patient's responsibility in maintaining health.

Definitions in Integrative Medicine

Many terms have been used to describe medical practices outside of the biomedical model. Many of these have been pejorative, such as "fringe medicine" and "unorthodox." "Nontraditional medicine" has been used to describe ancient traditional medical systems like Ayurveda or Chinese medicine; this choice of terminology seems somewhat paradoxical given that these systems have been used for several thousand years longer than has modern "traditional" medicine. "Alternative medicine," a term that appeared in the 1970s, implies the use of other healing practices in place of allopathic/biomedical medical treatments, and thus does not reflect the synthesis defined by the integrative approach. "Complementary" medicine suggests the addition of other healing practices to conventional biomedicine but relegates these therapies to a secondary role.

"Holistic" and "integrative" medicine are the commonly used terms closest in definition to integrative medicine, in that both imply a balanced, whole-person–centered approach and involve a synthesis of conventional medicine, CAM modalities, and/or other traditional medical systems, with the aim of prevention and healing as a basic foundation.

Integrative Medicine: An Approach with Many Tools

The integrative medicine practitioner is fortunate in having at his or her disposal a much wider variety of tools than are generally available to the conventional practitioner. Virtually any technique or intervention that is safe and effective—from both biomedicine/allopathic medicine and from other healing arts—is a potential tool in integrative practice. The use of any intervention is weighed in the context of the wishes of the patient, the objective of the visit, and the depth of the problem/disease that may or may not be present. For example, is the visit to address an acute condition or a chronic illness, or is this a visit designed to enhance health? Because much of the context of the integrative approach is oriented toward prevention, more time and effort is devoted to identifying lifestyle interventions that can lead to disease prevention, or at least to reducing the rate of progression of an established chronic condition. As the importance of the mind–body connection in influencing health, either positively or negatively, is considered critical in integrative medicine, therapies that engage this aspect of the individual are routinely included (Table 1–1).

▶ **TABLE 1–1** SOME COMMON TOOLS OF INTEGRATIVE MEDICINE

Traditional medical systems
Biomedicine or allopathic medicine
Ayurveda
Chinese medicine
East Asian medicine
Native American medicine
Manual medicine
Osteopathy
Chiropractic medicine
Massage
Lifestyle interventions
Diet
Exercise
Mind–body
Hypnosis
Biofeedback
Guided imagery
Spirituality
Religion
Botanical medicine
Western herbalism
Energy medicine
Homeopathy
Reiki

Key Concepts in Integration

Healing, Curing, and Health

Throughout human history the notion of nature's ability to restore itself to balance and wholeness has been a recurrent theme in philosophy, in religion, and in the practice of the healing arts. At the very roots of our allopathic training in the Hippocratic Collection, this perspective is expressed as a fundamental assumption informing the physician's decisions regarding which therapeutic interventions seem appropriate. Despite the importance of this idea in our past, the notion of nature's healing power has been largely neglected in modern medical education and practice.[33] Perhaps this is because our training has emphasized aggressive interventions and procedures that have very visible effects, and so the subtlety of the *restorative* process of that which has been affected has been overlooked.

"Healing" is the inherent quality of a living organism to become whole. It is a dynamic process involving restoration, adaptation to change, and repair. "Curing" implies a finite resolution to a condition, generally with a linear cause-and-effect reaction. To cure something in the context of medicine is an action to fix or alleviate a condition. To heal from something is a process through which a person reaches a new state of balance, whether or not the condition can be cured. Healing and curing are not interchangeable terms. In relation to health, and within the context of an integrative approach, this distinction is important.

The World Health Organization defines "health" as "a state of complete physical, mental, and social well-being and not merely the absence of disease or infirmity."[34] Because health is much more than the absence of disease, healing necessarily includes a restoration of the inner resources of the spirit, and a connection to one's community and environment. This is a much broader and more encompassing definition of health than that which is generally taught to modern physicians-in-training. As Weil and Rakel point out, the word "health" is derived from the Old English word "hal," which means wholeness, soundness, or a state of spiritual well-being. This traditional definition reaches beyond the realm of the physical body to include the "whole" being, including the spiritual side.

The following case illustrates the important distinction between "healing" and "curing." A patient diagnosed with pneumonia comes to the physician's office. The patient receives an antibiotic from the physician and over time the infection resolves. Although the antibiotic *cured* the pneumonia, it did not *heal* it. The immune system of the patient healed the condition; the antibiotic tipped the balance of control of the patient's infection in favor of a *restorative* response by the body. An integrative intervention by the physician to facilitate healing would *additionally* include addressing the contribution of stress, diet, and general conditioning that contributed to preexisting conditions that made that patient vulnerable to developing pneumonia. In this case, the integrative practitioner uses the conventional antibiotic but addresses the broader context of disease formation and its prevention. To highlight the importance of these other factors that enable healing consider the same scenario of a patient with pneumonia, but now this patient has terminal cancer. In this instance, despite the most sophisticated forms of antibiotics offered, the outcome of cure may not be possible. Does this mean that healing cannot occur? If the patient does not resolve the pneumonia, the patient is likely to perish and from the perspective of curing, the patient has failed. However, healing is still possible, in that as the patient is dying—realizing that the body does not have the capacity to restore itself—the patient can make peace with this transition. The patient can do this by deepening his relationship with his family, his community, and within himself spiritually before losing consciousness. The integrative practitioner can help facilitate this process of the patient's health, and thus from this broader context, the patient has *healed* in the process of *dying*.

The "Healing System"

The integrative practitioner acknowledges the intrinsic restorative capacity of the human organism. Activation of this process is critical to an integrative practitioner's decisions regarding which therapeutic choices are most beneficial for the patient. Weil has described the concept of a "healing system" operating in the human organism, not intrinsically different in nature from the "endocrine system," the "nervous system," the "immune system," or any other conventionally defined functional system in the human body.[35] Like these other systems, the healing system is not specifically located in any single organ, but functions via a subtle and complex web of intracellular signaling systems affecting all levels of the organism, from the cellular level to the tissue–organ level to the levels of mind and spirit. Weil gives an example of the process at the cellular level: when the DNA of a skin cell is damaged by ultraviolet radiation—potentially triggering mutation and unregulated replication, eventually leading to development of a skin malignancy—DNA ligase and a set of related enzymes within the damaged cell's nucleus are automatically activated, resulting in the identification and removal of the damaged sequence, with restoration of normal replication. If this level of "automatic healing" fails, then generally, once the cell has mutated and begun to replicate abnormally, immune cells will identify it as foreign and contain and destroy the affected group of cells—without any conscious action on the part of the person affected.

At the level of tissues or organs, the spontaneous healing of wounds is an obvious example of the healing system at work. The occurrence of an injury initiates a complex system of intracellular signaling, leading to local inflammation as a defense against infection, increased tissue perfusion to promote healing, and, ultimately, activation of fibroblasts and other cells to repair the damaged skin and subcutaneous tissues. Here again, although this process can potentially be influenced by certain inputs, including medications, botanicals, mind–body therapies, and others, the basic mechanisms of healing are intrinsic and require no intervention to be moved into action.

Finally, at the level of the mind, an excellent example of the healing system at work is in the process of grieving or recovery from loss. When a person experiences the death of a close friend or relative, for example, acute and intense pain is felt, often as if from a physical wound. This pain may persist for weeks or months and can impair functioning, disabling people from work, and even causing physical symptoms. However, over time, in the absence of past pathology or other obstacles to the healing process, the person will recover, gradually coming to terms with the loss. They will experience less pain, and return to normal functioning—they will heal. Although therapeutic inputs may speed this process or may help remove obstacles to the person's recovery, the healing takes place of its own accord.

This notion of a "healing system," and the practitioner's role in helping to activate that system in the patient, are what many of the traditional and CAM healing arts have in common. But this approach can apply equally well to the practice of any type of medicine.

Intuition

Intuition is an insight derived from past and present experience and from input from the senses but not necessarily from deductive reasoning. It is a process that incorporates details that may initially seem unimportant to the rational linear mind but which provide detail to complete a composite picture that manifests as a "hunch," "gut feeling," or "gestalt." This process is often nonlinear and without rationale. Although in everyday life each person has this capacity as a personal resource, and most people rely on intuition in making important decisions, in medicine it has been downplayed as a clinical tool. In recent years, evidence-based protocols have consumed our attention in medical decision-making. Yet often the most extraordinary outcomes can come from these "hunches." The use of intuition and

development of this aspect in ourselves as clinicians can add tremendous depth to our current primary source of knowledge—the scientific method. There are many ways to gain knowledge, and deductive reasoning is only one means by which to reach that goal. Intuition is a valuable tool that can bring great richness to the complex process that creates health. It allows us to use the full capacity of our clinical experience in making a clinical judgment.

Self-Care

Until recently, little attention was placed in medical education on the physical, emotional, and spiritual health of the physician. The result of the lack of attention to this important concept has been the entrainment of the graduating student physician to accept an unhealthy lifestyle as a model of professionalism. This has made physicians particularly vulnerable to failure and burnout—losing the original meaning of our work as we lose touch with ourselves and our feelings in order to accommodate the rigors of our training.[36] Rachel Naomi Remen comments on the educational process and its implications in neglecting self-care:

> Learning to serve requires education not training. The root word of education, *educari*, means to lead forth the innate wholeness of each student. Medical training often wounds and diminishes us. . . . As professionals we may not be fully connected to our lives. Distance may become a daily habit. In reality, most physicians lead far more meaningful lives than they realize.[37]

Physicians are educators of their patients; the root of the word "doctor" means to teach, or lead. It is difficult to see how a role model who ignores self-care can be effective in convincing patients to do otherwise. Integrative medicine is a model that supports time for self-care and exploration. The balance that we seek in this effort may never be entirely attained, but the process of working to remain attached to our loved ones and to our dreams and aspirations provides us with a powerful means for remembering the original intent of our call to serve in medicine. As Remen writes:

> Meaning is a human need. It strengthens us, not by numbing our pain or distracting us from our problems or even by comforting us. It heals us by reminding us of our integrity, who we are and what we stand for. Part of our responsibility as professionals is to fight for our sense of meaning—against fatigue and numbness and overwork. . . .[38]

Cultural Context of Treatment

Integrative medicine seeks to incorporate the diversity of many healing systems. We are a diverse body of peoples. Thus the meaning and significance of different patterns in our health can leave different impressions based on the culture in which we have been raised. If there is a willingness in the practitioner to recognize these differences and bridge these gaps, capitalizing on understanding the nuances of these differences can have far-reaching and positive outcomes. Therapeutic choices based on this enhanced understanding can match the belief system of the patient to that of the provider—a win-win situation.

▶ THE INTEGRATIVE VISIT

The integrative visit is a time for the practitioner to get to know the patient as much as it is about understanding the disease. Because as integrative practitioners we are interested in the full spectrum of being—mind, body, and spirit—understanding the nuances of each of these facets in our patients provides a rich context for understanding how and why they came to be where they are.

During the integrative interview, new insight is often gained, and patients may begin to understand the significance of particular past events in a new light. They learn how certain experiences may have affected their health as they listen to themselves speak, as many may never have had the opportunity to examine the effect of mind and spirit on their physical health. Inconsistencies in feelings and behaviors may be uncovered, thereby pointing to areas that need exploration and resolution. The discovery of these unrecognized areas may serve as a catalyzing event that creates great change. Patients may be surprised at their own conclusions. As Maizes, Koffler, and Fleishman have reflected, this insight in and of itself may provide a powerful form of healing.[39] The physician becomes the active listener, listening with empathy and without interruption. Empathetic listening has many benefits beyond fostering a deeper sense of trust in the patient: "The effectiveness of empathy promotes diagnostic accuracy, therapeutic adherence, and patient satisfaction while remaining time-efficient."[40]

As does the modern approach to clinical history-taking, the integrative interview relies heavily on open-ended questions such as, "What would you like to focus on today?" "What have been pivotal events in your life?" "Is there anything that has happened to you in the 6 months preceding the event that you think might be important?" "Is there anything that you would like to share with me that you have forgotten to mention (usually asked at the end of the visit)?" The use of deliberately open-ended questions allows the patient to freely choose the focus of the interview. The listener can synthesize with all of his or her senses and intuition what is said and what remains unspoken; by doing this, the listener learns who the patient is through use of verbal and nonverbal cues. The person sharing his or her "story" feels in control. Allowing the locus of control in conversation to remain with the patient has been shown to be important in establishing a sense of trust and hope.[41]

As the intent of integration is a synthesis, these questions do not replace a conventional history. They are designed to augment a traditional intake that would acquire information on past medical, surgical, family, and social history, and so forth. The intent of the augmented questions is threefold: to gain understanding of the person, of the medical condition, and of the goals of the visit.[42] Figure 1–2 provides a truncated version of a health assessment used at the Center for Health and Healing (CHH) at Beth Israel Medical Center.

This history tool is a synthesis of questions designed to explore the whole person and incorporates information on lifestyle and spirituality as well as elicits information on the presenting problem. This particular tool was developed by one of the authors (R.L.) based on a synthesis of materials developed at the Program in Integrative Medicine (PIM) at the University of Arizona and from significant input from the faculty of the CHH.

▶ EDUCATION IN INTEGRATIVE MEDICINE

As of this writing, more than 75% of US medical schools had at least some type of curricular offering in this area, and this number continues to increase every year.[43] In late 2002, *Academic Medicine,* the official journal of the American Association of Medical Colleges, devoted a special issue to the challenges of education in integrative medicine.[44] In January 2000, the Society of Teachers of Family Medicine published the first set of recommended curriculum guidelines for family practice residencies in this area.[45] The Consortium of Academic Health Centers for Integrative Medicine, a national group of 22 medical schools and academic health centers, is working on a similar set of curriculum guidelines for undergraduate education.[46] There are two residential fellowships in integrative medicine currently—at The University of Arizona and at Beth Israel Medical Center in New York—and a number of NIH-funded research fellowships at various institutions.

The question is no longer whether to teach about CAM and integrative medicine within conventional medical education, but how. The values described above as comprising the philosophy of integrative medicine are in many ways difficult to realize in conventional medical education as it is currently structured. How do we emphasize self-care when residents are expected to work 80 hours per week? How do we teach compassionate communication in an environment in which students and residents are typically treated with disrespect by their supervisors? How do we teach the importance of modeling a healthy lifestyle for our patients when we are not allowing our learners the opportunity to live that lifestyle?

These are the challenges we currently face in integrative medicine education. At the Beth Israel Fellowship Program, we use the fellowship as a laboratory in how to incorporate the values of integrative medicine into the teaching of this new discipline. Time is allotted in the fellows' weekly schedule for self-care. Attention to the process of the visit with patients is considered as important as attention to the content. In their work as teachers of our residents and students, the fellows are encouraged to keep these concepts in mind and to model them for the learners.

The core curriculum of the fellowship is divided into two major domains. The first is focused on developing an understanding of the basis for a healing-oriented perspective in medicine by developing a foundation of knowledge pertaining to healing as a process. The second is focused on developing skills and knowledge for the critical assessment of CAM. The latter involves not only the examination of scientific literature and didactic lectures but learning through an "immersion" process. Fellows are encouraged to receive treatments from their instructors so they can experience the healing process from the perspective of that traditional medical system or modality. In addition, the transition of these concepts in the abstract to direct clinical application within the context of a primary care model is a distinct focus of the Beth Israel Fellowship Program. As the fellowship was conceptualized in part by a graduate of the Program in Integrative Medicine at the University of Arizona (R.L.),

A CONDENSED INTEGRATIVE MEDICINE QUESTIONNAIRE

This is not a comprehensive list of integrative medicine questions but a supplemental condensation for those wishing to expand the usual medical evaluation.

Opening questions (choose one):
What brings you here today?
What would you like to focus on today?
Why are you here?
What would you like to accomplish with this visit?

Eliciting a history of present illness:
In addition to asking who, what, where, when, and why of the specific concern add the following:

Were there any stressful events (psychological, physical, or spiritual) preceding the concern?
Did you have any childhood trauma (psychological, physical, or spiritual) that preceded this event?
How do you see this event relating to your personal circumstances?
What meaning does this event have for you?
How do you put this all together?
Do you see yourself being affected by this event, if so, in what way?
Have you gained anything from this experience?
Have you lost anything from this experience?

Medications:
Add the following questions:
Are you on any dietary supplements or botanicals?
Who initiated your taking them and why?
How long have you been on these supplements?
Have you noticed any changes? (positive or negative)
Have you seen any alternative practitioners? For what length of time have you seen them?
Have your practitioners explained their reasoning for your treatment?
Have you shared this information with your primary care physician?

Eliciting a social history:
In addition to the routine social history questions add:

What do you do that gives you pleasure, happiness, or satisfaction?
Do you know how to relax? Do you do this (have a time to relax) every day?
Who are the significant people in your life? Do you spend time with them?
What is your spiritual perspective or belief?
Are you an active participant in your community?
Are there any significant environmental concerns in your community?
Is eating a meal an event that you enjoy?
What is your preventative health plan?

Closing the interview:
Any thing else you would like to share?
What would you like to focus on in the next visit?

Figure 1–2.   A truncated version of a health assessment.   *(Derived from the Integrative Medicine Fellowship Interview developed at the Program in Integrative Medicine at the University of Arizona.)*

similarities in the educational objectives at Beth Israel are acknowledged to be reflective of that training. Table 1–2 outlines the core components of the two curricula.

In looking toward the future, perhaps the most challenging question at hand is whether incorporating the principles of integrative medicine into our training of physicians in this country will ultimately require us to reexamine the criteria by which we select our future physicians. The availability of information on the Internet is reducing the importance of rote memorization of facts. Its ability to bring an exponential amount of information quickly to the clinician has made it a veritable "peripheral brain." Skills in critical thinking and in ability to rapidly access information from the bewildering array of possible sources—and intelligently critique that information—are now much more important. As patients continue to demand more compassionate and open-minded care from their physicians, medical educators will have to work harder to understand how to select for these particular qualities in applicants. The process of medical education—

particularly the clerkship and residency years—will need to be effectively reengineered in order not to then "train out" these qualities of compassion and open-mindedness in our students as they move through their education.

▶ GENERAL RESEARCH ISSUES

On the whole, the Western biomedical community only recently has taken an interest in researching complementary/alternative medicine practices and traditional healing systems. In large part, increased consumer interest and widespread use resulted in the call for more rigorous, scientific, evidence-based research in these fields to evaluate their safety and effectiveness.

Understanding Scientific Research and Study Design

To interpret research findings and evaluate their application to the treatment and prevention of disease, it is helpful to first understand the

---

▶ **TABLE 1-2** TABLE OF CORE CONCEPTS AND TOPICS IN INTEGRATIVE MEDICINE

Healing-oriented medicine concepts
- Healing-oriented medicine
- Philosophy of medicine
- Mind–body influences on health
- Self-healing
- Spirituality
- Relationship-centered care
- Philosophy of science

Curricular topics in integrative medicine
- Systems of medicine such as Chinese medicine, East Asian medicine, Ayurveda, Native American medicine, and homeopathy
- Nutritional medicine
- Manipulative medicine including osteopathic and chiropractic care
- Botanical medicine
- Mind–body therapies including hypnosis, meditation, and guided imagery
- Functional medicine
- Lifestyle influences in prevention—diet, exercise, and stress
- Chronic disease as a process
- Informatics and research

basic components of research design, general issues involved in all types of clinical research, and specific issues encountered in the study of alternative and complementary medicine. This may assist in gaining a perspective on the often contradictory and inconclusive results from different trials that study the same issue. In evaluating research in complementary medicine, it is important to remember that alternative medicine does not mean alternative science. The same rules of evidence must apply to both conventional and alternative medicine research, requiring the same study design characteristics to rule out other explanations of findings such as placebo effect and suggestion.

The gold standard for research design is the randomized, placebo-controlled, double-blind study. Although this has become standard practice in most medical research trials, it is simply not possible or even appropriate to accomplish all of these components of this gold standard for many types of interventions, whether conventional or alternative. This section discusses each of these requirements for good research design in terms of the special problems that are sometimes present when trying to study alternative therapy. Because randomization is an essential component of the gold standard research design, and because it is equally achievable regardless of the type of therapy being studied, it is not discussed further. There are special problems involving the use of placebo and masking, so we discuss these requirements by using acupuncture as the primary example of a therapy, but also making reference to other therapies. Other methodological problems that extend beyond the randomized, placebo-controlled, double-blind study are also discussed as they apply to research in some therapies, including homeopathy.

Studies include placebo conditions in order to control for the very powerful ability of the mind to affect the body through suggestion. Even in the placebo condition, the power of the mind is so strong that sometimes adverse reactions occur simply because they have been suggested as a possibility. Ideally, research should have a condition in which it appears that the participant is receiving the intervention but in fact is not, but this may not always be possible. New drugs are routinely compared to sugar pills or placebos, pills that look just like the real thing but which contain no active ingredients. Similarly, alternative therapies, such as herbs, need to have the same placebo condition for comparison, and most research that tests their effectiveness and safety use placebo controls. It is harder to create a placebo for some interventions than for others. A placebo for a standard surgical technique would involve cutting open the skin without actually performing any meaningful operation. Not only is this difficult to carry out in a credible fashion, it may be unethical as well. As a result, many surgical techniques have never been subjected to rigorous clinical trial research. Another example is physical manipulation of the body, such as physical therapy or massage. This is also difficult to simulate without the recipient becoming suspicious that nothing is really happening. With something like acupuncture, where the needle can be seen to penetrate the skin, it is very difficult to create a condition where the needle appears to go in, yet really does not. So this type of challenge exists in both conventional and complementary medicine.

With direct and observable manipulation such as acupuncture or chiropractic, it is very difficult to create credible placebos. Several sham needles (needles that appear to penetrate the skin, but actually do not) were recently developed for acupuncture placebo conditions, but suffer credibility if the subject has received acupuncture before and knows what it feels like when a needle penetrates the skin, particularly when the dull, aching sense, called de Qi (de chee), is elicited. The latter cannot occur with placebo needles. Other approaches include light needling, or needling on nonacupuncture points, but each of these approaches has its own set of drawbacks. Chiropractic manipulation can sometimes be mimicked by sham touching of the skin, but again, subjects who have had previous experience with the treatments may recognize that it is not a standard chiropractic therapy. So, although it is rather simple to create a drug placebo, where the pill looks like, feels like, and may even taste like the real thing, it is a much more difficult task to create credible placebos for most complementary therapies that do not involve ingesting a substance. Nevertheless, creative scientists are making rapid progress in the direction of developing credible sham interventions.

Finally, it is important for a clinical trial to be double blind. To be "blinded" or "masked" means that you do not know which experimental condition you are in, the real one or the placebo control. "Double-blinded" means that neither the researcher nor the patient knows which condition the patient is in. When doing research on drugs or herbals, this is relatively easy to accomplish. The placebo pill looks just like the active pill, so the patient does not know which pill he or she is receiving. The researcher does not know, because another person, an administrator otherwise not involved with the study, keeps track of this information, and all the drug containers are identified by a code that only the administrator knows. With interventions like surgery, physical therapy, or acupuncture, it is often quite difficult to create any blinding. Surgery leaves a scar, so even if patients are anesthetized they will still guess which condition they were in unless a sham surgery is performed to create a scar without doing anything. And the surgeon will obviously know whether it is the real thing or not. With acupuncture, you may be able to conceal the condition from the patient by putting needles into nonacupuncture points, but this is still difficult to accomplish successfully, because the body may react in a generalized manner whenever a needle penetrates the skin. And it is almost impossible to blind the acupuncturist as to whether it is real or sham acupuncture.

Masking or blinding is an obvious part of the classic gold standard research. Again, when the intervention involves something like a pill,

masking is easy to accomplish. However, for interventions that are administered by a practitioner, such as an acupuncturist or a chiropractor, it is almost impossible to mask the provider, just as it would be very difficult if not impossible to mask a surgeon performing a surgical procedure. The practitioner would know whether it was the real thing or not. As a result, double blinding is uncommon in studies involving this type of intervention, and is likely to remain so. Unfortunately, overzealous critics who like to judge the quality of research by simply counting the number of "required" conditions that should be present if you used the gold standard (the randomized double-blind, placebo-controlled study) often conclude that these single-blinded studies are of low methodological quality, when in fact they meet most other criteria of good science.

Within the context of the general considerations for good research design, each alternative therapy has its own set of characteristics that require special attention in conducting research. These include the individualized nature of many diagnostic systems and treatments; varying guidelines for the number of treatments depending on the condition; different treatment approaches within a modality with differing treatment protocols; a long time frame to determine effects; combinations of treatments in traditional medicine systems such as traditional Chinese medicine and Ayurveda; and difficulty in objectively studying the spiritual side of this approach. New methods and variations of old methods are beginning to emerge that reflect the growth of methodology in response to the need to evaluate these new therapies. A good example of this issue can be found in acupuncture. In keeping with the fixed-dose concept of a drug intervention (the drug or therapy is the same for all subjects), early trials of acupuncture (where the protocol was not specified or varied from subject to subject) were criticized if they did not follow this dictum of a fixed intervention. In response to this concern, a series of studies appeared in the research literature that used fixed protocols (meaning the same acupuncture points on the body were needled every treatment period for every subject). However, acupuncturists rightly complained that this did not represent true acupuncture, where the discretion of the acupuncturist was an integral part of the treatment, especially because the treatment might be modified a number of times as the symptoms of the patient changed. Often the treatment in one session would be completely different from the treatment in the next session for the same condition. What has emerged in recent years is a process whereby a treatment protocol is defined within a *range* of parameters, usually including several points that must be needled each time and a specified set of other points that may be treated at the acupuncturist's discretion. This idea of limited flexibility in treatment protocols has not yet been accepted in all scientific circles, but progress is occurring in this direction.

One of the most insidious effects of trying to do high-quality research can occur when the inappropriate application of classic research design elements gives the appearance of good science, when in fact it introduces methodological artifacts that make it difficult or impossible to determine if the true intervention is actually having any benefit compared to placebo. Research that attempts to test the homeopathic proving model—where healthy subjects will show symptoms in the presence of a homeopathically prepared substance—is a case in point. These studies are likely to have crossover designs, inadequate washout periods, possible introduction of order effects, the use of lists of symptoms that maximize suggestion, and attention factors for both placebo and verum conditions that introduce higher noise-to-signal ratios.[47] Unfortunately, these factors reduce the chances of finding statistical significance.

Bell et al.[48] have pointed out that in an integrative model

> whole system includes the patient–provider relationship, multiple conventional and CAM treatments, and the philosophical context of care as the intervention. The systemic outcomes encompass the simultaneous, interactive changes within the whole person. Within this conceptualization, the whole may exhibit properties that its separate parts do not possess.

The implications of this conceptualization are enormous. It not only demands a new definition of the clinical endpoint (still objectively measured, of course), but it also requires a more comprehensive definition of the actual intervention. No longer is an intervention "just the drug." Now, it is the drug in the context of the doctor–patient relationship, the expectations of the patient, the stressors and other environmental factors impacting the patient, and concomitant bodily factors that may be modulating the conventionally defined intervention. This approach also argues that, for any given condition, an intervention might occur at any one of several locations in a causal chain leading from environmental factors, behavioral factors, nutrition, psychosocial factors, or the underlying mechanisms of action on the condition in question. In fact, the "best" treatment may well be an integrated combination of several different interventions, including, for example, stress-reduction therapy and dietary changes in addition to the pharmacologic agent. The effect of the drug is likely to change depending on the nature of the other interventions (or lack thereof). In this context, an attempt to characterize the isolated effects of any of the intervention components may be an exercise in futility at best, and meaningless at worst.

The radical idea of considering a person as a whole, that is as a *person* with needs, thoughts, and feelings, and the extent to which a clinical trial actually reflects this life experience, comes to the forefront. In other words, to what extent can we expect the results of a clinical trial to generalize to the general population, given the role of beliefs and expectations inherent in any treatment? In a clinical trial, a subject is informed of everything under the sun, including the nature of the other arms of the study, the probability of receiving the drug or a placebo, the nature of and likelihood of a host of possible adverse events, and the right to leave the study at any time. Soon the patient will also be informed that a large number of people, including employees of the FDA and the National Institutes of Health (NIH), have the right to see their results and be asked to authorize the release of such information to those individuals. All of this is accomplished by two long and highly legalistic documents, administered by a researcher who is doing everything possible to be as neutral (perhaps interpreted as "cold" or "uncaring" by the patient) as possible. In short, a clinical trial does not really represent clinical experience, and the most rigorous intention-to-treat statistical analysis will not change that fact. Although many conventional drug trials are likely to continue to provide useful and valid information, it is becoming clear that for many conditions, and for many interventions, different results and conclusions can be drawn, depending on all of the factors in a patient's or subject's life that influence the way the primary intervention is processed, biologically as well as mentally and emotionally.

As our conceptualization of what constitutes a person and what the object of treatment is (a "condition" versus a "person"), our conceptualization of what the treatment *is*, and what it should be, will change to reflect that fact. In turn, the nature of the outcome will change to reflect the fact that complex systems may have a property of wholeness or synergy that is difficult to "tease out" in a reductionistic model.

► CONCLUSION

Healing and its development into the science of medicine are the legacy of physicians passed down from one generation to another for centuries. Embedded in this legacy is the belief that the mind, body, and spirit are essential facets that first must be in balance to achieve true health. Today, integrative medicine and holistic medicine are the terms used to define this healing-oriented perspective. Though the terms used will continue to change, the call to relieve the suffering of our patients will not. In our zeal to address this call, we have become dependent on technology to fix and to conquer disease in the least amount of time possible. However, a consensus[19–52] is building among medical educators and concerned practitioners that this focus on disease and on technology needs to be broadened in order to provide the best medical care for all. Ultimately, the point at which integrative medicine will achieve its greatest success will be when this constellation of modalities is no longer referred to as integrative medicine but rather as good medical practice. The inclusion of traditional medical systems and other proven modalities in a healing-oriented framework brings us back to a more balanced stance that serves the physician, the patient, and, ultimately, the health care system.

REFERENCES

1. Lyons A, Petrucelli J. *Medicine: An Illustrated History.* Hong Kong: Harry N Abrams Inc, Abradale Press; 1997:215.
2. Lyons A, Petrucelli J. *Medicine: An Illustrated History.* Hong Kong: Harry N Abrams Inc, Abradale Press; 1997:216.
3. www.philosophypages.com/ph/desc.htm.
4. Rakel D, Weil A. Philosophy of integrative medicine. In: Rakel D, ed. *Integrative Medicine.* Philadelphia: WB Saunders; 2003: .
5. Whorton JC. The history of complementary and alternative medicine. In: Jonas W, Levin JS, eds. *Essentials of Complementary and Alternative Medicine.* Philadelphia: Lippincott Williams & Wilkins; 1999:16–30.
6. Haller J. *A Profile in Alternative Medicine: The Eclectic Medical College of Cincinnati, 1845–1942.* Kent, OH: The Kent State University Press; 1999:6–8.
7. Weil A. *Health and Healing.* Boston: Houghton Mifflin; 1983:21.

8. Starr P. *The Social Transformation of American Medicine*. Cambridge, MA: Persius Publishing; 1982:384.

9. Flexner A. *Medical Education in the United States and Canada*. New York: Carnegie Foundation for the Advancement of Teaching; 1910.

10. Kohatsu W. History of complementary and alternative medicine in the US. In: Kohatsu W, ed. *Complementary and Alternative Medicine Secrets*. Philadelphia: Hanley & Belfus; 2002:4.

11. Lyons A, Petrucelli J. *Medicine: An Illustrated History*. Hong Kong: Harry N Abrams Inc, Abradale Press; 1997:215.

12. Dale H.H. Medicinal treatment: its aims and results. *Br Med J*. 1957; Aug 24:423–428.

13. Rakel D, Weil A. Philosophy of integrative medicine. In: Rakel D, ed. *Integrative Medicine*. Philadelphia: WB Saunders; 2002:3.

14. Starr P. *The Social Transformation of American Medicine*. Cambridge, MA: Persius Publishing; 1982:143–145.

15. National Center for Health Statistics. Life expectancy. Available at: http://www.cdc.gov/nchs/fastats/lifesepec.htm. Accessed March 6, 2003.

16. Weil A. *Health and Healing*. Boston: Houghton Mifflin; 1983:82–83.

17. Pizzorno J. *Total Wellness*. Rocklin, CA: Prima Publishing; 1996.

18. Rakel D, Weil A. Philosophy of integrative medicine. In: Rakel D, ed. *Integrative Medicine*. Philadelphia: WB Saunders; 2002:3.

19. Starr P. *The Social Transformation of American Medicine*. Cambridge, MA: Persius Publishing; 1982:384–385.

20. Rakel D, Weil A. Philosophy of integrative medicine. In: Rakel D, ed. *Integrative Medicine*. Philadelphia: WB Saunders; 2002:3.

21. National Center for Health Statistics. http://www.cdc.gov/nchs/fastats/hexpense.htm. Accessed March 6, 2003.

22. Starr P. *The Social Transformation of American Medicine*. Cambridge, MA: Persius Publishing; 1982:381.

23. Starr P. *The Social Transformation of American Medicine*. Cambridge, MA: Persius Publishing; 1982:384–385.

24. Ray P, Anderson S. *The Cultural Creatives: How 50 Million People are Changing the World*. New York: Random House; 2000:110.

25. Ray P, Anderson S. *The Cultural Creatives: How 50 Million People are Changing the World*. New York: Random House; 2000:110.

26. Eisenberg DM, Kessler RC, Foster C, et al. Unconventional medicine in the United States—prevalence, costs and patterns of use. *N Engl J Med*. 1993;328(4):246–252.

27. Eisenberg D, Davis RB, Ettner SL, et al. Trends in alternative medicine use in the United States, 1990–1997: results of a follow-up national survey. *JAMA*. 1998;280(18):1569–1575.

28. Astin JA. Why patients use alternative medicine: results of a national study. *JAMA*. 1998;279(19):1548–1553.

29. National Center for Complementary and Alternative Medicine. http://NCCAM.nih.gov. Accessed March 7, 2003.

30. Bell I, Caspi O, Schwartz G, et al. Integrative medicine and systemic outcomes research: issues in the emergence of a new model for primary healthcare. *Arch Intern Med*. 2002;162:133–140.

31. Rakel D. *Integrative Medicine*. Philadelphia. WB Saunders; 2002:6.

32. Gaudet TW. Integrative medicine: the evolution of a new approach to medicine and to medical education. *Integr Med*. 1998;1(2):67–73.

33. Weil A. *Health and Healing*. Boston: Houghton Mifflin; 1983:41–51.

34. World Health Organization. *Preamble to the Constitution of the World Health Organization. WHO Basic Documents*. 26th ed. Geneva: World Health Organization; 1976.

35. Weil A. *Spontaneous Healing: How to Discover and Enhance Your Body's Natural Ability to Heal Itself*. New York: Alfred Knopf; 1995.

36. McKegney CP. Medical education: a neglectful and abusive family system. *Fam Med*. 1989;21(6):452–457.

37. Remen R. Recapturing the soul of medicine. *West J Med*. 2001:174:4–5.

38. Remen R. Recapturing the soul of medicine. *West J Med*. 2001:174:4–5.

39. Maizes V, Koffler K, Fleishman S. Integrative assessment. In: Rakel D, ed. *Integrative Medicine*. Philadelphia: WB Saunders; 2003.

40. Coulehan JL, Platt FW, Egener B, et al. "Let me see if I have this right . . .": words that help to build empathy. *Ann Intern Med*. 2001;135(3):221–227.

41. Astin JA, Shapiro SL, Lee R, Shapiro DH. The construct of control in mind–body medicine. Im-

plications for healthcare. *Altern Ther Health Med.* 1999;5(2):42–47.

42. Maizes V, Koffler K, Fleishman S. Integrative assessment. In: Rakel D, ed. *Integrative Medicine.* Philadelphia: WB Saunders; 2003:11–16.

43. Wetzel MS, Eisenberg DM, Kapchuck TJ. Courses involving complementary and alternative medicine at US medical schools. *JAMA.* 1998;280: 784–787.

44. Whitcomb M. The general professional education of the physician: is four years enough time? *Acad Med.* 2002;77(9):845–846.

45. Kligler B, Gordon A, Stuart M, et al. Suggested curriculum guidelines on complementary and alternative medicine recommendations of the Society of Teachers of Family Medicine Group on Alternative Medicine. *Fam Med.* 2000;31: 30–32.

46. Kligler B, V Maizes. Personal communication conducted by R. Lee.

47. Vickers AJ, Van Haselen R, Heger M. Can homeopathy prepared mercury cause symptoms in health volunteers? A randomized, double-blind placebo-controlled trial. *J Altern Complement Med.* 2001;7:141–148.

48. Bell I, Caspi O, Schwartz G, et al. Integrative medicine and systemic outcomes research: issues in the emergence of a new model for primary healthcare. *Arch Intern Med.* 2002;162: 133–140.

49. Rakel D, Weil A. Philosophy of integrative medicine. In: Rakel D, eds. *Integrative Medicine.* Philadelphia: WB Saunders; 2003:3.

50. Gaudet T, Synderman R. Integrative medicine and the search for the best practice of medicine. *Acad Med.* 2002;77(9):861–863.

51. Sierpina VA, Philips B. Need for scholarly, objective inquiry into alternative therapies. *Acad Med.* 2001;76:863–864.

52. Maizes V, Schneider C, Bell I, et al. Integrative medical education: development and implementation of a comprehensive curriculum at the University of Arizona. *Acad Med.* 2002;77(9):851–860.

CHAPTER 2

Psychosocial Determinants of Health and Illness: Reintegrating Mind, Body, and Spirit

JOHN A. ASTIN AND KELLY FORYS

Presented in this chapter is a review of some of the evidence linking psychosocial factors to a variety of health outcomes. Drawing upon the work of the philosopher Ken Wilber, we begin with a consideration of some of the historic roots of the mind–body split. As will be seen, Wilber argues that in the premodern era, "mind" and "body" were essentially fused (i.e., thought of as not separate); with the dawn in the West of the Enlightenment and the emergence and subsequent dominance of the empiric–scientific mode of inquiry, the mind and body became separate; and in the postmodern world, the task now is one of reintegrating mind and body, an undertaking with obvious implications for the field of medicine. With the goal of helping in this mind–body reintegration, in this chapter we first summarize the epidemiological findings examining the relation between various psychosocial factors (personality, mood states, and cognitive factors) and physical health. We then review some of the physiological and mechanistic data that link mental–emotional factors (e.g., psychosocial stress) with physical function and health. Finally, we discuss the therapeutic implications of these findings.

▶ THE MIND–BODY SPLIT: "BLESSING OR CURSE"

In a series of more than 20 books,[1–3] the modern-day philosopher Ken Wilber has developed a grand theory or model that attempts to incorporate the research findings and theories of scholars across a multitude of disciplines. Toward this end, he has drawn from the wisdom and insights of numerous scientists, thinkers, social critics, scholars, and philosophers, and then set about to integrate their seemingly irreconcilable differences and disagreements regarding what is "true" about life and human beings. Based upon his extraordinarily comprehensive analysis of scholars and of research findings and theories, Wilber has essentially "divided" the universe (and the quest for knowledge) into four quadrants, what he refers to as "the four corners of the known universe" or "the four faces of the Kosmos": (1) the interior dimensions of individuals (feelings, meaning, concepts, and beliefs); (2) the interior dimensions of the collective (shared meetings, cultural beliefs, worldviews, and value subcultures); (3) the exteriors of individuals (organs, tissues, cells, and behavior); and (4) the exteriors of the collective (social structures, families/tribes, ecosystems, and modes of production). Figure 2–1 illustrates these different domains as four quadrants: the upper two referring to the individual level (left and right being interior and exterior dimensions, respectively), whereas the lower quadrants refer to the collective levels. Essentially, these different domains or dimensions of the known world rely on different modes of inquiry, as well as use different languages to describe them. The interiors of individuals are described primarily in "I" language (*I* feel joyful, sad), the interiors of the collective in "we" language (*We* understand one another), and the exteriors of

both the individual and the collective in "it" language (*It* weighs 2 pounds).

Because they can both be described in objective "it" language, Wilber suggests that if the two exterior dimensions are collapsed into one, these broad categories parallel Plato's "The Beautiful" (interior, individual), "The Good" (interior, collective), and "The True" (exterior, individual *and* collective); Karl Popper's three worlds: subjective (I), cultural (We), and objective (It); and Jurgen Habermas' three validity claims: subjective sincerity (I), intersubjective justness (We), and objective truth (It) (see Figure 2–1).

Wilber argues that in premodern cultures and civilizations, these three value spheres, which he terms "The Big Three"—art (I), morals (We), and science (It)—were essentially fused or undifferentiated. Wilber points out, for example, that in the Middle Ages, Galileo could not freely look through his telescope and honestly report on what he saw because his findings contradicted the Church's official doctrine.

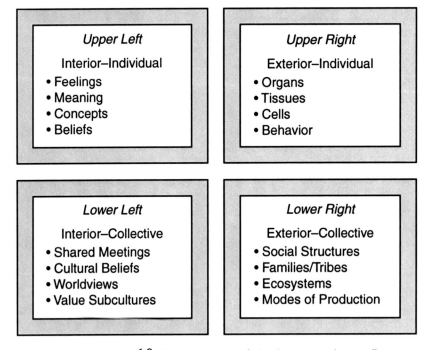

Figure 2-1. Wilber's[1-3] "four corners of the known universe."

Because these spheres were not clearly differentiated, the Church essentially dictated what science could or could not investigate and say. But with the rise of modernity, these spheres became more clearly differentiated. Thus, a Kepler or a Galileo could now study the world empirically regardless of whether their findings contradicted Church doctrine. Similarly, with the differentiation of these three spheres, artists were free to paint nonreligious, or even sacrilegious, images without fear of punishment, and public discourse regarding what was just or moral was no longer constrained by what the Bible decreed to be true or right in these areas.

Wilber argues that this differentiation of the "The Big Three" (art, science, and morals) is the real and enduring legacy and gift of modernity, its "dignity" if you will. He suggests that such differentiation is the hallmark of evolution and development (be it at the individual or collective level). For example, without it, rationality would have never been freed from the chains of mythic belief or personal whim, and objective science as we know it would never have flowered as it has. Although this differentiation was essential for humankind's evolution and progress, this differentiation all too quickly became *dissociation,* a state of affairs in which the empiric–scientific perspective came to dominate. The "I" and the "We" interior domains were essentially reduced to mere exteriors (the upper-right and lower-right quadrants in Figure 2–1). What was really "true" about life was that which could be described in objective, "it" language. And, as Wilber argues, if the world is reduced to that which is observable (e.g., behaviorism, positivistic science), then it is essentially stripped of all meaning, value, or depth. One is left with a "collapsed Kosmos," what Wilber refers to as "Flatland." This parallels Max Weber's "disenchantment of the world, the reduction of the cosmos to objective observables or exteriors." To quote Wilber:

> At the very least, then, the mind and the brain are two different views of your individual awareness, one from within, one from without; one interior, one exterior. Each has a very different phenomenology—they "look" quite different. The brain looks like a crumpled pink grapefruit; the mind looks like all the joys and desires and sorrows and hopes and fears and goals and ideas that fill your awareness from within. No doubt the brain and mind are intimately connected . . . but they also possess some profound differences that prevent either from being reduced, without remainder, to the other.

So although the differentiation of The Big Three represents the *dignity* of modernity, dissociation on the other hand represents its *disaster.* And Wilber states that what is now needed is a reintegration of these three major value spheres, a recognition of not just the value but the necessity of each, and the ways in which each sphere can and does inform the others.

In terms of medicine, the differentiation of the spheres of body (upper-right quadrant) and mind (upper-left quadrant) has in many respects facilitated the emergence of a medicine grounded in the physical and biological sciences. The remarkable biomedical and technological discoveries and advances witnessed in the last century certainly testify to the advantages of such a differentiated approach. However, as Wilber and many others have pointed out, the disaster of modernity is that this positive differentiation has, unfortunately, led to a kind of dissociation or fracturing of mind from body, resulting in a medicine that is not really "integral" precisely because it too often fails to consider factors other than those in the upper-right quadrant. In other words, in an effort to free itself from what may have been rightly seen as antiquated, premodern notions that the nonmaterial world (e.g., gods, spirits, personal beliefs, and superstitions) could influence the material world, the proverbial baby was thrown out with the bath water. For example, while it may represent an evolution in thinking and practice to realize that certain diseases are caused by physical phenomena rather than the whim of the gods, human beings and cultures *do* have interior dimensions that are not, as Wilber points out, reducible to the right-hand, material quadrants. These dimensions of human and cultural experience do not have "simple location"; that is, they cannot be seen with the physical senses or their extensions (e.g., microscopy or magnetic resonance imaging).

Needless to say, this conceptual/philosophical severing of mind from body has had unfortunate practical consequences for medicine. To give but one simple illustration, imagine a patient who comes to his internist for a checkup. The doctor discovers that the patient has hypertension. Now, although that particular physician may have some awareness or appreciation of the potential role of mental–emotional factors in the development of high blood pressure, the physician gives it passing attention, instead focusing exclusively on the upper right of Wilber's quadrants, determining that the treatment of choice is to manage the condition pharmacologically. The patient proceeds to take the medication but experiences significant side effects (lost sexual desire) and as a result fails to comply regularly with his treatment regimen. As a result his hypertension is not managed very well, and while the physician experiments with other drugs, the same pattern of side effects and poor compliance is repeated. Five years later, the patient suffers a massive and debilitating stroke, undoubtedly caused at least in large part by his poorly controlled hypertension. Now, because this patient's internist gave only minimal credence to the potential role of the upper-left quadrant in contributing to his hypertension, he failed to perceive the fairly obvious cues provided by this patient, cues that the patient was experiencing significant amounts of psychological stress and had not managed it well, as evidenced by periodic bouts of depressive symptoms and free-floating anxiety. Had the potential role of the upper-left quadrant (in terms of both its contribution to the hypertension itself and the patient's poor compliance) been more fully acknowledged and addressed, this patient

may very well have been protected from the effects of a terribly disabling stroke.

As becomes evident in the remainder of this chapter, there is now a compelling body of empirical evidence that has emerged over the past several decades that points to the limitations of reducing the causes and cures of physical health problems to the upper-right quadrant (e.g., biochemistry, molecular biology, and pathophysiology). This evidence suggests that what is now called for is in fact an *integral* medicine that considers the very important role that the other three quadrants— psychological or upper left, cultural or lower left, and social or lower right—play in determining health and wellness. Owing to space limitations, we focus our review primarily on the evidence that links phenomena in Wilber's upper-left quadrant to health outcomes, with some brief discussion of the relevance of cultural (lower left) and social (lower right) factors in health.

▶ THE UPPER-LEFT QUADRANT: PSYCHOLOGICAL FACTORS AND HEALTH

In modern times, the historical origins of mind–body medicine can be traced to the early theories of Freud, who proposed that unconscious mental processes could produce definite physiological symptoms. The notion that physical illnesses could be traced to unresolved psychic conflicts (Freud's so-called conversion hysteria) was subsequently carried on in the work of psychiatrists such as Franz Alexander and others in the 1930s and 1940s, who were instrumental in shaping the field of psychosomatic medicine. These writers argued that certain bodily disorders, for example, ulcers, rheumatoid arthritis, and hypertension, were actually caused by emotional conflicts and described the characteristic psychological patterns and profiles of these different diseases. For example, a 1936 journal described the "diabetic personality type" as "apathetic, hypochondriacal, clingy and passive, and immature and masochistic." The "rheumatoid arthritis personality type" was typically characterized as perfectionistic, compliant, subservient, restless, and angry.

While the notion that specific personality types actually *cause* specific illnesses has not held up to scientific scrutiny, evidence emerging over the past several decades *does* suggest that certain psychological (Wilber's upper-left quadrant) factors may play an important role in influencing physical health and illness. In the next section, we briefly summarize the evidence examining the role of three of the most heavily researched constructs in health— hostility, anxiety, and depression. We then consider the extent to which certain positive psychological states may influence physical health and well-being. Finally, we discuss the clinical implications of these relationships between Wilber's upper-left and upper-right quadrants by summarizing some of the evidence that demonstrates the efficacy of mind–body therapies for a variety of different health conditions.

Anger/Hostility

Numerous epidemiological and clinical studies suggest a strong link between hostility and negative health outcomes. Although the construct has been variously defined, hostility can be thought of as consisting of negative beliefs about and attitudes toward others, including cynicism and mistrust (the belief that others are motivated by selfish concerns and that they are likely to be either hurtful or provoking in some way).[1] Anger is also a component of the hostility construct and in this section we also review literature that examines the health effects of anger.

In one of the earliest epidemiological studies, Barefoot et al. found that physicians with the highest scores on the hostility scale of the Minnesota Multiphasic Personality Inventory (MMPI) at age 25 were seven times more likely to have died by age 50 of all causes, including heart disease, than those with lower hostility scores.[5] Although some research has failed to demonstrate a link between hostility and cardiovascular disease, Miller et al., in their meta-analysis of 45 studies,[1] reported that the cumulative evidence to date suggests that hostility *is*, in fact, an independent risk factor for coronary heart disease.

Studies also indicate that hostility is associated with behavioral risk factors such as smoking, alcohol, and dietary fat intake. It has, therefore, been suggested that research examining the hostility–health link that has statistically controlled for such lifestyle risk factors may actually be *underestimating* the health implications of hostility, since its effects may in part be mediated by these same risk factors (e.g., persons high in hostility are more likely to smoke, which, in turn, makes them more prone to various health problems).

Other data support the hostility/anger–poor health connection. For example, a recent study found that baseline cynical hostility was predictive of coronary artery calcification in young adults (N = 374) 10 years later after adjusting for demographic and lifestyle factors.[6] In another study, greater proneness toward anger appeared to place normotensive men and women at greater risk for coronary heart disease (CHD) morbidity/mortality, independent of established biological risk factors. In this study, high trait anger was associated with a two times greater risk of CHD and nearly three times greater risk of hard events, when compared with low levels of self-reported anger. Interestingly, these relationships did not hold for hypertensive individuals.[7]

In a study of Finnish men (N = 2,074), those who reported the highest levels of expressed anger had twice the risk of stroke (average follow-up time of 8 years) after adjusting for demographic and biological risk factors.[8] Kawachi et al. found that among a sample of 1,305 men who were free of CHD at baseline, those reporting the highest levels of anger were three times as likely to experience either non-fatal myocardial infarction or fatal CHD at 7-year follow-up.[9]

Along with its relationship to known behavioral risk factors, hostility may also exert direct pathophysiological effects that contribute to poor health. For example, studies show that hostility is associated with greater cardiovascular reactivity to laboratory stressors (e.g., highly hostile individuals show greater catecholamine responses as well as higher heart rate and blood pressure levels during exposure to mental stress). Hostile individuals also tend to show greater ambulatory blood pressure responses during daily life activities,[10] as well as increased platelet reactivity and diminished mononuclear leukocyte β-adrenergic receptor function.[11]

Anxiety

Substantial evidence points to a link between anxiety (including anxiety disorders) and negative health outcomes. In the case of cardiovascular disease, where the bulk of the research has been done, several large-scale community-based studies[12] show significant relationships between anxiety disorders and cardiac death (the effects appear to occur through sudden cardiac death but not myocardial infarction). Prospective studies also show positive associations between both anxiety disorders and worry (defined in this case as a subcategory of generalized anxiety disorder) and coronary artery disease.[11]

Several mechanisms have been suggested to explain the observed relationship between anxiety and cardiovascular disease. Research shows that individuals with anxiety disorders tend to have reduced heart rate variability, which, as noted by Rozanski et al.,[11] could suggest excessive sympathetic nervous system activation (possibly leading to arrhythmias and a greater incidence of sudden cardiac death) or impaired vagal control.

A meta-analysis by Friedman and Booth-Kewley[13] examined epidemiological data linking an array of psychological factors to different disease states. In the case of anxiety, their analysis revealed significant positive correlations between anxiety and headache disorders, asthma, arthritis, and ulcers. Because the majority of these studies were not prospective in design, it is difficult to determine definitively the causal direction of the observed correlations (i.e., it is possible that having these different health conditions tends to increase people's anxiety levels).

Studies also suggest that anxiety has implications for immune function. For example, Fehder[14] argues that anxiety brought about by anesthesia during surgery may, through its immunosuppressive effects, slow recovery and impair wound healing. This theory is consistent with the emerging body of literature from the field of psychoneuroimmunology[15] that demonstrates a broad array of negative health effects resulting from increased mental–emotional stress, including delayed wound healing, prolonged infection, and increased production of proinflammatory cytokines, which may explain the far-reaching and negative health consequences of psychosocial distress.[16]

Depression

Data from multiple prospective studies in both healthy populations and in patients with coronary artery disease have demonstrated a significant link between the incidence of major depression and future cardiac events. For example, in a study of 1,190 male medical students, Ford et al.[17] found that the incidence of clinical depression was a significant risk factor for subsequent coronary artery disease. This risk was present even for myocardial infarcts occurring 10 years after the onset of the patients' first episode of depression. Research also suggests that depressive symptoms, even in the absence of major depression, are associated with an increased risk of cardiovascular disease.[11]

The related constructs of hopelessness (negative expectations about the future and one's goals) and helplessness have also been shown to have significant relationships with both cardiovascular disease and cancer. In a study of 616 normotensive Finnish men, Everson et al.[18] found that those with high levels of baseline hopelessness were three times more likely to become hypertensive in the intervening 4 years. It should be noted that the investigators controlled for depressive symptoms in their study, suggesting that these two constructs may represent independent risk factors.

In a recent prospective study of 578 women with early stage breast cancer, researchers found that those patients who responded to the diagnosis with more pronounced feelings of hopelessness/helplessness were significantly more likely to have relapsed or died at 5-year follow up. In this study, higher levels of depression at baseline also predicted higher mortality rate at 5 years.[19]

Although the clinical implications are not currently well understood, it is now well documented that both clinical depression and depressed mood are associated with poorer immune function (e.g., decreased natural killer cell activity and proliferative response to mitogens).[16] There is also some evidence to suggest that immune dysregulation may help explain the observed relationships between depression and heart disease.[20]

Stress

The social psychologist Lazarus defined stress as the "particular relationship between the person and the environment that is appraised by the person as taxing or exceeding his or her resources and endangering his or her well-being." The physiological effects of acute and chronic stress have long been known through the pioneering efforts of such researchers as Hans Selye and Walter Cannon. We have long known that under either perceived or actual internal or external challenge or pressure, the body responds to meet such challenges. Although necessary and adaptive in many circumstances (e.g., the fight or flight response enables humans to respond to threats in the environment by mobilizing the body for intense physical activity), researchers over the past several decades have examined the potential health consequences resulting from an overexposure to stress and the resulting overactivation of the neurohormonal stress response. A large body of research now exists that demonstrates that exposure to acute and chronic levels of stress can elicit profound physiological changes (e.g., on the cardiovascular, immune, and neuroendocrine systems) that can, in turn, lead to negative health consequences.[11,16,21,22]

In many respects, one can look at the states of hostility/anger, anxiety, and depression/hopelessness as the emotional and behavioral *consequences* of stress—the cognitive/affective result when one perceives that one does not have the internal/external resources to meet a given demand or challenge in life. Understanding these emotional states as the consequence of, as well as contributor to, an overactive stress response might help explain why they so consistently correlate with a broad array of negative health outcomes.

Positive Psychological States

Although the majority of research to date linking psychological factors to physical health has focused primarily on "negative emotions," a number of studies have also explored the extent to which certain positive mental–emotional states can exert a corresponding beneficial effect on health. For example, research has examined the construct of optimism—the generalized expectation that outcomes will be positive or favorable.[23] Several prospective studies show that optimism predicts improved quality of life in cancer patients,[24] functional status in the elderly,[25] recovery from surgery and myocardial infarction,[26] and management of pain.[27]

Another positive psychological state that has received considerable research attention is "sense of control." Animal and human studies show that when subjects can exert (or perceive they can exert) some measure of control over a psychosocial stressor, they evidence less immune suppression. Research also suggests that individuals experience less of the physiological and psychological effects of environmental stress when they can predict when a negative event is going to occur, if they have (or perceive they have) some measure of control over the administration of a stressor, or if they know they have the capacity to stop the stressor.[28,29]

A construct related to sense of control is "self-efficacy," the subjective assessment that one has the internal–external resources to cope with a given or hypothetical situation (what might be construed using the Lazarus definition as the opposite of stress). Studies suggest that positive outcomes (e.g., in pain and disability) resulting from mind–body and behavioral interventions such as the Arthritis Self-Help Program are mediated by changes in self-efficacy.[30–32] Both laboratory and clinical studies indicate that perceived self-efficacy is an important cognitive factor in pain tolerance and control. Self-efficacy also predicts pain tolerance in normal subjects and these effects appear to be mediated by endogenous opioid mechanisms.[33]

The Complexity of the Upper-Left Interior Quadrant

This chapter paints a somewhat simplistic picture of the relationship between mind and body, one that (at least on the surface) would suggest that positive emotions contribute to positive physical health, whereas negative emotions contribute to poorer health. However, we feel it important to emphasize that the picture is probably considerably more complex and subtle than this (and evidence suggests it is). A few examples may be helpful.

First, as noted previously, there is an extensive body of research pointing to the mental and physical health-enhancing effects of sense of control. However, evidence also suggests that the relationship between psychological control and health is not a simple, linear one (i.e., more control = better health; less control = poorer health). In fact, there appear to be circumstances under which being given greater control (either perceived or actual) is experienced as aversive by some individuals.[28,29,34,35] For example, although some patients desire more information and control over health care decision-making, others do not want such control and report that it makes them more, rather than less, anxious. In addition, efforts to gain a sense of control may not always be health promoting or adaptive. For example, evidence suggests that letting go of active control efforts can under certain circumstances (e.g., those over which we have little actual control) contribute to positive mental and physical health outcomes.[36]

A second example that points to the complexity of the emotion–health link is the role of "negative affect." The body of evidence presented previously would suggest that negative affect (e.g., depression, anxiety, and stress) is, in the long run, ultimately damaging to one's health. However, research suggests that there may be situations in which the experience or expression of negative affect is therapeutic and correspondingly associated with *positive* physical health outcomes. One of the best examples of this comes from a recent randomized trial by Smyth et al.[37] in which individuals with either asthma or arthritis were asked to write about stressful life experiences. In this study, the researchers found that this emotional disclosure exercise was associated with significant improvements in symptoms in both groups of patients. However, the writing intervention appeared to be effective *to the extent that participants experienced negative affect*. In other words, the pattern, at least in this study, was that greater short-term distress immediately following the intervention was associated with more pronounced positive changes in physical symptoms (and ultimately less distress) by the end of the study.

A final example that illustrates the complexity of the relationships between phenomena in the upper-left quadrant and health is optimism. On the basis of her extensive research, the health psychologist Shelley Taylor argues that maintaining both positive illusions (e.g., about one's degree of personal control) and unrealistically optimistic beliefs (e.g., about the future) is health promotive.[38] However, an optimistic disposition could, theoretically, cause people to deny emotional and/or physical problems (e.g., "everything will turn out fine . . ."), which could in turn result in a failure to take appropriate action (e.g., self-care and visits to a physician) to prevent or treat an illness. Evidence also suggests that the tendency to either overlook, deny, or be unaware of negative affective states (i.e., what has been termed "repressive coping") is associated with a variety of negative health outcomes.[39]

► THE LOWER-LEFT QUADRANT: CULTURAL FACTORS AND HEALTH

The interpretation (by both patients and health care practitioners) of physical symptoms as well as emotional response to illness and the meanings given to these experiences are all embedded in and influenced by cultural beliefs and assumptions (Wilber's lower-left quadrant).[10] Although diseases of the physical body certainly have material/biological (upper-right quadrant) components and causes, they are also to some extent socially and culturally constructed phenomena. The actions and behavior of individuals when they are ill are also strongly influenced by culture. For example, cultures consider certain behaviors to be more or less socially appropriate or acceptable ways to respond to particular physical symptoms. Also, the types of health care decisions (e.g., the choice to use complementary and alternative therapies) and lifestyle choices we make are frequently influenced by the cultural groups we live in and with which we identify.[11]

An example that points to the important role of culture in shaping our experience of and response to bodily symptoms is menopause. As discussed by the cultural anthropologist Deikman in *The Illness Narratives*, women of most non-Western societies pass through the period of "menopause" with few real complaints or reported symptoms and with virtually no concept that this "life transition" is an illness. He notes that the same is true for premenstrual syndrome, a "medical condition" that is virtually unheard of in much of the world. Now whether it is the case that women experience actual symptoms during these periods and simply fail to report them (e.g., because there is not cultural permission to do so) or do not in fact experience symptoms because the conditions have not been culturally reified is not entirely clear. However, the point is that concepts of "health" and "illness" very much exist in rich and complex cultural contexts that must be appreciated and understood if our practice of medicine is to become truly integral.[10]

► THE LOWER-RIGHT QUADRANT: SOCIAL FACTORS AND HEALTH

There are numerous examples that point to the important role that social factors (Wilber's lower-right quadrant) play in shaping physical health. These include studies showing a linear correlation between lower socioeconomic status (particularly level of education[12]) and poorer health; the health benefits of social support;[13] the role of environmental factors (e.g., pollutants and hormones in the food supply) in health; and the impact upon individuals' health and well-being of public health initiatives such as improved sanitation, immunization, and education regarding lifestyle risk factors (e.g., smoking). For example, in terms of social support, a 1979 study[14] of 4,775 adults in California found that those individuals with fewer social connections or ties were more than twice as likely to die over the next 9 years (after controlling for health status, age, race, and socioeconomic status). More recently, Kawachi et al.[45] studied men who were free from coronary heart disease over a 4-year period. Those who were not married or with few friends or relatives and who were not members of community groups were at increased risk for cardiovascular death after adjusting for known biological risk factors.

The relationship between lower socioeconomic status and poor health remains one of the most robust in the epidemiological literature.[46–48] The exact reasons for these observed relationships (e.g., between less education and poorer health), however, remain somewhat unclear. One mechanism might be reduced access to quality health care, although some studies show a statistical relationship between socioeconomic status and health even after controlling for various "access to care" variables. It also has been suggested that these relationships may be mediated by psychoneuroimmunological factors; for example, people with less economic means experience greater psychosocial stress which, in turn, exacts a greater physiological toll through neuroimmune mechanisms such as increased cortisol or cytokine production. A recent study by Steptoe et al.[49] lends some credence to this latter theory. These investigators examined the relationship between responsiveness to stress and socioeconomic status (measured by grade of employment). Subjects lower in socioeconomic status evidenced significantly more delayed recovery in cardiovascular function (blood pressure and heart rate variability) following exposure to a series of mental stressors in a laboratory setting. The authors suggested that their findings may point to a potential mechanism to explain the observed relationship between lower socioeconomic status and increased risk for cardiac disease.

▶ CLINICAL IMPLICATIONS

The cumulative evidence presented in this chapter strongly supports the notion that an array of psychosocial factors can contribute to physical health and illness in significant ways. It points to the profound importance not only of Wilber's upper-right quadrant (i.e., biology, physiology, and genetics), which has been the primary focus of medical research and practice in the nineteenth and twentieth centuries, but of the other three quadrants in the Wilber model: psychological, cultural, and social. Given this body of epidemiological and laboratory findings, it would, therefore, be logical to hypothesize that if we intervened clinically at the level of the other three quadrants (e.g., through teaching individuals to manage stress more effectively, to reduce anxiety, to manage anger more effectively, to increase sense of control, and so on) we would be able to significantly influence health outcomes.

We recently reviewed evidence for the effectiveness of an array of mind–body/psychosocial interventions including relaxation, meditation, imagery, stress-management, and cognitive–behavioral therapy.[50] Based on the positive findings of meta-analyses and randomized controlled trials, we concluded that there was strong evidence to support the incorporation of mind–body approaches in (1) the treatment of chronic low back pain, (2) coronary artery disease, (3) headache, (4) insomnia, (5) preparation for surgical procedures, (6) management of the treatment and disease-related symptoms of cancer, (7) arthritis, and (8) urinary incontinence.

Additional clinical conditions that merited further research based on either promising findings from randomized trials or strong theoretical links to psychosocial stress included asthma, tinnitus, diabetes, gastrointestinal disorders (e.g., irritable bowel syndrome), and HIV.[50] Areas of future research identified by Astin et al.[50] included mechanisms of action of mind–body therapies, the potential value of such approaches in primary and secondary prevention, and clarifying the role of individual differences in terms of determining patient responsiveness to mind–body interventions.

Based on the relatively infrequent and mini-mal side effects associated with such treatments and the emerging evidence that these approaches may also result in significant cost savings, it is clear that the integration of psychosocial/mind–body approaches, particularly in the clinical areas highlighted above, should be considered a priority for medicine.

REFERENCES

1. Wilber K. *The Collected Works of Ken Wilber: Volumes 1–8.* Boston: Shambhala; 1999/2000.
2. Wilber K. *Sex, Ecology, Spirituality: The Spirit of Evolution.* Boston: Shambhala; 1995.
3. Wilber K. *A Brief History of Everything.* Boston: Shambhala; 1996.
4. Miller TQ, Smith TW, Turner CW, Guijarro ML, Hallet AJ. A meta-analytic review of research on hostility and physical health. *Psychol Bull.* 1996;119(2):322–348.
5. Barefoot JC, Dahlstrom WG, Williams RB Jr. Hostility, CHD incidence, and total mortality: a 25-year follow-up study of 255 physicians. *Psychosom Med.* 1983;45(1):59–63.
6. Iribarren C, Sidney S, Bild DE, et al. Association of hostility with coronary artery calcification in young adults: the CARDIA study. Coronary Artery Risk Development in Young Adults. *JAMA.* 2000;283(19):2546–2551.
7. Williams JE, Paton CC, Siegler IC, Eigenbrodt ML, Nieto FJ, Tyroler HA. Anger proneness predicts coronary heart disease risk: Prospective analysis from the Atherosclerosis Risk in Communities (ARIC) study. *Circulation.* 2000;101(17):2034–2039.
8. Everson SA, Kaplan GA, Goldberg DE, Lakka TA, Sivenius J, Salonen JT. Anger expression and incident of stroke: prospective evidence from the Kuopio Ischemic Heart Disease Study. *Stroke.* 1999;30(3):523–528.
9. Kawachi I, Sparrow D, Spiro A 3rd, Vokonas P, Weiss ST. A prospective study of anger and coronary heart disease. The Normative Aging Study. *Circulation.* 1996;94(9):2090–2095.
10. Jamner LD, Shapiro D, Goldstein IB, Hug R. Ambulatory blood pressure and heart rate in paramedics: effects of cynical hostility and defensiveness. *Psychosom Med.* 1991;53(4):393–406.
11. Rozanski A, Blumenthal JA, Kaplan J. Impact of psychological factors on the pathogenesis of cardiovascular disease and implications for therapy. *Circulation.* 1999;99(16):2192–2217.
12. Kawachi I, Sparrow D, Vokonas PS, Weiss ST. Symptoms of anxiety and risk of coronary heart disease. The Normative Aging Study. *Circulation.* 1994;90(5):2225–2229.
13. Friedman HS, Booth-Kewley S. The "disease-prone personality." A meta-analytic view of the construct. *Am Psychol* 1987;42(6):539–555.
14. Fehder WP. Alterations in immune response associated with anxiety in surgical patients. *CRNA.* 1999;10(3):124–129.
15. Kiecolt-Glaser JK, Page GG, Marucha PT, MacCallum RC, Glaser R. Psychological influences on surgical recovery. Perspectives from psychoneuroimmunology. *Am Psychol.* 1998;53(11):1209–1218.
16. Kiecolt-Glaser JK, McGuire L, Robles TF, Glaser R. Emotions, morbidity, and mortality: new perspectives from psychoneuroimmunology. *Annu Rev Psychol.* 2002;53:83–107.
17. Ford DE, Mead LA, Chang PP, Cooper-Patrick L, Wang NY, Klag MJ. Depression is a risk factor for coronary artery disease in men: the Precursors Study. *Arch Intern Med.* 1998;158(13):1422–1426.
18. Everson SA, Kaplan GA, Goldberg DE, Salonen JT. Hypertension incidence is predicted by high levels of hopelessness in Finnish men. *Hypertension.* 2000;35(2):561–567.
19. Watson M, Haviland JS, Greer S, Davidson J, Bliss JM. Influence of psychological response on survival in breast cancer: a population-based cohort study. *Lancet.* 1999;354(9187):1331–1336.
20. Murr C, Ledochowski M, Fuchs D. Chronic immune stimulation may link ischemic heart disease with depression. *Circulation.* 2002;105(14):e83.
21. Kiecolt-Glaser JK, McGuire L, Robles TF, Glaser R. Psychoneuroimmunology and psychosomatic medicine: back to the future. *Psychosom Med.* 2002;64(1):15–28.
22. Sapolsky RM. Glucocorticoids, stress, and their adverse neurological effects: relevance to aging. *Exp Gerontol.* 1999;34(6):721–732.
23. Scheier MF, Carver CS. Dispositional optimism and physical well-being: the influence of generalized outcome expectancies on health. *J Pers.* 1987;55(2):169–210.
24. Allison PJ, Guichard C, Gilain L. A prospective investigation of dispositional optimism as a predictor of health-related quality of life in head and neck cancer patients. *Qual Life Res.* 2000;9(8):951–960.
25. Achat H, Kawachi I, Spiro A 3rd, DeMolles DA, Sparrow D. Optimism and depression as predictors of physical and mental health functioning:

the Normative Aging Study. *Ann Behav Med.* 2000;22(2):127–130.

26. Seligman ME. Optimism, pessimism, and mortality. *Mayo Clin Proc.* 2000;75(2):133–134.

27. Kjellgren A, Sundequist U, Norlander T, Archer T. Effects of flotation-rest on muscle tension pain. *Pain Res Manag.* 2001;6(4):181–189.

28. Shapiro DH Jr, Schwartz CE, Astin JA. Controlling ourselves, controlling our world: psychology's role in understanding positive and negative consequences of seeking and gaining control. *Am Psychol.* 1996;51(12):1213–1230.

29. Astin JA, Shapiro SL, Lee R, Shapiro DH. The construct of control in mind–body medicine: implications for health care. *Altern Ther Health Med.* 1999;5:42–47.

30. Astin JA, Beckner M, Soeken K, Hochberg M, Berman B. Psychological interventions for rheumatoid arthritis: a meta-analysis of randomized controlled trials. *Arthritis Rheum.* 2002; 47:392–401.

31. Smarr KL, Parker JC, Wright GE, et al. The importance of enhancing self-efficacy in rheumatoid arthritis. *Arthritis Care Res.* 1997;10(1):18–26.

32. Hadhazy VA, Ezzo J, Creamer P, Berman BM. Mind–body therapies for the treatment of fibromyalgia. A systematic review. *J Rheumatol.* 2000;27(12):2911–2918.

33. Bandura A, O'Leary A, Taylor CB, Gauthier J, Gossard D. Perceived self-efficacy and pain control: opioid and nonopioid mechanisms. *J Pers Soc Psychol.* 1987;53(3):563–571.

34. Astin JA, Anton-Culver H, Schwartz CE, et al. Sense of control and adjustment to breast cancer: the importance of balancing control coping styles. *Behav Med.* 1999;25(3):101–109.

35. Shapiro DH Jr, Astin JA, eds. *Control Therapy: An Integrated Approach to Psychotherapy, Health, and Healing.* New York: John Wiley & Sons; 1998.

36. Astin JA, Shapiro SL, Schwartz CE, Shapiro DH. The courage to change and serenity to accept: further commentary on the relationship between "fighting spirit" and breast cancer. *Adv Mind Body Med.* 2001;17:142–146.

37. Smyth J, Stone AA, Hurewitz A, Kaell A. Effects of writing about stressful experiences on symptom reduction in patients with asthma or rheumatoid arthritis: a randomized trial. *JAMA.* 1999;281: 1304–1309.

38. Taylor SE, Kemeny ME, Reed GM, Bower JE, Gruenewald TL. Psychological resources, positive illusions, and health. *Am Psychol.* 2000; 55(1):99–109.

39. Jamner LD, Leigh H. Repressive/defensive coping, endogenous opioids and health: how a life so perfect can make you sick. *Psychiatry Res.* 1999;85(1):17–31.

40. Astin JA, Astin AW. An integral approach to medicine. *Altern Ther Health Med.* 2002;8:70–75.

41. Astin JA. Why patients use alternative medicine: results of a national study. *JAMA.* 1998;279 (19):1548–1553.

42. Pincus T, Callahan LF, Burkhauser RV. Most chronic diseases are reported more frequently by individuals with fewer than 12 years of formal education in the age 18–64 United States population. *J Chronic Dis.* 1987;40(9):865–874.

43. Eng PM, Rimm EB, Fitzmaurice G, Kawachi I. Social ties and change in social ties in relation to subsequent total and cause-specific mortality and coronary heart disease incidence in men. *Am J Epidemiol.* 2002;155(8):700–709.

44. Berkman LF, Syme SL. Social networks, host resistance, and mortality: a nine-year follow-up study of Alameda County residents. *Am J Epidemiol.* 1979;109(2):186–204.

45. Kawachi I, Colditz GA, Ascherio A, et al. A prospective study of social networks in relation to total mortality and cardiovascular disease in men in the USA. *J Epidemiol Community Health.* 1996;50(3):245–251.

46. Everson SA, Maty SC, Lynch JW, Kaplan GA. Epidemiologic evidence for the relation between socioeconomic status and depression, obesity, and diabetes. *J Psychosom Res.* 2002;53(4):891–895.

47. Krantz DS, McCeney MK. Effects of psychological and social factors on organic disease: a critical assessment of research on coronary heart disease. *Annu Rev Psychol.* 2002;53:341–369.

48. Poulton R, Caspi A, Milne BJ, et al. Association between children's experience of socioeconomic disadvantage and adult health: a life-course study. *Lancet.* 2002;360(9346):1640–1645.

49. Steptoe A, Feldman PJ, Kunz S, Owen N, Willemsen G, Marmot M. Stress responsivity and socioeconomic status. A mechanism for increased cardiovascular disease risk? *Eur Heart J.* 2002; 23(22):1757–1763.

50. Astin JA, Shapiro SL, Eisenberg DM, Forys K. Mind–body medicine: state of the science, implications for practice. *J Am Board Fam Pract.* 2003;16(2):131–147.

CHAPTER 3
Mind–Body Medicine

SUZANNE LITTLE

Mind–body medicine—the interplay of mind, emotions, and physical processes in health and illness—encompasses a philosophy of care, a body of research, and an approach to therapy. These domains, drawing on disciplines as diverse as neurobiology, developmental psychology, behavioral medicine, and spiritual healing, illustrate the breadth of this evolving field, as well as the challenge of forging a unifying framework for the practicing clinician.

Mind–body medicine is characterized by a philosophical commitment to whole-person care. Its origins are found in ancient and holistic healing traditions, which strive for unity of mind, body, and spirit. The catalytic shift from the biomedical to the biopsychosocial perspective[1] reflected growing public interest in humanistic health care approaches that foster self-healing. These factors, along with the failure of conventional medicine to prevent chronic illness, increased recognition of psychosocial factors as mediating variables in health and disease, and the need for improved ways to address physical complaints without clear organic pathology, gradually paved the way for acceptance of mind–body interventions into mainstream medical practice.

The mind–body connection has been documented by 30 years of laboratory, epidemiologic, and evidence-based clinical research. Cognitive and emotional processes are predisposing and perpetuating factors in a number of medical conditions, and there is accumulating evidence that mind–body interventions are effective in hypertension and coronary artery disease,[2,3] headaches,[4] gastrointestinal disorders,[5] presurgical procedures,[6] chronic pain,[7,8] anxiety,[9] and cancer.[10,11] A remedy for the impersonal, high cost, specialty-driven modern health care system, mind–body medicine offers safe, natural, noninvasive, empirically validated, and cost-effective therapy options for preventing and managing chronic conditions and promoting patient self-reliance.

This chapter describes mind–body medicine from the perspective of the mind–body psychologist in an integrative medical practice. Since the emergence of health psychology and behavioral medicine in the 1970s, psychologists have played an active role in medical settings—hospitals, pain clinics, obstetric and gynecologic services, and integrative health centers. Working in concert with physicians and other health providers, the psychologist sees an array of medical conditions, including mood dysregulation, acute and chronic illness, persistent pain syndromes, posttraumatic stress conditions, psychophysiological disorders, and nonspecific somatic distress. All illness is understood to have predisposing psychological and physical factors that can be profitably addressed with mind–body intervention. Many chronic medical problems are triggered and exacerbated by stressful life events, maladaptive coping, and poor lifestyle choices. Somatic distress can also be shaped by emotional perturbations in the individual's inner life, some of which may spring from loss or misattunements in early primary relationships. Lingering illnesses, particularly those that involve pain, disability, and body image disturbance, can be further aggravated by a rupture between actual and perceived bodily experience that the individual may not be aware of. All this poses a significant challenge to the development of an integrated mind–body consciousness. The mind–body psychologist employs mind–body interventions in tandem with knowledge of health and illness behaviors, pathophysiology, personality psychology, interpersonal and family dynamics, and psychotherapy skills to mobilize the resources of the individual.

Health practitioners in mainstream medicine are recognizing that the mind's powerful resources—cognitive skills, emotional responses, behavioral competencies, and spiritual faith—can stimulate the body's internal healing capacity. But with some important exceptions,[12–15] the medical literature offers a relative dearth of applied, practical writings on mind–body integration from the *clinician's* perspective. There is a need for more effective mind–body treatment guidelines—how to address individual differences in stress reactivity or emotional understanding; how to enhance somatic well-being; how to capitalize on the regulatory functions inherent in therapeutic relationships; how to bridge the seemingly separate realities of mind and body by translating bodily perceptions into conscious experience, or by converting words and images into healing physiological processes; and, finally, how to develop more sophisticated approaches that integrate psychotherapy principles with mind–body interventions to optimize medical care and maximize response to treatment.

▶ MIND–BODY MEDICINE: THEORY

What Is Mind–Body Medicine?

Mind–body medicine is "an approach to health that focuses not just on the physical body and the conscious mind, but also incorporates unconscious emotional life and an individual's spiritual dimension."[16] Although the interconnectedness of mind and body is a central tenet of mind–body medicine, the mechanisms underlying the various therapies differ. Some mind–body therapies (e.g., acupuncture) exert their healing effects, initially at least, through somatic mechanisms. Others, such as hypnosis, more explicitly emphasize the impact of psychological factors (e.g., response expectancies, and qualities of attention) on physiologic change. And still others, such as yoga, may exert simultaneous physical and psychological effects.

The Three Domains of Mind–Body Medicine

Mind–body medicine reflects three areas of concern in health and illness: psychosomatic medicine, the behavioral aspects of illness, and therapeutic care. The theme of mind–body unity, that is, psychosomatic interaction, can be found throughout the mind–body medicine literature, from the psychoanalytic research on the physical consequences of emotional repression in the 1940s and 1950s,[17,18] to placebo studies[19] that sparked interest in the medicinal power of belief, to the empirical study of stress and psychophysiology,[20,21] and the field of psychoneuroimmunology. Mind–body medicine is also the study of illness behavior. It provides insight into how patients construct illness (cognitive appraisal) and cope with its effects. By providing a counterpoint to the impersonal, technologically driven encounter, mind–body medicine contributes to humanizing conventional medical practice. It offers perspectives on the medical therapeutic relationships that are drawn from psychotherapy research,[22] patient-centered interviewing practices, and participatory decision-making physician–patient models.[23]

Scientific Underpinnings of Mind–Body Medicine

The scientific underpinnings of mind–body medicine are found in the links between stress, behavior, and health, and in the field of psychoneuroimmunology.[24] Psychoneuroimmunology is the study of interactions between mind, nervous system, and the immune system.[25] These systems function as a complex, cooperative network of communication within the body—an integrated circuit that protects against infection and disease. Psychoneuroimmunology has led to a new understanding of the mind, as being not solely involved in hard-wired synaptic neurotransmission, but engaged in a biochemical information flow of neuropeptides, steroids, and cytokines along intercellular channels.[26] It has highlighted the interdependence of major body systems once thought to operate autonomously but now governed by the central nervous system. The central nervous system regulates the body's behavioral, physiological, and immunological defenses via two neuroimmunomodulatory pathways—autonomic and neuroendocrine—that work together to defend against disease.

Self-Regulation

Self-regulation is the endeavor to modify voluntarily one's own physiological activity, behavior, or process of consciousness.

J.M. STOYA[27]

A basic biological principle, self-regulation is intrinsic to mind–body health and psychoneuroimmunology. Self-regulation is the cybernetic process of homeostasis,[28] whereby systems of the body maintain stability (e.g., automatic regulation of body temperature, and oxygen concentration). The concept of biological regulation originated in Bernard's discovery of the "milieu interior," the intracellular fluid (e.g., lymph) in which cells live, whose stabilizing mechanism Cannon[29] termed homeostasis. Self-regulation was first understood to be a function of the autonomic nervous system, but neu-

roendocrine regulation, which is implicated in the human stress response ("fight–flight"), also ensures physiological competence. The hypothalamic–pituitary–adrenal (HPA) axis and the sympathetic nervous system (SNS) together represent a critical neuroendocrine pathway in maintaining the homeostatic regulatory processes of the body. Psychoneuroimmunology—the bidirectional flow of chemical signals between the central nervous system and the organs of the immune system (spleen, lymph nodes, thymus, and bone marrow)—is the means by which mind and body regulate immunity. Damasio refers to this homeostatic state as "dynamic sameness,"[30] the way in which the brain detects minute changes in the body's internal chemical profile.

The body's prototypical defense mechanism is its own homeostatic regulatory system against infection, inflammation, autoimmune disorders, and emotional distress. Homeostatic breakdown is manifested in behavioral disturbances, metabolic changes, and autonomic reactivity, as well as immune dysregulation. Defense as a self-protective mechanism operates on multiple levels—from the cellular (the proliferation of cytokines to spur wound healing; the release of catecholamines and cortisol in the initiation of the fight–flight response) to the psychological (use of unconscious defense mechanisms, such as denial or projection, or intentional coping strategies, such as prayer and vigorous exercise).

Stress Response

Stress plays a key role in chronic and psychophysiological illness, including cellular immunity.[31–34] A stressor is any environmental or psychic disturbance that disrupts homeostatic equilibrium. The "stress response" is the body's survival mechanism in the face of perceived or actual threat—highly effective in acute situations, but physically deleterious when the sources of stress (stressors) do not abate over time. The brain release of catecholamines and glucocorticoids triggers a set of activating neurophysiological responses—increased respiration rate, cardiovascular tone, arousal, muscle tension—that mobilize the individual to fight, flee, or freeze in order to restore homeostatic balance. The interplay amongst the hypothalamus, the pituitary, and the adrenal glands, and the hormones they secrete (corticotrophin-releasing hormone [CRH], adrenocorticotrophin hormone [ACTH], and the stress hormone cortisol), are illustrated in Figure 3–1.

Health appears to be most compromised when the stress response is either repeatedly switched on or cannot shut down. Repeated exposure to stressful events results in a response of surrender, associated with helplessness, depression, and down regulation of the immune system. The chronically stressed individual reacts

to minor daily problems as if they were major catastrophes, and it is possible that these microstresses (minor aggravations or hassles) which afflict us on a regular basis are more deleterious to the immune system than responses to major single life events, such as bereavement.

Although the fight–flight response is the primary neuroendocrine response to stress, women can, in some instances, show a different biobehavioral pattern. Taylor et al. are studying a phenomenon termed "Tend and Befriend,"[35] a self-regulatory response that draws on the attachment-caregiving system and is mediated by oxytocin in conjunction with female reproductive hormones and endogenous opioid peptide mechanisms. More so than men,

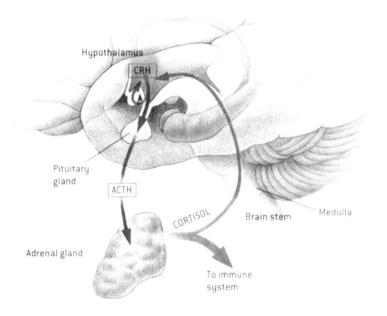

Figure 3-1. The stress response system. HPA axis—the interplay among the hypothalamus, the pituitary, and the adrenal glands—is a central component of the brain's neuroendocrine response to stress. The hypothalamus, when stimulated, secretes corticotropin-releasing hormone (CRH) into the hypophyseal portal system, which supplies blood to the anterior pituitary. CRH stimulates the pituitary to secrete adrenocorticotropin hormone (ACTH) into the bloodstream. ACTH causes the adrenal glands to release cortisol, the classic stress hormone that arouses the body to meet a challenging situation. But cortisol then modulates the stress response by acting on the hypothalamus to inhibit the continued release of CRH. Also a potent immunoregulator, cortisol acts on many parts of the immune system to prevent it from overreacting and harming healthy cells and tissue. *(From Sternberg EM, Gold PW. The mind–body interaction in disease.* Scientific American, *August 31, 2002, page 85.)*

women appear to seek solace and safety in nurturant activities designed to protect the self and offspring ("tending"), and are more likely to create and sustain social networks to aid in this process ("befriending"). Such research contributes to the literature on the health-protective influences of social support discussed in Chapter 2.

The Diathesis-Stress Model of Psychophysiological Disorders

How does stress influence the outcome of illness or disease? In the diathesis-stress conception of illness,[36] constitutional and environmental factors interact to produce physical illness. Applying this model to psychophysiological disorders, Sternbach[37] proposed that three factors must be present for a psychophysiological disorder to occur: (1) an individual response stereotypy, defined as the person's constitutional predisposition for a specific physiological response; (2) inadequate homeostatic restraints (such as a preexisting infection or trauma) that lead to a stress-induced breakdown; and (3) activation by a specific situational stressor. Examples of activating stressors are a reoccurrence of the predisposing homeostatic restraint (reinjury); internal cognitive distress; or a new stressful circumstance, such as loss. The first two factors correspond to Galland's concept of "antece-dents," and the third to his concept of "triggers," as discussed in Chapter 4.

The idea of response stereotypy suggests there may be individual differences in physiological reactivity[38] which can influence the outcome of illness in different ways. The more prominent physiological response patterns under stress include:

- Autonomic reactivity (anxiety and hypertension)
- Musculoskeletal disorders (temporomandibular joint dysfunction and tension headaches)
- Immune-related disorders (allergies, infections, and autoimmune disorders)

Mason[39,40] further suggests that different stressors produce different mixes of autonomic activation and hormone release, such as, heightened autonomic nervous system activity but minimal adrenal gland hormone release, or vice versa. Differences can be attributed, in part, to the influence of psychological modulators. Among the more potent of these psychological variables in mediating stress and immunity is emotional response: emotional inhibition (e.g., repressive coping style) has been linked to increased autonomic activity[41] and higher antibody titers to Epstein-Barr virus (EBV).[42] Emotional expressiveness (as measured in Pennebaker et al.'s emotional disclosure exercise)* is associated with increased lymphocyte proliferation in response to mitogens[43] and decreased antibody or titer, levels to EBV-viral capsid antigen.[44]

Allostasis and Allostatic Load

Allostasis is the body's capacity to maintain stability (homeostasis) through change.[45] As an explanatory biobehavioral construct, allostasis portrays the complex interaction between environmental challenge and biological response more accurately than does homeostasis (which assumes a single optimum per physiological parameter) because "different circumstances demand different homeostatic set points."[46] Over time, exposure to increased secretion of stress hormones may produce a debilitating allostatic load.[47] Allostatic load describes the long-term results of "accumulative strain on the body"—the sum of stress-induced metabolic and physiological changes in the body—and their pathophysiological consequences. Individual differences in stress perception,

---

*In Pennebaker's emotional disclosure task, subjects are asked to write continuously over consecutive sessions about traumatic experiences in their lives, while their reactivity is assessed on both subjective (e.g., self-reported physical symptoms) and physiological measures. Symptom improvements from this writing exercise have been found in individuals diagnosed with asthma and rheumatoid arthritis.[43] It is not known whether the benefits derive from emotional disinhibition, exposure to a feared stimuli, cognitive restructuring, or some other mechanism.

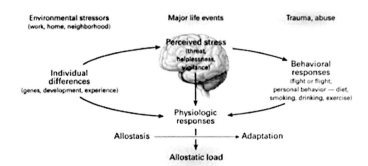

Figure 3–2. The stress response and development of allostatic load. Perception of stress is influenced by one's experiences, genetics, and behavior. When the brain perceives an experience as stressful, physiologic and behavioral responses are initiated, leading to allostasis and adaptation. Over time, allostatic load can accumulate, and the overexposure to neural, endocrine, and immune stress mediators can have adverse effects on various organ systems, leading to disease. *(Reprinted from McEwen with permission from* The New England Journal of Medicine. *Copyright 1998 Massachusetts Medical Society. All rights reserved.)*

genetics, and life experience determine the "price" the body pays. "There is a cascading effect of genetic predisposition and early developmental events, such as abuse and neglect or other forms of early life stress, to predispose the organism to overreact physiologically and behaviorally to events throughout life."[48] In one prospective study, higher allostatic loads are associated with poor cognitive and physical functioning, and a significantly higher risk of cardiovascular disease—independent of demographic and other health status risk factors (Figure 3–2).[47,49]

Emphasis on the long-term impact of stress (allostatic load) as a major contributing factor in physical illness and emotional distress distinguishes mind–body approaches from mental health approaches, which put a premium on psychogenic factors in psychophysiological or functional somatic illnesses. The mind–body therapist recognizes that emotions are embodied, that distress is normally experienced in the body, and that psychophysiological processes that emerge during stressful life events should not be summarily dismissed as a somatized version of neurosis. Mind–body therapies seek nonpejorative ways to locate the range of body experiences—both positive and negative—into larger conceptions of physical functioning and somatic well-being.

Current Perspectives on Self-Regulation and Emotion

The primacy of emotional experience in physical health and healing has yet to be recognized by mainstream medicine. Nor has it been fully integrated into psychoneuroimmunological investigations, which often contribute to compartmentalization by focusing on molecular substrates or physiological interactions, to the exclusion of subjective experience, or vice versa. The challenge of today's mind–body science and medicine is to forge more deeply— to expand investigations of mind–body unity on the cellular level while designing studies that simultaneously evaluate the psychospiritual domain: the feelings that accompany molecular events.

PERT, DREHER, AND RUFF[50]

An explosion of research from neuroscience as well as infant observation studies and attachment models has highlighted the centrality of emotions in human behavior and relationships. The limbic region, the older part of the mammalian brain, encompassing the amygdala, hypothalamus, and related areas, is key to understanding how we perceive bodily functions, regulate affect and arousal, form bonds, and organize and integrate experience.[51] An emerging view suggests that the mind is not an entity but a continuous flow of mental patterns or information;[52] that consciousness, memory, and emotions are inseparable; and that affect regulation learned in the context of early relationships is pivotal to the organization of the self.[53]

Neurobiology of Emotion

Neurobiologists exploring the links between memory and emotions have demonstrated that some emotional responses are not represented by cognition, thus confirming Freud's contention that a large part of emotional life operates unconsciously. They suggest that a subcortical level of emotional processing (which explains how primitive emotions, such as fear, become learned) must be integrated into accounts of self-experience.

In experimental research on rats, pairing sounds and electric shocks, LeDoux[54] showed that fear is a classically conditioned response mediated directly by thalamic sensory processing. That learning can take place via noncortical neural mechanisms may clarify why symptoms associated with anxiety, phobias, and trauma are so refractory. The body retains an enduring "emotional memory" of the physiological symptoms (e.g., sympathetic nervous system arousal, muscle contraction) activated by the traumatic experience, which renders the fear response highly susceptible to being reexperienced and very difficult to extinguish or resolve.

In his work on the biology of consciousness, Damasio[30,54a] asserts that the brain closely monitors the body's internal milieu and registers a memory of subtle changes in its physiological state in the form of "somatic markers." Based on this somatic feedback, the brain makes associations between stimulus events and bodily responses, which are stored in implicit memory. An internal stimulus (image or memory) can thus activate an "as-if marker," engendering the same kind of physiological response as if the stimulus were a real event. Although both actual and as-if markers arise without consciousness, their effects are palpable. These body signals help to construct a primitive sense of self—"a feeling of knowing"—that precedes self-awareness, but nevertheless influences how one responds, plans, and anticipates. Clinical uses of the signs and signals of the body's internal workings are discussed in a later section on body awareness and in the case studies.

Neurobiology of Attachment

Linking psychobiological research with findings from infant observation studies, scientists and psychoanalysts suggest homeostatic regulation begins as an *interactional* process between mother (caregiver) and infant.[55,56] Socioemotional regulatory experiences with the mother facilitate the development of postnatal brain structures, particularly the orbitofrontal cortex,[57] a cerebral system directly involved in homeostatic regulation, controlling ACTH and corticosteroid levels, especially in the right hemisphere.

Attachment as a psychobiological process has been studied in animal populations. Harlow[58] demonstrated the importance of body contact when monkeys, seeking solace after maternal separation, chose terry cloth-covered wire "mothers" to the plain wire "mothers" that dispensed milk. Hofer[56] found that mother rats nurture and stabilize infant pups through "hidden (sensorimotor) regulators." When rat pups are separated from their mothers, these nutritional, olfactory, thermal, and vestibular mechanisms can be experimentally manipulated (replaced with stabilizing surrogates), which suggests that homeostatic regulation is a complex system governed by differentiated (versus global) responses to loss.

The human mother also provides basic functions (thermoregulation, fluid balance) necessary to the infant's survival. She regulates the infant's immunity by providing the humoral antibodies and immunoglobulins in breast milk. Field,[59] in a study of premature infants with low birth weights, demonstrated that tactile– kinesthetic stimulation, another important regulatory function, resulted in greater weight gain, increased head circumference, and behavioral improvement over control infants. Such research prompted Hofer to argue that in human infants these psychobiological regulators may be "the building blocks" on which emotional attachments and intrapsychic processes are built.[49]

Psychoanalytic theorists maintain that the emotional *quality* of early mother–infant experiences predicts successful development of a self-regulatory capacity, including the ability to modulate affects and the subsequent ability to feel empathy. Early empathic ruptures, such as premature loss or separation, as well as misattunements in reciprocal mother–infant interactions, can lead to developmental delays that hinder the acquisition of autoregulation, and thus impede the child's development of a cohesive self. One explanatory model of illness that draws on psychobiological and attachment research is discussed in the next section.

Disorders of Self-Regulation: Affect Dysregulation in Illness

Taylor[60,61] hypothesizes that affect dysregulation—difficulty managing mood, arousal, and tension states—arising as a consequence of early life disruptions may be key to understanding stress reactivity and disturbances in the limbic–hypothalamic–pituitary axis that put one at risk for physical illness. An infant's response to loss or separation is influenced both by "the breaking of an attachment bond" (emotional regulation) and "the withdrawal of the previous biological and behavioral regulation supplied by the mother." Withdrawal of these regulatory functions lead to physiological disturbances that can precipitate the onset of a somatic disorder, or increase later susceptibility to disease.

Patients who somatize distress often show an impaired capacity for affective expression and cognitive processing—a characteristic identified as "alexithymia" (Table 3–1).[62,63] Taylor[61] suggests that in alexithymic individuals, "the normal developmental transition from interactional regulatory processes" (via sensorimotor pathways) "to self-regulatory processes that are primarily psychological" is disrupted.

Although it is unclear whether alexithymia is an affective style or a stress response, patients with disordered emotional regulation have a difficult time identifying and communicating feelings and appear susceptible for developing somatic disorders, such as essential hypertension,[65,66] diabetes mellitus,[67] eating disorders,[68] posttraumatic stress syndrome,[69] and substance use disorders.

The close relationship between alexithymia and somatization suggests that preoccupation with somatic distress may defend against painful emotions resulting from traumatic experiences.[70] In patients exposed to trauma, neural processes in the orbitofrontal cortex, the associational regions of the brain, become blocked. Disturbing memories elicit stress hormone and catecholamine release, which appears to impair hippocampal and amygdala circuits connected with memory processing, and reduced hippocampal volume has been found in patients diagnosed with posttraumatic stress disorder.[71]

In a study of somatically distressed individuals, Blaustein and Tuber[72] found a significant correlation between upsetting interpersonal life events and number of reported symptoms, and suggested that "an inability to tolerate the affective dimension of relational challenges may account for the distress of many somatizing pa-

▶ **TABLE 3-1** FEATURES OF ALEXITHYMIA

- Difficulty identifying feelings
- Difficulty distinguishing feelings from bodily sensations of emotional arousal
- Difficulty describing feelings to others
- Constricted imaginal processes (dearth of fantasies)
- An externally oriented cognitive style

Source: Taylor GJ, Bagby RM, Parker JDA. The alexithymia construct: A potential paradigm for psychosomatic medicine. Psychosomatics *1991;32:153–164*

tients." Feelings that remain at a presymbolic (i.e., bodily level) elude reflection and introspection. It is the reflective capacity that allows one to not only organize emotional and cognitive experience but to form stable attachments to significant others.[73] Stable attachments are integral to the capacity to translate somatic experience into personal symbols, to allow for the expression of more complex blends of feelings[71]—a precondition for the development of an integrated sense of self.

Therapeutic Implications

Mastery of self-regulation skills—an important therapeutic goal in managing chronic and stress-related illness—must encompass an understanding of how the expression of emotions facilitates or impedes regulatory activity and social interactions. By using mind–body techniques—hypnosis, biofeedback, imagery techniques, body awareness, and meditation—one can alter and control autonomic functions associated with stress reactivity (increased heart rate, respiration rate, vasodilation, gastrointestinal motility, and blood pressure), as well as influence muscle response and motor activity, and even intentional immunomodulation.[75] Mind–body therapists engage patients in becoming aware of the emotional dimension of bodily experience, in expressing unresolved or inchoate feelings, and in finding ways to release psychophysiological tension, all of which facilitate the realization of self-regulatory competence.

▶ MIND–BODY MEDICINE: CLINICAL PRACTICE

The Mind–Body Therapist in the Medical Setting

How can something as ethereal and immaterial as a thought have such dramatic effects on the material body?

LARRY DOSSEY[76]

Given the growing recognition that many medical conditions are best understood from an integrative mind–body perspective, the scope of practice for the mind–body therapist has broadened (Table 3–2). Individuals are increasingly learning how to integrate self-healing and health maintenance strategies into their lives.

The mind–body therapist in clinical practice typically sees patients with chronic illness and stress-related medical conditions (psychophysiological disorders), which can include persistent pain, gastrointestinal problems, essential hypertension, inflammatory bowel syndrome, migraine and tension headaches, habit disorders, and women's sexual health concerns. An estimated 70% of visits in the primary care setting are for medical or emotional problems related to stress, relationship, and lifestyle factors.[77] Yet physicians and other health care providers, lacking training in psychopathology, personality development, and psychological defense, can be hindered in their ability to recognize how psychosocial factors interact with physical illness; that is, how psychosocial factors can function as precipitants, as well as predisposing and perpetuating forces, in disease process. Medical education training in mind–body medicine can be additionally enhanced by training physicians to understand the relationship between psychosomatic disorders, physical disease susceptibility, and disruptions in the human attachment system.

Clinical Assessment

The dual tasks of the mind–body therapist are to provide clinical assessment and mind–body treatment. In mind–body assessment, the individual is viewed in the context of overall psychobiological functioning. Health and illness are considered products of interacting genetic, physiological (e.g., temperament), psychological, and social (e.g., ritual and community) factors, all of which make up the totality of the person. In an assessment of psychological determinants, the intrapersonal (cognitive style and emotional expressiveness), interpersonal (quality and stability of relationship), and transpersonal (spiritual belief) components are evaluated.

▶ **TABLE 3–2** COMMON MEDICAL PROBLEMS ADDRESSED BY MIND–BODY THERAPISTS

- Psychophysiological disorders
- Mood dysregulation
- Stress-related, including "chronic stress" or "sick building syndrome"
- Medically unexplained disorders; that is, disorders with no evidence of structural organic disease (also called somatoform disorders or functional somatic disorders)
- Problems unresponsive to standard medical intervention for emotional factors (treatment avoidance complicated by unresolved psychological issues)
- Undiagnosed or unmanaged DSM-IV Axis II personality disorders (e.g., borderline personality disorder)
- Posttraumatic stress disorder, which is often first identified by primary care physicians or obstetricians/gynecologists

Abbreviation: DSM-IV = *Diagnostic and Statistical Manual of Mental Disorders,* 4th ed. Washington, DC: American Psychiatric Association; 1994.

The mind–body therapist develops a clinical formulation by using a variety of tools, including (1) clinical interviewing and observation; (2) patient self-inquiry, which may involve personal narrative, diaries, and art; and (3) objective evaluation, which can include a biofeedback-assisted psychophysiological evaluation and/or standardized inventories, such as the Hypnotic Induction Profile. An additional resource is the clinician's own intuitive awareness; that is, "hunches" that pick up on incongruities in the patient's presentation, or derive from sympathetic body feelings in the therapist (e.g., shortened breath associated with implicit awareness of a patient's anxiety), and the subtle energies that are "sensed" outside the mind's perceptual apparatus.[78] The primary objective is to capture the integrity of the patient's experience, to find ways to activate intrinsic healing forces, and to help other providers see the patient's medical problems in the context of personal struggles and larger aspirations, thereby fostering greater empathy for the patient's suffering.

Although patients with chronic illness find the mind–body connection intuitively appealing, some are skeptical that a change in attitude or the adoption of a healthier behavior can have a physiological or immunological impact. To the average person, mind "stuff" (anxious thoughts, hopes, and wishes) looks and feels different from body "stuff" (itchy sensations, burning pain, and tight muscles). The chronically fatigued patient is more apt to think about his or her exhaustion in functional terms—"I can't get up in the morning"—than to ponder possible interactions of metabolic imbalance and negative cognitive style.

The mind–body therapist meets this challenge by translating clinical knowledge (what we know from research and observation) into therapeutic practice; this involves developing a rationale and strategies for health maintenance that patients can incorporate into daily life. For example, patients with chronic pain syndromes can gain a greater sense of health self-reliance by monitoring their symptoms. This may entail using a pain diary to track symptom course, or another method of self-inquiry to increase awareness of possible links between pain, life habits, body posture, and negative mood.

Mixed Physical and Psychological Presentations

Chronically ill patients may show overlapping mood and physical presentations. Mood disorders, such as depression, can be secondary to systemic medical conditions, including endocrine disorders, coronary artery disease, cancer, and end-stage renal disease.[79] Depressed patients commonly seek help in medical settings, and yet their condition often goes undetected. In one study of 98 primary care adults with current major depression, Rost et al.[80] found that in 32% of these patients the depression remained unidentified for up to 1 year. When combined with medical illness, depressive illness can increase nonadherence, a sense of fatalism, and can increase mortality in some disorders, such as postmyocardial infarction.[81]

Posttraumatic Stress Disorder

Posttraumatic stress disorder (PTSD) is often undetected in the medical setting, in part because the delayed physical and emotional consequences of the original trauma make it difficult to identify. Although PTSD presenting in medical practice is commonly associated with physical and/or sexual abuse, it can also be caused by an acute or life threatening medical illness, such as acute respiratory distress syndrome or cancer, or it may occur in the aftermath of surgery. The central features of PTSD are (1) reliving of the traumatic event; (2) emotional numbness; and (3) hyperarousal, usually in the form of increased vigilance or startle reaction. Other signs that may indicate a traumatic response include an exaggerated, negative response to a medical procedure (an intense loss of control), persistent preoccupation with illness, or reckless avoidance of medical care, either caused by anxiety about or denial of illness.[82] Cognitive behavioral therapy (CBT) is the best-studied psychological intervention in the treatment of PTSD: a review of 17 controlled trials found that psychotherapeutic treatment produced a better outcome than either supportive management or no treatment.[83]

Undifferentiated Complaints

A large majority of the chronic problems in medical settings are vague or undifferentiated physical complaints: chest pain, fatigue, dizziness, headache, and edema. Thirty to seventy-five percent of physical symptoms lack a precise organic cause, and standard treatments are often ineffective.[84] Physical symptoms appear to be a more common expression of distress than are emotional complaints, and the number of somatic symptoms presented by a patient is highly correlated with the likelihood of an accompanying psychiatric disorder.[85]

Lipowski defined somatization as "the tendency to communicate psychological distress in the form of physical symptoms" and to seek medical help for such symptoms.[86] Psychodynamically oriented mental health practitioners have traditionally viewed somatization as a problem of classic conversion (e.g., hysteria), in which the somatic symptom replaces a warded-off effect of emotional trauma, such as guilt. As noted earlier, the construct of alexithymia, a deficit in capacity for expressing emotions and processing cognitions, is associated with somatization.[87]

Cognitive–behavioral therapists view somatization as a problem of faulty information processing, an error of perception that results in symptom amplification. Barsky[88] found that somatizers, who tend to show heightened self-scrutiny (bodily hypervigilance), are likely to experience benign bodily sensations as unpleasant or noxious, and to infer that those sensations are symptomatic of disease. Some somatizers—repressive copers—minimize or ignore symptoms. Wickramasekera[89] measured susceptibility to distress and somatization on the trait of hypnotizability (nonvolitional suggestibility), and found that patients high in hypnotic ability tend to amplify somatic symptoms, and to show sympathetic hyperactivity, whereas those low in this trait are more apt to ignore the symptoms and to show dysregulation of the parasympathetic nervous system during periods of stress or trauma. Individuals at greatest risk for somatization appear to be those high in both hypnotizability and negative affect. The challenge in treating individuals who routinely convert emotional distress into somatic symptomatology is that they generally reject a psychobiological basis to their illness, even as psychophysiological measures, such as skin conductance or electromyography show heightened levels of tension. This incongruity between implicit and explicit perception is found in Damasio's concept of somatic markers,[30,54a] physiological reactions that become embodied memories not readily available in conscious awareness.

Somatization appears to be a universal human response to unpleasant or stressful stimuli. People commonly express their emotional distress in bodily symptoms, and this may not always be maladaptive. Some mind–body theorists criticize somatization (somatoform in the American Psychiatric Association's *Diagnostic and Statistical Manual of Mental Disorders,* 4th ed. [1994] [DSM-IV]) as a pejorative label, which privileges a psychogenic view of embodying distress. Often called a diagnosis of exclusion, somatization does not necessarily rule out the presence of an organic condition.[90,91] These theorists contend that, to avoid dualistic classifications, nonspecific illnesses are better viewed as functional somatic disorders, because all medical complaints have physical and psychological components. As Sharpe and Wessley note,[91] "Until the medical and psychiatric diagnostic systems are successfully combined the clinician should consider the use of descriptive diagnoses from both systems ... [their] combination conveys more information than either alone."

Mind–Body Therapy: An Overview of Approaches

Mind–body therapy of the medically ill patient is an eclectic practice that encompasses diverse treatment approaches, from behavioral (stress management), to psychological (CBT and interpersonal therapy), to spiritual approaches to healing (meditation, Qigong, and transpersonal psychology).

The concept of healing, whether seen in its simplest form as symptom resolution, or, more dramatically, as spontaneous remission, is deeply embedded in the treatment philosophy of the mind–body therapist. Healing is also found in psychological states, such as self-forgiveness, the gradual acceptance of a fatal disease, or an awareness of spiritual reality. However conceived, mind–body therapy offers

immense heuristic value for medically ill patients, and provides a source of mutual motivation for provider and patient.

Mind–body therapies embody both self-regulatory and spiritual objectives. They are de-signed to instill awareness by teaching voluntary control of cognitive, emotional, and physiological processes, and by fostering self-exploration and a larger intentionality of purpose. Treatment can be brief and problem-focused (a three-visit hypnosis for hyperemesis) or—if psychotherapy is indicated, such as in cases where unresolved trauma complicates medical recovery or personality factors subserve somatic distress—more intensive and longer-term.

The prevailing mind–body models in clinical practice are (1) behavioral medicine (clinical psychophysiology) and (2) psychospiritual healing, which has origins in psychotherapeutic traditions as well as energetic healing approaches.

The premise of behavioral medicine is that stress reactivity and autonomic imbalance are associated with many chronic medical problems, which can be effectively addressed by using psychophysiological education, stress management, cognitive restructuring, and behavioral strategies (see Ref. 91a for a comprehensive overview).

The efficacy of short-term psychotherapy for physically ill patients was established in the early 1980s, when brief intervention with patients following heart attacks reduced the average hospital length of stay by 2 days compared to controls who did not receive the intervention.[91b] The usefulness of combining psychotherapy and mind–body techniques for treatment of medical conditions is less well-documented. A recent meta-analysis of clinical trials on a variety of medical conditions (chronic pain, insomnia, hypertension, anxiety, obesity, and duodenal ulcer) showed a significant treatment effect when hypnosis is used as an adjunct to CBT for treatment of these conditions.[92] Although biofeedback practitioners tend not to integrate their work with psychotherapy, Moss and Lehrer[92a] argue that psychophysiological psychotherapy, a biofeedback-assisted approach, can enhance receptiveness to CBT protocols. The blending of mind–body techniques with brief dynamic and interpersonal approaches, although less-well documented, is also practiced. Many contemporary mind–body approaches, including the energy parapsychologies, owe intellectual allegiance to the earlier body-focused therapies as Bioenergetics, Gestalt therapy, and Feldenkrais, as well as the human potential movement and growth therapies of the 1960s and 1970s (Rogers and Maslow), which heralded self-actualization and personal transformation.

Psychospiritual healing, as practiced in mind–body medicine, derives from two principal sources. The first source is the humanistic psychologies, specifically transpersonal psychotherapy and psychosynthesis. Transpersonal therapy views self not in the traditional psychotherapeutic sense of personal ego, but as self in relation to spirit or soul, and emphasizes purification of being through awakened consciousness (including altered states) as the primary vehicle for therapeutic change. Transpersonal therapists see psychological and spiritual growth in terms of distinct, but often overlapping, lines of development, and regard the intention and consciousness of the therapist as a potent resource in fostering such development.

Mental or spiritual healing involves the activation of subtle energies or powerful forces, which may either reside in the healer and/or be elicited in the healee (the person to be healed). Common interventions include focused intention, hand contact, nontouch "passes," or activating Qi energy through chanting.[93]

Although spiritual traditions informing mind–body practice encompass both theistic (personal divine) and nontheistic (impersonal divine) philosophies (Cortright[93a]), the nondual nature of reality inherent in Buddhist and Vedanta meditative practices appeals to many mind–body practitioners. Kabat-Zinn's variant of mindfulness-based meditation,[93b] for example, arises from Buddhist traditions that teach the illusory nature of self.

Theories of subtle energy medicine have been proposed by a number of clinicians and researchers. A continuum of consciousness, articulated by the Indian mystic Sri Aurobindo, embraces the idea that matter is spirit made manifest and spirit is matter transformed, and that the fundamental facets of human reality—Sat Chit Ananda (existence, consciousness, and bliss)—are all indivisible aspects of larger spiritual unity.[91,95] Tart[95a] early on explored levels of consciousness in a psychospiritual framework, and Wilber[95b] continues to deepen our understanding of the psychological and spiritual dimensions of human consciousness by interweaving theories of self, personality, and development into his larger paradigm (see Chapter 2 for an elucidation of Wilber's overall theory). Benor maintains that the energetic basis of consciousness and healing is action through intent.[96] Distant healing (nonlocal mind) is thought to occur via nonneural mechanisms or divine energy means, and may account for the healing effects of prayer (see Chapter 14). Mind–body therapists working within a spiritual tradition embrace a paradigm in which "energy" or "consciousness" is seen as the vehicle for growth and change, and can be seen as moving from a psychosomatic network to a theosomatic network to encompass the spiritual dimensions of healing.[97]

Characteristics of Mind–Body Therapy

People seek mind–body therapy to find new ways to promote health, reduce illness, and effect positive, life-sustaining change, and to become more active in self-care and personal transformation. The central features of mind–body therapy are education, experience, and collaboration.

- Mind–body therapy is *educational:* The first goal, self-care, a precondition for self-healing, is attained by achieving greater balance in the mental, physical, and emotional dimensions of life. The mind–body connection is "discovered" through the acquisition of specific skills and strategies, a deeper grasp of unique patterns of stress reactivity, coping responses, and unconscious bodily and emotional defenses, all of which can elucidate links between somatic experience and emotional understanding.

- Mind–body therapy is *experiential:* One learns through *doing* and *being.* The body as it undergoes physiological shifts is experienced holistically, not in terms of discrete sensations or symptoms.[98] Developing a body consciousness—"a living, sensing, internalized perception of oneself"—is part of this learning, as is attaining a pranic or a nonphysical consciousness, found in the immutability of the present moment.
- Mind–body therapy is *collaborative:* All therapeutic relationships are based on principles of trust and rapport. The mind–body therapist assists the self-healing process in direct and participatory ways. To encourage spiritual awareness, a provider may act more as a guide or advisor; work with breathing or bioenergy fields may involve touch, which extends the bounds of conventional psychotherapeutic relationships.

Mind–body therapy without benefit of psychological expertise would be contraindicated in cases of debilitating mood dysregulation, personality dysfunction, relationship conflict, or psychic trauma. Table 3–3 outlines situations for which the physician may want to consider referral to a mind–body medicine practitioner.

Table 3–4 outlines the spectrum of mind–body/psychotherapeutic approaches typically applied in an integrative practice.

Energy Psychology

The field of mind–body therapy actually has evolved considerably from its origins as a simple relaxation technique. It encompasses nonconventional therapies such as eye-movement desensitization response (EMDR), applied kinesthesiology, and thought field therapy (TFT). In the past few years, there has been a proliferation of therapies, many considered derivatives of therapeutic touch or TFT, which fall under the rubric of energy psychology[99] and work through the "human vibrational matrix"— the biofield (auras), energy centers (chakras), and energy pathways (meridians). The Association for Comprehensive Energy Psychology

▶ **TABLE 3–3** SUGGESTED GUIDELINES FOR REFERRAL FOR PSYCHOLOGICAL MIND–BODY INTERVENTION

1. Patient exhibits significant emotional distress or impairment that warrants therapeutic intervention.
2. Physician identifies a trauma history that impedes self-care.
3. Patient asks for help to surmount treatment resistance, problems with adherence.
4. Relationship or family dysfunction is an impediment to successful health outcome.
5. Chronic pain is precipitated or exacerbated by maladaptive pain behaviors (symptom amplification).
6. The patient's emotional or behavioral response suggests undetected trauma.
7. The physician suspects that nonresponsiveness to treatment is emotionally triggered or stress-related.
8. Patient uses multiple medical providers and pursues conflicting medical agendas that adversely impact overall care.

▶ **TABLE 3-4** MIND–BODY AND PSYCHOLOGICAL THERAPIES

Mind–Body Approaches	Conventional Psychotherapy	Spiritual-based Therapies	Energy Psychology
• Somatic experiencing • Relaxation training • Hypnosis • Eye-movement desensitization response • Focusing • Biofeedback • Guided imagery • Meditation • Body-focused therapies	• Cognitive-behavioral therapy • Brief dynamic • Interpersonal • Hypnotherapy • Group therapy • Family systems	• Qigong • Dahn healing • Psychosynthesis • Transpersonal psychology • Mental healing	• Thought field therapy • EFT—Emotional freedom technique • Tapas acupressure technique

(ACEP), founded in 1999, is actively engaged in education, training, and research to promote these energy-balancing approaches. Many of these methods use verbal affirmation protocols, and subjective scales (e.g., subjective units of distress [SUDs]), in tandem with tapping methods targeted at meridians or chakras, and they promise rapid somatoemotional release for a wide range of physical and emotional problems, including addiction disorders, PTSD, effects of environmental toxins, and allergies. Tapas acupressure technique (TAT) and the emotional freedom technique (EFT) are two of the better-known methods. Empirical evidence of the safety and efficacy of many energy psychology approaches is still being established.

Awareness in Mind–Body Practice

Contemporary mind–body therapists maintain that qualities of awareness, attentional focus, and intentionality—how and where we direct our thinking—can enhance how we know ourselves, and, in turn, guide how self-regulatory strategies are used to prevent illness and protect health. Many psychotherapists who work with physically ill patients do not fully use the range or subtleties of awareness, in part because they tend to categorize consciousness along binary (implicit–explicit and unconscious–conscious) lines, and limit inquiry to a narrow sample of mental states. Perspectives on the therapeutic potential of self-awareness are examined later in this chapter.

We come to know ourselves in different ways—sensing, observing, and intuition. All three sources of knowledge—direct, inferred, and inspired—rely on the use of emotions and emotional experience as self-organizing guides. This theory is consistent with Damasio's concept[30] of a neural self, where cognitions and emotions coexist within the brain system to coordinate bioregulation. It is also consistent with the idea, intrinsic to mind–body work, that self-regulation—the capacity to modulate one's psychophysiological state—is contingent on effectively managing emotions; that is, maintaining equilibrium in the face of mounting arousal, tension, or distress. The theory further encompasses an intuitive form of knowing or consciousness that appears to be reliant on nonphysical or spiritual mechanisms. Helping a patient deepen awareness of the physical body, cultivate a capacity for psychological reflection, and become receptive to transpersonal dimensions of self and experience are all integral parts of the integrative approach to mind–body psychotherapy.

Body Awareness

Soma is a Greek word that from Hesiod onward has meant "living body." This living, self-sensing, internalized perception of oneself is radically different from the externalized perception of what we call a "body."

THOMAS HANNA[100]

Body awareness provides access to the internal feelings and movements that underlie symptoms. The breath is perhaps the most direct way to become attuned to, as well as to regulate, bodily and related emotional experience. Other somatic signals (heart rate and stomach acidity) are also associated with changes in arousal or body state. The temporal dimensions of bodily feelings—the "bursts" and "waves" of different emotional states such as anger or sadness—provide useful data as well. There are many powerful experiential methods of bodily self-monitoring (e.g., Gendlin's focusing, Levine's somatic experiencing, and Hakomi). Patients with bioenergy training can attend more deeply to shifting subtle energies in channels known as meridian pathways or can activate chakra centers aligned with the major neuroendocrine areas of the body.[101] Such awareness is generally activated through directed focus or meditation and breath work.

A heightened sensitivity to bodily feelings is akin to what psychologist Donald Bakal calls "somatic awareness"[95]—the mind's perception of the inner sensations of the body, using sensory and kinesthetic information from the viscera (internal organs) and the musculoskeletal system. Somatic awareness is an "emergent property" of the nervous system, readily discernible in the background of consciousness, and yet capable of directly influencing bodily processes. Although a common response during pain is to ignore or distance oneself from unpleasant sensations, these feelings often shift when one moves intentionally into the very core of them. By attending to such sensations one can experience them as meaningful stimuli or signals which, once heeded, can be modified. The following description of a patient with migraines illustrates this point:

▶ SOMATIC AWARENESS

Beth has had biweekly full-blown migraines, usually with vomiting, for the past 8 months. She has now gone without a severe headache for 4 weeks. She attributes her success to mind–body work (biofeedback, visualization and breathing), which engendered a newfound ability to attend to, and accept, her body. Beth describes the early signs of her migraines as "a kind of grisly texture" (she stresses this is not a feeling) along the back of her spine which, if she were to use a color, would be "gray." This "texture" is accompanied, she says, by "a definite feeling of tightness crawling up on either side of my neck," reaching just under the occipital ridge. Beth recognizes that emotional stress often triggers her headaches, but, in the past, she spurred them on with self-punitive messages—"I can't have this headache now" or "this isn't happening to me"—resulting in subtle muscle bracing, as well as surging dread. She recently prevented a migraine by paying attention to the incipient body signs with a more open, less fearful attitude. As a result, Beth became aware of what she actually needed at that moment: "I want to go slow"; "I don't want to do three things at once"; "I want to put ice on my neck." These thoughts helped her relax, let go, and breathe calmly, all of which contributed to dissipating the sensations.

Shortly after that episode, Beth's migraines recurred, but she reported she was able to forestall three attacks, one of them major, in a 2-week period. "I now lean into the pain rather than avoid it." Bakal[95] contends that avoidance of sensory information is directly related to the pattern of headache-related thoughts that occur prior to and during a specific migraine episode. The integration of sensory and bodily information into consciousness can result in a more confident feeling of self-control.

Self-Reflection—Psychological Self

Psychotherapists use the term "psychological mindedness" to describe the ability to reflect thoughtfully on one's actions or experiences. The self-reflective capacity (psychological mindedness) is evoked in Freud's "observing ego" and is a precondition for developing insight, and for the ability to "contain" rather than "act out" emotional arousal or distress.

▶ SELF-REFLECTION

Yvonne says passing a kidney stone is as painful as childbirth. A veteran of many hospital trips, her first anxious response is, "Do I need to go to the ER? The pain 'feels like a Tsunami.'" If she shifts her posture, if she cries out, or if she fixates on her frustration, the stabbing intensifies, boring into her body like a drill. She tells herself she can bear the feeling, however excruciating, because it will eventually go away: "I know I can ride the crest of this wave, I find a way to stay somehow on top of the pain, and there I wait for the first tiny sign that it is subsiding."

Psychoanalytic writers have broadened the concept of self-awareness to encompass the mind's unique capacity to observe and experience itself simultaneously. William James (1889) was the first to articulate this dual stance—self as "I" and self as "Me"—as a fundamental feature of consciousness. Yvonne's capacity to both observe and experience acute discomfort at the same time, while simultaneously managing arousal and anticipating relief, illustrates the regulatory aspects of what analysts call self-reflective functioning[102] or mentalization.[103] Hypnosis, in particular, amplifies and uses the dissociative aspects of such dual awareness, with therapeutic benefit for conditions of pain, trauma, and ego fragmentation.

More recently, psychoanalysts have described affective mentalizing,[104] the capacity to know one's own (and therefore another's) inner emotional state. Psychotherapists view the mind as a self-regulating system, for which affect regulation (the outward expression of emotions) is integral. The psychoanalytic "self" plays a dominant role in emotional development, and affects and emotions are considered a precondition for self-understanding. The relationship between body and emotions begins in infancy, where affects are first felt as bodily sensations, which then become "increasingly elaborated, differentiated, and desomatized into subjective emotional states."[105] Reflective self-awareness transforms affects from sensations into "signals to oneself" that can help in the project of developing self-care and self-regulation. The "core of the self," Schore writes, "lies in patterns of affect regulation that integrate a sense of self across state transitions, thereby allowing for the continuity of inner experience."[106]

Self-reflective capacity fosters personal integration. Somatic awareness can be seen as a form of self-reflective functioning focused on body sensations. The ability to reflect on inner bodily experience, to cultivate somatic awareness, may be a key stage in this integrative process. But it is not equivalent to being able to represent one's emotional experience in language or symbols in order to reflect on it, share it, and transform it.

Conscious Awareness— Transpersonal Self

> *The fundamental task . . . is the silence of the mind. . . . All kinds of discoveries are made, in truth, when the mental machinery stops, and the first is that if the power to think is a remarkable gift, the power not to think is even more so*
>
> SATPREM[107]

In mind–body therapy, higher states of awareness can be attained through contemplative practice. This entails both focused breathing and meditation (concentration techniques such as transcendental meditation and the relaxation response, as well as insight approaches, such as mindfulness). Sri Aurobindo, who wrote extensively on supramental states, notes, "Mental consciousness . . . no more exhausts all the possibilities of consciousness than human sight exhausts all the gradations of color or human hearing all the gradations of sound."[108] Possible ways to vitalize consciousness work in mind– body practice include (following Evans[108a]):

- Concentration on the breath
- Emptying of consciousness
- Enhanced receptivity to spirit (chanting, chakra visualization)
- Being open to spontaneous changes in consciousness (shamanic awareness)
- Access to creativity

Breath Practices

Focused breathing is a practice of great benefit in the treatment of respiratory problems, anxiety, panic, or any disorder involving sympathetic arousal. Meditative breathing does not simply involve gas exchange in the lungs, but the release and control of powerful energies in the brain— vital life forces (Prana, Chi, Ki) that enhance development of consciousness. Such practices include yogic breath (pranayama), which energizes the nadis, the body's network of subtle energy channels, and prepares the mind for meditation; tonglen, a Buddhist meditative practice designed to instill compassion (acceptance and letting go) for human suffering via the rhythmic inhalation– exhalation cycle of breath; and dahn-hak, a Korean mind–body practice that combines breathing and visualization to increase oxygen circulation and natural sensations of bioenergy flow (Ki) to restore health. Specific brain respiration exercises energize key components of the brain—cerebral cortex, limbic system, and brain stem—to achieve overall integration, while mind–body harmony is further achieved through moving and stimulating the body parts associated with the brain areas.

- Inner body breathing

> *Sit or lie down and close your eyes. Locate your breath (where it originates in your body).*
>
> *Draw the breath gradually down to the lower part of your body (where you feel your gut).*
>
> *Allow the breath to gently massage the inner organs—the stomach, the kidneys, and the intestines. Feel the organs move, rise, and shift with the rhythm of your breathing.*
>
> *When you stand, retain a sense of this core part of your body, now vitalized and invigorated.*

Mindfulness and Intentional Systemic Mindfulness

The therapeutic benefits of meditation are well-documented.[109,110] Mindfulness (sati), a pure, soft-focused awareness, is the foundation for developing the South Asian meditation practice of vipassana (insight meditation), which involves examining mental contents—thoughts, perceptions, and sensations—with a direct, nonjudgmental knowing, a "mirror-thought" that reflects only what is presently happening in exactly the way it is happening.[111]

One of the more robustly studied of mind–body practices, as well as one of the first to accompany psychotherapy,[112] meditation induces hypometabolic changes, autonomic stability, and calming of an overstimulated limbic system.[113] Goleman[110] suggests that meditation can serve as a general stress-management strategy, unlike biofeedback or behavior therapy, which can target specific physiologic conditions. Meditators show a differentiated arousal pattern with specific stressors (cortical activation and limbic inhibition) but, when anticipating stress, show a more global arousal, followed by a more rapid limbic inhibition.

> Thus the meditator [who] is more alert but composed in response to threat cues, may seem more "stressed" in anticipation, and recovers more efficiently. To the degree that the recovery phase of stress confrontation is the key to chronic anxiety symptoms and psychosomatic disorders, meditation may function as a stress therapy . . . facilitating more rapid recovery from the psychologic and physiologic coping processes mobilized in stress situations. As such, meditation may prove a useful adjunct to any modern psychotherapy.[110]

Recent research using functional magnetic resonance imaging (fMRI) images and advanced electroencephalographic (EEG) analysis suggests that mindfulness training can shift an individual's general emotional state. Davidson[114] believes that this training may activate neuronal activity in the left prefrontal cortex, thus damping limbic activity in the right prefrontal cortex, which is associated with emotional distress states.

Intentionality—directing one's attention toward a specific end—is increasingly used in self-regulatory strategies. A variant on mindful-

ness, and an antidote to reductionistic mind–body practices, intentional systemic mindfulness (ISM)[14] views awareness as evolving along personal, interpersonal, and transpersonal lines. The practice of a self-regulation technique within the model of ISM allows for "one's intentions [to] move through concern for the specific symptom" (elevated heart rate) "to concern for the larger context of one's symptoms,"[14] from an ability to feel gratitude to "a sense of interconnectedness with all beings." ISM endows awareness with emotional meaning to more fully enrich the practice of self-regulation and to enhance health on multiple levels.

- Listening Meditation

Find a quiet place where you won't be disturbed and invite your mind to become still and calm.

Close your eyes, and focus your attention on ambient sounds—the sounds that surround you.

Listen to each sound until it fades. Rest until another sound rises into awareness. Let it come, let it go.

Now extend the listening to more distant sounds—sounds outside your immediate area.

Let the listening become very large, very open.

Find the farthest, most distant sound. Listen to it until it completely fades away.

Open your eyes. Say to yourself: I am here in this moment. I am here.

Mind–body therapy is often described as "a set of tools" or "techniques." While in one sense true, the description is also misleading. Any technique must be understood in the context of its therapeutic goal and its specific intent to heal. Breathing can be a simple form of relaxation (counting on the exhale) or a meditative practice (alternate nostril breathing) that activates the nadis. It is the healing framework that informs how it will be used and received. The essence of therapy, in the words of one transpersonal theorist, "lies not in what the therapist says or does but in the *silent frame* that operates behind the therapist's actions, informing and giving meaning to the specific interventions. It is that wider container which can hold all other theoretical orientations in it."[115]

Empathic Resonance: Where Minds Meet

The greatest gains in meditative work are achieved in solitude. Therapy, in contrast, is an interpersonal endeavor, and the empathic therapist, in particular, offers a form of affect regulation. The roots of empathy—"limbic resonance"[116]—are found in early caregiver experiences, which shape the ways the child learns to experience, share, and communicate affects. This, in turn, engenders the adult capacity to simultaneously reflect on and experience one's inner emotional state—mentalized affectivity[104]—and to use such embodied reflection for mutual understanding.

> James, a divorced lawyer, takes Lorazepam to sleep. He dislikes being dependent on a drug, but insists, somewhat legalistically, he can't sleep without it. He is irked because I focus on his "anxiety" when he needs help. I ask him to remove his glasses, lie back, and to turn, after a cycle of deep breaths, his sight inward. I ask if he sees differently without his glasses, and he says yes, he worries less. "When I wear my glasses I worry I might break them." I suggest, with his glasses off, he may find an inner seeing (insight) that might interest him. He relaxes. He

experiences his head dropping into the pillow, while thoughts drift out of him. He feels light, empty. I suggest he can warm his left foot (which is cold from walking in the snow). He is amazed he can warm it several degrees, while his right foot remains cool. A feeling of peace moves through him. Later, he says the experience, deeply pleasurable, reminds him of when he massages his 14-year-old son's head to help him go to sleep—it's their ritual, a time when Danny, whom he sees on alternate weekends, "says what's on his mind." He wonders what it would be like to have his son massage his head in the same way. He decides he will ask and find out.

Mind–body therapists are exploring the ways in which therapy performs a regulatory function.[55] The provider's contemplative presence, the rhythmic regularity of visits, a hypnotic voice, may all, in different ways, have a stabilizing, psychobiological effect. A young woman, having experienced months of erratic menses (from 36 to 48 days) following the removal of her intrauterine device, announced, after 6 months of therapy, that her periods had become consistently 28 days. This is a corollary to Hofer's[117] observation that the menses cycles of cohabitating women tend to become synchronous. Similarly, participation in social groups has been found to regulate adrenal cortical levels.[118]

A central tenet of psychotherapy is that an affective experience in the presence of the therapist is necessary for change. Despite compelling evidence that social support protects health, and, specifically, that an empathic relationship is more conducive to health outcomes than other forms of social support,[119] mind–body medicine is only just beginning to address and study the healing dimensions of social and emotional relatedness in mind–body treatment, especially the ways positive affective experiences in the context of the therapeutic dyadic or group relationship may promote health.

► CASE EXAMPLES IN MIND–BODY PSYCHOTHERAPY

Four cases in mind–body psychotherapy are presented. The first two cases are brief, symptom-focused interventions that address functional chest pain and urinary incontinence, respectively. When focusing on targeted problems in a time-limited format, mind–body therapists have more modest goals than those of more extended psychological treatments. The objective, however, is not simply to effect symptom relief, but to provide insight into the self-healing processes through psychological and experiential work. At times, significant shifts can happen without extensive cognitive or emotional elaboration. The third and fourth case studies describe longer mind–body psychological treatments; they address essential hypertension, in one patient, and the residual impact of a traumatic surgery/hospitalization in the other. Both are presented in an abbreviated form to highlight specific therapeutic dynamics.

► Case Example 1: The Sound of Silence

God breaks the heart again and again and again until it stays open.

HAZRAT INAYAT KHAN

Anxiety and Chest Pain

Roger, a British man age 54 years, was referred for anxiety related to functional chest pain. He had moved to New York 8 months ago, leaving behind his wife and youngest child, to assist in a 3-year start-up project for an Internet company. A competent consultant, Roger found his work stressful because of the brash arrogance and chaotic work habits of the CEO, 25 years his junior. He dreaded weekly staff meetings, which typically started at 11 P.M., with ill consequences for his sleep. He missed his family very much.

Roger first noticed chest pain 3 weeks previously, while flying back from London after a brief visit home. In addition to a "piercing feeling" deep in his chest, he experienced cold sweats, blurry vision, and shortness of breath. After a second frightening episode, he went to the local emergency room, but an extensive cardiac work-up showed no abnormality. Roger was healthy, of moderate build, and had no family history or risk factors for coronary heart disease (CHD). He did not smoke, drank little, ate sensibly, and exercised three times a week. His sleep, which was poor to begin with, began to deteriorate after the first panic episode; he often woke at 3 A.M. with his mind racing, and worrying about unfinished tasks. Roger had a stoic, self-reliant demeanor, and he was not inclined to complain. He struck me as a sensitive man, who was empathic and sad.

The symptoms Roger described met criteria for DSM-IV panic disorder, but, except for concern about his chest, he did not feel particularly anxious. However, he was hypersensitive to noise, and showed a marked startle reaction. Roger was curious about what a mind–body intervention could offer him. He asked "if there were a technique that could give him cognitive control."

Despite a difficult, lonely childhood (his mother died when he was 3 years old), Roger had done well for himself. He was happily married and newly a grandfather. He also mentioned that his father had recently died. That the death occurred just prior to the onset of Roger's chest pain did not particularly impress him. When he was 7 years old, his father, "a cruel, selfish man," went off to Brazil to live on family property.

Roger was left alone on the English estate under the guardianship of a tenant farmer who beat him during alcoholic rages. He remembers trying to phone his father many times, feeling comforted by the sound of the dial tone. Their relationship was never warm.

Although mind–body therapy was foreign to Roger, he was open to learning pranayama breathing and meditative techniques to induce relaxation and increase awareness of possible links between anxiety and chest pain. With focused breathing, he became more curious about the different sensations in his chest area, and seemed uncertain as to how to interpret the feelings evoked. At times, with Roger, I felt an acute loneliness. He tried to please me. His breathing—jerky and laborious—frustrated him. His mind wandered. He worried that his wife didn't want to leave her life in London, and then said, inexplicably, "I would rather punish myself than see another person hurt."

During the next visit, he reported his sleep had improved, and that he had successfully used breathing to alleviate tension in his chest. The discomfort was more muted now. He explored listening to his heartbeat, and noticed how the sensations changed when he placed his hand on his chest and inhaled warmth into the cardiac wall. In one exercise, he shifted between internal and external awareness, settling on sound as an object of meditative focus. Roger could readily attend to sounds inside the room (the hum of lights), then outside (children in the corridor or a door shutting), eventually extending his awareness to fainter sounds— workers talking on a scaffold below, a truck shifting gears, or a distant horn. His ability to extend his listening beyond the body opened up a sense of hope and possibility. He looked forward to the day he could pursue fly-fishing. This led to a surprising outburst—a realization that his father had died before knowing his infant great-grandson. Roger wept, clutching a tissue in his hand,

apologizing profusely for the emotional display. He said he and his younger brother were arguing about what to do with his father's ashes. Neither wanted to bear the burden of planning the burial.

When he returned, Roger said his chest felt better. There was one "tightening episode," which he breathed through. This was a good sign; he felt more in control of his symptoms. During this meditation session, I asked Roger to observe the space between thoughts. We sat together in meditation for 4 minutes whereupon he abruptly stood up. "I can't do this." He complained his chest was tightening, and he couldn't swallow or breathe. He appeared to be having a panic attack. He said twice: "I can't stand silence; I can't stand silence."

Roger later explained that meditation evoked a painful memory of adolescence. Often, when his guardian beat him, he sought refuge on a particular rock on the moors. But on this day he could not console himself, and the ambient silence became so excruciatingly loud—"a screaming in my head"—that he decided only by dying could he end his suffering. He was thinking how to do this, when a wild pony, grazing nearby, ambled toward him. Several other ponies followed, and soon he was surrounded by a small group of horses standing about, watching him. "They spoke to me," Roger told me, without embarrassment. "They said I must not take my life." At the time he felt oddly jolted, and then a warm sensation spread all over his body. He never seriously thought of suicide again.

Roger was subdued at the end of our session. "It's interesting," he said, "how things happen in life." He had stopped bickering with his brother. They agreed to meet up in a small coastal town to scatter their father's ashes into the Atlantic. He felt peaceful about this; it meant he could mark his father's passing in a dignified way. After that visit, I did not hear from Roger again.

▶ Case Example 2: Unbearable Urges

Urinary Incontinence

A tall, anxiously depressed, 27-year-old woman called her excessive need to urinate "the old lady's disease." This was a striking comment for someone so lovely, with her mane of dark curly hair, and a voluptuous body (of which she was unaware). Natalia recited her medical history like a child confessing something unsavory. "I've always peed a lot, for years," she said, "but this past year, I don't know, the urge has become unbearable."

Although her urologist had ruled out genitourinary abnormality, Natalia was convinced her problem was anatomical. She was also treated for hypothyroidism and dysthymia, and complained of a disturbing lack of focus ("brain fog"), which aggravated her anxiety at her corporate job. There was a past history of panic attacks, and an ongoing fractious relationship with an unemployed, older boyfriend whom she financially supported.

Natalia tried hard to comply with her urologist's injunction to "resist the urge," but was impatient with a lack of progress. She was seen by a primary care physician, a homeopath who prescribed Sepia, and an acupuncturist who diagnosed "quick bladder" exacerbated by damp heat in the lower burner related to "leaky gut syndrome." She was recommended dietary changes and herbs, and was treated with acupuncture. She had a positive response and was continent without medication, but would relapse with specific kinds of stress. The acupuncturist decided her incontinence might have a psychogenic aspect that would benefit from mind–body treatment.

Natalia most often had the urge to urinate during stressful presentation meetings. She would hold it in, no matter how long, and then "sprint" down a long corridor to the bathroom. "I can feel it dripping out in little spurts," she said. "It never comes in a steady flow." Her "accidents" were most common at work or on the subway.

Although she had achieved rapid success as a marketing executive, Natalia drove herself hard and felt inadequate. She skipped meals and stayed up late. She resented having to wear dark clothes to conceal the frequent leaks. In our interactions, she would oscillate between quick, clipped speech and a slower, drawn-out spaciness in which she would trail off in mid-sentence while staring at a painting on my wall. Sitting with her, I felt tugged about by the shifting emotions, yet conscious of her brittle defiance that suggested a commingled desire for and fear of change.

Hypnosis seemed an ideal intervention, not only because it would help soothe Natalia—she once told me, "I never *ever* feel completely relaxed"—but because it could counteract the urologist's problematic recommendation to control the urge, which, as a behavioral strategy, I felt, undermined efforts to gain charge of her life.

I initiated hypnosis indirectly by way of conversational trance—using wordplay and confusional techniques to induce a mildly dissociative state. The words *press/push* (physical act), *pressure* (emotional state), and *impressive* (ideal state) helped build "a case" for transformation.

Therapist: I imagine you feel *pressed* at times to do things you don't feel like doing.
Patient: What do you mean?
Therapist: Well, like *pushing* yourself to perform at work. . . .
Patient: [Sigh] I do resent it, especially last minute presentations . . . [irritably]. They just expect me to drop everything!
Therapist: Hmm . . .
Patient: [Pause] It isn't any pressure I don't already put on myself.

Therapist: Exactly. . . . I wonder if you can consider feeling less *pushed to press* yourself, is that possible? . . . You can even *impress* yourself you can function without *pressure,* can you not? . . . And if there were less *pressure* you might *flow* . . . more freely . . . more comfortably . . and *that* would be *impressive.* . . .

Patient: [Musingly] I used to run after work. It helped calm me. Maybe I should get back into that.

The next session began with a formal hypnotic induction with indirect suggestions for *setting her own pace.* Building on her reference to jogging, I introduced the metaphor of the long distance runner. I told a story about a marathoner famed for running laps to build endurance. Each lap along the way represented a different "milestone," which enabled the runner to feel more in stride, more in control: *This is a lap for strength* . . . *This is a lap for stamina* . . . (I uttered the phrases in a monotonous tone to which Natalia responded with a slight, rocking motion) . . . *This is a lap for patience* . . . *This is a lap for courage.* . . .

Utilization, an Ericksonian[119a] technique, helped reinforce those qualities she associated with a positive self-image.

At the end of the session, Natalia lay curled up in the chair, and was reluctant to open her eyes, taking time to stretch her arms and legs, and yawn with catlike pleasure. "That was amazing," she said. "I can't believe it, I actually feel relaxed."

She returned, irritated by a fight with her boyfriend. They argue, go to bed, and wake up angry. She sees a link with her somatic problems—muscle tension, exhaustion, and moodiness. She wonders whether it aggravates her urinary problem. "I feel so anxious, like I'm in constant crisis." Natalia's urgency became a useful metaphor for helping her reflect on her inner state:

And Natalia . . . perhaps you can see a window of time . . . a wide open space in your future mind . . . opening . . . you to the possibility that in a way known only to you . . . you can separate the urge . . . and the urgency . . . because they are not the same . . . there is all the space . . . time . . . distance . . . in the world between them . . . that's how far apart they are . . .

In the fourth session she noticed a big difference: she had had fewer episodes during the past week and she felt more in charge, although she now worried she'd disappoint "us" by failing. She said she was more direct with her boyfriend, not "caving in" as much. I saw her newfound assertiveness as a consequence of a posthypnotic suggestion used in an earlier visit: *If you hold back less, you can let go more.*

Natalia remarked: "I think I'm getting better, I don't know why. Frankly, it's baffling." She went to a movie and was able for the first time in a long while to drink a small soda. She made only one bathroom trip near the end of the film. "Now if I hold it in," she said. "I have a weird pain, an internal muscle pain; the act of holding it in now hurts." Later, in a rare moment of expansiveness, she bought an expensive cream-colored suit "to wear when I'm better."

In the fifth session, Natalia made two bathroom trips in a 5- to 6-hour period. This was momentous. She made a major presentation to her corporate group without experiencing strain, maintaining composure even when the projector jammed and she had to ad lib without slides. After the talk she did go to the bathroom, but there was no rush. *She took her time.* In the next session, she said she could report a greater than 80% reduction in symptoms. We met a few times more, at which time the problem was almost completely resolved.

▶ Case Example 3: A Blooming Heart

Essential Hypertension

Peter, age 60 years, a tall, lanky owner of a garden nursery, was referred to an integrative nutritionist and to myself to wean off pharmaceuticals for treatment of lifelong essential hypertension. He was also diagnosed with mixed hyperlipidemia and considered at increased risk for cardiovascular disease. Although he had never smoked, he drank at least three scotches a night. The nutritionist noted a high intake of saturated animal fats and nitrites, and put him on a plant-based Mediterranean diet, along with supplements: garlic, ginger, and essential fatty acids. He was asked to increase cardiovascular exercise (stationary bike) to 4 hours weekly and to cut down on alcohol consumption.

Peter was eager to reduce his many medications—Pravachol, Lopressor, Norvasc, Accuretic, multivitamin with iron, and, later, Zocor. He reported unspecified anxiety, lethargy, apathy, and dulled libido, but he denied depression. Peter had tried many regimens, including yoga, biofeedback, and exercise, with varying success. His blood pressure could soar as high as 170/110 but was generally 136/90 with medication. I explained to him that blood pressure elevation in hypertensive patients can be worsened by psychological stress, whereas practicing relaxation techniques may allow for a reduction in the dosage of antihypertensive medications.

A second-degree Reiki practitioner, Peter described himself as a spiritual man who cared deeply about nature and animals. But he also called himself a loner, who used biting humor, and was mystified by the disparity between what he felt and how others reacted. He would say: "My wife tells me I am angry" ("not that I am aware of") or "my daughter says I'm depressed" ("I don't think I am"). Peter said he loved animals more than people because "they don't ask for anything in return."

Our early interactions were formal and impoverished in content. Although gracious, he showed a muted curiosity in his inner life, more characteristic, I felt, of helplessness than lack of interest. There was a quality of cognitive rigidity, an implicit stubbornness to stick to his way of doing things, most notable around alcohol use and social contacts. He lacked an ability to reflect on his thoughts, and often responded quizzically to my comments: "I never thought of that. I will have to take time to ponder that."

Peter's favorite activity was coming home after work and reading the paper while drinking a scotch, with his dog by his side. His aloofness was a source of distress to his wife, and they bickered frequently. He even avoided his shop employees. One incident haunted him: He had befriended a man whom he had engaged as a contractor who reneged on their deal and stiffed him out of a substantial amount of money. Peter felt betrayed and still had fantasies of vengeance.

Peter had characteristics associated with alexithymia—a decreased ability to communicate or identify feelings, a cognitive tendency to report detail, and a diminishment in ability to recall dreams or to evoke imaginative fantasy. His childhood, like Roger's, was one of pain and neglect. His parents, both hardworking in a blue collar midwestern town, fought bitterly, and he was often sent to his grandmother's while they ironed out their differences. His mother belittled his father's timidity, and once, when Peter and his father were building a toy log cabin, kicked down the logs. He said his mother "squashed his spirit."

Although Peter spoke sparingly, he seemed to respond to our encounters. He became able to label emotions and to reflect on their impact. He saw that his sarcasm "masked" feelings of anger and hurt. He created life goals, and kept a "flexibility" journal, which recorded his progress in becoming less rigid and defensive with his wife. He visualized his heart as slowly blooming, and brought me a Lady's Mantle from his garden. In one cathartic session he recalled he once was a promising outfielder on his high school baseball team. Despite immense athleticism and very real professional prospects, Peter gave up playing because he couldn't bear his mother's critical taunts. At home with his wife, he cried for several hours, and was deeply comforted by her concern. Shortly after, his dog died, and Peter asked his wife to volunteer with him at an agency helping runaway dogs. It was their first activity together outside the store in many years.

The success that Peter saw in lowering his blood pressure medications is noted below:

1. 3/01:   1st appointment: 138/90 with medication
2. 12/01:   128/80
3. 2/28/02: 140/84
4. 3/19/02: 140/77; cut Lopressor by 50% to 25 mg
5. 4/18/02: 139/low 80s to 84 with some spikes 165/97, 109/67; cutting back drinking
6. 6/20/02: 126/82
7. 7/1/02: 126/79—"broke barrier—that's where I want to be"

▶ Case Example 4: Healing from Medical Trauma

Tonglen reverses the usual logic of avoiding suffering and seeking pleasure. . . . When we get in touch with our pain and that of others, the circle of compassion expands. . . .

—PEMA CHODRUN[120]

All patients offer gifts—hard insights, wise thoughts, hurting truths, and sometimes expressions of love. To feel the abundance in another's burgeoning awareness, to join in mutual acknowledgment of life's inevitable sorrows and unalloyed joys is part of the therapeutic enterprise.

Nina survived a 3-month coma in an upstate hospital after her rectum was perforated during a gynecologic procedure. She nearly died, and she awoke to the terrifying, choking sensation of feeding tubes jammed in her throat. During her hospitalization, she had a colostomy and a hysterectomy, among other procedures. By the end of it she had lost most of her abdominal muscles, which are now replaced by a mesh. Virtually every organ in her body (lungs, kidneys, colon, and intestines) was affected, except, interestingly, her heart. When Nina finally left that hospital, she could still barely speak or walk. Months of arduous physical rehabilitation have not restored her full strength, and she continues to suffer daily pain.

Nina is an intelligent, commanding person—a journalist, mother of two boys, and a woman with a big heart. When she first walked into my office, some months after leaving the hospital, I was intimidated by her tall, glowering presence. She wore dark glasses and made forcefully clear she would not countenance "traditional therapy." Nina was edgy in initial meetings, afraid to really talk. It was clear she felt acutely alone in her pain. Later she would say she was haunted by the terror in the eyes of her boys as they stood by her bedside, uncertain if she would live or die.

Nina has worked with multiple providers and healers, and consistently practices yoga. In the course of our work, we have used sound chants, Tibetan bowls, breath meditations, energy work, guided imagery, and interpersonal psychotherapy. She was especially drawn to the breathing meditation, tonglen, a powerful method for working with compassion and suffering. In its initial stages, one breathes in a feeling of dark, hot, and heavy, and exhales a feeling of bright, cool, and light. Gradually, one includes a personal pain or sorrow in the rhythm of gathering in and releasing, and then, perhaps, a sense of another's pain, using the circulating breath all the while to facilitate taking in and letting go.

Nina's therapy reflected an ongoing pilgrimage for self-acceptance—from coping with residual trauma from her hospitalization, anger, and forgiveness, to an ongoing struggle to care for the self (soul), and a liberating new sense of her own power. Nina was also deeply moved by the events of September 11, 2001, and reached out to the firemen and their families, as well as to other survivors of accidents, illness, and trauma, with whom she shares a deep affinity.

The theme of tonglen surfaced at different points in our work. To awaken feeling in her body, which sometimes feels "encased in rubber." To ease intense pain in her feet at night. When her younger son wept at his brother's departure for college, Nina sat with him on his bed:

> I taught him tonglen. I didn't call it that, of course. I just said, "If you feel sad, you can take in the feeling with your breath and then let it out, knowing that others also feel sad, and that you might even feel the sadness of others, because they may be suffering too. . . ."

After some months, Nina began to have a series of dreams. In one dream she returned to the house of her childhood friend and visited the basement room where they used to sing and play guitar. In a dark corner, huddled a sacred figure. Nina brought in a line drawing she had made of this dream image—a figure in prayer, holding in clasped hands a long, slender reed (Figure 3–3). To me the dream symbolized Nina's gradual

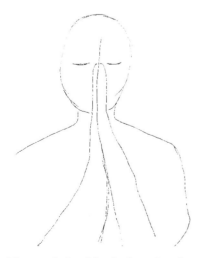

Figure 3–3. Nina's line drawing.

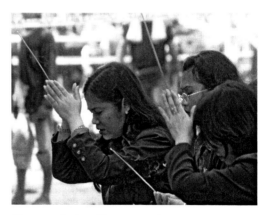

Figure 3–4. Photograph to accompany editorial on Balinese women. *(Courtesy of AP/Wide World Photos.)*

reentry into the world through spiritual awakening, and it was filled with images of death, suffering, recovery, and sacrifice.

Several days after Nina had this dream, she and a colleague were choosing a photograph to accompany an editorial on Balinese women who were protesting the recent terrorist bombing. A staff-mate brought in an AP photo (see Fig. 3-4). Its resemblance to her dream image stunned Nina—women holding slender reeds in graceful hands. We talked about the communion of minds, and the mystery of shared consciousness. Nina's work on her recovery continues. She continues to show courage in the midst of pain and aloneness, and still doesn't ask for very much support.

Over the holidays, Nina gave me a photograph of a canopy of trees over water, with a few red leaves in the rough shape of a triangle tucked into the dense green foliage. There was a note as well:

> I know you like green. So here's some green with some red at heart and a spring-fed lake beneath to give it life. For the longest time I had this picture at my bedside upside down. It was that red-root-heart that mattered. It is a vision of what you give . . . seeing the forest for the trees, the forest and the trees, the heart shining deep and a clear spring running through.

Chodrun[120] writes, "Tonglen awakens our compassion and introduces us to a far bigger view of reality." How characteristic of Nina to see things not as they might appear but as they are—a triangle turned round into a heart.

► CONCLUSION

Mind–body therapy, like any therapeutic method, endeavors to change, in beneficial ways, how people think, feel, and act. This involves a marshaling of both the regulatory and creative functions of mind, not simply the ability to reflect on self-experience—which is integral to all psychotherapies—but to cultivate qualities of attention and intention; to foster a more embodied emotional awareness; to engender an empathic knowing that extends the bounds of consciousness beyond the self; and to actively engage imaginative processes in the service of healing.

Mind–body work appeals to many psychotherapists because it offers a conceptual framework about health more expansive than the mental health models in which many of them have trained. Yet mind–body medicine, as it is currently practiced and taught, has limitations. It lacks a cohesive theory of self-development, and, to a large extent, predicates therapeutic progress on the acquisition of skills and techniques that teach self-control. Although coping with stress can help surmount unhealthy and maladaptive behaviors, the mind–body approach too often neglects the motivating power of unconscious defense. Nor does it fully appreciate the therapeutic relationship as a vehicle for change. Indeed, the short-term, sometimes utilitarian nature of some mind–body encounters, fueled by patients seeking tools rather than insight, impedes use of the therapeutic transference, which, along with the therapist's countertransference, is one of the most emotionally potent aspects of psychotherapy.

But mind–body medicine does offer a compelling alternative—and adjunct—to mainstream medical care. Although the mechanisms underlying the links between mind, emotions, and physical body are not fully understood, the impact of this connection on health cannot be questioned. In embracing science and spirituality, the mind–body practitioner begins to bridge such far-flung concepts as cellular intelligence and cosmic consciousness.[121] Humans use only a fraction of their full cerebral capacity. The power of mind–body medicine is not only that it recognizes the vast healing potential of the mind, but that it seeks ways to use that potential to transform medical practice.

REFERENCES

1. Engel GL. From biomedical to biopsychosocial: 1. Being scientific in the human domain. *Psychother Psychosom*. 1997;66:57–62.

2. Cooper M, Aygen M. Effect of meditation on blood cholesterol and blood pressure. *J Israel Med Assoc*. 1978;95:1–2.

3. Patel C, Marmot MG, Terry DJ, et al. Trial of relaxation in reducing coronary risk: 4-year follow-up. *Br Med J*. 1985;290(6475):1103–1106.

4. Bakal D. *The Psychobiology of Chronic Headache*. New York: Springer; 1982.

5. Blanchard EB, Schwarz SP. Adaptation of a multicomponent treatment for irritable bowel syndrome to a small group format. *Biofeedback Self Regul*. 1987;12(1):63–69.

6. Fawzy FI, Fawzy NW, Hyun CS, et al. Malignant melanoma: Effects of coping and affective state on recurrence and survival 6 years later. *Arch Gen Psychiatry*. 1993;50(9):681–689.

7. Kabat-Zinn J, Lipworth L, Burney R, Sellers W. Four-year follow-up of a meditation-based program for the self-regulation of chronic pain. *Clin J Pain*. 1986;2:150–173.

8. Kabat-Zinn J, Lipworth L, Burney R. The clinical use of mindfulness meditation for the self-regulation of chronic pain. *J Behav Med*. 1985;8:163–190.

9. Kabat-Zinn J, Massion AO, Kristeller J, et al. Effectiveness of a meditation-based stress reduction program in the treatment of anxiety disorders. *Am J Psychiatry*. 1992;149(7):936–943.

10. Fawzy FI, Fawzy NW, Hyun CS, et al. Malignant melanoma: Effects of coping and affective state on recurrence and survival 6 years later. *Arch Gen Psychiatry*. 1993;50(9):681–689.

11. Spiegel D, Bloom J, Kraemer HC, Gottheil E. Effect of psychosocial treatment on survival of patients with metastatic breast cancer. *Lancet*. 1989;2:888–891.

12. Bakal D. *The Psychobiology of Chronic Headache*. New York: Springer; 1982.

13. Achterberg J. *Imagery in Healing: Shamanism and Modern Medicine*. Boston: New Science Library/Shambhala; 1985.

14. Shapiro S, Schwartz G. Intentional systemic mindfulness: an integrative model for self-regulation and health. *Adv Mind Body Med*. 1999;15:128–134.

15. Cunningham AJ. Healing through the mind: extending our theories, research, and clinical practice. *Adv Mind Body Med*. 2001;17:214–227.

16. Watkins A. Mind–body pathways. In: Watkins A, ed. *Mind–Body Medicine: A Clinician's Guide to Psychoneuroimmunology*. New York: Churchill Livingstone; 1997;1–25.

17. Reich W. *Character Analysis*. 3rd ed. New York: Noonday Press; 1962.

18. Alexander F. *Psychosomatic Medicine: Its Principles and Applications*. New York: Norton; 1950.

19. Roberts AH. The powerful placebo revisited. Magnitude of non-specific effects. *Adv Mind Body Med*. 1995;11(1):35–43.

20. Cannon WB. *The Wisdom of the Body*. New York: Norton; 1939.

21. Selye H. *The Stress of Life*. New York: McGraw-Hill; 1956.

22. Mitchell A, Cormack M. *The Therapeutic Relationship in Complementary Health Care*. London: Churchill Livingstone; 1998.

23. Kaplan S, Gandek B, Greenfield S, Rogers W, Ware J. Patient and visit characteristics related to physicians' participatory decision-making style: results from the medical outcomes study. *Med Care*. 1995;33(12):1175–1187.

24. Ader R, Felten DL, Cohen N, eds. *Psychoneuroimmunology*. 2nd ed. New York: Academic Press; 1991.

25. Maier SF, Watkins LR, Fleshner M. Psychoneuroimmunology: the interface between behavior, brain, and immunity. *Am Psychol*. 1994;49:1004–1017.

26. Pert C, Dreher H, Ruff M. The psychosomatic network: foundations of mind–body medicine. *Alter Ther Health Med*. 1998;4(4):30–41.

27. Stoya JM. Guidelines in cultivating general relaxation: Biofeedback and autogenic combined. In: Basmajian JV, ed. *Biofeedback: Principles and Practice for Clinicians*. 2nd ed. New York: Williams and Wilkins; 1983.

28. Wiener N. *Cybernetics: Control and Communication in the Animal and the Machine.* New York: Wiley; 1948.

29. Cannon WB. *The Wisdom of the Body.* New York: Norton; 1939.

30. Damasio A. *The Feeling of What Happens.* New York: Harcourt; 1999:18.

31. Glaser R, Kiecolt-Glaser J, Stout JC, et al. Stress-related impairments in cellular immunity. *Psychol Res.* 1985;16:233–239.

32. Kiecolt-Glaser JK, Glaser R. Stress and immune function in humans. In: Ader R, Felton D, Cohen N, eds. *Psychoneuroimmunology,* 2nd ed. San Diego, CA: Academic Press; 1991:849–867.

33. Kiecolt-Glaser JK, Glaser R, Strain EC, et al. Modulation of cellular immunity in medical students. *J Behav Med.* 1986;9(1):5–21.

34. Kiecolt-Glaser JK, Fisher LK, Ogrocki P, et al: Marital quality, marital disruption and immune function. *Psychosom Med.* 1987;49(1):13–34.

35. Taylor S, Klein LC, Lewis B, Gruenewald TL, Gurung R, Updegraff JA. Biobehavioral responses to stress in females: tend-and-befriend, not fight-or-flight. *Psychol Rev.* 2000;107(3):411–429.

36. Levi L. Psychosocial stress and disease: a conceptual model. In: Gunderson EK, Rahe RH, eds. *Life Stress and Illness.* Springfield, IL: Charles C. Thomas; 1974.

37. Sternbach RA. *Principles of Psychophysiology: An Introductory Text and Readings.* San Diego, CA: Academic Press; 1966.

38. Gatchel RJ, Blanchard EB. *Psychophysiological Disorders: Research and Clinical Applications.* Washington DC: American Psychological Association; 1993.

39. Mason J. Psychological influences on the pituitary adrenal cortical system. *Recent Prog Horm Res.* 1959;15:345–389.

40. Mason JW. A re-evaluation of the concept of "non-specificity" in stress theory. *J Psychiatr Res.* 1971;8:123–140.

41. Weinberger DA, Schwartz GE, Davidson RJ. Low-anxious, high-anxious, and repressive coping styles: psychometric patterns and behavioral and physiological responses to stress. *J Abnorm Psychol.* 1979;88:369–380.

42. Esterling BA, Antoni MH, Kumar MH, et al. Emotional repression, stress disclosure responses, and Epstein-Barr viral capsid antigen titers. *Psychosom Med.* 1990;52:397–410.

42a. Smythe JM, Stone A, Kaelli A. Writing about stressful events produces symptom reduction in asthmatics and rheumatoid arthritics: A randomized trial. *JAMA.* 1999;281:1304–1309.

43. Pennebaker JW, Kiecolt-Glaser JK, Glaser R. Disclosure of traumas and immune function: Health implications for psychotherapy. *J Consult Clin Psychol.* 1988;56:239–245.

44. Esterling BA, Antoni MH, Fletcher MA, et al. Emotional disclosure through writing or speaking modulates latent Epstein-Barr virus antibody titers. *J Consult Clin Psychol.* 1994;62:130–140.

45. MacArthur Foundation. McEwen B, Seeman T. *Allostatic Load and Allostasis* (electronic version). 11/1/02 from http://www.macses.ucsf.edu/research/allostatic/notebook/allostatic.html; 1999.

46. Sapolsky R. *Why Zebras don't get Ulcers: An Updated Guide to Stress-Related Disease.* New York: WH Freeman; 1998:7.

47. McEwen BS, Stellar E. Stress and the individual: Mechanisms leading to disease. *Arch Intern Med.* 1993;153:2093–2101.

48. MacArthur Foundation. McEwen BS, Seeman T. *Allostatic Load and Allostasis* (electronic version). 11/1/02 from http://www.macses.ucsf.edu/research/allostatic/notebook/allostatic.html; 1999:1–12.

49. Seeman TE, Singer BH, Rowe JW, et al. Price of adaptation—allostatic load and its health consequences. MacArthur studies of successful aging. *Arch Intern Med.* 1997;157:2259–2268.

50. Pert C, Dreher H, Ruff M. The psychosomatic network: foundations of mind–body medicine. *Altern Ther Health Med.* 1998;4(4):30–41.

51. Siegal DJ. *The Developing Mind: Towards a Neurobiology of Interpersonal Experience.* New York: Guilford Press; 2000.

52. Damasio A. *The Feeling of What Happens.* New York: Harcourt; 1999:18.

53. Schore AN. *Affect Regulation and the Development of the Self: The Neurobiology of Emotional Development.* Hillsdale, NJ: Erlbaum; 1994.

54. LeDoux JE. *The Emotional Brain: The Mysterious Underpinning of Emotional Life.* New York: Simon and Schuster; 1996.

54a. Damasio A. *Descartes' Error: Emotion, Reason, and the Human Brain.* New York: Putnam; 1994.

55. Taylor GJ. *Psychosomatic Medicine and Contemporary Psychoanalysis.* Madison, CT: International Universities Press; 1987.
56. Hofer MA. Relationships as regulators: a psychobiologic perspective on bereavement. *Psychosom Med.* 1984;46:183–197.
57. Schore AN. *Affect Regulation and the Development of the Self: The Neurobiology of Emotional Development.* Hillsdale, NJ: Erlbaum; 1994.
58. Harlow HF. Love in infant monkeys. *Sci Am.* 1959;200:68–74.
59. Field TM, Schanberg SM, Scafidid F, et al. Tactile/kinesthetic stimulation effects on preterm neonates. *Pediatrics.* 1986;77:654–658.
60. Taylor GJ. *Psychosomatic Medicine and Contemporary Psychoanalysis.* Madison, CT: International Universities Press; 1987.
61. Taylor GJ. Psychosomatics and self-regulation; In: Barron J, Eagle M, Wolitsky D, eds. *Interface of Psychoanalysis and Psychology.* Washington, DC: American Psychological Association; 1992: 464–488.
62. Sifneos PE. Alexithymia: past and present. *Am J Psychiatry.* 1996;153:137–142.
63. Nemiah JC, Sifneos PE. Affect and fantasy in patients with psychosomatic disorders. In: Hill OW, ed. *Modern Trends in Psychosomatic Medicine,* vol. 2. London: Butterworths; 1970:26–34.
64. Taylor GJ. Psychosomatics and self-regulation. In: Barron J, Eagle M, Wolitsky D, eds. *Interface of Psychoanalysis and Psychology.* Washington, DC: American Psychological Association; 1992: 472–474.
65. Todarello O, Taylor GJ, Parker JD, Fanelli M. Alexithymia in essential hypertensive and psychiatric outpatients: a comparative study. *J Psychosom Res.* 1995;39(8):987–994.
66. Jula A, Salminen JK, Saarijarvi S. Alexithymia: a facet of essential hypertension. *Hypertension.* 1999;33(4):1057–1061.
67. Fonagy P, Morgan G. Psychoanalytic formulation and treatment. In: Erskine A, Judd D, eds. *The Imaginative Body.* London: Whurr Publishers; 1994:60–86.
68. Bourke MP, Taylor GJ, Parker JD, Bagby RM. Alexithymia in women with anorexia nervosa: a preliminary investigation. *Br J Psychiatry.* 1992; 161:240–243.
69. Hyer L, Woods MG, Summers MN, Boudewyns P, Harrison WR. Alexithymia among Vietnam veterans with posttraumatic stress disorder. *J Clin Psychiatry.* 1990;51:243–247.
70. Krystal H. *Integration and Self-healing: Affect, Trauma, Alexithymia.* Hillsdale, NJ: The Analytic Press; 1988.
71. Siegel D. *The Developing Mind.* New York: Guilford Press; 1999.
72. Blaustein J, Tuber S. Knowing the unspeakable: Somatization as an expression of disruptions in affective-relational functioning. *Bull Menninger Clin.* 1998;62(3):351–365.
73. Fonagy P, Target M. Attachment and reflective function: their role in self-organization. *Dev Psychopathol.* 1997;9:679–700.
74. Lane RD, Schwartz GE. Levels of emotional awareness: a cognitive-developmental theory and its application to psychopathology. *Am J Psychiatry.* 1987;144:122–143.
75. Olness K. Contemporary context: Psychoneuroimmunology. In: Temes R, ed. *Medical Hypnosis: An Introduction and Clinical Guide.* New York: Churchill Livingstone; 1999:33–39.
76. Dossey L. *Reinventing Medicine: Beyond Mind–Body to a New Era of Healing.* San Francisco: Harper; 1999.
77. Boone JL, Christensen JF. Stress and disease, Chap. 29. In: Feldman M, Christensen JF, eds, *Behavioral Medicine in Primary Care.* Stamford, CT: Appleton & Lange; 1997:265–276.
78. Leskowitz E. Life energy and western medicine; a reappraisal. *Adv Mind Body Med.* 1982;8(1): 63–67.
79. Popkins MK, Andrews JE. Mood disorders secondary to systemic medical conditions. *Semin Clin Neuropsych.* 1997;2(4):296–306.
80. Rost K, Zhangm M, Fortney J, et al. Persistently poor outcomes of undetected major depression in primary care. *Gen Hosp Psychiatry.* 1998;20(1): 12–20.
81. Barefoot JC, Schroll M. Symptoms of depression, acute myocardial infarction, and total mortality in a community sample. *Circulation.* 1996;93(11): 1976–1980.
82. Shalev Ay, Schreiber S, Galai T, et al. Post-traumatic stress disorder following medical events. *Br J Psychology.* 1993;32:247–253.
83. Sherman JJ. Effects of psychotherapeutic treatments for PTSD: a meta-analysis of controlled clinical trials. *J Trauma Stress.* 1998;11:413–436.
84. Kroenke K, Spitzer RL, Williams JB, et al. Physical symptoms in primary care: Predictors of

psychiatric disorders and functional impairment. *Arch Fam Med* 1994;3:774–779.

85. Kroenke K, Spitzer RL, Williams JB, et al. Physical symptoms in primary care: Predictors of psychiatric disorders and functional impairment. *Arch Fam Med* 1994;3:774–779.

86. Lipowski J. Psychosomatic medicine: past and present, part I. Historical background. *Can J Psychiatry*. 1986;31:2–7.

87. Nemiah JC, Sifneos PE. Affect and fantasy in patients with psychosomatic disorders. In: Hill OW, ed. *Modern Trends in Psychosomatic Medicine*, vol. 2. London: Butterworths; 1970:26–34.

88. Barsky AJ. Palpitations, cardiac awareness, and panic disorder. *Am J Med*. 1992;92(suppl 1A): 31–35.

89. Wickramasekera I. *Clinical Behavioral Medicine: Some Concepts and Procedures*. New York: Plenum Press; 1988.

90. Servan-Schreiber D, Kolb NR, Tabas G. Somatizing patients: part I. Practical diagnosis. *Am Fam Physician*. 2000;61:1073–1078.

91. Sharpe M, Wessley S. Non-specific health: a mind–body approach to functional somatic symptoms. In: Watkins A, ed. *Mind–Body Medicine: A Clinician's Guide to Psychoneuroimmunology*. New York: Churchill Livingstone; 2000:174.

91a. Schrodt GR, Tasman A. In: Jonas WB, Levin JS, eds. *Essentials of Complementary and Alternative Medicine*. Philadelphia: Lippincott, Williams & Wilkins; 1999.

91b. Schlesinger HJ, Mumford E, Glass G, et al. Mental health treatment and medical care utilization in a fee-for-service system: Outpatient mental health treatment following the onset of chronic disease. *Am J Pub Health*. 1983;73: 422–429.

92. Kirsch I, Montgomery G, Sapirstein GJ. Hypnosis as an adjunct to cognitive-behavioral psychotherapy: A metaanalysis. *Consult Clin Psychol*. 1995;63(2):214–220.

92a. Moss D, Lehrer P. Body-work in psychotherapy before biofeedback. *Biofeedback News Mag*. 1998;26(1):4–31.

93. Benor DJ. *Healing Research*. Vol. 1: *Spiritual Healing: Scientific Validation of a Healing Revolution*. Southfield, MI: Vision; 2001.

93a. Cortright B. *Psychotherapy and Spirit: Theory and Practice in Transpersonal Psychotherapy*. Albany, New York: State University of New York Press; 1997:15–16.

93b. Kabat-Zinn J. *Full Catastrophe Living*. New York: Bantam Doubleday Dell; 1990.

94. Aurobindo S. *Letters on Yoga*. Pondicherry, India: Sri Aurobindo Ashram Press; 1971.

95. Bakal D. *Minding the Body: Clinical Uses of Somatic Awareness*. New York: The Guilford Press; 1999.

95a. Tart C. *States of Consciousness*. New York: E.P. Dutton; 1975.

95b. Wilber K. *Integral Psychology: Consciousness, Spirit, Psychology, and Therapy*. Boston: Shambhala; 2000.

96. Benor D. Energy medicine for the internist. *Med Clin North Am*. 2002;86(1).

97. Levin, JS. Esoteric vs. exoteric explanations for findings linking spirituality and health. *Advances*. 1983;9(4):54–56.

98. Hanna T. *Somatics*. Reading, MA: Addison-Wesley; 1988.

99. Gallo F. *Energy Psychology: Explorations at the Interface of Energy, Cognition, Behavior, and Health*. Boca Raton, FL: CRC Press; 1999.

100. Hanna T. *Somatics: Reawakening the Mind's Control of Movement, Flexibility, and Health*. Cambridge, MA: Perseus Books; 1988.

101. Leskowitz E.. Life energy and western medicine; a reappraisal. *Adv Mind Body Med*. 1982;8(1):63–67.

101a. James W. *1890. The Principles of Psychology*. Cambridge, MA: Harvard University Press; 1981.

102. Aron L. The clinical body and the reflexive mind. In: Aron L, Anderson F, eds. *Relational Perspectives on the Body*. New York: Analytic Press; 1998: 3–37.

103. Fonagy P, Target M. Attachment and reflective function: their role in self-organization. *Dev Psychopathol*. 1997;9:679–700.

104. Fonagy P, Gergely G, Jurist E, Target M. *Affect Regulation, Mentalization, and the Development of the Self*. New York: Other Press; 2002.

105. Krystal H. *Integration and Self-healing: Affect, Trauma, Alexithymia*. Hillsdale, NJ: The Analytic Press; 1988.

106. Kroenke K, Spitzer RL, Williams JB, et al. Physical symptoms in primary care: Predictors of psychiatric disorders and functional impairment. *Arch Fam Med*. 1994;3:774–779.

107. Satprem. *Sri Aurobindo or the Adventures of Consciousness*. New York: Harper and Row; 1969.

108. Aurobindo S. *Letters on Yoga.* Pondicherry, India: Sri Aurobindo Ashram Press; 1971:236.

108a. Evans D. A Shamanic Christian approach in psychotherapy. In: Boorstein S, ed. *Transpersonal Psychotherapy.* Albany, NY: University of New York Press; 1996.

109. Benson H, Beary JF, Carol MP. The relaxation response. *Psychiatry.* 1974;37:37–46.

110. Goleman D. Meditation and consciousness: an Asian approach to mental health. *Am J Psychother.* 1976;30:41–54.

111. Gunaratana H. *Mindfulness in Plain English.* Somerville: MA: Wisdom Publications; 1993.

112. Miller JJ, Fletcher K, Kabat-Zinn J. Three-year follow-up and clinical implication of a mindfulness meditation-based stress reduction intervention in the treatment of anxiety disorders. *Gen Hosp Psychiatry.* 1995;17(3):192–200.

113. Everly GSS, Benson H. Disorders of arousal and the relaxation response: speculations on the nature and treatment of stress-related diseases. *Int J Psychosom.* 1989;36:15–21.

114. Davidson RJ, Kabat-Zinn J, Schumacher S, et al. Alterations in brain and immune function produced by mindfulness meditation. *Psychosom Med.* 2003;65:564–570.

115. Cortright B. *Psychotherapy and Spirit: Theory and Practice in Transpersonal Psychotherapy.* Albany, New York: State University of New York Press; 1997:15–16.

116. Lewis T, Amini F, Lannon R. *A General Theory of Love.* New York: Vintage Books; 2000.

117. Hofer MA. On the nature and consequences of early loss. *Psychosom Med.* 1996;58(6):570–581.

118. Mason JW. Psychological influences on the pituitary adrenal cortical system. *Recent Prog Horm Res.* 1959;15:345–389.

119. Uchino BN, Cacioppo JT, Kiecolt-Glaser JK. The relationship between social support and physiological processes: a review with emphasis on underlying mechanisms and implications for health. *Psychol Bull.* 1996;119:488–531.

119a. Haley J. *Advanced Techniques of Hypnosis and Therapy: Selected Papers of Milton H. Erickson, MD.* New York: Grune and Stratton; 1967.

120. Chodrun P. *When Things Fall Apart.* Boston: Shambhala; 1997.

121. Taylor GJ, Bagby RM, Parker JDA. The alexithymia construct: a potential paradigm for psychosomatic medicine. *Psychosomatics.* 1991;32:153–164.

CHAPTER 4

A New Definition of Patient-Centered Medicine

Leo Galland

▶ THE EVOLUTION OF DISEASE-CENTERED MEDICINE

Conceptual Framework

A fundamental difference between contemporary Western medicine and all alternative systems is the way the patient is viewed in relationship to illness. Conventional medicine equates illness with disease. The diagnosis and treatment of disease entities are the foundation of medical education and research, the economic and legal structures of the health care system, and the concept of what constitutes scientific evidence. Diseases are understood as distinct clinical entities, each having its own pathophysiology, natural history, accepted treatments, and International Classification of Diseases (ICD) code. The major crises in conventional medicine today result from the disease-centered model of care. Impersonal care is a great source of dissatisfaction among patients. Cassell explains: "Disease theory has no logical relation to person—in disease theory it does not matter what person has the disease—therefore, the common complaint that patients are overlooked in the treatment of their diseases is another way of saying that in the intellectual basis of modern medicine patients and their diseases are not logically related."[1]

Other well-known problems that derive from a disease-centered approach to illness include the narrowness of specialization, the excessive use of tests and procedures to "rule out" diseases, the increasing use of drugs (with attendant side effects and cost), and the aggressive application of unwanted invasive therapies in dying patients. The malpractice litigation crisis is yet another result of disease-centered care. The likelihood that patients will sue has far more to do with the quality of the doctor–patient relationship than with the injury sustained, yet there is a near-total neglect of training in empathic communication in medical education.[2] Disease-centered care often ignores or undervalues important patient-specific variables that influence the pathogenesis of illness, prognosis, and recovery. These include dietary practices, beliefs and expectations, social and psychological support, the environment in which a person lives, and the patient's role as an active participant in his or her care.

Ancestral and modern alternative health systems, however much they differ in the details, all equate illness with imbalance or disharmony. The healer's job is to understand the imbalances that underlie illness in each patient and help restore harmony. Disease entities are not the primary focus, and their treatment usually depends upon the healing of the patient. In contemporary Western medicine, conversely, healing of the patient is believed to depend upon the treatment of the disease. This fundamental difference in perspective, not the specific modalities used, separates integrative from conventional medicine. Differences in treatment modalities are secondary manifestations that are subject to change. Acupuncture, massage, and spinal manipulation, for example, are gaining widespread acceptance within mainstream medical care in the United States. Colonic irrigation, frequently advocated by alternative health practitioners, has lost its acceptance. A century ago it was standard therapy for arthritis, hypertension, and other disorders thought to result from "autointoxication," and offered by institutions as respected as the Mayo Clinic.[3]

Historical Background

Concepts of imbalance and its genesis differ among the various healing systems. Some of the most important concepts are reviewed elsewhere in this text. They may be simple or intricate, naturalistic or metaphysical, but they all share a clinical vision that is centered on disharmonies of each unique person rather than diseases that fit groups of patients into sharply delineated categories. This is no less true for ancestral medicine in Europe—the traditions spawned by the Hippocratic writings, the works of Galen, and the Canon of Avicenna (Ibn Sinna). Greco-Roman physiology was based upon humoral theory, which was derived from Ayurvedic concepts of *doshas*.[1] Adapting the concept of humors to a culture that was pragmatic and materialistic, the Greeks saw humors as physical substances that were visibly discharged from the bodies of the sick, who bled, coughed, or excreted their humors. Different qualities of temperature and moisture attributed to each humor explained the effect of environ-

mental change and unsound habits in causing disease. Although Greek physicians were able to distinguish among different types of sickness in vague and broad terms, they saw, in effect, only one universal disease—an imbalance of the humors—the effects of which varied among different individuals, depending upon the unique circumstances of each case. Physicians trained in the Greco-Roman tradition did not concern themselves with identifying a disease, but with identifying the strengths and weaknesses of the patient. They relied on careful observation of symptoms, habits, and environment, from which was formulated practical advice about diet and activity, ever mindful that a disturbance in any organ was unlikely to be localized to that organ but instead corresponded to a disturbance in the whole person.

Dietetics was the cornerstone of Hippocratic therapy. The Greek concept of diet *(daiata)* incorporated a person's entire mode of living: the relationship between rest and exercise; sleep and waking; the choice and quantity of food; cleanliness; and patterns of excretion. The physician's art lay in knowing accurately the influence on each individual of food, rest, and exercise, and the proper prescription of each. Hippocratic researchers paid exacting attention to the effects of innumerable foods, solid and liquid, raw and cooked, on the human body in health and disease. They also observed the location of a patient's dwelling place; the winds to which it was exposed; the nearness of the sea, rivers, and swamps; and the quality of the water supply. In the Hippocratic worldview, environment was a major determinant of both health and sickness. Throughout the European Middle Ages and the Renaissance, physicians trained in the Hippocratic approach believed that terrible epidemic diseases, such as malaria and bubonic plague, resulted from environmental toxicity, or *miasmata*. Their conclusions, although often erroneous, were nonetheless based upon careful observation of the circumstances in which epidemics occurred.[5] Attention to *daiata* and environmental toxicity is common among integrative practitioners today and derives from the same holistic impulse that drove Greco-Roman medicine.

Modern Biomedicine

The movement away from the Greco-Roman tradition received its impetus and form from the Scientific Revolution, which began during the seventeenth century. No force had more impact than the development of pathological anatomy, the dissection of corpses to determine the nature and causation of disease. The change in medical vision engendered by the autopsy has itself been dissected in detail by Foucault in *The Birth of the Clinic: An Archaeology of Medical Perception.*[6] Revealed pathology was soon seen as the cause of disease, and a path was cleared for dividing diseases into *organic* and *functional* as well as *physical* and *psychological*, distinctions first made in the nineteenth century. Since its birth, this new medicine (as its French fathers named it), has continually asserted its claim to be a child of the Scientific Revolution and has consistently criticized all other healing arts for being unscientific. Yet, scientific observation finds that pathology is an inadequate explanation for sickness and frequently is unrelated to the presence or severity of signs or symptoms.[7,8] Numerous studies, for example, show that the degree of pain and disability experienced by patients with osteoarthritis bears little relationship to the amount of disease demonstrated on radiographs. Pain and disability are more strongly correlated with the patient's age, weight, general fitness, degree of anxiety or depression, and, in the case of knee pain, with quadriceps strength.[9,10] These observations apply not only to symptoms such as pain, but to physical signs and laboratory abnormalities. In nephrotic syndrome, for example, "minimal change disease" (i.e., an almost normal biopsy) is associated with the worst edema and greatest proteinuria. Furthermore, many patients who consult physicians have problems that cannot be attributed to revealed pathology. In one large published study, 74% of patients seen by general internists for various common symptoms were left with no medical or psychiatric diagnosis to explain the cause of their problems.[11]

The major tool by which disease-centered medicine has attempted to apply science directly to clinical practice is the randomized, controlled clinical trial. Randomized trials assume that it is possible to make interindividual differences negligible, so that the only significant variable influencing outcome is the specific treatment being offered for the specific disease. They often exclude patients with complex comorbidities, even though complex comorbidities are common among chronically ill patients. That randomized controlled trials yield data of higher quality than clinical observation is an unproven hypothesis. Although conclusions drawn from randomized controlled trials form the foundation for evidence-based medicine, the latest evolutionary stage of disease-centered medicine,[12] they have not been shown to produce more enduring truths than conclusions drawn from clinical observation. Historical reviews of the surgical literature (in which randomized trials are rare) from 1935 to 1994 led Hall and Platell to estimate that the half-life of truth for conclusions in the surgical literature was 45 years.[13] Poynard et al. found the same half-life for conclusions of controlled scientific studies on hepatitis and cirrhosis published between 1945 and 1999.[11] They were surprised to discover that "conclusions based on good methodology had no clear survival advantage." The results of high-quality randomized trials fared no better at discovering durable truths than those derived from nonrandomized studies. Although randomized controlled trials may be very useful in identifying short- or intermediate-term effects of medication in the treatment of disease, they may tell us little about what it takes to help patients heal.

▶ PATIENT-CENTERED DIAGNOSIS

When the term "patient-centered" is used in conventional medical circles, it generally refers to the doctor's eliciting and understanding the patient's concerns. This is a vital area that is often neglected. Observers at the University of Colorado were highly critical of the skills with which physicians elicited even basic information from patients:

> To our surprise all did not seem as it should be. Physicians at all levels who had previously been thought quite competent appeared defective in their interactions with patients. Our initial reaction was to distrust our observations, but repeated oservations have shown great consistency. . . .[15]

As a cornerstone of integrative medicine, "patient-centered" includes, but extends far beyond, acknowledgment of the patient's concerns. It represents a clinical vision that seeks the origins of illness and the paths to healing in individual characteristics of each patient. This is the ancient vision that emerges in shamanic healing, Ayurveda, traditional Chinese medicine, the Hippocratic texts, and the writings of Ibn Sinna. Writing from a modern psychobiological perspective, Thomas describes patient-centered care using the metaphor of a kaleidoscope:

> The kaleidoscope model . . . states that *many* genetic and environmental factors enter into the health equation. While some factors are more important than others, it is the overall pattern that determines the outcome. As life goes on, the kaleidoscope turns a little as each new positive or negative factor is added. Thus the pattern is constantly changing, and is susceptible to future change. The persistence of good health, or the development of disease, depends upon the particular configuration of factors in a given individual at a given time.[16]

The practice of patient-centered, integrative medicine must begin with a patient-centered approach to diagnosis. Diagnosis underlies all human problem-solving activities. Diagnostic systems are intended to sort through information, separating signal from noise. Conventional medicine is based upon the process of differ-

ential diagnosis, which answers the question, "What disease does this patient have?" Much information that patients consider important—or that may influence individual prognosis—is filtered out by the process of differential diagnosis. Reliance on narrow categories of differential diagnosis often leads doctors to ignore information that is important to patients or to understanding the totality of factors generating a state of disharmony.[17–19] Additionally, this ignorance can lead to considerable dissatisfaction among patients.[20–22]

It is the integrative physician's task to know the context in which sickness occurs, the physical and social environment, the dietary habits of the person who is sick, her beliefs about the illness, her hopes and fears, and the factors that aggravate and ameliorate symptoms and that predispose to illness or facilitate recovery. Collecting and organizing this knowledge so that it may be used therapeutically, is the purpose of patient-centered diagnosis.

▶ TRIGGERS, MEDIATORS, AND ANTECEDENTS

Patient-centered diagnosis unites the ancient perspective on illness with the fruits of modern biological and behavioral science. What modern science has taught us about the genesis of disease can be represented by three words: triggers, mediators, and antecedents. *Triggers* are discrete entities or events that provoke disease or its symptoms. Microbes are one example. The greatest scientific discovery of the nineteenth century was the microbial etiology of the major epidemic diseases. Triggers are usually insufficient in and of themselves for disease formation; however, host response is an essential component. Identifying the biochemical mediators that underlie host responses was the most productive field of biomedical research during the second half of the twentieth century. *Mediators*, as their name implies, do not "cause" disease. They are intermediaries that contribute to the manifestations of disease. *Antecedents* are factors that predispose to acute or chronic illness. For a person who is ill, they form the illness *diathesis*. From the perspective of prevention, they are risk factors. Knowledge of antecedents has provided a rational structure for the organization of preventive medicine and public health. Molecular biology, the most highly anticipated area of biomedical research at the present time, seeks to better understand chronic disease by identifying disease-related genes and their products. The application of molecular biology to clinical medicine requires the integration of antecedents (genes and the factors controlling their expression) with mediators (the downstream products of gene activation). Mediators, triggers, and antecedents are not only key biomedical concepts, they also are important psychosocial concepts, as is explained below. In patient-centered diagnosis, the mediators, triggers, and antecedents for each person's illness form the focus of clinical investigation, and a seamless welding of the biological and psychosocial dimensions of illness is enabled.

▶ MEDIATORS AND THE FORMATION OF ILLNESS

A mediator is anything that produces symptoms, damage to tissues of the body, or the types of behaviors associated with being sick. Mediators vary in form and substance. They may be biochemical (like prostanoids and cytokines), ionic (like hydrogen ions), social (like reinforcement for staying ill), or psychological (like fear). Table 4–1 lists common mediators. Illness in any single person usually involves multiple interacting mediators. Biochemical, psychosocial, and cultural mediators interact continuously in the formation of illness.

Cassell argues that suffering, an important manifestation of illness, results from fear of loss—loss of life, identity, independence, valued relationships, and hopes for the future.[23] The suffering of sickness, then, is mediated by fear, and by the associated thoughts and be-

▶ **TABLE 4-1** COMMON MEDIATORS OF ILLNESS

Biochemical
  Cytokines
  Free radicals
  Neuropeptides (e.g., beta-endorphin and substance P)
  Neurotransmitters (e.g., serotonin)
  Nitric oxide
  Prostanoids
  Stress hormones (e.g., catecholamines and cortisol)
Cognitive/emotional
  Beliefs about sickness, including cultural and spiritual
  Fear of loss (life, identity, independence, and relationships)
  Fear of pain
  Feelings about sickness (anxiety and depression)
  Poor self-esteem, low perceived self-efficacy
Social
  Behavioral conditioning
  Lack of resources (poverty and social isolation)
  Rewards for being ill
Subatomic
  Electrical and magnetic energy fields
  Electrons
  Ions

liefs, personal and communal, with which we label, explain, and evaluate the experience of being sick. These *cognitive mediators* determine how patients appraise symptoms and what actions they take in response to that appraisal.[24] They may even modulate the symptoms themselves. People in pain, for example, experience more pain when they fear that pain control will be inadequate than when they believe that ample pain management is available.[25,26]

Expectations may not only mediate symptoms, but mortality. To examine the effect of expectation of death on actual mortality, a

California research team examined the death records of 28,000 Chinese Americans and compared them with 400,000 death records of people who were described as "white." Chinese astrology predicts that the association between certain birth years and certain types of sickness dooms the victim to an early death. The death records indicated that individuals of Chinese ancestry who bore these unfortunate concordances died younger of the same causes than people whose birth years and diagnoses were not star crossed. The control group comprised people with no knowledge of or attachment to Chinese astrological doctrine. The researchers' conclusion

> Chinese Americans, but not whites, die significantly earlier than normal (1.3 to 4.9 years) if they have a combination of disease and birth year which Chinese astrology and medicine consider ill-fated. The more strongly a group is attached to Chinese traditions, the more years of life are lost. Our results hold for nearly all the major causes of death studied. The reduction in survival cannot be completely explained by a change in the behavior of the Chinese patient, doctor, or death registrar. . . .[27]

Percieved self-efficacy (the belief in one's ability to cope successfully with specific problems) is another cognitive mediator that molds the shape of illness. People with a high degree of health self-efficacy usually adapt better to chronic disease, maintaining higher levels of activity, requiring lower doses of pain medication, adopting healthier lifestyles, and complying more with prescribed therapies, than people with low self-efficacy.[28] Low self-efficacy contributes to the formation of sickness, increasing disability and decreasing the effectiveness of treatment. It is a treatment-responsive mediator of illness. Self-management education is designed to enhance self-efficacy,[29] and has been shown to improve the clinical outcome for patients with several types of chronic disease, including asthma,[30] arthritis,[31] and diabetes.[32]

Spiritual beliefs and practices have also been shown to mediate the impact of illness, thereby influencing clinical outcomes. Among elderly patients, religious faith improves functional status and decreases the frequency and severity of depression among disabled[33,34] or chronically ill individuals,[35] and is associated with decreased mortality after elective cardiac surgery.[36] Among students, religious commitment is positively associated with health enhancing behaviors[37] and negatively associated with visits to health care providers.[38] Numerous studies show that regular church attendance is associated with significant reductions in the prevalence of hypertension and cardiovascular mortality, even when other risk factors are controlled.[39]

It is not enough to elicit a patient's symptoms and uncover the pathological manifestations of disease that reveal themselves through physical examination, laboratory tests, and techniques of imaging and measurement. The integrative practitioner must discover the patients' beliefs about their illness, including its causes and treatment, and their beliefs about themselves and their world in relation to the illness. This extends the therapeutic dialogue beyond conventional notions of mind and body to embrace the interdependence of mind, body, and spirit, a cornerstone of integrative medicine that is discussed in detail in Chapters 2 and 3.

► BIOCHEMICAL MEDIATORS AND CELLULAR DAMAGE

The *biochemical* mediators of disease are best known for their ability to promote cellular damage. They include autocoids and cytokines, hormones and neurotransmitters, growth and transcription factors, and free radicals. Biochemical mediators are organized into circuits and cascades that subserve homeostasis and allostasis. In these networks, each mediator is multifunctional and most functions involve multiple mediators, so that redundancy is the rule, not the exception. The most striking characteristic of biochemical mediators is their *lack of disease specificity.* Each mediator can be implicated in many different, apparently unrelated diseases, and every disease involves multiple chemical mediators in its formation. Mediator networks that regulate inflammatory and neuroendocrine stress responses have been the subject of intensive research with important clinical implications. A detailed discussion of these networks is outside the scope of this chapter, but comprehensive reviews have appeared.[10–13]

Key components of mediation of the inflammatory cascade include nuclear factor-κB (NFκB), which activates many of the genes involved in inflammatory responses; peroxisome proliferator-activated receptors (PPARs), which are gene transcription factors that among other functions regulate NFκB production; proinflammatory cytokines such as interleukin (IL)-6, tumor necrosis factor-α (TNFα) and IL-1; prostaglandins; and leukotrienes. Inflammation is believed to play a critical role not only in response to infection and in the classic inflammatory diseases, but also in the pathogenesis of coronary artery disease, diabetes, cancer, and depression, and in the negative health effects associated with obesity and with aging.[41–50]

The hypothalamic–pituitary–adrenal (HPA) axis plays a central role in mediation of neuroendocrine stress-response circuits. Inflammatory cytokines stimulate the HPA axis, increasing adrenal cortical and medullary activity. Products of adrenal cortical activation downregulate inflammatory response. Cortisol is immune suppressive, especially for responses mediated by T-helper 1 (Th1) lymphocytes. Sulfated dehydroepiandrosterone (DHEA) (but not free DHEA) is a natural PPAR agonist with antiinflammatory effects, especially for responses mediated by T-helper 2 (Th2) lymphocytes.[51,52] The orchestration of mediator signals in the inflammation and neuroendocrine stress networks, as they interact with one another, is critical for normal physiological functions, like the architecture of sleep, the repair of injury and the response to infection, and for the dys-

functional physiology central to the pathogenesis of most of the major chronic diseases.[53–55]

For the integrative practitioner, the most important feature of biochemical mediators is the rhythm of mediator activity, which is strongly influenced by the common components of life: diet, sleep, exercise, hygiene, social interactions, solar and lunar cycles, age, and sex. For example, fatal myocardial infarction is most likely to occur at dawn, which is when platelet aggregability and cortisol levels are greatest.[56,57] Aging, illness, and chronic psychological distress upregulate activity of the inflammatory and neuroendocrine stress networks. Regular physical exercise downregulates both.

Platelet aggregability, which is upregulated by inflammation and by adrenal activation, is an important mediator of many disease processes. Aggregability increases with cigarette smoking and consumption of a meal high in saturated fat. It is decreased by consumption of fish, vegetables, garlic, and red wine, and by regular exercise.[58] Mediator-driven platelet activation may be one link between emotions, habits, and myocardial infarction,[59] and may explain why denial and minimizing of symptoms improve prognosis for patients with severe cardiovascular disease.[60]

Understanding the ways in which mediators are modulated by diet enables the practitioner to apply creative nutritional therapies. Salicylic acid, for example, which is the major metabolite of aspirin, has antiinflammatory effects that are independent of cyclooxygenase inhibition and which may be responsible for some effects of low-dose aspirin therapy.[61] Vegetables are rich sources of natural salicylates, and vegetarians may have serum concentrations of salicylic acid as high as those of people ingesting 75 mg of aspirin a day.[62]

Magnesium supplementation is another example of the potential use of nutritional therapies as modulators of mediator pathways. Dietary magnesium has a number of important effects on the neuroendocrine-stress response network, especially the response to adrenergic stimulation. Men with lower erythrocyte magnesium levels are more sensitive to noise stress, and under stress conditions, make more mistakes, become more irritable, secrete more norepinephrine, and excrete more magnesium in the urine, depleting intracellular magnesium stores. Increasing magnesium consumption through food and dietary supplements improves magnesium status, ameliorates stress-induced irritability, and diminishes adrenergic outflow.[63] Magnesium deficit has subtler effects on the inflammatory mediator cascade, tending to shift the operation of the network in a direction that favors hypersensitivity and allergy.[64] Individuals with low dietary magnesium are at increased risk for cardiac arrhythmia and asthma. Magnesium administration attenuates these effects.[65–70]

Dietary fatty acids may also have profound effect on the network of inflammatory mediators, altering prostanoid synthesis, PPAR activity, and the response to cytokines such as IL-1.[71,72] They have subtler effects on the neuroendocrine stress-response network, modulating neuronal responses to serotonergic and adrenergic transmission.[73] Detailed attention to nutritional status is warranted in all patients with chronic illness, regardless of diagnosis. Nutrients with likely clinical effects on the major human mediator response networks include, but are not limited to calcium; iron; selenium; zinc; vitamins A, C, D, E, and all the B vitamins; and a diverse group of dietary antioxidants such as the carotenoids and flavonoids.[74,75] A full discussion of these effects would require a separate textbook. A practical approach to assessing unmet needs for magnesium and essential fatty acids is presented below.

▶ ASSESSMENT AND TREATMENT OF MEDIATORS: COGNITIVE AND PSYCHOSOCIAL DIMENSIONS

Assessment of illness mediators begins with the clinical interview. The first step is to allow the patient to fully express his concerns. A study done at the University of Rochester found that most patients have three reasons for visiting a physician, are interrupted within 18 seconds of starting to tell their stories, and never get the chance to finish.[76] Although doctors excuse this behavior by citing lack of time, it takes an average of 1 minute and rarely more than 3 minutes for a complete list of problems to be elicited. Doctors who ignore the patient's concerns are likely to miss important medical information.[77]

The second step is to elicit the patient's beliefs about her illness. Every patient has her own ideas and feelings about her sickness. In most medical consultations, the patient and the doctor are not in full agreement about the nature of the principal problem and some form of negotiation is needed.[78] A study that carefully analyzed taped transcripts of visits to a medical clinic found that patients attempted to clarify or to challenge what the doctor said in 85% of cases. Usually their requests were ignored or interrupted.[79] Even when physicians are informed of their patients' concerns, they are loathe to recognize the patient's perspective.[80] Useful questions for eliciting a person's beliefs about her illness are the following:

- "What do you think has caused your problem?"
- "What do you most fear about your problem?"
- "How much control do you think you have over your symptoms?"

Remember that a person's beliefs are important mediators of illness. They influence symptoms and the patient's perception, satisfaction, and compliance with treatment, and in some cases, the outcome of care. Dysfunctional belief systems are those that increase anxiety, depression, and hopelessness or that interfere with the patient's ability to take an active role in her own care.

An appropriate therapeutic intervention for dysfunctional beliefs is the giving of information. Patients have an intense need for explanations about the causes of their diseases.[81] Doctors are usually content to name the disease and treat it. Patients want to know *how* they came to be sick, so that they can attach some meaning to the illness.[82] They want to know what to expect from the illness and what they can do to relieve symptoms or speed recovery. Information of this type can reduce anxiety, even when the diagnosis itself is frightening, and may increase feelings of personal control, and improve the ability to cope with pain. People change their behaviors more readily when they receive information about the importance and the nature of the changes they need to make, and help with setting goals and measuring progress. The amount of information given by physicians consistently correlates with the degree of satisfaction patients express concerning the treatment they have received.[83] Advice and information that would help patients change is often not given, however, in conventional medicine.[84–87] Doctors consistently underestimate the amount of information patients want and grossly overestimate the amount of information they actually give. In one study in a general practice, doctors spent less than 5% of their time informing patients, but believed they were spending 45% of their time giving information.[88]

The desire for information is universal and has no relationship to the patient's level of education or social class.[89] The discrepancy between the physician's expectations and the patient's desires is especially strong for the economically disadvantaged. The more information the patient receives and the more the patient is actively involved in making decisions about treatment, the higher the level of mutual satisfaction and the better the clinical outcome. Patients coaxed by assistants to ask more questions and participate in decisions about their care fared better in the outcome of chronic conditions such as high blood pressure, diabetes, and ulcers.[90] The kind of information needed is personal, not statistical. It must answer the question, "What can *I* do?" The answer to that question is *never,* "Nothing." Even when the outlook for recovery is bleak, there are powerful personal strategies for reducing the suffering of illness. Feelings of hopelessness contribute to sickness and death and inhibit cooperation with medical treatments.[91] Debilitating disease is always accompanied by feelings of guilt or inadequacy. Even in a terminal illness, the offering of hope is not deception. The doctor can encourage the patient by praising his determination to get better or his commitment to following the treatment plan. In her landmark work, *On Death and Dying,* Elizabeth Kubler-Ross observed that physicians can share in the hope of their dying patients that remission may occur and that they will outlive the statistics, without deceiving the patient.[92] Cassell reminds us that even when there is nothing more a physician can do for the body, there is a lot to be done for the person.[93]

The third step in assessing illness mediators involves evaluating the patient's spiritual beliefs and practices. Religion has been studied more extensively than spirituality, with the result that validated scales for quantifying religiousness have been published.[94,95] Kasl's Religious Index contains three questions that were shown to have prognostic implications for the ability of elderly men to cope with the stresses associated with aging and disabling illness[96]:

1. How often do you attend regular religious services during the year?
2. Aside from how often you attend regular religious services, do you consider yourself to be (a) very religious, (b) fairly religious, (c) only slightly religious, (d) not at all religious, or (e) against religion.
3. How much is religion (and/or God) a source of strength and comfort to you?

A fourth step in a comprehensive assessment of psychosocial mediators is inquiry into sources of family and social support, the existence of a network of mutual obligations which leads a person to believe she is cared for, loved, and esteemed.[97] Ornish[98] and Galland[99] recently reviewed the large body of data showing that lack of social support increases the rate of sickness and of death, and that strong family or community ties alleviate sickness and enhance cooperation with medical treatments. Because illness itself often contributes to isolation, an integrative physician must always inquire about a patient's social integration. Helpful questions include, "Are there people in whom you can confide?"; "How satisfied are you with your marriage/family/friends/social life?"; "How much support do you receive in dealing with your health problems?"; and "How often do you feel loved or cared for?"

The physician can help patients who are suffering from isolation by calling this isolation to the attention of family members or friends or by attempting to connect the patient with a support group or a community agency. Five studies have been published that evaluate the effect of support groups on cancer-related mortality. Spiegel[100] recently reviewed their disparate results. Four studies showed a positive effect of support group participation on psychological function and two showed prolonged survival. Studies published prior to 1993 were more likely to show survival benefit than are recent studies. One explanation is that cancer therapy has become more effective and that the social stigma associated with cancer has decreased significantly during the past decade.

Spiegel's group found that disruption of the normal diurnal pattern of cortisol secretion among women with metastatic breast cancer was associated with decreased natural killer (NK) cell cytotoxicity, shortened survival, and the presence of social stressors such as divorce or widowhood.[101] Among women with early breast cancer, support group participation decreased mean cortisol secretion[102]; patients with melanoma experienced an increase in natural killer cell function after support group participation.[103] These support groups were structured, led by experienced therapists, and succeeded in creating a supportive environment and improving patients' quality of life.

Varied mechanisms comprise the link between social support, health, and mortality. Satisfying relationships may buffer the impact of stress, actually lowering the levels of chemical mediators, and decreasing the strain on mind and body.[104] The rewards of friendship may include an increase in self-esteem and with it a boost to perceived self-efficacy.

Possibly, there is nothing that can be done to relieve the patient's isolation, but the doctor's awareness and acknowledgment of it can be important to the patient. Eisenberg wrote:

> The physician is one valuable source of social support . . . whether the physician wills it or no, all medical practice is a set of social and interpersonal transactions. Surely, if the patient is inevitably going to be affected in important ways by the relationship with the doctor, it is an imperative for good clinical care that the doctor increase the knowledge and the skill he or she brings to bear on that relationship, the one invariant in healing encounters, folk and professional, medical and surgical.[105]

For all patients, but especially for those who are socially isolated, a strong doctor–patient relationship can materially affect the outcome of care.

The impact of the doctor–patient relationship can be gauged from some variables reported in controlled clinical trials. Surgical patients report less pain, request less pain medications, and have a shortened hospital stay if the preoperative visit from the anesthesiologist lasts longer and includes information about the nature of pain, advice about simple techniques for coping with pain, and reassurance about the availability of backup medication if their pain is not adequately relieved.[106] For patients with chronic headache, the best predictor of symptom relief is the patient's satisfaction with the doctor's discussion of the nature of his problem.[107,108] Within a single trial with a uniform experimental design, placebo response varies from clinic to clinic. Drugs *and* placebos work better when given by a caring physician.[109] When a doctor enthusiastically supports a treatment, the placebo response may be greater than 80%.

Empathy is an important component of caring, and is a teachable skill. An empathic physician is able to share the patient's experience of being sick, an activity that enriches the experience of being a doctor. The physician then has the option of altering treatment to meet the patient's values and expectations rather than her own.[110,111]

▶ ASSESSMENT AND TREATMENT OF MEDIATORS: PHYSIOLOGIC AND BIOCHEMICAL DIMENSIONS

Knowledge of the psychosocial mediators of each patient's illness is necessary for the practice of integrative medicine, but not sufficient. Biochemical mediators must also be assessed on an individual basis, and here a great deal of technical knowledge is needed. Understanding the biochemical alterations that underlie a conventional disease diagnosis is very important, as in the following examples.

Patients with type 1 diabetes mellitus, Crohn's disease, or any other disorder categorized by granuloma formation or excessive cell-mediated immune responses, are likely to have an immune response to common triggers in which the Th1 component is upregulated and not subject to the normal downregulation provided by Th2 activity. Their mediator response to inflammatory stimulation produces excessive levels of interferon gamma (IFN-γ) and IL-12, key Th1-related cytokines.[112] Treatment strategies for these conditions should focus on the nature of the mediator imbalance.

As another example, patients with severe depression often show a loss of negative feedback in the HPA axis. Urine free cortisol is elevated; the diurnal pattern may be disrupted, with increased nighttime cortisol secretion and blunting of dexamethasone suppression. This phenomenon appears to be driven at the level of the hypothalamus, not the adrenals, because

spinal fluid corticotropin-releasing hormone (CRH) is elevated.[113] Several groups of researchers have speculated that impaired synaptic function because of a deficit of omega-3 fatty acids may contribute to the central nervous system dysfunction of patients with depressive illness. Their omega-3 fatty acid levels tend to be lower in blood samples than in control populations; placebo-controlled studies of patients with depression, schizophrenia, and attention deficit disorder show that administration of omega-3 supplements derived from fish oil is beneficial. The key component appears to be eicosapentaenoic acid.[114-117]

To use the vast database of available information about biochemical disease mediators, integrative clinicians should maintain up-to-date knowledge of disease pathophysiology by reading reviews in mainstream journals on mechanisms of disease or on specific mediators. In reading these, clinicians should pay special attention to the types of mediators mentioned and their functions within the networks that subserve inflammation, oxidative stress, and neuroendocrine balance. Integrative practitioners must also then employ their understanding of the most common biochemical imbalances in chronically ill North Americans, and the influence of diet, nutrition, and dietary supplements on these imbalances. The metabolic syndrome (syndrome X), for example, affects approximately 25% of the US population. Insulin resistance with a resultant increase in circulating insulin is a key feature. Conditions associated with the metabolic syndrome include type 2 diabetes mellitus, type IV hyperlipidemia, low levels of high-density lipoprotein (HDL) cholesterol, hypertension plus hyperuricemia, obesity, and polycystic ovarian syndrome.[118] There are many individuals without established disease who show mild or incomplete evidence of the metabolic syndrome. Impaired activity of PPAR-γ is an important feature of this syndrome, which may explain its association with upregulation of the inflammatory mediator network and increased risk of coronary heart disease.[119] The acute manifestations of the metabolic syndrome often respond to a diet of low glycemic index. A low glycemic index diet is one of the few interventions that actually raises the HDL cholesterol level without raising total cholesterol.[120] The long-term manifestations are more responsive to dietary lipids. Diets high in saturated fat increase the risk of insulin resistance. Consuming long-chain polyunsaturated fatty acids from fish can reverse insulin resistance.[121]

Therapy with omega-3 fatty acids provides an excellent example of nutritional modulation of disease activity though alteration of biochemical mediators. As mentioned above, long-chain polyunsaturated fatty acids (essential fatty acids) of both the omega-6 and omega-3 families have potent effects on the activity of the inflammatory and neuroendocrine mediator networks and show positive effects in controlled studies of patients with arthritis, inflammatory bowel disease, coronary artery disease, peripheral vascular disease, dysmenorrhea, cyclic mastalgia, cystic fibrosis, migraine headaches, bipolar disorder, schizophrenia, attention deficit disorder, atopic eczema, and multiple sclerosis.[122–131] Because the fatty acid composition of the contemporary Western diet differs significantly from that of Paleolithic and ancestral diets, reflecting a marked decrease in omega-3 consumption relative to total fat, the response of so many unrelated disorders to essential fatty acid (EFA) supplementation may indicate that EFAs are not merely working as nutriceutical agents, but that EFA dietary status is important for disease pathogenesis. The clinical evaluation of essential fatty acid status is, therefore, an important guide to understanding how dietary modulation may influence crucial mediator networks for prevention or treatment of illness.

Prasad stated that the best test for nutritional adequacy is a functional test: determine a parameter to follow and measure how administration of the nutrient(s) in question affects that parameter.[132] This method can be applied to the use of EFA therapy in clinical practice. Stevens et al., studying boys with at-tention deficit hyperactivity disorder and a randomly selected population of school children, found a correlation between low concentrations of omega-3 EFAs, learning and behavior problems, and symptoms associated with EFA deficiency (thirst, dry skin, and dry hair).[133,134] Evaluating the presence of these symptoms in patients and observing how they change with EFA supplementation is a quick guide to EFA status that may be used clinically to evaluate the EFA contribution to mediator imbalance. The author's method for doing this is described elsewhere.[135]

Magnesium is another nutrient with profound effects on mediator networks, especially those involved in producing or maintaining spasm disorders. Magnesium deficiency has been described in patients with variant angina, cardiac arrhythmia, migraine headache, asthma, mitral valve prolapse syndrome, chronic fatigue syndrome, attention deficit disorder with hyperactivity, irritable bowel syndrome, fibromyalgia, hearing loss, and hypertension.[136–138] Magnesium status influences the vascular response to carbon dioxide. Hypocarbia, which may result from hyperventilation or from metabolic acidosis, induces vasoconstriction, especially in the cerebral circulation, and may contribute to numerous disorders involving local ischemia. Breath-regulation techniques, highly valued by many integrative practitioners, can overcome the hypocarbia of chronic hyperventilation or induce resistance to its vasoconstrictor effects. Magnesium depletion increases and magnesium repletion decreases vascular sensitivity to carbon dioxide, so that magnesium enhances the self-regulation of vascular tone.[139]

Food consumption data indicate that about two-thirds of the US population consume less than two-thirds of the recommended daily allowance for magnesium.[140] Accurate assessment of magnesium status can be difficult, because magnesium is primarily an intracellular cation and its concentration within different tissues may not co-vary, so that erythrocyte magnesium is a poor index of skeletal muscle magnesium. Symptoms associated with magnesium deficit include fatigue, irritability, sleep disturbances, muscle tension and spasm, and palpitation. Inquiring about the presence of these common symptoms and assessing their response to dietary supplementation with magnesium allows the application of Prasad's rule to the assessment of magnesium as a modulator of the neuroendocrine stress network. The author's method for using common symptoms and signs to address the problem of magnesium insufficiency is described elsewhere.[141]

Ensuring optimal, individualized intake of long-chain fatty acids and magnesium are two examples of using nutritional therapies to modulate the function of biochemical mediators for prevention and treatment.

▶ TRIGGERS AND THE PROVOCATION OF ILLNESS

The search for triggers is where medical detective work is needed. For some conditions, the trigger is such an essential part of our concept of the disease that the two cannot be separated; the absence of the trigger negates the diagnosis. Examples include head trauma and concussion or *Mycobacterium tuberculosis* and tuberculosis. These are *essential triggers*. Triggers are often not disease-specific, however, and for many chronic ailments, multiple interacting triggers may be present. Asthmatic attacks, for instance, may be triggered by air pollution[142]; passive smoking[143]; thunderstorms[144]; exposure to dust, cats, or cockroaches[145,146]; viral respiratory infection[147]; feelings of anxiety[148]; cold temperature[149]; hyperventilation[150]; and strenuous exercise.[151] None of these triggers is considered to be the cause of asthma in most patients; these are *incidental triggers*. All triggers, however, exert their effects through the activation of host-derived mediators. In closed head trauma, for example, activation of N-methyl-D-aspartate receptors, induction of nitric oxide synthetase, and liberation of free intraneuronal calcium determine the late effects.

Intravenous magnesium at the time of trauma attenuates severity by altering the mediator response.[152,153] Sensitivity to different triggers often varies among persons with similar ailments. A prime task of the integrative practitioner is to help patients identify important triggers for their ailments and develop strategies for eliminating them or diminishing their virulence.

The most challenging triggers to identify are those for which the relationship to the condition being treated is not immediately obvious. *Helicobacter pylori* is an excellent model for this type of relationship. Originally isolated from the gastric mucosa of patients with gastritis and peptic ulcer disease, it has been implicated in the pathogenesis of nonsteroidal antiinflammatory drug gastropathy,[154] gastric carcinoma,[155] and lymphoma,[156] and a variety of extradigestive disorders, including ischemic heart disease,[157] ischemic cerebrovascular disorders,[158] rosacea,[159] Sjögren's syndrome,[160] Raynaud's syndrome,[161] food allergy,[162] vitamin B_{12} deficiency,[163] and open-angle glaucoma.[164] For elderly patients with open-angle glaucoma and incidental *H. pylori* infection of the stomach, eradication of *H. pylori* by antibiotics was associated with improved control of glaucoma parameters at the 2 years follow-up.[165] The mechanism by which *H. pylori* aggravates open-angle glaucoma is unknown, but may result from the ability of *H. pylori* colonization of the gastric tract to trigger the local and systemic release of platelet-activating factor, inflammatory cytokines, and vasoactive substances.

Although the identification and elimination of triggers, whether essential or incidental, can yield great benefits for patients, many physicians avoid the search. A study was conducted by telephone in which practicing physicians were asked how they would treat a new patient with abdominal pain, who had a recent diagnosis of gastritis made by a specialist in another town. Almost half were ready to put the patient on acid-lowering therapy without asking about the patient's use of aspirin, alcohol, or tobacco, all of which are potential triggers for gastritis. The authors of the study concluded, "In actual practice, ignoring these aspects of the patient may well have reduced or even negated the efficacy of other therapeutic plans implemented."[166]

A comprehensive search for triggers requires that you know the following about your patient: each drug—prescription, over-the-counter, or recreational—that the patient has used and when; nutritional habits and each dietary supplement used and when; what effects the patient noted from the use of each substance; and sources of stress—life events, environmental exposures, thoughts or memories, and social interactions—and when they occurred in relation to symptoms. Elicit the patient's own ideas about possible triggers by asking, "What do you think causes or aggravates your symptoms?" The patient's observations may be insightful and accurate in ascribing causality. Of course, the patient's—and the clinician's—observations can also mislead, or focus on nonessential factors. Teach patients to challenge their own observations by looking for consistency and replicability wherever possible. Suggest alternative theories for the patient to consider, and explain that the search for triggers works best as a collaborative effort between patient and doctor. The patient's ability to recognize triggers is an important step in self-care.

For example, a useful question in uncovering the microbial triggers for symptomatic illness is the previous response of a given symptom or symptom complex to antibiotics. In 1988, physicians at the University of Minnesota conducted a study in which they administered intravenous cephalosporins to patients with various types of arthritis who also manifested antibodies to *Borrelia burgdorferi*. Most of these patients were not thought to have Lyme disease. Some met diagnostic criteria for rheumatoid arthritis (both seropositive and seronegative), some for osteoarthritis, and some for spondyloarthropathies. As would be expected, the response to antibiotics was quite variable and ranged from no response to dramatic and sustained improvement. The authors noted that

improvement in arthritis following antibiotics was not related to the patient's clinical diagnosis or the level of anti-*Borrelia* antibody. The best predictor of a positive response to the experimental treatment was a previous history of improvement of arthritis associated with the use of antibiotics.[167]

The most comprehensive way to ask the antibiotic question is as follows: "During the time you have had symptom X, have you taken antibiotics for any reason? Which antibiotic? Did symptom X change while you were taking the drug?" Among patients with chronic diarrhea of unknown cause, for example, some will report that their gastrointestinal symptoms improved when taking a specific antibiotic, whereas others will report that they worsened. The former case suggests that bacteria or protozoa sensitive to the antibiotic may be causally related to the patient's gastrointestinal problems. Repeating the antibiotic prescription can establish if this response is replicable. If so, therapy can focus on treating the infection and understanding why a single course of antibiotics was ineffective. The latter case suggests that depletion of bacteria by antibiotics and concomitant increase in antibiotic-resistant strains may be contributing to diarrhea, and treatment can focus on restoration of normal intestinal flora.

Food and Environment as Common Triggers of Illness

Pollution

Food and environment were important sources of illness triggers in Hippocratic medicine; they continue to be so. Numerous studies conducted in US cities, demonstrate a close correlation between fine-particle air pollution and daily mortality rates, even at levels of pollution considered safe by the World Health Organization.[168,169]

In the industrialized world, most people spend most of their time indoors, and indoor air pollution is a serious cause of morbidity. Studies using experimental chambers show that volatile organic compounds (VOCs) released from building materials, furnishings, office machines, and cleaning products can cause irritation of the respiratory system in humans and animals at levels that are 100 times weaker than permissible exposure levels or the World Health Organization's *Indoor Air Guidelines*.[170] Controlled experiments with people who describe themselves as sensitive to VOCs confirm that VOC exposure causes headache, fatigue, and difficulty concentrating. People who deny such sensitivity also experience symptoms but do not experience mental impairment when exposed. Air samples of buildings with and without sick building complaints have established an association between VOC exposure and human sickness.[171]

A study conducted in Scotland found that people who lived in housing that was judged to be damp or that showed visible mildew had a higher rate of sickness than did people whose housing was free of dampness or visible mold growth. These differences were not dependent upon smoking habits, occupation, or income; they seemed to be related to the dampness itself.[172] Allergy is one possible mechanism. Molds and dust mites thrive in damp environments and are common causes of allergic symptoms that occur in damp environments.[173] Dust mites are not only triggers but also are antecedents of allergic reactivity. Heavy childhood exposure increases the incidence of allergy.[174,175] Exposure to airborne mycotoxins from indoor molds is implicated in both sick building syndrome and in the occurrence of cancer.[176,177] A questionnaire can elicit important information about environmental exposures at home and at work. The open-ended question "Has your work or home environment been a concern to you?" should be accompanied by a checklist of potential exposures. See Table 4–2.

Food Intolerance

Food intolerance is a very common phenomenon, reported by 33% of the population in one large study.[178] A minority of these reactions

▶ **TABLE 4-2** COMMON OCCUPATIONAL EXPOSURES OF POTENTIAL MEDICAL SIGNIFICANCE

Adhesives, glue
Asbestos
Chemical fumes (specify which, if known)
Cold, extreme
Combustion engines
Computer/video display terminal
Construction materials/new construction (type)
Copy machines
Dampness
Dust, coal
Dust, grain
Dust, other
Formaldehyde
Harassment (type)
Heat, extreme
Herbicides
Lifting, physical straining
Metals (specify which)
Mildew
Noise
Pesticides
Printers (type)
Radiation
Repetitive motion
Solder
Solvents
Space heaters
Tobacco smoke
Welding fumes

(4–14%) were caused by true food allergies. Most food intolerance has no clear immunologic basis. Mechanisms include sensitivity to the pharmacologic effect of alkaloids, amines, or salicylates in food.[179–182] Histamine poisoning from scombroid fish and tyramine-induced headache are dramatic examples.[183] Although most food intolerance is short-lived, severe chronic illness can occur, and the food trigger may elude identification unless the physician starts the investigation with a high index of suspicion. Gluten intolerance, with its protean manifestations, is probably the best example.

Affecting approximately 2% of people of European ancestry,[184] gluten intolerance is common and often unrecognized. In addition to being the essential trigger for celiac disease, gluten sensitivity may be manifest in patients with neurologic disorders of unknown cause,[185] cerebellar degeneration,[186] dermatitis herpetiformis,[187] failure to thrive,[188] pervasive developmental delay,[189] inflammatory arthritis,[190–194] psoriasis,[195,196] Sjögren syndrome,[197,198] and schizophrenia.[199,200] The different presentations of gluten sensitivity may derive from genetic differences among affected patients.[201]

Recognition of food intolerance as a cause of chronic illness is an important aspect of integrative medicine and requires an understanding of the patterns of food intolerance, which are reviewed elsewhere.[202] If the patient has a disease diagnosis, then a MEDLINE search may reveal previously observed associations between specific foods and the patient's condition. Access PubMed via the Internet (www.pubmed.gov) and run a search that cross-references the name of the patient's condition with "hypersensitivity, food" and with "food, adverse reactions." Both of these are Medline Subject Headings (MESH). There is no MESH listing for "food allergy" or "food intolerance." Your search will be more efficient if you list the patient's condition as it appears in MESH. A negative search does not eliminate food intolerance as a trigger for the condition being searched, but the number of positive findings may surprise you. Of course, if the patient does not have a diagnosis of a type listed in on MEDLINE, this strategy will not work.[203]

▶ Case Example 1: Cyclic Diarrhea and Vomiting and *Blastocystis Hominis*

A 15-year-old girl, first seen by the author in April 1989, had experienced cyclic vomiting, diarrhea, and abdominal pain every 3 to 6 weeks for the past 9 months. The symptoms would last about 5 days and were severe enough that she was unable to attend school. She was evaluated at a major tertiary care center, where no diagnosis was made. She was treated empirically with metronidazole and discharged to the care of her family physician. The drug made her acutely ill and her symptoms continued, but during her initial interview with the author, she and her parents recalled that the first two cycles of illness following the use of metronidazole had been milder and less frequent than others. Although multiple stool specimens failed to reveal pathogenic organisms, the previous partial response to metronidazole suggested the presence of a microbial trigger. Antimicrobial herbs with demonstrated activity against protozoa (extracts of *Artemisia annua*, goldenseal, and grapefruit seed) were prescribed and continued for several months. She remained asymptomatic for 6 months, but after discontinuation of the herbs suffered a mild relapse, during which a stool specimen showed small quantities of *Blastocystis hominis*, a protozoan that is associated with acute and chronic gastrointestinal symptoms. Although they had no symptoms of any kind, the patient's parents had stool tests for ova and parasites (this testing should have been done initially). They were each found to be colonized by *Entamoeba histolytica*, *B. hominis*, and *Dientamoeba fragilis*. They were treated with metronidazole and diiodoquinol and were free of infestation at subsequent examination. Their daughter received another 6 weeks of herbal therapy and has remained free of illness for the past 11 years.

▶ Case Example 2: Chronic Diarrhea and Antibiotics

A 57-year-old man developed diarrhea following a trip to India in the fall of 2001. In India, he was treated with metronidazole without improvement. Upon return to the United States, he underwent repeated stool examinations, which failed to demonstrate any pathogens. He was treated with several antibiotics, antifungal drugs, and probiotics, with no improvement. After 3 months, the frequency and severity of diarrhea diminished, leaving him with two to three soft or loose bowel movements daily. In February 2002, he received amoxicillin for a dental infection and his diarrhea worsened, so that he was again experiencing 10 to 12 explosive, watery bowel movements a day. Further treatment with antibiotics and antifungals produced acute exacerbations of his symptoms and no net improvement. Because antibiotics appeared to aggravate his symptoms, treatment was started with a probiotic, which is a preparation of concentrated normal intestinal bacteria. The preparation used in this case contains nine different organisms at a dose supplying about one trillion live bacteria per day. Within 4 days his diarrhea had improved, and within 10 days his bowel movements became normal. The lack of response and further aggravation of symptoms by antimicrobials suggest depletion of normal bacterial flora. This preparation restored normal intestinal flora.

▶ Case Example 3: Inflammatory Arthritis and Food

A 55-year-old woman sought nutritional advice for controlling joint pain. She had a 32-year history of Crohn's colitis and had experienced considerable relief of gastrointestinal symptoms over the past 10 years by following a diet that eliminated cereal grains, sucrose, and lactose. She had been using adrenal steroids for more than 20 years, but the dietary changes allowed her to remain free of gastrointestinal symptoms on prednisone 5 mg/d. Her daughter had received a diagnosis of regional ileitis 8 years ago and had gone into complete and permanent remission following the same diet. Despite dietary control of her disease and the continued use of low-dose prednisone, the patient had begun to experience symmetrical polyarthralgia of the small joints of all extremities about a year before. A rheumatologist was uncertain whether her condition was rheumatoid arthritis or a Crohns'-related arthropathy. Because she had done well with nutritional therapy for Crohn's colitis, she presented for a short consultation on nutritional therapy for her arthritis. A quick dietary history revealed that she had been living with a man who was a gourmet cook for 2 years; he enjoyed spicy food flavored with hot peppers (capsicum). Capsaicin, an alkaloid found in capsicum, is a potent secretagogue of substance P, an importance pain mediator, which is elevated in inflamed joints.[204] This effect has been used pharmacologically in the topical treatment of chronic pain, including arthritis pain. Continuous local application of capsaicin depletes the supply of substance P in small unmyelinated sensory neurons and gradually relieves pain.[205] Intermittent ingestion of capsaicin, however, may have the opposite effect. An observational study at Lehigh University of the effect of numerous foods on arthralgia in patients with different types of arthritis, identified a number

of food additives that were likely to increase pain; capsicum was high on the
list.[206] The patient was presented with the
results of this ongoing study and advised to
use it as an experimental manual to deter-

mine which dietary components she needed
to avoid. At follow-up 1 month later, she
was pain-free and had observed that capsicum and allspice were her main arthritic
triggers.

Antecedents and the Origins of Illness

Identifying triggers may be helpful in eliminating symptoms and ameliorating tissue pathology, but it does not explain why *this* person is
sensitive to *this* trigger. A thorough knowledge
of the illness *diathesis* (predisposition) may provide a working explanation. Antecedents are
those factors that existed before the patient's illness that contributed to the development of disease. Table 4–3 lists important antecedents, divided into congenital (genetic and ontogenetic)
and developmental factors. The most important
congenital factor is sex: women and men differ
markedly in susceptibility to many disorders.
The most important developmental factor is age:
what ails children is rarely the same as what ails
the elderly. These two differences are obvious.
Beyond them lies a diversity of factors as immense as the genetic differences and separate
life experiences that distinguish one person from
another. Fessel explains:

In most circumstances, disease is not an
inevitable outcome of a single event occurring
at a point in time but generally a probabilis-
tic result of many events, each impinging on
the organism at separate times and each producing its own sequence of biological reactions. The sum total of these events produces
sufficient discomfort to the person to be recognized as illness. . . . Although the [body's]
ultimate . . . reaction . . . may be the same in
different persons, suggesting a uniform illness
and, by extension, a disease entity in its own
right, each person nevertheless probably has
a unique and separate illness by virtue of the
probability that no one else has the same combination and permutation of antecedents and
their time relations. In this sense, every disease consists of multiple diseases; in this sense,
too, there are no diseases but only sick
people.[207]

Understanding the antecedents of illness helps
the physician understand the unique characteristics of each patient as they relate to his
current health status. Congenital factors may
be inherited or acquired in utero. They can
most readily be evaluated from a comprehensive family history, including mother's health
before and during pregnancy.

Some familial disorders may not be genetic.
Hypertension is often familial, and twin studies indicate a higher concordance for blood
pressure among identical twins than among
fraternal twins. However, identical twins with a
common placenta have a higher concordance
for adult hypertension than do identical twins
with separate placentas.[208] Presumably, events
occurring in utero can influence the tendency
toward chronic illness in adulthood. Low birth

▶ **TABLE 4–3** COMMON CATEGORIES OF ILLNESS ANTECEDENTS

Congenital
  Acquired in utero
  Genetic
Developmental
  Age-related
  Learned or conditioned
  Nutritional
  Pharmacologic
  Symbiotic
  Toxic
  Traumatic (emotionally or physically

weight, for example, is associated with an increased risk of hypertension, diabetes, hypercholesterolemia, myocardial infarction, and chronic pulmonary disease in adulthood.[209–211] This association may represent the effects of maternal nutrition, tobacco use, and alcohol consumption.[212]

Postnatal developmental factors that govern the predisposition to illness include nutrition, exposure to toxins, trauma, learned patterns of behavior, and the microbial ecology of the body. Sexual abuse in childhood, for example, is associated with an increased risk of abdominal and pelvic pain syndromes among women.[213,214] Recurrent otitis media increases the risk of a child developing attention deficit disorder,[215,216] an effect that is not associated with hearing loss but may result from antibiotics. The presence of these factors is detected through a detailed, chrono-logical history from birth to the present that includes information about the patient's diet, drug and medication use, previous illnesses, work, leisure activities, travels, family life, sexual experiences, habits, life stressors, and places of residence. Because gathering these data can be very time consuming, a self-administered questionnaire completed by the patient before the interview may help to prompt responses and improve memory of remote events. For many patients with complex, chronic health problems, understanding the present illness requires a thorough knowledge of its antecedents, and it may be useful to take a detailed life history before seeking detailed information about present symptoms.

▶ Case Example 4: Fibromyalgia Following Antibiotics

A 36-year-old woman presented with a 6-year history of muscle pain and fatigue, which followed an acute illness characterized by sore throat, swollen lymph nodes, and diarrhea. A diagnosis of fibromyalgia had been made in 1995; she received numerous therapies without benefit, including physical therapy, antidepressant drugs, psychotherapy, acupuncture, homeopathy, chiropractic care, various herbal medicines, and juice fasts. She stopped working, moved in with her parents, and was bedridden for the next several years. In early 2000, she started taking guaifenesin, verapamil, propoxyphene, and acetaminophen, and she began to follow a low-salicylate diet. This program is based upon the notion that calcium is a key mediator of fibromyalgia, that various organic acids are the primary triggers for calcium activation, and that the main antecedent is a genetic predisposition to the accumulation of noxious organic acids in muscle.[217] Over the next 14 months, she experienced a 20% reduction in pain and was encouraged enough to seek further consultation. At the time of consultation she was still disabled and complained of the following symptoms: fatigue, headache, neck and shoulder pain, mucus in her bowel movements, abdominal pain and distension, irritability, lightheadedness, and numbness and tingling in her extremities.

Key questions for gathering information about the illness diathesis were asked, including the following: What was your health like in childhood, adolescence, young adulthood? What health problems did you experience during these periods of your life? What significant events occurred? Her responses indicated that she was one of five siblings in a closely knit family with strong communal ties. Her siblings were healthy, but she had suffered from numerous health problems and had received antibiotics several times a year for most of her life. Other problems included enuresis until age 10 years; seasonal allergic rhinitis and recurrent sinusitis from the time of puberty; premenstrual mood changes and menstrual cramps from the time of menarche; dry skin and hair for as long as she could remember; depression at age 18 years; and oral ulcerations beginning at age 19 years. An allergist had told her she was allergic to apples, dust, and regional pollens. Attempted hyposensitization provoked respiratory symptoms and was discontinued. At age 21 years she entered into an "abusive" marriage that lasted for 3 years. She had always been a perfectionist and hard working, had worked successfully in retail sales, and had been very stressed by overtime work at the time she became ill.

On physical examination she had a resting pulse of 76 beats per minute, which increased to 108 beats per minute with orthostatic change. Her blood pressure was 100/70 mm Hg supine and 108/84 mm Hg standing.

Her skin was visibly dry with a rough texture on palpation; her breasts were tender with a diffuse, symmetric nodularity; her abdomen was diffusely mildly to moderately tender; and she had 24 tender points in muscles of the torso and extremities, 18 of which were in locations that satisfy the American Rheumatological Society's criteria for a diagnosis of fibromyalgia.[218]

The question answered by knowing the antecedents of this illness was not "What illness does this patient have?" but "What person has this illness?" The data indicate that it was a woman with preexisting depression, premenstrual dysphoria, dysmenorrhea, compulsive work habits, bad judgment in marriage, allergic respiratory problems, and recurrent antibiotic prescriptions. In fact, the acute illness that initiated her chronic illness had been treated with antibiotics.

This information permits the formulation of a theory of probable mediators and triggers. This theory has several dimensions:

1. Repeated use of antibiotics alters the microbial ecology of the body. One effect is depletion of indigenous bacterial flora and increased mucosal colonization with antibiotic-resistant organisms, including yeasts. The predominant mucosal yeast, *Candida albicans,* has significant potential as an endogenous allergen and has been implicated as an allergic trigger in irritable bowel syndrome,[219,220] urticaria,[221] asthma,[222,223] and chronic vaginitis.[224-226] The role of *Candida* as a trigger for chronic fatigue has been greatly disputed, but its potential role in premenstrual syndrome was demonstrated in one controlled study.[227] Like *Helicobacter pylori, Candida* species may trigger multiple types of illness through different mechanisms. The evidence supporting this concept has been reviewed.[228] Unlike *H. pylori,* definitive laboratory tests for colonization have not been established and empirical antifungal therapy may be beneficial. The role of *Candida* in systemic illness is discussed further in Chapter 21.

2. Depression, premenstrual syndrome, and dysmenorrhea suggest underlying neuroendocrine disturbances that are amenable to nutritional therapy. Omega-3 EFAs are beneficial for patients with dysmenorrhea[106] and major depression.[100] Calcium,[229] magnesium,[230,231] and γ-linolenic acid[232] have demonstrated value for treatment of premenstrual symptoms. The patient's orthostatic increase in systolic blood pressure is not a normal finding and suggests an excessive noradrenergic stress response, a possible sign of magnesium insuf-

fiency.[233] Her dry, scaly skin is a possible sign of EFA insufficiency.

3. Her bad marriage, perfectionism, and overwork suggest an external locus of control and a strong desire to please others. The effects of these may be buffered by her strong family and community ties, but they are characteristics that can interfere with self-care, slowing response to therapy, or setting her up for a relapse should she initially respond well to treatment.

The patient's treatment was based upon the analysis of antecedents and was as follows:

1. To correct the effects of antibiotics, she was given a probiotic, *(Lactobacillus plantarum)*, an antifungal medication (nystatin), and a low-sugar yeast-elimination diet.
2. To improve self-regulation of the neuroendocrine stress network, she was given dietary supplements of calcium (1000 mg/d), magnesium (400 mg/d), a

fish oil extract supplying eicosapentaenoic acid (720 mg/d), and a multivitamin supplying vitamin E (400 mg/d). Verapamil was discontinued because this drug can cause fatigue and constipation, symptoms which already troubled her.

There was a gradual improvement in all symptoms, including fatigue, pain, headache, gastrointestinal symptoms, mood, paresthesia, disequilibrium, dysmenorrhea, and dry skin. After 2 months, her major symptom was persisting premenstrual dysphoria. Evening primrose oil (3000 mg/d) was added as a source of γ-linolenic acid. After 4 months of treatment she was pain-free, and after 8 months she had found full-time employment. Her only remaining symptom was seasonal allergic rhinitis. The most important therapeutic consideration at this point was to help her maintain balance and perspective as she rebuilt her life in the workforce and as she developed new social relationships.

Critical Antecedents: The Precipitating Events

An important methodologic aspect of the case just presented was the therapeutic decision to prescribe an antifungal drug without a definite fungal infection being identified. The patient, incidentally, attributed most of her improvement to nystatin, especially for her cardinal symptom, which had been muscle pain. That decision was based not only on her previous history of frequent antibiotic use, but on the onset of her present illness following a course of antibiotics for an acute respiratory and gastrointestinal illness. This acute illness and its

treatment can be thought of as a precipitating event.

Precipitating events can frequently be identified in chronic illness. Sometimes the patient cites the precipitating event as the origin of the present illness. Sometimes the precipitating event occurs prior to the present illness. It can be elicited by asking the questions, "When is the last time you felt completely well?" and "During the 6 months or so before that time, were there any changes in your life? Acute illnesses, travel, stressors, changes in medications, diets, work, home, relationships?" The precipitating event is a boundary in time. Before it, the person was relatively healthy; after it, she had become a patient with a chronic illness.

► Case Example 5: Dizziness after a Caribbean Vacation

A 41-year-old woman presented with an 18-month history of dizziness, by which she meant both vertiginous sensations and disequilibrium. The onset had been gradual and she had become progressively more disturbed by the symptom. After consulting her primary physician, a neurologist, and an endocrinologist, she consulted a psychologist, who referred her for an integrative medicine assessment. Some weeks prior to the onset of dizziness, she and her husband had taken a Caribbean vacation, at the end of which she developed an acute diarrheal illness. The diarrhea subsided spontaneously and was replaced by constipation and some abdominal distension. Her gastrointestinal function never returned to normal, but she became so concerned by the symptom of dizziness that she never complained of changes in bowel function. The information was extracted from a search for a precipitating event. A stool specimen was examined microscopically for ova and parasites; cysts of *Giardia lamblia* were identified. Because she did not want prescription drug therapy, she was treated for giardiasis with an herbal preparation containing extract that combined artemisinin and berberine for a period of 4 weeks. Dizziness and constipation both cleared and the stool examination became negative. Acute giardiasis often produces a diarrheal illness, which may resolve spontaneously. Chronic giardiasis is as likely to cause constipation as diarrhea,[234] and may provoke a number of extraintestinal effects, including asthma,[235,236] urticaria,[237-243] arthritis,[244-247] uveitis,[248] and chronic fatigue.[249] *Giardia* infection was a likely trigger for this patient's intestinal and extraintestinal symptoms. It was found by looking for a precipitating event that preceded the onset of her present illness.

Sometimes the effects of a precipitating event cannot be readily reversed. A high level of emotional distress may predispose to conditions that persist after the stress subsides. Juvenile diabetes, Graves disease, acute appendicitis, and chronic headache are all associated with preceding stressors.[250-253] An increase in life stress during the third trimester of pregnancy more than doubles the rate of serious neonatal illness. Recent or pending marital separation is associated with suppression of several measures of immune function.[254] Understanding the precipitating event is nonetheless helpful in understanding the patient's illness. Discussing the event(s) can help patients who are chronically ill fulfill their need for explanations of the genesis of their illnesses. This is a common and compelling need of patients that is generally ignored in disease-centered medicine.[255]

REFERENCES

1. Cassell E. *The Nature of Suffering and the Goals of Medicine.* New York: Oxford University Press; 1991:138.
2. Forster HP, Schwartz J, DeRenzo E. Reducing legal risk by practicing patient-centered medicine. *Arch Intern Med.* 2002;162:1217–1219.
3. Smith JL. Sir Arbuthnot Lane, chronic intestinal stasis and autointoxication. *Ann Intern Med.* 1982;86:365–369.
4. Frawley D. *Ayurvedic Healing. A Comprehensive Guide.* Salt Lake City: Passage Press; 1989:12.
5. Galland L. *Power Healing.* New York: Random House; 1998:6–11.
6. Foucault M. *The Birth of the Clinic: An Archeology of Medical Perception,* Sheridan Smith AM, trans. New York: Pantheon Books; 1973.
7. Stoeckle J, Zola IK, Davidson G. The quantity and significance of psychological distress in medical patients. *J Chronic Dis.* 1964;17:959–970.

8. Kleinman A, Eisenberg L. Culture, illness, and care: clinical lessons learned from anthropology and cross cultural research. *Ann Intern Med.* 1978;88:251–257.

9. Hadler NM. Knee pain is the malady—not osteoarthritis. *Ann Intern Med.* 1992;116:598–599.

10. Salaffi F, Cavaliery F, Nolli M, Gerraciolo G. Analysis of disability in knee osteoarthritis. Relationship with age and psychological variables but not with radiographic score. *J Rheumatol.* 1991; 18:1581–1586.

11. Kroenke K, Arrington ME, Mangelsdorff D. Common symptoms in ambulatory care: incidence, evaluation, therapy and outcome. *Am J Med.* 1989;86:262–266.

12. Sackert DL, Rosenberg WM. The need for evidence-based medicine. *J R Soc Med.* 1995;88: 620–624.

13. Hall JC, Platell C. Half-life of truth in the surgical literature. *Lancet* 1997;350:1752–1759.

14. Poynard T, Munteanu M, Ratziu V, et al. Truth survival in clinical research: an evidence-based requiem? *Ann Intern Med.* 2002;136:888–896.

15. Platt FW, McMath JC. Clinical hypocompetence: the interview. *Ann Intern Med.* 1979;91:898–902.

16. Thomas CB. Stamina: the thread of life. *J Chronic Dis.* 1981;34:41–44.

17. Reiser SJ. The era of the patient. Using the experience of illness in shaping the missions of health care. *JAMA.* 1993;269:1012–1017.

18. Beckman HB, Frankel RM. The effect of physician behavior on the collection of data. *Ann Intern Med.* 1984;101:692–696.

19. Frankel R. Talking in interviews: a dispreference for patient-initiated questions in physician-patient encounters. In: Psathas G, ed. *Studies in Ethnomethodology and Conversation Analysis. No. 1.* Washington, DC: The International Institute for Ethnomethodology and Conversation Analysis and University Press of America; 1990:231–262.

20. Bartlett EE, Grayson M, Barker R, Levine DM, Golden A, Libber S. The effects of physician communications skills on patient satisfaction; recall and adherence. *J Chronic Dis.* 1984;37: 755–764.

21. Smith RC, Hoppe RB. The patient's story: integrating the patient- and physician-centered approaches to interviewing. *Ann Intern Med.* 1991; 115:470–477.

22. Sanchez-Menegay C, Stalder H. Do physicians take into account patients' expectations? *J Gen Intern Med.* 1994;9:404–406.

23. Cassell EJ. *The Nature of Suffering and the Goals of Medicine.* New York: Oxford University Press; 1991.

24. Kleinman A, Eisenberg L, Good B. Culture, illness and care. Clinical lessons from anthropologic and cross-cultural research. *Ann Intern Med.* 1978;88:251–258.

25. O'Leary A. Self-efficacy and health. *Behav Res Ther.* 1985;23:437–451.

26. Holden G. The relationship of self-efficacy appraisals to subsequent health related outcomes: a meta-analysis. *Soc Work Health Care.* 1991; 16:53–93.

27. Phillips DP, Ruth TE, Wagner LM. Psychology and survival. *Lancet.* 1993;342:1142–1145.

28. O'Leary A. Self-efficacy and health. *Behav Res Ther.* 1985;23:437–451.

29. Bodenheimer T, Lorig K, Holman H, Grumbach K. Patient self-management of chronic disease in primary care. *JAMA.* 2002;288:2469–2475.

30. Wilson SR, Scamagas P, German DF, et al. A controlled trial of two forms of self-management education for adults with asthma. *Am J Med.* 1993;94:564–576.

31. Mullen PD, LaVille EA, Biddle AK, Lorig K. Efficacy of psychoeducational interventions on pain, depression, and disability in people with arthritis: a meta-analysis. *J Rheumatol.* 1987;14(suppl 15):33–39.

32. Litzelman DK, Slemenda CW, Langefeld CD, et al. Reduction of lower extremity clinical abnormalities in patients with non-insulin dependent diabetes mellitus. A randomized, controlled trial. *Ann Intern Med.* 1993;119:36–41.

33. Koenig HG, Cohen HJ, Blazer DG, et al. Religious coping and depression among elderly hospitalized medically ill men. *Am J Psychiatry.* 1992;149:1693–1700.

34. Pressman P, Lyons JS, Larson DB, Strain JS. Religious belief, depression, and ambulation status is elderly women with broken hips. *Am J Psychiatry.* 1990;147:758–760.

35. Idler EL, Kasl SV. Religion, disability, depression and the timing of death. *Am J Sociol.* 1992;97: 1052–1079.

36. Oxman TE, Freeman DH, Mannheimer ED. Lack of social participation or religious strength or comfort as risk factors for death after cardiac surgery in elderly. *Psychosom Med.* 1995;57:5–15.

37. Olecko WA, Blackonniere MA. Relationship of religiosity to wellness and other health related behaviors and outcomes. *Psychol Rep.* 1991; 68:819–826.

38. Frankel BG, Hewitt WE. Religion and well-being among Canadian university students: the role of faith groups on campus. *J Sci Study Religion.* 1994;33,62–73.

39. Larson DB, Greenwald MA. Are religion and spirituality clinically relevant in health care? *Adv Mind Body Med.* 1995;1:147–157.

40. Habib KE, Gold PW, Chrousos GP. Neuroendocrinology of stress. *Endocrinol Metab Clin North Am.* 2001;30:695–728.

41. Miller DB, O'Callaghan JP. Neuroendocrine aspects of the response to stress. *Metabolism.* 2002; 51(6 suppl 1):5–10.

42. Petrovsky N. Towards a unified model of neuroendocrine-immune interaction. *Immunol Cell Biol.* 2001;79:350–357.

43. Chikanza IC, Grossman AB. Reciprocal interactions between the neuroendocrine and immune systems during inflammation. *Rheum Dis Clin North Am.* 2000;26:693–671.

44. Schmidt MI, Duncan BB, Sharrett AR, et al. Markers of inflammation and prediction of diabetes mellitus in adults (Atherosclerosis Risk in Communities study): a cohort study. *Lancet.* 1999;353:1649–1652.

45. Visser M, Bouter LM, McQuillan GM, et al. Elevated C-reactive protein levels in overweight and obese adults. *JAMA.* 1999;2823:2131–2135.

46. Ross R. Atherosclerosis: an inflammatory disease. *N Engl J Med.* 1999;340:115–126.

47. Abramson JL, Vaccarino V. Relationship between activity and inflammation among apparently healthy middle-aged and older adults. *Arch Intern Med.* 2002;162:1286–1292.

48. Maes M. Major depression and activation of the inflammatory response system. In: Danzer EA, ed. *Cytokines, Stress and Depression.* New York: Kluwer Academic/Plenum Publishers; 1999: 25–46.

49. Shacter E, Weitzman SA. Chronic inflammation and cancer. *Oncology.* 2002;16:217–226, 229.

50. Franceschi C, Ottaviani E. Stress, inflammation and natural immunity in the aging process: a new theory. *Aging (Milano).* 1997;9(suppl): 30–31.

51. Yen SS, Laughlin GA. Aging and the adrenal cortex. *Exp Gerontol.* 1998;33:897–910.

52. Rook GA. Glucocorticoids and immune function.

Baillieres Best Pract Res Clin Endocrinol Metab. 1999;13:567–581.

53. Elenkov IJ, Chrousos GP. Stress hormones, proinflammatory and anti-inflammatory cytokines, and autoimmunity. *Ann N Y Acad Sci.* 2002;966: 290–303.

54. Petrovsky N. Towards a unified model of neuroendocrine-immune interaction. *Immunol Cell Biol.* 2001;79:350–357.

55. Raber J, Sorg O, Horn TFW, et al. Inflammatory cytokines: putative regulators of neuronal and neuro–endocrine function. *Brain Res Rev.* 1998;26:320–326.

56. Muller JE, Ludmer PL, Willich SN, et al. Circadian variation in the frequency of sudden cardiac death. *Circulation.* 1987;75:131–138.

57. Tofler GH, Brezinski D, Schafer Al, et al. Concurrent morning increase in platelet aggregability and the risk of myocardial infarction and sudden cardiac death. *N Engl J Med.* 1987;316: 1514–1518.

58. Rauramaa R, Vaisanen SB. Interaction of physical activity and diet: implications for haemostatic factors. *Public Health Nutr.* 1999;2:383–390.

59. Markovitz JH, Matthews KA. Platelets and coronary heart disease: potential psychophysiologic mechanisms. *Psychosom Med.* 1991;53:643–668.

60. Levenson JL, Mishra A, Hamer RM, Hastillo A. Denial and medical outcome in unstable angina. *Psychosom Med.* 1989;51:27–35.

61. Giggs GA, Salmon JA, Henderson B, Vane JR. Pharmacokinetics of aspirin and salicylate in relation to inhibition of arachidonate cyclooxygenase and anti-inflammatory activity. *Proc Nat Acad Sci U S A.* 1987;84:1417–1420.

62. Blacklock CJ, Lawrence JR, Wiles D, et al. Salicylic acid concentrations in the serum of subjects not taking aspirin: comparison of salicylic acid concentrations in the serum of vegetarians, nonvegetarians and patients taking low-dose aspirin. *J Clin Pathol.* 2001;54:553-555.

63. Galland L. Magnesium, stress and neuropsychiatric disorders. *Magnes Trace Elem.* 1991–1992;10: 287–301.

64. Galland L. Magnesium and immune function: an overview. *Magnes Trace Elem.* 1988;7:290–299.

65. Britton J, Pavord I, Richards K, et al. Dietary magnesium, lung function, wheezing, and airway hyperresponsiveness in a random adult population sample. *Lancet.* 1994;344:357–362.

66. Burch GE, Giles TD. The importance of magne-

sium in cardiovascular disease. *Am Heart J.* 1977;94:649–657.

67. Woods Kl, Fletcher S, Roffe C, Haider Y. Intravenous magnesium sulphate in suspected acute myocardial infarction: results of the second Leicester Intravenous Magnesium Intervention Trial (LIMIT-2). *Lancet.* 1992;339:1553–1558.

68. Skobeloff EM, Spivey WH, McNamara RM, Greenspon L. Intravenous magnesium sulfate for the treatment of acute asthma in the emergency department. *JAMA.* 1989;262:1210–1213.

69. Okayama H, Okayama M, Aikawa T, et al. Treatment of status asthmaticus with intravenous magnesium sulphate. *J Asthma.* 1991;28:11–17.

70. Klevay LM, Milne DB. Low dietary magnesium increases supraventricular ectopy. *Am J Clin Nutr.* 2002,75:550–554.

71. Calder PC, Grimble RF. Polyunsaturated fatty acids, inflammation and immunity. *Eur J Clin Nutr.* 2002;56(suppl 3):S14–S19.

72. Diep QN, Touyz RM, Schiffrin EL. Docosahexaenoic acid, a peroxisome proliferator-activated receptor-alpha ligand, induces apoptosis in vascular smooth muscle cells by stimulation of p38 mitogen-activated protein kinase. *Hypertension.* 2000;36:851–855.

73. Chalon S, Vancassel S, Zimmer L, Guilloteau D, Durand G. Polyunsaturated fatty acids and cerebral function: focus on monoaminergic neurotransmission. *Lipids.* 2001;36:937–944.

74. Seaman DR. The diet-induced proinflammatory state: a cause of chronic pain and other degenerative diseases? *J Manipulative Physiol Ther.* 2002;25:168–179.

75. Grimble RF. Interaction between nutrients, proinflammatory cytokines and inflammation. *Clin Sci (Lond).* 1996;91:121–130.

76. Beckman DB, Frankel RM. The effect of physician behavior on the collection of data. *Ann Intern Med.* 1984;101:692–696.

77. Roter DL, Hall JA. Physician interviewing styles and medical information obtained from patients. *J Gen Intern Med.* 1987;2:325–329.

78. Fredidin RB, Goldin L, Cecil RR. Patient-physician concordance in problem identification in the primary care setting. *Ann Intern Med.* 1980; 93:490–493.

79. Tuckett D, Boulton M, Olson C, Williams A. *Meetings Between Experts: An Approach to Sharing Ideas in Medical Consultations.* London: Tavistock Publications; 1985.

80. Sanchez-Menegay C, Stalder M. Do physicians take into account patients' perspectives? *J Gen Intern Med.* 1994;9:404–406.

81. Korsch BM, Gozzi EK, Francis V. Gaps in doctor–patient communication. I: Doctor–patient interaction and patient satisfaction. *Pediatrics.* 1968; 42:855–871.

82. Williams GH, Wood PHN. Common-sense beliefs about illness: a mediating role for the doctor. *Lancet.* 1986;328:1435–1437.

83. Hall JA, Roter DL, Katz NR. Meta-analysis of correlates of provider behavior in medical encounters. *Med Care.* 1990;28:657–675.

84. Ades PA, Waldmann ML, McCann WJ, Weaver SO. Predictors of cardiac rehabilitation participation in older coronary patients. *Arch Intern Med.* 1992;152: 1033–1035.

85. Brody DS. Physician recognition of behavioral, psychological, and social aspects of medical care. *Arch Intern Med.* 1980;140:1286–1289.

86. Mullen PD, LaVille EA, Biddle AK, Lorig K. Efficacy of psychoeducational interventions on pain, depression, and disability in people with arthritis: a meta-analysis. *J Rheumatol.* 1987;14(suppl 15):33–39.

87. Lorig KR, Mazonson PD, Holman HR. Evidence suggesting that health education for self-management in patients with chronic arthritis has sustained health benefits while reducing health care costs. *Arthritis Rheum.* 1993;36:439–446.

88. Thomas KB. The placebo in general practice. *Lancet.* 1994;344:1066–1067.

89. Waitzkin H. Doctor-patient communication: clinical implications of social scientific research. *JAMA.* 1984;252:2441–2446.

90. Kaplan SH, Greenfield S, Ware JE Jr. Assessing the effects of physician-patient interactions on the outcomes of chronic disease. *Med Care.* 1989;27(suppl 3):S110–S127.

91. Engel GL. Psychologic stress, vasodepressor (vasovagal) syncope, and sudden death. *Ann Intern Med.* 1978;89:403–412.

92. Kubler-Ross E. *On Death and Dying.* New York: Macmillan; 1969.

93. Cassell E. *The Nature of Suffering and the Goals of Medicine.* New York: Oxford University Press; 1991:245.

94. Hogue DR. A validated intrinsic motivation scale. *J Sci Study Religion.* 1972;11:369–376.

95. Strayhorn JM, Weidman CS, Larson DB. A measure of religiousness and its relation to parent

and child mental health variables. *J Community Psychol*. 1990;18:34–43.

96. Zuckerman DM, Kasl SV, Ostfield AM. Psychosocial predictors of mortality among the elderly poor. *Am J Epidemiol*. 1984;119:410–423.

97. Cobb S. Social support as a moderator of life stress. *Psychosom Med*. 1976;38:300–314.

98. Ornish D. *Love and Survival: 8 Pathways to Intimacy and Health*. New York: Harper Collins; 1999:279.

99. Galland L. *Power Healing*. New York: Random House; 1997:115–135.

100. Spiegel D. Effects of psychotherapy on cancer survival. *Natl Rev Cancer*. 2002;2:1–7.

101. Sephton SE, Sapolsky RM, Kraemer HC, Spiegel D. Diurnal cortisol rhythm as a predictor of breast cancer survival. *J Natl Cancer Inst*. 2000; 92:994–1000.

102. Cruess DG, Antoni MH, McGregor BA, et al. Cognitive-behavioral stress management reduces serum cortisol by enhancing benefit finding among women being treated for early stage breast cancer. *Psychosom Med*. 2000;62: 304–308.

103. Fawzy FI, Kemeny ME, Fawzy NW, et al. A structured psychiatric intervention for cancer patients. II. Changes over time in immunological measures. *Arch Gen Psychiatry*. 1990;47:729–735.

104. Bucher HC. Social support and prognosis following first myocardial infarction. *J Gen Intern Med*. 1994;9:409–417.

105. Eisenberg L. What makes persons "patients" and patients "well." *Am J Med*. 1980;69:277–286.

106. Egbert LD, Battit GE, Welch CE, et al. Reduction of post-operative pain by encouragement and instruction of patients: a study of doctor–patient rapport. *N Engl J Med*. 1964;270:825–827.

107. The Headache Study group of the University of Western Ontario. Predictors of outcome in headache patients presenting to family physicians—a one-year prospective study. *Headache*. 1986;26: 285–294.

108. Benson H, McCalie DP. Angina pectoris and the placebo effect. *N Engl J Med*. 1979;300:1424–1429.

109. Kleinen J, de Craen AJM, van Everdingen J, Leendert K. Placebo effect in double-blind clinical trials: a review of interactions with medications. *Lancet*. 1994;344:1347–1349.

110. Fine VK, Therrien ME. Empathy in the doctor–patient relationship. Skill training for medical students. *J Med Educ*. 1977;52:752–757.

111. Spiro H. What is empathy and can it be taught? *Ann Intern Med*. 1992;116:843–846.

112. Podolsky DK. Inflammatory bowel disease. *N Engl J Med*. 2002;347:417–429.

113. Wong ML, Kling MA, Munson PJ, et al. Pronounced and sustained central hypernoradrenergic function in major depression with melancholic features: relation to hypercortisolism and corticotropin-releasing hormone. *Proc Natl Acad Sci U S A*. 2000;97(1):325–330.

114. Maes M, Christophe A, Delanghe J, et al. Lowered omega-3 polyunsaturated fatty acids in serum phospholipids and cholesteryl esters of depressed patients. *Psychiatry Res* 1998;85: 275–291.

115. Adams PB. Arachidonic acid to eicosapentaenoic acid ratio in blood correlates positively with clinical symptoms of depression. *Lipids* 1996; 31(suppl):S157–S161.

116. Peet M, Murphy B, Shay J, Horrobin D. Depletion of omega-3 fatty acid levels in red blood cell membranes of depressive patients. *Biol Psychiatry*. 1998;43:315–319.

117. Stoll AL, Locke CA, Marangell LB, Severus WE. Omega-3 fatty acids and bipolar disorder: a review. *Prostaglandins Leukot Essent Fatty Acids*. 1999;60:329–337.

118. Roth JL, Mobarhan S, Clohisy M. The metabolic syndrome: where are we and where do we go? *Nutr Rev*. 2002;60(10 pt 1):335–337.

119. Olefsky JM, Saltiel AR. PPAR gamma and the treatment of insulin resistance. *Trends Endocrinol Metab*. 2000;11(9):362–368.

120. Pelkman CL. Effects of the glycemic index of foods on serum concentrations of high-density lipoprotein cholesterol and triglycerides. *Curr Atheroscler Rep*. 2001;3(6):456–461.

121. Rivellese AA, De Natale C, Lilli S. Type of dietary fat and insulin resistance. *Ann N Y Acad Sci*. 2002;967:329–335.

122. Belch JJF, Ansell D, Madhok R, O'Dowd A, Sturrock RD. Effects of altering dietary essential fatty acids on requirements for non-steroidal anti-inflammatory drugs in patients with rheumatoid arthritis: a double blind placebo controlled study. *Ann Rheum Dis*. 1988;47:96–104.

123. Appel LJ, Miller ER, Seidler AJ, Whelton PK. Does supplementation with "fish oil" reduce blood pressure? A meta-analysis of controlled clinical trials. *Arch Intern Med*. 1993;153:1429–1438.

124. Gapinski JP, VanRuiswyk V, Heudebert GR, Schectman GS. Preventing restenosis with fish

oils following coronary angioplasty. *Arch Intern Med.* 1993;153:1595–1601.

125. Stenson WF, Cort D, Rodgers J, et al. Dietary supplements with fish oil in ulcerative colitis. *Ann Intern Med.* 1992;116:609–614.

126. McCaren T, Hitzeman R, Smith R, et al. Amelioration of severe migraine by fish oil (n-3) fatty acids. *Am J Clin Nutr.* 1985;41:874.

127. Harel Z, Biro FM, Kottenhahn RK, Rosenthal SL. Supplementation with omega-3 polyunsaturated fatty acids in the management of dysmenorrhea in adolescents. *Am J Obstet Gynecol.* 1996;174(4): 1335–1338.

128. Stenson WF, Cort D, Rodgers J, et al. Dietary supplements with fish oil in ulcerative colitis. *Ann Intern Med.* 1992;116:609–614.

129. Nordvik I, Myhr KM, Nyland H, Bjerve KS. Effect of dietary advice and n-3 supplementation in newly diagnosed MS patients. *Acta Neurol Scand.* 2000;102(3):143–149.

130. Fenton WS, Dickerson F, Boronow J, Hibbeln JR, Knable M. A placebo-controlled trial of omega-3 fatty acid (ethyl eicosapentaenoic acid) supplementation for residual symptoms and cognitive impairment in schizophrenia. *Am J Psychiatry.* 2001;158(12):2071–2074.

131. Bates D, Cartlidge NEF, French JM, et al. A double-blind controlled trial of n-3 polyunsaturated fatty acids in the treatment of multiple sclerosis. *J Neurol Neurosurg Psychiatry.* 1989;52:18–22.

132. Prasad AS. Clinical manifestations of zinc deficiency. *Annu Rev Nutr.* 1985;5:341–363.

133. Stevens LJ, Zentall SS, Deck JL, et al. Essential fatty acid metabolism in boys with attention deficit hyperactivity disorder. *Am J Clin Nutr.* 1995;62:761–768.

134. Stevens LJ, Zentall SS, Abate ML, et al. Omega-3 fatty acids in boys with behavior, learning and health problems. *Physiol Behav.* 1996;59:75–90.

135. Galland L. *Power Healing.* New York: Random House; 1997:156–162.

136. Cohen L, Kitzes R. Characterization of the magnesium status of elderly people with congestive heart failure, hypertension and diabetes mellitus by the magnesium-load test. *Magnes Bull.* 1993; 15:105–109.

137. Romano TJ, Stiller JW. Magnesium deficiency in fibromyalgia syndrome. *J Nutr Med.* 1994;4: 165–167.

138. Gordin A, Goldenberg D, Golz A, Netzer A, Joachims HZ. Magnesium: a new therapy for id-iopathic sudden sensorineural hearing loss. *Otolaryngol Neurootol.* 2002;23(4):447–451.

139. Fehlinger R, Seidel K. The hyperventilation syndrome: a neurosis or a manifestation of magnesium imbalance? *Magnesium.* 1985;4(2–3): 129–136.

140. Morgan KJ, Stampley GL, Zabik ME, Fischer DR. Magnesium and calcium dietary intakes of the US population. *J Am Coll Nutr.* 1985;4:195–206.

141. Galland L. *Power Healing.* New York: Random House; 1997:162–169.

142. Schwartz J, Slater D, Larson TV, et al. Particulate air pollution and hospital emergency room visits for asthma in Seattle. *Am Rev Respir Dis.* 1993;147:826–831.

143. Chilmonczyk BA, Salmun LM, Megathlih KN, et al. Association between exposure to environmental tobacco smoke and exacerbations of asthma in children. *N Engl J Med.* 1993;328:1665–1669.

144. Rossi OVJ, Kinnula VL, Tienari J, Huhti E. Association of severe asthma attacks with weather, pollen and air pollutants. *Thorax.* 1993;48: 244–248.

145. O'Byrne PM, Dolovich J, Hargreave FE. Late asthmatic responses. *Am Rev Respir Dis.* 1987;136: 740–751.

146. Gelber LE, Seltzer LH, Bouzoukis JK, et al. Sensitization and exposure to indoor allergens as risk factors for asthma among patients presenting to hospital. *Am Rev Respir Dis.* 1993;147: 573–578.

147. Lemanske RF Jr, Dick EC, Swenson CA, Vrtis RF, Busse WW. Rhinovirus upper respiratory infection increases airway hyperactivity and late asthmatic reactions. *J Clin Invest.* 1989;83:1–10.

148. Rumbak MJ, Kelso TM, Arheart KL, Self TH. Perception of anxiety as a contributing factor of asthma: indigent versus nonindigent. *J Asthma.* 1993;30:165–169.

149. Eschenbacher WL, Moore TB, Lorenzen TJ, Weg JG, Gross KB. Pulmonary responses of asthmatic and normal subjects to different temperatures and humidity conditions in an environmental chamber. *Lung.* 1992;170:51–62.

150. Morgan MD. Dysfunctional breathing in asthma: is it common, identifiable and correctable? *Thorax.* 2002;57(suppl 2):II31–II35.

151. Mahler DA. Exercise-induced asthma. *Med Sci Sports Exerc.* 1993;25:554–561.

152. Cernak I, Savic VJ, Kotur J, Prokic V, Veljovic M, Grbovic D. Characterization of plasma magnesium concentration and oxidative stress following

graded traumatic brain injury in humans. *J Neurotrauma.* 2000;17(1):53–68.

153. Vink R, Nimmo AJ, Cernak I. An overview of new and novel pharmacotherapies for use in traumatic brain injury. *Clin Exp Pharmacol Physiol.* 2001;28(11):919–921.

154. Chan FK, To KF, Wu JCY, et al. Eradication of *Helicobacter pylori* and risk of peptic ulcers in patients starting long-term treatment with non-steroidal anti-inflammatory drugs: a randomized trial. *Lancet.* 2002;359:9–13.

155. Uemara N, Okamoto S, Yamamoto S, et al. *Helicobacter pylori* and the development of gastric cancer. *N Engl J Med.* 2001;345:784–789.

156. Wotherspoon AC, Dogliani C, Diss TC, et al. Regression of primary low-grade B-cell lymphoma of mucosal-associated lymphoid tissue after eradication of *Helicobacter pylori*. *Lancet.* 1993;342:575–577.

157. Mendall MA, Goggin OM, Molineaux N, et al. Relation of *Helicobacter pylori* infection and coronary heart disease. *Br Heart J.* 1994;71:437–439.

158. Markus HS, Mendel MA. *Helicobacter pylori*: a risk factor for ischemic cerebrovascular disease and carotid atheroma. *J Neurol Neurosurg Psychiatry.* 1998;64:104–107.

159. Szlachcic A, Liwowski Z, Karczewska E, Bielans P. *Helicobacter pylori* and its eradication in rosacea. *J Physiol Pharmacol.* 1999;50:777–786.

160. Aragona P, Magazzu G, Macchia G, et al. Presence of antibodies against *Helicobacter pylori* and its heat-shock protein 60 in the serum of patients with Sjögren's syndrome. *J Rheumatol.* 1999;26:1306–1311.

161. Gasbarrini A, Franceschi F, Arnuzzi A, et al. Extradigestive manifestations of *Helicobacter pylori* gastric infection. *Gut.* 1999;45(suppl):I9–I12.

162. Matysiak-Budnik T, Heyman M. Food allergy and *Helicobacter pylori*. *J Pediatr Gastroenterol Nutr.* 2002;34:5–12.

163. Kaptan K, Beyan C, Ural AU, et al. *Helicobacter pylori*: is it a novel causative agent in vitamin B_{12} deficiency? *Arch Intern Med.* 2000;160:1349–1353.

164. Kountouras J, Mylopoiulos N, Boura P, et al. Relationship between *Helicobacter pylori* infection and glaucoma. *Ophthalmology* 2001;108:599–604.

165. Kountouras J, Mylopoulos N, Chatzopoulos D, et al. Eradication of *Helicobacter pylori* may be beneficial in the management of chronic open-angle glaucoma. *Arch Intern Med.* 2002;162:1237–1244.

166. Avorn J, Everitt DE, Baker MW. The neglected medical history and therapeutic choices for abdominal pain: a nationwide study of 799 physicians and nurses. *Arch Intern Med.* 1991;151:694–698.

167. Caperton EM, Heim-Duthoy KL, Matske GR, et al. Ceftriaxone therapy of chronic inflammatory arthritis: a double-blind placebo-controlled trial. *Arch Intern Med.* 1990;150:1677–1682.

168. Schwartz J, Dockery DW. Particulate air pollution and daily mortality in Steubenville, Ohio. *Am J Epidemiol.* 1992;135:12–19.

169. Dockery DW, Pope A, Xu X, et al. An association between air pollution and mortality in six US cities. *N Engl J Med.* 1993;329:1753–1759.

170. Hodgson MJ, Frohlinger J, Permar E, et al. Symptoms and microenvironmental measures in non-problem buildings. *J Occup Environ Med.* 1991;35: 527–533.

171. Hodgson MJ. Buildings and health. *Health Environ Dig.* 1993;7:1–3.

172. Platt SD, Martin CJ, Hunt SM, Lewis CW. Damp housing, mould growth and symptomatic health state. *BMJ.* 1989;198:1673–1678.

173. Verhoeff AP, van Strien RT, van Wijnen JH, et al. Damp housing and childhood respiratory symptoms: the role of sensitization to dust mites and molds. *Am J Epidemiol.* 1995;141:103–110.

174. Platts-Mills TAE, Tovey ER, Mitchell EB, et al. Reduction of bronchial hyperreactivity during prolonged allergen avoidance. *Lancet.* 1982;320:675–678.

175. Sporik R, Holgate ST, Platts-Mills TAE, Cogswell JJ. Exposure to house-dust mite allergen and the development of asthma in childhood. A prospective study. *N Engl J Med.* 1990;323: 502–507.

176. Croft WA, Jarvis BB, Yatawara CS. Airborne outbreak of trichothecene toxicosis. *Atmosphere Environ.* 1986;20:549–552.

177. Wray BB, O'Steen KG. Mycotoxin-producing fungi from house associated with leukemia. *Arch Environ Health.* 1975;30:571–573.

178. Bender AE, Matthews DR. Adverse reactions to foods. *Br J Nutr.* 1981;46:403–407.

179. Moneret-Vautrin DA. Food antigens and additives. *J Allergy Clin Immunol.* 1986;78:1039–1046.

180. Kniker WT, Rodriguez M. Non-IgE mediated and delayed adverse reactions to food or additives. In: Breneman JC, ed. *Handbook of Food Allergies.* New York: Marcel Dekker; 1987:125–161.

181. Perry CA, Dwyer J, Gelfand JA, et al. Health ef-

fects of salicylates in foods and drugs. *Nutr Rev.* 1996;54(8):225–240.

182. Lovenberg W. Some vaso- and psychoactive substances in food: amines, stimulants, depressants and hallucinogens. In: Committee on Food Protection, Food & Nutrition Board, National Research Council, eds. *Toxicants Occurring Naturally in Foods.* 2nd ed. Washington, DC: National Academy of Sciences Press; 1973:170–188.

183. Somogyi JC. Natural toxic substances in food. *World Rev Nutr Diet.* 1978;29:42–59.

184. Catassi C, Ratsch I-M, Fabiani E, et al. Coeliac disease in the year 2000: exploring the tip of the iceberg. *Lancet.* 1994;343:200–203.

185. Hadjivassiliou M, Gibson A, Davies-Jones GAB, et al. Does cryptic gluten sensitivity play a part in neurological illness? *Lancet.* 1996;347:369–371.

186. Hadjivassiliou M, Grunewald RA, Chattopadhyay AK, et al. Clinical, radiological, neurophysiological, and neuropathological characteristics of gluten ataxia. *Lancet.* 1998;352:1582–1585.

187. Collin P, Reunala T. Recognition and management of the cutaneous manifestations of celiac disease: a guide for dermatologists. *Am J Clin Dermatol.* 2003;4(1):13–20.

188. Burgin-Wolff A, Berger R, Gaze H, Huber H, Lentze MJ, Nussle D. IgG, IgA and IgE gliadin antibody determinations as screening test for untreated coeliac disease in children, a multicentre study. *Eur J Pediatr.* 1989;148(6):496–502.

189. Jyonouchi H, Sun S, Itokazu N. Innate immunity associated with inflammatory responses and cytokine production against common dietary proteins in patients with autism spectrum disorder. *Neuropsychobiology.* 2002;46(2):76–84.

190. Ramos-Remus C, Bahlas S, Vaca-Morales O. Rheumatic features of gastrointestinal tract, hepatic, and pancreatic diseases. *Curr Opin Rheumatol.* 1997;9(1):56–61.

191. Falcini F, Ferrari R, Simonini G, Calabri GB, Pazzaglia A, Lionetti P. Recurrent monoarthritis in an 11-year-old boy with occult coeliac disease. Successful and stable remission after gluten-free diet. *Clin Exp Rheumatol.* 1999;17(4):509–511.

192. Kallikorm R, Uibo O, Uibo R. Coeliac disease in spondyloarthropathy: usefulness of serological screening. *Clin Rheumatol.* 2000;19(2):118–122.

193. Slot O, Locht H. Arthritis as presenting symptom in silent adult coeliac disease. Two cases and review of the literature. *Scand J Rheumatol.* 2000;29(4):260–263.

194. Bagnato GF, Quattrocchi E, Gulli S, et al. Unusual polyarthritis as a unique clinical manifestation of coeliac disease. *Rheumatol Int.* 2000;20(1):29–30.

195. Lindqvist U, Rudsander A, Bostrom A, Nilsson B, Michaelsson G. IgA antibodies to gliadin and coeliac disease in psoriatic arthritis. *Rheumatology.* 2002;41(1):31–37.

196. Michaelsson G, Gerden B, Hagforsen E, et al. Psoriasis patients with antibodies to gliadin can be improved by a gluten-free diet. *Br J Dermatol.* 2000;142(1):44–51.

197. Teppo AM, Maury CP. Antibodies to gliadin, gluten and reticulin glycoprotein in rheumatic diseases: elevated levels in Sjögren's syndrome. *Clin Exp Immunol.* 1984;57(1):73–78.

198. Collin P, Korpela M, Hallstrom O, et al. Rheumatic complaints as a presenting symptom in patients with coeliac disease. *Scand J Rheumatol.* 1992;21(1):20–23.

199. Dohan FC. Is celiac disease a clue to the pathogenesis of schizophrenia? *Ment Hyg.* 1969;53(4):525–529.

200. Vlissides DN, Venulet A, Jenner FA. A double-blind gluten-free/gluten-load controlled trial in a secure ward population. *Br J Psychiatry.* 1986;148:447–452.

201. Karell K, Korponay-Szabo I, Szalai Z, et al. Genetic dissection between coeliac disease and dermatitis herpetiformis in sib pairs. *Ann Hum Genet.* 2002;66(pt 6):387–392.

202. Brostoff J, Challacombe SJ, eds. *Food Allergy and Intolerance.* London: Baillieres-Tindall; 1987.

203. Medical cybrarian Valerie Rankow (vgr99@optonline.net) has assisted the author with this search strategy and with numerous other, more complex searches.

204. Sluka KA, Wright A. Knee joint mobilization reduces secondary mechanical hyperalgesia induced by capsaicin injection into the ankle joint. *Eur J Pain.* 2001;5(1):817–820.

205. Robbins W. Clinical applications of capsaicinoids. *Clin J Pain.* 2000;16(2 suppl):S86–S89.

206. *Foods Found to Cause Pain, Swelling and Stiffness: Results of the Latest Detailed Food Studies.* Wharton, NJ: Arthritis Help Centers; 2000.

207. Fessel JW. The nature of illness and diagnosis. *Am J Med.* 1983;75:555–560.

208. Phillips DW. Twin studies in medical research [letter]. *Lancet.* 1993;342:52.

209. Barker DJP, Winter PD, Osmond C, et al. Weight

in infancy and death from ischaemic heart disease. *Lancet.* 1989;2:577–580.

210. Barker DJP. *Fetal and Infants' Origins of Adult Disease.* London: BMJ; 1992.

211. Barker DJP, Bull AR, Osmond C, Simmonds SJ. Fetal and placental size and risk of hypertension in adult life. *BMJ.* 1990;301:259–262.

212. Goldberg GR, Prentice A. Maternal and fetal determinants of adult diseases. *Nutr Rev.* 1994;52: 191–200.

213. Romans S, Belaise C, Martin J, Morris E, Raffi A. Childhood abuse and later medical disorders in women. An epidemiological study. *Psychother Psychosom.* 2002;71(3):141–150.

214. Lampe A, Solder E, Ennemoser A, Schubert C, Rumpold G, Sollner W. Chronic pelvic pain and previous sexual abuse. *Obstet Gynecol.* 2000; 96(6):929–933.

215. Hagerman RJ, Falkenstein AR. An association between recurrent otitis media in infancy and later hyperactivity. *Clin Pediatr (Phila).* 1987;26(5): 253–257.

216. Adesman AR, Altshuler LA, Lipkin PH, Walco GA. Otitis media in children with learning disabilities and in children with attention deficit disorder with hyperactivity. *Pediatrics.* 1990;85(3 pt 2):442–446.

217. Marek C. *What Your Doctor May Not Tell You About Fibromyalgia: The Revolutionary Treatment That Can Reverse the Disease.* New York: Warner Books; 1999.

218. Greene WB, ed. *Essentials of Musculoskeletal Care.* Rosemont, IL: American Academy of Orthopedic Surgeons; 2001:33.

219. Gordon EH, Klaustermeyer WB. Hypersensitivity to *Candida albicans. Immunol Allergy Pract.* 1986;8:29–34.

220. Holti G. Candida allergy. In: Winner HL, Hurley R, eds. *Symposium on Candida Infections.* London: E. & S. Livingstone Ltd; 1966:73–81.

221. James J, Warin RP. An assessment of the role of *Candida albicans* and food yeast in chronic urticaria. *Br J Dermatol.* 1971;84:227–237.

222. Akiyama K, Yui Y, Shida T, Miyamoto T. Relationship between the result of skin, conjunctival and bronchial tests and RAST with *Candida albicans* in patients with asthma. *Clin Allergy.* 1981;11:323–351.

223. Gumowski P, Lech B, Chaves L. Chronic asthma and rhinitis due to *Candida albicans, Epider-*

mophyton and *Trichophyton. Ann Allergy.* 1987; 59:48–51.

224. Witkin SS. Immunology of recurrent vaginitis. *Am J Reprod Immunol.* 1987;15:34–37.

225. Mathur S, Goust JM, Horger EO, Fudenberg HH. Immunoglobulin E anti-*Candida* antibodies and candidiasis. *Infect Immun.* 1977;18:257–259.

226. Palacios HJ. Hypersensitivity as a cause of dermatologic and vaginal moniliasis resistant to topical therapy. *Ann Allergy.* 1976;37:110–113.

227. Schinfeld JS. PMS and candidiasis: study explores possible link. *Female Patient.* 1987;12:66–74.

228. Galland L. The effect of intestinal microbes on systemic immunity. In: Jenkins R, Mowbray P, eds. *Post-Viral Fatigue Syndrome.* London: John Wiley and Sons; 1991:405–430.

229. Thys-Jacobs S, Starkey P, Bernstein D, Tian J. Calcium carbonate and the premenstrual syndrome: effects on premenstrual and menstrual symptoms. Premenstrual Syndrome Study Group. *Am J Obstet Gynecol.* 1998;179(2):444–452.

230. Walker AF, De Souza MC, Vickers MF, Abeyasekera S, Collins ML, Trinca LA. Magnesium supplementation alleviates premenstrual symptoms of fluid retention. *J Womens Health* 1998;7(9): 1157–1165.

231. De Souza MC, Walker AF, Robinson PA, Bolland K. A synergistic effect of a daily supplement for 1 month of 200 mg magnesium plus 50 mg vitamin B_6 for the relief of anxiety-related premenstrual symptoms: a randomized, double-blind, crossover study. *J Womens Health Gend Based Med.* 2000;9(2):131–139.

232. Goodwin PJ, Neelam M, Boyd NF. Cyclical mastopathy: a critical review of therapy. *Br J Surg.* 1988;75(9):837–844.

233. Lichodziejewska B, Klos J, Rezler J, et al. Clinical symptoms of mitral valve prolapse are related to hypomagnesemia and attenuated by magnesium supplementation. *Am J Cardiol.* 1997;79(6): 768–772.

234. Chester AC, MacMurray FG, Restifo MD, Mann O. Giardiasis as a chronic disease. *Dig Dis Sci.* 1985;30(3):215–218.

235. Fossati C. Manifestazioni broncopulmonari in corso di infestazione da Giardia lamblia. *Revista Iberica de Parisitologia.* 1971;31:283–298.

236. Lopez-Brea M, Sain ZT, Camarero C, Baquero M. Giardia lamblia associated with bronchial asthma and serum antibodies, and chronic diarrhoea in

a child with giardiasis. *Trans R Soc Trop Med Hyg.* 1979;73:600–601.

237. Harris RH, Mitchell JH. Chronic urticaria due to *Giardia lamblia. Arch Dermatol Syphilol.* 1949; 59:587–589.

238. Wilhelm RE. Urticaria associated with giardiasis lamblia. *J Allergy.* 1958;28:351–353.

239. Webster BH. Human infection with *Giardia lamblia. Am J Dig Dis.* 1958;3:64–71.

240. Dellamonica P, Le Fichoux X, Monnier B, Duplay H. Syndrome dysenterigue et urticaire, au cours d'une giardiase. *Nouvelle Presse Med.* 1976;5: 913–914.

241. Weisman BL. Urticaria and *Giardia lamblia* infections. *Ann Allergy.* 1979;49:91–93.

242. Kennou ME. Skin manifestation of giardiasis. Some clinical cases. *Arch Institut Pasteur Tunis.* 1980;51:257–260.

243. Farthing MJG, Chong SKF, Walker-Smith JA. Acute allergic phenomena in giardiasis. *Lancet.* 1983; 2:1428–1429.

244. Goobar JP. Joint symptoms in giardiasis. *Lancet.* 1977;1:1010–1011.

245. Woo P, Panayi GS. Reactive arthritis due to infestation with *Giardia lamblia. J Rheumatol.* 1984;11:719–721.

246. Shaw RA, Stevens MB. The reactive arthritis of giardiasis. A case report. *JAMA.* 1987;258: 2734–2735.

247. Galland L. Intestinal protozoan infection is a common unsuspected cause of chronic illness. *J Adv Med.* 1989;2:529–552.

248. Carroll ME, Anast BP, Birch CL. Giardiasis and uveitis. *Arch Ophthalmol.* 1961;65:775–778.

249. Galland L, Lee M, Bueno H, Heirnowitz C. *Giardia lamblia* infection as a cause of chronic fatigue. *J Nutr Med.* 1990;2:27–32.

250. Hagglof B, Blom L, Dahlquist G, Lonnenberg G, Sahlin B. The Swedish Childhood Diabetes Study: indication of severe psychological stress as a risk factor for type 1 (insulin-dependent) diabetes mellitus in childhood. *Diabetologia.* 1991;34: 579–583.

251. Winsa B, Adami H-O, Bergstrom R, et al. Stressful life events and Graves' disease. *Lancet.* 1991;338:1475–1479.

252. Creed F. Life events and appendectomy. *Lancet.* 1981;i:1381–1388.

253. De Benedittis G, Lorenzetti A, Pieri A. The role of stressful life events in the onset of chronic primary headache. *Pain.* 1990;40:65–75.

254. Kiecolt-Glaser JK, Glaser R. Psychosocial moderators of immune function. *Ann Behav Med.* 1987;9:16–20.

255. Williams GH, Wood PHN. Common-sense beliefs about illness: a mediating role for the doctor. *Lancet.* 1986;328:1435–1437.

PART II

Therapeutic Modalities

CHAPTER 5

Botanical Medicine: Overview

ROBERTA LEE

A brief history of medicine
I have an earache.
2000 B.C. Here, eat this root.
1000 A.D. That root is heathen, say this prayer.
1850 A.D. That prayer is superstition, drink this potion.
1940 A.D. That potion is snake oil, swallow this pill.
1985 A.D. That pill is ineffective, take this antibiotic.
2000 A.D. That antibiotic is artificial. Here, eat this root.

ANONYMOUS

In this chapter, the general history of botanicals in medicine, types of preparations, and recommendations for evaluation and use are described. Specific botanicals are not discussed here, as information on specific botanicals is provided throughout the text where relevant. Table 5–1 is a list of recommended resources for the reader who is interested in a more comprehensive discussion of specific botanicals.

The use of plants by humans dates back many centuries. Archeologists have found prehistoric graves dating back to the Neolithic era, with evidence of botanical artifacts used for medicinal purposes.[1] Medical texts have documented the use of herbals in ancient cultures around the world beginning as early as 3000 B.C. One of the oldest Chinese texts (c. 2800 B.C.), the *Pen-tsao*, compiled information on the effects of 365 herbal medicines. Its author,

Shen Nung—also known as the Red Emperor—was said to have personally tested each of these herbs.[2] In Mesopotamia, around 2200 B.C., a Sumerian physician's collection of empiric prescriptions written on cuneiform tablets, recorded the use of plants, minerals, and animal substances to be given by mouth, in salves and in fomentations. These preparations were blown into orifices, inhaled as vapors, and inserted as suppositories or enemas.[3] Ayurveda—East Indian medicine, deriving its roots from the Vedic writings dating back to 1500 B.C.—had an extensive formulary as well, involving more than 500 medicinal plants.[1]

The ancient Egyptian pharmacopoeia contains one of the largest collections of medications used (as many as 400 plants); some of these substances were imported from elsewhere: "saffron and sage from Crete; cinnamon

Texts

Blumenthal M. *The ABC Clinical Guide to Herbs.* Austin, TX: American Botanical Council; 2003.

Blumenthal M, et al., eds. *The Complete German Commission E Monographs—Therapeutic Guide to Herbal Medicines.* Austin, TX: American Botanical Council; 1998.

Blumenthal M, Goldberg A, Brinckmann J, eds. *Herbal Medicine: Expanded Commission E Monographs.* Newton, MA: Integrative Medicine Communications; 2000.

Bratman S, Girman A. *Mosby's Handbook of Herbs and Supplement and Their Therapeutic Uses.* St. Louis, MO: Mosby; 2003.

Brinker F. *Herb Contraindications and Drug Interactions.* 3rd ed. Sandy, OR: Eclectic Medical Publications, 2001.

Duke JA. *The Green Pharmacy.* Emmaus, PA: Rodale/St. Martin's Press; 1997.

Fugh-Berman A. *The 5-Minute Herb and Dietary Supplement Consult.* Philadelphia: Lippincott Williams & Wilkins; 2003.

Hocking GM. *A Dictionary of Natural Products.* Medford, NJ: Plexus Publishing; 1997.

Huan KC. *The Pharmacology of Chinese Herbs.* 2nd ed. Boca Raton, FL: CRC Press; 1999.

Kapoor LD. *CRC Handbook of Ayurvedic Medicinal Plants.* Boca Raton, FL: CRC Press; 1990.

McCaleb RS, Leigh E, Morien K. The Encyclopedia of Popular Herbs. Roseville, CA: Prima Health; 2000.

McGuffin M, Hobbs C, Upton R, Goldberg A. eds. *American Herbal Product Associations Botanical Safety Handbook.* Boca Raton, FL: CRC Press; 1997.

Schultz V, Hansel R, Tyler V. *Rational Phytotherapy: A Physician's Guide to Herbal Medicine.* Berlin: Springer-Verlag; 1998.

Internet Resources

AGRICOLA. Agricultural Online Access is a bibliographic database of citations to the agricultural literature by the US National Agricultural Library. www.nal.usda.gov/ag98

AltMedDex. The US Pharmacopoeia herbal monographs. www.micromedex.com

Native American Ethnobotany. Foods, drugs, dyes and fibers of Native American peoples. http://herb.umd.umich.edu

FDA Poisonous Plant Database. Resource on plant names and citations accessible by alphabetical listing. http://vm.cfsan.fda.gov/~djw/readme.html

HerbMed. HerbMed hyperlinks to evidence on contraindications, toxic and adverse effects, and drug–herbal interactions. www.herbmed.org

MedWatch. The FDA safety information and adverse events reporting program. www.fda.gov/medwatch

NAPRALERT. Natural Products ALERT. Large database of worldwide literature on ethnomedical information, chemistry, and pharmacology of plants, and more. www.ag.uiuc.edu/~ffh/napra.html

National Institutes of Health, Office of Dietary Supplements database. www.nal.usda.gov/fnic/IBIDS

Natural Medicines Comprehensive Database. A proprietary database with reliable information. www.naturaldatabase.com

Phytonet. European Scientific Cooperative on Phytotherapy (ESCOP) contains adverse effects data. www.escop.com

US Department of Agriculture Agricultural Research Service (ARS) phytochemical and ethnobotanical databases. Dr Duke's Phytochemical and Ethnobotanical Databases. www.ars-grin.gov/duke

Organizations

American Botanical Council, 6200 Manor Rd., Austin, TX 78723 (www.Herbalgram.org).

American Herbalists Guild, 1931 Gaddis Rd., Canton, GA 30115 (www.americanherbalist.com).

Herb Research Foundation, 1007 Pearl St., Suite 200, Boulder, CO 80302 (www.herbs.org).

from China; perfumes and spices from Arabia; and sandalwood, gums, and antimony from Abyssinia."[5] It is said that many of these medications and plants found their way into the herbals of Dioscorides, Galen, and Pliny, as well as into Arabic and Persian formularies. Additionally, in the Egyptian formulary, as early as the second millennium B.C., products from the opium poppy *(Papaver somniferum)* were used, along with substances such as hyocyamine and scopolamine derived from the mandrake plant *(Mandragora officinarum L).*[6] These tablets also record some of the unfortunate earliest accounts of clinical trials, in which slaves were used to test the efficacy and the nonlethal doses of poisonous plants before they were used to treat royalty.[7] In this way, "very poisonous plants like the Deadly Nightshade"[8] could be used to understand how they counteracted bladder spasms, persistent coughs, and other troubling clinical problems.

Galen (130–200 A.D.) practiced and taught pharmacy and medicine in Rome. He is remembered for his complex compounding medicines and is credited for developing many methods for mixing, extracting, and refining botanical medicines. In fact, his techniques reflect the roots of many of the compounding formulas used today.[9] Dioscorides (first century A.D.) is credited by many (including Galen) with having elevated the use of botanicals from the status of a trade to that of a science. He traveled with the Roman armies throughout the world, recording what he observed and writing about how to collect, store, and use botanicals. Dioscorides' texts were considered as written resources in basic sciences up to the sixteenth century.[10]

In the Middle Ages, with the fall of the Roman empire, remnants of this knowledge were preserved in cloisters in England, Ireland, France, Switzerland, and Germany. Marcus Aurelius Cassiodorus (490–585 A.D.), a Benedictine monk and chancellor to Theodoric the Great (c. 454–526 A.D.), is credited with the first efforts to systematize this knowledge. He ordered the texts of Hippocrates, Galen, Dioscorides, and others, to be recorded and translated. His efforts to preserve these works prevented them from being completely lost during the Dark Ages. Interestingly, during that time, the monasteries became the institutions primarily associated with medical care. The medical texts translated from Latin were preserved, but the knowledge of well-developed medical procedures reflected in the works of these great physicians was lost. Pharmacology in its experimental aspects was abandoned, and the medicine practiced by the monastic orders "regressed to a simple herbalism characteristic of many types of folk medicine."[11] However, in every monastery across Europe, a library, an infirmary, and scribes for translation of these texts were considered indispensable. Meanwhile, Arabic medicine under development during the first five centuries of the Christian era became a "fountainhead of Greco-Roman knowledge."[12] Abu Ali al-Husain ibn Abdallah ibn Sina, also known as Avicenna (c. 980–1037 A.D.), the Persian equivalent of Galen, wrote the *Canon Medicinae*. This text had extensive pharmaceutical sections that were accepted as the definitive scientific resource in the West up to the seventeenth century.[13]

The seventeenth century is considered the grand era of English herbalists, in which Nicolas Culpeper, John Gerard, and John Parkinson wrote on the use of herbal medicine in healing. However, somewhere around 1650, a rift emerged between herbalists and physicians who favored drugs. An increasing number of physicians began to favor isolates of plant constituents that could be made into drugs rather than the plant itself.[14] Furthermore, practices of herbalists not licensed as physicians began to be held in contempt by the existing English medical community. In fact, the English medical community "did their utmost to prevent the sacred secrets of medicine from leaking out even to apothecaries: every professional medical work, like the *London Pharmacopoeia* itself, was printed in Latin,"[15] a language that few could read except the educated elite.

Nicolas Culpeper (1616–1654), found this attitude contemptuous. He was lucky enough to be educated at Cambridge University, as he was the son of a Surrey rector. Able to read and write Latin, he eventually translated the *London Pharmacopoeia* into English as the *Physicall Directory*. Included in this translation were many editorials expressing his disdain for the medical community's arrogance and poor treatment of indigents. He suffered much criticism for his scathing comments in the translated work but went on to publish *The English Physician,* which was an enormous success in England. It still endures as an archival text, and is considered representative of the strong English tradition of domestic herbal medicine of that time.

However, breakthroughs in chemistry—first beginning with the isolation of morphine by Serturner, a young German apothecary in 1816, followed by the isolation of quinine from species of the *Cinchona*—continued to highlight the value of single plant constituents isolated as drugs as potentially more effective medicines than the whole plants from which they were derived. Later, the discovery of bacteria as a cause of many diseases and the discovery of many antibiotics to conquer these ailments provided the continued impetus to value the precision and effectiveness of pharmaceutical agents over herbals.

In the 1800s, the Thomasonian and Eclectic movements attempted to preserve the use of herbal medicine as heroic practices (bloodletting, use of mercury, etc.) increased in popularity in the United States. Subsequently, the Flexner report of 1910 dramatically changed the direction of medical training; with it came further interest in pharmaceutical preparations and a loss of interest in herbalism. Still, despite the advances of modern medicine, Western herbalism has been preserved through the continued practices of a variety of "alternative" specialties such as naturopathic medicine and anthroposophical medicine.

In England, herbalists are recognized as clinical professionals with a code of ethics and disciplinary procedures for practices that are beyond the recognized scope of practice. They are covered by full professional insurance. The body of practicing herbalists in the United States is represented by the American Herbalist Guild. Within this body, licensure and credentialing remain ongoing topics of discussion. In Germany and other countries, there are strict regulations on botanical substances with detailed monographs on all aspects of botanical use. Special commissions exist that review the evidence for efficacy and safety of botanicals in these European countries. One example is the German Commission E, which evaluates all botanical products on the German formulary. Other traditional medical systems, such as the practices in Native American medicine, Chinese medicine, and Ayurveda, have unique formularies that remain in active use. Through this variety of systems, botanical medicine remains a dynamic approach of great interest to many patients.

At present, it is estimated that more than 40% of prescription drugs sold in the United States contain at least one ingredient derived from a natural source.[16] Up to 25% of prescription drugs contain an ingredient derived from a flowering plant; common examples include the use of the periwinkle *(Catharanthus roseus)* for chemotherapy and foxglove *(Digitalis purpurea)* for production of cardiac glycosides. Table 5–2 provides additional examples.

Until about the 1930s, herbs and herbal products constituted a sizable proportion of the materia medica of North America.[17] Herbs and their associated monographs were at their peak in 1870, comprising 670 substances, but by 1926, the total number fell to 203.[18] Interest in botanical preparations continued to fall—mostly as a consequence of their less-dramatic pharmacologic actions.

In 1888, the American Pharmaceutical Association published the National Formulary (NF). This was a formulary comprised mostly of botanical-based medicines. In 1975, the publication of the NF was shifted to the United States Pharmacopoeia (USP). In 1980, the USP-NF was created. After the Dietary Supplement and Health

▶ **TABLE 5-2** PLANT SOURCES OF COMMONLY ENCOUNTERED DRUGS

Drug	Common Name	Latin Name
Colchicine	Autumn crocus	*Colchicum autumnale*
Digoxin	Foxglove	*Digitalis* spp.
Tubocurarine	Curare	*Chondrodendron tomentosum*
Physostigmine	Calabar bean	*Physostigma venenosum*
Scopolamine	Jimsonweed	*Datura stramonium*
Taxol	Pacific yew	*Taxus brevifolia*

Source: Compiled from information presented in Fransworth NR, Akerle O, Bingel AS, Soejarto DD, Guo ZG. Medicinal plants in plant therapy. Bull WHO; *1985: 965–981.*

and Education Act (DSHEA) of 1994 was passed, the USP began creating monographs that established identity and purity standards for selected botanicals; to date, the USP has published 86 standard monographs.

The prevalence of botanical medicine use was thought to be insignificant until David Eisenberg's first study in 1990 revealed that botanical medicine was the sixth most commonly used alternative therapy.[19] By 1997, botanical medicine use became the second most commonly used alternative therapy.[20] This represented a baseline use of 2.5% in the adult population, as measured in 1990, that grew to 12% in the subsequent study. Reflecting this trend, botanical retail sales in the United States reached their highest point in 1998, totaling $688,352,192,[21] and gradually declining to $377,207,360 by 2001.[22]

▶ ARE BOTANICAL MEDICINES CONSIDERED DRUGS?

In the United States, until 1994, from a legal standpoint, the status of botanical products was unclear. That year, the Dietary Supplement Health Education Act (DSHEA) legally recognized botanical products as "dietary supplements" rather than as drugs. The DSHEA describes botanical products as follows:

. . . containing combinations of many numerous naturally occurring plant chemicals; herbals generally act in a wider more general, less specific way than most single ingredient pharmaceutical drugs. Their actions are more gentle than conventional medicine and work usually in more long-term situations.[23]

On the basis of this view, the DSHEA requires restrictions on product labeling: botanical labels could claim only general physiologic or therapeutic effects rather than efficacy for a specific disease or medical condition. The DSHEA asserted that "unlike many drugs, the role of herbal dietary supplements is to enhance the diet by adding safe and natural plants and their constituents to support and protect bodily functions and processes." The categorization of botanical products as supplements has created great confusion for some people as to whether botanical substances behave as drugs. Because they are not classified as drugs, the public does not view them with the same level of caution. Consequently, most patients—as many as 70%—fail to mention to their doctors that they are taking these products.[21]

The DSHEA places the responsibility for ensuring supplement safety on the manufacturers. It dictates how literature may be used in connection with sales, specifies labeling requirements, and provides for the establishment of good manufacturing practices, stating that "companies marketing products outside of the [United States] with products licensed as Traditional Herbal Medicines in Canada or as Therapeutic Goods in Australia must meet the [good manufacturing practice] requirements of those countries respectively."[25] However, proposed rules for dietary supplement good manufacturing practices are not yet published; these are expected in the near future.[26] One reason for passing the DSHEA was to ensure consumers access to natural products and truthful information regarding those products. However, under the DSHEA—because they are dietary supplements rather than medicines—these products are not subjected to the same rigorous testing required for drugs by the FDA. Although most practitioners applaud the access to herbals that the DSHEA ensured, many feel that the decision to exempt this class of medicines from a more rigorous level of FDA scrutiny was not in the best long-term interests of the public health.

However, despite the assertions of the DSHEA, it is well recognized that many plants have powerful pharmacologic actions. A controversial aspect of the DSHEA is the issue of safety in protecting the public from unsafe dietary supplements. Once a supplement is on the market, the FDA must prove that it is unsafe before imposing restrictions on its use: "the burden of proof has now shifted from the manufacturer proving safety to the FDA proving that a substance poses an imminent health hazard."[27] There has been considerable debate over whether the FDA has adequate authority to remove unsafe supplements and protect the American public from dangerous or otherwise unsafe herbs.

As increased use and awareness of use by professionals grow, so do reports of interactions and adverse effects in the news and in medical journals. This process has eroded consumer and professional confidence in herbal preparations.[28] Some professionals assert that the standards for safety held for botanicals are higher than those for pharmaceuticals; others argue, based on increasing reports of drug interactions, that the standards are too lax. A recent systematic review of herb–drug interactions concluded that of the 108 interactions evaluated, 74 cases (68.5%) could not be evaluated because of a lack of adequate information, whereas 14 (13%) were "well documented." The authors of this review emphasized the need for better documentation of all relevant data for future case studies of potential interactions.[29]

Chapter 6 contains a full discussion on adverse effects in botanical medicines and on adverse effect reporting.

Regulatory assessment and evaluation of botanicals remain a problem in the United States, as there is no official system that evaluates and tracks the benefits and hazards of herbal preparations. Consequently, reports in the news of adverse reactions to herbal products—in the absence of formal risk–benefit assessment—creates the "opportunity for disproportionate exaggerations" relative to their health implications.[30] This is in distinct contrast to over-the-counter (OTC) and prescription drugs in which some formal risk–benefit assessment has been made.

Some legislators and industry leaders are looking for guidance in this area to countries with established herbal medicine regulatory bodies such as the German Commission E. There, botanical preparations are regulated as conventional drugs and have established criteria for safety and quality similar to those required for all drugs. However, in Germany, botanicals are approved by a standard of "reasonable certainty" versus the stricter standard applied to pharmaceutical drugs. The Commission E is a federally mandated panel of 24 experts from various disciplines associated with medicinal plants including physicians and pharmacists.[31] From 1978 to 1995, 300 herbal preparations or fixed herbal combinations were reviewed; 380 monographs were finally published—254 for botanicals considered positive and 120 for botanicals considered neutral or negative.[32] It remains to be seen whether this system, or one like it, will be used in the United States. Meanwhile, as medical professionals continue to evaluate the use of herbals in the absence of this type of assistance, rational scientific evaluation remains difficult, confusing, and time-consuming.

▶ HERBS AND DRUGS: IMPORTANT DISTINCTIONS

Herbs are different from the substances we recognize as pharmacologic drugs. The active constituents in herbs are present in much lower concentrations than those in their pharmacologic counterparts. This is not the only difference, however; botanical medicines may also contain "secondary" active constituents that may be closely related chemically to the constituent regarded as the primary active ingredient. One example of this is the digitalis leaf *(Digitalis purpurea)*. Various species of this herb may contain as many as 30 closely related glycosides, all with cardiotonic properties at different concentrations and with different half-lives and peak and trough activity levels.[33] Proponents of whole-plant products have made assertions that the complexity of plant compounds and their concentrations create a potential for physiologic synergy that may enhance therapeutic effects. In some cases, because a single plant can contain hundreds of biologically active compounds, there may be more than one physiologic effect. Others, more comfortable with identifying and isolating active constituents, are convinced that standardizing herbal preparations is the best way to ensure their therapeutic activity.

Standardization is a process by which one or more marker compounds are identified as the active ingredients responsible for activity in the herb. A manufacturer will measure these constituents and guarantee that a certain amount of these constituent(s) are present in each product. In some cases, this may involve fortifying the product with the marker compound(s). Advocates of the use of whole-plant products believe that standardization is unnecessary because nature has already formulated the correct proportions for medicinal use. Furthermore, these advocates argue that standardization cannot not address all of the potential factors influencing the quality of a product. The exact timing of harvesting, including tasting and smelling of the plant parts (techniques

previously used by herbalists) has been abandoned as plant cultivation has become more mechanized. Whole plant advocates argue that abandoning these harvesting practices produces the risk of a mediocre botanical crop. In some cases, the identified so-called active ingredients were later found to be less active than previously thought, as in the case of St. John's wort *(Hypericum perforatum)*. Initially, hypericin was identified as the active ingredient; later, hyperforin was found to be equally, if not more, physiologically influential.[34] In weighing both sides of the argument between advocates of standardized products and advocates of whole-plant preparations, it seems clear that the data providing a definitive answer to this issue are still lacking. As a compromise, many companies have chosen to include whole-plant parts in a standardized product. In the cases of certain botanicals, the exact active ingredients have not been identified and thus the products remain without standardization to a specific constituent. Saw palmetto *(Seranoa repens)* is an example of this; although the actives are known to reside in the lipophilic fraction, the specific constituents primarily responsible for the therapeutic action have not been identified, and so the products are generally standardized to simply contain 80–90% fatty sterols.[35]

▶ BOTANICALS: PERSPECTIVES IN TRADITIONAL MEDICINE AND ALLOPATHIC MEDICINE

There are different perspectives on the use of herbs in allopathic medicine, Western herbalism, and traditional medical systems. The allopathic physician, trained to value pharmaceuticals for specific indications, has the tendency to gravitate toward the use of singular botanical preparations. It can be easy to use botanical preparations as a pharmaceutical substitute to "fix" a clinical problem. On the one hand, the single herbal used as a botanical "silver bullet" for treatment of a specific disease may be desirable, as it is more natural and less likely to cause side effects than some pharmaceuticals. But this approach is not necessarily "integrative." An integrative physician will use botanicals as part of treatment of the whole person, with the perspective of removing the causes of disease and promoting health.

A traditional herbalist will typically combine many herbs in one formula, incorporating their use as an individualized treatment with a whole-person approach in mind. Traditional healing systems, such as Chinese medicine, East Asian medicine, Ayurveda, Unani, and Native American medicines, may use "herbs to support the systems of the body and to protect and enhance their function."[36] More often than not, these traditional healing systems also use preparations containing combinations of many plants. The idea is that many plants blended together in lower concentrations may be more effective and potentially less toxic than either a pharmaceutical or a single botanical used in an extremely concentrated formulation. The current movement in herbal medicine toward extraction and standardization may be helpful—even crucial for the physician—but it is important to recognize that this perspective is distinctly different from a holistic traditional view of herbal healing practices.

▶ IDENTIFICATION OF QUALITY PRODUCTS

There are a number of simple strategies for identifying quality botanical products, including reading about the companies that manufacture the products and specifically about their quality control procedures; knowing the botanical names (Latin name or Latin binomial) and checking whether these plants are identified as being used in the product; and knowing which plant parts in particular are believed to create the desired effect(s). For example, a consumer with this knowledge of active plant parts can look on the label to see if the correct plant parts are pro-

vided. If incorrect plant parts are used, potency and efficacy may be jeopardized. In addition, buying organic herbs, if possible, to minimize pesticide exposure seems prudent. Because of the more rigorous standards by which German botanical products are produced, it has been suggested that seeking brands that are derived from these companies may increase assurance of a quality product. Table 5–1 lists other organizations that can help in product assessment.

Knowing the Latin names can be extremely helpful. Common names can lead the unaware consumer to the wrong plant. Ginseng is a case in point—various species are all commonly known as ginseng, including Chinese or Korean ginseng *(Panax ginseng)*, American ginseng *(Panax quinquefolius)*, and Siberian ginseng *(Eleutherococcus senticosus)*. All differ in their pharmacologic actions; the latter is in a completely different plant family (Araliacea) from the other ginsengs.

▶ INTERPRETING A PRODUCT LABEL

Interpreting a product label can be challenging. Figure 5–1 includes key points to be noted by professionals and consumers.

▶ HERBAL PREPARATIONS

There are many forms of herbal preparations. Depending on the indication and the specific herb, botanicals can be prepared as tinctures, liquid or solid extracts, capsules, tablets, lozenges, teas, concoctions, poultices, compresses, vapor treatments, salves, creams, and oils.

Tinctures

An herb extracted in alcohol or another solvent is a tincture or liquid extract. The alcohol concentrates the active constituents of the plant and preserves the contents. A tincture is typi-

① Brand name

② Product/herb name

③ Herbal products and other "dietary supplements" may make "statements of nutritional support," often referred to as "structure/function claims," as long as they are truthful and not misleading, a documentable by scientific data, and do not claim to diagnose, cure, treat, or prevent any disease, and carry a disclaimer on the product label to this effect. The disclaimer must also note that FDA has not evaluated the claim.

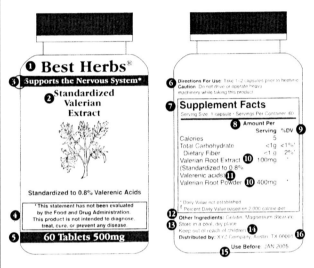

④ A structure/function claim requires this disclaimer when it appears on the label of a dietary supplement.

⑤ Number of tablets, capsules, and net weight of each in package.

⑥ Directions for Use and Cautions.

Items 7–11 are part of the "Supplement Facts" panel.

⑦ "Serving Size" is the suggested number of tablets, capsules, softgels, tea bags, liquid extract, or tincture to take at one time.

⑧ "Amount per Serving" first indicates the nutrients present in the herb and then specifies the quantity. The following items must be declared if in excess of what can legally be declared as zero: calories, fat, carbohydrates, sodium, and protein. In addition, the following nutrients must also be declared if present in quantities exceeding what can legally be declared as zero: vitamins A, C, D, E, K, B-1, B-2, B-3, B-6, B-12, folic acid, biotin, calcium, iron, phos-

phorus, iodine, magnesium, zinc, selenium, copper, manganese, chromium, molybdenum, chloride, and potassium.

⑨ "Percent Daily Value" (%DV) indicates the percentage of daily intake provided by the herb. An asterisk under the "Percent Daily Value" heading indicates that a Daily Value is not established for that dietary ingredient.

⑩ Herbs should be designated by their standardized common names as listed in the book *Herbs of Commerce*, published in 1992 by the American Herbal Products Association. If the common name is not listed in *Herbs of Commerce*, then the common name must be followed by the herb's Latin name. The plant part must be listed for each herb. The amount in milligrams of each herb must be listed unless the herbs are grouped as a proprietary blend—then only the total amount of the blend need be listed. For herbal extracts, the following information must be disclosed: 1. the ratio of the weight of the starting material to the volume of the solvent (even for dried extracts where the solvent has been removed, the solvent used to extract the herb must be listed); 2. whether the starting material is fresh or dry; and 3. the concentration of the botanical in the solvent.

⑪ Standardization. If a product is chemically standardized, the product label may list the component used to measure standardization (e.g., ginsenosides in Asian ginseng, etc.) and the level to which the product is standardized (e.g. 4% ginsenosides). Therefore, if a product contained 100 mg of Asian ginseng extract per capsule and the extract was standardized to 4% ginsenosides, one capsule would contain 4 mg of ginsenosides.

⑫ A list of all other ingredients, in decreasing order by weight, must appear outside the Supplement Facts box. In herb formulas containing multiple herbal ingredients, the herbs must be listed in descending order of predominance.

⑬ The proper location for storage of herbal products is typically labeled as a cool, dry place.

⑭ All herbal products and other dietary supplements should be kept out of the reach of children.

⑮ The herb should be used before the expiration date for maximum potency and effectiveness. Expiration dates are often arbitrarily established by the manufacturer, regardless of the ingredients and their relative stability. Such dates are routinely set at two years from the date of manufacture.

⑯ The product must list the manufacturer or distributor's name, city, state, and zip code.

Figure 5–1. Interpreting Product Labels. *(From Blumenthal,[17] with permission.)*

cally made at a 1:5 (or 1:10) concentration. This means that one part herb (in grams) is soaked in five (or ten) parts of the solvent (in milliliters). This means that in the final product there is five (or ten) times the amount of solvent (alcohol) as there is plant material.

Liquid Extracts

Liquid extracts are more concentrated than tinctures. Typical fluid extract ratios are 1:1.

Solid Extracts

Solid extracts are typically a 4:1 concentration. This means that one part of the extract is equivalent to four parts of crude herb. One gram of a 4:1 solid extract is equivalent to 4 mL of a 1:1 fluid extract. Some solid extracts can be much more concentrated (100:1). This means that 1 g of a 100:1 extract is equal to 100 g of crude herb or 100 mL of fluid extract (1:1) or 1 L of a tincture (1:10).

Solid extracts are derived from liquid extracts and have the alcohol or water removed. These preparations usually have large amounts of filler (soy or millet powder). Fillers add bulk and stabilize the active constituents. Tablets may contain binders such as magnesium stearate or dicalcium phosphate. Binders can help to increase absorption of water or facilitate breakdown in the intestinal system. A disadvantage of both capsules and tablets is the difficulty in assessing the herbal content, as the fillers tend to mask odor and color.

Teas

Teas can be used for many things and come in the form of decoctions and infusions. A decoction is made by boiling the herb for 10–15 minutes. This is the preferred method for roots, barks, and berries. An infusion is made by adding plant material to hot water and steeping for 3–5 minutes. Brewing a cup of tea is an example of an infusion.

Poultices and Compresses

Poultices are crushed herbs that are made into a paste. The mixture is applied directly to the skin, using cloth or gauze to keep the mixture on the skin. A compress is made for direct application to the skin and usually involves soaking a cloth in a strong tea, tincture, or oil.

Essential Oils

Essential oils contain concentrated essences of plants. Many are potentially toxic and readily absorbed into the skin. Before applying to the skin they should be diluted in carrier oils.

▶ TECHNIQUES USED IN THE PRODUCTION OF HERBALS

An enormous range in sophistication is present in the preparation of plants to become standardized products. Here is a synopsis of commonly encountered stages:

Collection/Harvesting

Plants collected "in the wild" are said to be "wildcrafted." Some practitioners believe these plants are superior because they are taken from their natural environment. Most commercial products are cultivated and come from all over the world.

Drying

After harvesting, plants contain a moisture content up to 80% and cannot be stored without drying; storing them without drying encourages molding or decomposing. Most plants are dried within a temperature range of 100–140°F. After drying, the usual moisture content is approximately 14%.[37]

Garbling

This is the process of mincing an herb. Different particle sizes can be made depending on the machinery employed.

Extraction

Extraction is the process of using physical or chemical means to remove the desired product. It can involve the use of alcohol, hypercritical carbon dioxide, or lipophilic solvents. This process can be quite elaborate and expensive. High or low temperatures can be employed, as well as low or high pressures.

Concentration

This is the process of condensing. In the process of making a solid extract, solvent vapors are condensed and returned to a liquid for reuse.[38]

▶ ANALYTICAL METHODS

There are many analytical methods used to determine product purity, quality, and identity. The main techniques are organoleptic analysis, microscopic analysis, chemical analysis, and biological analysis. Organoleptic inspection involves the use of the senses to inspect the plant material by smell, taste, or touch. Microscopic evaluation is self-explanatory and often will reveal crude contaminants such as mold and insects. Chemical analysis provides a wealth of information on a variety of aspects of the botanical including alkaloid content, percentage of active material present, and fat content. One of the more sophisticated analytical techniques involves thin layer chromatography, high-pressure liquid chromatography, or nuclear magnetic resonance. The latest technology to emerge is DNA fingerprinting; this is still being commercially developed.

▶ QUALITY CONTROL

Quality control remains one of the largest dilemmas for health professionals who seek to implement herbal medicines in their clinical practice. Within the United States, no organization or government body exists that cer-tifies that an herbal product is labeled correctly. Several reports issued in the last 10 years have revealed wide variances in the actual constituents contained in similarly labeled products. Increasing attention has been focused on this problem. Information from independent laboratory testing is available on a limited basis and is usually costly. ConsumerLabs.com is one of the older labs known to provide this service; it also provides information on the quality of a variety of commercial products for a nominal fee. Another independent testing site, sponsored by the US Pharmacopoeia, is still in development.

▶ CLINICAL TRIALS

Until recently, active support for research in this area was quite limited in the United States. With the continued interest by the public in botanical use, the National Center for Complementary and Alternative Medicine (NCCAM) has begun appropriating more funds to study the efficacy of selected botanical supplements, but the majority of the studies continue to be produced in Europe, where there is acceptance of herbal use and more active support for herbal research. The inability to patent an herbal limits the incentive to fund expensive, large, random, controlled trials. Furthermore, the question of appropriate protocols for which to test ingredients that have more than one active constituent remains an issue of scientific debate. Table 5–3 lists the 10 most common herbal products used in clinical trials in Europe and elsewhere.

▶ **TABLE 5-3** TEN CLINICALLY RESEARCHED BOTANICALS AND THEIR US BRAND EQUIVALENTS

Herb	Foreign Trade Name/ Manufacturer	US Trade Name/ Importer	Use
Black cohosh (*Cimicifuga racemosa*)	Remifemin/ Lichtwer	Remifemin/ Glaxo Smith Kline	Menopause
Chamomile (*Matricaria recutita*)	Kamillosan/ Asta Medica	CamoCare/ Abkit	Dermatologic
Chaste tree (*Vitex agnus-castus*)	Agnolyt/ Madaus	Femaprin/ Nature's Way	Premenstrual syndrome
Echinacea (*Echinacea purpurea*)	Echinacin/ Madaus AG Echinaforce/ Bioforce AG	Echinaguard/ Nature's Way Echinaforce/ Bioforce	Flu and upper respiratory infections
Garlic (*Allium sativum*)	Kwai/ Lichtwer Pharma Kyolic/ Wakunaga	Kwai/ Abkit Kyolic/ Wakunaga	Circulatory Circulatory; chemopreventive
Ginkgo (*Ginkgo biloba*)	Tebonin/ Schwabe	Ginkgold/ Nature's Way Ginkoba/ Pharmaton Ginkai/ Abkit	Circulatory; cognitive
Ginseng (*Panax ginseng*)	Ginsana/ Pharmaton	Ginsana/ Pharmaton	Tonic
Saw palmetto (*Seranoa repens*)	Permixon/ Pierre Fabre Prostagutt/ Schwabe Prostaserene/ Indena	Not available in the US ProsActive/ Nature's Way available in several brands (e.g., Enzymatic Therapy/ Phytopharmika Solaray)	Benign prostatic hyperplasia
Milk thistle	Legalon/ Madaus	Thisylin/ Nature's Way	Hepatoprotectant
St. John's wort	Jarsin (LI 160) Lichtwer Pharma LI 160 WS Lichtwer-Schwabe Kira/ Lichtwer Pharma Neuroplant Schwabe Remotive Bayer	Kira/ Abkit Formerly Quanterra/ Warner Lambert Not imported; different from US brand Perika/Nature's Way Movana/Pharmaton St. John's wort (Ze117)/ GNC	Depression Emotional balance

Source: Compiled from Bratman S, Girman A. Mosby's Handbook of Herbs and Supplements and Their Therapeutic Uses. St. Louis, MO: Mosby; 2003, and Blumenthal M. Clinically researched brands of commercial herbal products: the issue of phytoequivalence and borrowed science. Presented at: Columbia University Course on Botanical Medicine in Modern Clinical Practice, May 2002.

REFERENCES

1. Litynska-Zajac M. Polish archaeobotanical studies in North Africa: Armant (Egypt). *Wiadomosci Botaniczne.* 1993;37(3–4):171–172.
2. Lyons A, Petrucelli RJ. *Medicine: An Illustrated History.* New York: Harry N. Abrams; 1978:121.
3. Lyons A, Petrucelli RJ. *Medicine: An Illustrated History.* New York: Harry N. Abrams; 1978:63.
4. Bellamy D, Pfister A. *World Medicine: Plants, Patients and People.* Oxford, UK: Blackwell Publishers; 1992:50.
5. Lyons A, Petrucelli RJ. *Medicine: An Illustrated History.* New York: Harry N. Abrams; 1978:97.
6. Moldenke H, Moldenke BA. *Plants of the Bible.* New York: Ronald Press; 1952:137–138.
7. Bellamy D, Pfister A. *World Medicine: Plants, Patients and People.* Oxford, UK: Blackwell Publishers; 1992:23.
8. Bellamy D, Pfister A. *World Medicine: Plants, Patients and People.* Oxford, UK: Blackwell Publishers; 1992:23.
9. Bender G. *Great Moments in Pharmacy: A History of Pharmacy in Pictures.* Detroit, MI: Parke, Davis & Co; 1966.
10. Bender G. *Great Moments in Pharmacy: A History of Pharmacy in Pictures.* Detroit, MI: Parke, Davis & Co; 1966.
11. Lyons A, Petrucelli RJ. *Medicine: An Illustrated History.* New York: Harry N. Abrams; 1978:283.
12. Lyons A, Petrucelli RJ. *Medicine: An Illustrated History.* New York: Harry N. Abrams; 1978:295.
13. Bender G. *Great Moments in Pharmacy: A History of Pharmacy in Pictures.* Detroit, MI: Parke, Davis & Co; 1966.
14. Damian P, Damian K. *Aromatherapy: Scent and Psyche.* Rochester, VT: Healing Arts Press; 1995:8.
15. Griggs B. *Green Pharmacy: The History and Evolution of Western Herbal Medicine.* Rochester, VT: Healing Arts Press; 1981:92–93.
16. Foster S, Duke J. *A Field Guide to Medicinal Plants: Eastern and Central North America.* Boston: Houghton Mifflin; 1990.
17. Blumenthal M. *The ABC Guide to Herbs.* Austin, TX: American Botanical Council; 2003.
18. Boyle W. *Official Herbs: Botanical Substances in the United States Pharmacopoeia 1820–1990.* East Palestine, OH: Buckey Naturopathic Press; 1991.
19. Eisenberg DM, Kessler RC, Foster C, et al. Unconventional medicine in the United States: prevalence, costs and patterns of use. *N Engl J Med.* 1993;328:246–252.
20. Eisenberg DM, Davis RB, Ettner SL, et al. Trends in alternative medicine use in the United States, 1990–1997. *JAMA.* 1997;280:1569–1575.
21. Blumenthal M. Herb market levels after five years of boom: 1999 sales in mainstream market up only 11% in first half of 1999 after 55% increase in 1998. *HerbalGram.* 1999;47:64–65.
22. Blumenthal M. Herb sales down in mainstream market, up in natural food supermarkets. *HerbalGram.* 2002;55:60.
23. United States Congress. Dietary Supplement Health and Education Act of 1994. Pub L. No. 103–117, 108 Stat. 4325–4333.
24. Eisenberg DM, Davis RB, Ettner SL, et al. Trends in alternative medicine use in the United States, 1990–1997. *JAMA.* 1997;280:1569–1575.
25. Blumenthal M. *The ABC Guide to Herbs.* Austin, TX: American Botanical Council; 2003:12.
26. Blumenthal M. *The ABC Guide to Herbs.* Austin, TX: American Botanical Council; 2003:13.
27. Blumenthal M. *The ABC Guide to Herbs.* Austin, TX: American Botanical Council; 2003:14.
28. Blumenthal M. *The ABC Guide to Herbs.* Austin, TX: American Botanical Council; 2003:15.
29. Fug-Berman A, Ernst E. Herb–drug interactions: review and assessment of report reliability. *Br J Clin Pharmacol.* 2001;52:587–595.
30. Blumenthal M. *The ABC Guide to Herbs.* Austin, TX: American Botanical Council; 2003:16.
31. Blumenthal M, Busse WR, Goldberg A, et al. *The Complete German Commission E Monographs: Therapeutic Guide to Herbal Medicines.* Austin, TX: American Botanical Council; 1998.
32. Blumenthal M, Busse WR, Goldberg A, et al. *The Complete German Commission E Monographs: Therapeutic Guide to Herbal Medicines.* Austin, TX: American Botanical Council; 1998.
33. Tyler V. *Herbs of Choice.* New York: Hayworth; 1994.
34. Bennet DA, Phun L, Polk JF, et al. Neuropharmacology of St. John's wort *(Hypericum). Ann Pharmacol Ther.* 1998;32:1201–1208.
35. Fugh-Berman A. *The Five-Minute Herb and

Dietary Supplement Consult. Philadelphia: Lippincott Williams & Wilkins; 2003.

36. Lee R. Botanical medicine. In: Kohatsu W, ed. *Complementary and Alternative Medicine Secrets.* Philadelphia: Hanley & Belfus; 2002.

37. Pizzorno J, Murray M. *Textbook of Natural Medicine.* Vol. 1. 2nd ed. Edinburgh, UK: Churchill–Livingstone; 1999:274.

38. Pizzorno J, Murray M. *Textbook of Natural Medicine.* Vol. 1. 2nd ed. Edinburgh, UK: Churchill-Livingstone; 1999:275.5

CHAPTER 6

Issues Concerning the Safety of Herbs and Phytomedicinal Preparations

MARK BLUMENTHAL

Like so many subjects being examined in this textbook, the issues surrounding the relative safety and potential risks of herbs and phytomedicinal preparations are significantly larger than can adequately be explained in one chapter. Entire books have been written on the subjects of herbal toxicology,[1] the adverse effects of herbs,[2–4] their contraindications and drug interactions,[5] and their general safety from a commercial product labeling perspective.[6] Safety concerns have been evaluated as well in numerous official monographs developed by recognized experts in herbal medicine such as the German Commission E[7] and the World Health Organization.[8,9]

As with conventional drugs, the risks and safety concerns related to herbs are relative. Conventional pharmacology and toxicology recognize that the safety of *any* substance is dependent on a number of variables, including, but not limited to, the dosage, the route of administration, the "biochemical individuality" of the patient, additive or antagonistic effects of other simultaneously administered substances (including drugs, foods, and herbs, and other dietary supplements), as well as the intended use of the therapeutic agent.

The issue of intended use (benefit) is a key factor in determining safety. For this reason, conventional drugs are subjected to formal risk–benefit assessments to determine to what extent the potential or actual risk can be tolerated in view of the perceived benefit. In the United States, however, herbs and related phytomedicinal preparation are marketed as "dietary supplements" and are thus technically considered foods. Thus, no formal preapproval process is usually required for these products to enter the market, nor is there any formal process for the assessment of their potential benefits. The lack of officially recognized benefits for herbs creates a situation in which health care professionals and the general public are often exposed to reports of adverse effects or herb–drug interactions in such a way as to exaggerate the actual risk associated with use of the herb.

When Congress passed the Dietary Supplement Health and Education Act of 1994 (DSHEA),[10] it recognized that consumers need additional guidance and information on how to use these products responsibly. Thus, Section 10 of the DSHEA allows for virtually unlimited disclosure of potential risk on the labels of herb and other dietary supplement products, including contraindications, pregnancy and lactation warnings, adverse effects, and herb–drug interactions, without such warnings constituting drug labeling, as had previously been the case. The DSHEA contains definitions of safety standards as shown in Table 6–1. From a regulatory perspective, DSHEA shifted the burden of proof of safety to the FDA, giving it additional authority to remove an unsafe dietary supplement from the market that was deemed by the Secretary of Health and Human Services as an imminent hazard to the public health, but only if the agency was able to prove this in an administrative hearing. This provision has been mischaracterized as weakening the FDA's ability to protect the public, but legal experts have noted that FDA does have adequate authority to protect the public from unsafe herbs and other dietary supplements.[11]

Although no formal mechanism has yet been established by the FDA to assess the safety of herbs and other dietary supplements, the FDA has contracted with the Institute of Medicine (IOM) at the National Institutes of Health (NIH) to develop a framework for such an evaluation. In 2002, the IOM published a proposed framework for review and public comment[12] and subsequently published two draft monographs according to its extensive process: chaparral leaf *(Larrea divaricata)* and saw palmetto berry *(Serenoa repens)*. The extent to which the IOM safety framework may be adopted by the FDA to evaluate herbs has not been determined at the time of this writing. Furthermore, there is increased discussion in the United States regarding the establishment of mechanisms for the reporting of serious adverse events associated with herbs and other dietary supplements. In Western Europe,

▶ **TABLE 6–1** LEGAL STANDARDS FOR SAFETY OF DIETARY SUPPLEMENTS AS ESTABLISHED BY THE DSHEA

Section 4: Safety of Dietary Supplements and Burden of Proof of Safety on FDA
DSHEA amends existing sections of the Food and Drug Act [§402 (21 U.S.C. 342)] by adding the following language:

(1)(A) If it is a dietary supplement or contains a dietary ingredient that—presents a significant or unreasonable risk of illness or injury under—(i) conditions of use recommended or suggested in labeling, or (ii) if no conditions of use are suggested or recommended in the labeling, under ordinary conditions of use;

(B) is a new dietary ingredient for which there is inadequate information to provide reasonable assurance that such ingredient does not present a significant or unreasonable risk of illness or injury;

(C) the Secretary declares to pose an imminent hazard to public health or safety, except that the authority to make such declaration shall not be delegated and the Secretary shall promptly after such a declaration initiate a proceeding in accordance with sections 554 and 556 of title 5, United States Code to affirm or withdraw the declaration; or

(D) is or contains a dietary ingredient that renders it adulterated under paragraph [402](a)(1) under the conditions of use recommended or suggested in the labeling of such dietary supplement.

In any proceeding under this paragraph, the United States shall bear the burden of proof on each element to show that a dietary supplement is adulterated. The court shall decide any issue under this paragraph on a de novo basis.

(2) Before the Secretary may report to a United States attorney a violation of the paragraph (1)A for a civil proceeding, the person against whom such proceeding would be initiated shall be given appropriate notice and the opportunity to present views, orally and in writing, at least 10 days before such notice, with regard to such proceeding.

Source: From the Federal Food, Drug, and Cosmetic Act, P.L. 75-717 §402, as amended 21 U.S.C. §342(f), 2001.

adverse events for herbs and phytomedicines are routinely reported within the existing framework for conventional drugs. The evidence gleaned from this system of pharmacovigilance demonstrates that the rate of adverse events related to herbs and phytomedicines is significantly lower (per capita usage) than those for conventional medications, suggesting that the herbals are generally milder acting and safer than conventional drugs.

► SELF-REGULATORY SAFETY LABELING INITIATIVES

Industry Initiative: AHPA Botanical Safety Handbook Rating System

With no formal guidelines yet in place from the FDA for the labeling of commercial herbal products with respect to their potential risks, much of the responsibility for consumer guidance in this area has fallen on either the herb industry or nonprofit educational organizations. The most ambitious attempt from the herb industry to standardize the labeling of commercial herb products with respect to safety issues was created by the American Herbal Products Association (AHPA), the leading trade association for the herb and botanicals industry, which

published the *Botanical Safety Handbook*, a listing of more than 600 herbs and botanical products sold in the US market with a rating of the relative safety of each herb.[13] This compilation of safety data is based on 29 authoritative general references plus additional references (e.g., clinical studies, toxicological and pharmacological studies, and case reports) for each botanical. The *Botanical Safety Handbook* encourages the standardization of the declaration of safety and potential risks associated with use of herbal products by creating four classes of herbs with respect to their relative safety/potential toxicity (Table 6–2).

The *Botanical Safety Handbook*[11] has various limitations, as acknowledged by the authors; the book does not include potential risks that may arise from any of the following conditions:

- Excessive consumption of an herbal preparation; the safety data relates to consumption of herbs at relatively normal levels.
- Safety or toxicity concerns based on isolated constituents; individual phytochemical constituents of an herb (e.g., plant-derived pharmaceutical drugs) are not considered herbs or phytomedicinals and thus they were not included.
- Toxicity data based solely upon intravenous or intraperitoneal administration; only oral

---

► **TABLE 6–2** SAFETY CLASSIFICATIONS FOR HERBAL PRODUCTS BY THE HERB INDUSTRY

Class 1: Herbs which, when used appropriately, can be consumed safely without specific use restrictions.
Class 2: Herbs for which the following use restrictions apply:
   (2a) For external use only;
   (2b) Not to be used during pregnancy. No other use restrictions apply, unless noted;
   (2c) Not to be used while nursing. No other use restrictions apply, unless noted;
   (2d) Other specific use restrictions, as noted.
Class 3: Herbs for which significant data exists to recommend the following labeling:
   "To be used only under the supervision of an expert qualified in the appropriate use of this substance." Labeling must include proper use information: dosage, contraindications, potential adverse effects and drug interactions, and any other relevant information related to the safe use of this substance.
Class 4: Herbs for which insufficient data are available for classification.

Source: Reproduced with permission of the American Herbal Products Association from McGuffin et al.[6]

consumption and/or topical application was considered as neither IV nor intraperitoneal administration is consistent with self-selected herbal dietary supplements in the United States nor with the limited use of herbs by health care practitioners in the United States.

- Traditional Chinese medicine and Ayurvedic contraindications. (The authors limited their scope not to include these areas because they are often based on traditional, energetically based systems that do not correspond directly to the Western pharmacological classifications.)
- Gastrointestinal disturbances; these are so common with use of many pharmacologically active agents that it seemed unreasonable to include them here, unless there is a real possibility that serious gastrointestinal disturbances are predictable.
- Potential drug interactions; only those drug interactions that are relatively well documented or are published in official compendia are included (e.g., those documented by Commission E, despite the fact that some of those in Commission E monographs are speculative and are not well documented).
- Idiosyncratic reactions; obviously, there is no way to predict this type of problem.
- Allergic reactions; unless a pattern of allergic reactions is well documented, there is always a possibility that sensitive individuals may react to any herb, conventional food, or conventional pharmaceutical drug.
- Contact dermatitis; limited for same reasons as allergic reactions above.
- Well-known toxic plants that are not found in trade (e.g., *Aconitum napellus, Colchicum autumnale, Conium maculatum, Datura* spp., *Hyoscyamus niger,* and *Strychnos nux-vomica*).
- Essential oils.
- Herbal products to which chemically defined active substances, including chemically defined isolated constituents of an herb, have been added.

- Environmental factors, additives, or contaminants.

Independent Safety Initiative: The American Botanical Council's Safety Labeling Program

To help consumers use herbal products in a responsible manner, the American Botanical Council (ABC), the leading independent non-profit educational organization on herbal medicine, initiated a program, in 2002, that provides significant consumer guidance in this area. The Safety Labeling Program is designed to convey a rational interpretation of the scientific and medical literature on specific herbs directly on the labels of commercial herb products. The program is designed to benefit both consumers and health care professionals, who can use such information to help assess the potential risk and appropriateness of many popular herbs.

The Safety Labeling Program is based on an extensive literature review and evaluation of the scientific and clinical literature on a particular herb. The ABC develops Safety Information Sheets from the data, and then licenses to qualifying manufacturers the use of this safety information. The Safety Information Sheets can then be adapted by the manufacturer into the text of the product label, including accordion-style labels, peel-out labels, package inserts, and/or on the panel of a box.

The peer-reviewed Safety Information Sheets present a rational interpretation of the literature on the safety aspects of a particular herb, and provide accurate, current information on contraindications, adverse effects, potential interactions with prescription and over-the-counter (OTC) drugs, as well as pregnancy and lactation warnings and other guidelines.

The primary source of information for the initial set of Safety Information Sheets is *The ABC Clinical Guide to Herbs,*[15] a reference book that includes comprehensive monographs, abbreviated clinical overviews, patient information sheets, and extensive references for 29 of the most commonly used herbs and 13 proprietary products and herb combinations. In addition, ABC has accessed and reviewed safety information that may not be included in *The Guide* to help ensure that the Safety Information Sheets accurately reflect a comprehensive view of each herb's safety considerations. This includes, but is not limited to, various authoritative sources, including official and nonofficial monographs, *The Complete German Commission E Monographs,*[7] the WHO *Monographs on Selected Medicinal Plants,*[8,9] the ESCOP *Monographs on the Medicinal Uses of Plants,*[16] and the AHPA's *Botanical Safety Handbook,*[17] plus primary references (clinical trials, case reports, pharmacological studies, meta-analyses, etc.), and other literature. As part of the ongoing activity of the Safety Labeling Program, key safety information in the Safety Information Sheets is updated on an as-needed basis, and the updated Safety Information Sheets are forwarded to participating manufacturers so that they may consider whether to revise their product labels.

In general, the ABC employs the following criteria stipulated by the FDA for warnings on OTC drug products in determining what types of information should be considered for risk disclosure. The information should be (1) scientifically documented, (2) clinically significant, and (3) important for the safe and effective use of the product by consumers.[18] The ABC is using these criteria with full awareness that dietary supplements are *not* drugs as defined by the DSHEA. However, the ABC also recognizes that the FDA's OTC drug-labeling policy provides some rational guidelines for consideration of how to evaluate risks in the development of label warnings. There are many challenges that the ABC and manufacturers face in this process, including questions regarding what is "scientific" documentation of adverse event reports, to what extent are some adverse event reports adequately documented, and what is the clinical significance of in vitro experiments on potential drug interactions. In

other words, although the FDA policy provides guidelines, there is still the need for rational evaluation and interpretation of the existing safety information on each herb.

The Safety Labeling Program was developed with the assistance of the Pharmavite Corporation, manufacturer of a line of about two dozen herbal supplements under the Nature's Resource brand. It is estimated that ABC-based safety information will be printed on approximately 5–6 million Nature's Resource labels in 2003 and thereafter. Other companies will also carry the ABC safety information. (Information from selected ABC Safety Information Sheets is given below.)

► SAFETY ISSUES

Toxic Medicinal Plants

It is universally recognized that various plants contain numerous naturally occurring chemical compounds that are potentially toxic. Some of these provide the basis for many modern plant-derived pharmaceutical drugs. Many of these compounds are alkaloids (e.g., atropine, colchicine, scopolamine) or glycosides (e.g., digoxin, Lanoxin). In general, with a few exceptions, such toxic medicinal plants are usually not found as herbal dietary supplements in the market in the United States.

Adulteration and Misbranding

There has been considerable concern expressed over the years about the quality of various herbal preparations. Because herbal materials are by nature chemically complex, it is usually much more difficult to produce products of consistent chemical profiles than is the case with pharmaceutical drugs, which are almost always a purified single chemical entity. In the past few decades, there has been much progress in the area of standardization of herbal materials, whereby specific components in herbal extracts are "standardized," "adjusted," or "normalized" to specific ranges. This is done for the sake of quality control and/or to produce a more consistently reliable product from a pharmacological perspective.

In some cases, safety concerns regarding herbs have been the result of poor quality control.[19] There have been numerous cases in which safety concerns have arisen with herbal products when the products were either (1) misidentified and a different (toxic) plant from a different genus was substituted (ether accidentally or intentionally), (2) the herb material contained toxic heavy metals, or (3) conventional drugs were added into the herbal mixture, creating a potential adverse effect or interaction. Recently, various independent organizations have developed quality control seals to help identify products from reliable manufacturers. These include initiatives by the United States Pharmacopoeia (USP), NSF (formerly the National Sanitation Foundation, the leading certifier of drinking water and water filters), and ConsumerLab.com (a for-profit company that tests dietary supplements). Additionally, as required by the DSHEA in 1994, in 2003 the FDA issued proposed Good Manufacturing Practices (GMPs) for dietary supplements, which are intended to increase the quality and purity of these products; these GMPs are more stringent than the GMPs to which manufacturers previously had to adhere (i.e., GMPs for conventional foods), although many leading manufacturers had already developed advanced GMPs well in advance of FDA's proposal.

► EPHEDRA: CONTROVERSIAL TRADITIONAL HERB

One of the most controversial herbs in the marketplace has been ephedra, also known by its Chinese name *ma huang (Ephedra sinica)*, a traditional Chinese herb that has been used successfully and safely for centuries to treat pulmonary conditions. Ephedra is the source of the sympathomimetic alkaloids ephedrine and pseudoephedrine, both well known as approved nonprescription drug ingredients, one as a decongestant for cold and flu symptoms and the other as a bronchodilator for some allergic reactions. In the past several decades, herbal dietary supplements containing ephedra have been used (some would say misused) for enhancing athletic performance and for weight loss. Concerned about a significant number of serious adverse effects reportedly associated with supplements containing ephedra, the FDA and the Office of Dietary Supplements at the National Institutes of Health commissioned an independent scientific analysis of the literature on ephedra.[20] Known as the RAND report, the researchers found that there was some evidence of moderate weight loss (approximately 0.9 kg [2 lb] per month) associated with clinical trials conducted on ephedra supplements, but that there were no data supporting its use in athletic performance.

The researchers reported that there was sufficient evidence to conclude that ephedrine and ephedra are associated with an increase of two to three times normal in the risk of psychiatric symptoms, autonomic symptoms, upper gastrointestinal symptoms, and heart palpitations. An evaluation of more than 16,000 reports (dealing with adverse events and "incident reports" to manufacturers) revealed 5 deaths, 5 heart attacks, 11 cerebrovascular accidents, 4 seizures, and 8 psychiatric cases; these were termed "sentinel events" associated with prior consumption of ephedra or ephedrine.[21] However, the RAND report found that the evidence was insufficient to find a *causal* relationship between the serious adverse effects and the use of ephedra. It is also conceivable that the number of serious adverse events reported with ephedra may represent the occurrence of these incidents in a general population. In February 2003, the FDA proposed that an extensive warning be affixed to all ephedra product labels. Since 1994, herb and supplement industry associations have voluntarily provided warnings on ephedra products that are similar to those on nonprescription drug products.

Safety Considerations for Ginger

The primary concerns regarding the safety of ginger root in recent years have centered on its use in pregnancy.

Commission E, for example, contraindicates the common spice as a remedy for morning sickness during pregnancy. However, there is no evidence that the therapeutic dosage for antinauseant activity cited by Commission E (1 g/d of dried root) produces any harm to either the fetus or the mother. The Commission presumably based its caution on two studies published in the 1980s in Japan on 6-gingerol, one of the compounds isolated from ginger rhizome. In vitro tests indicated that 6-gingerol had mutagenic activity in vitro at high doses.[25,26] However, other compounds in ginger have been found to exhibit antimutagenic activity.[27] The following is used with permission from the American Botanical Council's Safety Information Sheet on Ginger as part of ABC's Safety Labeling Program:[22]

> Safety of Ginger *(Zingiber officinale)* in pregnancy:
>
> > Pregnancy and Lactation Section
> >
> > Based on the available evidence, it appears that pregnant women may be able to safely use moderate amounts of fresh and dried ginger for morning sickness during the first trimester of pregnancy.[23] Pregnant women should use caution when taking excessive doses of either fresh or dried ginger (e.g., more than 1 g/d dried ginger) and should consult with their health care practitioner before using any herbal product or conventional medication.
> >
> > The [German] Commission E's contraindication of ginger as, "No administration for morning sickness during pregnancy," bears clarification. ABC's translation of the Commission E monographs[24] contains the following parenthetical editor's note: "A review of the clinical literature could not justify this caution. There is no evidence that ginger causes harm to the mother or fetus."

Ginger is also widely used in traditional Chinese medicine (TCM), but without contraindications in pregnancy. "On the contrary, ginger has been traditionally used for nausea and vomiting in pregnancy, though as in typical TCM usage, rarely by itself. There is no lack of remedies for these conditions using ginger. Also, there is no contraindication of ginger in any of the recent issues of the *Pharmacopoeia of the People's Republic of China*.[28] The dosage is 3–9 g (per day) for both fresh and dried ginger."[29] A literature review of all available clinical studies on ginger could find no scientific or medical evidence for Commission E's contraindication during pregnancy.[30] Prof. Schilcher agrees with this assessment of ginger's presumed safety during pregnancy.[31]

Additional research has also demonstrated antimutagenic activity in ginger components as well as ginger juice.[25]

The scientific literature contains references to ginger's having abortifacient activity, but this action is presumably based on relatively high doses. Barnes et al.[31a] write that "uteroactivity has been documented for a related species" without noting the identity of the species, leading to the caution that ginger doses "that greatly exceed the amounts used in foods should not be taken during pregnancy or lactation." It is generally acknowledged that mutagenic substances are commonly found in much of the food eaten in American diets. Research on relatively high doses of isolated components in vitro have relevance to human experience only if correlative effects have already been identified in oral doses in vivo. In general, the normally used dosage for ginger for nausea and motion sickness is 2–4 g/d (as recommended by the German Commission E), a level that may be equal to or greater than the amount of ginger commonly used to flavor foods, although such comparisons are difficult to assess.

Safety Considerations for Ginkgo

Ginkgo *(Ginkgo biloba)* is one of the most popular herbal preparations in North America and

Western Europe. The ginkgo product most commonly used is a highly concentrated (usually 50:1) extract made from the leaves. Ginkgo has been well recognized for its ability to increase cognitive function in cognitively impaired adults, as well as to provide benefits in peripheral arterial occlusive disease, and, to a lesser extent, tinnitus of vascular origin.[32] A meta-analysis of 33 controlled trials on cognitively impaired adults concluded that ginkgo extract showed "promising evidence" for treatment of dementia related to early stages of Alzheimer disease and related dementia syndromes.[33]

Use of ginkgo preparations in clinical trials and in actual use has been relatively uneventful, with minor adverse effects in a very small percentage of patients.[34] According to the ABC's Safety Information Sheet on Ginkgo, based on a peer-reviewed assessment of the literature:

> In general, the results from various clinical trials and meta-analyses of clinical trials and pharmacoepidemiological data suggest that ginkgo extract is safe when used appropriately. Results from clinical trials and meta-analyses show that adverse effects to ginkgo standardized extract are mild and consistent with adverse effects experienced by patients taking a placebo. One postmarketing surveillance study on one of Europe's leading standardized ginkgo extracts resulted in only 1.7 percent of 10,815 subjects reporting adverse events.[35]

There is some concern about the implications of potential bleeding problems associated with ginkgo, as it has a potential blood-thinning action. According to the American Botanical Council's Safety Information Sheet on Ginkgo:

> Ginkgo is also contraindicated in people with bleeding disorders due to increased bleeding potential associated with regular use (6–12 months). Ginkgo should not be used at least 36 hours before elective surgery, and to help ensure a wider margin of safety, should be discontinued at least 1 week prior. Some

sources recommend discontinuing ginkgo 2 weeks prior to elective surgery. This caution is based on isolated case reports, as actual INR (International Normalization Ratio, a measurement of bleeding time) measures have not been done.[36]

Safety Considerations on St. John's Wort

St. John's wort *(Hypericum perforatum)* has become popular in the United States since news of a meta-analysis in the *British Medical Journal* in 1996 showed that the herb was useful in treating cases of mild-to-moderate depression.[37]

The relative safety of St. John's wort has been fairly well established through controlled clinical trials and general use. In controlled clinical trials, the frequency of adverse effects for St. John's wort has been the same as placebo (ranging from 4–12%), significantly less than that encountered with use of standard antidepressants.[38] (These adverse effects include mild gastrointestinal upset, dry mouth, nervousness, and skin rash.) A meta-analysis of 13 placebo-controlled, double-blind clinical trials on St. John's wort documented approximately 4.1% adverse effects.[39] Between October 1991 and December 1999, only 95 reports of side effects were documented from a pool of more than 8 million patients in Germany. Reported side effects included allergic skin reactions, increased prothrombin time (i.e., increased clotting time), minor gastrointestinal complaints, breakthrough bleeding for women taking oral contraceptives, lethargy, and restlessness.[40]

The main concerns regarding safety of St. John's wort pertains to potential drug interactions. Like many effective pharmaceutical agents, St. John's wort has interactions with other substances, for which there should be precautions. The primary documented mechanisms for St. John's wort interactions is based on its ability to induce certain isozymes (particularly CYP3A4) of the cytochrome P450 enzyme system and the P-glycoprotein transporter system.[41] Based on the induction of these enzyme systems, there is increased metabolic clearance and a reduction in serum levels— and, therefore, usually the activity of drugs that are metabolized by these mechanisms. Thus, persons who contemplate the use of St. John's wort and are taking standard OTC or prescription medications should check with their physician, pharmacist, or other qualified health practitioner to determine if these medications are metabolized by these mechanisms prior to using St. John's wort.[42]

For further information on herb safety, see Tables 6–3 through 6–7.

▶ **TABLE 6–3** LITERATURE SOURCES OF HERB SAFETY AND HERB–DRUG INTERACTION DATA

Only recently have there been systematic documentation of herb–drug interactions published in the professional literature. For example, as a result of a 16-year review of the literature, the Commission E, a special expert panel, has published monographs documenting the therapeutic aspects of over 300 herbal drugs and herb combinations sold in pharmacies in Germany (Blumenthal et al., 1998). In addition, the European Scientific Cooperative on Phytotherapy (ESCOP, 1997), a pan-Western European group of medicinal plant experts, has published monographs on herbal therapeutics, with most of the herb–drug interactions listed closely reflecting those listed by Commission E. The World Health Organization[8,9] has also published monographs listing interactions (WHO, 1999, 2003). Additionally, articles are beginning to appear in both alternative (Brinker, 1999) and mainstream medical journals (Miller, 1998; Fugh-Berman, 2000), as well as books focusing on this subject[5] (Brinker, 2001). Other sources have published cases of herb–drug interactions, or in some cases, situations where the interactions are presumed based on theoretical biochemical interactions.

AHPA Botanical Safety Handbook (BSH). As noted above, a comprehensive review of the literature pertaining to the safety of about 540 popular herbs in the US marketplace was published in the *American Herbal Product Association's Botanical Safety Handbook* (McGuffin et al., 1997). The authors rank the relative safety of herbal products according to four classes of safety. The information upon which this assessment was based was gleaned from 38 authoritative general sources as well as from hundreds of published studies and case resports on the respective individual herbs.

Brinker's *Herb Contraindications and Drug Interactions.* A new publication,[5] *Herb Contraindications and Drug Interactions, 3d ed.* (Brinker, 2001), written by a research-oriented naturopathic physician, provides a hierarchy of evidence for each interaction and corresponds this evidence to each cited reference for each interaction. Current information on herb–drug interactions has relied on authoritative sources like the German Commission E Monographs, ESCOP Monographs, WHO (see below) and other authoritative primary and secondary sources. Interactions noted by Commission E and/or ESCOP, for example, sometimes are based either on specific known interactions, and in some cases, *theoretical* interactions based on *suspected* activities of primary active compounds in botanicals, interacting with a presumed interaction with the particular conventional drug. However, a cogent, well-documented, evidence-based database has been lacking, until the publication of this book.

German Commission E Monographs. More than any other Western industrialized nation thus far, in Germany, the German Federal Institute of Drugs and Medical Devices (equivalent to the Canadian Health Protection Branch or the US FDA) conducted a risk–benefit assessment of over 300 herbs and herb combinations sold as drugs in German pharmacies. A panel of medical and pharmacy experts, known as the Commission E, evaluated all the relevant scientific and clinical literature on each herb and published the findings as monographs between 1983 and 1995.

Continued

▶ **TABLE 6–3** LITERATURE SOURCES OF HERB SAFETY AND HERB–DRUG INTERACTION DATA *(Continued)*

These monographs have been systematically translated and cross-referenced in English[7] (Blumenthal et al., 1998). They were intended as package inserts for herbal drugs sold in German pharmacies and include the uses, dosages, duration of use, side effects, contraindications, interactions, etc.

Natural Standard. A relatively recent entry into the herbal medicine reporting field is Natural Standard (NS), an organization that produces evidence-based monographs on a variety of herb and dietary supplement ingredients. Natural Standard is a collaborative effort of health professionals and herbal experts who have systematically rated the levels of evidence in the literature on the safety and efficacy of herbs. The NS information is found on its website on a subscription basis (www.naturalstandard.com).

World Health Organization (WHO) Monographs. The World Health Organization[8,9] has published 58 monographs on medicinal plants of importance around the world (WHO, 1999; WHO, 2003). Unlike the Commission E and ESCOP monographs, those from WHO contain both standards and identity information as well as information on therapeutics. Adverse effects, contraindications and herb–drug interactions are noted where the documentation merits inclusion of such data.

Other literature. In addition to the aforementioned sources, various publications are beginning to include systematic data on safety concerns on herbs, including suspected and/or actual herb–drug interactions. These include monographs from the American Herbal Pharmacopoeia (Upton, 1999a; 2000–2002), and various online databases and CD-ROMs available for health professionals and consumers, e.g., HealthNotes Online (www.HealthNotes.com).

References: Brinker F, Stodart N. *Herb Contraindications and Drug Interactions,* 2nd ed. Eclectic Medical Publications; December 1998. Miller LG. Herbal medicinals: Selected clinical consideration focusing on known or potential drug–herbs interactions. 1998 *Arch Inter Med.* 1998;158((20):2200–2211. Fugh-Berman A. Herb-drug interactions. *Lancet.* 2000;355(9198):134–138. Upton R, ed. *American Herbal Pharmacopoeia Monographs and Therapeutic Compendium Series 1.* Santa Cruz: American Herbal Pharmacopoeia; 1999. Upton R, ed. *American Herbal Pharmacopoeia Monographs Series 2–4.* Santa Cruz: American Herbal Pharmacopoeia; 2000–2002.

▶ **TABLE 6–4** HERBS CONTRAINDICATED DURING PREGNANCY ACCORDING TO GERMAN COMMISSION E

Aloe (*Aloe vera*)
Autumn crocus (*Colchicum autumnale*)
Black cohosh root (*Actaea race mosa*)
Buckthorn bark and berry (*Rhamnus frangula; Rhamnus cathartica*)
Cascara sagrada bark (*Rhamnus purshiana*)
Chaste tree fruit (*Vitex agnus-castus*)
Cinchona bark (*Cinchona* spp.)
Cinnamon bark (*Cinnamomum zeylanicum*)
Coltsfoot leaf (*Tussilago farfara*)
Echinacea purpurea herb (*Echinacea purpurea*)*
Fennel oil (*Foeniculum vulgare*)
Combination of licorice, peppermint and chamomile
Combination of licorice, primrose, marshmallow, and anise
Combination of senna, peppermint oil, and caraway oil
Ginger root (*Zingiber officinale*)**
Indian snakeroot (*Rauwolfia serpentina*)

Continued

▶ **TABLE 6–4** HERBS CONTRAINDICATED DURING PREGNANCY ACCORDING
TO GERMAN COMMISSION E *(Continued)*

Juniper berry (*Juniperus communis*)
Kava kava root (*Piper methysticum*)
Licorice root (*Glycyrrhiza glabra*)
Marsh tea (*Ledum palustre*)
Mayapple root (*Podophyllum peltatum*)
Petasite root (*Petasites* spp.)
Rhubarb root (*Rheum palmatum*)
Sage leaf (*Salvia officinalis*)
Senna (*Cassia senna*)

The Commission E monographs were published from 1983 and 1995. Since that period, new data have been published that would probably temper the decisions of the commissioners, if they were still publishing monographs, originally intended as package inserts for herbal drug products in Germany. The monographs for echinacea and ginger contraindicated the use of these herbs during pregnancy. However, in light of subsequent published data, these contraindications would probably be rescinded.

*The contraindication of echinacea for pregnancy was made for speculative reasons; there were no data at the time of the publication of the monograph (early 1990s) that supported such a contraindication. A recent clinical study supports the general safety of preparations made from species of the genus *Echinacea* during pregnancy (Gallo et al., 2000).

**A subsequent review of the clinical literature could find no basis for the contraindication of ginger, a common spice, during pregnancy (Fulder & Tenne, 1996). A recently published study from Thailand on pregnant women in the first trimester of pregnancy indicated the general safety of ginger root for the effective treatment of nausea and morning sickness during the first trimester of pregnancy, with no adverse effects on the course of the pregnancy or the newborn child (Vutyavanich et al., 2001). Another study on a ginger syrup also suggested the safety of ginger on the mother and fetus (Keating & Chez, 2002).

References: Gallo M, Sarkar M, Au W, et al. Pregnancy outcome following gestational exposure to echinacea: a prospective controlled study. *Arch Intern Med* 2000:160(20):3141–3143. Fulder S, Tenne M. Ginger as an anti-nausea remedy in pregnancy: the issue of safety. *Herbal Gram* 1996;38:48–50. Vutyavanich T, Kraisarin T, Ruangsri R. Ginger for nausea and vomiting in pregnancy: randomized, double masked, placebo controlled trial. *Obstet Gyn* 2001;97(4):577–582. Keating A, Chez RA. Ginger syrup as an antiemetic in early pregnancy. *Altern Ther Health Med* 2002; Sep-Oct, 8(5):89–91.

Adapted with permission from Blumenthal et al.,[7] 1998, courtesy of the American Botanical Council.

▶ **TABLE 6–5** HERBS CONTRAINDICATED
DURING LACTATION ACCORDING
TO GERMAN COMMISSION E

Aloe (*Aloe vera*)
Basil (*Ocimum basilicum*)
Buckthorn bark and berry (*Rhamnus frangula; Rhamnus cathartica*)
Cascara sagrada bark (*Rhamnus purshiana*)
Coltsfoot leaf (*Tussilago farfara*)
Combinations of senna peppermint oil and caraway oil
Kava kava root (*Piper methysticum*)
Petasite root (*Petasites* spp.)
Indian snakeroot (*Rauwolfia serpentina*)
Rhubarb root (*Rheum palmatum*)
Senna (*Cassia senna*)

Adapted with permission from Blumenthal et al., 1998, courtesy of the American Botanical Council.

▶ **TABLE 6-6** POPULAR HERBS ON THE US MARKET THAT SHOULD BE RESTRICTED
IN CHILDREN

Herb	Restriction
Aloe (*Aloe capensis*)	Children under 12; stimulant laxative (dried leaf extract as stimulant laxative; not aloe gel)
Bitter orange peel (*Citrus aurantium* var. *amara*)	Large doses (contains stimulant alkaloid synephrine)
Cascara sagrada bark (*Rhamnus purshiana*)	Children under 12; stimulant laxative
Cat's claw root (*Uncaria tomentosa*)	Children under 3
Ephedra (*Ephedra sinica*)	Children under 18; large doses, nervous system stimulant
Eucalyptus leaves (*Eucalyptus globulus*)	Children under 2; essential oil, nasal area
Fennel fruit (*Foeniculum vulgare*)	Children under 2; essential oil
Peppermint leaves (*Mentha X piperita*)	Children under 2; essential oil, nasal area; nervous system
Red clover plant or flower (*Trifolium pratense*)	Children under 12; large doses; chronic use
Senna leaves, pods (*Cassia senna*)	Children under 12; stimulant laxative
Tea leaves (*Camellia sinensis*)	Children under 6; nervous system; may block absorption of important nutrients, esp. minerals
Uva ursi leaves (*Arctostaphylos uva-ursi*)	Children under 12; chronic use

From Brinker[5] 2001 (used with permission of the author).

▶ **TABLE 6-7** REFERENCES AND RECOMMENDED RESOURCES ON HERB SAFETY,
TOXICOLOGY, AND CLINICAL BENEFITS

Title	Author, Year
The ABC Clinical Guide to Herbs	Blumenthal et al., 2003
American Herbal Pharmacopoeia	Upton, 1999
American Herbal Products Association's Botanical Safety Handbook	McGuffin et al., 1997
The Complete German Commission E Monographs—Therapeutic Guide to Herbal Medicines	Blumenthal et al., 1998
Herbal Medicine: Expanded Commission E Monographs	Blumenthal et al., 2000
Herbal Medicine, 2d ed.	Fintelmann, Weiss 2000
Herb Contraindications and Drug Interactions, 3d ed	Brinker, 2001
ESCOP Monographs	ESCOP, 1997
Rational Phytotherapy: A Physician's Guide to Herbal Medicine, 4th ed.	Schulz et al., 2000
WHO Monographs	WHO, 1999, 2003

Blumenthal M, Hall T, Goldberg A, Kunz T, Dinda K, Brinckmann J, Wollschlaeger B. *The ABC Clinical Guide to Herbs.*
Austin, TX: American Botanical Council, 2003). [Reference book and CME module accredited for physicians,
pharmacists, nurses, dietitians, and other health professionals.]
Herbal Medicine: Expanded Commission E Monographs. Newton, MA: Integrative Medicine Communications, 2000.
[Additional material based on new studies on ca. 107 herbs from the previous Commission E book.]
Blumenthal M. et al. (eds.). *The Complete German Commission E Monographs—Therapeutic Guide to Herbal Medicines.*
Austin, TX: American Botanical Council, 1998. [The 2nd ranked medical book of 1998; covers ca. 300 herbs.]
Brinker F. *Herb Contraindications and Drug Interactions, 3rd ed.* Sandy, OR: Eclectic Medical Publications, 2001. [One
of the most lucid publications on this important subject.]
European Scientific Cooperative on Phytotherapy. Monographs on the Medicinal Uses of Plant Drugs. [60 detailed
therapeutic monographs on leading herbs, published from 1996–1999.]
Fintelmann V and Weiss RF. *Herbal Medicine* (2nd English edition). New York: Thieme Publishers, 2000. [The revised
version of the classic German textbook used to train physicians for 40 years.]
McGuffin M. et al. (eds.). *American Herbal Products Association's Botanical Safety Handbook.* Boca Raton, FL: CRC
Press, 1997.

REFERENCES

1. Brinker F. *The Toxicology of Herbal Medicines.* 3rd ed. Sandy, OR: Eclectic Medical Publications; 2000.
2. DeSmet PAGM, Keller K, Hänsel R, Chandler F. *Adverse Effects of Herbal Drugs.* Vol. 1. New York: Springer; 1993.
3. DeSmet PAGM, Keller K, Hänsel R, Chandler F. *Adverse Effects of Herbal Drugs.* Vol. 2. New York: Springer; 1993.
4. DeSmet PAGM, Keller K, Hänsel R, Chandler F. *Adverse Effects of Herbal Drugs.* Vol. 3. New York: Springer; 1993.
5. Brinker FJ. *Herb Contraindications and Drug Interactions.* 3rd ed. Sandy, OR: Eclectic Medical Publications; 2001.
6. McGuffin M, Hobbs C, Upton R, Goldberg A. *American Herbal Product Association's Botanical Safety Handbook.* Boca Raton, FL: CRC Press; 1997.
7. Blumenthal M, Busse WR, Goldberg A, eds. *The Complete German Commission E Monographs— Therapeutic Guide to Herbal Medicines.* Klein S, Rister RS, trans. Austin, TX: American Botanical Council; 1998.
8. WHO. *Monographs on Selected Medicinal Plants.* Vol. I. Geneva: World Health Organization; 1999.
9. WHO. *Monographs on Selected Medicinal Plants.* Vol. II. Geneva: World Health Organization; 2003.
10. 103rd Congress. Public Law 103–417. Dietary Supplement Health and Education Act of 1994 (21 USC).
11. McNamara SH. FDA has adequate power and authority to protect the public from unsafe dietary supplements. *HerbalGram.* 1996;38:25–27.
12. Committee on the Framework for Evaluating the Safety of Dietary Supplements, Food and Nutrition Board, Board on Life Sciences, Institute of Medicine and National Research Council, July 2002.
13. McGuffin M, Hobbs C, Upton R, Goldberg A. *American Herbal Product Association's Botanical Safety Handbook.* Boca Raton, FL: CRC Press; 1997.
14. McGuffin M, Hobbs C, Upton R, Goldberg A. *American Herbal Product Association's Botanical Safety Handbook.* Boca Raton, FL: CRC Press; 1997.
15. Blumenthal M, Hall T, Goldberg A, Dinda K, Brinckmann J, Wollschlaeger B. *The ABC Clinical Guide to Herbs.* Austin, TX: American Botanical Council; 2003.
16. ESCOP. *Monographs on the Medicinal Uses of Plants.* Exeter, England: European Scientific Cooperative on Phytotherapy; 1997.

17. McGuffin M, Hobbs C, Upton R, Goldberg A. *American Herbal Product Association's Botanical Safety Handbook.* Boca Raton, FL: CRC Press; 1997.
18. Soller RW. When to warn. *Regulatory Affairs Focus.* 1997;2(10):18–21.
19. Farnsworth NR. The relative safety of herbal medicines. *HerbalGram.* 1993;29:36S.
20. Shekelle P, Morton S Maglione M, et al. *Ephedra and Ephedrine for Weight Loss and Athletic Performance Enhancement: Clinical Efficacy and Side Effects.* Evidence Report/Technology Assessment No. 76. AHRQ Publication No. 03-EO22. Rockville, MD: Agency for Healthcare Research and Quality; 2003.
21. Anonymous. Comprehensive report provides evidence that links use of ephedra with risk for heart, psychiatric and gastrointestinal problems [press release]. American Medical Association, March 10, 2003.
22. Blumenthal M, Engels G. *Ginger Safety Information Sheet.* Austin, TX: American Botanical Council; January 2003.
23. Vutyavanich T, Kraisarin T, Ruangsri RA. Ginger for nausea and vomiting in pregnancy: randomized, double-masked, placebo-controlled trial. *Obstet Gynecol.* 2001;97(4):577–582.
24. Blumenthal M, Hall T, Goldberg A, Dinda K, Brinckmann J, Wollschlaeger B. *The ABC Clinical Guide to Herbs.* Austin, TX: American Botanical Council; 2003.
25. Namakura H. Yamamoto T. Mutagen and anti-mutagen in ginger, *Zingiber officinale. Mutat Res.* 1982; 103(2):119–126.
26. Nagabhyshan M, Amonkar A, Bhide S. Mutagenicity of gingerol and shogaol and antimutagenicity of zingerone in Salmonella/microsome assay. *Cancer Lett.* 1987;36(2):221–223.
27. Kada T, Morita K, Inoue T. Anti-mutagenic action of vegetable factors on the mutagenic principle of tryptophan pyrolysate. *Mutat Res.* 1978;53(3): 351–353.
28. *Pharmacopoeia of the People's Republic of China* (PPRC English Edition, 1997). Beijing, China: Chemical Industry Press; 1997.
29. Leung A, Foster S. *Encyclopedia of Common Natural Ingredients Used in Food, Drugs and Cosmetics.* 2nd ed. New York: John Wiley & Sons; 1996.
30. Fulder S, Tenne M. Ginger as an anti-nausea remedy in pregnancy: the issue of safety. *HerbalGram.* 1996;38:47–50.

31. Schilcher H. The present state of phytotherapy in Germany. *Deutsche Apotheker Zietung*. 138 Jahragang No. 3. 1998;15:144–149.

31a. Barnes J. Complementary therapies in pregnancy. *Pharma J*. 2002;270:402–404.

32. Blumenthal M, Hall T, Goldberg A, Dinda K, Brinckmann J, Wollschlaeger B. *The ABC Clinical Guide to Herbs*. Austin, TX: American Botanical Council; 2003.

33. Birks J, Grimley Evans J, Van Dongen M. Ginkgo biloba for cognitive impairment and dementia (Cochrane Review). In: The Cochrane Library, Issue 4, 2002. Oxford: Update Software.

34. Blumenthal M, Hall T, Goldberg A, Dinda K, Brinckmann J, Wollschlaeger B. *The ABC Clinical Guide to Herbs*. Austin, TX: American Botanical Council; 2003.

35. Blumenthal M, Engels G. *Ginkgo Safety Information Sheet*. Austin, TX: American Botanical Council, January 2003.

36. Blumenthal M, Engels G. *Ginkgo Safety Information Sheet*. Austin, TX: American Botanical Council, January 2003.

37. Linde K, Ramirez G, Mulrow C, Pauls A, Weidenhammer W, Melchart D. St. John's wort for depression—an overview and meta-analysis of randomized clinical trials. *BMJ*. 1996;313(7052):253–258.

38. Rotblatt M, Ziment I. *Evidence-Based Herbal Medicine*. Philadelphia: Hanley & Belfus; 2001.

39. Linde K, Ramirez G, Mulrow C, Pauls A, Weidenhammer W, Melchart D. St. John's wort for depression—an overview and meta-analysis of randomized clinical trials. *BMJ*. 1996;313(7052):253–258.

40. Schulz V, Hänsel R, Tyler VE. *Rational Phytotherapy: A Physician's Guide to Herbal Medicine*. 4th ed. New York: Springer Verlag; 2000.

41. Blumenthal M, Hall T, Goldberg A, Dinda K, Brinckmann J, Wollschlaeger B. *The ABC Clinical Guide to Herbs*. Austin, TX: American Botanical Council; 2003.

42. Blumenthal M, Engels G. *Ginkgo Safety Information Sheet*. Austin, TX: American Botanical Council, January 2003.

CHAPTER 7

Integrative Approach to Nutrition

MaryBeth Augustine

The use of dietary modification both for prevention and for treatment of specific conditions is a cornerstone of the integrative approach to health care. This chapter reviews several of the most useful and commonly applied therapeutic diets, their indications, and the evidence for their utility.

As with all lifestyle change, dietary change can be challenging for many patients. Our choices regarding food are emotionally complex, and enabling change in our patients often means encouraging them in developing their awareness of the role of eating in their personal emotional and psychological life. Family dynamics are also a significant influence, particularly in applying therapeutic dietary change in children. Motivation is critical, as is a supportive relationship with the health care practitioner. Recognizing where a patient is on the continuum of change—from precontemplation to contemplation to action to maintenance—is a critical first step for the provider wanting to effectively use dietary change as a therapeutic tool.

▶ ELIMINATION DIET

Description

The elimination diet is considered to be a *hypoallergenic diet*. It involves strict avoidance/ elimination of the foods that are the most "allergenic"—dairy, soy, eggs, corn, wheat, citrus, nuts, shellfish, rye, pork, chocolate, peanuts, white sugar, caffeine, tomatoes, eggplant, peppers, mushrooms, white potatoes, yeast, and beef, or varying combinations thereof. Any food that is eaten more than three times per week is also eliminated. An elimination diet consists of the *exclusion/elimination phase*, which generally lasts from 14–30 days, and is followed by the *reintroduction/provocation phase*. Some conditions, such as rheumatoid arthritis or menstrual disorders, may require a much longer exclusion phase (as long as 2–3 months) to see an effect, depending upon their severity and/or the cyclic nature of the symptoms.

The dramatic improvement that occurs with relatively mild symptoms may not happen for those with a serious long-term condition such as rheumatoid arthritis because of the past damage to the joints that cannot be quickly repaired. In these cases, a marked but partial improvement is an acceptable sign of food contributing to the illness. It is critical to reintroduce only one suspected "allergenic" food at a time during the reintroduction/provocation phase, eating that food two to three times daily for 3–7 days. If a "positive" reaction occurs, as evidenced by worsening of symptoms, then a 4-day elimination diet period must be observed before reintroducing another food. If there is no reaction after 7 days, another food may be reintroduced. Usually, a "food/mood/symptom diary" is kept by the patient to record significant symptoms so they can be linked to the correct food(s).

Rationale/Indications

The purpose of the diet is to evaluate the role of food allergy/hypersensitivity as a contributor to the severity of a patient's chronic medical condition. It makes sense then that the foods eaten most frequently (chronically) are the foods most likely to be the culprit. If the patient eats sweet potato once a year at Thanksgiving, then it is highly unlikely that food intolerance to sweet potato is contributing to the severity of their chronic medical condition.

Almost any unresolved complaint that is refractory to conventional medical approaches can be potentially responsive to an elimination-diet approach, including migraine, bowel disturbances, nausea and indigestion, joint pain, fatigue and malaise, recurrent mouth ulcers, gastric or duodenal ulcers, asthma, eczema or urticaria, rhinitis, arthritis, menstrual complaints, inflammatory bowel disease, weight-loss resistance, and mood disorders. The important point to remember is that each of these symptoms and conditions can have another etiology, and that thorough diagnostic evaluation is required before defining a symptom as "food-sensitivity" and treating it with an elimination diet. The proposed physiology behind the use

of elimination diets is discussed in detail in Chapter 21. Applications of elimination diets to many of these conditions is described throughout this text in the discussions of the specific conditions and is not reiterated here. One particular constellation of symptoms—joint pain, atopic disorders, gastroesophageal reflux, and altered gastrointestinal motility (diarrhea, constipation, or irritable bowel)—is highly characteristic of food intolerance, and a trial elimination diet should be done to evaluate the contributory role of food sensitivities in this case.

Evidence

Food sensitivity can manifest symptoms in the gastrointestinal, respiratory, neurological, and cutaneous systems, and is linked in some cases to asthma, autism, arthritis, gastroesophageal reflux, recurrent abdominal pain, diarrhea, eczema, psoriasis, headache, and recurrent otitis media. In particular, discussion of the evidence for the elimination diet appears in the sections of this text on asthma, allergy, atopic dermatitis, colic, autism, inflammatory bowel disease, and functional bowel disorders.

▶ LOW GLYCEMIC INDEX DIET

Description

This diet is characterized by the exclusion of foods ranked high in glycemic index, and the inclusion of foods ranked low or moderate in glycemic index. The fat profile of the diet is high in monounsaturated fatty acid, with a low polyunsaturated-to-saturated fatty acid ratio, and low trans fatty acid content. It is high in fiber and provides adequate protein. One variation of the diet adjusts the macronutrient content of the diet to approximately 40% carbohydrates, 30% protein, and 30% fat, and calories can be adjusted accordingly as indicated. Refined grains are eliminated and whole grains are emphasized in limited amounts. Low fat dairy is restricted. Starchy vegetables are re-stricted, but nonstarchy vegetables are unre-stricted. Fruits with high glycemic index are eliminated and low and moderate glycemic in-dex fruits are allowed in restricted amounts to minimize glycemic load. Legumes are empha-sized because of their low glycemic index. Lean proteins, fatty fish, low glycemic index vegeta-bles and fruits, and nuts are emphasized. Low glycemic diet guidelines are given in Table 7–1.

▶ **TABLE 7–1** EXAMPLES OF DIETARY GUIDELINES FOR LOW GLYCEMIC INDEX

Legumes
Average serving size: ½ cup cooked beans, ¼ hummus/bean spreads, ¾ cup bean soups.
Servings: 1–2 per day.

Foods: Split peas, green peas, lentils (all varieties), aduki, mung (all varieties), garbanzo, pinto, kidney, black, lima, cannellini, navy, mung beans, soy beans.

Nuts and Seeds
Average serving size: 1 oz (equals approximately 2 T whole nuts or 2 T nut butters).
Servings: 1 per day.

Foods: Almonds, walnuts, pecans, macadamia, brazil, hazelnut, peanuts, cashews, pistachios, sunflower, pumpkin, or sesame seeds; any sugar-free/"natural" nut butter or tahini.

Dairy
Average serving size: 6 oz milk or milk substitute, ½ cup yogurt.
Servings: 1–2 as indicated per calorie needs. Avoid known allergens/intolerances.
Note: Soft "white" cheeses are considered proteins based on glycemic index.

Foods: Plain low fat or fat-free yogurt, nonfat, 1 or 2% milk, and calcium-enriched soy milk, rice milk, or almond milk.

Low Glycemic Index Vegetables
Average servings size: ½ cup cooked, 1 cup raw and leafy, ¾ cup fresh vegetable juice
Servings: unlimited, with a minimum of 3–5.

Foods: Asparagus, artichokes, bamboo shoots, bean sprouts, peppers, broccoli, broccoflower, Brussels sprouts, cauliflower, celery, chives, onion, leeks, garlic, cucumber, cabbage (all varieties), eggplant, green beans, bok choy, escarole, Swiss chard, kale, collard, greens, spinach, dandelion, mustard, or beet greens, lettuce (all varieties), watercress, and chicory, mushrooms, okra, radishes, snow peas, sprouts, tomatoes, water chestnuts, zucchini, yellow squash, sea vegetables (all varieties).

Moderate Glycemic Index Vegetables
Average serving size: ½ cup or 3 oz cooked weight
Servings: 1–2 per day.
Note: White potatoes, whether fried, mashed, or baked are high glycemic index.

Foods: Sweet potatoes/yams, carrots, beets, winter squashes, corn.

Low-Moderate Glycemic Index Fruits
Average serving size: 1 medium piece fresh fruit, 1 cup cut fruit or berries, as indicated.
Servings: 2–3 per day as indicated per calorie needs.
Note: Dried fruits, tropical fruits, and fruit juices are higher in glycemic index.

Foods: Apple, orange, peach, pear, all berries, 1 grapefruit, 2–3 medium apricots, 15 cherries, 2 fresh figs, 15 grapes, ¼ small honeydew melon, 2 small nectarines, 2 small plums, 2 small tangerines.

Continued

► **TABLE 7-1** EXAMPLES OF DIETARY GUIDELINES FOR LOW GLYCEMIC INDEX *(Continued)*

Whole Grains
Average serving size: ½ cup whole grain, 1 oz bread, ¾ cup high fiber cereal, ½–1 oz high-fiber low-fat crackers, or as indicated.
Servings: 2–3 per day.
Note: Minimum grams fiber per serving of processed grains: breads 2 grams per slice, cereals 5 grams, crackers 1 gram.

Foods: Amaranth, teff, or quinoa, barley, buckwheat, millet, spelt, wheat berries, kamut berries, bulgur (cracked wheat), brown rice, wild rice, basmati rice, ⅓ cup of whole raw oats, ¾ cup of cooked long-cooking oatmeal, 100% whole-wheat/spelt/kamut pastas.

Lean Protein Sources
Average serving size: 3 oz meat/poultry/fish after cooking, or as indicated.
Servings: 3 per day, ideally 1 at each meal (or the equivalent of 1 gram protein per kilogram body weight).
Note: Meat poultry, and fish should be grilled, baked, roasted or poached. Keep cheese and lean red meat intake low due to saturated fat content.

Foods: Chicken, Cornish hen (breast only), turkey, fish or shell fish, lean pork, leg of lamb, lean roast beef, venison, elk, buffalo, 2 whole eggs, 3 egg whites, ⅔ cup egg substitute, or 6 oz canned tuna or salmon in water, 1 cup cubed tofu, ½ cup tempeh, 4 oz soy burger, ¾ cup of nonfat or low fat cottage cheese, ½ cup part skim ricotta cheese, 2 oz or ½ cup shredded part skim mozzarella, 2 T grated Parmesan cheese equals ½ serving, 1 cup textured vegetable protein concentrate.

Oils
Average serving size is 1 tsp or as indicated.
Servings: 6 tsp per day, or approximately 25–30% of total calories
Note: Oils should be cold pressed and refrigerated.

Flaxseed oil, walnut oil, extra virgin or virgin olive oil, canola oil, 1 T mayonnaise made with canola or soy oil, 8–10 ripe or green medium olives, ⅛ avocado.

Beverages
Servings: unlimited.
Note: Artificial sweeteners are to be avoided, as bitter artificial sweeteners have been shown in animal studies to stimulate insulin release from pancreatic islet cells. Small amounts of stevia for sweetening are permitted.

Decaffeinated, herbal, or green teas; decaffeinated coffee, water: seltzer, plain or unsweetened flavored.

Condiments
Servings unlimited.

Fresh, powdered, dried herbs and spices, mustard, tamari soy sauce, vinegar, lime, lemon, unsweetened flavored extracts (e.g., vanilla, or almond)

The following dietary guidelines are examples of foods low to moderate in glycemic index. Foods excluded are either high in glycemic index (example white bread, white rice, watermelon, banana), or omitted due to space restraints in text. Detailed food lists of glycemic index and glycemic load should be consulted to expand food choices. When choosing foods based on glycemic index, choose low glycemic index (GI) foods (with a GI of 1–50) often, moderate glycemic index foods (with a GI of 71–100) seldom. Additionally, glycemic load should be considered when choosing foods. Choose low glycemic load (GL) foods (with a GL of 1–10) often, moderate glycemic load foods (with a GL of 11–20) in moderation, and high glycemic load foods (with a GL of greater than 20) seldom.

Rationale/Indications

When we eat a meal containing a carbohydrate, our blood glucose and insulin levels rise and fall. The extent to which they rise and remain high is critically important to health. Both the amount and type of carbohydrate predict blood glucose response to individual foods and a meal.

The glycemic index (GI) is a ranking of foods on a scale from 0 to 100 according to the extent to which they raise blood glucose and insulin levels after eating. Carbohydrate foods that break down quickly during digestion have the highest glycemic indexes. Their blood glucose response is fast and high. Carbohydrates that break down slowly release glucose gradually into the bloodstream, and have low glycemic indexes. To determine a food's GI rating, measured portions of the food containing 50 g of carbohydrate are fed to people after an overnight fast. Fingerstick blood glucose samples are taken at 15–30 minute intervals over the next 2 hours. These samples are used to construct a blood sugar response curve. The area under the curve (AUC) is calculated and reflects the total rise in blood glucose levels after eating the test food. The GI rating of the test food is calculated by dividing the AUC for the test food by the AUC for the reference food (white bread or glucose) and multiplying by 100. The average of the GI ratings from all subjects is published as the GI of that food. Factors that influence the GI value of a food include starch gelatinization, physical entrapment, amylose-to-amylopectin ratio, particle size, viscosity of fiber, acidity, and protein, sugar, and fat content.[1]

A low GI diet can increase insulin sensitivity, help control diabetes, aid weight loss, and lower blood lipids, and may even be of benefit in cancer risk reduction by decreasing insulin-like growth factor hormones. Insulin-like growth factor-1 (IGF-1) has anti-apoptotic and mitogenic effects on various cell types, and raised IGF-1 levels are increasingly being implicated as potential risk factors for cancer.

The glycemic load of a food or meal can be calculated by multiplying the GI value of a food by the amount of carbohydrate per serving and dividing by 100.

Indications for the use of a low glycemic index diet include diabetes, coronary heart disease, obesity, breast cancer, prostate cancer,[2–5] cervical, ovarian, and endometrial cancers,[6] colon cancer,[7] polycystic ovary syndrome,[8–12] hyperinsulinemia, hyperlipidemia, hypertriglyceridemia, appetite control, carbohydrate craving, recurrent yeast infections, weight management, compulsive/binge eating, and depression.[13]

Evidence

The risks of type 2 diabetes and coronary heart disease are strongly related to the GI of the overall diet.[11–16] The World Health Organization (WHO) and Food and Agriculture Organization of the United Nations (FAO) recommend that people in industrialized countries base their diets on low GI foods in order to prevent chronic diseases of affluence, such as coronary heart disease, diabetes, and obesity.[17] A case-control study of dietary glycemic index and glycemic load on breast cancer risk found moderate, direct associations between glycemic index or glycemic load and breast cancer risk, and a possible role of hyperinsulinemia/insulin resistance in breast cancer development.[18] In patients with type 2 diabetes, a low-GI diet lowered the glucose and insulin responses throughout the day and improved the lipid profile and capacity for fibrinolysis.[19]

Diets of differing GIs (low versus high) were investigated to evaluate the effect of GI on overeating in obese adolescent males. Voluntary energy intake after the high GI meal was 53% greater than after the medium GI meal, and 81% greater than after the low GI meal. In addition, compared with the low GI meal, the high GI meal resulted in higher serum insulin levels, lower plasma glucagon levels, lower postabsorptive plasma glucose and serum fatty acids levels, and elevation in plasma epinephrine.[20] The flexible nature of the low GI diet, as compared to the measured carbohydrate exchange ("carbohydrate counting") advocated by the American Diabetes Association and the American Dietetic Association, improves glycosylated hemoglobin (HbA1c) levels without increasing the risk of hypoglycemia, and enhances the quality of life in children with diabetes.[21] Low GI diets improve high-density lipoprotein (HDL) metabolism significantly versus high GI diets in patients with non–insulin-dependent diabetes mellitus.[22]

▶ DIETARY APPROACH TO STOPPING HYPERTENSION DIET

Description

The dietary approaches to stop hypertension (DASH) diet is based on the Dietary Approaches to Stop Hypertension (DASH) study. The DASH diet is low in sodium, saturated fat, cholesterol, and total fat, and is rich in magnesium, potassium, and calcium, as well as in protein and fiber. The diet emphasizes fruits, vegetables, and low-fat dairy foods, and includes whole-grain products, fish, poultry, and nuts, while reducing red meat, sweets, and sugar-containing beverages.

Rationale/Indications

Populations eating mainly vegetarian diets have lower blood pressure levels than do populations eating omnivorous diets, and epidemiologic findings suggest that eating fruits and vegetables lowers blood pressure. The mechanism via which this diet affects blood pressure is unclear. High potassium content, low sodium content, increased fiber, increased calcium, and a number of other mechanisms have been proposed. Most likely, the effect of this dietary approach is mediated through a combination of these factors.

Indications for this diet include systolic hypertension with or without hyperlipidemia, and hyperhomocysteinemia.[23]

Evidence

The DASH study involved 459 adults with systolic blood pressures of less than 160 mm Hg and diastolic pressures of 80–95 mm Hg.[24,25] Twenty-seven percent of the participants had hypertension. Approximately 50% were women and 60% were African Americans. The DASH study compared three eating plans: a plan similar in nutrients to what many Americans consume; a plan similar to what Americans consume but higher in fruits and vegetables; and the DASH diet. All three plans used about 3,000 milligrams of sodium daily. Results were dramatic. Both the fruit and vegetable plan and the DASH diet reduced blood pressure, but the DASH diet had the greatest effect, especially for those with high blood pressure. Overall, blood pressure in the DASH group fell from 146/85 to 134/82 mm Hg. The DASH diet lowered systolic blood pressure significantly in the total group by 5.5/3.0 mm Hg, in African Americans by 6.9/3.7 mm Hg, in whites by 3.3/2.4 mm Hg, in hypertensives by 11.6/5.3 mm Hg, and in nonhypertensives by 3.5/2.2 mm Hg. The fruit and vegetable diet also reduced blood pressure in the same subgroups, but to a lesser extent. The DASH diet lowered blood pressure similarly throughout the day and night. Furthermore, the blood pressure reductions came within 2 weeks of starting the plan.

A second study, called DASH-Sodium, was done. It looked at the effect on blood pressure of a reduced dietary sodium intake as participants followed the DASH diet.[26] DASH-Sodium involved 412 participants. Their systolic blood pressures were 120–159 mm Hg and their diastolic blood pressures were 80–95 mm Hg. Approximately 41% percent had high blood pressure. Approximately 57% were women and 57% were African Americans. Participants were randomly assigned to three sodium levels: 3,300 mg per day (the level consumed by many Americans); 2,400 mg per day; and 1,500 mg per day. The biggest blood pressure reductions were for the 1,500 mg per day level. The researchers concluded that sodium reduction and the DASH diet together may lower blood pressure to an extent not as yet demonstrated for nonpharmacologic treatment.

Also of note, the DASH diet resulted in lower total cholesterol (−0.35 mmol/L, or −13.7 mg/dL), low-density lipoprotein (−0.28 mmol/L, or −10.7 mg/dL), and HDL (−0.09 mmol/L, or −3.7 mg/dL) concentrations (all $P < 0.0001$), without significant effects on triacylglycerol. HDL levels decreased more in participants with higher baseline HDL cholesterol concentrations than in those with lower baseline HDL cholesterol concentrations.

▶ PALEOLITHIC DIET

Description

The Paleolithic diet is also known as the "hunter-gatherer," "stone age," or "evolutionary" diet. In comparison with today's standard Western diet, the Paleolithic diet is characterized by lower total fat and lower saturated fat; a balanced intake of omega-6 and omega-3 essential fatty acids; and small amounts of naturally occurring trans fatty acids contributing less than 2% of dietary energy. The diet is also high in vitamins E and C, calcium, potassium, antioxidants, and fiber, and lower in sodium than the typical Western diet. The Paleolithic diet is richer in animal protein derived from very lean wild meat, with consumption of wild ruminant fat representing the primary lipid source for preagricultural humans. The lipid composition of Paleolithic ruminants is different from today's domesticated grain-fed cattle, with pasture/grass-fed ruminants having a lower polyunsaturated-to-saturated fat ratio and higher omega-3 fatty acid content than grain-fed cattle.[27] The Paleolithic diet is higher in

low-energy density and high-nutrient density uncultivated vegetable foods (excludes starchy vegetables), green leafy vegetables, fruits, and nuts. Sucrose, lactose, and alcohol play no roles. The major food groups that are eliminated are all forms of dairy, grains (whole or otherwise), tubers, and legumes. Processed and refined foods of any sort are eliminated.

Rationale/Indications

Proponents of this dietary pattern postulate that from the emergence of the genus *Homo*, over 2 million years ago, until the agricultural revolution of roughly 10,000 years ago, our ancestors were hunter-gatherers, so the adaptive pressures inherent in that environment have exerted a defining influence on the human genetic makeup. It is thus theorized that a Paleolithic era diet may be the best defense against diseases of affluence. The basic nutritional anthropologic premises are as follows:

1. The human genome was selected in past environments far different from those of the present.
2. Cultural evolution now proceeds too rapidly for genetic accommodation, resulting in dissociation between our genes and our lives.
3. The mismatch between biology and lifestyle fosters development of today's chronic degenerative diseases.[28]

Indications for the use of the Paleolithic diet include obesity, altered glucose tolerance, hyperinsulinemia, non–insulin-dependent diabetes mellitus, hyperlipidemia, and cardiovascular disease.

Evidence

Much of the evidence in support of the Paleolithic diet comes from research examining changes in the health status of traditional indigenous populations that are suddenly or rapidly exposed to a Western diet. For example, cardiovascular disease risk factors dramatically increase in Australian Aborigines when they make the transition from their traditional hunter-gatherer diet to a Westernized diet.[29] When Westernized diabetic Aborigines reverted temporarily to a traditional hunter-gatherer diet, fasting glucose and triglyceride levels fell markedly, glucose tolerance and insulin secretion improved, weight loss occurred, blood pressure decreased, and bleeding time increased.

Kung San men living in the Bushmanland district of Namibia and consuming a traditional hunter-gatherer diet exhibit decreased levels of saliva testosterone when supplementing the diet with domestic and Western food products and alcohol.[30]

A particularly striking example is the case of the Pima Indians. When 168 Pima Indians were studied over 6 years, it was shown that the risk of developing non–insulin-dependent diabetes mellitus for those Pima Indians following an "Anglo" (Westernized) diet was 2.5 times that for the Pima Indians following a traditional Pima diet, after adjusting for age, sex, body mass index, and total calories.[31] For those Pima Indians eating a "mixed" diet (primarily traditional diet supplemented with some Western foods), the risk of non–insulin-dependent diabetes mellitus increased by 1.3 times that of Pima Indians consuming a traditional Pima diet.

▶ SPECIFIC CARBOHYDRATE DIET

Description

The specific carbohydrate diet (SCD) is a low disaccharide diet. All disaccharides and polysaccharides are eliminated. Thus, all lactose-containing dairy, all grains, and all legumes are eliminated. This diet is most commonly applied in the treatment of inflammatory bowel disease (IBD).

Rationale/Indications

The pathophysiologic basis of IBD is thought to involve a hypersensitive cellular immune response to components of the indigenous intestinal flora. Diet influences the nature of the intestinal flora, and several studies show that specific foods can trigger symptoms in patients with both ulcerative colitis and Crohn's disease.

Of the dietary macronutrients—protein, fat, and carbohydrates—carbohydrates have the greatest influence on the intestinal microbes that are believed to be involved in intestinal disorders. Inflammatory bowel disorders, in particular, are thought to involve a hypersensitive cellular immune response to components of the indigenous intestinal flora. The SCD is based on the principle that specifically selected carbohydrates—monosaccharides—requiring minimal digestion are well absorbed, leaving nothing for pathogenic intestinal microbes to feed on. As the microbes decrease because of a lack of food, their harmful by-products also diminish, leading to improvement in gut flora. The mucus-producing cells stop producing excessive mucus, malabsorption decreases, and carbohydrate digestion is improved. In a "vicious cycle" of carbohydrate malabsorption, pathogenic microbes proliferate, altering intestinal pH, disrupting digestion, impairing systemic immunity by their negative interaction with gut-associated lymphoid tissue, and fostering fermentive degradation of certain hard-to-digest foods, leading to mucus in the stool, melena, and steatorrhea. According to SCD proponents, the main dietary culprits are disaccharides, polysaccharides, and other enzymatically resistant carbohydrates found in grains, certain starchy vegetables, certain fruits, table sugar, and lactose-rich dairy products, thus leading to their elimination.

Indications for the SCD include ulcerative colitis, Crohn's disease, irritable bowel syndrome, celiac disease, diarrhea, and digestive disorders of unknown etiology. Proponents of the SCD also advocate it for autistic spectrum disorders and cystic fibrosis.

Evidence

As Hart et al. noted, "The gut flora is a vast interior ecosystem whose nature is only beginning to be unraveled. Lifelong crosstalk between the host and the gut flora determines whether health is maintained or disease intervenes. An understanding of these bacteria–bacteria and bacteria–host immune and epithelial cell interactions is likely to lead to a greater insight into disease pathogenesis."[32]

In a study of carbohydrate expression in the intestinal mucosa, a study of gut-associated lymphoid tissue was undertaken to test the hypothesis that lymphocyte–epithelial interactions influence the glycosylation of cells overlying Peyer patches. The study demonstrated that interactions between diet and flora alter the mucosal architecture and the activity of endocrine cells, and that dietary changes are influential in modifying epithelial mucin predominantly in the small intestine, while the microbial flora influences the mucosal architecture predominantly in the large intestine.[33]

Studies confirm that carbohydrate consumption is significantly higher in patients with IBD than in healthy controls.[34–36] The pathogenetic significance of these findings, however, remains unclear. Patients with Crohn's disease have a higher dietary intake of sucrose, refined carbohydrates, and omega-6 fatty acids, and a reduced intake of fruits and vegetables. In a study of 204 patients with Crohn's disease, 69 were randomized to a low-carbohydrate diet (84 g/d), with 54% gaining benefit for as long as they maintained the diet.[37]

Elemental and exclusion diets are known to be effective in Crohn's disease,[38] lending credence to the inclusion of monosaccharides in the SCD, with exclusion of disaccharides and polysaccharides. In a study of 33 patients with Crohn's disease, 29 patients reported specific food intolerances, and 21 of these remained in remission on diet alone (elimination diet or elemental diet), with the mean length of remission being 15.2 months.[39] The most important foods provoking symptoms were wheat and dairy products.

In a study presented at the Fourth Annual Symposium on Alternative Therapies, 20 patients with Crohn's disease demonstrated a decrease in symptoms and reduction in medication use with the SCD approach.[10] Six patients experienced complete clinical remission, discontinued all medication, and maintained remission for 5 to 80 months.

Although a significant body of research evidence for the SCD in the management of IBD is lacking, anecdotal evidence is overwhelmingly positive. A 6-week trial of this diet should be considered for any patient who is refractory to conventional approaches, who desires a reduction in symptoms or decrease in use of medications, or who has diminished quality of life or activities of daily living on their current management plan.

▶ ANTIINFLAMMATORY DIET

Description

An antiinflammatory diet is characterized by modifying intake in five crucial dietary "categories": fat, sugar, antioxidants, allergenic foods, and antiinflammatory culinary spices.

Dietary fat modifications include increasing omega-3 fatty acids, and decreasing omega-6 fatty acids, saturated fat, and trans fatty acids. Furthermore, polyunsaturated fatty acid–rich vegetable oils should be used only in cold dishes as they are not heat stable, and heating them causes chemical and molecular changes that promote inflammation and carcinogenesis.

Dietary sugar modifications include eliminating foods high in glycemic index, choosing foods low and moderate in glycemic index, and calculating total glycemic load for meals (see Table 7–1). High carbohydrate, highly refined diets, lacking in fiber, increase postprandial insulin levels and indirectly promote inflammation by their effect on essential fatty acid metabolism and prostaglandin synthesis. Dietary antioxidants can be increased through emphasis on yellow–orange–red-colored vegetables and fruits; red–purple–blue-colored vegetables and fruits; dark, leafy greens; cruciferous vegetables; allium vegetables; citrus fruits; and green and black teas.

Known allergenic foods should be avoided, and a trial elimination diet should be considered to rule out food hypersensitivity/allergy for any patient with an inflammatory disorder who also has clinical manifestations of food hypersensitivity/allergy, including symptoms of the gastrointestinal, cutaneous and respiratory systems (see "Elimination Diet").

Finally, research suggests that many common culinary spices exhibit antiinflammatory, analgesic, and thrombolytic activity, such as ginger, rosemary, turmeric, oregano, cayenne, garlic, onion, clove, and nutmeg.[41–45] These culinary spices should be used liberally in the antiinflammatory diet.

Rationale/Indications

Essential fatty acids (EFAs) are beneficial in the prevention and management of heart disease, hypertension, type 2 diabetes, renal disease, ulcerative colitis, Crohn's disease, chronic obstructive pulmonary disease, depression, cystic fibrosis, cancer, menstrual disorders, and pain.[46] Omega-6 EFAs increase inflammation, platelet aggregation, vasospasm, vasoconstriction, cell proliferation, and allergic reactions, and decrease bleeding time. In contrast, omega-3 EFAs are antithrombotic, antiarrhythmic, hypolipidemic, vasodilatory, and antiinflammatory. Omega-6 to omega-3 EFA ratios ideally should be in the 4–1:1 range to mimic that of the Paleolithic diet (1–2:1),[47] the traditional Greek diet of Crete (1:1),[47] the Mediterranean diet (4:1),[48] and the Okinawan diet (1:1),[48] where the population has the highest plasma α-linolenic acid in the world. In contrast, the standard American diet has an omega-6 to omega-3 ratio of 20-30:1.[48]

The omega-6 to omega-3 ratio of the American diet is this high as a consequence of the decrease in saturated fatty acids because of the substitution of omega-6–rich vegetable oils, and because of decreased fish consumption. Additionally, food production of domesticated animals fed omega-6–rich grains versus omega-3–rich grass has altered the tissue lipid composition of meat, resulting in lower omega-3 fatty acids than in grass-fed animals. Farm-raised fish and hen eggs are also lower in omega-3 fatty acids than are wild fish[49] and free-range hen eggs,[50] respectively. The high consumption of packaged foods and the low-fat/fat-free food craze also contributes to the high omega-6 to omega-3 ratios in the standard American diet. An EFA deficiency or imbalanced omega-6 to omega-3 ratio negatively influences prostaglandin synthesis, thereby leading to increased proinflammatory prostaglandin (PG) E_2 series prostaglandins and increases the risk of chronic degenerative diseases. Altered prostaglandin function, such as deficiency of PGE_1 and excess of PGE_2, may play a major role in autoimmunity.[51] Preliminary animal and human research suggests that omega-3 fatty acid–rich fish oil may delay the onset and progression of certain autoimmune diseases.[52–57]

Low GI diet modifications are indicated to minimize the effects of elevated postprandial insulin levels on EFA metabolism. One of the many effects of elevated insulin levels is the upregulation of the enzyme delta-5-desaturase, which converts dihomo-gamma-linolenic acid (DGLA) into arachidonic acid. DGLA is a potent antiinflammatory EFA (converted to PG_1 series prostaglandins), whereas arachidonic acid is a proinflammatory EFA (converted to PG_2 series prostaglandins).

There is ample evidence that allergic disorders, such as asthma, rhinitis, and atopic dermatitis, are mediated by oxidative stress, and that augmenting endogenous antioxidant defenses might be beneficial.[58] It has been demonstrated that low serum levels of antioxidants result in enhanced cytokine production and effects.[59] Free radicals formed during inflammation can be counteracted by a diet high in antioxidants. Studies show arthritic patients to have low levels of vitamins C, E, and other antioxidants.

Clinical experience suggests that many common inflammatory conditions may involve food allergy or sensitivity reactions, and that eliminating these foods may result in improvement.

The antiinflammatory diet is commonly recommended for a wide range of disorders characterized by increased systemic inflammatory activity, including chronic pain syndromes; syndrome X; non–insulin-dependent diabetes mellitus; insulin resistance; autoimmune diseases, particularly rheumatoid arthritis and systemic lupus erythematosus; and allergic disorders.

Evidence

The antiinflammatory diet described previously is a relatively new therapeutic approach and thus has not been well-researched to date. The individual components of the approach—such as the use of omega-3 EFAs in rheumatoid arthritis and other conditions, the impact of low GI diets on insulin metabolism, and the impact of vitamin C and other antioxidant substances on exercise-induced asthma—have been validated in clinical research, and many are discussed elsewhere in this text.

▶ GLUTEN-FREE DIET, GLUTEN-FREE CASEIN-FREE DIET, AND GLUTEN-FREE CASEIN-FREE SOY-FREE DIET

Descriptions

Gluten is a general name given to the storage of proteins (prolamins) present in wheat, rye, barley, and oats. This diet eliminates all foods containing wheat, rye, barley and oats. The specific names of the cereal prolamins that are toxic in celiac disease are gliadin in wheat, secalin in rye, hordein in barley, and avenin in oats. The storage proteins of corn and rice do not contain the toxic cereal prolamins and are not harmful to individuals with celiac disease. Research is underway to determine the safety of oats in a gluten-free diet, but the results are not yet conclusive.

According to WHO/FAO guidelines, a gluten-free food may contain no more than 200-ppm prolamin on a dry weight basis. Foods labeled as gluten-free in the United States and Canada do not allow the presence of any gluten-containing ingredients. Carefully reviewing ingredient lists on food and drug labels to determine if gluten-containing ingredients are present is important. The food manufacturer must be contacted for product information if an ingredient list is not available. Because many additives, stabilizers, and preservatives may contain gluten, it is best to check with each manufacturer for clarification. In addition, some medications, toothpaste, and mouthwashes may contain gluten. Individuals should be advised to check with their physicians or pharmacist before taking any prescribed or over-the-counter medications. The *Compendium of Pharmaceuticals and Specialties* (CPS) contains a list of pharmaceutical manufacturers that do not use gluten as an excipient.

Traditionally, the gluten-free diet is used in the management of celiac disease. In this inherited autoimmune disorder, an immune system response to eating gluten (or more specifically, the storage proteins gliadin and prolamine in gluten) results in damage to the small intestine of people with gluten intolerance. According to the Gluten Intolerance Group of North America, when following a gluten-free diet, the following grains are not allowed: wheat, rye, barley, spelt, triticale, and kamut; and the following grains are allowed: buckwheat, rice, corn, sorghum, amaranth, quinoa, millet, and teff. Label reading for derivatives of the prohibited grains (often used as stabilizers, thickeners, and natural flavorings) is critical to dietary compliance.

Of great debate in the medical and research communities is the acceptability of oats in a gluten-free diet. Oats have traditionally been considered to be toxic to celiacs, but recent scientific studies suggest otherwise, including a

5-year followup study with histologic, histomorphometric, and immunologic methods, and antigliadin antibody (AGA), antireticulin antibody (ARA), and antiendomysial antibody (EMA) serologic test results of those in the oat group that showed no negative effects that could be linked to eating oats.[60] To include oats or not to include oats is a source of ongoing debate among celiac organizations and health care providers who believe it is too early to draw definitive conclusions and make recommendations. There is also concern by the medical and research communities that the level of possible contamination of oats with gluten from unacceptable sources is too high. The Gluten Intolerance Group of North America does not recommend the use of oats by the celiac community, nor does the Celiac Sprue Association of America.

According to the Celiac Sprue Association of America, some patients with celiac disease also have demonstrated toxicity or sensitivities to the following cereals: quinoa, amaranth, teff, buckwheat, and millet. Use of these grains by persons with celiac disease should be determined on the basis of individual tolerance.

Two variants of the gluten-free diet exist in the complementary/alternative medicine community. They are the gluten-free casein-free diet, and the gluten-free casein-free soy-free diet. Both diets are used by integrative medicine providers in the management of autoimmune disorders.

The gluten-free casein-free diet eliminates gluten sources, milk, and the milk protein casein and all products derived from it. All forms of cow's milk, yogurts, and cheeses must be eliminated. Ingredients on food labels that may indicate the presence of casein include casein, sodium caseinate, calcium caseinate, curds, whey, lactose, milk solids, lactalbumin, and lactoglobulin.

The gluten-free casein-free soy-free diet eliminates gluten sources, casein sources, and soy foods including miso, edamame, tofu, soy milk, soy beans, dry-roasted soy "nuts," tempeh, and soy derivatives: lecithin, soy-bean oil, soy curd, soy flour, soy protein isolate, textured vegetable protein, modified food starch, vegetable gum, vegetable oil, vegetable starch, natural flavoring, and hydrolyzed plant protein. See Table 7–2 for gluten-free diet guidelines.

Rationale/Indications

The treatment for celiac disease is the complete elimination of these grains and their by-products from the diet. Risks of untreated celiac disease include gastrointestinal carcinoma or lymphoma. If a person with the disorder continues to eat gluten, studies show that he or she will increase their chances of gastrointestinal cancer by a factor of 40 to 100 times that of the normal population.[61] Because of the broad range of symptoms celiac disease presents, it can be difficult to diagnose. The symptoms can range from "mild weakness, bone pain, and aphthous stomatitis to chronic diarrhea, abdominal bloating, and progressive weight loss."[62] It is this broad range of presenting symptoms that makes a gluten-free diet an acceptable trial diet to assess the contribution of gluten to the severity of any gastrointestinal disorder, or gastrointestinal distress of unknown etiology, that is refractory to conventional treatment. Celiac disease does not just "develop overnight." Prior to the presence of serologic antibodies to gluten (antiendomysial antibody, antigliadin antibody, and tissue transglutaminase) or confirmed intestinal biopsy, there is a "preceliac" stage of subclinical illness, much as there is a "prediabetes" stage marked by increasing insulin resistance prior to abnormal glucose values. Thus the absence of a "positive" test does not necessarily rule out functional impairments in gluten tolerance.

Many providers of integrative medicine recommend a "zero tolerance" approach to evaluation of gluten intolerance, with at least a 3–6-month trial to evaluate for reduction in symptomatic complaints. However, "dietary

Food Products	Foods Allowed	Foods to Question	Foods Not Allowed
Milk Products			
Elimination of casein (milk protein) and soy protein should be considered in conjunction with gluten-free diet or three months after gluten-free diet initiated to evaluate "hypersensitivity" to these two commonly allergenic proteins.	Milk, cream, buttermilk, plain yogurt, cheese, cream cheese, processed cheese. Processed cheese foods, cottage cheese	Milk drinks, flavored yogurt, frozen yogurt, sour cream	Malted milk
Grain Products			
Breads	Bread and baked products made from corn, rice soy, arrowroot, pea flour, corn starch, potato starch, potato flour, whole-bean flour, tapioca, sago, rice bran, cornmeal, buckwheat, millet, flax, teff, sorghum, amaranth, and guinoa		Breads and baked products containing ingredients not allowed: wheat, rye, triticale, barley, oats, wheat germ, wheat bran, graham flour, gluten flour, durum flour, wheat starch, oat bran, bulgur, farina, wheat-based semolina, spelt, and kamut; and imported foods labeled "gluten-free," which may contain ingredients not allowed, e.g., wheat starch
Cereals	*Hot:* Cream of rice, soy cereal, hominy, hominy grits, brown and white rice, buckwheat groats, millet, cornmeal, and quinoa flakes *Cold:* Puffed corn, puffed rice, puffed millet, rice flakes	Rice and corn cereals, rice and soy pablum	Cereals made from wheat, rye triticale, barley, and oats; cereals with added malt extract and malt flavoring
Pastas	Macaroni, spaghetti, and noodles from rice, corn, soy, quinoa, beans, potato, pea, or other allowed flours		Pasta made from wheat, wheat starch, and other ingredients not allowed

Continued

▶ TABLE 7-2 GLUTEN-FREE DIET GUIDELINES (Continued)

Food Products	Foods Allowed	Foods to Question	Foods Not Allowed
Miscellaneous grain products	Corn tacos, corn tortillas	Rice crackers, some rice cakes, and popped corn cake	Wheat flour tacos, wheat tortillas
Meats and Alternatives			
Meat, fish and poultry	Fresh, frozen, canned, salted, and smoked	Prepared or preserved meats, such as luncheon meat, ham, bacon, meat and sandwich spreads, meat loaf, frozen meat patties, sausages, pate, wieners, bologna, salami, imitation meats or fish products, and meat product extenders	Fish canned in vegetable broth containing hydrolyzed vegetable protein (HVP) or hydrolyzed plant protein (HPP) from ingredients not allowed; turkey basted or injected with HVP/HPP
Eggs	Eggs	Eggs substitutes, dried eggs, and egg whites	
Others	Lentils, chickpeas, peas, beans, nuts, seeds, and tofu	Baked beans, dry roasted nuts, and peanut butter	
Fruits and Vegetables			
Fruits	Fresh, frozen, and canned fruit juices	Fruit pie fillings and dried fruits	Scalloped potatoes (containing wheat flour)
Vegetables	Fresh, frozen, dried, and canned	French-fried potatoes (especially those in restaurants)	Battered dipped vegetables
Soups	Homemade broth, gluten-free bouillon cubes, cream soups and stocks made from ingredients allowed	Canned soups, dried soup mixes, soup bases, and bouillon cubes	Soups made with ingredients not allowed; bouillon and bouillon cubes containing HVP or HPP
Fats	Butter, margarine, lard, vegetable oil, cream, shortening, homemade salad dressing with allowed ingredients	Salad dressing and some mayonnaise	Packaged suet

Desserts

Ice cream, sherbet, water, ice whipped toppings, egg, custards, gelatin desserts, cakes, cookies, and pastries made with allowed ingredients	Milk puddings, custard powder, and pudding mixes	Ice cream with ingredients not allowed, cake, cookies, muffins, pies and pastries made with ingredients not allowed, ice cream cones, wafers, and waffles

Miscellaneous

Beverages	Tea (instant or ground), coffee (regular or decaffeinated), cocoa, soft drinks, cider, distilled alcoholic beverages such as rum, gin, whisky, and vodka, wines, and pure liqueurs	Instant tea, coffee substitutes, fruit-flavored drinks, chocolate drinks, chocolate mixes, and flavored and herbal teas	Beer, ale, and lager; cereal and malted beverages
Sweets	Honey, jam, jelly, marmalade, corn syrup, maple syrup, molasses, and sugar (brown and white)	Icing/powdered sugar, spreads, candies, chocolate bars, chewing gum, marshmallows, and lemon curd	Licorice, candies with ingredients not allowed
Snack foods	Plain popcorn and nuts	Dry roasted nuts, flavored potato chips, and tortilla chips	Pizza, unless made with ingredients allowed
Condiments	Plain pickles, relish, olives, ketchup, mustard, tomato paste, pure herbs and spices, pure black pepper, all vinegars, gluten-free soy sauce	Worchestershire sauce, mixed spices and seasonings (e.g., chili powder, curry powder)	Soy sauce (made from wheat), mustard pickles (made from wheat flour), and imitation pepper
Other	Sauces and gravies made with ingredients allowed, pure cocoa, pure baking chocolate, carob chips and powder, chocolate chips, monosodium glutamate (MSG), cream of tartar, baking soda, yeast, brewer's yeast, aspartame, and coconut	Baking powder	Sauces and gravies made from ingredients not allowed such as HVP/HPP, oat gum, and communion wafers

responders" may respond in even shorter periods. Of note, an association between celiac disease and other autoimmune disorders has been described.[62a] Whether the gluten intolerance autoimmune correlation is coincidence or a pathogenic relationship, there is no harm in medically supervised trial(s) of gluten-free, gluten-free casein-free, and gluten-free casein-free soy-free diets.

The use of the gluten-free casein-free and the gluten-free casein-free soy-free diets for autoimmune disorders is based on the premise of "molecular mimicry"—a pathological process wherein structural similarities between external antigen and self components are believed to be a possible cause of autoimmunity, in this instance between tripeptide sequences in gliadin, casein, and, to a lesser extent, soy protein and mammalian tissue tripeptide sequences. One hypothesis for the etiology and pathogenesis of celiac disease lies in the speculation that molecular mimicry between one or more gliadin peptides and some, as yet unidentified, bacterial or viral superantigen plays a role in celiac disease pathogenesis.[63] One study describes the presence of similar structures shared by gliadin and enterocyte surface molecules recognized by antigliadin monoclonal antibodies.[64]

Cow's milk is thought to be an environmental trigger for autoimmune response in type 1 diabetes. In one study aimed at investigating the antibody response to bovine beta-casein in different immune- and non-immune–mediated diseases, significantly increased levels of antibodies to beta-casein were found in patients with type 1 diabetes, celiac disease and in latent autoimmune diabetes in adults compared to age-matched controls.[65]

Common indications for the use of this diet include celiac disease, ulcerative colitis, Crohn's disease, irritable bowel syndrome, autoimmune disorders including insulin-dependent diabetes, Addison's disease, systemic lupus erythematosus, rheumatoid arthritis, alopecia areata, Hashimoto's thyroiditis, autism, and autoimmune myocarditis.

Evidence

The incidence of celiac disease in various autoimmune disorders is increased 10- to 30-fold in comparison to the general population, although in many cases celiac disease is clinically asymptomatic or silent.[66] Patients with celiac disease are at high risk of having other autoimmune disorders, with untreated celiacs having been found to have a higher than expected prevalence of organ-specific autoantibodies. One prospective study of 90 patients with celiac disease found that the prevalence of diabetes and thyroid-related serum antibodies was 11.1% and 14.4%, respectively. Like antiendomysial antibodies, these organ-specific antibodies seem to be gluten-dependent and tend to disappear during adherence to a gluten-free diet.[66a]

In alopecia areata, it has been suggested that antigliadin and antiendomysial antibodies should be included in the workup of patients. Based on this idea, a prospective screening program for celiac disease using antigliadin and antiendomysial antibodies was therefore set up in 256 consecutive outpatients with alopecia areata. Three patients, all completely asymptomatic, were found to be positive and underwent biopsy, confirming the diagnosis of celiac disease. The authors concluded that the association between these two conditions is a real one because the observed frequency of association is much greater than that expected by chance.[66b]

In a study of 14 patients with Hashimoto's thyroiditis without serologic evidence of celiac disease, who underwent immunohistochemical analysis of jejunal biopsies, 43% showed signs of mucosal T-cell activation. The authors concluded that a significant proportion of patients with Hashimoto thyroiditis present signs of "potential celiac disease." In another study of 241 newly diagnosed patients with celiac disease, thyroid disease was found to be threefold higher in patients than in controls ($P < 0.0005$).[66c] The hypothyroidism diagnosed in 13% of the patients was subclinical and of nonautoimmune origin in 9%; autoimmune thyroid disease with euthyroidism was present in 16%. In most patients who strictly followed a 1-year gluten-free diet as confirmed by intestinal mucosa recovery, there was a normalization of subclinical hypothyroidism. Of note, 25% of patients with euthyroid autoimmune disease shifted toward either a subclinical hyperthyroidism or subclinical hypothyroidism; in these subjects, dietary compliance was poor. The authors concluded that in distinct cases of thyroid disease among patients with celiac disease, gluten withdrawal may reverse the abnormality.[67] In an unusual case of a woman diagnosed with Hashimoto's thyroiditis, autoimmune Addison's disease, and karyotypically normal spontaneous premature ovarian failure, an intestinal biopsy confirmed the diagnosis of celiac disease. On a gluten-free diet the patient showed a marked clinical improvement accompanied by a progressive decrease in thyroid and adrenal replacement therapies. After 6 months, serum EMA became negative and after 12 months a new jejunal biopsy showed complete mucosal recovery. After 18 months on a gluten-free diet, the patient's antithyroid antibody titers decreased significantly, and thyroid substitutive therapy was discontinued.[67a]

In an interesting study of 187 patients with autoimmune myocarditis, 4.4% of them were positive for celiac disease, while celiac was observed in 0.3% of 306 normal controls ($P < 0.003$). Of the nine patients with myocarditis, five had myocarditis associated with heart failure, and four had myocarditis with ventricular arrhythmias. The five patients with myocarditis and heart failure received immunosuppression and a gluten-free diet, which elicited recovery of cardiac volumes and function. The four patients with arrhythmia, after being put on a gluten-free diet alone, showed improvement in the arrhythmia. The researchers concluded that a common autoimmune process toward antigenic components of the myocardium and small bowel can be found in >4% of the patients with myocarditis. In these patients, immunosuppression and

a gluten-free diet can be effective therapeutic options.[67b]

The use of gluten-free, gluten-free casein-free, and gluten-free casein-free soy-free diets has been investigated in autistic spectrum disorders, and is a common therapeutic approach among integrative medicine providers. In a small study of children with autistic spectrum disorder (ASD), researchers measured interferon-γ, interleukin-5, and tumor necrosis factor-α against representative dietary proteins, including gliadin from gluten grains, cow's milk protein, and soy by peripheral blood mononuclear cells (PBMCs) from ASD and control children. Also measured was endotoxin (lipopolysaccharide [LPS]), a microbial product of intestinal flora and a surrogate stimulant for innate immune responses. ASD PBMCs produced elevated interferon-γ and tumor necrosis factor-α and increased proinflammatory cytokine responses with endotoxin LPS at high frequency, with positive correlation between proinflammatory cytokine production with LPS and interferon-γ and tumor necrosis factor-α production against dietary proteins. The authors concluded that immune reactivity to dietary proteins may be associated with dietary protein intolerance and gastrointestinal inflammation in children with ASD that may be partly associated with aberrant innate immune response against endotoxin produced by the gut bacteria.[68] In another small study of 36 ASD children in Italy,[69] researchers noticed a marked improvement in the behavioral symptoms of patients after a period of 8 weeks on an elimination diet, and found high levels of immunoglobulin (Ig) A antigen-specific antibodies for casein, lactalbumin, and β-lactoglobulin, and IgG and IgM for casein. The levels of these antibodies were significantly higher than those of a control group of 20 healthy children.

▶ CONCLUSION

Dietary manipulation is a powerful therapeutic tool that plays a critically important role in the integrative approach to health and illness. The therapeutic diets described in this chapter provide a number of examples of specific dietary therapies and their potential applications; there are many more. In practice, the dietary therapies described here are often combined for complex patients. For example, a patient seeing an integrative nutritionist for hypertension and a chronic pain syndrome might be prescribed a diet plan incorporating elements of both the DASH diet and the antiinflammatory diet.

The therapeutic potential of dietary manipulation is greatly underestimated and underused by conventional practitioners, perhaps in part because of a widespread belief that change in diet is too difficult for patients to actually undertake, and so will rarely be successful. Although granting that behavioral change is difficult to achieve and even more difficult to sustain, the integrative model—founded as it is on a belief in the intrinsic healing systems of the human organism—finds nutritional interventions an invaluable tool, which, if applied in the hands of a supportive and sensitive practitioner, can be successful and sustainable in a substantial proportion of patients.

REFERENCES

1. Brand-Miller J, Foster Powell K, Burani JC, Colagiuri S, Wolever TMS. *The New Glucose Revolution.* New York: Marlowe & Co; 2003.
2. Miyata Y, Sakai H, Hayashi T, Kanetake H. Serum insulin-like growth factor binding protein-3/prostate-specific antigen ratio is a useful predictive marker in patients with advanced prostate cancer. *Prostate.* 2003;54(2):125–132.
3. Barnard RJ, Aronson WJ, Tymchuk CN, Ngo TH. Prostate cancer: another aspect of the insulin-resistance syndrome? *Obes Rev.* 2002;3(4): 303–308.
4. Ismail AH, Pollak M, Behlouli H, Tanguay S, Begin LR, Aprikian AG. Insulin-like growth factor-1 and insulin-like growth factor binding protein-3 for prostate cancer detection in patients undergoing prostate biopsy. *J Urol.* 2002;168(6): 2426–2430.
5. Bubley GJ, Balk SP, Regan MM, et al. Serum levels of insulin-like growth factor-1 and insulin-like growth factor-1 binding proteins after

radical prostatectomy. *J Urol.* 2002;168(5): 2249–2252.
6. Druckmann R, Rohr UD. IGF-1 in gynaecology and obstetrics: update 2002. *Maturitas.* 2002;41: 565–583.
7. Giovannucci E. Obesity, gender, and colon cancer. *Gut.* 2002;51(2):147.
8. Legro RS, Kunselman AR, Dodson WC, Dunaif A. Prevalence and predictors of risk for type 2 diabetes mellitus and impaired glucose tolerance in polycystic ovary syndrome: a prospective, controlled study in 254 affected women. *J Clin Endocrinol Metab.* 1999;84(1):165–169.
9. Marshall K. Polycystic ovary syndrome: clinical considerations. *Altern Med Rev.* 2001;6(3): 272–292.
10. Legro RS. Detection of insulin resistance and its treatment in adolescents with polycystic ovary syndrome. *J Pediatr Endocrinol.* 2002;15(suppl 5): 1367–1378.
11. Legro RS. Insulin resistance in polycystic ovary syndrome: treating a phenotype without a genotype. *Mol Cell Endocrinol.* 1998;145(1–2):103–110.
12. Lefebvre P, Bringer J, Renard E, Boulet F, Clouet S, Jaffiol C. Influences of weight, body fat patterning and nutrition on the management of PCOS. *Hum Reprod.* 1997;12(suppl 1):72–81.
13. Moyad MA, Pienta KJ. Mind-body effect: insulin-like growth factor-1; clinical depression; and breast, prostate, and other cancer risk—an unmeasured and masked mediator of potential significance? *Urology.* 2002;59(4 suppl 1):4–8.
14. American Diabetes Association. Dietary fiber, glycemic load, and risk of NIDDM in men. *Diabetes Care.* 1997;20(4):545–555.
15. Dietary fiber, glycemic load, and risk of non-insulin-dependent diabetes mellitus in women. *JAMA.* 1997;277(6):472–477.
16. Liu S, Willett WC. Dietary glycemic load and atherothrombotic risk. *Curr Atheroscler Rep.* 2002; 4(6):454–461.
17. FAO/WHO. Carbohydrates in human nutrition. Report of a joint FAO/WHO expert consultation. Rome, 14–18 April 1997. FAO Food and Nutrition. Paper 66, 1998.
18. Augustin LSA, et al. Dietary glycemic index, glycemic load and ovarian cancer risk: a case study in Italy. *Ann Oncol.* 2003;14(1):78–84.
19. Jarvi AE, Karlstrom BE, Granfeldt, et al. Improved glycemic control and lipid profile and normalized fibrinolytic activity on a low-glycemic index diet in type 2 diabetic patients. *Diabetes Care.* 1999;22(1):10–18.

20. Ludwig DS, Majzoub JA, Al-Zahrani A, et al. High glycemic index foods, overeating, and obesity. *Pediatrics.* 1999;103(3):E26.

21. Gilbertson HR, Brand-Miller JC, Thorburn AW, et al. The effects of flexible low glycemic index dietary advice versus measured carbohydrate exchange diets on glycemic control in children with type 1 diabetes. *Diabetes Care.* 2001;24(7): 1137–1143.

22. Luscombe ND, Noakes M, Clifton PM. Diets high and low in glycemic index versus high monounsaturated fat diets: effects on glucose and lipid metabolism in NIDDM. *Eur J Clin Nutr.* 1999; 53(6):473–478.

23. Anonymous. DASH diet lowers homocysteine levels. *Harv Heart Lett.* 2000;11(3):6–7.

24. Moore TJ, Conlin PR, Ard J, Svetkey LP. DASH (Dietary Approaches to Stop Hypertension) diet is effective treatment for stage 1 isolated systolic hypertension. *Hypertension.* 2001;38(2):155–158.

25. Sacks FM, Appel LJ, Moore TJ, et al. A dietary approach to prevent hypertension: a review of the Dietary Approaches to Stop Hypertension (DASH) study. *Clin Cardiol.* 1999;22(7 suppl): III6–III10.

26. Svetkey LP, Sacks FM, Obarzanek E, et al. The DASH Diet, Sodium Intake and Blood Pressure Trial (DASH-Sodium): rationale and design. DASH-Sodium Collaborative Research Group. *J Am Diet Assoc.* 1999;99(8 suppl):S96–S104.

27. Cordain L, Watkins BA, Florant GL, Keller M, Rogers L, Li Y. Fatty acid analysis of wild ruminant tissues: evolutionary implications for reducing diet-related chronic disease. *Eur J Clin Nutrition.* 2002;56(3):181–191.

28. Eaton SB, Strassman BI, Nesse RM, et al. Evolutionary health promotion. *Prev Med.* 2002;34(2): 109–118.

29. O'Dea K. Cardiovascular disease risk factors in Australian Aborigines. *Clin Exp Pharmacol Physiol.* 1991;18(2):85–88.

30. Christiansen KH. Serum and saliva sex hormone levels in Kung San men. *Am J Physical Anthropol.* 1991;86(1):37–44.

31. Williams DE, Knowler WC, Smith CJ, Hanson RL, Roumain J, Saremi A, Krisska AM, Bennett PH, Nelson RG. The effect of Indian or Anglo dietary preference on the incidence of diabetes in Pima Indians. *Diabetes Care.* 2001;24(5):811–816.

32. Hart AL, Stagg AJ, Frame M, et al. The role of the gut flora in health and disease, and its modification as therapy. *Aliment Pharmacol Ther.* 2002;16(8):1383–1393.

33. Sharma R. Schumacher U. Carbohydrate expression in the intestinal mucosa. *Adv Anat Embryol Cell Biol.* 2001;160:III–IX, 1–91.

34. Persson PG, Ahlbom A, Hellers G. Diet and inflammatory bowel disease: a case-control study. *Epidemiology.* 1992;3(1):47–52.

35. Mayberry JF, Rhodes J, Newcombe RG. Increased sugar consumption in Crohn's disease. *Digestion.* 1980;20(5):323–326.

36. Tragnone A, Valpiani D, Miglio F, et al. Dietary habits as risk factors for inflammatory bowel disease. *Eur J Gastroenterol Hepatol.* 1995;7(1):47–51.

37. Lorenz-Meyer H, Bauer P, Nicolay C, et al. Omega-3 fatty acids and low carbohydrate diet for maintenance of remission in Crohn's disease. A randomized controlled multicenter trial. *Scand J Gastroenterol.* 1996;31(8):778–785.

38. Sanderson IR, Boulton P, Menzies I, Walker-Smith JA. Improvement of abnormal lactulose/rhamnose permeability in active Crohn's disease of the small bowel by an elemental diet. *Gut.* 1987;28(9):1073–1076.

39. Workman EM, Alun Jones V, Wilson AJ, Hunter JO. Diet in the management of Crohn's disease. *Hum Nutr Appl Nutr.* 1984;38(6):469–473.

40. Galland L. Presentation at: Fourth Annual Symposium on Alternative Therapies. New York: Marriott World Trade Center; 28 March 1999.

41. Petersen M, Simmonds MS. Rosmarinic acid. *Phytochemistry.* 2003;62(2):121–125.

42. Katiyar SK, Agarwal R, Mukhtar H. Inhibition of tumor promotion in SENCAR mouse skin by ethanol extract of *Zingiber officinale* rhizome. *Cancer Res.* 1996;56(5):1023–1030.

43. Rao UJ, Lokesh BR. Presence of an acidic glycoprotein in the serum of arthritic rats: modulation by capsaicin and curcumin. *Mol Cell Biochem.* 1997;169(1–2):125–134.

44. Olajide OA, Ajayi FF, Ekhelar AI, Awe SO, Makinde JM, Alada AR. Biological effects of *Myristica fragrans* (nutmeg) extract. *Phytother Res.* 1999;13(4):344–345.

45. Sharma JN, Srivastava KC, Gan EK. Suppressive effects of eugenol and ginger oil on arthritic rats. *Pharmacology.* 1994;49(5):314–318.

46. Simopoulos AP. Essential fatty acids in health and chronic disease. *Am J Clin Nutr.* 1999;70(3): 560S–569S.

47. Simopoulos AP. Evolutionary aspects of omega-3 fatty acids in the food supply. *Prostaglandins Leukot Essent Fatty Acids.* 1999;60(5–6):421–429.

48. Simopoulos AP. Essential fatty acids in health

and chronic disease. *Am J Clin Nutr.* 1999;70(3): 560S–569S.

49. van Vliet T, Katan MB. Lower ratio of n-3 to n-6 fatty acids in cultured than in wild fish. *Am J Clin Nutr.* 1990;51:1–2.

50. Simopoulos AP, Salem N Jr. n-3 fatty acids in eggs from range-fed Greek chickens. *N Engl J Med.* 1989;331:1412.

51. Das UN. Prostaglandins and immune response. *J Assoc Physicians India.* 1981;29(10):831–833.

52. McCarty MF. Upregulation of lymphocyte apoptosis as a strategy for preventing and treating autoimmune disorders: a role for whole-food vegan diets, fish oil and dopamine agonists. *Med Hypotheses.* 2001;57(2):258–275.

53. Venkatraman JT, Chu WC. Effects of dietary omega-3 and omega-6 lipids and vitamin E on serum cytokines, lipid mediators and anti-DNA antibodies in a mouse model for rheumatoid arthritis. *J Am Coll Nutr.* 1999;18(6):602–613.

54. Aug Ergas D, Eilat E, Mendlovic S, et al. n-3 Fatty acids and the immune system in autoimmunity. *IMAJ.* 2002;4(1):34–38.

55. Jolly CA, Muthukumar A, Reddy Avula CP, Fernandes G. Maintenance of NF-kappaB activation in T-lymphocytes and a naive T-cell population in autoimmune-prone (NZB/NZW)F(1) mice by feeding a food-restricted diet enriched with n-3 fatty acids. *Cell Immunol.* 2001;213(2): 122–133.

56. Fernandes G, Troyer DA, Jolly CA. The effects of dietary lipids on gene expression and apoptosis. *Proc Nutr Soc.* 1998;57(4):543–550.

57. Fernandes G. Dietary lipids and risk of autoimmune disease. *Clin Immunol Immunopathol.* 1994;72(2):193–197.

58. Bowler RP, Crapo JD. Oxidative stress in allergic respiratory diseases. *J Allergy Clin Immunol.* 2002;110(3):349–356.

59. Grimble RF. Nutritional modulation of cytokine biology. *Nutrition.* 1998;14(7–8):634–640.

60. Janatuinen EK, Kemppainen TA, Julkunen RJ, Kesmo VM, Maki M, Heikkinen M, Uusitupa MI. No harm from five year ingestion of oats in coeliac disease. *GUT.* 2002;50:332–335.

61. Goggins M, Kelleher D. Celiac disease and other nutrient related injuries to the gastrointestinal tract. *Am J Gastroenterol.* 1994;89(8):S2–S13.

62. Halsted CH. The many faces of celiac disease. *N Engl J Med.* 1996;334(18):1190–1191.

62a. Cuoco L, Certo M, Jorizzo RA, et al. Prevalence and early diagnosis of coeliac disease in autoimmune thyroid disorders. *Ital J. Gastroenterol Hepatol.* 1999;31(4):283–287.

63. Barbeau WE, Novascone MA, Elgert KD. Is celiac disease due to molecular mimicry between gliadin peptide-HLA class II molecule-T cell interactions and those of some unidentified superantigen? *Mol Immunol.* 1997;34(7):535–541.

64. Tuckova L, Tlaskalova-Hogenova H, Farre MA, et al. Molecular mimicry as a possible cause of autoimmune reactions in celiac disease? Antibodies to gliadin cross-react with epitopes on enterocytes. *Clin Immunol Immunopathol.* 1995;74(2): 170–176.

65. Monetini L, Cavallo MG, Manfrini S, et al. Antibodies to bovine beta-casein in diabetes and other autoimmune diseases. *Horm Metab Res.* 2002;34(8):455–459.

66. Kumar V, Rajadhyaksha M, Wortsman J. Celiac disease-associated autoimmune endocrinopathies. *Clin Diagn Lab Immunol.* 2001;8(4):678–685.

66a. Ventura A, Neri E, Ughi C, et al. Gluten-dependent diabetes-related and thyroid-related autoantibodies in patients with celiac disease. *J Pediatr.* 2000;137(2):263–265.

66b. Corazza GR, Andreani ML, Venturo N, et al. Celiac disease and alopecia areata: report of a new association. *Gastroenterology.* 1995;109(4):1333–1337.

66c. Valentino R, Savastano S, Maglio M, et al. Markers of potential coeliac disease in patients with Hashimoto's thyroiditis. *Eur J Endocrinol.* 2002; 146(4):479–483.

67. Sategna-Guidetti C, Volta U, Ciacci C, Usai P, Carolino A, De Franceschi L, Camera A, Pelli A, Brossa C. Prevalence of thyroid disorders in untreated adult celiac disease patients and effect of gluten withdrawal: an Italian multi center study. *Am J Gastroenterol.* 2001;96(3):751–757.

67a. Valentino R, Savastano S, Tommaselli AP, et al. Unusual association of thyroiditis, Addison's disease, ovarian failure and celiac disease in a young woman. *J. Endocrinol Invest.* 1999;22((5):390–394.

67b. Frustaci A, Cuoco L, Chimenti C, et al. Celiac disease associated with autoimmune myocarditis. *Circulation.* 2002;105(22)2611–2618.

68. Jyonouchi H, Sun S, Itokazu N. Innate immunity associated with inflammatory responses and cytokine production against common dietary proteins in patients with autism spectrum disorder. *Neuropsychobiology.* 2002;46(2):76–84.

69. Lucarelli S, Frediani T, Zingoni AM, et al. Food allergy and infantile autism. *Panminerva Med.* 1995;37(3):137–141.

CHAPTER 8

Chiropractic and Osteopathic Care

KAREN ERICKSON, ANTHONY ROSNER, AND FRANCINE RAINONE

Life is the expression of intelligence through matter.

R. W. STEPHENSON (*CHIROPRACTIC TEXTBOOK.* DAVENPORT,
IA: PALMER SCHOOL OF CHIROPRACTIC; 1948)

Integrative health care focuses on how to restore health by the use of diet, supplements, herbs, medications, the mind–body connection, and environmental modifications. Manipulative medicine is concerned with restoring optimal health and well-being by addressing the relationship between the structure and the function of the body. Reestablishing normal structure and function of the neuromusculoskeletal system has a profound effect on optimizing health on many levels.

Evidence of hands-on healing is found in every ancient culture. Ayurvedic, Egyptian, Chinese, Greek, and Native American healing traditions all understood the relationship between the structure and function of the body. Hippocrates describes manipulative techniques in detail in his writings dating back to 400 B.C.[1] In this chapter we discuss two uniquely American healing arts that incorporate some of these ancient healing principles: chiropractic and osteopathy.

Chiropractic and osteopathy are manipulative healing arts that have several commonalities. Both are hands-on therapies that facilitate neuromusculoskeletal and visceral function, improve circulation and lymphatic drainage, release endorphins, reduce stress, and harness the body's own innate healing potential. This chapter focuses on the history, philosophy, education, research, and clinical use of chiropractic and osteopathy.

▶ CHIROPRACTIC CARE

Chiropractic is the third largest health care profession in the United States after medicine and dentistry. It is a patient-centered healing art concerned with restoring and optimizing health by manipulating the relationship between the structure and function of the body, without the use of drugs or surgery. The vitalistic philosophy of chiropractic is based on the "innate" ability of the body to maintain homeostasis and heal itself.

Chiropractic comes from the Greek *praxis* and *chier,* meaning practice or treatment by hand. Chiropractors diagnose, treat, and prevent disorders of the neuromusculoskeletal system. Chiropractic adjustment uses manual treatments to the spine and related structures, including spinal manipulations to *subluxations* of the spine. Chiropractors assign special importance to the synovial joints of the spinal column because unlike other joints, spinal vertebrae house the spinal cord and spinal nerves that coordinate the neurologic function of the body. The definition of a subluxation has evolved over the past 100 years as the scientific basis of joint biomechanics and neurology has become more sophisticated. No longer defined as a static "misalignment of a vertebrae," a subluxation or a subluxation complex is now characterized by an abnormal biomechanical function of a joint and its associated structures including muscle, ligaments, bone, nerve, and discs. Subluxations can be characterized by reduction in normal joint motion; inflammation, muscle spasm and pain; and changes in motor control. Vertebral subluxations are believed to cause interference with the proper function of the nervous system, which can limit the body's innate ability to maintain homeostasis and heal. Chiropractors assert that the restoration of proper function to the joints and associated structures, not solely the reduction of pain, is the ultimate clinical goal of chiropractic care.

Chiropractic techniques embody many adjusting styles. Some involve the "traditional" precisely applied high-velocity–low-amplitude adjustment to a synovial joint, in which a "release" sound is heard. Other techniques are low force or nonforce and have the same goal of restoring normal neuromusculoskeletal function, including joint range of motion, and reducing pain, inflammation, and myospasm. Some chiropractic techniques are appropriate for lumbar disc herniations; other approaches incorporate cranial adjusting techniques. Specific, nonforce, chiropractic adjustment techniques are appropriate for all patients, but can be especially helpful to patients for whom traditional osseous manipulation might be contraindicated such as infants; women with osteoporosis; high-risk pregnancy; and patients with bleeding disorders, bone fractures, or metastases. In addition to vertebral adjustments, chiropractors use many natural noninvasive treatments, including soft-tissue therapies such as massage, physical therapy modalities, craniosacral therapy, nutrition, exercise and rehabilitation programs, stress reduction, lifestyle modification, orthotics, and orthopedic support braces. Increasingly health care providers of all types are becoming more educated about the range of chiropractic techniques and the evidence basis for its use for a wide variety of clinical conditions.

Chiropractic was founded in 1895 by D. D. Palmer in Davenport, Iowa. He and his son, B. B. Palmer, developed chiropractic into a formal profession with Chiropractic Colleges, a distinct philosophy of health, and a continuously strengthening clinical rationale. According to the World Federation of Chiropractic based in Toronto, Canada, there are now 65,000 doctors of chiropractic practicing in the United States alone. There are 6,000 chiropractors in Canada and 90,000 internationally.[2] In many parts of the world, the potential for chiropractic to relieve suffering is great. Because it relies on manual therapy, chiropractic is "low tech," with a relatively low overhead and cost.

The growing sophistication of chiropractic education and research in the past 20 years has ushered chiropractic into a more respectful relationship with mainstream medicine. There are now many examples of physician–chiropractor collaborations at hospitals and institutions, as well as in private group practices. Another emerging trend is the establishment of doctors of chiropractic as "gatekeepers" for insurance companies. Chiropractic also brings its patient-centered, hands-on, holistic healing philosophy to the emerging integrative paradigm.

Chiropractic Education and Licensing

In the United States, admission to chiropractic college requires an undergraduate education that includes successful completion of courses in biology, general chemistry, organic chemistry, physics, psychology, English/communications, and the humanities. A chiropractic college curriculum consists of four or five academic years with at least 4,200 hours of supervised classroom, laboratory, and clinical experience. During the first 2 years, classroom and laboratory work focus on basic sciences, such as anatomy, physiology, public health, microbiology, pathology, and biochemistry. The second 2 years stress courses in manipulation and spinal adjustments, and provide clinical experience in physical and laboratory diagnosis, neurology, orthopedics, geriatrics, pediatrics, gynecology, physiotherapy, radiology, and nutrition. Different schools stress varying amounts of chiropractic philosophy.

Standards for chiropractic education have been established by the Commission on Accreditation of the Council on Chiropractic Education (COA-CCE) since 1974. The CCE monitors curriculum, faculty, staff, facilities, patient care, and research and is recognized by the US Department of Education and the Council for Higher Education Accreditation as the specialized accrediting agency for chiropractic education. Table 8–1 lists the 16 chiropractic programs and institutions in the United States

▶ **TABLE 8–1** ACCREDITED COLLEGES OF CHIROPRACTIC IN THE UNITED STATES

Cleveland Chiropractic College—Kansas City
Cleveland Chiropractic College—Los Angeles
Life University College of Chiropractic
Life Chiropractic College West
Logan College of Chiropractic
National University of Health Sciences
New York Chiropractic College
Northwestern Health Sciences University
Palmer College of Chiropractic
Palmer College of Chiropractic—West
Parker College of Chiropractic
Sherman College of Straight Chiropractic
Southern California University of Health Sciences (formerly LACC)
Texas Chiropractic College
University of Bridgeport College of Chiropractic
Western States Chiropractic College

accredited by the CCE. Ten of the 16 colleges were established prior to 1945. Graduates who successfully complete their requirements receive a Doctor of Chiropractic degree (DC). Licensing boards require that graduates receive their DC from an accredited chiropractic college.

The practice of chiropractic is licensed and regulated in all 50 states and in the District of Columbia in the United States, and in more than 30 countries worldwide. State licensing boards regulate the education, experience, and moral character of candidates for licensure, and protect the public health, safety, and welfare. The National Board of Chiropractic Examiners (NBCE), established in 1963, maintains consistency and fairness among state licensing boards. The NBCE administers the national board examination, which is necessary to pass for practice as a chiropractor. The examination is divided into four parts covering basic sciences, clinical sciences, clinical competency, and practical skills. Most state boards rely on all or part of the NBCE examination for licensure. State examinations may supplement the NBCE tests, depending on individual state requirements. Chiropractors can only practice in states in which they are licensed.

As with MDs, most states require DCs to complete a specified number of hours of continuing education each year to maintain licensure. Some chiropractic associations offer extensive postgraduate programs leading to "diplomate" certification in clinical specialties such as orthopedics, neurology, sports injuries, occupational and industrial health, nutrition, diagnostic imaging, internal disorders, and pediatrics.

Chiropractic is an emerging force in health care internationally. There are chiropractic schools in Canada, Australia, England, France, and Denmark, as well as in Brazil, Japan, Korea, New Zealand, South Africa, and Wales. Some schools in these countries have reciprocal agreement status with the United States CCE, which imposes the highest standards for chiropractic education and licensing in the world.

► CHIROPRACTIC CARE FOR SPECIFIC CONDITIONS

Low Back Pain

Clinical Trials

More than 50 clinical trials on spinal manipulation for low back pain can be identified to date; in 1992, Shekelle et al. reviewed 25 of these trials,[3] and Bronfort reviewed an additional 9 in 1997,[4] with the balance reviewed thereafter. The earlier trials—many of which were seriously flawed in their design—tended to suggest only short-term benefits for spinal therapy, eliciting a widespread belief from many quarters that spinal manipulative therapy was beneficial in the alleviation of acute pain, but that there existed insufficient documentation of its efficacy with chronic pain.[5–7] More recent studies would seem to indicate a role for chiropractic in treating chronic low back pain as well.

Beginning with the publication of a prospective study by Kirkaldy-Willis and Cassidy in 1985,[8] and continuing through the landmark *New England Journal of Medicine* study in 1998, there has been a consistent overall trend suggesting that the improvement in acute low back pain produced by manual therapy at least equals that achieved by standard medical treatment, but without the potential side effects of conventional medications.

Probably one of the most important current trends is that, in contrast to some of the earlier trials in which the relief provided by spinal manipulation appeared to be short-lived (less than 3 weeks),[9–11] some of the more recent larger trials demonstrate that the beneficial effects of spinal manipulative therapy are uniquely *long* lived, persisting for as long as 12 months[12–14] to 3 years.[15]

Several systematic reviews and meta-analyses have added to the body of literature on chiropractic for low back pain. In Anderson et al.'s study of 23 randomized clinical trials, in most cases, spinal manipulative therapy was compared to alternative therapies rather than to true no-treatment placebos. Although the effectiveness of spinal adjustments per se could not be clearly evaluated, they consistently proved more effective in the treatment of low-back pain than any of the comparative interventions.[16] Shekelle et al.'s meta-analysis retrieved 58 articles representing 25 trials and supported the short-term benefit of spinal manipulation in some patients, particularly those with uncomplicated, acute low back pain. Data regarding *chronic* low-back pain at the time of this publication were judged insufficient to evaluate the efficacy of spinal manipulation in managing this particular condition.[17]

Over the 9 years since this meta-analysis was done, a significant body of literature has accumulated supporting the use of spinal manipulation in managing chronic low-back pain. However, controversy remains regarding this literature. In a systematic review by van Tulder and colleagues of 16 randomized controlled trials involving manipulation, the evidence supporting manipulation for chronic low-back pain is found to be actually *stronger* than that for acute conditions. This conclusion, however, was based largely on findings from only 2 of the 16 studies, which were the only studies deemed of sufficient quality to draw conclusions. A somewhat different interpretation was reached in Bronfort's systematic review.[18] Here, the evidence supporting spinal manipulation for managing either acute or chronic low-back pain was judged to be "moderate," while that for a *mix* of chronic and acute low-back pain was considered to be "inconclusive." Yet another systematic review of randomized clinical trials cites adequate follow-up periods, avoidance of cointerventions, and avoidance of dropouts as frequent strengths in the manipulation literature; significant recurrent weaknesses, however, include randomization procedures, sample sizes, and blinded assessments of outcomes—the latter being virtually impossible to perform in a trial involving manual therapy.[19] Finally, a meta-analysis of 51 literature reviews of spinal manipulative therapy suggests that, although the overall methodologic quality was low, 9 of the 10 methodologically best reviews reached positive conclusions regarding spinal adjustments.[20,21]

Government agencies in the United States,[22] Canada,[23] Great Britain,[24] Sweden,[25] Denmark,[26] Australia,[27] and New Zealand[28] have all done evaluations of the evidence for manipulation as treatment for back pain and reached very similar conclusions. For example, according to the assessment of back pain treatment by the Agency for Health Care Policy and Research, the strength of the evidence found to support manipulation was rated sufficiently high to place this intervention among the first of two options (together with the use of analgesics and nonsteroidal antiinflammatory drugs), to be considered from 22 different types of interventions reviewed.[29] The British guidelines stated that "there is considerable evidence that manipulation can provide short-term symptomatic benefits" in certain patients,[24] while the Danish report echoed this sentiment by declaring that "manual treatment can be recommended for patients suffering from acute low-back symptoms and functional limitations of more than 2–3 days duration."[30]

One final area deserving mention in terms of the research on chiropractic treatment for back pain is the area of patient satisfaction. For matched conditions dealing with back pain, patient satisfaction with chiropractic treatment is invariably greater than that with conventional management (i.e., administered by a primary care physician, an orthopedist, or an HMO provider).[31,32] Satisfied patients are far more likely to be compliant in their treatment,[33] theoretically giving chiropractic patients an advantage over those of other therapists in terms of their outcomes.

The RAND Appropriateness and Utilization Study

Several years and millions of dollars in the making, the RAND Appropriateness and Utilization Study has sought to provide "a comprehensive set of indications for performing spinal manipulation with low back pain," the guidelines being based upon (1) a review of the literature, (2) appropriateness ratings by both multidisciplinary and all-chiropractic panels of experts, and (3) field studies abstracted from five geographical sites.

The literature review of 67 articles and 9 books published between 1952 and 1991 established that chiropractors within the United States performed 94% of all the manipulative care for which reimbursement was sought, with osteopaths delivering 4% and general practitioners and orthopedic surgeons accounting for the remainder.[31] The conclusions of this report were that the use of spinal manipulation is an effective treatment for patients with acute low-back pain and an absence of other signs or symptoms of lower limb nerve-root involvement. The evidence regarding efficacy of manipulation when lower limb neurologic findings or sciatica was present was conflicting. There was no systematic report on the frequency of complications.

Lumbar Disc Herniation

The currently available options for treating disc herniations are surgery or conservative care, the latter often involving spinal manipulation. There are no controlled trials to date directly comparing these two options.

Two randomized trials currently support the wisdom of considering spinal manipulation as a treatment option for this condition. One study involving 51 cases of myelographically confirmed disc herniation compared rotational mobilization to conventional physical therapy (e.g., diathermy, exercise, and postural education). The manipulation group demonstrated greater improvement in range of motion and straight leg raising compared to the physical therapy cohort, leading Nwuga to conclude that manipulation was superior to conventional treatment.[35]

The second trial examined 40 patients with unremitting sciatica diagnosed as caused by lumbar disc herniation with no clinical indication for surgical intervention. Subjects were randomized into two treatment groups:

chemonucleolysis (chymopapain injection under general anesthesia) and manipulation (15-minute treatments over 12 weeks, including soft-tissue stretching, low-amplitude passive maneuvers of the lumbar spine, and the judicious use of side-posture manipulations). Back pain and disability were appreciably lower in the manipulated group at 2 and 6 weeks with no improvement or deterioration in the chemonucleolytic group. By 12 months there were improvements in both groups, with a tendency toward superiority in the manipulated cohort. Costs of treatment in the manipulated group were less than 30% of that encountered by the injected patients.[36]

Further support for manipulation in the treatment of disc herniations is provided from several prospective studies.[37–41] The largest involved 517 patients who were diagnosed with lumbar disc protrusion, 77% of these having favorable response from pain after manipulative therapy. A literature review from Cassidy et al.[42] suggests that an additional 14 of 15 patients with lumbar disc herniations experienced significant relief from pain and experienced clinical improvement after a 2- to 3-week course of side-posture manipulation.

The safety of rotational manipulation in the treatment of lumbar disc herniations is supported by Cassidy et al., who dispute the assertion by Farfan and colleagues that rotational stress causes disc failure. This is because their work demonstrates that, in rotation, normal discs withstand an average of 23 degrees and degenerated discs an average of 14 degrees rotation before failure.[43] However, posterior facet joints limit rotation to only 2 to 3 degrees and would have to fracture to allow further rotation to occur;[44] any disc failures produced experimentally by torsion are caused by peripheral tears in the annulus, rather than by prolapse or herniation.

Neck Pain and Upper Extremity Disorders

In addition to addressing manipulation as a treatment for low-back pain, the RAND study also included an extensive literature review and a multidisciplinary panel appropriateness study for cervical spine and upper extremity disorders. The RAND review suggested that manipulation or mobilizations gave short-term pain relief and enhancement of range of motion for chronic or subacute neck pain. However there was a paucity of data on acute neck pain in the literature.[45,46]

In chronic and subacute neck pain, there is evidence in the literature of a trend toward improvement in pain after adjustment or manipulation. In a study of 100 subjects with unilateral neck pain with referral into the trapezius, Cassidy et al. noted that 85% of the manipulated group and 69% of the mobilized group reported pain improvement. The decrease in pain intensity was more than 1.5 times greater in the manipulated patients.[47] Another study receiving high ratings for chronic and subacute neck and back pain together showed that improvements in the severity of pain were greater for manipulation than for physical therapy; for neck pain only, the mean improvement in neck pain after manipulation was greater than for the physical therapy group, as shown by the visual analog scale.[48] Most chiropractors report that spinal adjustments are helpful in whiplash injuries, although more research in this area is needed.

Because chiropractic techniques restore normal joint range of motion, the application of manipulation for acute whiplash is in keeping with the current concept that mobility early in care—as opposed to the immobilization recommended in earlier times—more effectively restores the structure and function of the cervical spine after whiplash injury. Morphologically, immobilization of the neck following soft-tissue injury of muscles, joint capsules and ligaments causes scar formation or adhesions. Restoring motion to the spine and soft tissues following injury produces improved collagen concentration, which is superior to scar tissue. Improved tensile strength occurs when proper rehabilitation takes place after injury.[49–51]

Carpal tunnel syndrome (CTS), and a number of other repetitive-stress syndromes of the upper extremity, are often responsive to manipulation. Studies of CTS show that adjustment to the wrist reduced pressure on the transverse carpal ligament resulting in measurable improvements including decreased pain, improved electrical conduction on electromyelogram, and magnetic resonance image changes revealing increased anteroposterior and transverse dimensions of the carpal canal after treatment.[52,53a,53b] Although steroid injections may provide more rapid pain reduction in some severe cases, patients who underwent manipulation in one study ($N = 22$) showed that decreased pain levels were sustained at a 6 month follow-up.[54]

Headache

The International Headache Society classifies headaches into three types: cervicogenic, tension, and migraine/other headaches.

Cervicogenic headaches are most commonly caused by injury or trauma to the neck. Frequently, this is caused by motor vehicle accidents and subsequent whiplash injuries. Other causes are sports injuries, adult and childhood falls, and repetitive stress injuries. Additionally, degenerative joint disease can be a significant cause of cervicogenic headache. Diagnosis of cervicogenic headache is based upon a normal neurologic examination and the patient's description of the headache.

A number of studies strongly favor chiropractic care for cervicogenic headaches. A randomized controlled trial in 1995 compared patients receiving chiropractic treatments to a control group receiving massage and low-level laser treatments.[55] This study showed that chiropractic care decreased headache intensity, analgesic use, and frequency. A second study showed improved headache scores: headache intensity diminished to 40% of pretreatment levels, frequency was reduced to 39% of pretreatment levels, and duration was reduced to 23% of the original value.[56] Vernon's review of manipulation for headaches found it to be an effective therapy.[57] The systematic review by Bronfort et al., in 2001,[58] concludes that spinal manipulative therapy has a comparable effect to the first-line prophylactic prescription medications for tension and migraine headaches, and is more efficacious than massage for treatment of cervicogenic headache.

Tension headache is the most common type of headache, experienced by an estimated 60–70% of the population in any given year. Some clinicians feel that muscle spasm in the shoulder, neck, and head are the cause of tension headaches. It is believed that for many patients, neurotransmitter imbalance or stress may also contribute to tension headache. The diagnosis of tension headache is based on the patient's description of the headache and a normal neurological examination. Pain is usually bilateral, and there is a pressing or squeezing feeling around the head. There are tight neck and shoulder muscles. Photophobia may also be present. There are overlaps in symptomatology between tension and cervicogenic headache in some cases.

Chiropractic care can be extremely helpful for tension headache patients. Spinal manipulation restores normal range of motion, relaxes muscle spasm, and reduces local inflammation. Additionally, chiropractors may use soft-tissue therapies such as massage, ultrasound, manual distraction, and lifestyle modifications, including stress management and diet. Chiropractic care generally reduces the frequency, length, and severity of headaches.

In a 1995 study, a group of 70 patients receiving chiropractic care for tension headache were compared to a cohort of 56 patients who were treated with amitriptyline over the same period.[59] Four outcome measures showed chiropractic care was statistically favorable: frequency, pain intensity, over-the-counter medication use, and general health. Most importantly, the chiropractic patients sustained these improvements after the treatment period, whereas the headaches of the medically treated patients returned when the medication was withdrawn.[59a]

Migraine headache affects nearly 11 million adults in the United States. As with tension headache, the research on migraine shows a positive response to chiropractic adjustments with reductions in frequency, duration, and intensity.[60] Other studies show a decrease in motion restriction, dizziness, and pain.[61,62] Nelson et al. compared the treatment of three groups: one receiving chiropractic care, one receiving amitriptyline, and the third receiving both treatments. The 8-week study showed improvement in outcomes in all three groups over time, but the chiropractic groups seemed to maintain the improvement into the 4-week posttreatment period. There was no advantage to using the medication and chiropractic together; chiropractic alone was just as effective.[63]

Aerobic exercise, stretching, and proper ergonomic support and posture are important parts of headache management. Cradling a telephone with the neck and shoulder or having a poor computer set-up can, over time, become a headache trigger. Bed pillows that are too thick or thin, or stomach sleeping with head rotated to the side, can also contribute to cervicocranial structural imbalances that might be a contributing trigger to a headache. Clenching or grinding teeth at night may cause temporomandibular joint dysfunction and myospasm of the masseter and temporal muscles, which can be a trigger for headaches.

► CHIROPRACTIC AND VISCERAL DISORDERS

With the widening acceptance of chiropractic care for musculoskeletal dysfunction in the eyes of medical researchers and managed care administrators, there is a tendency to overlook the somatovisceral research on chiropractic. All chiropractors have had the experience of having patient's visceral or nonmusculoskeletal symptoms resolve while they were receiving concurrent chiropractic care. Chiropractors are carefully trained to differentially diagnose, re-

> *. . . So much depends in each case on the structural factors, the type of patient, and the competence of the practitioner, but it is still true as ever, whatever the patient's disease, that he will have a better chance of recovery if he is mechanically sound. . . . Mechanical lesions are etiological in many diseases because the lesions weaken those viscera which are reflexly and segmentally linked with them.*
>
> A. STODDARD (*MANUAL OF OSTEOPATHIC PRACTICE*. 2ND ED. LONDON, ENGLAND: HUTCHINSON & CO, 1983)

fer to medical specialists, and comanage patients with physicians. Clearly, when treating serious visceral symptoms, patients should have prior or concurrent medical evaluation and/or supervision.

There is a tradition of research on the visceral effects of chiropractic care dating back to the founding of chiropractic care. There is a growing consensus that restoring normal function to spinal joints can effect somatovisceral reflex arcs that control organ function.[64] Currently, the Federation for Chiropractic Education and Research supports research on many visceral disorders.

Integrative health care tends to explore the subtle interrelationships between a person and their many health issues. This whole-person approach has been a cornerstone of chiropractic philosophy. How does low-back dysfunction relate to postmenstrual stress or inflammatory bowel syndrome? Does poor posture cause musculoskeletal problems alone, or could it contribute to the onset of cardiac arrhythmias, digestive disturbances, or poor immune response? Are there other biological markers that are changed by chiropractic adjustments? These are areas that are ripe for future research.

Sinusitis

Although there are many etiologies of sinusitis, we have found that chiropractic care and cranial adjusting techniques are extremely helpful at reducing symptoms and bringing this often painful condition to resolution more quickly. Etiology may include bacterial, viral, and fungal causes, anatomic anomalies, such as deviated septum, and turbinate anomaly or pathology. Adjusting the spine, particularly the upper cervical, and the cranium improves sinus drainage and lymphatic flow. Ancillary techniques, such as craniopathy, sinus reflex point stimulation, temporomandibular joint work, suboccipital and trapezius myofascial release or trigger point work, lymphatic massage, and the use of essential oils, such as eucalyptus and others, may be helpful.

Two studies show that joint manipulation and endonasal- and nasal-specific techniques, as well as physiotherapy and nutrition, all of which are employed by chiropractors, can be useful adjuncts or alternatives to common medical treatments for sinusitis.[65,66]

Asthma and Chronic Obstructive Pulmonary Disease

Research on chiropractic care for asthma has not consistently shown efficacy. It seems that some people respond extremely well, whereas other patients do not have relief of symptoms. The key is to determine which patients are most likely to respond, and this should be the direction of future research. Asthma is characterized by recurrent inflammation, and smooth-muscle spasm of the medium and small bronchi in the lungs, causing difficulty in breathing. Many factors may trigger such a reaction, including environmental allergens such as mold, pollen, dust mites, cigarette smoke, and pollution, as well as exercise and respiratory infection. Other factors, such as stress, emotion, and diet, may also play a role in the hypersensitivity that the body develops to these triggers. The underlying causes of these sensitivities may include neurologic or physiologic imbalance.

Chiropractors call the dysfunction of a vertebral segment motion and the attending nerve irritation and intrinsic muscle spasm at the level of dysfunction a *vertebral subluxation complex* (VSC). The chiropractic model for treatment of asthma looks at the mechanical and neurological imbalances that may be a cause or contributing factor in asthma. The clinical rationale is that in some patients, restricted movement of spinal joints causing a VSC can compromise the proper function and regulation of the autonomic nervous system, thus affecting the chest wall and airway function. Chiropractic adjustment of the vertebral subluxation restores normal mechanical function and corrects the neurological dysregulation which may be an underlying cause of hypersensitivity in some patients. Studies done by Miller on 44 patients with chronic obstructive pulmonary disease (COPD) showed that the most frequent abnormal spinal function was found at T2–5. The conclusion of this study was that the treatment group that received manipulation did not experience a statistically significant improvement in lung volume over the control group; in fact, both treatment and control groups improved. Patients in the treatment group reported subjective improvements, including less coughing, less dyspnea, fewer colds, and the ability to walk greater distances.[67] Havid reported manipulation improved peak expiratory flow rates and vital capacity for asthmatics,[68] but Balon et al.[69] and Bronfort et al.[70] found only subjective improvements in dyspnea and less dependence on medication. Sham procedures that are "hands-on" and too closely mimic manipulation techniques constitute a troublesome design flaw in many studies. A new major study is underway in Australia that hopes to shed more light on this topic.[71]

Masarsky and Weber theorize that vertebral subluxation complex may "increase the work of breathing before frank obstruction develops. By the same token, correction of the VSC may reduce the physiologic cost of deep breathing before any measurable improvement in volume occurs, especially in cases of chronic pulmonary disease. Therefore, unlike pain, at the current state of the art, dyspnea may be an early indicator, while objective respiratory measurements may be lagging indicators."[71] In addition to addressing subluxation, a chiropractor working with a patient with chronic respiratory issues often uses other techniques, including myofascial release of the trapezius, rhomboid, sternocleidomastoid, scalene, and pectoral muscles; manual pressure to the shiatsu lung points; and craniosacral therapy with special emphasis on respiratory diaphragm, thoracic inlet, and suboccipital regions.

The process of breathing involves an elegant blend of somatovisceral function. It is prudent to evaluate cervical and thoracic function in patients with asthma and COPD to determine if manipulation may improve symptoms by normalizing vertebral function and autonomic regulation.

Digestive Disorders

Chiropractic can play a role in addressing various digestive symptoms including colic, constipation, duodenal ulcer, and irritable bowel syndrome (IBS).[72] Because the digestive tract has a diverse distribution of innervation, it often is a good indicator of autonomic disturbance.

Although trials to date are somewhat equivocal as a consequence of methodologic weaknesses, anecdotal clinical experience supports the effectiveness of chiropractic care for infantile colic. Colic is described as persistent, rigorous crying for no apparent reason in an otherwise healthy and thriving infant. It usually begins at weeks 1–4 of age, and resolves at 3 months of age. The source of pain is unclear, but assumed to be digestive or spinal. The hypothesis for the role of manipulation in treating colic is that adjusting vertebral subluxation complexes modulates the normal function of the autonomic nervous system and improves both digestive function and nervous system

function overall. It is not fully understood why some babies have vertebral subluxations, but certainly difficult pregnancies, labors, or births could be a contributing factor. The research literature on chiropractic manipulation for colic is reviewed in Chapter 31.

Three studies demonstrated the ability of chiropractic manipulation to help the remission or healing of duodenal ulcers.[73–75] In one study, 16 patients with spinal dysfunction and duodenal ulcer confirmed by endoscopic examination were manipulated (most frequently in the T9–12 region) for 3 weeks. They showed ulcer remission in 16.4 days. This was 10 days earlier, or 40% faster, than in the control group of 40 patients, who received a standard medication and dietary regimen for 4–7 weeks.[73] Basic science research by DeBoer et al. suggested a possible mechanism for the role of manipulation in treating ulcers. DeBoer et al. showed that a surgically induced misalignment of T6 produced inhibited duodenal and stomach smooth muscle function in rabbits.[76]

Although clinical trials for treatment of constipation with chiropractic are lacking to date, many clinicians believe that spinal adjustments can effectively treat severe constipation in both adults and children. There are two published case reports supporting the role of manipulation in the alleviation of constipation.[77,78] In addition to addressing the VSC that may be impinging on proper digestive function, many chiropractors use soft tissue techniques, such as gentle pressure on the ileocecal and Houston valves, and myofascial release on the iliotibial bands, which is a neurolymphatic reflex muscle for the large intestine, as adjunctive measures to help stimulate peristalsis.

Otitis Media

In addition to the classic signs and symptoms, children with otitis media, upon chiropractic examination, are often found to have a subluxation or fixation of the occiput, atlas, and axis. Cranial palpation often reveals a restriction in movement in the temporal, occiputital, and/or parietal bones. In infants and toddlers eustachian tubes are still horizontal and vulnerable to accumulation of fluid. It is believed that osseous adjusting and soft tissue techniques, including craniosacral therapy, sinus reflex points, and lymphatic massage help drain the eustachian tubes. In one of the best studies, Fallon looked at the role of chiropractic care for 332 children between the ages of 27 days and 5 years who had otitis media.[79] This study demonstrated that nearly 80% of the children treated were free of ear infections for at least the 6-month follow-up period, which included maintenance treatments every 4–6 weeks. Other studies show chiropractic to improve the condition of up to 93% of children with otitis media.[80–82] It is thought that by restoring joint and neurophysiologic function to the occipital–atlas junction and upper cervical spine, manipulation enables the eustachian tubes and lymphatic system to drain more effectively.

► SAFETY ISSUE/ADVERSE EFFECTS OF CHIROPRACTIC CARE

As with any therapeutic intervention, complications, however rare, do occur in the course of chiropractic manipulation. The two primary complications that have been reported are (1) cauda equina syndrome following manipulation in patients with lumbar disc herniation, consisting of neurogenic bowel and bladder disturbances, saddle anesthesia, bilateral leg weakness, and sensory changes, and (2) cerebrovascular accidents (CVAs) as the result of cervical manipulations.

The symptoms of cauda equina syndrome have been described extensively.[83] A review of the worldwide medical literature indicates that 16 of the 26 reported cases occurred with the far more vigorous manipulation applied under anesthesia. Of the remaining 10 cases, only 4 have been reported in North America.[84] Estimates of the frequency of cauda equina syndrome range from 2 per million[85] to 1 per 100 million adjustments.[86]

As established by researchers from both the medical and chiropractic professions, the risk of CVA following manipulation is somewhere between 2 and 4 per million adjustments[87,88] and one case per 5.85 million treatments.[89] The more recent data from the RAND Corporation suggests the rate of vertebrobasilar accident or other complications (cord compression, fracture, or hematoma) to be 1.46 per million manipulations, with the rates of serious complications and death from cervical spine manipulation estimated to be 0.64 and 0.27 per million manipulations, respectively.[90]

Interestingly, in a comprehensive review of 107 known cases of CVA, nearly a third were reported to have involved care by practitioners other than chiropractors.[91] In addition, in clinics representing highly trained practitioners from at least one major chiropractic college performing more than 5 million manipulations over the past 15 years, not a single CVA case has been reported.[92]

It would appear that any head movement that produces occlusion of a vertebral artery in cases in which the flow in the contralateral artery is already compromised has the potential to lead to a CVA. Thus, it is no surprise that a large variety of *non*-manipulative movements of the head are reported to be associated with CVAs, the occurrence of which may be no less frequent than those receiving cervical manipulations. These nonmanipulative movements include yoga,[93] calisthenics,[94] overhead work,[95] turning the head while driving a car,[96,97] stargazing,[98] archery,[99] and bending the neck for extension radiographs or a bleeding nose.[100] Indeed, the rates of *spontaneous* vertebral artery dissection have been reported to be 1–3 per 100,000 patients.[101] By using an estimated value of 10 from the literature to represent an average number of manipulations per patient per episode,[102] it becomes apparent that the proposed exposure rate for CVAs attributed to spinal manipulation is equivalent to the spontaneous rates for cervical arterial dissections as reported.[103] It is important to keep in mind that death rates caused by medication side effects are estimated by the Institute of Medicine to range from 230,000–280,000 per year.[104] Those deaths caused by commonly used NSAIDs such as ibuprofen are reported to approach an annual rate of 16,000[105]—dwarfing any estimates of chiropractic-related fatalities by several orders of magnitude. In any case, it seems clear that the real but extremely rare complications of chiropractic care should be viewed by physicians as serious but recognized risks of an effective procedure—much like the known and accepted risks of a medication or of a surgical procedure—and not as an absolute contraindication to chiropractic referral.

Table 8–2 provides a useful overview of the relative risks encountered in medical or chiropractic treatment as compared to those in everyday living. In terms of accident rates reported, one must take into account three major considerations:

1. The most recent and precise estimate of serious complications from cervical manipulations is 6 per 10 million manipulations with death rates at 3 per 10 million manipulations.[106,107] This is a real concern, but must be viewed in the context of a known rare risk for an accepted medical procedure.

2. With the recent association of cerebrovascular accidents with rotational maneuvers applied to the upper neck,[108,109] the accident rate produced by spinal manipulations may be anticipated to decrease with modifications of practice and training.

3. The literature shows that the actual number of iatrogenic complications specifically ascribed to chiropractic care is significantly overestimated, because the practitioner actually involved is often *not* a chiropractor. Rather, a major portion of these accidents occur at the hands of a practitioner with inadequate professional training, but who is incorrectly represented in the medical literature as a chiropractor.[110]

▶ RESEARCH ISSUES AND CHALLENGES IN CHIROPRACTIC CARE

In 1997, the Consortial Center for Chiropractic Research (CCCR) came into being with funding from the National Institutes of Health National

▶ **TABLE 8–2** RISKS OF CHIROPRACTIC MANIPULATION IN COMPARISON TO OTHER COMMON RISKS

Risk	Frequency
Morbidity	
Risk of serious neurologic complication from cervical manipulation	0.6 in 1,000,000[90]
Developing cauda equina syndrome from lumbar manipulation	1 in 100,000,000[26]
Mortality	
Death from neurologic complications from cervical manipulation	0.3 in 1,000,000[83]
Overall mortality rate for spinal surgery	700 in 1,000,000[101,102]
Death per year from gastrointestinal bleeding caused by NSAID use	400 in 1,000,000[103]
Smoking 20 cigarettes per day	1 in 200[104]
Automobile driving (United Kingdom)	1 in 5,900[104]
Soccer, football	1 in 25,500[104]

Center for Complementary and Alternative Medicine. The CCCR now represents six chiropractic colleges as well as one private and five state-supported universities, including National University of Health Sciences, New York Chiropractic College, Northwestern Health Sciences University, Southern California University of Health Sciences, Western States Chiropractic College, and Canadian Memorial Chiropractic College, Kansas State University, McMaster University, State University of New York, University of Iowa, University of Calgary, and Harvard Medical Center. An advisory committee provides scientific and chiropractic expertise in setting research priorities, making final decisions on the support of specific research projects, and directing the CCCR in various other programmatic aspects. Finally, a program staff provides input in consulting, training, biostatistics and data management, and scientific review.

Table 8–3 lists 19 CCCR-supported research projects. The CCCR program encompasses both outcome studies and the basic sciences, providing insight into the mechanisms of both spinal manipulation and the disorders that it is intended to treat. It is only through such an integrated approach that significant progress regarding the chiropractic alternative to health care may be realized.

A number of criticisms have been raised of much of the early chiropractic literature; some of these are unique to the challenge of studying chiropractic, whereas others are common to all clinical research. All will need to be addressed more effectively in future studies. Some of the most important issues are as follows:

1. Often lacking an adequate description of manipulation, these trials commonly described mobilization rather than manipulation. Furthermore, the methods often lacked adequate descriptions to permit their precise replication.
2. There was ambiguity in the clinical characterizations of the sample population.

▶ **TABLE 8–3** RESEARCH PROJECTS SUPPORTED BY THE CCCR AS OF OCTOBER 2002

Gert Bronfort, DC, PhD	Cost effectiveness of chiropractic care
	A pilot study of conservative therapies for sciatica
	Conservative treatments for neck pain: a pilot study
Lisa A. Caputo, DC	Changes in health measures in HIV+ chiropractic patients
Donald Dishman, DC, MSc	Spinal manipulation and motor systems physiology
David Eisenberg, MD	Chiropractic Rx for chronic otitis media with effusion
Anita Ruth Gross, MSc	Conservative management for neck disorders: a series of Cochrane Reviews
Mitchell Haas, DC	Dose response in chiropractic care for low-back pain
	Clinical utility of cervical end-play assessment
Cheryl K. Hawk, DC, PhD	Evaluation of a chiropractic manual placebo
	Multisite pilot study of chiropractic for chronic pelvic pain
Stephen Injeyan, DC, PhD	Studies on effects of spinal manipulations on the immune response
Partap S. Khalsa, DC, PhD	Facet joint capsule strains during spinal manipulation
	Facet capsule biomechanics from physiological spinal motion
Steven J. Kirstukas, PhD	Load distribution during bilateral manipulation
Joel G. Pickar, DC, PhD	Changes in paraspinal muscle spindle sensitivity
	Effect of vertebral loading on sympathetic nerve regulation
Veronica M. Sciotti, PhD	Trigger point metabolic and microcirculatory imbalances
Esther Suter, PhD	Changes in muscle excitability after spinal manipulation

3. Qualifications of those administering treatment were not reported.
4. Physician–patient contact times were not uniform across compared groups.
5. Sample sizes were often too small to approach statistical significance.
6. The failure to observe or control baseline characteristics was common.
7. Experimental bias was often introduced into the trial and often implicit in the recruitment process.
8. In a laboratory setting under tightly controlled conditions, the interventions tended to be very individualized and as such were difficult if not impossible to generalize to the clinical situation.

▶ MODELS OF INTEGRATION

In contrast to many of the other healing arts discussed in this text, chiropractic is, in many domains, thoroughly integrated into the mainstream of health care service delivery and reimbursement. Medicare has reimbursed for chiropractic care for several years. Many states have passed laws requiring other insurers to reimburse for chiropractic. Based on a pilot project that provided for chiropractic care at 10 selected Department of Defense treatment sites across the United States, which indicated that patients under chiropractic as compared to medical care were more likely to report improvements in health by using five separate scales over the 4-week survey period, in addition to reporting fewer days away from work or active duty, the Defense Authorization Act of 2001 recently mandated that chiropractic services be accessible to all active duty personnel in the US armed forces. The Veterans' Health Administration as well is moving to offer chiropractic as a benefit to all veterans.

One unusual experiment in integration of chiropractic is Alternative Medicine, Inc. (AMI), a managed care plan unique in that it uses doctors of chiropractic as full primary care gatekeepers and as such represents a blueprint for the future integration of health care services. It has provided strong justification for this position with a wealth of cost-effectiveness data that, for the first 12–18 months of implementation, demonstrated (1) the reduction of hospitalizations by 80%, (2) the reduction of outpatient procedures and surgeries by 85%, and (3) cuts in the use of pharmaceuticals by 56%. Patient satisfaction was reported to be nearly 100%.[111] Comparable data have been released for extended periods, with the key demonstration that the profile of condition (International Classification of Diseases [ICD]-9) codes for patients at AMI matches that of the general population.[112] This change in the role requested of chiropractors by our health services delivery system will bear further exploration and study; its cost-effectiveness and satisfaction data may provide a strong impetus for other third-party payers to seriously consider the integration of chiropractic services with its full scope of practice.

▶ OSTEOPATHIC CARE

To find health should be the object of the doctor. Anyone can find disease.

ANDREW TAYLOR STILL, MD (1828–1917)[113]

Osteopathic medicine began as a revolutionary approach to American health care. The founder of osteopathy, Andrew Taylor Still, MD, was a physician, farmer, and ardent abolitionist.[114–116] Medical treatments in his time involved laxatives, purgatives, bloodletting, calomel (a mercury compound), narcotics, and remedies containing a large amount of alcohol. Mercury poisoning and alcohol and drug addiction were common complications of these treatments. After an epidemic of meningitis in 1864, during which three of his children died, Still became disenchanted with allopathic measures. He saw the medicine he had been taught as both irrational and ineffective. His goal was to establish a system of treatment that addressed the mechanisms of disease, rather than treating the symptoms. An expert mechanic, Still began to see the body as a complex machine created by God, and good health as the proper, integrated functioning of all its systems. In other words, almost a century ahead of his time, he studied health in order to understand disease.

By 1874 he had created a system of osteopathic manipulative treatment (OMT). He was rejected by his church, which regarded his system as a form of "laying on of hands" permitted only to Christ.[117] When he was also repudiated by his allopathic colleagues and unable to teach in their schools, he established his own medical school in 1892, which granted a new degree, the Doctor of Osteopathy (DO).[118] Currently, there are 20 schools of osteopathic medicine in the United States. Although there are schools of osteopathy in other countries that do not grant medical degrees, the graduates of American schools are fully licensed physicians, like Dr. Still.

The Philosophy of Osteopathy

Three principles are commonly accepted as the basic tenets of the philosophy of Osteopathy. They have been interpreted in a number of complementary ways. In what follows, the words that express the author's interpretation are written in italics.

1. The body is a unit *designed to move.*

   Dr. Still makes it clear that referring to the body as a unit implies that the systems of the body work together in an integrated way, and that each part affects every other part. Osteopaths pay particular attention to the fascia, the fibrous tissue that surrounds and supports each part of the body, uniting them in a continuous whole from head to foot. A unique tenet of osteopathy is that each part of the body, including each organ, has the structure it does because it moves in relation to all the other structures. Anticipating the holistic medicine of today, Dr. Still regarded the person as a unity of "mind, matter, and spirit," any one of which could either adversely or positively affect the others.

2. Structure and function are reciprocally interrelated by *motion.*

   The motion of the body may be extrinsic (voluntary) or intrinsic (involuntary). Whenever a part of the body is restricted from moving in the way it was designed, there is the potential for disease. Dr. Still developed a system of correcting disordered functions by adjusting disordered structures. He considered knowledge of anatomy the key to understanding, preventing, and treating the mechanisms of disease.

3. The body possesses self-regulatory and self-healing mechanisms, based on the unrestricted motion of blood, lymph, and neurohormonal substances.

   Throughout his writings, Dr. Still refers to the importance of the circulation of endogenously produced substances. Without the advantage of our contemporary knowledge, he expressed his thought in approximations. He says that disease is an effect of "a partial or complete failure of the nerves to properly conduct the fluids of life,"[119] that disease may be created through "irritation and abnormal response of the nerve and blood supply to other organs,"[120] and also refers to the effects of the lymphatic and glandular systems.[121] Anticipating current thinking, Dr. Still emphasized the need for preventive medicine.

Osteopathic Techniques

Dr. Still never wrote a textbook of techniques. He believed that techniques followed from an understanding of anatomy. He also realized that because the body is a unit with a continuous connection through the fascia, the same symptoms could be produced by radically different anatomic disarrangements. For example, right upper extremity pain may be the result of restricted motion of the clavicle, scapula, or the liver, among other possibilities.

Today, there are standardized texts of a broad range of techniques, many of which were developed during the last three decades. Their basis in functional anatomy, which can be viewed as the study of how structures move in relation to one another, is the common language that underlies them all. Precise localization of the key structure maintaining the restriction, and application of just enough force to effect normalization, are the syntax of that language.

The types of techniques can be classified in many ways.[122] One such classification is based on the way the practitioner engages the patient's body. In this view, the types of technique are counterstrain, muscle energy, facilitated positional release, thrusting techniques, myofascial release techniques, cranial osteopathy, ligamentous articular strain, visceral manipulation, functional techniques, articulatory techniques, and fluid-motion techniques. Counterstrain involves passive shortening of contracted muscles while holding tender points on muscle, ligament, or tendon. The muscle returns to its resting length and the tenderness is relieved. In muscle-energy techniques, the practitioner holds a joint at its restrictive barrier. The patient is asked to use a small amount of force in the opposite direction for a couple of seconds, and then to relax. After a couple of repetitions, the practitioner passively stretches the involved muscles, and joint motion is restored to its physiologic limits. In facilitated positional release, the spine is placed in a position in which its facets are disengaged. The practitioner adds a facilitating force of compression and/or torsion, holds for a few seconds, and then passively moves the joint to its resting position. Thrusting techniques involve placing the affected joint at its restrictive barrier and then adding force to move it through the barrier. Myofascial or fascial release techniques involve passive positioning of the body so that patterns of strain are relieved. The patient may be asked to assist by breathing in a certain way, but otherwise expends no energy. Cranial osteopathy consists of techniques specifically developed to normalize involuntary motion of the bones of the cranium and restore balance to the tension membranes of the central nervous system. Most practitioners use mere grams of force to effect these changes. Ligamentous articular strain techniques resemble cranial techniques, but were developed to normalize motion by restoring balance to the ligaments that stabilize a joint. Visceral manipulation, as the name implies, is aimed at restoring the normal, involuntary motion of the viscera. Functional techniques are based on the recognition that tissues express the condition of the joints they connect to, as they respond to the need to move and position the body. The practitioner applies gentle, low-velocity stress to restricted joints and moves them in a way that decreases tissue resistance. Articulatory techniques create forces that overcome tissue resistance by gradually moving a joint through its full range of motion. Finally, fluid-motion techniques move fluid, particularly by directly addressing the lymphatic system and draining the sinuses.

Research on Osteopathic Care

There are both historical and methodological reasons for the relative paucity of clinical trials of OMT. From the start, painstaking studies of anatomy and physiology were an integral part of osteopathy. But since the osteopathic profession had to struggle to attain the acceptance it now enjoys,[123] emphasis was placed on education and providing medical care rather than on clinical research. Perhaps this is one reason that some of the foundations of research, such as interexaminer reliability, have not been definitively established.[124–127] As mentioned above, the same symptoms may have radically different anatomic etiologies, so standardization of treatment protocols can be challenging.

In addition, there are always several techniques that can be used to make any particular adjustment, and there are no data about which type works best under which circumstances. Regardless of the technique chosen, no trial can be conducted in a double-blind fashion. Nonetheless, a growing number of clinicians are conducting clinical trials, many of which are well designed.

The Pulmonary System

Historically, the most famous evidence for the efficacy of osteopathy is a case series of more than 6,000 patients in the United States with influenza complicated by pneumonia that was collected during the influenza epidemic of 1918. Reportedly, the mortality rate among patients given standard of care was 25%, while the mortality rate among those who received OMT was 10%.[128] Recently, a group of elderly patients hospitalized with pneumonia received either standard of care, sham OMT, or real OMT. The mean duration of leukocytosis, intravenous antibiotic treatment, and days of hospitalization were shortest in the group receiving OMT, but not to a statistically significant degree. This may be a result of the small sample size.[129]

In a randomized controlled trial of 42 cholecystectomy patients, OMT was compared to incentive spirometry for preventing postoperative atelectasis. There was no difference in incidence of atelectasis in the two groups. However, the group receiving OMT had a statistically significant shorter recovery and return to preoperative forced vital capacity and forced expiratory volume in 1 second values. Aside from its small size, this study is flawed by the length of follow up (only 3 days), lack of data on clinically important outcomes, and the fact that the authors excluded those who withdrew from the study (number unknown), rather than include them in an intention-to-treat analysis.[130]

The Immune System

Most osteopaths believe that lymphatic techniques improve immune function. Two recent studies provide some concrete evidence to support this view. In an animal model of antigen-induced arthritis, Haller and colleagues showed that rats treated with OMT and exercise had a statistically significant better improvement on computerized motion analysis, knee circumference, stride length, and ankle lift than did animals that were not treated.[131] A group of healthy medical students developed a transient but statistically significant increase in serum basophils, compared to their baseline values, after treatment with lymphatic techniques.[132] Another interesting study compared two groups of medical students who received the hepatitis B vaccine series. One group ($N = 20$) received lymphatic techniques after each vaccine, while the other ($N = 19$) did not. At 13 weeks, 50% of those receiving OMT developed protective titers, as compared to 16% in the control group. The mean titer in the group treated with OMT was higher at every measurement, including the final measurement at 34 weeks. However, perhaps because of the small sample size, the difference was not statistically significant except at the 25-week measurement.[133] Neither of these studies clearly demonstrates a clinical difference achieved by using OMT, but they do suggest promising avenues of future research.

Other Conditions

In two small studies, patients with carpal tunnel syndrome who were treated with OMT improved both symptomatically and electrodiagnostically.[134,135] Another small study found that after a single session of OMT, patients experiencing tension headache reported a significantly reduced amount of pain immediately after treatment. No long-term follow up was conducted.[136]

A blinded, randomized controlled trial of 14 patients hospitalized with pancreatitis showed that those treated with OMT spent statistically significant fewer days in the hospital. The mean reduction was 3.5 days. There were no significant differences in use of pain medications or time to oral feeding. Unfortunately, the authors do not specify the objective criteria used to establish that the two groups had comparable severity of disease, although the exclusion criteria suggest that they did.[137]

Jarski and colleagues conducted a prospective, single-blinded, match-controlled study comparing outcomes after elective knee or hip arthroplasty. The intervention group ($N = 38$) received OMT on postoperative days 2 through 5. The control group ($N = 38$) received standard care. The intervention group performed better to a statistically significant degree on the following outcomes: negotiating stairs (mean of 4.3 ± 1.2 versus 5.4 ± 1.6 days), distance ambulated on the third postoperative day (mean 24.3 ± 18.3 versus 13.9 ± 14.4 m). There were also trends toward requiring less analgesia, staying in hospital fewer days, and ambulating further on postoperative days 1, 2, and 4.[138]

Lower Back Pain

The efficacy of osteopathic and other types of spinal manipulation in the treatment of back pain is controversial. In 1995, the US Agency for Health Care Policy and Research recommended manipulation as a safe and effective treatment for acute lower back pain, but concluded that its efficacy for patients with radiculopathy remained unproven.[139] A full discussion of the difficulties of design and interpretation are beyond the scope of this chapter. However, lower back pain is probably the most common complaint for which people seek spinal manipulation.

Common Clinical Applications

There is general consensus among osteopaths that OMT is effective for a wide range of medical problems and conditions. It is impossible to create a definitive list of indications. No surveys have been done to identify the problems most commonly treated. What follows reflects the literature, including case series and theoretical writings. In the musculoskeletal system, OMT is used for acute and chronic back pain, acute and chronic sprains (for which counterstrain, facilitated positional release, and articular ligamentous release are particularly effec-

tive), noncardiac chest pain, acute and chronic neck pain, carpal tunnel syndrome, and tendinitis. Pain is relieved by releasing strain patterns in the soft tissues and restoring normal joint motion.

Acute and chronic sinusitis, otitis media (for which cranial osteopathy is widely used), and acute viral pharyngitis are often treated with OMT. Fluid motion techniques are commonly used to enhance lymphatic flow and, along with cranial osteopathy, to restore balanced motion of the cranial bones, whose involuntary motion provides drainage of the sinuses and ear canals. In the respiratory system, OMT is used to treat acute and chronic bronchitis, asthma, and sometimes COPD. Restoring motion of the structures of the chest affects intrathoracic pressure, compliance, and range of expansion. Correcting spinal alignment affects afferent and efferent signals to the nerves innervating the lungs and diaphragm, as well as improves blood supply to the chest.

Visceral manipulation, which was developed in France, is most commonly used by osteopaths in the United States for gastrointestinal and genitourinary dysfunctions, such as gastroesophageal reflux disease, irritable bowel syndrome, incontinence, and dysmenorrhea.

Dr. Still emphasized preventive medicine. No greater opportunity for prevention exists than when treating pregnant women, the newborn, and young children. Various case series[140] suggest that OMT during pregnancy results in lower rates of complications of labor and delivery. Cranial osteopathic treatment of the infant is believed to prevent scoliosis, prevent or relieve colic, and decrease the development of allergies, among other benefits.

▶ CONCLUSION

The basic concept informing manipulative medicine in general is that structure can have a significant influence on function. Concurrently, new methodologies are developing to address the challenges in studying individualized manipulative approaches used in osteopathic and chiropractic care. These more rigorously designed studies are enhancing our understanding of the scientific basis of why structure effects function in health. All clinicians have encountered patients who present with a set of symptoms that clearly do not fit into an established conventional diagnosis—in most cases, they have been given the label of "somatic" or "functional" with no clear therapeutic direction to improve the situation. In these cases, by incorporating the concept that form (structure) and function are integrated, it makes sense that correcting structural imbalances in bones, tendons, muscles, and fascia can be an effective treatment option. As patient demand for the regular incorporation of manipulative medicine continues to grow, we can expect a continuing integration of these modalities into both preventive care and treatment of specific conditions over the coming years.

REFERENCES

1. Lomax E. Manipulative therapy: a historical perspective from ancient times to the modern era. In: Goldstein M, ed. *The Research Status of Spinal Manipulative Therapy*. Bethesda, MD: HEW/NINCDS; 1975:11. Monograph No. 15.
2. Chapman-Smith D. Chiropractic Report: Origin and Professional Organization. Last day accessed 9/24/03. www.chiropracticreport.com/chiropractic.htm.
3. Shekelle PG, Adams AH, Chassin MR, Hurwitz EL, Brook RH. Spinal manipulation for low-back pain. *Ann Intern Med*. 1992;117:590–599.
4. Bronfort G. *Efficacy of Manual Therapies of the Spine*. Amsterdam: Thesis Publishers; 1997.
5. Bigos S, Bowyer O, Braen G, et al. *Acute Low Back Pain in Adults. Clinical Practice Guideline No. 14*. Rockville, MD: Agency for Health Care Policy and Research, Public Health Service, U.S. Department of Health and Human Services; 1994. AHCPR Publication No. 95–0642.
6. Shekelle PG, Adams AH, Chassin MR, Hurwitz EL, Brook RH. Spinal manipulation for low-back pain. *Ann Intern Med*. 1992;117:590–599.
7. Jayson MIV. A limited role for manipulation. *BMJ*. 1986;293:1454–1455.
8. Walter GW. *The First School of Osteopathic Medicine: A Chronicle, 1892–1992*. Kirksville, MO: Thomas Jefferson University Press; 1992.
9. Hadler NM, Curtis P, Gillings DB, Stinnett S. A benefit of spinal manipulation as adjunctive therapy for acute low-back pain: a stratified controlled trial. *Spine*. 1987;12:702–706.
10. Kirkaldy-Willis WH, Cassidy JD. Spinal manipulation in the treatment of low back pain. *Can Fam Phys*. 1985;31:535–540.
11. Hoehler FK, Tobis JS, Buerger AA. Spinal manipulation for low back pain. *JAMA*. 1981;245:1835–1838.
12. Koes BW, Bouter LM, van Mameren H, et al. Randomised clinical trial of manipulative therapy and physiotherapy for persistent back and neck complaints: results of one-year follow-up. *BMJ*. 1992;304:601–605.
13. Skargren EI, Oberg BE, Carlsson PG, Gade M. Cost and effectiveness analysis of chiropractic and physiotherapy treatment for low back and neck pain. *Spine*. 1997;22:2167–2177.
14. Meade TW, Dyer S, Browne W, Townsend J, Frank AO. Low back pain of mechanical origin: randomised comparison of chiropractic and hospital outpatient treatment. *BMJ*. 1990;300:1431–1437.
15. Meade TW, Dyer S, Browne W, Frank AO. Randomised comparison of chiropractic and hospital outpatient management for low back pain: results from extended follow-up. *BMJ*. 1995;311:349–351.
16. Anderson R, Meeker WC, Wirick BE, Mootz RD, Kirk DH, Adams A. A meta-analysis of clinical trials of spinal manipulation. *J Manipulative Physiol Ther*. 1992;15(3):181–194.
17. Shekelle PG, Adams AH, Chassin MR, Hurwitz EL, Brook RH. Spinal manipulation for low-back pain. *Ann Intern Med*. 1992;117:590–599.
18. Bronfort G: *Efficacy of Manual Therapies of the Spine*. Amsterdam: Thesis Publishers; 1997.
19. Foreman SM, Croft AC. *Whiplash Injuries: The Cervical Acceleration/Deceleration Syndrome*. 2nd ed. Baltimore: Williams & Wilkins; 1995.
20. Assendelft WJJ, Koes BW, Knipschild PG, Bouter LM. The relationship between methodological quality and conclusions in reviews of spinal manipulation. *JAMA*. 1995;274(24):1942–1948.
21. Spitzer WO, Skovron ML, Salmi LR, et al. Scientific monograph of the Quebec Task Force on whiplash-associated disorders: refining

"whip-lash" and its management. *Spine*. 1995; 20(8S):1S–73S.

22. Eisenberg DM, Davis RB, Ettner SL, et al. Trends in alternative medicine use in the United States, 1990–1997. *JAMA*. 1998;280(18):1569–1575.

23. Manga P, Angus D, Papadopoulos C, Swan W. *The Effectiveness and Cost-effectiveness of Chiropractic Management of Low-back Pain*. Richmond Hill, Ottawa, Canada: Kenilworth; 1993.

24. Rosen M. *Back Pain: Report of a Clinical Standards Advisory Group Committee on Back Pain*. London: HMSO; 1994.

25. Commission on Alternative Medicine, Social Departmentete. Legitimazation for Vissa Kiropraktorer. Stockholm, Sweden. 1987;12:13–16.

26. Danish Institute for Health Technology Assessment. Low-back pain, frequency, management, and prevention from an HTA perspective. *Danish Health Tech Assess*. 1999;1(1):63.

27. Thompson CJ. Chiropractic. In: *Second Report, Medicare Benefits Review Committee*. Canberra, Australia: Commonwealth Government Printer; 1986:152.

28. Hasselberg PD. *Chiropractic in New Zealand: Report of a Commission of Inquiry*. Wellington, NZ: Government Printer; 1979.

29. Bigos S, Bowyer O, Braen G, et al. *Acute Low Back Pain in Adults. Clinical Practice Guideline No. 14*. Rockville, MD: Agency for Health Care Policy and Research, Public Health Service, U.S. Department of Health and Human Services; 1994. AHCPR Publication No. 95-0642.

30. Danish Institute for Health Technology Assessment. Low-back pain, frequency, management, and prevention from an HTA perspective. *Danish Health Tech Assess*. 1999;1(1):63.

31. Williams B. Patient satisfaction: a valid concept? *Soc Sci Med*. 1994;509–516.

32. Rosner A. Letter to the editor. *Spine*. 1995;20(23): 2595–2598.

33. Cherkin DC, MacCornack FA. Patient evaluations of low back pain care from family physicians and chiropractors. *West J Med*. 1989;150:351–355.

34. Shekelle PG, Adams AH, Chassin MR, Hurwitz EL, Phillips RB, Brook RH. *The Appropriateness of Spinal Manipulation for Low Back Pain: Project Overview and Literature Review*. Santa Monica, CA: RAND; 1991. Monograph No. R-4025/1-CCR/FCER.

35. Nwuga VCB. Relative therapeutic efficacy of vertebral manipulation and conventional treatment in back pain management. *Am J Physical Med*. 1982;61(6):273–278.

36. Burton AK, Tillotson KM, Cleary J. Single-blind randomised controlled trial of chemonucleolysis and manipulation in the treatment of symptomatic lumbar disc herniation. *Eur Spine J*. 2000; 9:202–207.

37. Henderson RS. The treatment of lumbar disk intervertebral disk protrusion: an assessment of conservative measures. *BMJ*. 1952;2: 597–598.

38. Mensor MC. Non-operative treatment, including manipulation, for lumbar intervertebral disc syndrome. *J Bone Joint Surg Am*. 1955;37:925–936.

39. Chrisman OD. A study of the results following rotary manipulation in the lumbar intervertebral disc syndrome. *J Bone Joint Surg Am*. 1964;46: 517–524.

40. Kuo PP-F, Loh Z-C. Treatment of lumbar intervertebral disc protrusions by manipulation. *Clin Orthop*. 1987;215:47–55.

41. d'Ornano J, Conrozier T. Effets des manipulations vertebrales sur la hernie discale lombaire. *Rev Med Orthop*. 1990;19:21–25.

42. Cassidy JD, Thiel HW, Kirkaldy-Willis KW. Side posture manipulation for lumbar disc herniation. *J Manipulative Physiol Ther*. 1993;16(2):96–103.

43. Farfan HF, Cossette JW, Robertson GH, Wells RV, Kraus H. The effects of torsion on the lumbar intervertebral joints: the role of torsion in the production of disc degeneration. *J Bone Joint Surg Am*. 1970;52:468–497.

44. Adams MA, Hutton WC. Mechanics of the intervertebral disc. In: Ghosh P, ed. *The Biology of the Intervertebral Disc*. Vol. 2. Boca Raton, FL: CRC Press; 1988:39–71.

45. Coulter I, Shekelle P, Mootz, R, Hansen D. The use of expert panel results: the RAND panel for appropriateness of manipulation and mobilizations of the cervical spine. *Top Clin Chiropractic*. 1995;2(3):54–62.

46. Coulter I, Hurwitz E, Adams A, et al. The appropriateness of spinal manipulation and mobilizations of the cervical spine: Literature review, indications and ratings by a multidisiplinary expert panel. Santa Monica, CA: RAND; 1995. Monograph No. DRU-982-1-CCR.

47. Cassidy JD, Lopes A, Yong-Hing K. The immediate effect of manipulation versus mobilization on pain and range of motion in the cervical spine: a randomized controlled trial. *J Manipulative Physiol Ther*. 1992;15(9):570–575.

48. Koes B, Bouter L, Van Mameren H, et al. A randomized clinical trial of manual therapy and physiotherapy for persistent back and neck complaints: subgroup analysis and the relationship between outcome measures. *J Manipulative Physiol Ther.* 1993;16(4):211–219.

49. Long M, Frank C, Schachlan N, Dittrick D, Edwards, G. The effects of motion on normal healing ligaments [abstract]. *Proc Orthop Res Soc.* 1982;7:43.

50. Fronek J, Frank C, Amiel D, Woo SL-Y, Coutts R, Akeson W. The effects of intermittent passive movement (IMP) in the healing of medical collateral ligament [abstract]. *Proc Orthop Res Soc* 1983;8:31.

51. Akenson, W, Amiel D, Mechanic C, Soo SL-Y, Harwood F, Hamer M. Collagen cross-linking alternations in joint contractures. Changes in the reducible cross-links in periarticular connective tissue after nine weeks of immobilization. *Connective Tissue Res* 1977;5:15–19.

52. Davis P, Hulbert J, Kassak K, Meyer J. Comparative efficacy of conservative medical and chiropractic treatments for carpal tunnel syndrome: a randomized clinical trial. *J Manipulative Physiol Ther.* 1998;21(5):317–326.

53. Davis P, Hulbert J. Carpal tunnel syndrome: conservative and nonconservative treatment: a chiropractic physician's perspective. *J Manipulative Physiol Ther.* 1998;2(5):356-362.

53a. Sucher BM. Myofascial manipulative release of carpal tunnel syndrome. *J Am Osteopath Assoc.* 1994;94(8): 647–663.

53b. Winters J, Sobel J, Groenier K, Arendzen H, Meyboom-de-Jong B. Comparison of physiotherapy, manipulation and corticosteroid injection for treating shoulder complaints in general practice: randomised, single-blind study. *BMJ.* 1997;314: 1320–1325.

54. Bonebrake, A, Fernandez J, Dahalan J, Marley R, A treatment for carpal tunnel syndrome: results of a follow-up study. *J Manipulative Physiol Ther.* 1993;93(12):1273–1278.

55. Nilsson N. A randomized controlled trial of the effect of spinal manipulation in the treatment of cervicogenic headache. *J Manipulative Physiol Ther.* 1995;18:435.

56. Wittingham W, Ellis WB, Milyneux TP. The effect of manipulation (toggle recoil) for headaches with upper cervical joint dysfunction: a pilot study. *J Manipulative Physiol Ther.* 1994;17:369.

57. Vernon HT. The effectiveness of chiropractic manipulation in the treatment of headache: an exploration of the literature. *J Manipulative Physiol Ther.* 1995;18:611.

58. Bronfort G, Assendelft WJJ, Evans R, Haas M, Bouter L. Effects of spinal manipulation for chronic headache: a systematic review. *J Manipulative Physiol Ther.* 2001;24(7):457–466.

59. Boline P, Kassak K, Bronfort G, et al. Spinal manipulation vs. amitriptyline for the treatment of chronic tension-type headaches: a randomized clinical trial. *J Manipulative Physiol Ther.* 1995;18: 148–154.

59a. Williams B. Patient satisfaction: a valid concept? *Soc Sci Med.* 1994;38:509–516.

60. Parker G, Tupling H, Pryor D. A controlled trial of the effect of spinal manipulation for migraine. *Aust NZ J Med.* 1978;8:589–593.

61. Wight JS. Migraine: a statistical analysis of chiropractic treatment. *Chiro J.* 1978;12:363.

62. Stodolny J, Chmielewski H: Manual therapy in the treatment of patients with cervical migraine. *Manual Med.* 1989;4:49.

63. Nelson CF, Bronfort G, Evans R, Boline P, Goldsmith C, Anderson AV. The efficacy of spinal manipulation, amitriptyline and the combination of both therapies for the prophylaxis of migraine headache. *J Manipulative Physiol Ther.* 1998;21: 511–519.

64. Mennell MD: *Joint Pain: Diagnosis and Treatment Using Manipulative Techniques.* Boston, MA: Little Brown; 1964.

65. Oliver SE, LeFebvre R. Sinusitis and sinus pain: conservative chiropractic care. *Top Clin Chiropractic.* 1998;5(1):39–47, 62–65, 73–75.

66. Folweiler DS, Lynch OT. Nasal Specific technique as part of a chiropractic approach to chronic sinusitis and sinus headaches. *J Manipulative Physiol Ther.* 1995;18(1):38–41.

67. Miller WD. Treatment of visceral disorders by manipulative therapy. In: Goldstein M, ed: *The Research Status of Spinal Manipulative Therapy.* Bethesda, MD: National Institute of Neurological and Communicative Disorders and Stroke; 1975: 295.

68. Havid C. A comparison of the effect of chiropractic treatment on respiratory function in patients with respiratory distress symptoms and patients without. *Bull Eur Chiro Union.* 1978;26:17–34.

69. Balon J, Aker PD, Crowther ER, et al. A comparison of active and simulated chiropractic

manipulation as adjunctive treatment for childhood asthma. *N Engl J Med*. 1998;339:1013–1020.

70. Bronfort G, Evans R, Cubic P, Filkin P. Chronic pediatric asthma and chiropractic spinal manipulation. A Prospective Clinical Series and Randomized Clinical Pilot Study. *J Manipulative Physiol Ther*. 2001;24:B369–B377.

71. Daniel Redwood, ed. *Contemporary Chiropractic*. New York: Churchill Livingstone; 1997:194.

72. Wagner T, Owen J, Malone E, Mann K. Irritable bowel syndrome and spinal manipulation: a case report. *Chiropr Tech*. 1995;7:139.

73. Pikalov AA, Kharin VV. Use of spinal manipulative therapy in the treatment of duodenal ulcer. *J Manipulative Physiol Ther*. 1994;17:310.

74. Rychlikova E. Schmerzen im gallonblazan bereich auf grund vertebragenger storungen. *Deutches Gesundheitswesen*. 1975;29:2092.

75. Lewit K. Ein fall von auftahrunfall. *Manuelle Med*. 1975;13:71.

76. DeBoer KF, Schultz, M, McKnight ME. Acute effects of spinal manipulation on gastrointestinal myoelectric activity in conscious rabbits. *Manual Med*. 1988;3:85.

77. Eriksen K. Effects of upper cervical correction on chronic constipation. *Chiropr Tech*. 1994;7:139.

78. Falk JW. Bowel and bladder dysfunction secondary to lumbar dysfunctional syndrome. *Chiropr Tech*. 1990;2:45.

79. Fallon J. The role of chiropractic adjustment in the care and treatment of 332 children with otitis media. *J Clin Chiropr Pediatr*. 1997;2(2):167–183.

80. Frohle RM. Ear infection: a retrospective study examining improvement from chiropractic care and analyzing for influencing factors. *J Manipulative Physiol Ther*. 1996;19(3):169–177.

81. Degenhardt BF, Kuchera ML. Efficacy of osteopathic evaluation and manipulative treatment in reducing the morbidity of otitis media in children. *J Am Osteopath Assoc*. 1994;94(8):673.

82. Schmidt M. Otitis media in children. *J Naturopathic Med*. 1994;5(1):17–26.

83. Laderman JP. Accidents of spinal manipulations. *Ann Swiss Chiro Assoc*. 1981;7:161–208.

84. Haldeman S, Rubinstein SM. Cauda equina syndrome in patients undergoing manipulation of the lumbar spine. *Spine*. 1992;17(12):1469–1473.

85. Terrett AGL, Kleynhans AM. Complications from manipulations of the low back. *Chiro J Austr*. 1992;22(4):129–140.

86. Hosek RS, Schram SB, Silverman H, Myers JB, Williams SE. Cervical manipulation [letter]. *JAMA*. 1981;245:922.

87. Hamann G, Haas A, Kujat C, Felber S, Strittmatter M, Schimrigk K, Piepgras U. Cervicocephalic artery dissections due to chiropractic manipulations. *Lancet*. 1993;341:114.

88. Dvorak J, Orelli F. How dangerous is manipulation of the cervical spine? *Manual Med*. 1985; 2:1–4.

89. Haldeman S, Carey P, Townsend M, Papadopoulos C. Arterial dissections following cervical manipulation: the chiropractic experience. *Can Med Assoc J*. 2001;165(7):905–906.

90. Hurwitz EL, Aker PD, Adams AH, Meeker WC, Shekelle PG. Manipulation and mobilization of the cervical spine: a systematic review of the literature. *Spine*. 2000;21(15):1746–1760.

91. Terrett AGJ. Vascular accidents from cervical spine manipulation: report on 107 cases. *J Aust Chiro Assoc*. 1999;17(1):15–24.

92. Jaskoviak PA. Complications arising from manipulation of the cervical spine. *J Manipulative Physiol Ther*. 1980;3:213–219.

93. Hanus SH, Homer TD, Harter DH. Vertebral artery occlusion complicating yoga exercises. *Arch Neurol*. 1977;34:574–575.

94. Nagler W. Vertebral artery obstruction by hyperextension of the neck: report of three cases. *Arch Phys Med Rehabil*. 1973;54:237–240.

95. Okawara S, Nibbelink D. Vertebral artery occlusion following hyperextension and rotation of the head. *Stroke*. 1974;5:640–642.

96. Easton JD, Sherman DG. Cervical manipulation and stroke. *Stroke*. 1977;8:594–597.

97. Sherman DG, Hart RG, Easton JD. Abrupt change in head position and cerebral infarction. *Stroke*. 1981;12:2–6.

98. Barty GM. Expert testimony. In: *Klippel v Alchin*. Wagga Wagga, Australia: 12 1983:33.

99. Barty GM. Expert testimony. In: *Klippel v Alchin*. Wagga Wagga, Australia: 12 August 1983:33.

100. Fogelhom R, Karli P. Iatrogenic brainstem infarction. *Eur Neurol*. 1975;13:6–12.

101. Shievink WT, Mokri, B, O'Fallon WM. Recurrent spontaneous cervical-artery dissection. *N Engl J Med*. 1994;330(6):393–397.

102. Carey TS, Garrett J, Jackman A, et al, and the North Carolina Back Pain Project. The outcomes and costs of care for acute low back pain among patients seen by primary care practitioners, chiropractors, and orthopedic surgeons. *N Engl J Med*. 1995;333(14):913–917.

103. Shievink WT, Mokri B, O'Fallon WM. Recurrent spontaneous cervical-artery dissection. *New Engl J Med.* 1994;330(6):393–397.
104. Schuster M, McGlynn E, Brook R. How good is the quality of health care in the United States? *Milbank Q.* 1998;76:517–563.
105. Wolfe MM, Lichenstein DR, Singh G. Gastrointestinal toxicity of nonsteroidal antiinflammatory drugs. *N Engl J Med.* 1999;340(24):1888–1899.
106. Haldeman S, Carey P, Townsend M, Papadopoulos C. Arterial dissections following cervical manipulation: the chiropractic experience. *Can Med Assoc J.* 2001;165(7):905–906.
107. Hurwitz EL, Aker PD, Adams AH, Meeker WC, Shekelle PG. Manipulation and mobilization of the cervical spine: a systematic review of the literature. *Spine.* 2000;21(15):1746–1760.
108. Klougart N, Leboeuf-Yde C, Rasmussen LR. Safety in chiropractic practice, part II: treatment to the upper neck and the rate of cerebrovascular incidents. *J Manipulative Physiol Ther.* 1996;19(9):563–569.
109. Klougart N, LeBoeuf-Yde C, Rasmussen LR. Safety in chiropractic practice, part I: the occurrence of cerebrovascular accidents after manipulation to the neck in Denmark from 1978–1988. *J Manipulative Physiol Ther.* 1996;19(6):371–377.
110. Terrett AGJ. Misuse of the literature by medical authors in discussing spinal manipulative therapy. *J Manipulative Physiol Ther.* 1995;18(4):203–210.
111. Eldridge LE. Improving quality of care lowers employer and employee costs. *Health Care or Wealth Care?* British Columbia Chiropractic Association conference, Vancouver, September 16, 2002.
112. Eldridge LE. Improving quality of care lowers employer and employee costs. *Health Care or Wealth Care?* British Columbia Chiropractic Association conference, Vancouver, September 16, 2002.
113. Still AT. *The Philosophy of Osteopathy.* Kirksville, MO: 1899. Reprinted. Indianapolis: American Academy of Applied Osteopathy; 1946:40.
114. Still AT. *Autobiography of Andrew T. Still.* Rev ed. Kirksville, MO: Published by the author; 1908:28.
115. Trowbridge C. *Andrew Taylor Still, 1828–1917.* Kirksville, MO: Thomas Jefferson University Press; 1991.
116. AT Still Pension File. Still National Osteopathic Museum, Kirksville, MO. Cited in: Trowbridge C. *Andrew Taylor Still, 1828–1917.* Kirksville, MO: Thomas Jefferson University Press; 1991.
117. Trowbridge C. *Andrew Taylor Still, 1828–1917.* Kirksville, MO: Thomas Jefferson University Press; 1991.
118. Walter GW. The first school of osteopathic medicine: a chronicle, 1892–1992. Kirksville MO: Thomas Jefferson University Press; 1992.
119. Trowbridge C. *Andrew Taylor Still, 1828–1917.* Kirksville, MO: Thomas Jefferson University Press; 1991:94.
120. Still AT. *Autobiography of Andrew T. Still.* Rev ed. Kirksville, MO: Published by the author. Distributed Indianapolis: American Academy of Osteopathy; 1908:94.
121. Peterson BA. Major events in osteopathic history. In: Ward RC, ed. *Foundations for Osteopathic Medicine.* Baltimore: Williams & Wilkins; 1997: 15–21.
122. See, e.g., DiGiovanna EL. Osteopathic manipulation. In: DiGiovanna EL, Schiowitz S, eds. *An Osteopathic Approach to Diagnosis and Treatment.* 2nd ed., Philadelphia: Lippincott-Raven; 1997:13–16.
123. Peterson BA. Major events in osteopathic history. In: Ward RC, ed. *Foundations for Osteopathic Medicine.* Baltimore: Williams & Wilkins; 1997: 15–21.
124. Beal MC, Patriquin DA. Interexaminer agreement on palpatory diagnosis and patient self-assessment of disability: a pilot study. *J Am Osteopath Assoc.* 1995;95:97–105.
125. Kappler RE. A comparison of structural examination findings obtained by experienced physician examiners and student examiners on hospital patients. *J Am Osteopath Assoc.*1980;79:468–471.
126. Beal MC. Incidence of spinal palpatory findings: a review. *J Am Osteopath Assoc.* 1989;89: 1027–1035.
127. McConnell DG, Beal MC, Dinnar U, et al. Low agreement of findings in neuromusculoskeletal examinations by a group of osteopathic physicians using their own procedures. *J Am Osteopath Assoc.* 1980;79:441–450.
128. Thorpe R. Osteopathic manipulation for infection. *Osteopath Ann.* 1980;9:253.
129. Noll D, Shores J, Bryman PN, Masterson CV. Adjunctive osteopathic manipulative treatment in the elderly hospitalized with pneumonia: a pilot study. *J Am Osteopath Assoc.* 1999;99:143.
130. Sleszynski SL, Kelso AF. Comparison of thoracic manipulation with incentive spirometry in preventing postoperative atelectasis. *J Am Osteopath Assoc.* 1993;93(8):834–845.

131. Haller B, Lehman S, Bosak A, et al. Establishment of behavioral parameters for the evaluation of osteopathic principles in a rat model of arthritis. *J Am Osteopath Assoc.* 1997;97:207–214.

132. Messina J, Hampton D, Evans R, et al. Transient basophilia following the application of lymphatic pump techniques: a pilot study. *J Am Osteopath Assoc.* 1998;98(2):91–94.

133. Jackson KM, Steele TF, Kukula G, Blue W, Roberts A. Effect of lymphatic and splenic pump techniques on the antibody response to hepatitis B vaccine: a pilot study. *J Am Osteopath Assoc.* 1998;98:155–160.

134. Sucher BM. Palpatory diagnosis and manipulative management of carpal tunnel syndrome. *J Am Osteopath Assoc.* 1994;94:647–663.

135. Sucher BM. Palpatory diagnosis and manipulative management of carpal tunnel syndrome; "double crush" and thoracic outlet syndrome. *J Am Osteopath Assoc.* 1995;95:471–479.

136. Hoyt WH, Shaffer F, Bard DA. Osteopathic manipulation inn the treatment of muscle-contraction headache. *J Am Osteopath Assoc.* 1979;78:322–325.

137. Radjieski JM, Lumley HA, Cantieri MS. Effect of osteopathic manipulative treatment on length of stay for pancreatitis: a randomized pilot study. *J Am Osteopath Assoc.* 1998;98:264–272.

138. Jarski RW, Loniewski EG, Williams J, et al. The effectiveness of osteopathic manipulative treatment as complementary therapy following surgery: a prospective, match-controlled outcome study. *Altern Ther Health Med.* 2000;6(5): 77–81.

139. Bigos S, Bowyer O, Braen G, et al. *Acute Low Back Pain in Adults. Clinical Practice Guideline No. 14.* Rockville, MD: Agency for Health Care Policy and Research, Public Health Service, U.S. Department of Health and Human Services; 1994. AHCPR Publication No. 95–0642.

140. King HH. Osteopathic manipulative treatment in prenatal care. *JAAO.* 2000;10(1):25–31.

CHAPTER 9

Acupuncture and East Asian Medicine

ARYA NIELSEN AND RICHARD HAMMERSCHLAG

Acupuncture with moxa, a system of medical treatment that developed in a civilization quite different from that of the West, was already 2,000 years old when modern science was born.[1] This perspective begs the question as to which systems of medicine are traditional, and which are alternative, and explains why the title "complementary and alternative medicine" is being replaced by "integrative medicine" when referring to collaborative care.

Until recently, conventional medicine has maintained a cultural authority over sanctioned institutions of care, effectively containing practices like acupuncture within the private setting. When consumers have exhausted conventional options, they have sought other available forms of care such as acupuncture. Thus, it is the consumer who has been the primary integrator of conventional and unconventional forms of care.

Partly as a consequence of consumer demand, interest in acupuncture has been piqued within institutional settings. Research is expanding on the biological mechanisms of acupuncture. The National Institutes of Health (NIH)

recognized acupuncture in its consensus statement of efficacy in 1997.[2] In its pain strategy initiative, the Joint Commission on Accreditation of Healthcare Organizations (JCAHO) has mandated that patients be asked about pain, and be educated about effective pain management, including nonpharmacologic approaches. Acupuncture is named as one "example of implementation for other pain management techniques successfully demonstrating compliance with JCAHO standard[s]."[3]

The training and licensing of acupuncturists continues to grow in the United States, with 46 accredited acupuncture colleges, and some medical schools adding programs for physician certification. Indeed, traditional systems of health care, such as East Asian medicine, have not only survived modernity, but thrive into the twenty-first century, and continue to inspire the movement for integrative care.

The following pages discuss traditional East Asian medicine generally, acupuncture specifically, and their relevance to the emerging integrative medicine model of health care. Frequently asked questions are answered in Table 9-1.

▶ **TABLE 9-1** SHORT ANSWERS TO FREQUENTLY ASKED QUESTIONS ABOUT ACUPUNCTURE

What is acupuncture?	Acupuncture is a modality of treatment deriving from East Asian medicine that involves stimulation of specific body points by insertion and manipulation of fine needles. When practiced in a context informed by East Asian medicine, acupuncture is often used in combination with other techniques, as well as therapeutic recommendations.
	An acupuncture treatment involves cutaneous and subcutaneous stimulation at multiple intentional sites, the inclusion of which for type of stimulation is based on the presenting disorder(s).
Does acupuncture hurt?	If done properly, a patient feels sensation at a needled point. Called "de Qi" in Chinese, it means the Qi has arrived, feeling heavy, achy, or tingly. East Asians typically do not perceive this as pain, so they say acupuncture is *bu tong*, or painless. Westerners who are less familiar with acupuncture may experience mild discomfort. There is no discomfort once the needles are in place. Communication between provider and patient facilitates comfortable treatment.
What does acupuncture treat?	Acupuncture facilitates innate healing. Acupuncture aids the body in resolving acute disorders like a cold, flu, or bronchitis, avoiding recurrence or chronicity.
	Any chronic problem, such as allergies, asthma, fatigue, arthritis, and gynecologic, urinary, or digestive disorders, as well as musculoskeletal and neurologic problems, may improve or resolve completely with acupuncture treatment. Acupuncture treats pain by reducing inflammation, promoting healing, and enhancing immune response.
What is an acupuncture point?	There are 365 ancient points, as well as common "extra" points, that are effectively used in the treatment of specific disorders. These points lie on channels mapped by the Chinese more than 2,000 years ago. Research has shown that bioelectrical and biomechanical activity at acupuncture points distinguish these sites from surrounding tissue. An acupoint's potential for therapeutic value is reflected in its state of sensitivity.
How does an acupuncturist know which points to treat?	Points are chosen based on the patient's symptoms and their association with East Asian medicine's common patterns of disharmony, as well as empirical knowledge of disease states and their relationship to specific channels, organs, and areas of the body. Palpation along channels enhances precise location of important known points and patterns of points requiring needling.
How deep do the needles go?	The depth of the needle varies depending on the disorder; where the point is located on the body; the amount of body fat at a particular location; the size, age, and state of the patient; as well as the acupuncturist's style of practice. Most body points require a minimum penetration of 0.25 inches; ear or scalp points are more superficial, whereas points on the buttocks are deeper.
Are the needles sterile?	Acupuncturists in the United States today use pre-sterilized, individually packaged, disposable needles. The National Commission for the Certification of Acupuncture and Oriental Medicine (NCCAOM) requires acupuncturists to pass a National Board Exam and Clean Needle test, using the Centers for Disease Control and Prevention's standards of sterile procedure.
How does acupuncture work?	From a traditional perspective, the body is seen as having channels of streaming Qi, blood, and fluid that express internal organ function. When Qi, blood, and fluid move freely, vital processes are fostered and health is maintained. If obstructed, there is pain, congestion, and eventually illness. Acupuncture stimulates the movement of Qi, blood, and fluids. Its effect is to supply where there is deficiency, drain where there is excess, and move through where there is obstruction.

How does acupuncture work in modern biomedical terms?

Research is confirming that acupuncture stimulates changes in neural and extraneural, biomechanical, and biochemical states. We have known for some time that acupuncture stimulates the nervous system's release of endorphins, but release of these endogenous opioids alone cannot account for acupuncture's therapeutic effect. Reflex stimulation is a sympatholytic effect that spreads throughout a body segment releasing vasoconstriction caused by muscle shortening common to pain and spasm. When the muscles relax, the pain and spasm resolve. Extraneural changes are responses outside of the nervous system. When a needle is inserted into a point it penetrates the connective tissue causing a tiny wound, discharging an injury potential, and stimulating collagen formation in the connective tissue. The effect of this stimulation lasts several days until the microtrauma heals. Because connective tissue is a contiguous fabric wrapping the entire body as well as every organ, muscle, vessel, and nerve, down to each cell, it is theorized that the channel system emanates within the connective tissue network.

Do acupuncturists only insert needles?

Acupuncture practice in the context of East Asian medicine includes recommendations on diet, work, and lifestyle habits that augment outcome. Acupuncture is often used in combination with other cutaneous techniques such as gua sha, cupping, direct or indirect moxibustion, electrical stimulation, plum blossom, and tui na. Some acupuncturists are also trained in prescribing herbal medicine.

Are there different styles of acupuncture?

Yes. Although acupuncture originated in China, it has migrated to many other regions, including Japan, Korea, Vietnam, Europe, Russia, and the United States, each adapting it to their uniquely evolving cultural and medical needs. This has resulted in different styles and application of practice. For example, acupuncture for drug detoxification and withdrawal has seen wider use in the United States than in East Asia.

How many treatments will a patient need?

This depends on the duration and severity of the complaint. The patient or referring practitioner should ask the acupuncturist what their experience is with this particular problem. It is recommended that a patient receive at least three sessions. The patient and the practitioner then evaluate need for further treatment. A prognosis is positive if the presenting problem is changed in any way, even if it briefly worsens. Subsequent treatment is timed to retain the effect of the prior treatment.

How will I feel after acupuncture?

Most patients feel deeply relaxed during and after acupuncture treatment. Alcohol, recreational drugs, heavy labor or workouts, and fasting or feasting are discouraged on the day of a treatment.

What is the best way to choose an acupuncturist?

The patient and/or the referring practitioner should ask for a referral from other health care providers or knowledgeable friends. One may also contact the state professional acupuncture organization or licensing board to find a licensed acupuncturist in the area. Contact the National Commission for Certification of Acupuncture and Oriental Medicine at www.NCCAOM.org to find a board-certified acupuncturist. NCCAOM certification requires 3 years of training and passage of a board examination. For referral to a medical doctor who uses acupuncture in practice, contact the American Association of Medical Acupuncture (AAMA) at www.medicalacupuncture.org. In most states, physicians who use acupuncture are not required to receive any specialized training, although many do complete a 300-hour course designed for physicians.

▶ BIOLOGICAL MECHANISMS OF ACUPUNCTURE

The healing mechanisms of cutaneous- and subcutaneous-mediated therapies, including acupuncture, moxibustion, gua sha, and cupping, are complex and variable depending on the potential within the points or areas treated, which, in turn, depends on the nature of the illness, the patient's age, hydration, type and appropriateness of stimulation, and the sensitivity response.

Practitioners palpate for the precise location of points using anatomic topography. Points are often found in a slight crook or depression, corresponding to the convergence of connective tissue planes.[4] The exact location and potential are confirmed as the patient senses tenderness or pain more at the point than in surrounding tissue, explained by small hypersensitive loci in myofascial structures when said points correspond to trigger points.[5] This oc-curs at 70% of common acupuncture sites.[6] A point's potential for therapeutic value is reflected in its state of sensitivity, or lack thereof. Point potential has been attributed to an abundance of nerve endings and sensory receptors[7,8]; neurochemical mechanisms[9-12]; decreased electrical conductivity, the potential of which changes with illness[13,14]; and altered connective tissue matrix and signal transduction.[15]

The effect of needle insertion and manipulation has been attributed to a variety of mechanisms, including the stimulation of response within the site via current of injury[16]; concentration and activity of mast cells[17]; bioelectric effect[18]; sensory mechanoreceptor stimulation along connective tissue planes; and connective tissue fiber winding and/or contraction of fibroblasts, with cellular activation/gene expression leading to restored connective tissue matrix composition and signal transduction (see Figs. 9–1, 9–2, and 9–3);[19] and activation

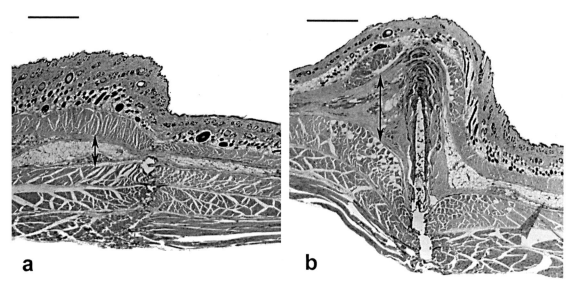

a   **b**

Figure 9-1. Rat abdominal wall tissue histology. An acupuncture needle was inserted into the abdominal wall of live anesthetized rats, followed by no rotation **(a)** or unidirectional rotation **(b)**. Immediately after needling, the animal was killed, tissues were formalin-fixed, sectioned roughly parallel to the needle track (labeled with ink) and stained with hematoxylin/eosin. Abdominal wall layers include dermis, subcutaneous muscle, subcutaneous tissue (arrow), and abdominal wall muscle. Marked thickening of subcutaneous tissue is seen with needle rotation. Scale bars: 1 mm. *(From Langevin H, Churchill D, Wu J, et al. Evidence of connective tissue involvement in acupuncture. FASEB J. 2002;8:872–874.)*

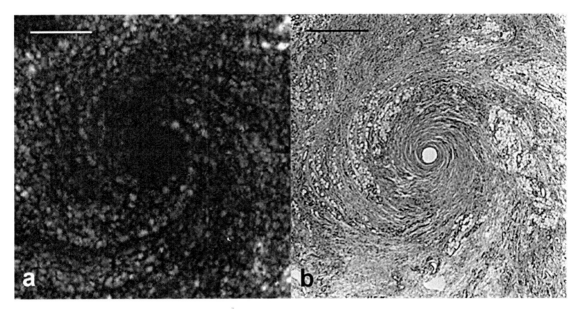

Figure 9-2. Acoustic and optical images of subcutaneous tissue with unidirectional needle rotation. **(a)** Fresh tissue sample imaged with ultrasound scanning acoustic microscopy. **(b)** The same tissue sample was formalin fixed after ultrasound imaging, embedded in paraffin, sectioned, and stained for histology with hematoxylin/eosin. Scale bars: 1 mm. *(From Langevin H, Churchill D, Wu J, et al. Evidence of connective tissue involvement in acupuncture. FASEB J. 2002;8:872–874.)*

of relevant structures in the brain as shown on a functional magnetic resonance imaging (fMRI) study of the brain during point stimulation.[20]

While "research on the physiology of acupuncture has been contributing to the development of neuroscience from the molecular level to the behavioral,"[21] the questions posed by the scientific community are grounded in a worldview that functions mostly outside the demands of an acupuncture clinical encounter. Associating acupuncture with endorphins discovered in the 1970s came at a time of initiatives related to drug addiction, when researchers aspired to discover safe and lucrative pharmacologic answers to negative drug dependency.[22] This setting defined acupuncture as analgesia, while the other numerous and valuable effects of acupuncture were dismissed as "patriotic zeal."[23] Because additional biological mechanisms were not understood at that

time, the misconception that acupuncture only treats pain became well established. To this day, insurance companies may require a pain code to reimburse for acupuncture.

While most studies still seek efficacy in relation to problems where pain is a primary feature, evidence that acupuncture, for example, prevents recurrent cystitis in susceptible women,[21] and shortens initial stages of labor, in addition to reducing labor pain (see Table 9–5), points to the healing effect of acupuncture beyond analgesia.

Ongoing efforts on the part of both acupuncturists and conventional health care providers to bridge the paradigm and linguistic gap is serving the integration of acupuncture into the conventional setting. While the traditional East Asian construct that has informed acupuncture practice is simple and based on naturally occurring phenomena, the

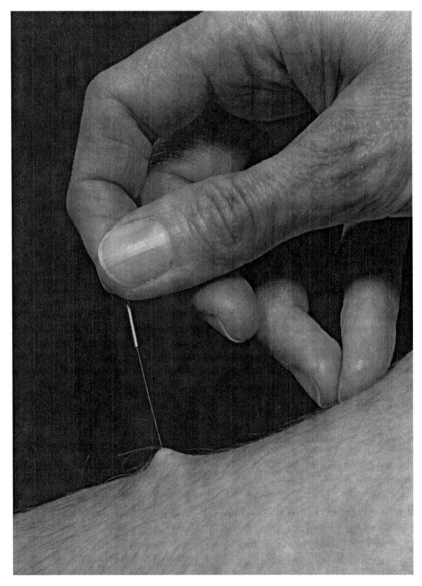

Figure 9–3. Tenting of skin observed during needle grasp. An acupuncture needle (seirin; 0.25 mm diameter) was inserted into the forearm of a human volunteer. After insertion, the needle was rotated until needle grasp was observed. Pulling back on the needle resulted in visible tenting of the skin. *(From Langevin H, Churchill D, Cipolla MJ. Mechanical signaling through connective tissue: a mechanism for the therapeutic effect of acupuncture. FASEB J. 2001;15: 2275–2282.)*

▶ **TABLE 9-2** SUMMARY OF PROPOSED MODEL OF PHYSIOLOGICAL EFFECTS
SEEN IN ACUPUNCTURE

Traditional Chinese Medicine Concepts	Proposed Anatomic/Physiologic Equivalents
Acupuncture meridians	Connective tissue planes
Acupuncture points	Convergence of connective tissue planes
Qi	Sum of all body energetic phenomena (e.g., metabolism, movement, signaling, and information exchange)
Meridian Qi	Connective tissue biochemical/bioelectrical signaling
Blockage of Qi	Altered connective tissue matrix composition leading to altered signal transduction
Needle grasp	Tissue winding and/or contraction of fibroblasts surrounding the needle
De Qi sensation	Stimulation of connective tissue sensory mechanoreceptors
Propagated De Qi sensation	Wave of connective tissue contraction and sensory mechanoreceptor stimulation along connective tissue planes
Restoration of flow of Qi	Cellular activation/gene expression leading to restored connective tissue matrix composition and signal transduction

Source: Langevin H, Yandow J. Relationship of acupuncture points and meridians to connective tissue planes. Anat Rec. 2002;269(6):257–265.

Western-trained reader might like to refer to Table 9–2, which provides proposed anatomic and physiologic equivalents to some traditional East Asian concepts.[25]

▶ THE SHARED AND DIVERGENT HISTORIES OF EAST ASIAN AND EARLY WESTERN MEDICINE

The early Chinese medical texts of the first and second centuries correspond in large measure to the *Hippocratic Corpus.*[26] Interestingly, while Hippocrates is considered the father of Western medicine, his practice was thought to be Egyptian in origin: the principles of the Hippocratic Oath date to the Egyptian Ebers papyrus, written in 1553 B.C.[27]

Medical practice across early civilization shared similar classification dyads, which were used to sort illness presentations into, for example, hot/cold, damp/dry, and full/empty (see "The Clinical Encounter" below). These may have been communicated from China to the other ancient civilizations with the distribution

of trade. Trade was so fluent along the Silk Road connecting China with Egypt, Rome, Greece, Persia, Arabia, and India that a relative homogeneity of the germ pool among the early civilizations is thought to have been maintained by the first century A.D.[28]

▶ EASTERN AND EARLY WESTERN TREATMENT

All early health care systems predate technology-determined diagnoses. Surviving traditional systems are based in the "ability to maintain health by manipulating conditions perceived by ordinary human sensory awareness."[29] Eastern and early Western medicine similarly associated illness signs into identifiable, if fluctuating, entities of imbalance, with treatment aiming to counteract errant or pathogenic substantive humors, and/or to strengthen the body's resistance: *vis medicatrix naturae.*[30] Direct attack of pathogens, as well as supporting innate immunity, remain a focus of medicine today, yet particular manual interventions distinguish early practice from modern, and traditional East Asian from conventional Western medicine. These physical interventions involve cutaneous and subcutaneous forms of stimulation, and while acupuncture is the best known of East tui na Asian therapies, moxibustion, gua sha, cupping, plum blossom, and internal and external application of herbs are also widely used, and are discussed below in "The Clinical Encounter."

Counteraction, Bloodletting, and Allopathy

Early Western medicine is referred to as Hippocratic or counteractive medicine. Therapies counteracted illness features.[31] Direct counteraction warmed the person who was cold, cooled a person who was too hot, nourished the hungry, hydrated the thirsty, and so on. More complicated problems were addressed by carefully observing the patient and illness signs through time. "The cause of disease should be sought in nature, the cure due to nature." What distinguished Hippocrates' practice was his careful recording of illness features.

Noting that illness often resolved after a crisis point, Hippocrates understood that the crisis precipitated the cure. Therapies were developed that mimicked these crises to hasten recovery. Thus, because vomiting was the crisis that cured nausea, emetics were prescribed for this symptom. The discomfort of constipation was relieved with defecation, so purgatives were administered. The crisis point of fever intensifies to sweating, so diaphoretics were used in cases of fever.

It was observed that local infections healed when they burst and bled, so lancing was used to reduce local infection, referred to as an excess or "plethora" in Hippocratic terms.[32] Similarly, bloodletting used to reduce extreme fevers was called antiphlogistic bloodletting. Antiphlogistic bloodletting and therapeutic seasonal bloodletting were common to many early traditional systems. Bloodletting fell out of practice in the West in the early twentieth century[33]

as a consequence of overzealous practice: the sicker the patient, the more the letting. Western local specific bloodletting devolved to venisection,[34] where the patient was typically bled until they passed out. With Western medicine's shift from humors to microbes, and with the emergence of useful drugs such as quinine, codeine, and salicin, the value of venisection was challenged, and Western bloodletting was considered misinformed.[35] However, bloodletting is retained in East Asian practice. Blood is let specific to a channel until the color turns from dark to bright, which usually involves a few drops. The site is then closed with pressure.

Last in the counteractive approach is the strategy of countering existing infections by introducing a second, more superficial, inflammation, as in the counteractive practice used in the West called a "seton." Here a thread or horse hair was imbedded just under the skin and left in place to intentionally develop a superficial infection. The superficial infection from the embedded thread countered in this case a deeper more persistent infection nearby, as in Figure 9–4.

This was the closest early Western medical practice came to acupuncture therapy. The practice is called threading, and can be found in contemporary Chinese texts.[36]

It is interesting to note that the definition of allopathy stems from this lineage of counteractive medicine. "Allopathy is a therapeutic system in which a disease is treated by producing a second condition that is incompatible with or antagonistic to the first."[37] While conventional medicine is often referred to as allopathic, it is a distinction that fails because East Asian medicine is also an allopathic system.

Consider, for example, bronchitis associated with a pathogenic bacteria. This condition would be countered in a conventional setting with antibiotics, fluids, and bed rest. East Asian medicine would sort the disorder not by pathogen but by presentation, color of mucus, sound of cough, and so on. Herbs would be administered, as well as forms of cutaneous and subcutaneous stimulation, such as acupuncture, gua sha, or cupping, with an equal emphasis on fluids and bed rest. In the end,

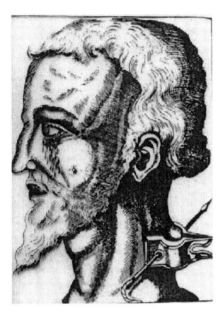

Figure 9-4. Early Western medicine's seton or threading. Skin is pinched at the back of the neck, and a thread or horse hair is inserted and left in place. Subsequent inflammation counters running eye sores. This is the closest early Western medical practice came to acupuncture therapy, 1583. *(From Brockbank W. Ancient therapeutic arts. In:* Fitzpatrick Lectures, Royal College of Physicians. *London: William Heineman Medical Books; 1954.)*

most patients receiving either therapy recover, but recovery in East Asian medicine does not just mean resolution of acute symptoms; it also means the clearing of residual heat and resolution of all forms of stasis, including phlegm, fluid, blood, and Qi. The benefit is prevention of relapse or risk of a secondary problem.

Acupuncture and Bloodletting

Acupuncture needling most likely derived from therapeutic bloodletting. The Ma-Wang-Tui texts found in the Han tombs buried in 165 B.C., thought to be recorded around 200 B.C., indicate points for bloodletting and direct moxibustion, with no reference to acupuncture needling.[38] Because the original meaning of Qi

is rising vapor[39] and because Qi warms, application of moxa heat was used to supplement Qi. On the other hand, bloodletting was used to reduce pathogenic nature of stasis and excess.

Early channels or meridians followed the path of apparent veins, and the first acupoints were those anatomically available for therapeutic bloodletting, proximal to a problem site, as in lancing for boils, or distal along vascular zones. Over time, therapeutic changes were observed when intentional points were pierced but no blood was let. Bloodletting evolved to needling of points with finer instruments. Moxibustion cautery had been applied to distal sites, but also to the body trunk. When the transition was made to include acupuncture needling, these trunk sites were also employed, increasing the number of sites then incorporated into an acupuncture point formulary. While the first text to refer to needling was written in 90 B.C.,[40] it is thought that acupuncture was adopted somewhere in the late second or first century B.C.[41]

Isomorphism

In early medicine of the East and West, the influence of demons or spirits preceded threatening elements of climate as cause of illness. The principles that came to guide health and healing were observable in the natural world, and the body construct isomorphic with nature. The elements of wind, cold, heat, dry, damp, and their combinations "act inside the body like they act outside."[42, 42a] Exposure to cold beyond the body's ability to warm itself leads to obstruction of substances, and slowing of function. Heat speeds things up increasing overall or local temperature, redness, and restlessness. Dampness is seen in collection of fluid, or "leaking" as in pouring down diarrhea or discharge. Dryness may associate with dehydration, dry skin, or a cracked tongue. Wind penetration results in obstruction of Qi, causing aching or shooting pain. Deficiency conditions are distinguished by a decrease of function and strength, and tend to be moderate but protracted. Excess conditions are often more acute, and stronger in symptomatology.

While pain is the first and most compelling sign of illness, it is not the only object of treatment in East Asian medicine, any more than it is in a modern Western clinic. Typhoid, cholera, or appendicitis were claimed to remit or be cured with East Asian treatment long before the use of modern antibiotics.[43] In both the Daoist and Confucian traditions in China, "perception is a form of response."[44] That a patient has pain, and how and where they experience the sensation, are as important to the provider of East Asian medicine as an MRI is to a Western clinician. Understanding the traditional East Asian perception of pain elucidates the manner of therapeutic response.

Pain Stasis

Pain is first defined as "stuck Qi," reflected in the third century B.C. Confucian work *Lu-shih ch'un-ch'iu*[45] and expressed in the aphorism, *Bu tong ze tong, tong ze bu tong,* meaning "no free-flow, there is pain; free flow, there is no pain."[46] Protracted or significant Qi stasis leads to stasis of other substances. In the clinical encounter, the symptom of pain triggers an exploration of what is stuck; where is it stuck; what is the stasis associated with; what helps; what hinders; and when it changes, how does it change.

Various forms of cutaneous and subcutaneous stimulation, which will be considered shortly, move Qi in specific channels that relate to specific organ function. The recovery of function is determined not only by improvement in pain status, but by changes in pulse, tongue, digestion, urine, stool, sleep, libido, flexibility, mood, and so on.

▶ SYNCRETISM AND EAST ASIAN MEDICINE

There are varied and valuable subsystems within East Asian medicine that contradict one another in part, and yet are active within the syncretic whole.[47] As groups adapted medicine to their cultural needs, and to changing illness presentations, a diversity of approaches remained necessary to meet the concrete demands of the clinical moment. Despite the homogeneity that often appears in Western translations of East Asian texts, East Asian medicine is a multimodal system of healing with multiple competing explanatory models.[48] This polyparadigmism[49] allows for versatility of choice in responding to illness. The goal is virtuosity[50] in honing a treatment that matches the illness, and the test of the method is in the patient response. If there is no response, another approach is tried.

It is an acceptable, favorable state of affairs that there is not a diagnostic truth aspired to in East Asian medicine. This is difficult to reconcile when modern Western treatment relies on correct diagnosis. In East Asian medicine, diagnosis evolves by interacting with an illness, "understood in all its dimensions only after it has been worked with for awhile."[51] This principle is actually in keeping with a basic tenet of science articulated by modern research theorists that, "in order to understand a thing, one must change it."[52]

▶ THE CLINICAL ENCOUNTER

The clinical encounter in East Asian medicine differs from a Western clinical encounter in significant ways. In an acupuncture encounter based in East Asian practice, the practitioner and the patient look at the problem together. Called "kanbing"[53] in Chinese, the patient narrative, their experience of their problem, is central to the process. What is the nature of your pain? How does it respond to movement or rest? Do you feel hot or cold? These questions require patient participation and body location. "The doctor does not have the power to reject any sign reported by the patient. Patients retain a sense of being expert, the authority of last resort, on their illness."[54] In addition, the patient becomes cued to the nuance of change that is inherent to any problem.

Western medical determinations rely less on interaction with the patient than on clinically significant test findings that occur outside the encounter, with the exception of psychoanalysis or psychotherapy. In East Asian medicine, it is the encounter itself, the somatic interaction as well as the cognitive discourse, that informs the shift toward healing. Whereas in Western medicine theory forms practice, in East Asian medical knowing, it is the practice, the somatic rapport of treatment and assessing sensation and changes in the problem within the session and through time, that after the fact forms theory.[55]

Discovery

Looking, listening, asking, and palpating are the four categories of kanbing. Use of all four areas ensures a thorough kanbing, and prevents a biased emphasis on one symptom or sign. For example, a fast pulse may indicate a state of overheating; however, the conclusion that there is overheating must be corroborated by other signs of fullness and heat. The practitioner associates signs and symptoms as expressions of either a disorder's branch or root, not to be confused with cause. The branch refers more to the expression as symptoms, while the root of an illness

> . . . is the state of play between yin and yang forces that gives rise to its symptoms . . . the yin yang condition exists at the same moment in time with the manifestations it produces. It is not a temporally or mechanically prior factor inducing an illness sequence; rather, it is the hidden condition that continually generates the perceptible forms of the moment.[56]

Yin and yang are understood in relation to each other. The original translation of yin was the shady side of a slope; yang was the sunny side. Where stillness is yin, movement is yang.

Yet there is movement in stillness, and stillness in movement. So yin and yang reside in each other. Something is not yin or yang of itself, but only in relation to something that gives context. The paired yin and yang organs are listed in "Location, Quality, Mutability" below.[57]

Looking

Looking is observation directed generally at a person's posture, gait, pallor, and demeanor, and specifically at any problem area. Unique to East Asian medicine is looking at the tongue.[58,58a-58d] The tongue's changing flesh color, shape, and coating clarify the quality, depth, and direction of a disorder.[59] Two patients may have what appears to be the same flu, but delineation by four examinations can reveal distinct root situations that require different treatment.

Because any encounter serves as a slice of life, the patient's countenance, behavior, attitude, and beliefs may be noted. A patient who is chronically late, hurried, frustrated, or angry— signs of difficulty in the liver channel—might be questioned about other liver channel signs involving digestion, sleep, and regularity of stool.

Asking

Asking inquires about 11 basic areas, including:

1. Pain: location frequency, severity, and responsiveness
2. Body temperature, per patient's sensation, as well as provider's touch
3. Digestion: what, when, and how food is eaten, and to what satisfaction
4. Fluid metabolism: thirst, sweat, saliva, tears, and movement
5. Urination: frequency, color, sensation, and stream
6. Stool: regularity, shape, color, smell, and sensation
7. Sleep: amount, timing, dreaming, waking, if restful
8. Menses: regularity, length, quality, color, and sensation related to cycle

9. Vitality: work, activity, capacity, and pleasure
10. Sensing: seeing, hearing, tasting, touching, thinking, feeling, and imagining
11. Sexual desire and activity

Listening

Listening is focused on the responses to questions posed and on the changing nature and strength of body sounds: breath, voice, cough, sneeze, wheeze, peristalsis, and voluntary movement sound. For example, a voice, cough, or sneeze that is forceful and loud implies strength of illness as well as strength in underlying constitution or terrain. Treatment must include clearing the excess. If the voice, cough, or sneeze is weak, treatment must include strengthening the underlying weakness. The latter treatment is contraindicated for the former condition, as it could make the illness stronger.

Palpation

In Western medicine, the problem associated with pain is often thought to be at the site of pain, or at the area of spine that enervates it. In East Asian medicine, palpation examines which areas are hot, cold, tight, ropey, or flaccid. Does the pain refer or traject, and which points, channels, organs, or muscles affect intensity? Palpation joins the practitioner and patient in a shared somatic experience of sorting and redefining the problem, in the moment, by sensation, touching areas that relate to and/or relieve original pain. If the pain is relieved by manipulation alone, it is the Qi that is stuck. If manipulation comforts but does not resolve the pain, it is the blood that is stuck.

Acupuncture systems active in China, Japan, Korea, and the United States use palpation of channels and points, as well as the pulse, as an important assessment and treatment technique.[60,60a–60f]

Classical Chinese acupuncture predates the modern Chinese emphasis on herbal medicine and internal organ pathology popularized in what is called traditional Chinese medicine (TCM).[61] While classical practice included herbs, there was more employment of manual techniques, discussed below, and consequently palpation for precise active areas or points informed practice. This is true for Japanese acupuncture where abdominal, or hara,[62] as well as channel palpation, is regularly employed.[63] Korean "amma" incorporates manual irrigation of the channels as assessment and treatment.[64] Fortunately, providers in the United States persist in East Asian medicine's syncretic tradition of drawing on multiple styles, including TCM and classical practice.

Palpating the pulse is one of the most exoticized aspects of East Asian medicine, with almost psychic abilities assigned to certain historical pulse takers. In general practice, the radial pulse is touched to assess overall strength and rate. The upper, middle, and lower pulses relate to the upper, middle, and lower sections of the body, called *jiaos*. The literal translation of jiao is burner. The san jiao is the organ corresponding to the three burners. The upper burner includes the heart and lung area; the middle burner includes the midsection abdomen; and the lower burner includes the lower abdomen. Each pulse position is touched for its surface and deep strength, indicating the state of internal organs that occupy the corresponding body section. For example, the lung pulse is the upper part of the radial pulse, just proximal to the right wrist crease. It feels large or disturbed in cases of acute bronchitis. Beginning students are taught to seek out family or friends with upper respiratory infections because the changing quality of the lung pulse is readily discernible.

▶ PATTERNS OF DISHARMONY, SYSTEM OF CORRESPONDENCES, AND DIAGNOSES IN EAST ASIAN MEDICINE

The well-known patterns of disharmony and system of correspondences,[65] which are represented as the heart of East Asian medical diagnostics in contemporary theoretical texts, guide, but by no means determine, treatment.[66] To illustrate, consider patient records in China, which are, incidentally, often retained by the patient alone. In them, the provider will record the patient's presenting signs, reported symptoms, tongue, pulse, important history, acupuncture points used, techniques applied, herbs prescribed, and any labs or tests ordered. Syndromes, diagnoses, and treatment principles go unrecorded.[67] Similarly, in the West, clinicians do not record an East Asian diagnosis in the patient chart.

Kanbing assessment seeks to identify the fundamental responsive nature of a problem rather than its cause. Where cause implies something in the past, the responsive nature presents in the moment, open to interaction. An illness is described best not in a diagnosis but in the quality, location,[68] and mutability[69] of its present nature. The changes that result from the therapeutic interaction within the session and over time direct further acupuncture treatment, herbal prescribing, recommendations, and follow-up.

It is interesting to note that in the past, East Asian practitioners were taught through observation of senior clinicians' practices and through case studies. Dividing texts into volumes of theory and practice is relatively recent,[70] and while these didactic formats permeate contemporary pedagogy, it is still not the theoretical framework that trains the clinician; it is practice itself—clinical experience. Hence the phrase often used in China, "we take practice to be our guide,"[71] the practice of interacting with "location, quality, and mutability."

Location, Quality, Mutability

Locations in East Asian medicine are overlapping anatomical and/or functional "sites." They include, but are not limited to, the channels, organs, essences, substances, spirits, levels, and curious places. The *jing* channel vessels include the 12 bilateral vertical channels that are associated with internal organs in addition to the ventral and dorsal central channels, known as the conception and governing vessels, respectively. The luo vessels emanate in the body flesh, connecting the flesh, and the jing vessels to one another and to the internal organs.

Organs are entities of vital function, material in form but not limited to Western anatomical location. They resist parallel categorization to Western physiology because the organs in East Asian medicine operate not as distinct entities but in contextual interrelationship with the other organs, substances, and potentials of becoming and declining. In the following list the yin *(zang)* organs are on the left with their paired yang *(fu)* organs on the right:

Heart ~ Small Intestine
Lung ~ Large Intestine
Liver ~ Gallbladder
Spleen ~ Stomach
Kidney ~ Bladder
Pericardium ~ Triple Burner

The *jiaos*, or burners, represent upper, middle, and lower sections of the body (see Figure 9–5A). They are connected and maintained by the organ that has no Western twin, the san jiao, or triple burner.

The *levels* can refer to general outer/inner areas. There are also the six levels associated with the stages of illness involving progression of cold induction. The four levels refers to stages of illness involving progression of heat induction.

The *substances* are Qi, blood, jing, fluid, phlegm, and food. Qi is the most fundamental concept of East Asian cosmology and is associated with the early Western medicine's "pneuma."[72] Its original definition was air, or vapor rising from cooking rice, like the Greek winds or humours caused by what remains after the digestion of food.[73] (see Figure 9–5B)

Qi is inclusive of material form and function, and is not synonymous with energy. Qi moves, protects, stabilizes, transforms, and warms. The Qi of my hand implies the material form of my

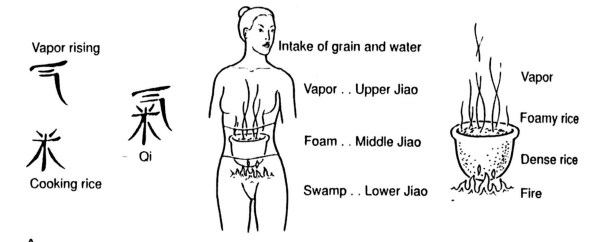

Vapor rising

Cooking rice

Qi

Intake of grain and water

Vapor . . Upper Jiao

Foam . . Middle Jiao

Swamp . . Lower Jiao

Vapor

Foamy rice

Dense rice

Fire

A

Figure 9–5A. One form of Qi rises from food rendered or spoiled by fire. Each of the upper, middle, and lower jiao (or burner) has a role in the transformation and circulation of Qi. The ancients regarded the San Jiao, or three burners, as an organ. (From Nielsen A. *Gua Sha. A Traditional Technique for Modern Practice.* Philadelphia: Elsevier; 1995:36.)

hand and it's ability to move as I type. Qi is divided into subcategories associated with place or function: *zang-fu* or organ Qi, *jing-luo* or channel Qi, *ying* or nutritive Qi, *zhong* or Qi of the chest, also called ancestral, and *wei* or protective Qi. In pathology, Qi becomes errant, stuck, or deficient.

Blood nourishes, moistens and warms by circulating in the vessels and channels. It is produced by the transformation of food combining with the "clear" air of the lungs, and is propelled in circulation by the heart and *zhong* Qi of the chest. In pathology, the blood becomes deficient, stuck, or out of place. Aspects of the blood support comfort, memory, and self-esteem. Blood stasis pain is persistent and aggravating, and when focal is stabbing, boring, or searing. Figures 9–6 and 9–7 illustrate a method of palpation called "press and blanche" to identify blood stasis in the surface tissues.

Jing, or essence, is sourced from the essence of one's parents, called "prenatal," and maintained through the contribution of transformation of food and harmonious living resulting in

appropriate maturation and passing of life stages. Pathology of the jing can manifest in problems of maturation and development. The jing may be considered when major life or

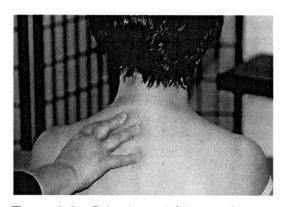

Figure 9–6. Palpating painful areas for surface blood stasis called sha, the practitioner presses her fingers onto the flesh. (Reprinted from Nielsen A. *Gua Sha. Eine traditionelle technik fur die moderne medizin.* Koetzting, Germany: Verlag fur Ganzheitliche Medizin; 2000; with permission from Verlag fur Ganzheitliche Medizin.)

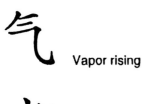 Vapor rising

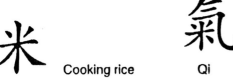 Cooking rice   Qi

φ ῡσαι ἕχ τⱨν πεοιττωιιάτⱨν

Winds or humors caused by what remains after the digestion of food

B

Figure 9-5B. The ideogram of Qi depicts vapor rising from cooking rice. Hippocratic medicine had a similar concept dating from 400 B.C.[39] The Greeks also assumed a heat source in the body. (From Nielsen A. *Gua Sha. A Traditional Technique for Modern Practice.* Philadelphia: Elsevier; 1995:18.)

"destiny" issues such as choice of career, sexuality, reproduction, and so on challenge a patient.

Fluids are divided into the *jin* and *ye,* the lighter/clearer versus the heavier/thicker. The fluids include the visibly expressed tears, saliva, sweat, and urine. Internally, fluids moisten and nourish, and while there is some synchronicity with the blood, the fluids are not as dense or nourishing as the blood. In pathology, fluids become stuck, deficient, or absent, resulting in edema, drying, or withering.

The *shens* are the psychospiritual aspects associated with the yin organs, and in their common, but not inclusive, translation are

Heart shen: consciousness
Spleen yi: thinking
Liver hun: noncorporeal soul
Lung po: corporeal soul, animal body
Kidney zhi: destiny or will of heaven

The special sites include the orifices or senses, and the six curious organs: brain, bone, marrow, blood vessels, uterus, and gallbladder.

The qualities of wind, hot, cold, damp, dry, moving, stuck, deficient, and full act in the body like they act outside in nature. Wind, hot, dry, moving, and full are yang qualities. Cold, damp, and deficient are yin qualities. Stuckness can be yin in its not-moving nature, but yang in the excess of what is stuck.

Wind is said to penetrate at the surface of the body, and is associated with muscle aches, headache, and early stages of the flu. Hot, cold, damp, or dry can accompany wind penetration. When wind is generated internally, it may be associated with headache, spasms, paralysis, shooting pain, and even seizure.

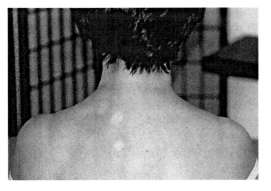

Figure 9-7. Sha is indicated when finger pressure causes blanching that is distinct and disappears slowly. (Reprinted from Nielsen A. *Gua Sha. Eine traditionelle technik fur die moderne medizin.* Koetzting, Germany: Verlag fur Ganzheitliche Medizin; 2000; with permission from Verlag fur Ganzheitliche Medizin.)

A heat-dominated state or location is warm to the touch, and will likely be associated with agitation, restlessness, redness, and inflammation, and perhaps reactivity. Pain with heat is comforted but not necessarily resolved by application of cold.

A cold-dominated state or location is cool to the touch, and will likely be associated with cramping, contraction, chill, and depressed function. Pain with cold is comforted but not necessarily resolved by application of heat.

A damp-dominated state or location is boggy to the touch, and feels clogged or heavy to the patient. Dampness pours down in diarrhea, leukorrhea, or weeping from sites. Pain from dampness is comforted but not necessarily resolved by passive or active movement. A dry-dominated state or location is deficient of fluid and wants moistening. It may be accompanied by itch and agitation, and be comforted but not resolved by hydrating or external moistening.

Moving is characterized by proper functioning but can lapse in pathology to under- or overactivity. Stillness or stasis is a necessary counter to movement, but can lapse in pathology to inertia and/or pooling of stuck things. Either may be comforted but not completely resolved by simple physical movement or rest. Hence manual or internal medicine may be required specific to these problems.

Finally, deficiency describes a lack of substance or function. Fullness describes an excess. When a log falls across a running stream, above it one finds excess, below one finds deficiency. So, too, in the body, excess in one place or function may imply deficiency in another.

Mutability: Waxing and Waning

East Asian medicine does not operate in a cause–effect nexus but rather as expression of source–manifestation.[74] "Things are already changing"[75]—becoming, declining, and/or resting between becoming and declining. The clinical question is not how to diagnose and then fix a problem, but how to associate features of presentation to reveal where and how to enter, to influence innate waxing and waning. Rarely is an illness static, or the same each day. What comforts the problem? What exacerbates it?

When we add to that the feedback loop of the clinical encounter's somatic interaction—where "to understand a thing you must change it"[76]—then treatment becomes evaluation, and evaluation becomes treatment.[77]

Consider a stomachache. Cold at the belly, with clear vomit can be called obstruction in the middle burner, or cold in the stomach and spleen. Without cold signs it may be noted as rebellious stomach Qi, or liver Qi constraint with liver invading the stomach. If the pain is boring and severe, there may be blood stasis corroborated by blue or purple on the tongue. The honing process that locates, describes qualities, and assesses mutability leads to action; what matters is the effectiveness of the action and the ability to respond to the unfolding.

▶ TREATMENT

Treatment has already begun in the kanbing process of discussing, defining, and reframing. The somatic interaction not only gives "diagnostic" information, but actually begins to shift the problem. Choosing points or areas of the body to treat depends on empirical point knowledge, and familiarity with historical literature of point application through time for particular illnesses. Multiple sites are chosen as the treatment proceeds, and treated with different forms of stimulation.[78]

Acupuncture Needling

Needling techniques vary depending on the explanatory model of acupuncture used. Dominant Chinese acupuncture technique intends to congest, disperse, tonify, or sedate Qi, and may be used with other manual procedures such as moxibustion, gua sha, cupping, tui na, plum blossom, or herbal medicine. A needle may be inserted and manipulated for the de Qi response, which is mandatory in Chinese acupuncture. De Qi means the Qi has arrived at the point. The provider feels it as movement—a pulling, grasping or sinking of the needle.[79] The patient experiences de Qi as a sensation of jumping or fasciculation; aching, heaviness, tingling, trajecting, or referring locally; or in another area altogether. After one or several de Qi at the same site, needles may be removed or left in place for 5–30 minutes. Types of stimulation are associated with the point, the depth of needling, practice style and intention. Most needles seek a depth of 0.25 inches, to reach the surface of the subcutaneous fascia. However, if not satisfied with the response, the provider will not hesitate to obtain de Qi from deeper connective tissue, to a depth of an inch or more. Some needling techniques call for a 3-inch depth, but this is uncommon. Some needling does not even pierce the skin. There are systems that treat exclusively at the ear (Nogier), the hand (Korean), or the wrist or ankle (Lao), all of which serve as responsive holographs of the body.[80]

Trigger-point needling has become popular in the United States through the work of Janet Travell and Mark Seem,[81] and a resurgence of classical Chinese acupuncture as taught by Drs. James Tin Yao So[82,82a] and Yi Tian Ni.[83] Trigger-point reduction needling involves first pressing or lifting the trigger points or bands, called "ah shi" areas in Chinese. "Reduction" in the area is as a result of de Qi fasciculation, which may be repeated many times with the same needle insertion until the point is reduced, and the banding disbanded. Then the needle is either withdrawn or set to rest in the point for 10–20 minutes. Areas are then repalpated to assess the condition of the constraint pattern aptly referred to by Travell as the "mytotic conspiracy."

Distal points on the limbs are needled, but not aggressively unless there is banding involved locally. In distal needling, a de Qi is obtained, but may involve a feeling of heaviness, ache, or ping, rather than fasciculation. The needles may be withdrawn or set for 10–20 minutes.

Additional techniques described below may be used during a session. Recommendations may be given during and at the end of treatment and might include an herbal prescription, dietary changes, exercise, and meditation, and adjustments in work or activity. The presentation in follow-up sessions may be entirely different, necessitating a modification in approach.

Moxibustion

Cautery was the early Western medical counterpart to moxibustion. Moxa might be used after acupuncture needling of a point, or independent of needling treatment. Moxibustion involves burning the fiber precipitate from *Artemisia vulgaris* either directly on a point, called direct moxibustion, or just above and over an area, called indirect moxibustion. Indirect moxa is used to warm a person who is deficient and cold. Direct moxa is a stronger treatment that is used for long-standing focal or channel stasis.

Moxa is most often contraindicated in hot conditions such as fever, hypertension, or distended inflammation. However, when indicated, moxibustion resolves focal stasis that cannot be addressed in any other way. Unfortunately, because of the smoke generated by moxibustion, its use is limited in modern clinical settings.

Gua Sha

Gua sha is a technique commonly used in Asia by practitioners of traditional medicine in the clinical setting and in the home. In gua sha, the skin is pressured in strokes by a round-edged instrument resulting in red, raised petechiae called sha. With gua sha, blood extravasates from the peripheral vasculature, but is not let from the skin. The petechiae resemble the end-stage petechial crisis seen in cholera, hence sha

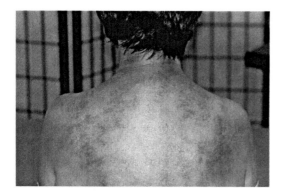

Figure 9–8. Sha petechiae raised after gua sha on patient palpated in Figures 9–6 and 9–7. (Reprinted from Nielsen A. *Gua Sha. Eine traditionelle technik fur die moderne medizin.* Koetzting, Germany: Verlag fur Ganzheitliche Medizin; 2000; with permission from Verlag fur Ganzheitliche Medizin.)

is also translated as cholera. Gua sha was historically used in China to treat cholera[84] and cholera-like disorders.[85] The early Western counterpart used to treat cholera was frictioning.[86]

Gua sha is considered adaptogenic, warming those who are cold, cooling those who are hot, supporting deficiency and clearing excess. By moving blood stasis, pain is resolved immediately. Gua sha removes metabolic waste congesting the surface tissue, promotes circulation, and normalizes metabolic processes.[87] Figures 9–6, 9–7, and 9–8 show palpation indications for blood stasis congesting the surface, and the resulting sha petechiae raised from gua sha. (Pain associated with blood stasis is resolved immediately with gua sha.)

Cupping

Popular in both the East and West, many patients remark that they had cupping done when they were young by a grandmother, mother, or aunt. A vacuum is created in a glass, bamboo, or gourd cup by lighting a ball of alcohol-soaked cotton and passing it inside the cup, then immediately placing it on the skin. This is called fire cupping. The vacuum cup creates

suction at the surface, producing sha petechiae as in gua sha. Modern cups create a vacuum effect by using a suction pump, which is equally moving but less warming than fire cupping.

Like gua sha, cupping is used to remove blood stasis. One technique is only preferred over the other depending on the area to be treated and the personal preference of the provider. While gua sha easily accesses a wider area, it cannot be applied over an existing rash, where cupping would be preferred if indicated.

Tui Na

Tui na involves surface and musculoskeletal manipulation resembling Western massage. However, Tui Na incorporates many unique hand movements specific to a desired effect and therefore has a wider range of therapeutic value in the context of East Asian practice than Western massage currently experiences in the West.

Plum Blossom

Plum blossom refers to either a seven-star needle, or the technique that uses a seven-star needle, or a number of needles clustered together in the forefinger grip and tapped with equal pressure at the skin surface. The tiny cutaneous pinpricks may bleed slightly. They create a cascade of responses locally and along an applied channel. Plum blossom is also used in the care of children who generally do not require acupuncture. Plum blossom is also used, for example, in cases of eczema, where the tapping is thought to break the obstruction in the *biao,* skin, healing the lesion site.

Herbal Medicine

The Ma-Wang-Tui texts buried in 165 B.C. contained charts marking the channels or meridians with prescriptions for moxibustion, bloodletting, herbal poultices, and herbal decoctions.[88] Herbs have also been and continue to be used in the Western clinical settings, with many pharmaceutical drugs being synthetic versions of ingredients derived from medicinal plants. Chapters 5 and 6 detail some of the plants used in the modern conventional setting.

East Asian herbology is a subject beyond the scope of this book. However, there are several important issues worth mentioning concerning herbs. Herbs may or may not be prescribed in an acupuncture session. The NCCAOM that board certifies acupuncturists in the United States, also board certifies herbalists in the East Asian tradition. However, not every acupuncturist chooses to study herbs, while some are board certified and prescribe herbs as often as acupuncture. Most states do not regulate the prescribing of herbal medicine, so US herbology retains some of its early Western domesticity. That is, herbs, like vitamins, are a part of home health care, as yet not controlled by the professional sector.[89]

Where Western herbs are often prescribed alone as "simples," East Asian herbs are given in combinations as archetypal responses to illness, and modified to treat the unique features of a person's presentation. Combining and individualizing herbs is said to enhance the indicated effects and greatly reduce side effects common to Western drug therapy. Formulas are adjusted based on the patient's changing presentation. The expectation is that the action of herbs will build over time, but that recovery is possible, at which point the herbs will be discontinued. Rarely, if ever, are herbs prescribed with the expectation that they are needed in any permanent way. While outcome studies can be done for herbal combinations, research to isolate active ingredients is challenged by the variability of complex formulas.

▶ CLINICAL RESEARCH IN ACUPUNCTURE

The following subsections present an overview of randomized controlled trials published since the NIH Consensus Conference on Acupuncture.

NIH Consensus Conference on Acupuncture

In the fall of 1997, the NIH convened a landmark Consensus Conference on Acupuncture that was, arguably, the most extensive evaluation of controlled trials of acupuncture ever undertaken.[90] The conference represented a coming of age of acupuncture in the West because it signaled the interest of the biomedical community in assessing the therapeutic effectiveness of this millennia-old practice. Of considerable significance were the ground rules of the conference: Acupuncture was not to be assessed in terms of its origins as *experience-based* medicine and there would be no presentations of clinical records or testimony from patients. Instead, it would be evaluated according to the newly emerging criteria of *evidence-based* medicine, as applied to results of published clinical trials. In essence, the NIH panel asked two interrelated questions: Is there convincing evidence that acupuncture is more effective than placebo or other control treatment? Has acupuncture been tested in a manner sufficiently rigorous and adequate to consider results of the trials as valid?

Both issues were directly addressed in the Consensus Conference report. First, based on review of the research findings, guarded approval was given to the clinical practice of acupuncture. Conditions for which results were considered "promising" were limited to adult postoperative and chemotherapy-related nausea and vomiting, and postoperative dental pain. Other conditions for which acupuncture was deemed "may be useful," as either adjunctive or alternative care, comprised a broad list, including addiction, stroke rehabilitation, headache, menstrual cramps, tennis elbow, fibromyalgia, myofascial pain, osteoarthritis, low back pain, carpal tunnel syndrome, and asthma. Second, the overall design and reporting of acupuncture trials were considered, in no uncertain terms, to be of poor quality. The frequent occurrence of a low sample size, omission of random assignment of study participants to treatment groups, and lack of blinding of treatment evaluator were noted, as was the confusing diversity of so-called placebo, sham, and minimal acupuncture control procedures.

The Post-Consensus Conference Climate for Acupuncture Research

Since the NIH conference the biomedical community has increasingly applied the standards of evidence-based medicine to evaluate its own treatments, as well as those of acupuncture and the numerous other modalities and systems of complementary and alternative medicine. In this context, it is important to examine whether and how the quality of acupuncture research has improved. Before reviewing recent studies that have tested efficacy of acupuncture for specific conditions, several warming trends should be noted that have markedly improved the climate for acupuncture research.

Directly following the NIH Consensus Conference report, the NIH Office of Alternative Medicine, predecessor of the present National Center for Complementary and Alternative Medicine (NCCAM), earmarked funds specifically for research to develop rigorous designs for acupuncture trials.[91] This resulted in a small but important group of clinical trials that systematically examined the effectiveness of acupuncture when compared to acupuncture-like needling at sites inappropriate to the condition studied or to noninvasive "needling" techniques. An example of the latter is light stimulation at predetermined sites on the skin surface with a toothpick, placed within a plastic tube commonly used as a guide for an acupuncture needle.[92] This group of studies also stressed the importance of validating the research design by questioning each "blinded" subject receiving acupuncture or control needling as to which treatment they believed they had been given.[93,94] Only if the guesses are close to the chance level is the blinding considered successful and thus the study considered valid.

A second important trend is the direct encouragement from NCCAM for practitioners of complementary and alternative medicine (including acupuncture and Oriental medicine) to receive training in research design. This occurs through training grants to individual practitioners and to NCCAM-funded research centers. This approach helps to ensure the twin goals of acupuncture research: to meet appropriate standards of design and to best reflect the traditions of its practice.

The years since the NIH Conference have also seen the application of systematic reviews to the field of acupuncture research.[95] A systematic review is a rigorous exercise in quality assessment of controlled clinical trials of a specific treatment (e.g., acupuncture) for a specific condition (e.g., osteoarthritis or migraine) or general condition (e.g., pain). It has largely replaced the earlier form of narrative review, in which the author(s) is free to review selected strengths and weaknesses of a preferentially chosen group of clinical trials. In contrast, the systematic review requires a thorough search of the scientific literature for articles meeting predetermined inclusion criteria, followed by evaluation of all included articles according to a predetermined set of quality assurance criteria. Many of the better systematic reviews of acupuncture have been performed under the auspices of the Cochrane Collaboration, an international organization with a mission to collect and review controlled clinical trials in every area of medicine.[96] Interestingly, some 40 systematic reviews of acupuncture[97] have revealed the same set of design flaws that the NIH conference panel had highlighted (see above). One additional finding is the positive correlation between number of acupuncture treatments and efficacy in clinical trials of pain conditions.[98] This observation suggests that many clinical trials have underevaluated acupuncture. The main, generally accepted conclusion is the need for a temporary cessation of systematic reviews of acupuncture and the corresponding need for well-designed new trials.[99]

A fourth occurrence, aimed at improving acupuncture research is a set of Standards for Reporting Interventions in Controlled Trials of Acupuncture (STRICTA)[100] that modifies the biomedical guidelines of Consolidated Standards for Reporting of Trials (CONSORT)[101] to better apply to acupuncture trials. What systematic reviews would do to improve the design of clinical trials, STRICTA and CONSORT would do to improve the reporting of methodology and results. STRICTA, drafted for use by reviewers who determine whether submitted research reports are acceptable for publication, was initially adopted by five US and British journals that publish acupuncture trials.

Clinical Trials of Acupuncture: 1998-2002

Having highlighted the improved climate for acupuncture research since the NIH Consensus Conference on Acupuncture, we can consider the clinical research itself, published during the 5-year postconference period. Examples of recent studies for conditions on the "A List" (deemed "promising") and "B List" ("may be useful") are briefly reviewed, as are studies of the rapidly expanding area of acupuncture for women's reproductive health, for which a paucity of studies existed at the time of the NIH conference. While neither the selection nor the analyses of the trials covered in this review are meant to be inclusive or systematic, a short list of criteria (Table 9–3) was followed in selecting the articles presented in Tables 9–4 and 9–5.

As mentioned at the start of this section, the only conditions considered by the NIH panel as having an acceptable evidence-base are adult postoperative- and chemotherapy-related emesis and postoperative dental pain. Table 9–4 lists more recent controlled clinical trials of acupuncture for these conditions. A major contribution to the emesis literature is the demonstration that adjunctive acupuncture significantly improves the effectiveness of antiemetic medications in women receiving high-dose

▶ **TABLE 9-3** SELECTION CRITERIA FOR ACUPUNCTURE TRIALS LISTED IN TABLES 9–4 AND 9–5*

1. Controlled clinical trial
2. English language
3. Full article
4. Publication date 1998–2002
5. Inclusion and exclusion criteria for patient selection presented
6. Assignment to treatment groups described as randomized*
7. Baseline demographics across treatment groups presented
8. Patients and/or outcome evaluator described as blinded
9. Protocols for acupuncture and control groups adequately described*

---

*A few trials included in Tables 9–4 and 9–5 are exceptions to these criteria; for example, trials in which acupressure, transcutaneous electrical nerve stimulation, or laser at acupuncture points was used instead of acupuncture; or where matched pairs or case-controlled designs were used instead of randomization assignment. In such cases, the design feature in question is italicized in the *Research Design* column.

chemotherapy subsequent to breast cancer-related stem cell transplants.[102] In this rigorously designed study, the acupuncture plus medication protocol also proved significantly more effective than adjunctive sham acupuncture. As the study was nearing completion, however, an improved class of antiemetic medication was approved, and new trials have begun to test whether acupuncture will again prove useful as complementary care. The management of postoperative nausea by acupuncture or acupressure (at a single acupuncture point on the inner forearm just below the wrist) has been confirmed in several well-designed placebo-controlled studies.[103,104] As has been pointed out in a systematic review of acupuncture for nausea and vomiting, a major variable in the design of these studies is the timing of treatment.[105] Trials for which acupuncture was found ineffective were mainly those in which it was performed during anesthesia; in virtually

▶ **TABLE 9-4** CONTROLLED CLINICAL TRIALS OF ACUPUNCTURE, 1998–2002: CONDITIONS FOR WHICH ACUPUNCTURE WAS CONSIDERED "PROMISING" BY THE 1997 NIH CONSENSUS CONFERENCE PANEL

Reference	Condition Treated	Research Design	Group Size	Results
Shen et al.[102]	Chemotherapy-related emesis	Three groups: (1) electroacu acu + meds; (2) sham electroacu + meds; (3) meds alone	34–37	Electroacu > sham > meds alone (median number of emesis episodes: 5, 10, and 15, respectively).* Differences among groups not significant at day 9 of follow-up.
Harmon et al.[103]	Postoperative emesis	Acu vs sham acu	52	Incidence of nausea or vomiting reduced from 42% (sham) to 19% (acu).
Kotani et al.[104]	Postoperative emesis	Acu vs noninvasive sham acu	38–50	Relative to controls, acu reduced supplemental IV morphine 50%, postoperative nausea 20–30%, and plasma cortisol and epinephrine levels 30–50%.*
Lao et al.[106]	Postoperative dental pain	Acu vs noninvasive sham acu	19–20	Acu increased pain-free postoperative time and decreased consumption of pain meds.*

Abbreviations: acu = acupuncture; electroacu = electroacupuncture; meds = medicines; IV = intravenous.
*Statistically significant.

all successful trials, acupuncture was provided once the patients had regained consciousness.

The evidence base for acupuncture as effective pain management in postoperative dental care has been strengthened by a larger study[106] confirming the initial findings.[107] Again, the postsurgery, pain-free time for patients randomly assigned to receive acupuncture was significantly greater than for patients assigned to receive a noninvasive sham acupuncture procedure. Also, as in the earlier trial, the findings were validated because patients were unable to guess their treatment group at a level greater than chance.

Table 9–5 lists selected post-1997 clinical trials covering the range of conditions for which the NIH panel rated acupuncture as "may be useful." As in the previous section, the articles do not represent an inclusive list but do meet the inclusion criteria in Table 9–3 and were selected independent of trial outcome. (The seemingly arbitrary order of conditions follows that of the NIH conference report.)

Addiction

Of particular note are two trials demonstrating effectiveness of acupuncture for smoking cessation,[108,109] a positive outcome trial of acupuncture for treatment of methadone-maintained cocaine addicts,[110] and a negative outcome, large-scale multicenter trial, again for treating methadone-maintained cocaine abusers.[111] In puzzling out the possible design differences between the latter two trials, which may have bearing on their respective outcomes, it seems important to recognize the importance of basing the research protocol as much as possible on clinical practice. In this regard, virtually all substance abuse programs involving acupuncture use it as adjunctive treatment to 12-step or other psychotherapeutic counseling sessions, and not as a stand-alone treatment, as it was

▶ **TABLE 9-5** CONTROLLED CLINICAL TRIALS OF ACUPUNCTURE, 1998–2002: CONDITIONS FOR WHICH ACUPUNCTURE WAS CONSIDERED "MAY BE USEFUL" BY THE 1997 NIH CONSENSUS CONFERENCE PANEL

Reference	Condition Treated	Research Design	Group Size	Results
He et al.[109]	Nicotine addiction	Acu vs invasive sham acu	23	Acu decreased cigarette consumption relative to sham at completion of treatment and at 8-month follow-up.* No between-group difference at 5-year follow-up
Bier et al.[108]	Nicotine addiction	3 groups: ear acu; ear acu + edu; invasive sham ear acu + edu	38–58	Posttreatment cigarette consumption decreased for all groups; acu + edu had the greatest effect*; trend continued at follow-up.
Avants et al.[110]	Cocaine addiction	3 groups: ear acu; invasive sham ear acu; relaxation	27–28	Acu decreased cocaine-positive urine samples relative to sham acu and to relaxation.*
Margolin et al.[111]	Cocaine addiction	3 groups: ear acu; invasive sham ear acu; relaxation	195–222	Urine samples showed a significant overall reduction in cocaine use,* but no differences by treatment condition. Counseling sessions in all 3 conditions were poorly attended.
Gosman-Hedstrom et al.[118]	Stroke rehab	3 groups: electroacu; superficial acu; no acu; all received usual care	33–37	No between-group differences on neurologic score, ADL index, or use of health care and social services, at 3 and 12 months.
Wong et al.[121]	Stroke rehab	TENS at acupoints + usual rehab care vs rehab care only	59	TENS had shorter duration of hospital stay for rehab, better neurologic and functional outcomes, and improved scores for self-care and locomotion.*
Johansson et al.[119]	Stroke rehab	3 groups: electroacu; acu; TENS; sham TENS	48–51	No clinically important or significant between-group differences for any of the outcome variables at 3-month and 1-year follow-up.
Sze et al.[120]	Stroke rehab	Acu + usual care vs usual care	53	No significant between-group differences for any outcome measure.
Karst et al.[124]	Tension headache	Acu vs. noninvasive sham acu	34–35	No significant between-group differences in VAS or frequency of headaches. Acu improved QOL.*
Karakurum et al.[125]	Tension headache	Trigger-point acu vs minimal acu	15	Headache indices improved in both groups.* Neck ROM and tenderness improved only in acu group.*

(Continued)

▶ **TABLE 9-5** CONTROLLED CLINICAL TRIALS OF ACUPUNCTURE, 1998–2002: CONDITIONS FOR WHICH ACUPUNCTURE WAS CONSIDERED "MAY BE USEFUL" BY THE 1997 NIH CONSENSUS CONFERENCE PANEL (*Continued*)

Reference	Condition Treated	Research Design	Group Size	Results
White et al.[126]	Tension headache	Brief acu vs non-invasive sham acu	25	No significant between-group differences for any outcome variable.
Liguori et al.[128]	Migraine	Acu vs meds	60	Acu at least as effective as meds in decreasing migraine frequency at 6- and 12-month follow-up.
Allais et al.[127]	Migraine	Acu vs flunarizine	80	On-treatment frequency of attacks and use of symptomatic meds decreased in both groups.* Acu more effectively reduced number of attacks at 2- and 4-month follow-up.* Fewer side effects in acu group.*
Carlsson et al.[132]	Pregnancy nausea	Crossover: acu vs invasive sham acu	16–17	Faster reduction of nausea VAS and decreased vomiting with acu relative to sham.*
Knight et al.[131]	Pregnancy nausea	Acu vs noninvasive sham acu	27–28	Nausea significantly decreased in both groups*; no between-group difference.
Smith et al.[130]	Pregnancy nausea	4 groups: individualized acu; standardized acu (P6 only); invasive sham acu; no acu	148–149	Acu, P6 acu, and sham acu decreased nausea and dry retching as compared to no acu.*
Wedenberg et al.[134]	Pregnancy back pain	Acu vs PT	30	Acu more effective than physiotherapy for relieving VAS pain and disability.*
Tempfer et al.[137]	Duration of labor	*Matched pairs:* acu vs no acu	40	Acu reduced duration of labor,* with no effects on serum levels of IL-8, PGF_2alpha, or beta-endorphin.
Zeisler et al.[136]	Duration of labor	*Case-control study:* acu vs no acu	57–63	Acu shortened duration of first stage of labor.*
Rabl et al.[138]	Duration of labor	Acu vs no acu	20–25	Acu supports cervical ripening at term and shortens the interval between estimated date of confinement and actual time of delivery.*
Skilnand et al.[135]	Labor-related pain	Acu vs invasive sham acu	102–106	Acu lowered pain scores,* decreased need for pharmacologic analgesia,* and decreased time in active labor.*

(*Continued*)

Reference	Condition Treated	Research Design	Group Size	Results
Stener-Victorin et al.[140]	In vitro fertilization	Electroacu vs standard care (alfentanil)	74–75	Electroacu as effective as meds in reducing pain and nausea. Electroacu had higher rates of implantation, pregnancy, and take home baby per embryo transfer.*
Paulus et al.[141]	In vitro fertilization	Acu vs no acu	80	Pregnancy rate: 43% for acu vs 26% for control.
Fink et al.[142]	Tennis elbow	Acu vs invasive sham acu	22–23	Acu > sham for reducing pain, and improving arm function and strength at 2-week follow-up.* Acu > sham for function,* but not pain or strength, at 2-months.
Tsui and Leung[143]	Tennis elbow	Electroacu vs manual acu	10	VAS pain and pain-free hand grip strength improved in both groups.*
Birch and Jamison[145]	Neck pain	3 groups: acu; invasive sham acu; NSAIDS	15–16	Greater pre-to-post differences in pain with acu than sham or meds.* Confidence in treatment and past experience with acu correlated with decreased pain.* No between-group differences.
David et al.[144]	Neck pain	Acu vs physiotherapy	35	Both groups improved in all criteria at 6 weeks on treatment and 6-month follow-up. Acu > physiotherapy in patients with higher baseline pain scores.*
Irnich et al.[146]	Neck pain	3 groups: massage; acu; sham laser	56–61	Acu = sham laser > massage for motion-related pain at 1-week posttreatment.*
Irnich et al.[147]	Neck pain	3 groups: single-treatment cross-over: distal acu; trigger-point acu; sham laser acu	33–34	Distal acu reduced motion-related pain scores, improved ROM, and improved patient-assessed change as compared to the other 2 groups.*
Dyson-Hudson et al.[148]	Shoulder pain	Acu vs Trager integration	9	Shoulder pain decreased in both groups*; no between-group difference.
Kleinhenz et al.[149]	Rotator cuff tendonitis	Acu vs noninvasive sham acu	25–27	Acu > sham for pain relief.*
Jensen et al.[150]	Knee pain	Acu vs no treatment	34–36	Acu decreased knee pain and improved function at 12-month follow-up when compared to control.*
Berman et al.[151]	Osteoarthritis	Acu + usual care vs usual care alone	36–37	Acu group improved on two osteo-arthritis indices when compared to usual care at 4 and 8 weeks on treatment and at 4-week follow-up.*

(Continued)

▶ **TABLE 9-5** CONTROLLED CLINICAL TRIALS OF ACUPUNCTURE, 1998–2002: CONDITIONS FOR WHICH ACUPUNCTURE WAS CONSIDERED "MAY BE USEFUL" BY THE 1997 NIH CONSENSUS CONFERENCE PANEL (*Continued*)

Reference	Condition Treated	Research Design	Group Size	Results
Haslam[152]	Osteoarthritis	Acu vs advice + exercise	12–16	Acu decreased pain indices posttreatment and at 8-week follow-up, over time and between groups.*
Tillu et al.[153]	Osteoarthritis	Acu on most-affected knee vs acu on both knees	22	Both groups significantly reduced symptoms at posttreatment and 6-month follow-up*; no significant between-group difference.
Fink et al.[154]	Osteoarthritis	Acu vs invasive sham acu	32–33	Both groups improved from baseline on VAS pain, function, and ADL at 2 weeks and 2 months posttreatment*; no significant between-group difference.
Giles and Muller[155]	Low/upper back and neck-related spinal pain	3 groups: acu; NSAIDS; chiropractic	20–36	Chiropractic achieved statistically significant improvements on all pain scales.* No significant improvement for acu or meds on any scale.
Cherkin et al.[156]	Low back back	3 groups: acu; massage; self-care education	78–94	At 10 weeks, massage was superior to education on symptom and disability scales and to acupuncture on the disability scale.* At 1 year: massage = edu > acu.
Leibing et al.[157]	Low back pain	3 groups: PT + acu; PT + invasive sham acu; PT only	40–46	Acu superior to PT for pain intensity, pain disability, and psychological distress.* Compared to sham acu, acu reduced psychological distress.* The trends decreased at 9-month follow-up.
Carlsson and Sjolund[158]	Low back pain	3 groups: manual acu; electroacu; sham TENS	16–18	Pain decreased over time in both acu groups relative to control.* Both acu groups had improvements in return to work, quality of sleep, and analgesic intake.*
Molsberger et al.[159]	Low back pain	3 groups: VC + acu; VC + invasive sham acu; VC only	60–65	Acu decreased VAS pain posttreatment as compared to sham acu* and at 3-month follow-up as compared to both groups.*
Ceccherelli et al.[160]	Low back pain	Superficial acu vs deep acu	21	Pain reduced in both groups posttreatment; no between-group difference. Deep acu > superficial acu for pain reduction at 3-month follow-up.*

(*Continued*)

Reference	Condition Treated	Research Design	Group Size	Results
Naeser et al.[161]	Carpal tunnel syndrome	Crossover: laser acu + TENS vs sham laser acu + sham TENS	11	Improvements in pain score, median nerve sensory latency, and Phalen and Tinel signs in treatment group as compared to sham.* Patients could perform previous work and were stable for 1–3 years.
Biernacki and Peake[163]	Asthma	Crossover: acu vs invasive sham acu	11–12	No improvement in respiratory function after either treatment.
Shapira et al.[162]	Asthma	Crossover: acu vs invasive sham acu	19	No change in lung functions, bronchial hyperreactivity, or patient symptoms for either group.
Joos et al.[164]	Asthma	Acu vs invasive sham acu	18–20	Acu > sham in improving general well-being,* and immune system biomarkers (e.g., CD3/4 and IL-8).*

Abbreviations: acu = acupuncture; ADL = activities of daily living; edu = education; electroacu = electroacupuncture; IL = interleukin; meds = medicines; NSAIDS = nonsteroidal antiinflammatory drugs; PGF$_2$alpha = prostaglandin F$_2$-alpha; PT = physiotherapy; QOL = quality of life; rehab = rehabilitation; ROM = range of motion; TENS = transcutaneous electrical nerve stimulation; VC = visual care; VAS = Visual Analog Scale.
*Statistically significant.

essentially provided in the multicenter trial.[112,113] The added cost notwithstanding, the multicenter study results would have been far more useful to the public health community if acupuncture and sham acupuncture groups had been compared to a third group receiving acupuncture plus counseling sessions, based on "real-world" treatment protocols.

Stroke Rehabilitation

The conclusion of the NIH Consensus panel that acupuncture "may be useful" for recovery from poststroke paralysis was based on the promising outcomes of at least four controlled trials of acupuncture as adjunctive care, two treating in the acute phase, less than 2 weeks poststroke,[114,115] and two in the subacute phase, 2 weeks to 3 months poststroke.[116,117] However, since 1997, most of the evidence has weighed in against the efficacy of acupuncture for stroke rehabilitation. Three well-designed trials, providing acute-phase adjunctive acu-

puncture rehabilitation treatment, resulted in little if any improved motor function.[118–120] In contrast, transcutaneous electrical nerve stimulation (TENS) at acupoints plus usual rehabilitation care improved neurologic and functional status to a significantly greater extent than did usual care alone.[121] The conclusion of a recent meta-analysis of 14 trials of acupuncture for stroke rehabilitation is that acupuncture has no added effect to that of conventional physical therapy and occupational therapy treatment.[122] While no obvious study design variable (e.g., type or number of treatments, or choice of control groups) appears to correlate with treatment outcomes, it seems important to design future research to evaluate whether specific patient-related factors and/or subtype of stroke may be predictive of positive acupuncture outcome.[123]

Headache

Clinical trials over the preceding 5 years have produced equivocal results. Treatment of tension-type headache with a standardized acupuncture point protocol was no more effective than placebo needling,[121] whereas intramuscular acupuncture and subcutaneous (shallow) acupuncture, performed at the *same* fixed set of trigger points, were both effective in reducing mean tension-type headache indices.[125] (In the latter study, shallow needling was inappropriately considered as placebo treatment. The study can be viewed, instead, as having compared Chinese-style deep needling to Japanese-style superficial needling, finding both to be effective.) In a third study on tension-type headache, brief acupuncture at a combination of acupoints and local tender points was no more effective than noninvasive placebo treatment.[126] Two randomized controlled trials for patients with migraine without aura reported acupuncture at least as effective as pharmacologic treatment.[127,128] Of additional interest is a large-scale (400 subjects) randomized, pragmatic trial comparing acupuncture to standard care for migraine and headache, currently underway in the United Kingdom.[129] Pragmatic trials assess "real-world" treatment options, recording all details of the individualized treatments chosen by the practitioner.

Women's Reproductive Health
Evaluation of acupuncture for obstetric- and gynecologic-related conditions is a rapidly growing area of clinical research. The past 5 years have seen a range of trials testing its efficacy for reducing nausea and vomiting in early pregnancy, relieving low back and pelvic pain during pregnancy, and decreasing the duration and pain of labor. Acupuncture has also been tested as adjunctive care in trials of fertility-promoting techniques. Overall, the results have been promising. Acupuncture, either at a single traditionally used acupoint or at multiple acupoints informed by individualized Chinese medicine differentiations, consistently produced reductions in early pregnancy-related nausea,[130–132] although it significantly outperformed sham acupuncture in only one of these trials.[133] When tested for relieving pregnancy-related low back and pelvic pain, acupuncture was significantly

more effective than physiotherapy.[134] Acupuncture reduced the time of active labor in three trials;[135–137] in a fourth trial the overall time from "estimated date of confinement" to delivery was shortened but not the duration of labor.[138] Acupuncture was also more effective than sham needling in reducing labor-related pain.[139] In in vitro fertilization trials, women receiving electroacupuncture had significantly higher rates of implantation and pregnancy than those receiving the opioid analgesic, alfentanil;[140] a higher rate of clinical pregnancy was also documented in women receiving acupuncture relative to those in a no-acupuncture group.[141]

Tennis Elbow
Two controlled trials provide additional suggestive evidence for acupuncture's effectiveness in treating chronic epicondylitis or tennis elbow. Acupuncture significantly reduced pain and improved arm strength and function in comparison to needling at nonacupoint sites.[142] While group differences in all three measures were detected at 2 weeks posttreatment, only the group difference in arm function was maintained at 2-month follow-up. In a separate trial, electroacupuncture was superior to manual acupuncture for reducing pain and improving pain-free hand grip strength.[143]

Fibromyalgia
No new controlled clinical trials of acupuncture for fibromyalgia patients were identified.

Myofascial Pain
Review of six randomized controlled trials for chronic neck, shoulder, or knee pain reveal inconsistent benefits of acupuncture. While chronic neck pain was as effectively relieved by acupuncture and physiotherapy,[144] no significant differences were detected between groups treated at relevant or irrelevant acupoints for the same condition.[145] In other trials, neck pain was significantly reduced by acupuncture in comparison to massage but not to sham laser at acupoints,[146] whereas a single treatment of individualized TCM-based acupuncture was more effective than a single treatment of sham laser

at the same TCM-selected acupoints or a single acupuncture treatment at local trigger points.[117] Shoulder pain developed by wheelchair users was effectively reduced in groups receiving either acupuncture or Trager bodywork therapy,[118] while pain of rotator cuff tendonitis responded significantly better to acupuncture than to patient-blinded treatment with a specially designed "retractable" placebo needle.[119] In a trial for chronic knee pain, the group randomly assigned to receive acupuncture responded significantly better than did the no-treatment group, as assessed at 1-year follow up.[150]

Osteoarthritis

Four randomized controlled trials, each with a markedly different control or comparison group, provide suggestive evidence of acupuncture effectiveness for osteoarthritis of the knee or hip. In an adjunctive care design, patients randomized to acupuncture improved on several self-reporting scales of pain and disability to a significantly greater extent than patients receiving standard care alone.[151] Acupuncture also outperformed advice and exercises,[152] was equally effective when applied to the most affected knee only or to both knees,[153] and provided as much benefit when performed at specific acupoints as at local nonspecific sites.[151] Of considerable interest is a current large-scale, randomized controlled trial (525 patients, at the University of Maryland School of Medicine) comparing acupuncture, sham acupuncture, and an education/attention group for treating knee osteoarthritis.

Low Back Pain

Despite six recent good-quality trials of acupuncture for ameliorating chronic low back pain, the evidence for efficacy remains equivocal. In randomized comparative outcome studies, acupuncture was markedly outperformed by spinal manipulation[155] and by therapeutic massage.[156] When provided as adjunctive care to physiotherapy, acupuncture treatment was significantly more effective when compared to physiotherapy alone, but not when compared to adjunctive sham acupuncture,[157] suggesting a

stronger placebo effect associated with acupuncture than with physiotherapy. In contrast, both acupuncture and electroacupuncture were more effective than placebo treatment (inactive transcutaneous electrical nerve stimulation) at 1- and 6-month follow-up.[158] As well, acupuncture plus "conservative orthopedic treatment" outperformed sham acupuncture plus conservative orthopedic treatment, as well as conservative orthopedic treatment alone, as evidenced by reduction in Visual Analog Scale (VAS) pain at end of treatment and at 3-month follow-up.[159] A comparison of superficial and deep acupuncture revealed no difference in effectiveness posttreatment, but significantly better results from deep acupuncture at 3-month follow-up.[160]

Carpal Tunnel Syndrome

A single small-scale crossover trial found low-level laser and microampere TENS stimulation at acupuncture points to be significantly more effective than sham laser treatment in decreasing pain and median nerve sensory latency in patients who had failed to respond to conservative biomedical treatment for carpal tunnel syndrome.[161]

Asthma

Three recent, small-scale controlled trials have done little to resolve the conflicting claims of acupuncture efficacy for asthmatics. Respiratory function was not significantly improved relative to sham acupuncture in patients with moderate persistent asthma.[162,163] In contrast, patients with "mild to moderately severe bronchial allergic asthma" benefited to a significantly greater extent from acupuncture at asthma-specific points than at acupoints not specific for asthma.[161] Improvement was in general well-being, as well as in several biomarkers of immune system function.

Conclusions

A more rigorous review of the 50 recently published controlled clinical trials of acupuncture (Tables 9–3 and 9–4) than that presented above is likely to reveal an overall improvement in research design relative to the trials available for review by the 1997 NIH Consensus Development panel. Improved methodology notwithstanding, the evidence base for this traditional health care practice does not appear to have greatly expanded for most conditions. Two trends, however, are of particular interest: a higher proportion of *positive* outcomes in trials when acupuncture was compared to either *noninvasive* sham needling or standard care, and a higher proportion of *negative* outcomes (wherein acupuncture and sham acupuncture appeared equally effective, *not* where neither treatment was effective) when acupuncture was compared to *invasive* sham needling. These trends, which were also noted in earlier reviews,[165,166] suggest that a large benefit of acupuncture may derive from nonspecific physiologic effects of needling.[167] One testable hypothesis, for example, is that these nonspecific effects are quicker acting than the specific effects.

Of general importance for future trials is that the selection of acupuncture treatment parameters be given greater attention, with particular consideration focused on whether there is a justifiable expectation that the proposed treatment protocol will be adequate for the condition under study. Unlike pilot drug trials, where the norm is to include dose–response testing, the varying of acupuncture treatment parameters within a given trial is notable for its absence. As mentioned in an earlier section, a positive correlation between number of treatments and trial outcome was noted in a systematic review of acupuncture for pain.[168] For these reasons, STRICTA (the recently published guidelines for reporting clinical trials of acupuncture) includes an item calling for, at the least, presentation of the rationale for acupuncture point selection and choice of treatment parameters.[169]

As evidenced in the trials considered in this section, the main problems today for health care stakeholders faced with the task of assessing acupuncture efficacy are essentially the same as those facing the 1997 NIH panel: First, how to make sense of the confusing array of intertrial variability in acupuncture style and treatment on the one hand and the broad spectrum of control and comparison groups on the other. Second, how to judge whether trial designs are appropriate, adequate, and sufficiently rigorous so that the trial outcomes can be considered to be valid. These dilemmas will be gradually resolved by several approaches, including the training of acupuncturists in the language and strategies of clinical research, increasing the involvement of experienced acupuncturists in the design phase of clinical trials, and a commitment by the health care community to improve its understanding of the unique features of acupuncture practice.

▶ ACUPUNCTURE REGULATION, TRAINING, AND LICENSURE

Acupuncture practice is well established in the United States and Europe. Forty-two states and the District of Columbia regulate acupuncture, specifying education requirements and scope of practice. Laws vary from state to state and are available in print[170] and online.[171] Acupuncture schools are accredited by the Accreditation Commission for Acupuncture and Oriental Medicine (ACAOM),[172] which is recognized by the US Department of Education as a "specialized and professional" accrediting agency for Masters degree and Masters level acupuncture programs and programs in Oriental medicine. Recognition by the US Department of Education qualifies students in accredited acupuncture programs to receive federal financial aid. There are 46 colleges that are accredited or have candidacy status.[173]

Students applying to acupuncture school must have completed at least 2 years, 60 semester credits or the equivalent, of accredited postsecondary education. Some states require applicants to have 4 years undergraduate education prior to or in addition to acupuncture education. Professional acupuncture training that leads to licensure must be at least 3 academic years in length, providing at least 1,725 hours (93 semester credits) of instruction over a period of at least 27 months. The professional program in East Asian or Oriental medicine must be at least 4 academic years in length, providing at least 2,175 hours (123 semester credits) of instruction over a period of at least 36 months.[174] The course of study is didactic with supervised clinical internship. Minimum hours and credits have been established for specific areas such as clinical training, biomedical clinical science, and herbal medicine. Training may also include therapeutic forms of bodywork, diet, and exercise. Curriculum requirements are revised periodically to reflect the ongoing evolution and indigenization of acupuncture and East Asian medicine, with some schools developing doctoral programs.

After completion of the standard 3 or 4 years of full-time study, an acupuncture candidate must pass a qualifying board exam. Most states use the exam developed by the National Commission for the Certification of Acupuncture and Oriental Medicine.[175]

Currently, there are approximately 10,000 licensed acupuncturists in practice in the United States who are NCCAOM board certified; with approximately 1,500 new candidates certified each year. In most states, once candidates have been NCCAOM board certified, and then become state licensed, they need only maintain their state license. Thus, overall there are many more acupuncturists licensed to practice than remain NCCAOM active with estimates exceeding 25,000. There are approximately 3,000 practitioners that are board certified in Chinese herbal medicine. NCCAOM's website (www. NCCAOM.org) provides information on board-qualified acupuncture and herbal practitioners.

Physician Acupuncture Practice

Laws regulating physician practice of acupuncture vary by state. Only eight states have some form of registration for physicians incorporating acupuncture into their practice. In all others, physicians may include acupuncture in their practice without any form of separate training or documentation to the state. Some states require medical doctors who use acupuncture in their practice to complete a 300-hour course of study designed for the physician. By contrast, in most states, medical doctors can perform chiropractic care without any study or certification.

There is no way to assure an accurate count of the numbers of physicians practicing acupuncture in the United States because there is no uniform requirement that they be certified, licensed, or registered with any agency or entity. Approximately 6,000 physicians have completed the 300-hour course in a US training program, with another 1,000 physicians educated in programs outside the United States, all of whom may be practicing.[176] Information on physician acupuncture practice may be found at the website of the American Academy of Medical Acupuncture (AAMA).[177] The courses for physician certification in acupuncture do not include herbs, and there are no abbreviated courses on East Asian herbs for physicians. To be NCCAOM board certified in East Asian herbology requires 2 years of coursework in an approved program and passage of herbal examination.

Hospital Privileges

It is difficult to assess how many hospitals privilege acupuncture or acupuncture providers because there are no organizations that codify this information or promote advancing acupuncture privileges in hospital. Few nonphysician providers are credentialed by hospitals; however, community-based hospitals appear more open than medical teaching facilities to credentialing nonphysician acupuncture providers. Nonphysician providers that are credentialed by a hospital are likely to have that privilege limited to providing acupuncture care. They would not have admission or discharge privileges, because those decisions are based on conventional assessments.

► FEE FOR SERVICE AND REIMBURSEMENT

The first question patients have for acupuncture providers is whether acupuncture will help their problem. The second is "will my insurance company pay for it." Most acupuncture care provided by licensed acupuncturists, those who have completed the 3-year course of study in a Masters-level acupuncture program, is paid out of pocket. This means the patient pays the provider directly. Fees generally range from $50 to $150 per follow-up session, with new patient sessions being slightly higher. Because acupuncture is a low-tech time-based service, and occurs primarily in private practice settings, overhead costs can be controlled.

While it appears that more insurance carriers are reimbursing for acupuncture, it is often via a limited network of providers with no reimbursement for out-of-network care. While a 2000 study found 4 of 6 new managed care organization respondents said they pay for acupuncture care, coverage is inadequate and offered mainly to attract enrollees.[178] Additionally, in some cases, insurance companies pay for acupuncture only if performed by a medical doctor, although they may not be required to have specific acupuncture training.

Increasing market demand is the primary motivator for insurance companies to cover alternative medicine such as acupuncture.[179] Acupuncture, chiropractic, and osteopathy are stated as being the most frequently covered "unconventional" services, with naturopathy, massage, homeopathy, chelation, and stress management covered less frequently. Only 8 states mandate reimbursement for acupuncture, as compared to 41 for chiropractic, 35 for podiatry, 17 for osteopathy, 15 for midwifery, and 10 for physical therapy.[180]

Some insurers will reimburse a limited number of acupuncture treatments with a letter of medical necessity, often limited to particular diagnoses, usually associated with pain. This stems from an early misconception of limited biological mechanism assigned to acupuncture by Western physicians.[181] In some states, auto insurance, as well as workers compensation insurance, will reimburse for acupuncture, but preauthorization may be necessary. Overall, although the popular media reports that an increasing number of insurers are offering coverage for "unconventional" therapies such as acupuncture, the current status of reimbursement is quite limited.[182]

Reluctance to reimburse for acupuncture may have more to do with the culture of medicine and consensus practice in the West than with proven efficacy. Insurers and providers, as well as the public, perceive conventional medicine as science based, and proven safe and effective. However, most conventional Western medical procedures and interventions fail to conform to this standard of quality.[183] Ignorance about efficacy and the nature of acupuncture service are the stated major obstacle to insurance reimbursement, even while many conventional medical practices are not grounded in evidence-based medicine—nevertheless, they are reimbursed.[184]

Finally, although acupuncture is not widely reimbursed, the Internal Revenue Service did rule, in 1972, that fees for acupuncture services qualify as medical expenses, and can be deducted. More currently, legislation is being considered to secure acupuncture reimbursement for federal employees and for Medicare and Medicaid recipients.

It is recommended that patients contact their insurance carriers to inquire about coverage for acupuncture care by a licensed acupuncturist or medical doctor. It may be helpful to provide the insurance carrier with a letter of medical necessity. For patients who need acupuncture care but who cannot afford a provider in a private setting, consult the website for the Accreditation Commission for Acupuncture and Oriental Medicine (www.acaom.org) for a list of accredited acupuncture schools. Similar to medical and dental schools, acupuncture schools offer treatment in supervised student clinics for a small fee.

► CLINICAL PRACTICE IN THE INTEGRATIVE SETTING

At this time, most medical doctors and insurance companies are not familiar with acupuncture's safety or efficacy, operate under the misconception that acupuncture only treats pain,[185] do not know qualified providers for referral, and have little or no exposure to qualified traditional systems practice in a modern clinical setting.[186] Although most patients do present to an acupuncturist with a Western diagnosis, they come without informing their conventional medical provider. This concerns conventional providers who fear patients may postpone or forego conventional diagnosis and care.

Integrative medical practice affords providers of these different systems of medicine the opportunity to collaborate through the course of treating the patients they share. The atmosphere of cooperation and inclusion greatly enhances quality of care, research, and best practice. Patients experience ease of access to qualified providers it might otherwise take months to find and/or appoint. This is especially true when a patient presents with an acute painful illness or injury, such as back or musculoskeletal strain or sprain, headache, nausea, cramping, diarrhea, asthma, bronchitis, influenza, dysmenorrhea, menorrhagia, insect bite, poison ivy, or shingles. These problems respond well to immediate acupuncture care, reducing protracted discomfort and the need for medication; in the integrative setting where physician and acupuncturist work together, this type of same-day referral and treatment can be very effective.

The Joint Commission on Accreditation of Healthcare Organizations has mandated in its pain strategy initiative that patients be asked about pain, and that they be educated about effective pain management, including nonpharmacologic approaches.[187] This was done "because of literature replete with studies documenting the undertreatment by physicians of pain,"[188] and that "education alone was not going to change practice" because the "willingness of physicians to relinquish control to a collaborative process is often lacking."[189,190] Acupuncture has been included as one "example of implementation for other pain management techniques successfully demonstrating compliance with JCAHO standard."[191] The Group Health Cooperative Gap Analysis on nonpharmacologic approaches to pain management in the hospital setting found that ". . . the main reasons/barriers for not offering different modalities (including acupuncture) were lack of training of existing personnel and/or lack of resources."[191]

► WHEN SHOULD A PHYSICIAN REFER TO AN ACUPUNCTURIST?

Texts on East Asian medicine have treatment protocols for nearly every type of problem including inflammatory disorders and infection such as septicemia, hepatitis, meningitis, pneumonia, dysentery, cholera, and diphtheria, as well as everyday bronchitis, influenza, and acute or chronic sinusitis. Degenerative diseases such as multiple sclerosis, Parkinson's, and postpolio have been treated, as well as common problems such as hemorrhoids, dysmenorrhea, diarrhea, and constipation, and even impotency, better known as "withering of the penis."

A physician should consider referral to a qualified provider of East Asian medicine when the patient expresses interest in acupuncture care and their problem is one that may respond to it. If their problem fluctuates in intensity, there is a good chance that East Asian medicine can help to maximize their improvement.

How many treatments are needed is a question that is likely to be posed by anyone seeking a referral. The answer varies according to presentation. Because acupuncture has a cumulative effect it is best to have at least three sessions no more than 1 week apart. Three sessions are sufficient to assess whether the problem being treated is responding, and to agree upon a treatment plan, if more treatment is needed.

A physician can inquire as to what experience an acupuncture provider has with a given disorder. Seeking acupuncture care for oneself, even as a preventive measure is a first-hand way for a physician to become familiar with acupuncture providers in a community. Being open to communicating with providers with whom you share patients serves good practice. Finally, listening to patients who receive acupuncture and East Asian medicine with an ear open to their experience will give any physician broader knowledge of how patients integrate their care options.

Acknowledgment

Special thanks to Ryan Milley for help in drafting Tables 9–4 and 9–5.

REFERENCES

1. Needham J, Lu Gwei-Djen. *Celestial Lancets. A History and Rationale of Acupuncture and Moxa.* Cambridge, UK: Cambridge University Press; 1980:318.
2. NIH Consensus Conference on Acupuncture. *JAMA.* 1998;280:1518–1524.
3. Weeks J. The Joint Commission's pain standards: an opportunity for integration? *The Integrative Medicine Consult. Quarterly Business Report.* 2002; January:R1–8.
4. Langevin H, Yandow J. The relationship of acupuncture points and meridians to connective tissue planes. *Anat Rec.* 2002;269:257–265.
5. Travell J, Simmons D. *Myofascial Pain and Dysfunction. The Trigger Point Manual.* Baltimore, MD: William and Wilkins; 1983.
6. Melzak R, Stillwell DM, Fox EJ. Trigger points and acupuncture points for pain: correlations and implications. *Pain.* 1977;3:3–23.
7. Dung HC. Anatomical features contributing to the formation of acupuncture points. *Am J Acupuncture.* 1984;12:139–143.
8. Gunn CD, Ditchburn FG, King MH, Renwhick GJ. Acupuncture loci: a proposal for their classification according to their relationship to known neural structures. *Am J Chinese Med.* 1976;4:183–195.
9. Han J. Physiology of acupuncture: review of thirty years of research. *J Altern Complement Med.* 1997;3(suppl 1):S101–S108.
10. Pomeranz R, Stux G, eds. *Scientific Bases of Acupuncture.* New York: Springer-Verlag; 1989.
11. Cheng RS, Pomeranz BH. Electroacupuncture analgesia is mediated by stereospecific opiate receptors and is reversed by antagonists of type I receptors. *Life Sci.* 1980;26:631–638.
12. Han JS, Terenius L. Neurochemical basis of acupuncture analgesia. *Annu Rev Pharmacol Toxicol.* 1982;22:193–220.
13. Su J. Electrodermal response during spell of dizziness. *Am J Acupuncture.* 1979;7(4):305–309.
14. Steinberger A. Specific irritability of acupuncture points as an early symptom of multiple sclerosis. *Am J Chinese Med.* 1986;14:175–178.
15. Langevin H, Yandow J. The relationship of acupuncture points and meridians to connective tissue planes. *Anat Rec.* 2002;269:257–265.
16. Stux G, Pomeranz B. *Basics of Acupuncture.* Berlin: Springer-Verlag; 1995.
17. Zhong A, Wu J, Hu Y, Feng Y, Deng X. Study on correlation between the mast cell and the acupoint. *World J Acup-Mox.* 1994;4(4):53–58.
18. Oschmann JL. *Connective Tissue and Myofascial Systems.* Berkeley, CA: Aspen Research Inst; 1987.
19. Langevin M, Churchill D, Cipolla M. Mechanical signaling through connective tissue: a mechanism for the therapeutic effect of acupuncture. *FASEB J.* 2001;15:2275–2282.
20. Cho ZH, Chung SC, Jones JP, et al. New findings of the correlation between acupoints and corresponding brain cortices using functional MRI. *Proc Natl Acad Sci U S A.* 1998;95:2670–2673.
21. Han J. Physiology of acupuncture: review of thirty years of research. *J Altern Complement Med.* 1997;3(suppl 1):S106.
22. Pert C. *Molecules of Emotion. Why You Feel the Way You Feel.* New York: Scribner; 1997.
23. Wolpe P. The maintenance of professional authority: acupuncture and the American physician. *Soc Prob.* 1985;32(5):409–424.
24. Alraek T, Soedal L, Fagerheim S, et al. Acupuncture treatment in the prevention of uncomplicated recurrent lower urinary tract infection in adult women. *Am J Public Health.* 2002; 92(10):1609–1611.
25. Langevin H, Yandow J. The relationship of acupuncture points and meridians to connective tissue planes. *Anat Rec.* 2002;269:257–265.

26. Needham J, Lu GD. *Celestial Lancets. A History and Rationale of Acupuncture and Moxa.* Cambridge, UK: Cambridge University Press; 1980:9.

27. Atkinson D. *Magic, Myth, and Medicine.* New York: New World Publishing; 1956.

28. McNeil W. *Plagues and Peoples.* New York: Anchor Press; 1989:109.

29. Kaptchuk T. Acupuncture: theory, efficacy, and practice. *Ann Intern Med.* 2002;136(5):374–383.

30. Needham J, Lu Gwei-Djen. *Celestial Lancets. A History and Rationale of Acupuncture and Moxa.* Cambridge, UK: Cambridge University Press; 1980:7.

31. Epps J. *Counteraction Viewed as a Means of Cure with Remarks on the Use of the Issue.* London: Renshaw and Rush; 1832.

32. King L. The Bloodletting Controversy: A Study in the Scientific Method. *Bull Hist Med.* 1961;35(1): 1–13.

33. Haller J. Decline of bloodletting: a study in 19th-century ratiocinations. *South Med J.* 1986;79: 469–475.

34. Klugler M. The history of bloodletting. *Nat Hist.* 1978;87:78–83.

35. Castiglione A. *History of Medicine.* Krumbhaar EB, trans-ed. New York: Knopf; 1941.

36. Shanghai College of Traditional Medicine, 1974; O'Connor J, Bensky D, trans; Bensky D, ed. *Acupuncture: A Comprehensive Text.* Chicago: Eastland Press; 1981:464.

37. *Stedman's Pocket Medical Dictionary.* Baltimore, MD: Williams & Wilkins; 1987.

38. Epler DC. Bloodletting in early Chinese medicine and its relation to the origin of acupuncture. *Bull Hist Med.* 1980;54:337–367.

39. Unschuld P. *Medicine in China: A History of Ideas.* Berkeley, CA: University of California Press; 1985:97.

40. Unschuld P. *Medicine in China. A History of Ideas.* Berkeley, CA: University of California Press; 1985:97; also see Huang Fu Mi. *Systematic Classic of Acupuncture with Annotations by Shandong Institute of Traditional Chinese Medicine.* Beijing: People's Press; 1979 (first published, 282 CE.).

41. Unschuld P. *Medicine in China: A History of Ideas.* Berkeley, CA: University of California Press; 1985:97.

42. Nielsen A. *Gua Sha. A Traditional Technique for Modern Practice.* Edinburgh: Churchill Livingstone, 1995.

42a. Nielsen A. *Gua Sha. Eine Traditionelle Technik Fur die Moderne Medicine.* Koetzting, Germany: Verlag fur Ganzheitliche Medicine; 2000.

43. Needham J, Lu Gwei-Djen. *Celestial Lancets. A History and Rationale of Acupuncture and Moxa.* Cambridge, UK: Cambridge University Press; 1980:7.

44. Kuriyama S. Between mind and eye: Japanese anatomy in the eighteenth century. In: Leslie C, Young A, eds. *Paths to Asian Medical Knowledge.* Berkeley, CA: University of California Press; 1992:39.

45. Unschuld P. *Medicine in China: A History of Ideas.* Berkeley, CA: University of California Press; 1985:82.

46. Nielsen A. *Gua Sha. A Traditional Technique for Modern Practice.* Edinburgh, UK: Churchill Livingstone, 1995:46.

47. Unschuld P. *Medicine in China: A History of Ideas.* Berkeley, CA: University of California Press; 1985:57.

48. Birch S. Diversity and acupuncture: acupuncture is not a coherent or historically stable tradition. In: Vickers A, ed. *Examining Complementary Medicine. "The Skeptical Holist."* Cheltenham, UK: Stanley Thorne Publishers; 1998;45–63.

49. Unschuld P. *Medicine in China: A History of Ideas.* Berkeley, CA: University of California Press; 1985:51.

50. Farquhar J. Time and text: approaching Chinese medical practice through analysis of a published case. In: Leslie C, Young A, eds. *Paths to Asian Medical Knowledge.* Berkeley: University of California Press; 1992;72.

51. Farquhar J. Time and text: approaching Chinese medical practice through analysis of a published case. In: Leslie C, Young A, eds. *Paths to Asian Medical Knowledge.* Berkeley: University of California Press; 1992;70.

52. Mies M. Women's research or feminist research? The debate surrounding feminist science and methodology. In: Fonow M, Cook J, eds. *Beyond Methodology: Feminist Scholarship as Lived Research.* Bloomington: Indiana University Press; 1991:60–84.

53. Farquhar J. *Knowing Practice. The Clinical Encounter in Chinese Medicine.* Boulder, CO: Westview Press; 1994:45–46.

54. Farquhar J. *Knowing Practice. The Clinical Encounter in Chinese Medicine.* Boulder, CO: Westview Press; 1994:45–46.

55. Farquhar J. *Knowing Practice. The Clinical Encounter of Chinese Medicine*. Boulder, CO: Westview Press; 1994:5.

56. Farquhar J. *Knowing Practice. The Clinical Encounter of Chinese Medicine*. Boulder, CO: Westview Press; 1994:91.

57. For theoretical discussion of Yin and Yang, see Kaptchuk T. *The Web That Has No Weaver*. Chicago, IL: Contemporary Books; 2000.

58. Song T. *Atlas of the Tongue and Lingual Coatings in Chinese Medicine*. Beijing, Strasbourg: Peoples Medical Publishing House, Editions Sinomedic; 1986. Chinese, English, French, Spanish, German, Italian.

58a. Chen Z, Chen M. *The Essence and Scientific Background of Tongue Diagnosis*. Long Beach, CA: Oriental Healing Arts Institute; 1989.

58b. Maciocia G. *Tongue Diagnosis in Chinese Medicine*. Seattle, WA: Eastland Press; 1995, 1997.

58c. Nielsen A. *Immediate and Significant Tongue Changes as a Direct Result of Gua Sha*. Amsterdam: Anglo-Dutch Institute or Oriental Medicine. November; 1999. Chinese Medicine in the 21st Century. Defining the Profession www.guasha.com; last accessed September 2003.

58d. Kirschbaum B. *Atlas of Chinese Tongue Diagnosis*. Seattle, WA: Eastland Press; 2001.

59. Nielsen A. *Immediate and Significant Tongue Changes as a Direct Result of Gua Sha*. Presented at the International Symposium: Oriental Medicine at the Dawn of the 21st Century. Defining the Profession. Amsterdam: November, 1999. Anglo-Dutch Institute of Oriental Medicine www.guasha.com; last accessed Sept 2003.

60. Travell J, Simmons D. *Myofascial Pain and Dysfunction: The Trigger Point Manual*. Baltimore, MD: William & Wilkins; 1983.

60a. Matsumoto K, Birch S. *Hara Diagnosis. Reflections on the Sea*. Brookline, MA: Paradigm Publications; 1988.

60b. So J. *Treatment of Disease with Acupuncture. Volume Two of a Complete Course in Acupuncture*. Brookline, MA: Paradigm Publications. 1987.

60c. Seem M. *A New American Acupuncture. Acupuncture Osteopathy. The Myofascial Release of the Bodymind's Holding Patterns*. Boulder, CO: Blue Poppy Press. 1993.

60d. Denmai S. *Japanese Classical Acupuncture. Introduction to Meridian Therapy*. Brown S, trans. Seattle, WA: Eastland Press; 1990.

60e. Finando D, Finando S. *Informed Touch. A Clinicians Guide to the Evaluation and Treatment of Myofascial Disorders*. Rochester, VT: Healing Arts Press, 1999.

60f. Ni YT. *Navigating the Channels of Traditional Chinese Medicine*. San Diego, CA: Oriental Medicine Center; 1996.

61. Farquhar J. *Knowing Practice. The Clinical Encounter of Chinese Medicine*. Boulder, CO: Westview Press; 1994;11–13.

62. Matsumoto K, Birch S. *Hara Diagnosis. Reflections on the Sea*. Brookline, MA: Paradigm Publications; 1988.

63. Denmai S. *Japanese Classical Acupuncture. Introduction to Median Therapy*. Brown S, trans. Seattle WA: Eastland Press; 1990.

64. Finandos D, Finando S. *Informed Touch. A Clinician's Guide to the Evaluation and Treatment of Myofascial Disorders*. Rochester, VT: Healing Arts Press; 1999.

65. Kaptchuk T. *The Web That Has No Weaver*. Chicago, IL: Contemporary Books; 2000:239–281.

66. Farquhar J. *Knowing Practice. The Clinical Encounter of Chinese Medicine*. Boulder, CO: Westview Press; 1994:168.

67. Farquhar J. *Knowing Practice. The Clinical Encounter of Chinese Medicine*. Boulder, CO: Westview Press; 1994:43.

68. Farquhar J. *Knowing Practice. The Clinical Encounter of Chinese Medicine*. Boulder, CO: Westview Press; 1994:72.

69. Nielsen A. Why we do not diagnose in Chinese medicine. *The Anglo-Dutch Institute of Oriental Medicine Magazine*. 1999;7:24–26. www.guasha.com; last accessed Sept 2003.

70. Farquhar J. *Knowing Practice. The Clinical Encounter of Chinese Medicine*. Boulder, CO: Westview Press; 1994:38.

71. Farquhar J. *Knowing Practice. The Clinical Encounter of Chinese Medicine*. Boulder, CO: Westview Press; 1994:1.

72. Needham J, Lu G-D. *Celestial Lancets. A History and Rationale of Acupuncture and Moxa*. Cambridge, UK: Cambridge University Press; 1980:15.

73. Nielsen A. *Gua Sha. A Traditional Technique for Modern Practice*. Edinburgh: Churchill Livingstone, 1995:18.

74. Farquhar J. *Knowing Practice. The Clinical Encounter of Chinese Medicine*. Boulder, CO: Westview Press; 1994:32.

75. *The I Ching or Book of Changes.* 3rd ed. Princeton: Princeton University Press; 1950, 1967.

76. Mies M. Women's research or feminist research? The debate surrounding feminist science and methodology. In: Fonow M, Cook J, eds. *Beyond Methodology: Feminist Scholarship as Lived Research.* Bloomington: Indiana University Press; 1991:61.

77. Nielsen A. Why we do not diagnose in Chinese Medicine. *The Anglo-Dutch Institute of Oriental Medicine Magazine.* 1999;7:25.

78. *Needling colloquium.* New York: Tri-State College of Acupuncture; 15 February 2003.

79. Langevin H, Churchill D, Cipolla M. Mechanical signaling through connective tissue: a mechanism for the therapeutic effect of acupuncture. *FASEB J.* 2001;15:2275–2282.

80. Birch S, Ida J. *Japanese Acupuncture. A Clinical Guide.* Brookline, MA: Paradigm Press; 1998: 46–47.

80a. Nogier P, Nogier R. *The Man in the Ear.* Sainte-Ruffine, FR: Masonneuve; 1985.

80b. Yoo TW. *Korean Hand Therapy-Korean Hand Acupuncture,* 2nd rev ed. Seoul, SK: Eum Yang Mek Hin Pub; 1988.

80c. Lao HH. *Wrist Ankle Acupuncture. Methods and Application,* 2nd ed. Brookline, MA: Redwing; 1999.

81. Seem M. *A New American Acupuncture. Acupuncture Osteopathy. The Myofascial Release of the Bodymind's Holding Patterns.* Boulder, CO: Blue Poppy Press; 1993.

82. So J. *The Book of Acupuncture Points, Vol. 1. Complete Course in Acupuncture.* Brookline, MA: Paradigm Press; 1984.

82a. So J. *Complete Course in Acupuncture. Treatment of Disease with Acupuncture, Vol 2.* Brookline, MA: Paradigm Press; 1987.

83. Ni Y. *Navigating the Channels of Traditional Chinese Medicine.* San Diego, CA: Oriental Medicine Center; 1996.

84. Nielsen A. Gua Sha. *A Traditional Technique for Modern Practice.* Edinburgh: Churchill Livingstone; 1995:44.

85. So J. *Complete Course in Acupuncture. Treatment of Disease with Acupuncture, Vol 2.* Brookline, MA: Paradigm Press; 1987:315.

86. Jackson H. On efficacy of certain external applications. Inaugural Dissertation printed in *Medical Theses.* Philadelphia: University of Pennsylvania and TW Bradford; 1806.

87. Nielsen A. *Gua Sha. A Traditional Technique for Modern Practice.* Edinburgh: Churchill Livingstone; 1995;48–50.

88. Epler DC. Bloodletting in early Chinese medicine and its relation to the origin of acupuncture. *Bull Hist Med.* 1980;54:337–367.

89. Kleinman A. *Patients and Healers in the Context of Culture.* Berkeley: University of California Press; 1980:52–59.

90. NIH Consensus Conference. *JAMA.* 1998;280: 1518–1524.

91. Hammerschlag R. Funding of acupuncture research by the National Institutes of Health: a brief history. *Clin Acupunct Oriental Med.* 2000;1:133–138.

92. Sherman KJ, Hogeboom CJ, Cherkin DC, et al. Description and validation of a noninvasive placebo acupuncture procedure. *J Altern Complement Med.* 2002;8:11–19.

93. Vincent C. Credibility assessment in trials of acupuncture *Complement Med Res.* 1990;4:8–11.

94. Lao L, Bergman S, Langenberg P, et al. Efficacy of Chinese acupuncture on postoperative oral surgery pain. *Oral Surg Oral Med Oral Pathol.* 1995;79:423–428.

95. Linde K, Vickers A, Hondra M, et al. Systematic reviews of complementary therapies—an annotated bibliography. Part 1: acupuncture, BMC. *J Complement Altern Med.* 2001;1:3. Available at: http://www.biomedcentral.com/1472–6682/1/3. Last access 9/14/03.

96. Ezzo J, Berman BM, Vickers AJ. Complementary medicine and the Cochrane Collaboration. *JAMA.* 1998;280:1628–30.

97. Linde K, Vickers A, Hondra M, et al. Systematic reviews of complementary therapies—an annotated bibliography. Part 1: acupuncture, BMC. *J Complement Altern Med.* 2001;1:3. Available at: http://www.biomedcentral.com/1472–6682/1/3. Last access 9/14/03.

98. Ezzo J, Berman BM, Hadhazy VA, et al. Is acupuncture effective for the treatment of pain? A systematic review. *Pain.* 2000;86:217–225.

99. White A, Trinh K, Hammerschlag R. Performing systematic reviews of clinical trials of acupuncture: problems and solutions. *Clin Acupunct Orient Med.* 2002;3:26–31.

100. MacPherson H, White A, Cummings M, et al. Standards for reporting interventions in controlled trials of acupuncture: the STRICTA recommendations. *J Altern Complement Med.* 2002;8:85–89.

101. Altman DG, Schulz KF, Moher D, et al. The revised CONSORT statement for reporting randomized trials: explanation and elaboration. *Ann Intern Med.* 2001;134:663–694.

102. Shen J, Wenger N, Glaspy J, et al. Electroacupuncture for control of myeloablative chemotherapy-induced emesis: a randomized controlled trial. *JAMA.* 2000;284:2755–2761.

103. Harmon D, Gardiner J, Harrison R, Kelly A. Acupressure for the prevention of nausea and vomiting after laparoscopy. *Brit J Anaesth.* 1999;82:387–390.

104. Kotani N, Hashimoto H, Sato S, et al. Preoperative intradermal acupuncture reduces postoperative pain, nausea and vomiting, analgesic requirement, and sympathoadrenal responses. *Anesthesiology.* 2001;95:349–356.

105. Vickers AJ. Can acupuncture have specific effects on health? A systematic review of acupuncture antiemesis trials. *J R Soc Med.* 1996;89:303–311.

106. Lao L, Bergman S, Hamilton GR, et al. Evaluation of acupuncture for pain control after oral surgery: A placebo-controlled trial. *Arch Otolaryngol Head Neck Surg.* 1999;125:567–572.

107. Lao L, Bergman S, Langenberg P, et al. Efficacy of Chinese acupuncture on postoperative oral surgery pain. *Oral Surg Oral Med Oral Pathol.* 1995;79:423–428.

108. Bier ID, Wilson J, Studt P, et al. Auricular acupuncture, education, and smoking cessation: a randomized, sham-controlled trial. *Am J Public Health.* 2002;92:1642–1647.

109. He D, Medbo JI, Hostmark AT. Effect of acupuncture on smoking cessation or reduction: an 8-month and 5-year follow-up study. *Prev Med.* 2001;33:364–372.

110. Avants SK, Margolin A, Holford TR, et al. A randomized controlled trial of auricular acupuncture for cocaine dependence. *Arch Intern Med.* 2000;160:2305–2312.

111. Margolin A, Kleber HD, Avants SK, et al. Acupuncture for the treatment of cocaine addiction: A randomized controlled trial. *JAMA.* 2002;287:55–63.

112. Margolin A, Avants SK, Holford TR. Interpreting conflicting findings from clinical trials of auricular acupuncture for cocaine addiction: does treatment context influence outcome? *J Altern Complement Med.* 2002;8:111–121.

113. Kaptchuk TJ. () Acupuncture for the treatment of cocaine addiction. *JAMA.* 2002;287:1801–1802.

114. Johansson K, Lindgren I, Widner H, et al. Can sensory stimulation improve the functional outcome in stroke patients? *Neurology.* 1993;43:2189–2192.

115. Hu HH, Chung C, Liu TJ, et al. A randomized controlled trial on the treatment for acute partial ischemic stroke with acupuncture. *Neuroepidemiology.* 1993;12:106–113.

116. Sallstrom S, Kjendahl A, Osten PE, et al. Acupuncture in the treatment of stroke patients in the subacute stage: a randomized controlled trial. *Complement Ther Med.* 1964:193–197.

117. Naeser MA, Alexander MP, Stiassny-Eder D, et al. Real vs. sham acupuncture in the treatment of paralysis in acute stroke patients: a CT scan lesion site study. *J Neurol Rehabil.* 1992;6:163–173.

118. Gosman-Hedstrom G, Claesson L, Klingensteirna U, et al. Effects of acupuncture treatment on daily life activities and quality of life: a controlled, prospective, and randomized study of acute stroke patients. *Stroke.* 1998;29:2100–2108.

119. Johansson BB, Haker E, von Arbin M, et al. Acupuncture and transcutaneous nerve stimulation in stroke rehabilitation: a randomized controlled trial. *Stroke.* 2001;32: 707–713.

120. Sze FK-H, Wong E, Yi X, et al. Does acupuncture have additional value to standard poststroke motor rehabilitation? *Stroke.* 2002;33:186–194.

121. Wong AMK, Su T-Y, Tang F-T, et al. Clinical trial of electrical acupuncture on hemiplegic stroke patients. *Am J Phys Med Rehabil.* 1999;78:117–122.

122. Sze FK, Wong E, Or KK, et al. Does acupuncture improve motor recovery after stroke? A meta-analysis of randomized controlled trials. *Stroke.* 2002;33:2604–2619.

123. Louw SJ. Research in stroke rehabilitation: confounding effects of the heterogeneity of stroke, experimental bias and inappropriate outcomes measures. *J Altern Complement Med.* 2002;8:691–693.

124. Karst M, Reinhard M, Thum P, et al. Needle acupuncture in tension-type headache: a randomized, placebo-controlled study. *Cephalalgia.* 2001;21:637–642.

125. Karakurum B, Karaalin O, Coskun O, et al. The "dry-needle technique": intramuscular stimulation in tension-type headache. *Cephalalgia.* 2001; 21:813–817.

126. White AR, Resch KL, Chan JC, et al. Acupuncture for episodic tension-type headache: a multicentre

randomized controlled trial. *Cephalalgia*. 2000;20: 632–637.

127. Allais G, De Lorenzo C, Quirico PE, et al. Acupuncture in the prophylactic treatment of migraine without aura: a comparison with flunarizine. *Headache*. 2002;42:855–861.

128. Liguori A, Petti F, Bangrazi A, et al. Comparison of pharmacological treatment versus acupuncture treatment for migraine without aura. *J Trad Chin Med*. 2000;20:231–240.

129. Vickers A, Rees R, Zollman C, et al. Acupuncture for migraine and headache in primary care: a protocol for a pragmatic, randomized trial. *Complement Ther Med*. 1999;7:3–18.

130. Smith C, Crowther C, Beilby J. Acupuncture to treat nausea and vomiting in early pregnancy: a randomized controlled trial. *Birth*. 2002;29:1–9.

131. Knight B, Mudge C, Openshaw S, et al. Effect of acupuncture on nausea of pregnancy: a randomized, controlled trial. *Obstet Gynecol*. 2001;97: 184–188.

132. Carlsson CP, Axemo P, Bodin A, et al. Manual acupuncture reduces hyperemesis gravidarum: a placebo-controlled, randomized, single-blind, cross-over study. *J Pain Symptom Manage*. 2000; 20:273–279.

133. Carlsson CP, Axemo P, Bodin A, et al. Manual acupuncture reduces hyperemesis gravidarum: a placebo-controlled, randomized, single-blind, cross-over study. *J Pain Symptom Manage*. 2000; 20:273–279.

134. Wedenberg K, Moen B, Norling A. A prospective randomized study comparing acupuncture with physiotherapy for low-back and pelvic pain in pregnancy. *Acta Obstet Gynecol Scand*. 2000;79: 331–335.

135. Skilnand E, Fossen D, Heiberg E. Acupuncture in the management of pain in labor. *Acta Obstet Gynecol Scand* 2002;81:943–948.

136. Zeisler H, Temfer C, Mayerhofer K, et al. Influence of acupuncture on duration of labor. *Gynecol Obstet Invest*. 1998;46:22–25.

137. Tempfer C, Zeisler H, Heinzl H, et al. Influence of acupuncture on maternal serum levels of interleukin-8, prostaglandin F2alpha, and beta-endorphin: a matched-pair study. *Obstet Gynecol*. 1998;92:245–248.

138. Rabl M, Ahner R, Bitschnau M, et al. Acupuncture for cervical ripening and induction of labor at term—a randomized controlled trial. *Wien Klin Wochenschr*. 2001;113:942–946.

139. Skilnand E, Fossen D, Heiberg E. Acupuncture in the management of pain in labor. *Acta Obstet Gynecol Scand* 2002;81:943–948.

140. Stener-Victorin E, Waldenstrom U, Nilsson L, et al. A prospective randomized study of electro-acupuncture versus alfentanil as anaesthesia during oocyte aspiration in in-vitro fertilization. *Hum Reprod*. 1999;14:2480–2484.

141. Paulus WE, Zhang M, Strehler E, et al. Influence of acupuncture on the pregnancy rate in patients who undergo assisted reproduction therapy. *Fertil Steril*. 2002;77:721–724.

142. Fink M, Wolkenstein E, Karst M, et al. Acupuncture in chronic epicondylitis: a randomized controlled trial. *Rheumatology*. 2002;41:205–209.

143. Tsui P, Leung MC. Comparison of the effectiveness between manual acupuncture and electroacupuncture on patients with tennis elbow. *Acupunct Electrother Res*. 2002;27:107–117.

144. David J, Modi S, Aluko AA, et al. Chronic neck pain: a comparison of acupuncture treatment and physiotherapy. *Br J Rheumatol*. 1998;37: 1118–1122.

145. Birch S, Jamison RN. Controlled trial of Japanese acupuncture for chronic myofascial neck pain: assessment of specific and nonspecific effects of treatment. *Clin J Pain*. 1998;14:248–255.

146. Irnich D, Behrens N, Molzen H, et al. Randomised trial of acupuncture compared with conventional massage and "sham" laser acupuncture for treatment of chronic neck pain. *BMJ*. 2001;322:1–6.

147. Irnich D, Behrens N, Gleditsch JM, et al. Immediate effects of dry needling and acupuncture at distant points in chronic neck pain: results of a randomized, double-blind, sham-controlled crossover trial. *Pain*. 2002;99:83–89.

148. Dyson-Hudson TA, Shiflett SC, Kirshblum SC, et al. Acupuncture and Trager psychophysical integration in the treatment of wheelchair user's shoulder pain in individuals with spinal cord injury. *Arch Phys Med Rehabil*. 2001;82:1038–1046.

149. Kleinhenz J, Streitberger K, Windeler J, et al. Randomised clinical trial comparing the effects of acupuncture and a newly designed placebo needle in rotator cuff tendonitis. *Pain*. 1999;83: 235–241.

150. Jensen R, Gothesen O, Liseth K, et al. Acupuncture treatment of patellofemoral pain syndrome. *J Altern Complement Med*. 1999;5:521–527.

151. Berman BM, Singh BB, Lao L, et al. A randomized trial of acupuncture as an adjunctive therapy

in osteoarthritis of the knee. *Rheumatology*. 1999; 38:346–354.

152. Haslam R. A comparison of acupuncture with advice and exercises on the symptomatic treatment of osteoarthritis of the hip—a randomised controlled trial. *Acupunct Med*. 2001;19:19–26.

153. Tillu A, Roberts C, Tillu S. Unilateral versus bilateral acupuncture on knee function in advanced osteoarthritis of the knee—a prospective randomised trial. *Acupunct Med*. 2001;19:15–18.

154. Fink MG, Wipperman B, Gehrke A. Non-specific effects of traditional Chinese acupuncture in osteoarthritis of the hip. *Complement Ther Med*. 2001;9:82–89.

155. Giles LG, Muller R. Chronic spinal pain syndromes: a clinical pilot trial comparing acupuncture, a nonsteroidal anti-inflammatory drug, and spinal manipulation. *J Manipulative Physiol Ther*. 1999;22:376–381.

156. Cherkin DC, Eisenberg D, Sherman KJ, et al. Randomized trial comparing traditional Chinese medical acupuncture, therapeutic massage, and self-care education for chronic low back pain. *Arch Intern Med*. 2001;161:1081–1088.

157. Leibing E, Leonhardt U, Koster G, et al. Acupuncture treatment of chronic low-back pain—a randomized, blinded, placebo-controlled trial with 9-month follow-up. *Pain*. 2002;96:189–196.

158. Carlsson CP, Sjolund BH. Acupuncture for chronic low back pain: a randomized placebo-controlled study with long-term follow-up. *Clin J Pain*. 2001;17:296–305.

159. Molsberger AF, Mau J, Pawelec DB, Winkler J. Does acupuncture improve the orthopedic management of chronic low back pain—a randomized, blinded, controlled trial with 3 months follow up. *Pain*. 2002;99:579–587.

160. Ceccherelli F, Rigoni MT, Gagliardi G, et al. Comparison of superficial and deep acupuncture in the treatment of lumbar myofascial pain: a double-blind randomized controlled study. *Clin J Pain*. 2002;18:149–153.

161. Naeser MA, Hahn KA, Lieberman BE, Branco KF. Carpal tunnel syndrome pain treated with low-level laser and microamperes transcutaneous electric nerve stimulation: a controlled study. *Arch Phys Med Rehabil*. 2002;83:978–988.

162. Shapira MY, Berkman N, Ben David G, et al. Short-term acupuncture therapy is of no benefit in patients with moderate persistent asthma. *Chest*. 2002;121:1396–1400.

163. Biernacki W, Peake MD. Acupuncture in the treatment of stable asthma. *Respir Med*. 1998;92: 1143–1145.

164. Joos S, Schott C, Zou H, et al. Immunomodulatory effects of acupuncture in the treatment of allergic asthma: a randomized controlled study. *J Altern Complement Med*. 2000;6:519–525.

165. Ezzo J, Berman BM, Hadhazy VA, et al. Is acupuncture effective for the treatment of pain? A systematic review. *Pain*. 2000;86:217–225.

166. Lewith G, Vincent C. On the evaluation of the clinical effects of acupuncture: a problem reassessed and a framework for future research. *J Altern Complement Med*. 1996;2:79–90.

167. Birch S, Hammerschlag R, Trinh K, Zaslawski C. The non-specific effects of acupuncture treatment: when and how to control for them. *Clin Acupunct Orient Med*. 2002;3:20–25.

168. Ezzo J, Berman BM, Hadhazy VA, et al. Is acupuncture effective for the treatment of pain? A systematic review. *Pain*. 2000;86:217–225.

169. Biernacki W, Peake MD. Acupuncture in the treatment of stable asthma. *Respir Med*. 1998;92: 1143–1145.

170. Mitchell B. *Acupuncture and Oriental Medicine Laws*. Washington, DC: National Acupuncture Foundation; 2001.

171. http://www.acupuncturealliance.org or http://www.aaom.org.

172. American Commission for Acupuncture and Oriental Medicine, http://www.acaom.org.

173. http://www.ccaom.org/members3.asp.

174. http://www.acaom.org.

175. http://www.NCCAOM.org.

176. American Association of Medical Acupuncture, http://www.medicalacupuncture.org. C. James Dowden, personal correspondence.

177. http://www.medicalacupuncture.org/.

178. Pelletier K, Astin J. Integration and reimbursement of complementary and alternative medicine by managed care and insurance providers. 2000 Update and cohort analysis. *Altern Ther Health Med*. 2002;8(1):46.

179. Pelletier K, Astin J. Integration and reimbursement of complementary and alternative medicine by managed care and insurance providers. 2000 Update and cohort analysis. *Altern Ther Health Med*. 2002;8(1):46.

180. Pelletier K, Astin J. Integration and reimbursement of complementary and alternative medicine by managed care and insurance providers. 2000

Update and cohort analysis. *Altern Ther Health Med.* 2002;8(1):47.

181. Wolpe P. The maintenance of professional authority: acupuncture and the American physician. *Soc Prob.* 1985;32(5):409–424.

182. Pelletier K, Astin J. Integration and reimbursement of complementary and alternative medicine by managed care and insurance providers. 2000 Update and cohort analysis. *Altern Ther Health Med.* 2002;8(1):42.

183. Pelletier K, Astin J. Integration and reimbursement of complementary and alternative medicine by managed care and insurance providers. 2000 update and cohort analysis. *Altern Ther Health Med.* 2002;8(1):46.

183a. Office of Technology Assessment. Assessing the Efficacy and Safety of Medical Technologies. Congress of the United States. September 1978: Library of Congress Catalog Card Number 78-600117.

183b. White KL. International comparisons of health care systems. *Milbank Mem Fund Q.* 1968; 46:117.

184. Pelletier K, Astin J. Integration and reimbursement of complementary and alternative medicine by managed care and insurance providers.

185. Wolpe P. The maintenance of professional authority: acupuncture and the American physician. *Soc Prob.* 1985;32(5):409–424.

186. Seattle Group Health Cooperative GAP analysis in: Weeks J. The Joint Commission's pain standards: an opportunity for integration? *Integrative Med Consult Quart Bus Rep;* January 2002:1–8.

187. http://www.jcaho.org/standard/pain_hap. html.

188. Quoting Don Nielsen, MD. In: Weeks J. The Joint Commission's pain standards: an opportunity for integration? *The Integrative Medicine Consult. Quarterly Business Report.* 2002; January:2.

189. Quoting June Dahl, PhD. In: Weeks J. The Joint Commission's pain standards: an opportunity for integration? *The Integrative Medicine Consult. Quarterly Business Report.* 2002; January:2.

190. Cabana M, Rand C, Powe N, Wu A, et al. Why don't physicians follow clinical practice guidelines? A framework for improvement. *JAMA.* 1999;282(15):1458–1465.

191. Weeks J. The Joint Commission's pain standards: an opportunity for integration? *Integrative Med Consult.* January:R2.

CHAPTER 10

Ayurvedic Medicine

SUNIL PAI, VIVEK SHANBHAG, AND SRINIVASA ARCHARYA

▶ AYURVEDA: A HOLISTIC APPROACH

Ayurveda (pronounced aa-yoor-vay-da), which originated in India around 5,000 B.C., is one of the world's oldest and most complete systems of medicine. The word Ayurveda means "the science of life" or "life knowledge." Ayurveda is a science in which the knowledge of the body *(sarira)*, senses *(indriya)*, mind *(sattva)*, and soul *(atma)* are defined into one meaningful system. Ayurveda was one of the first systems of medicine to offer a holistic approach to health care. It emphasizes the uniqueness of the individual, promotes prevention, and offers natural methods of treatment. Furthermore, it stresses one's responsibility for one's own well-being, which makes for a very cost-effective approach for the management of disease states. This system is as practical and timely now as it was 5,000 years ago.[1]

The concept of life as the harmonious blending of the body, mind, and spirit is well defined in Ayurveda. The aggregate of these three, like a tripod, establishes the balance for human life. Health is not just the absence of disease but the state of enjoying uninterrupted physical, mental, and spiritual happiness. By achieving optimum health one can enjoy the ultimate goals of life; namely virtue *(Dharma)*, wealth *(Artha)*, enjoyment *(Kama)*, and salvation *(Moksha)*.[2]

Ayurveda is one of the first systems of medicine to recognize the concept of individual mind-body types (see "Individual Constitution: *Prakriti*" below) and the importance of the mind–body connection. Each person differs in relation to their physical and mental makeup. Humans are considered to be psychosomatic individuals. This unique makeup of body and mind influences all aspects of one's life, including body structure, emotional makeup, predisposition to illnesses, and reactions to various treatments. This ancient idea of individuality resembles the modern ideas of functional medicine. Either in a diseased or healthy state, the body and mind of an individual are never studied in isolation; thus Ayurveda emphasizes the importance of mind–body medicine. Adapting an unhealthy lifestyle without knowing one's individual constitution may create imbalances, and, therefore, lead to illness. Thus, specific dietary regimens and behavioral patterns are advised in Ayurveda for different persons having different mind–body constitutions called *doshas*.[3]

The inner intelligence of the body and its natural strengthening and healing ability is described in detail in Ayurveda. Through the practice of proper dietary, physical, and mental exercises, an individual can improve his or her resistance power and prevent diseases.[4] Ayurveda emphasizes lifestyle behavioral modification and biopurification *(Panchakarma)* procedures that strengthen the indigenous immune system. The treatment that eradicates the illness from its root, minimizing the risk of relapses, and side effects, is considered to be the noble principle of medical practice in Ayurvedic science. This concept in Ayurveda is known as *Swabhavoparama.*

In India, the duration of training to become an Ayurvedic physician is similar to Western medical training. Ayurvedic medical training ranges from 4–6 years with postgraduate training in different specialty areas in medicine and surgery, such as dermatology and gynecology. The education includes training in both Ayurveda and Western medical concepts of anatomy, biochemistry, pathology, pharmacology, physiology, and preventative and public health, as well as laboratory medicine. Clinical training includes at least 3–5 years of inpatient hospital wards and outpatient clinic care.

Currently in India, there are more than 200 Ayurvedic undergraduate schools and 53 postgraduate schools including such well-known Ayurvedic schools as the Banaras Hindu University, University of Poona, and Gujarat Ayurved University. To date, more than 200,000 Ayurvedic physicians have been trained. Most of the clinical research in Ayurveda has been performed as postdoctoral thesis work at the universities. Unfortunately, for multifaceted reasons, such as lack of funding, nonstandardized catalog systems, and lack of computerization, such research is difficult for the Western world to access. Currently, with the emerging growth of Ayurveda worldwide, certain private organizations, such as Maharishi University, as well as governmental organizations such as the National Center for Complementary and Alternative Medicine (NCCAM) of the National Institutes of Health (NIH), are performing clinical studies to demonstrate the use and efficacy of Ayurveda.

In the United States, there is no official licensing process for Ayurvedic physicians. Although there are certification programs by various Ayurvedic organizations and schools, there exists no national approval of licensure or state certification boards. Presently, most training in the United States ranges from 1–4-year programs. These programs are open to everyone, although mainly attended by people in the health care field or services that support them (doctors, osteopaths, naturopaths, chiropractors, nurses, dietitians, and massage and physical therapists). Some Ayurvedic physicians practice under other licenses such as naturopathic licenses (in states that license naturopathy). After completing a training program, one can be certified as a "health instructor" or "Ayurvedic specialist/consultant," which permits one to educate on diet and use of herbs, and to teach the importance of lifestyle and behavioral changes.

▶ HISTORICAL OVERVIEW AND CLASSICAL TEXTS

Ayurveda has it roots in the four oldest documented scriptures written in Sanskrit, known as the *Vedas.* Ayurveda is considered a subsidiary subject of one of the Vedas—the Atharva Veda. The Vedas not only address the topics of health, spirituality, and ethical living, but also describe the science of archery, fine arts, architecture *(Vastu),* astrology *(Jyothish),* and yoga.

With the influence of Vedic knowledge, three important classical texts emerged: the *Charak Samhita,* the *Sushruta Samhita,* and the *Ashtanga Samgraha.* Charak and Sushruta were two well-recognized physicians whose texts transformed into the working guidelines of the practice of Ayurvedic medicine. From their texts, two schools of Ayurveda evolved over the centuries: the school of physicians *(Atreya)* and the school of surgeons *(Dhanvantari).* These schools transformed Ayurveda into a scientifically verifiable and classifiable medical system.[5]

The *Charak Samhita* was written in 700 B.C. on the subject of general medicine and is considered to be the first classical text. The *Charak Samhita* defines disease from its etymology, etiology, clinical presentation, pathophysiology, and prognosis.[6] Furthermore, it describes treatment for the diseases, including herbal medicines, dietary recommendations, and behavioral lifestyle changes, encompassing a holistic approach.

The second classical text written on the subject of general surgery is called the *Sushruta Samhita* (600 B.C.). It is named after the author who is considered the "father of plastic surgery." The *Sushruta Samhita* describes in detail various operative techniques and procedures, such as abdominal operations for intestinal obstruction and removal of bladder stones, as well as plastic surgery. In fact, the forehead skin flap to reconstruct the deformed nose was first described by Sushruta, and even today is named after him. Other described procedures include operations for delivery of a fetus, amputation of a limb, and use of prosthetic devices. Sushruta describes 101 different types of blunt surgical instruments and 24 different types of sharp surgical instruments. Sushruta also mentions nearly 760 botanical sources of medicines.[6] The *Sushruta Samhita* describes the first science of massage therapy, as a therapeutic and rehabilitative modality of treatment, along with treatment of *marma points*, or vital body points, which were later adopted into Chinese acupuncture.[7]

The third classical text is called *Ashtanga Samgraha*, which means "collection of the eight branches or specialties" of Ayurvedic medicine, which was written by Vagbhata around the seventh century A.D.[8] (see Table 10–1). These branches are parallel to the fields of modern medicine that we practice today.

Since its inception, Ayurveda has had global appeal. Its influence flourished in places like Tibet, Greece, Egypt, and China. As a consequence of the Mogul invasion of India (1400–1800) and later the British occupation (1800–1948), there was a significant decline in the practice of Ayurveda in India. Finally, in the late twentieth century Ayurveda has reemerged.

▶ **TABLE 10–1** EIGHT BRANCHES OF AYURVEDA

Kayachitkitsa—internal medicine
Balaroga Chikitsa—pediatrics and obstetrics and gynecology
Salyachikitsa—general surgery
Shalakya Chikitsa—ear, nose, throat, and ophthalmology
Agandatantra—toxicology
Rasayana Chikitsa—geriatrics and rejuvenation
Vajikarana Chikitsa—fertility and sexual health
Bhuta Vidya—psychiatry

Source: Vagabhatacharya.[8]

The oldest system of medicine is now the last to be rediscovered.

▶ COMPONENTS OF THE AYURVEDIC APPROACH

To arrive at the identification and diagnosis of disease, Ayurveda proposes a thorough clinical examination that includes a detailed medical history and an eightfold physical examination. The eight factors involved are pulse diagnosis *(Nadi Pariksha)*; tongue diagnosis; examination of voice/speech, skin, eyes and general appearance; and specific characteristics of the urine and stool. With this methodical Ayurvedic approach, one can diagnose and treat even the most complex diseases.[9]

Below is an example of what a comprehensive and customized Ayurvedic natural health program may consist of when referring a patient to an Ayurvedic health specialist/educator.[10]

1. Natural diet to suit the individual's body type.
2. Therapeutic botanical herbs and nutritional supplements.
3. Detoxification by gentle cleansing, which is called *Panchakarma* therapy.

4. Ayurvedic bodywork and massage.
5. Physical exercise and stretches, including yoga postures.
6. Stress management through relaxation exercises, breathing techniques *(Pranayama),* music, aromatherapy, focusing exercises, and meditation.
7. Rejuvenation therapy, called *Rasayana,* to delay aging and to promote longevity.
8. Special daily routines that include natural oral hygiene; preventive care of eyes, ears, nasal passages, sinuses, and throat; and nourishing treatment of skin, hair, and nails.
9. Special seasonal routines for year-round health by adapting to the seasons.
10. Counseling and health education on healthy lifestyles.

▶ HEALTHY ENVIRONMENT AND HEALTHY LIVING

An influential relationship between public health *(Hitayu)* and personal health *(Sukhayu)* is clearly defined by Ayurveda. An individual and the society in which they live influence each other. Thus, individuals living in a healthy society will have additional support for their healthy living with a nourishing effect. Likewise, individuals living in an unhealthy environment may have unhealthy influences upon them. Kind behaviors toward fellow beings are also an important part of health. Thus, Ayurveda describes *Sukhayu* and *Hitayu* as an obligation on the part of individuals to be useful and purposeful for the society in which they live, for the nation of which they are a citizen, and for the world of which they are a part. This is the understanding of complete health described in Ayurveda.[11]

▶ HERBAL MEDICINE

Presently in areas that practice Ayurveda in India, if it is determined that medicines are to be used in treatment, then herbal medicines along with medicines containing minerals and/or metals are preferred. With the influence of Western medicine upon India, many Ayurvedic hospitals and physicians use allopathic medicines, such as antibiotics, for acute situations; however, they still rely mainly on the herbal medicines for most chronic conditions. These herbal medicines act as general tonics for strengthening the overall health of the individual and do not just focus on the specific disease.

Sometimes in Western medicine there is a tendency to treat the symptoms with minimal emphasis on the causative factors, which may prolong the clinical condition. By using an Ayurvedic approach, not only are the symptoms considered, but greater emphasis is given to the management of the causative factors of the clinical condition. For example in allopathic medicine, when a patient presents with symptoms of heartburn, an acid-blocking agent is commonly prescribed. This tends to give immediate relief of symptoms, but does not address the cause. This may prompt the recurrence of the symptoms and prolongation of therapy. An Ayurvedic approach would address the heartburn with medical herbs, for immediate relief, that have fewer potential side effects, yet will mainly focus attention on educating the patient on the contributing factors of diet and lifestyle changes, which would then shorten the duration of the clinical condition and its dependency on medicines.

Unlike some schools of Western herbalism that hold that standardized extracts are the most effective way to use an herb medicinally, Ayurvedic herbal tradition holds that nature has compounded and balanced all the important ingredients in different parts of the herbal plant. These ingredients often act synergistically with each other to enhance potency and reduce the potential side effects by their blending.[12] Ayurvedic practitioners tend to feel that removal or concentration of the active ingredient by itself—as in the standardization practices common in Western herbalism—may actually cause harm, and that efficacy may be lost as a result of removal of various beneficial and balancing cofactors.

On the contrary, the whole herbal drug may have slower onset of action to get the therapeutic effect in comparison to the isolated active principle of the drug (pharmaceutical) or the extracted active ingredient (standardized extracts), but usually has less risk of side effects. Most herbal formulas are considered to be "balanced" formulas using multiple herbal ingredients. These include not only the herbs that are the active main ingredients for the treatment, but also adjuncts in aiding absorption, digestion, and assimilation, and herbs that counterbalance any known potential unwanted effect.

Currently in India there is a rapid growth of exportation of Ayurvedic herbal medicines worldwide. The total exports of Ayurvedic products have grown from $62 million in 2000–2001 to $155 million in 2001–2002 and is projected to rise to $1.03 billion by 2005.[13] Because of such growth, the WHO (World Health Organization) and the government of India recently implemented strict guidelines for the Good Manufacturing Practices (GMP) of Ayurvedic companies who export to the United States and abroad. These new guidelines will ensure the purity, potency, and bioavailability of the herbal medicines. Presently, there are more than 700 manufacturing companies, of which only 70 adhere to the manufacturing guidelines of the WHO.[13] Based on the philosophy of Ayurvedic herbalism, it is recommended to use formulas that use specific and appropriate plant parts rather than standardized extract formulas when possible and also to use traditional "formulas" rather than using single ingredients alone. There are many US and non-US importing companies that sell Ayurvedic products, but one should only purchase products from those that document GMP, as well as other safety testing, such as for pesticide residues, heavy metals, and biological contaminants. Although traditional Ayurvedic medicines are less expensive than pharmaceutical drugs in the United States, with the implementation of the new guidelines, the costs of Ayurvedic herbal medicines will increase. However, these medicines still may be a cheaper substitute or alternative to allopathic pharmaceuticals when appropriately used.

▶ NUTRITION: THE SIX TASTES

Ayurveda places great importance on nutrition in the prevention of disease and sustenance of a healthy body and mind. Balancing of foods is not by food groups but by their taste qualities. There are six tastes: sweet, salty, sour, bitter, pungent, and astringent. Examples of the six tastes are as follows: Sweet tastes include sugar, carbohydrates (such as pasta, rice, and wheat), milk, and sweet fruits. Sour tastes include yogurt, cheese, vinegar, sour and citrus fruits. Salty tastes include table salt and seaweed. Bitter tastes include spinach, kale, and other dark-green, leafy vegetables. Pungent tastes include spices such as garlic, onions, ginger, black pepper, chili, and jalapeños. Astringent tastes include tea leaves, fruit peels, unripe bananas, and certain beans and lentils. Each *dosha* has three tastes that increase and three tastes that decrease the *dosha* characteristics[12] (Table 10–2). For example, if a person has a condition that is caused by an aggravated *Vata dosha* or excessive *Vata* characteristics, then they need to take in more foods that have *Vata* decreasing qualities and vice versa.

▶ **TABLE 10–2** EFFECTS OF TASTES ON THE THREE DOSHAS

Vata decreasing	Vata increasing
Sweet	Pungent
Sour	Bitter
Salty	Astringent
Pitta decreasing	**Pitta increasing**
Sweet	Pungent
Bitter	Sour
Astringent	Salty
Kapha decreasing	**Kapha increasing**
Pungent	Sweet
Bitter	Sour
Astringent	Salty

Source: From Shanbhag.[14] Reproduced with permission.

The key to optimum health is to balance the *doshas* by counterbalancing the excess or deficiency with the tastes that have opposite or similar qualities. Although an individual will emphasize certain tastes in the diet to help pacify the *dosha* if aggravated, it is recommended that the most balanced meal for health maintenance contain all six tastes in moderation. Dietary recommendations should be followed according to an individual's *prakriti* to maintain the balance of their inherent psychophysiological nature.[15]

Another therapeutic approach in Ayurveda is the proper blending of herbs and spices used in food to enhance or balance the *doshas*. The following are examples of herbs and spices that can be used in cooking.[16]

1. *Vata-balancing herbs and spices:* basil, bay, black pepper, cardamom, ginger, marjoram, nutmeg, salt, and savory.
2. *Pitta-balancing herbs and spices:* cilantro, coriander, cumin, dill, fennel, lemongrass, licorice, mint, and sugar.
3. *Kapha-balancing herbs and spices:* basil, black pepper, caraway, cardamom, cayenne, cinnamon, dill, fenugreek, ginger, mint, mustard, nutmeg, parsley, rosemary, and sage.

Most general books on Ayurveda contain lists grouped by *doshas* and describe which foods one should emphasize, should eat in moderation, and should avoid. In summary, if any factor is increased in the body, it can be reduced by the intake of substances having opposite qualities. If any factor in the body is deficient, it can be rectified by the supplementation of the substances having similar properties.

► YOGA

Yoga comes from the Sanskrit word that means "yolk" or "union." In the Vedic literature, many texts have been written about various types of yoga. Although Western culture has long viewed yoga as stretching exercises or mere physical postures, yoga also incorporates the mind and spirit. Currently, approximately 12 million Americans practice yoga.[17] The most common type of yoga is Hatha yoga, which incorporates postures (asanas), breath work (pranayama), and meditation. Hatha yoga incorporates various subtypes such as Ashtanga, Bikram, Integral, and Iyengar yoga. Hatha yoga, in general, incorporates physical postures, breath work, sensory methods, affirmations, visualizations, mantra, and meditation.[18] Similar to the prescribing of physical therapy for certain conditions, Ayurveda incorporates yoga as part of the health plan of prevention and treatment and has specific yoga postures, routines, and exercises indicated for specific diseases.

In Hatha yoga there is a simple practice that is recommended in Ayurveda as part of a daily routine. It is called *surya namaskar* or "sun salutation." This practice is *tridoshic*, which means it is good for all *doshas*. This comprises a series of 10 or 12 yoga postures done in a systematic sequence (flexion and extension with breath work). It is recommended that it be performed twice a day, during sunrise and sunset, for general health maintenance. It can be performed slowly or if one is well trained, it can be performed quickly to become an aerobic workout (see Figure 10–1).

► FUNDAMENTAL PRINCIPLES OF AYURVEDA

Five Basic Elements: Pancha Maha Bhuta

A fundamental concept in Ayurveda is that an individual (human body/mind/spirit) is the epitome of the universe. If the universe is the macrocosm, the individual (human body/mind/spirit) is the microcosm. This relationship between the universe and the individual can be defined on the basis of their physical elements and generic properties. All matter in the universe or within the mind–body is basically made of the five basic elements, popularly

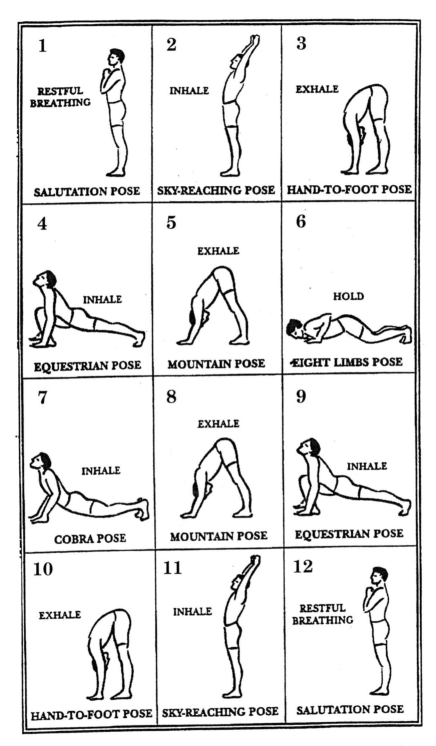

Figure 10–1. The 12 postures of sun salutation (surya namaskar) yoga.

known as the doctrine of *Pancha Maha Bhuta.*
These five elements are known as: space
(akasha), air *(vayu),* fire *(teja),* water *(jala),*
and earth *(prithivi).*[19]

Each basic element has its own distinctive
qualities. Space represents the field in which
all other matter is accommodated. Air represents the mobile gaseous state. Fire represents
the transforming force within matter. Light emission is also a physical character of fire. Water
is represented by the cohesive liquid state and
the earth represents the structural solid state.
Furthermore, this theory of five basic elements
is extended to explain the perception of sensations in the body. In the body, space is characterized by sound, air by touch, fire by vision,
water by taste, and earth by odor.

Structural and Functional Units of the Body: Tridosha, Saptadhatu, and Mala

The human body is composed of three fundamental units: *tridosha, saptadhatu,* and *mala.*
Doshas are three specific combinations of the
five basic elements and can be regarded as psychophysiological characteristics or mind–body
principles of an individual. The *saptadhatus* or
"seven tissues" form the structure of the body.
The activity of the body is governed by the
doshas and is mediated through the structure or
the *dhatu* (the "tissue"). The interaction between *doshas* and the *dhatu* results in the generation of metabolic waste. These wastes are
collectively known as *mala. Doshas* are the
characteristics of the mind–body and are best
assessed by their functions rather than their
structure. *Dhatus* build the gross body structure
and are best studied by the physical properties
and functions. The balanced state of these *dosha,
dhatu,* and *mala* is referred to as health, and
imbalance of these three is known as disease.[20]

Six stages of the disease process are described in Ayurveda according to the development and movement of the aggravated *doshas*
(see Table 10–3). The first two stages refer to

▶ **TABLE 10–3** THE SIX STAGES OF DISEASE

1. Accumulation (sancaya)
2. Aggravation (prakopa)
3. Overflow (prasara)
4. Relocation (sthana samsraya)
5. Manifestation (vyakti)
6. Diversification (bheda)

*Source: From Sutrasthana. Sushruta Samhita. Varanasi,
India; Chaukhambha Surbharati prakasan; 1994:91.*

the increase of *doshas* in their respective sites,
and if preventive lifestyle behaviors and biopurification procedures are performed, the disease condition may be completely eliminated.
The other four stages show the progressive
worsening of the disease and its spread to different parts of the body.[21] At these later stages,
the disease is harder to control and thus worsens the prognosis. Therefore, the importance
of early prevention rather than late intervention is emphasized in Ayurveda.

Individual Constitution: Prakriti

Prakriti is defined as one's individual constitution or linked to one's own physiopsychologi-
cal makeup. It is as distinctive for an individual as his or her own fingerprint. *Prakriti* is
said to be determined at the time of conception itself. It is the relative predominance and
culmination of the *dosha* in the *shukra* (sperm)
and *shonita* (ovum) of the parents at the time
of the fertilization and this inherent ratio will
remain throughout one's life. Thus, depending
upon the relative dominance of the *doshas,*
one may have any of the following major seven
types of the *prakriti.* This is a general simpli-
fication. Further, depending on the various ratios of the dominant *doshas,* several combinations can be defined. One can have a *prakriti*
with a relative dominance of any one *dosha:
Vata, Pitta,* or *Kapha.* Having this single predominance is quite common. One also can
have a *prakriti* with a relative dominance of
two *doshas: Vata-Pitta, Vata-Kapha,* or *Pitta-*

Kapha. Having these two predominant *doshas* is very common. Finally, one can have an equal dominance of all three *doshas* (tridoshic): *Vata-Pitta-Kapha.* Having this predominance of all three *doshas* is a rare occurrence.

When using *dosha* for assessment of health and lifestyle behaviors, there is no "correct" or "perfect" *dosha.* Each *dosha* has its own benefits. The goal of Ayurveda is to maintain one's current psychophysiological state *(vikruti)* in balance with one's inherent constitution *(prakriti).* Understanding an individual's *Prakriti* will give an insight to one's actions and can give clues for self improvement.[22] *Doshas* have a tendency to be influenced by various factors such as food, ambient temperature, season, sensory input, and mental state, and for the same reason, all these factors have to be considered to maintain the balance of these *doshas.*

Psychophysiological Characteristics or Mind–Body Principles: The Doshas

The five basic elements *(Pancha Maha Bhutas)* have been condensed into three *doshas—Vata, Pitta,* and *Kapha*—to conform to the functional attributes (see Table 10–4). These *doshas* are reflective of the various physical as well as mental characteristics that represent the elements.

Vata Dosha

Air *(vayu)* and space *(akasha)* are the basic elements that make up the *Vata dosha.* It shows its action in the body through its kinetic energy and is the principle of movement. Therefore, the structures and functions of *Vata* are responsible for transportation and communication of all aspects of the body, as well as the mind. Physical movements include cardiovascular

▶ **TABLE 10–4** ATTRIBUTES OF VATA, PITTA, AND KAPHA DOSHAS

Attributes	Vata	Pitta	Kapha
Basic element composition	Space and air	Fire and water	Earth and water
Physical characteristics	Dry Light Cold Quick Rough Unstable	Hot Moist Fluid Sharp Intense Sour-smelling	Heavy Cold Wet Slow Oily Smooth
Major physiological functions	Transport Communication Movement	Biotransformation Digestion Temperature	Structure Growth Storage
Major mental functions	Creativity Imagination Indecisiveness	Intelligence Confidence Leadership	Memory Tranquility Devotion
Major emotions	Exhilaration Fear Insecurity	Excitement Anger Jealousy	Love Patience Greed
Location—general	Lower trunk: Thighs Hips Bones Ears Bladder Organs of touch	Mid-trunk: Stomach Liver Gallbladder Pancreas Sweat glands Organs of vision	Upper chest: Throat Head Sinuses Tongue Lymph Nose Adipose tissues
Location with digestive system	Colon	Small intestine	Stomach

Source: Shanbhag.[14] Reproduced with permission.

circulation, respiration, gastrointestinal motility, elimination, and neuromuscular movements. Mental functions include creativity, imagination, intuition, sensitivity, spontaneity, indecisiveness, and emotions such as fear, insecurity, doubt, and exhilaration. Physical characteristics of *Vata* include being dry, light, cold, rough, and quick. Although ubiquitously distributed in the body, *Vata dosha* is primarily located in the lower half of the digestive system—the colon. The influence of *Vata dosha* on the body is said to be maximum during old age and during the fall season. All micro and macro movements (i.e., ovum to the womb to motion of limbs) in the body, as well as all voluntary and involuntary movements (i.e., rhythm of heart and peristalsis in intestines), are mediated through the *Vata dosha*. Because *Vata* is the "airy" principle of movement, disorders similarly have the same "airy" component (i.e., emphysema). Examples of conditions caused by imbalance of *Vata dosha* are arthritis, cracking joints, ticks and tremors, spasms, anxiety, dry skin, dry hair, flatulence, constipation, and insomnia.[23]

Pitta Dosha

Fire *(teja)* predominately and water *(jala)* are basic elements that make up the *Pitta dosha*. All the metabolic activity including anabolism and catabolism of all materials of the body and mind are attributed to *Pitta dosha* and hence it is considered the principle of biotransformation. The structures and functions of *Pitta* are responsible for the digestive enzymes secreted in the gastrointestinal system, the cellular enzymes and the stimulating hormones. Physical biotransformation includes digestion, assimilation, visual perception, mental discrimination, temperature regulation, coloration and pigmentation as well as all metabolism of food into energy and thoughts into understanding. Mental functions include intelligence, leadership, confidence, organization and emotions like excitement, joy, courage, anger, jealousy, and hatred. Physical characteristics of *Pitta dosha* are being hot, moist, light, intense, and sour smelling. *Pitta* behavior is usually sharp

and direct. Although pervading the whole body, *Pitta dosha* is primarily located in the middle portion of the trunk and in the small intestine. Furthermore, the influence of the *Pitta dosha* is greatest during the middle age of an individual and during late spring and summer season (hot and humid, thus increasing *Pitta* as like increases like). Because *Pitta* is predominantly the "fiery" principle of biotransformation, disorders usually have a heat component, that is, fever or inflammatory properties. Examples of conditions caused by imbalance of *Pitta dosha* are heartburn, hyperacidity, skin rashes, infections, ulcers, and inflammation.[21]

Kapha Dosha

Earth *(prithivi)* and water *(jala)* are the basic elements that make up the *Kapha dosha*. All activities responsible for growth, stability, lubrication, and storage within the body are attributed to the *Kapha dosha* and hence it is the principle of cohesion, structure, and lubrication. *Kapha* physical structures and functions include the myelin sheath covering the axons of some neurons in the nervous system, connective tissues, muscular support, taste and smell perception, digestive tract protection, respiratory tract and joint lubrication, water and fat regulation, and tissue building and wound healing. Mental functions include memory, tranquility, faith, forgiveness, loyalty, and devotion, and emotions such as love, patience, sympathy, attachment, and greed. The physical properties of *Kapha* are being heavy, cold, wet, slow, oily, smooth, dense, and stable. *Kapha dosha* actually provides structural strength and protects the body against diseases. Although it pervades the whole body, *Kapha dosha* is primarily located in the upper chest region and in the digestive system, predominantly the stomach. The influence of *Kapha dosha* is maximal during the childhood of a person and during the winter season and early spring. Because *Kapha* is the "watery" or the structural and lubrication principle, disorders usually have a component of these qualities that is in excess. Examples of conditions caused by imbalanced *Kapha dosha* are swelling, obesity, diabetes, lethargy, and excess mucus production.[21]

Imbalance: Signs and Symptoms of Increased (Aggravated) Doshas

When a *dosha* is increased or aggravated causing imbalance, various physiological and psychological manifestations occur. Table 10–5 lists the various manifestations of imbalanced *doshas*. An individual may show one or more of these imbalances, depending on the severity of the imbalance.[25]

To summarize, *prakriti* is a system of determining an individual's unique mind–body constitutions so that one can understand their nature, immunity, susceptibility to illness, and prognosis of a particular disease, as well as tolerance for the different therapeutic procedures. The predominant *dosha* in a *prakriti* because of genetic inheritance dictates certain demands in terms of diet, behavioral pattern, and environment. Individuals can prevent disease if they adjust their diet and their daily and seasonal lifestyles according to their *prakriti*. As these adjustments are made according to the *prakriti*, it tunes the *doshas* to one's inherent balanced ratio, and optimizes the physiological activities.

Seven Basic Structural Elements: Saptadhatu

The seven *dhatus* form the whole structure of the body and these are the basic tissue elements described in Ayurveda. *Dhatu* supports the body by forming its infrastructure. It derives its nourishment by the ingested food by way of biotransformation in the body at various levels. Quite similar to the other body constituents, this is also made up of *Pancha Maha Bhuta*. Activities of the *dhatus* are tuned by *doshas* in the body. These seven *dhatus* are placed in a specific hierarchy starting from

the plasma *(rasa)* and ending at the level of the reproductive tissue *(shukra)* (see Table 10–6). Each of the seven tissues has a relationship with each other. When a disease presents at a certain level, it has passed through the previous levels to get there. Thus, when treating a disease or condition it must not just be localized to the level of the problem; rather, the overall treatment should consider addressing all of the tissues in the above levels in order to bring the individual back to an optimal healthy state.[26]

Metabolic Waste: Mala

The word *mala* refers to the waste or inferior by-products in the body. These include all the by-products produced during the digestion of food as well as produced during the biotransformation of the *dhatus*. For example, secretions of the body orifices, such as earwax, mucus in the nose, and lacrimal secretions, are all known as the inferior waste by-products from the metabolism of the *mamsa dhatu*. Another example is sweat, which is the waste from the metabolism of the *meda dhatu*. The build-up of toxins and waste products in the body is referred to as *ama* and can block the communicating channels (*srotas*; see "Communicating Channels: Srotas" below). When in normal amounts, these waste products help in the maintenance of health; if the wastes are either excessive or deficient, then they are likely to upset the equilibrium of the *doshas* and *dhatus*, and hence cause disease.[27]

Metabolic Transformation: Agni

The word *agni* refers to "biofire," or the digestive strength and power of the mind–body to metabolize input from emotions to actual food products. The concept is very important in Ayurveda as an individual's state of health is also determined by the level and presence of *agni*. There are four levels of *agni*, which go

▶ **TABLE 10–5** SIGNS AND SYMPTOMS OF IMBALANCE DOSHAS

Physical Manifestations	Psychological Manifestations
Imbalanced Vata Increase	
Loss of weight, emaciation	Overactivity of the mind
Loss of energy and stamina	Inability to relax
Severe and acute pain	Inability to concentrate
Muscle spasms	Anxiety
Back pain, especially lower back	Worry
Joint aches or arthritis	Restlessness
Chapped skin, lips	Impatience
Constipation	Depression
Flatulence, intestinal gas	Insomnia
Irritable bowel syndrome	Fatigue
Increased blood pressure	Loss of appetite
Intolerance to wind and cold	
Menstrual cramps	
Imbalanced Pitta Increase	
Sharply increased hunger or thirst	Hostile behavior
Increased acidity and heartburn	Irritability
Ulcers	Anger
Intolerance to heat	Rage
Hot flashes	Impatience
Skin inflammations	Criticism of oneself and others
Rashes	Arrogant argumentation
Acne	Aggressive and domineering behavior
Sour body odors	
Bad breath	
Rectal burning, hemorrhoids	
Sunburn, sunstroke	
Bloodshot eyes	
Dark yellow feces and urine	
Imbalanced Kapha Increase	
Congested chest, throat	Lethargy
Congested nose, sinuses	Dullness
Cough with mucus	Mental inertia
Sore throat and runny nose	Oversleeping
Frequent colds	Daytime drowsiness
Intolerance to cold and dampness	Depression
Allergies, asthma	Lack of motivation
Obesity and increased cholesterol	Procrastination
Edema and fluid retention	Overattachment
Bloating	Greed
Pale and cold skin	Possessiveness
Cysts and other growths	
Diabetes	

Source: Shanbhag.[25] Reproduced with permission.

▶ **TABLE 10–6** THE SEVEN TISSUES—
SAPTADHATU

1. Rasa (plasma)
2. Rakta (blood)
3. Mamsa (muscle)
4. Meda (adipose tissue)
5. Asthi (bone)
6. Majja (bone marrow)
7. Shukra (reproductive tissue)

Source: Vagabhatacharya.[8]

from the gross digestion of food to the molecular metabolism and transformation. For an individual to be healthy, their digestion and metabolism of all materials must be in balance; if they are not in balance, treatments are given to correct the imbalances.

Communicating Channels: Srotas

Srotas are the special intricate communication systems in the body used by the *doshas* and *dhatus* that includes both micro- and macrochannels. These channels are also where the nourishment of the body tissues and biotransformation takes place. For example, the passage of food in the body, the oxygen we breathe, and the formation and excretion of urine, feces, and sweat all occur through the *srotas* according to Ayurveda.[28] Circulation of blood and nutrients and the activities of other *dhatus* are also through the *srotas* and are named after the respective dhatu (i.e., *rasa vaha srotas, rakta vaha srotas*). Similarly there are *srotas* related to the *mala*. The free flow of the *dosha* and *dhatu* without any obstruction is required for the maintenance of a healthy state. If the circulation is obstructed or the substance circulating is impaired in the *srotas,* an abnormal accumulation occurs, thereby affecting tissue metabolism. If any of these *srotas* are blocked or function impaired, disease results.

Fundamental Qualities of the Mind: Sattva, Rajas, and Tamas

The three fundamental qualities of the mind, or *gunas,* are known as *Sattva, Rajas,* and *Tamas.* The *Sattva* qualities of the mind are clarity, alertness, love, and compassion. The *Rajas* quality of the mind maintains and renders it very active and agile. Contrary to this, the *Tamas* qualities of the mind are lethargic and dull. In Ayurveda, these three are popularly known as the three *gunas* of the mind akin to the *Vata, Pitta,* and *Kapha* of the body. The balanced state of these three *gunas* is physiological, and the imbalance is suggestive of a pathological state. The imbalance in these properties leads to psychological and physiological illness. It is also true that food possesses these qualities in variable amplitudes and is likely to influence the property of the mind. The type and quality of food one eats affects the mind as well as the body. For example, if foods possessing the *Sattva guna* properties are consumed, it adds to the *Sattva* property of the mind.[29] Examples of Sattvic foods are those which are sweet such as fruits.

▶ PANCHAKARMA THERAPIES

Kerala Panchakarma

A unique aspect of Ayurveda is its detoxification or biopurification treatments known as *Panchakarma,* which means the "five cleansing therapies." There are two traditional predominant schools of thought on *Panchakarma* technique. The Charak technique recommends the use of emesis, purgation, medicated enemas, both unctuous (oily) and nonunctuous (nonoily), and medicated nasal oils. The Sushruta technique suggests the same therapies but includes the use of bloodletting. The detailed procedures of *Panchakarma* indicated specifically in each and every disease are enumerated in the Ayurvedic texts. Currently in

India various kinds of *Panchakarma* are performed, but two types are the most popular: *Classical Panchakarma,* which includes both Charak and Sushruta approaches and mainly stronger internal treatments, and *Kerala Panchakarma,* which is mainly milder external treatments that are used more for rejuvenation, detoxification, and health-maintenance purposes. *Classical Panchakarma* refers to the original five internal treatments (as described above) and *Kerala Panchakarma* refers to more external treatments focusing on the preparatory treatments. Although within each category of treatment there are several procedures and applications, for the purpose of this chapter, a general summary of the most common is given below.

The goal of *Panchakarma* therapies is to eliminate toxins from the body, allowing healing and restoration of the tissues, channels, digestion, and mental functions.[30] The stronger treatments of expelling the imbalanced *doshas* in *Panchakarma* are known as *Shodana.* Prior to the beginning of *Panchakarma* therapies, preparatory therapies known as *Poorva Karma* must be completed. *Poorva Karma* includes 10 therapies, which are also known as palliation or *Shamana* (see Table 10–7).[31] Depend-

▶ **TABLE 10–7** POORVA KARMA: TEN PREPARATORY THERAPIES PRIOR TO PANCHAKARMA

1. Oleation (Snehan)
2. Sudation/fomentation (Swedana)
3. Herbal tonics
4. Oils and ghee
5. Exercise
6. Food
7. Aromatherapy
8. Colors, meals, and environment
9. Lifestyle
10. Meditation (Sadhana)

Source: Tirtha.[31] Modified with permission.

Note: Oleation and Sudation are the most common Panchakarma (Kerala style) procedures performed in the United States.

ing on the chronicity of the condition, these preparatory procedures last from 1 week to up to 3 months. Healthy persons undergoing *Panchakarma* for prevention or maintenance may skip the palliation therapies, but optimal outcomes using the *Poorva Karma* therapies are always preferred. Of these 10 therapies, oil massage or oleation *(snehana)* and sweat therapy or sudation/fomentation *(swedana)* are the most commonly performed main treatments used in *Kerala Panchakarma.*[32] Of the *Panchakarma* therapies, these preparatory procedures of oleation, sudation, and *Kerala*-style *Panchakarma* are performed most commonly in the United States, rather than the *Classical* style, because of medicolegal issues (see "Emesis Therapy [Vamana]" and "Bloodletting [Raktamokshana]" below) and lack of authentic *Panchakarma* training, as well as cultural acceptance (see "Enema Therapy [Basti]" below).

Oleation (Snehan)

Snehan uses herbal medicated oils externally and internally to help loosen and liquefy the toxins in the body. *Snehan* helps to dislodge the toxins from the smallest channels, allowing them to be excreted through the skin or gastrointestinal tract. Examples of herbs used in the medicated oils are plants such as Eranda *(Ricinus communis),* Tila (sesame), and Sarshapa *(Brassica nigra),* and animal products such as ghee (clarified butter). Although there are very different types of oil for each condition and *prakriti* of an individual, sesame oil is most commonly used. Sesame oil is known to have antibacterial, antifungal, and anti-inflammatory, as well as antioxidant, properties. *Snehan* can be used internally, and there are specific protocols for each condition reflecting the size of the dose and duration of the administration of oils. Externally, *snehan* can be used to treat specific areas of the body such as the head as seen with the popular treatment called *shirodhara. Shirodhara* consists of the continuous pouring of medicated oils of varying temperatures over the forehead in the supine position. Further treatments to the head include wrapping a cloth soaked in medicated oil over the head *(picu)* to wearing a tall hat-like apparatus filled with oil *(shiro basti)*. These applications of oils to the head region are useful for the treatment of neurological conditions,[33] headaches,[34] and sleep disorders such as insomnia.[35,36] It is also useful in stress reduction, relaxation, and decreasing anxiety.[37] Oils can also be added to treat conditions of the ears *(karna purana)* and eyes *(netra basti)*.

Snehan is most commonly used externally. It is applied with a special massage called *Abhyanga*. This distinct type of oil massage is well known and has a multitude of beneficial effects on the body. Traditionally four massage practitioners attend to one individual. Two practitioners massage from the shoulders to the navel and the other two from the navel to the feet. The massage is performed with synchronistic movements with not only specific motion of direction but also pressure and depth. This type of massage improves blood circulation, facilitates removal of toxins from tissues and relieves physical and mental fatigue. It also strengthens the musculoskeletal system and improves the elasticity of the skin.[38] clears stiffness and heaviness in the body, and leads to feelings of lightness and well-being. It assists development of a healthy body, helps in the improvement of body figure, recuperates body tissues and reduces body weight as well as fat. *Abhyanga* has a curative effect on a plethora of diseases by the pharmacologic actions of the herbal drugs used in the processing of the oil. Finally, the use of *marma* points (similar points from which Chinese acupuncture was derived but less in number and without the use of needles) or "energy points" are used in the therapies to help create balance between the body, mind, and spirit. *Snehan* has been extensively used in treating various *Vata* imbalances and diseases, which include arthritis, nervous exhaustion, constipation, mental illness, and wasting disorders such as anorexia and weight loss.[39]

Sudation/Fomentation (Swedan)

The word "sweda" in Sanskrit means "sweat," which is described as one of the metabolic wastes that needs to be expelled from the body. After oleation, Ayurveda recommends *swedan,* which are therapeutic sweating or steam therapies. Dozens of different types of *swedan* therapies are used. Most commonly, the procedure includes the use of a sweatbox *(ushma)*. Here the individual is either sitting or lying down with their head exposed outside the box (made of wood or fiberglass) while the steam from a boiling medicinal decoction is pumped inside the box. Another common *swedan* treatment is the placing of heated cloths on the body *(Tapa)* similar to what is commonly known as a "body wrap" or "herbal wrap." Finally one of the most important types of *swedan* (*Kerala Panchakarma* style) is called *Pinda Sweda*. In this procedure, hot medicated cooked special rice boluses bound in cloth pouches are applied on the body rhythmically and massaged to induce sudation. Numerous herbs have been mentioned in Ayurvedic texts for the different *swedan* procedures. Examples of the herbal medicines used in *swedana* procedures are plants like Nirgundi *(Vitex nigundo)*, Arka *(Calotropis procera)*, Punarnava *(Boerrhavia diffusa)*, Vasa *(Adhatoda vasica)*, Eranda *(Ricinus communis)*, and Karanja *(Pongamia glabra)*. This therapy can be administered to the whole body or to a specific site on the body and is said to enhance the digestive fire, ensure proper and unobstructed circulation, improve functioning of joints, and aid in expulsion of the morbid *doshas*. It is beneficial in *Vata* and *Kapha* disorders. It is usually done with caution in *Pitta* disorders.[40]

Classical Panchakarma

Emesis Therapy (Vamana)

Of the five classical *Panchakarma* therapies, only therapeutic emesis, or *Vamana,* needs to be performed by a qualified *Panchakarma* specialist. It is a highly systematized procedure for treatment of *Kapha* and *Pitta* disorders through the oral route by way of induction of emesis. Specific protocols are given on the administration and medications that are used. Examples of *Vamana* herbal medicines include Madanapala *(Randia dumetorum)*, Kutaja *(Wrightia tinctoria)*, Vacha *(Acorus calamus)*, Yashtimadhu *(Glycyrrhiza glabra)*, milk, sugar cane juice, and salts. To complete the full procedure, the individual is afterward subjected to a specific dietary regimen.[41]

Purgation Therapy (Virecana)

Virecana therapy is the administration of herbal medicines to lubricate the intestines and colon. This induces purgation with its mild laxative effects. It is used primarily for *Pitta* disorders, such as psoriasis.[42] Examples of herbal drugs that are used for *Virecana* are Trivrit *(Operculina turpethum)*, Aragwadha *(Cassia fistula)*, Snuhi *(Euphorbia nerifolia)*, Jayapala *(Croton tiglium)*, and Eranda *(Ricinus communis)*.[43]

Enema Therapy (Basti)

Amongst all the *Panchakarma* therapies, *Basti* occupies the foremost position because it is the treatment of choice for *Vata* disorders, which is defined in Ayurveda as responsible for 80% of all diseases. The colon is viewed as being related to all the other organs and tissues, and thus digestion and elimination are of utmost importance. Consequently, from routine cleansing and toning of the colon, the entire body can be healed and rejuvenated.[44] It can be used to treat conditions such as hemiparesis,[45,46] obesity,[47] hypertension,[48] and osteoarthritis.[49] *Basti* is also more practical and easier than the other therapies, as it neither requires elaborate preparatory procedures, as do *Snehana* and *Swedana,* nor the strict observance of post-*Panchakarma* dietary regimens. There are many types of *Basti,* ranging from those containing herbal medicinal decoctions in unctuous materials (oils) to those that are nonmedicated and non–oil-based. Examples of the drugs used for the various *Basti* preparation include plants such as Madanapala *(Randia dumetorum)*, Kutaja *(Wrightia tincto-*

ria), Punarnava *(Boerrhavia diffusa)*, Eranda *(Ricinus communis)*, and Trivrit *(Operculina turpethum)*.[50]

Nasal Therapy (Nasya)

Nasya is a nasal therapy, such as nasal drops and lavage, that cleanses the upper respiratory system. It can also be used to treat conditions from anxiety[51] to the pain of cervical spondylosis.[52] Various *Nasya* administrations exist and range from the use of medicated oils or extracted juices made from herbs (nasal drops), to inhalation of herbal powders (snuffing) and the inhalation of smoke from medicinal herbs *(dhuma)*. The "Neti Pot," which is presently popular in lavaging the nasal cavities to prevent sinus problems, was used in Ayurveda hundreds of years ago to deliver medicated nasal solutions. Examples of herbal medicines used in *Nasya* include Apamarga *(Achyranthes aspera)*, Pippali *(Piper longum)*, Vacha *(Acorus calamus)*, Shigru *(Moringa olifera)*, Haridra *(Curcuma longa)*, Tulasi *(Ocimum sanctum)*, and Aguru *(Aquallaria agallocha)*.[53]

Bloodletting (Raktamokshana)

This *Panchakarma* procedure was introduced by the Susruta school of thought. Therapeutic bloodletting or *Raktamokshana* (removal of 2–8 ounces) by leech or venipuncture is still used in India for certain conditions. Bloodletting is described as being ideal for certain *Pitta* disorders (blood disorders) and skin disorders, as well as for other conditions such as abscesses *(vidradhi)*.

In summary, *Panchakarma* are natural therapies used for preventative health, as well as treatment for chronic conditions. According to Ayurveda, the body has natural mechanisms for elimination of waste metabolites. If these metabolites are retained for any reason (including seasonal variation), it is likely to harm the body. This elimination may be further assisted by the administration of these biopurification procedures, thus maintaining a waste-free body. As part of a health-maintenance program an individual should undergo these therapies at regular intervals, depending upon the seasonal variations. *Panchakarma* is said to improve the digestive power, clear the sense organs, and promote intelligence. It also improves the complexion, while nourishing and strengthening the body's natural immunity to disease.[54] Currently in the United States, certain aspects of *Panchakarma* are offered in health centers, clinics, and spas.

▶ COMMON CONDITIONS: DEFINITIONS AND TREATMENTS ACCORDING TO AYURVEDA

Obesity (Sthoulya Roga)

Obesity or *Sthoulya Roga* is characterized by abnormal and excessive accumulation of fat in the body. It is important in Ayurvedic medicine because it leads to more serious and fatal disorders like cardiovascular disease, cerebrovascular disease, diabetes, and hypertension.[55]

Etiology

Obesity can be familial. Factors such as ingestion of foods that increase *Kapha dosha* (i.e., excessive sweets and oily foods) and lack of mental and physical exercise all cause imbalance with excessive accumulation in relation to utilization.[56]

Pathology

Obesity is related to the impaired biotransformation at the level of the *meda dhatu* and nourishment of the other *dhatus* in the *dhatu* hierarchy (see Table 10–6). This impairment is a result of the blockage and vitiation of the *Kapha dosha* causing excessive accumulation of fat in the body.

Clinical Features

Individuals suffering from the *Sthoulya Roga* have the following features: heavy with plumpness of the face, large protuberant abdomen, pendulous breasts, large buttocks, and broad thighs. Contrary to their body mass, the person shows hypokinetic physical activity with dyspnea on physical exertion. Extremities are said to be lax, and the person has little strength or stamina. Excessive hunger and thirst are common symptoms. Laziness and somnolence, as well as malodorous sweat and impairment of the libido, also are present. The Ayurvedic literature stresses that *Sthoulya Roga* reduces one's life span.

Treatment

The stimulation of the morbid *Vata dosha*, elimination of the vitiated *Kapha dosha*, and reduction of the accumulation of the *meda dhatu* forms the crux of the treatment of *Sthoulya Roga*. This may be achieved by reduction in food intake *(langhana)*, physical exercise *(vyayama)*, massage with dry herbal powders *(udvartana)*, and colonic lavage with herbal decoctions *(tiksna basti)*.[47] Herbal oral medications are usually administered for several months, until the desired results are obtained.[57,58] Examples of such herbs are Silajatu, Takrarista, Triphalakwath, Triusanadya loha, Navaka guggulu, Trimurthi rasa, and Vadavagni rasa. Triphalakwath, or popularly known as "Triphala," is one of the most prescribed Ayurvedic medicines. It aids in proper digestion and elimination, thereby cleansing and detoxifying the colon, which is best for Kapha disorders[58] and general health.[55]

Obesity is often difficult to treat with conventional medicines and surgical treatments, which carry high risks of side effects and complications. Once metabolic and physiological causes are ruled out using conventional diagnostics, Western physicians can refer to an Ayurvedic educator/specialist to aid in the management and teaching of lifestyle and behavioral changes that are needed. Although treatment of obesity using the Ayurvedic approach does not provide immediate results, the results occur gradually and the probability of maintaining the weight loss is increased.

Hypertension (Shonitha Dushti)

Hypertension or *Shonitha dushti* is described in Ayurveda as the abnormality of blood circulation.[59]

Etiology

Factors that cause this condition are excessive intake of oily and heavy foods, which include the intake of meat and dairy products, as well as alcoholic beverages. Various emotional and behavioral habits, such as anxiety, mental tension, anger, and daytime somnolence, also contribute to hypertension. It is also said to be aggravated more in the winter season.

Pathology

Abnormal accumulation of *Kapha dosha* and *meda dhatu* (adipose tissue) causes narrowing of the blood vessels called *margavarana*, which is akin to the modern condition of atherosclerosis. Narrowing due to *margavarana*, as well as reduced elasticity, of the blood vessels increases peripheral vascular resistance. Furthermore, the development of morbidity of the *rakta dhatu* (blood tissues) causes a set of clinical symptoms characterized by the alteration in the psychological and behavioral patterns of those with hypertension.[60]

Clinical Features

Headache, anger, overactivity, tremor, drowsiness, sleep, and fainting are some of the clinical manifestations that a person with hypertension presents in general. In Ayurveda, specific symptoms have been described and vary depending on the individual's predominant *dosha*.[61]

Treatment

Treatment is aimed at rectifying the abnormality of *Kapha dosha*, *Pitta dosha*, *rakta dhatu*, and *meda dhatu*. First dietary control, as well as physical exercise, meditation, and yoga (specific practices such *surya namaskar*, or "sun salutation;" see "Yoga" above) are prescribed. Various types of *Snehan* procedures such as *abhyanga* and *shirodhara*[62,63] (specific applications of oil to the body and head, usually with medicinal herbs; see "Panchakarma Therapies" above) are recommended for *Shonitha Dushti*.[64] These are helpful in reducing blood pressure by combating the anxiety and mental tension associated with hypertension and also by promoting restful sleep. Various types of mild laxatives *(Virecana)*[65] and colon-cleansing enemas *(Basti)* are also given to help those with hypertension[17] and atherosclerosis *(margavarana)*. Oral herbal medications are also given. Rauwolfia serpentine (also known as reserpine in modern medicine), or Sarpagandha, was one of the first antihypertensive medicines used. Other herbs used include bramhi, Vacha *(Acorus calamus)* and Jatamamsi *(Nardostachys jatamansi)*. Silajatu prayoga and combinations like Prabhakara vati, Chandraprabha vati, as well as Triushanadi loha, are also very effective.[66]

The referral of hypertensive patients to an Ayurvedic educator/specialist can be helpful to the Western physician because patients can be taught physical exercise, meditation, and yoga, all of which have been demonstrated in many clinical studies to reduce blood pressure. Along with these techniques, and along with following a healthy lifestyle, the use of herbal medicines in mild to moderate hypertension may be useful as a first-line treatment to control blood pressure. If a patient is given a trial of such education and use of herbal medicines, pharmaceutical drugs maybe avoided. If the patient is not responsive to the herbal medicines, then conventional medicine can be started but it is important to continue with the lifestyle and behavioral recommendations.

Heart Disease (Hridroga and Hritshula)

General heart-related disorders *(hridroga)*, such as congenital heart disease, valvular heart disease, infective heart disease, hypertensive cardiovascular disease, and cardiomyopathy, are all described in Ayurveda. More specifically, ischemic heart disease, known as *hritshula*, has been emphasized.[67]

Etiology
Excessive intake of meat and dairy products that are heavy for digestion are considered to be factors that cause heart disease. Other factors include lack of physical exercise, mental tension, and suppression of naturally manifesting urges.

Pathology
The above-stated etiological factors cause imbalance of the *doshas*, which, in turn, weakens the plasma *(rasa dhatu)* and is localized to the heart tissue. The prime pathology of *hritshula* may be defined as the obstruction of the blood vessels as a consequence of excessive accumulation of *meda dhatu* and *Kapha dosha* manifesting as *margavarana* (atherosclerosis).

Clinical Features
Chest pain is the cardinal symptom of *hridroga* and *hritshula*. In general, exertional dyspnea, orthopnea, cyanosis, anemia, edema, cough, syncope, and altered states of consciousness are all clinical symptoms that may present. According to the *dosha* of the individual, specific types of chest pain symptoms have been described which present and localize differently.

Treatment
Dietary and behavioral habits (lifestyle changes) of the patient should be planned according to one's *prakriti* to reduce *Kapha dosha* and *meda dhatu*. For additional benefits, the practice of yoga is recommended. The principal line of treatments includes both *Shodhana* and *Shamana*. In the *Shodhana* treatments, medicated enema *(Basti)* is the safest and most commonly used procedure; it has been shown to be effective in treating heart disease[68]. For example, *Manjistadi ksara basti* is indicated in *hritshula* and is effective in clearing the *margavarana*. Also, herbal medicines have been used in conjunction with these therapies to decrease the number of angina attacks.[69]

Examples of *Shamana* treatments include *abhyanga* and *shirodhara* (with the use of herbal medicated oils). These are used to relieve exhaustion, mental tension, and stress, and they also aid in lowering possible accompanying hypertension.[70] Finally, herbal medicines are also used; the most commonly used herb being Arjuna *(Terminalia arjuna)*. Other combinations that are proven effective include Prabhakara vati, Hridayarnava rasa, Silajatwadi loha, Triusanadi loha, Mrigasringa bhasma, and Dasamula khada.

Along with the diet and exercise recommendations, the referral to an Ayurvedic educator/specialist and the use of the various treatments described above maybe a helpful adjunct or alternative to those who can not tolerate conventional lipid-lowering medications such as statin drugs.

► CONCLUSION

Ayurveda brings a holistic approach to health by addressing the body, mind, and soul of an individual. By incorporating allied sciences such as astrology *(jyotish)*, exercise (yoga), stress reduction/spirituality (meditation), architecture *(vatsu)*, herbology, and energy medicine, Ayurveda has proven to be a unique and vital science.

An individualized approach to health is the hallmark of Ayurvedic medical practice. Identification of *dosha* or the mind–body constitution and formulation of therapy based on the above principle can provide treatment options that address the individuality of each patient and each situation. Integration of the principles of preventive medicine, self-healing, and judicious use of proper diet, exercise, and herbal medicines are the basic principles in the practice of Ayurveda.

REFERENCES

1. Bhagavan das. The unique features of ayurveda. In: *Handbook of Ayurveda*. New Delhi: Concept Publishing; 1983:8.

2. Bhagavan das. *The Unique Features of Ayurveda. Handbook of Ayurveda*. New Delhi: Concept Publishing; 1983:5.

3. Sharadini D, Urmila T. The rulers dosas. In: *Ayurveda Unraveled*. New Delhi: National Book Trust; 1998:46.

4. Dhyani S. *Ayurvedic Concept of Health. Salient Features of Ayurveda*. New Delhi: Chaukhamha Orientalia; 1987:5.

5. Tirtha S. Overview of Ayurveda. In: *The Ayurveda Encyclopedia: Natural Secrets to Healing, Prevention, and Longevity*. New York: Ayurveda Holistic Center Press; 1998:3.

6. Shanbhag V. *An Historical Overview of Ayurveda. A Beginner's Introduction to Ayurvedic Medicine: The Science of Natural Healing and Prevention Through Individualized Therapies. A Keats Good Health Guide*. New Canaan, CT: Keats Publishing; 1994:8.

7. Tirtha S. Overview of Ayurveda. In: *The Ayurveda Encyclopedia: Natural Secrets to Healing, Prevention, and Longevity*. New York: Ayurveda Holistic Center Press; 1998:6.

8. Vagabhalacharya. *Astanga hridayam*. Chaukhambha prakasan. Varansi, India: 1997:5.

9. Tirtha S. Overview of Ayurveda. In: *The Ayurveda Encyclopedia: Natural Secrets to Healing, Prevention, and Longevity*. New York: Ayurveda Holistic Center Press; 1998:8.

10. Shanbhag V. *An Historical Overview of Ayurveda. A Beginner's Introduction to Ayurvedic Medicine: The Science of Natural Healing and Prevention Through Individualized Therapies. A Keats Good Health Guide*. New Canaan, CT: Keats Publishing; 1994:10.

11. Dhyani S. *Ayurvedic Concept of Health. Salient Features of Ayurveda*. Delhi, India: Chaukhamha Orientalia; 1987:4.

12. Chopra D, Simon D. *The Chopra Center Herbal Handbook: Forty Natural Prescriptions for Perfect Health*. New York: Three Rivers Press; 2000:209.

13. Iype G. India abroad. October 19, 2002:B1, B3.

14. Shanbhag V. *An Historical Overview of Ayurveda. A Beginner's Introduction to Ayurvedic Medicine: The Science of Natural Healing and Prevention Through Individualized Therapies. A Keats Good Health Guide*. New Canaan, CT: Keats Publishing; 1994:29.

15. Kutumbaih P. The doctrine of Tridosa. In: *Ancient Indian Medicine* (revised ed.). Calcutta: Orient Longman:1974:113.

16. Simon D. *The Wisdom of Healing: A Natural Mind Body Program for Wellness*. New York: Three Rivers Press; 1997:133.

17. Kohatsu W, Greenfield R. Yoga. In: *Complementary and Alternative Medicine Secrets*. Philadelphia: Hanley & Belfus; 2002:54.

18. Frawley D. *Yoga and Ayurveda*. Twin Lakes, WI: Lotus Press; 1999:3.

19. Dwarakanath C. Outlines of Samkhya Patanjala system. In: *The Fundamental Principles of Ayurveda*. Varanasi, India: Krishnadas Academy; 1998:77.

20. Bhagavan das. Basic principles. In: *Handbook of Ayurveda*. New Delhi: India: Concept Publishing; 1983:17.

21. Frawley D. Six stages of disease. In: *Ayurvedic Healing: A Complete Guide*. Twin Lakes, WI: Lotus Press; 2000:50.

22. Sharadini D, Urmila T. The rulers dosas. In: *Ayurveda Unraveled*. New Delhi: National Book Trust; 1998:46.

23. Bhagavan das. Basic principles. In: *Handbook of Ayurveda*. New Delhi: Concept Publishing; 1983:17.

24. Kutumbaih P. The doctrine of Tridosa. In: *Ancient Indian Medicine* (revised ed.). Calcutta: Orient Longman; 1974:62.

25. Shanbhag V. *An Historical Overview of Ayurveda. A Beginner's Introduction to Ayurvedic Medicine: The Science of Natural Healing and Prevention Through Individualized Therapies. A Keats Good Health Guide*. New Canaan, CT: Keats Publishing; 1994: 23.

26. Kutumbaih P. The doctrine of Tridosa. In: *Ancient Indian Medicine* (revised ed.). Calcutta: Orient Longman; 1974:42

27. Bhagavan das. Basic principles. In: *Handbook of Ayurveda*. New Delhi: Concept Publishing; 1983:27.

28. Bhagavan das. Basic principles. In: *Handbook of Ayurveda*. New Delhi: Concept Publishing; 1983:36.

29. Dwarakanath C. Outlines of Samkhya Patanjala system. In: *The Fundamental Principles of Ayurveda*. Varanasi, India: Krishnadas Academy; 1998:77.

30. Tirtha S. Overview of Ayurveda. In: *The Ayurveda Encyclopedia: Natural Secrets to Healing, Pre-*

vention, and Longevity. New York: Ayurveda Holistic Center Press; 1998:169.

31. Tirtha S. Overview of Ayurveda. *The Advanced Encyclopedia: Natural Secrets to Healing, Prevention, and Longevity.* New York: Ayurveda Holistic Center Press; 1998:169.

32. Devaraj TL. *The Panchakarma Treatment of Ayurveda.* Bangalore, India: Dhanvantary Oriental Publications; 1980:1.

33. Muthukrishna M. *A Clinical Study of Shirobasti on Shirogatavata Roga.* Jamnagar, India: Institute for Post-graduate Teaching and Research in Ayurveda, Gujarat Ayurved University; 1973.

34. Sharma PK. *Clinical Evaluation of Shirodhara Chikitsa on Idiopathic Shirashula (Chronic Headache).* India: Faculty of Ayurveda: Institute of Medical Sciences, Banaras, India: Banaras Hindu University; 1989.

35. Trivedi K. *A Comparative Study of Shirodhara and Shirobasti in the Management of Anidra (Insomnia).* Jamnagar, India: Institute for Postgraduate Teaching and Research in Ayurveda, Gujarat Ayurved University; 1995:125–131.

36. Prakash NB, Chandola HM, Singh G, Ravishanker. Management of Aswapana (sleep disorders) with certain indigenous drugs and Ashwagandha taila dhara. Jammagar, India: *AYU.* 2001;12:17–23.

37. Sanjay C, Singh G. A clinical study on the role of Jaladhara and Sankhapushi (convolvulus chols) in the management of cittodvega (anxiety disorders). Jammagar, India: *AYU.* 2001;11:23–27.

38. Hejamadi S. *Study on Ayurvedic Management of Ageing (Jara).* Jamnagar, India: Institute for Postgraduate Teaching and Research in Ayurveda, Gujarat Ayurved University; 1990.

39. Shashidhar K. Sirobasti: panchakarma. *Ayurwave.* 1999;1(1):7–9.

40. Vayaskara NS. Pinda Sweda. In: *Ayurvedic Treatments of Kerala.* Kottayam, Kerala, India: OmVaidyasarathi Press; 1983.

41. Devaraj TL. *The Panchakarma Treatment of Ayurveda.* Bangalore, India: Dhanvantary Oriental Publications; 1980:21.

42. Joorawan PR, Shukla VD, Bhaghel MS. A clinical study of Ekakusta (psoriasis) and its management with Shodhana and Samana yoga. Jammagar, India: *AYU.* 2000;12:13–18.

43. Devaraj TL. *The Panchakarma Treatment of Ayurveda.* Bangalore, India: Dhanvantary Oriental Publications; 1980:78.

44. Tirtha S. Overview of Ayurveda. In: *The Ayurveda Encyclopedia: Natural Secrets to Healing, Prevention, and Longevity.* New York: Ayurveda Holistic Center Press; 1998:192.

45. Inamura SH. *A Clinical and Experimental Study on the Systemic Effect of Basti Therapy with Special Reference to Vata Vyadhi.* Jamnagar, India: Institute for Post-graduate Teaching and Research in Ayurveda, Gujarat Ayurved University; 1994.

46. Goyal R, Singh G. A clinical study on the role of Karma Basti (Masadi Kvatha and Masadi Taila) in the management of Pakshaghata (hemiplegia). Jammagar, India: *AYU.* 2001;9:5–9.

47. Bhatt SK. *Assessment of Efficacy of Lekhan Basti and Navaka Guggulu Yoga in Cases of Sthouyla (Obesity).* Jamnagar, India: Department of Kayachitisa, Shree Akhandanand Sarakari Ayurvedic College, Gujarat Ayurved University; 1991.

48. Vasasitha AG. *A Clinical Study of the Role of Basti Chikitsa in the Management of Essential Hypertension.* Jamnagar, India: Department of Kayachitisa, Shree Akhandanand Sarakari Ayurvedic College, Gujarat Ayurved University; 1994.

49. Jhinde K, Vyas S, Singh G. A clinical study on the role of Panchatikta Ghrita Matra Basti and Panchatikta Ksirapaka with Shudhha Ghrita in the management of Sandhigata Vata. Jammagar, India: *AYU.* 2001;1:19–22.

50. Haridas S. Basti Vijnana. In: *Ayurvediya Panchakarma Vijnana.* Nagpur, India: Vaidyanath Ayurveda Bhavan, 1979:389.

51. Sharma S, Chandola HM, Singh G, Acharya S. Role of Bramhi compound and Chaitas Ghrita Nasya in the management of anxiety disorders. Jammagar, India: *AYU.* 2001;3:23–26.

52. Shaligram DS, Baghel MS, Acharya SH. A study of Asthigatavata with special reference to cervical spondylosis and role of Snehana and Nasya Karma in its management. Jammagar, India: *AYU.* 1999;8:1–7.

53. Devaraj TL. *The Panchakarma Treatment of Ayurveda.* Bangalore, India: Dhanvantary Oriental Publications; 1980:227.

54. Haridas S. Basti Vijnana. In: *Ayurvediya Panchakarma Vijnana.* Nagpur, India: Vaidyanath Ayurveda Bhavan, 1979:560.

55. Krishna Kumar CD. Management of hyperlipidemia. *KAPL News.* 2000;111:5–13.

56. Sharma R. Fight fat to stay fit. *Ayurveda Vikas.* March/April 2001:26–28.

57. Varshneya S. *A Clinical Evaluation of Trigunadi Guggulu in Patients of Medoroga (Obesity)*. Thiruvanathapuram. Kottayam, Kerala, India: Government Ayurvedic College, Kerala University; 1983.

58. Raval DM. *To Assess the Efficacy of Triphala bhavita Shilajit in Obesity (Sthoulya)*. Jamnagar, India: Department of Kayachitisa, Shree Akhandanand Sarakari Ayurvedic College, Gujarat Ayurved University; 1994.

59. Kishore Kumar R, Acharya S. Charakas views of hypertension. 4th National Conference of Association of Anaesthetists of Indian Medicine. SDM College of Ayurveda, Udupi, India. November 24–26, 2000.

60. Pai S, Acharya S. Consciousness in Ayurveda. 4th National Conference of Association of Anaesthetists of Indian Medicine. SDM College of Ayurveda, Udupi, India. November 24–26, 2000.

61. Tubaki Basavaraj R, Acharya S. Case study of altered state of consciousness. 4th National Conference of Association of Anaesthetists of Indian Medicine. SDM College of Ayurveda, Udupi, India. November 24–26, 2000.

62. Dave AR. *A Comparative Study on the Role of Rasayana Drugs and Jaladhara in the Management of Uccha Raktachapa (Hypertension)*. Jamnagar, India: Institute for Post-graduate Teaching and Research in Ayurveda, Gujarat Ayurveda University; 1988.

63. Pathania SK, Vyas S. Role of Takradhara and Sarpagandha Vati in the management of Uccha Raktachapa (essential hypertension). Jammagar, India: *AYU*. 2001;8:11–21.

64. Gupta HC. *A New Care in Treatment of Hypertension*. Varanasi, India: Faculty of Ayurveda, Institute of Medical Sciences, Banaras Hindu University; 1990.

65. Jani J, Dhukls VF, Santawani MA. A Study on the aetiopathogenesis of essential hypertension and its management with certain Ayurvedic drugs. Jammagar, India: *AYU*. 2001;5:17–20.

66. Rai Anil Kumar, Acharya S. Treatment of Sonitaja mada. 4th National Conference of Association of Anaesthetists of Indian Medicine. SDM College of Ayurveda, Udupi, India. November 24–26, 2000.

67. Acharya S. Radical approach to the treatment of Ardita. *Ayurveda Chandrika*. 2001;17(9):39–45.

68. Krishna Kumar CD. Management of hyperlipidemia. *KAPL News*. 2000;111:5–13.

69. Chaudhari K. *A Clinical Study in the Management of Hridroga with Special Reference to Ischemic Heart Disease*. Institute for Post-Graduate Teaching and Research in Ayurveda. Jammagar, India: Gujarat University; 1989.

70. Yadayya DP. Snehana Karma. In: *Textbook on Clinical Panchakarma*. Akola, India: Jayaprakasan, 2000:10.

CHAPTER 11

Movement and Body-Centered Therapies

DAVID RILEY, DAGMAR EHLING, AND KENNETH SANCIER

Movement therapies in alternative medicine are a culturally diverse group of therapies that, like their conventional medical counterparts, involve active participation of the patient and a physical interaction between the provider and patient. Some such as yoga or Qigong, involve seemingly complicated series of movements, and others involve movement as subtle as breathing. In a wide variety of medical conditions—from low back pain to high blood pressure to cancer—movement therapies are often used both preventively and therapeutically. Patient moving and participating in a therapy being delivered is not only therapeutic in and of itself, but can also be a powerful stimulus of the self-healing response. Movement therapies are represented in virtually all cultural traditions and medical systems from India to China to the West. This chapter discusses several movement therapies: Hatha yoga, Qigong, Tai Chi, massage, and Feldenkrais.

▶ HATHA YOGA

History and Theory

This discussion of the potential medical application of yoga concentrates on the use of postures known as *asana*, breathing exercises known as *pranayama*, and meditation. Hatha yoga is part of the nonsectarian philosophical system of yoga that emerged from the Indian culture approximately 4,000 years ago and was designed to foster the attainment of self-awareness. Even though there are references to the postures of Hatha yoga dating back to the sixth century B.C. in the Upanishads, its major principles were first systematically reviewed in the classic text, *Yoga Sutras*, by Patanjali in 200 B.C. Originally, the postures of Hatha yoga, which have become so popular in the West, were designed to purify the body in preparation for higher states of consciousness and meditation. Several systematic

The Qigong material is adapted with permission from *Alternative Therapies in Health and Medicine.* 1996;2(1):40–45.

texts on Hatha yoga appeared between the sixth and fifteenth centuries A.D. including *Hatha Yoga Pradipika* by Swatmarama, *Goraksha Samhita* by Yogi Gorakhnath, *Gherand Samhita* by Gherand, and *Hatharatnavali* by Srinivasabhatta Mahayogindra. The practice of Hatha yoga in these texts often includes a series of steps beginning with *yama* or moral commandments, *niyama* or purification (such as fasting), asanas or postures, pranayama (breathing exercises), and then various stages of meditation leading to *samadhi,* a state where one merges with the object of meditation.

This chapter focuses on the aspects of Hatha yoga that involve the postures that are familiar to Westerners; these postures are intimately linked with breathing exercises (pranayama) and meditation. There are many styles of Hatha yoga available today; three of the primary schools are Iyengar yoga associated with BKS Iyengar, Viniyoga associated with TKV Desikachar, and Ashtanga yoga associated with Pattabhi Jois. All of these styles of Hatha yoga lead back to the Hatha yoga master Sri T. Krishnamacharya, and each of these schools pays great attention to the postures, breathing, meditation, and therapeutic possibilities of Hatha yoga. The Iyengar system of Hatha yoga is known for its emphasis on technical alignment; Viniyoga is known for its attention to the individualized nature of the yoga practice; and Ashtanga yoga is known for its vigorous flow in a standardized series of posture. There are, of course, many other styles of yoga, ranging from Kundalini yoga,[1] to Bikram yoga—a currently popular style in which the temperature of the room is kept quite high (often over 100°F)—to Kripalu and Integral yoga. For therapeutic purposes, particularly because most yoga practitioners do not have medical qualifications, Iyengar yoga and Viniyoga are probably most appropriate for those with specific medical conditions.

The postures of Hatha yoga involve standing, balancing, forward bending, back bending, and twisting; all strengthen the body and increase flexibility. The controlled breathing of pranayama helps the mind focus and is an important component of relaxation, a modulator of autonomic nervous system function. Dhyana, the meditative aspect of yoga, calms and focuses the mind. These three foundations of Hatha yoga (postures, breathing, and meditation) are interconnected and complement one another. Western physiological explanations of how Hatha yoga might be effective in the treatment of illness focus on two mechanisms. First is the modulation of autonomic nervous system tone, which commonly means a reduction in sympathetic tone. Second, the simultaneous activation of antagonistic neuromuscular systems, such as flexion and extension and intrafusal and Golgi tendon–organ feedback, may provide a way to maintain range of motion. Thus an increase in the relaxation response in the neuromuscular system is achieved.

Clinical Evidence

In a review of the research literature on the use of Hatha yoga as a medical intervention, it is often difficult to determine the type of yoga intervention and instruction given, particularly when the study was published in a non-Western scientific journal. Nevertheless, there are quite a few clinical trials of varying quality on the use of Hatha yoga (postures, breathing, and meditation) as a medical intervention. There is at least some positive clinical evidence in the medical literature for the effectiveness of Hatha yoga for a wide variety of conditions, including asthma, cardiovascular disease, diabetes, headaches, hypertension, mental disorders, osteoarthritis, pain, rheumatoid arthritis, seizures, and stress. Some evidence is convincing; however, the majority of it is preliminary and inconclusive. Two therapeutic strategies seem to emerge from the clinical data: Hatha yoga is useful for the treatment of musculoskeletal pain and for lowering sympathetic tone of the autonomic nervous system. The latter strategy may explain the reported benefits of yoga in asthma, idiopathic hypertension, and headaches.

A Hatha yoga intervention was shown to be useful for carpal tunnel syndrome in a randomized trial by Garfinkel et al. in 1998.[2] In this clinical trial, subjects with carpal tunnel syndrome in the treatment group were given 11 yoga postures to increase strength and flexibility of the upper body and, in particular, the arms. The control group was given a splint to augment their current treatment regimen. The yoga treatment group had significant improvement in grip strength, pain reduction, and range of motion. In another randomized controlled study on osteoarthritis, Garfinkel et al. also showed that 8 weeks of yoga instruction once a week provided relief in osteoarthritis of the hand. The treatment group improved significantly more than the control group with regard to pain, tenderness, and range of motion.

Several studies show that the regular practice of Hatha yoga is useful in the treatment of hypertension.[3–5] One study showed that Hatha yoga, done daily, was equally effective as a pharmacologic agent at reducing blood pressure. Another series of randomized controlled clinical trials studies by Latha[5a] demonstrated a significant reduction in headaches, use of medications, and perception of stress in the group receiving yoga therapy. Groups of Hatha yoga poses that are felt to be particularly beneficial for hypertension include forward bends and inversions and their modifications. Inversion poses in particular should be used with medical supervision, as they may be contraindicated in certain conditions such as cervical strain, glaucoma, and retinal detachment.

The slow, controlled breathing patterns of pranayama have a beneficial effect on disorders of the respiratory system, particularly asthma.[6–8] One study by Singh et al.,[7] a randomized, double-blind, controlled clinical trial on 18 asthmatic patients, showed a statistically significant increase in the dose of histamine required to provoke a reduction in forced expiratory volume at 1 second in the pranayama group, when compared to the dose of hista-mine needed in the control group. Studies show that people who do yoga regularly have lowered breathing rates and increased lung capacity.[9] The data seems to suggest that a primary action of the regular practice of Hatha yoga may be a resetting of the resting tone of the autonomic nervous system.[10]

There are many other medical applications of Hatha yoga. Several studies show some benefit of Hatha yoga, pranayama, and meditation for improving concentration, reducing stress, and promoting relaxation.[11–13] This, of course, may be linked with autonomic tone and helps explain how Hatha yoga may be useful for a wide range of medical conditions—from rheumatoid arthritis to diabetes.[14] This decreased tone and the concomitant decreases in blood pressure and heart rate may also explain the utility of yoga as part of the integrative approach to cardiovascular atherosclerosis developed by Dr. Dean Ornish. Table 11–1 summarizes some of the research on the clinical applications of Hatha yoga.

The postures of Hatha yoga, particularly when integrated with Ayurvedic medicine, are often useful in the treatment of musculoskeletal conditions, particularly low back pain. *Back Care Basics* by Mary Schatz, MD, is a physician's guide to a gentle yoga program for back and neck pain relief that illustrates the medical applications of yoga for musculoskeletal problems.[15] The Arthritis Foundation recently endorsed Hatha yoga as a potentially useful treatment for various forms of arthritis,[16] and there are many protocols available for the treatment of a wide range of musculoskeletal problems—from low back pain and sciatica to scoliosis. These specific series of postures are generally available through certified yoga instructors with training in therapeutic yoga.

Pranayama

Pranayama, the yogic science of control of various aspects of breathing (inhalation, exhalation, and the intervals between) is a highly refined art and an important part of the

▶ **TABLE 11-1** CLINICAL APPLICATIONS OF MOVEMENT THERAPY

Therapy Evaluated	Diagnosis	Citation	Type of Study
Hatha yoga	Carpal tunnel syndrome	Garfinkel M, Singhal A, Katz W, Allan D, Reshetar R, Schumacher H. Yoga-based intervention for carpal tunnel syndrome: a randomized trial. *JAMA.* 1998;280(18):1601–1603.	Randomized clinical trial
Hatha yoga	Osteoarthritis	Garfinkel M, Husain A, Levy M, Reshetar R. Evaluation of a yoga based regimen for treatment of osteoarthritis of the hands. *J Rheumatol.* 1994;21:2341–2343.	Observational study
Hatha yoga	Rheumatoid arthritis	Dash M, Telles S. Improvement in hand grip strength in normal volunteers and rheumatoid arthritis patients following yoga training. *Indian J Physiol Pharmacol.* 2001;45(3):355–360.	Controlled clinical trial
Hatha yoga	Hypertension	Haber D. Yoga as a preventive health care program for white and black elders: an exploratory study. *Int J Aging Hum Dev.* 1983;17(3): 17(3):169–176.	Uncontrolled clinical trial
Hatha yoga	Hypertension	Damodaran A, Malathi, Patil N, et al. Therapeutic potential of yoga in modifying cardiovascular risk profile in middle-aged men and women. *J Assoc Physicians India.* 2002;50(5):633–640.	Prospective clinical trial
Hatha yoga	Hypertension	Patel C, North W. Randomised controlled trial of yoga and bio-feedback in management of hypertension. *Lancet.* 1975;2(7925): 93–95.	Randomized, placebo-controlled clinical trial
Qigong	Hypertension	Kuang A, Wang C, Xu D, Qian Y. Research on the anti-aging effect of Qi Gong. *J Tradit Chin Med.* 1991;11(2):153–158.	Controlled prospective clinical trial
Qigong	Hypertension	Wang C, Xu D, Qian Y. Medical and healthcare Qi Gong. *J Tradit Chin Med.* 1991;11(4):296–301; Kuang A, Wang C, Xu D, Qian Y. Research on the anti-aging effect of Qi Gong. *J Tradit Chin Med.* 1991;11(2):153–158.	Prospective clinical trial
Hatha yoga (pranayama)	Asthma	Nagarathna R. Yoga for bronchial asthma: a controlled study. *Br Med J.* 1985;291:1077–1079.	Controlled clinical trial
Hatha yoga (pranayama)	Asthma	Singh V, Britton J, Tattersfield A. Effect of yoga breathing exercises (pranayama) on airway reactivity in subjects with asthma. *Lancet.* 1990;335:1381–1383.	Randomized, double-blind, placebo-controlled, crossover clinical trial
Hatha yoga and pranayama	Asthma	Vedanthan P, Kesavaly L, Murthy K, et al. Clinical study of yoga techniques in university students with asthma: a controlled study. *Allergy Asthma Proc.* 1998;18(1):3–9.	Randomized, controlled clinical trial
Hatha yoga	Asthma	Khanam A, Sachdeva U, Guleria R, Deepak K. Study of pulmonary and autonomic functions of asthma patients after yoga training. *Indian J Physiol Pharmacol.* 1996;40(4):318–324.	Prospective noncontrolled clinical trial
Hatha yoga	Headaches	Latha D. Efficacy of yoga therapy in the management of headaches. *J Indian Psychol.* 1992;10:41–47.	Randomized, controlled clinical trial

therapeutic application of yoga. Cultivation of breath awareness, its patterns, and the possibilities of its change are significant components of yoga therapy. The regular practice of yoga is associated with an enhanced vitality, endurance, and balance. Its deeper importance, however, seems to lie in the way it can train the mind and change autonomic nervous system tone. In the delicate interplay between mind and body, yoga is one of several techniques well suited to cultivate mental and physical health.

Hatha yoga and pranayama can be adapted for most patients. Almost any program of Hatha yoga will incorporate postures, breathing exercises, and relaxation or meditation into a 1- to 2-hour yoga class. It can be challenging to find a yoga teacher with the experience, patience, and communication skills to adapt the therapy to the patient. The referring health care providers should be aware that most yoga instructors are not medical professionals and that no state licensing is required to teach Hatha yoga. Certification can be obtained through some yoga schools and some yoga traditions, and it is best to seek out a teacher who has at least several years of teaching experience and who continues to study and practice yoga regularly. Certified yoga therapists with experience in both teaching yoga and working with patients are becoming more common as Hatha yoga is integrated more frequently with other medical therapies for a range of illnesses.

▶ MEDITATION

Meditation is most commonly used in a medical setting as a stress-reduction technique[17]; however, the rise and fall of the abdomen and chest during inhalation and exhalation is also a subtle movement therapy with the attention and focus on the movement of the breath. The intimate link among meditation, Hatha yoga, and other movement disciplines such as Tai Chi and Qigong gives meditation a place in the discussion of movement therapies. A regular meditation practice is likely to not only reduce

stress and promote relaxation, but may also improve a variety of medical conditions, ranging from hypertension to chronic pain.[18–20] Here, as in yoga practice, these benefits are probably mediated by the effects of meditation on the autonomic nervous system.

There are a wide variety of styles of meditation, most of which share a common theme of self-directed focusing of the mind; most commonly, that focus is on the breath. In most cases, one begins the process of meditation in a comfortable seated position, ideally with a straight back. The eyes may be closed or open, and the focus of attention is initially on the breath. Then, depending on the style of meditation, the focus may shift to a phrase or "mantra"—a word or series of words that are repeated over and over as one meditates—or may continue to simply follow the flow of the breath. Several approaches to meditation are described briefly below. A meditation session commonly lasts 15–30 minutes or longer, but even a few minutes daily of contemplative awareness may benefit one's health. Instruction can be helpful to many patients in beginning a meditation practice; this is available in individual or group classes, or by using tapes and books. Consistency of practice is the key to obtaining the benefits of meditation.

Vipasana Meditation

Vipasana meditation, often called mindfulness meditation, comes from the Theravada Buddhist tradition and uses breath awareness as a starting point in learning meditation. The student is instructed not to concentrate on any one thing, but to impartially observe the breath, bodily sensation, and thoughts that arise in the mind, and to note them as they occur in the present moment. The purpose is to be aware of physical sensations, thoughts, and emotions in the moment without trying to hold on to them; the state of attachment to a particular thought, emotion, or physical sensation seems to create a state of agitation. Once again, the state of meditative awareness is accompanied by changes in autonomic nervous system function and brain wave activity.[21]

Siddha Yoga Meditation

This meditation tradition was brought to the West in the early 1970s by Swami Muktananda and works with the inner energy of the body, sometimes referred to as the *Kundalini energy*.[22] The goal, if it can be called that, of meditation is to increase the subtlety of awareness and thereby facilitate a spiritual transformation. In Siddha yoga, the field of awareness in the process of meditation may include the breath, but eventually goes much further into the general field of awareness. Techniques, including breath awareness, chanting, or mantras, may be used to provide support for the mind and awareness, but are not an end in themselves.

Transcendental Meditation

This form of meditation was popularized by Maharishi Mahesh Yogi and incorporates the use of a mantra or repeated word or phrase to help focus the mind and increase concentration. Its medical applications have been studied in Iowa at Maharishi University under the auspices of the National Center for Complementary and Alternative Medicine at the National Institutes of Health.[23–28] Transcendental meditation is the practice initially studied in the 1970s by Benson in his landmark research on mind–body practice and hypertension, and has been successfully used in many settings as an adjunctive therapy in the treatment of hypertension, coronary artery disease, and stress reduction.

Mindfulness-Based Stress Reduction

Mindfulness-based stress reduction (MBSR) as developed by Jon Kabat-Zinn integrates mindfulness meditation with Hatha yoga in a 2-month program that began at the Stress Reduction Clinic at the University of Massachusetts Medical School in 1980. This 8-week program has treated thousands of patients with a variety of medical conditions—from chronic pain to cancer—and is now available throughout the country in many hospital-affiliated programs and through independent practitioners of MBSR. The program consists of weekly classes and daily practice of almost 1 hour, integrating meditation, Hatha yoga, and the "body scan," using a series of tapes designed to support home practice. Clinical research has demonstrated a role for MBSR in the treatment of numerous conditions, including anxiety disorders, pain syndromes, and psoriasis.[18–20]

▶ TAI CHI

Tai Chi, also known as *Taiji Quan,* is an ancient Chinese practice dating back almost 5,000 years and originating in a series of exercises and movements practiced after a strenuous day of work. Certain breathing and movement techniques were found to affect the flow of energy, or Qi, in the body, in specific ways. By refining these techniques, these ancient Chinese masters experienced increased vigor and mental sharpness and a sense of well-being and relaxation while exercising. These movements were the precursors to the Daoist meditation practices *Tai Chi* and *Qigong*.[29] Qigong is translated as "Qi exercise"; it is also known as "longevity method" or "breathing exercise."

Qi is believed to be the vital energy that is behind all processes pertaining to body, mind, and spirit. Other translations for Qi are energy-matter, ether, vital energy, or life force. Qi emanates through energy pathways or meridians, which cover the body like a network system; Qi is what animates us and what generates life. In a simplified way, it is generated from the air we breathe and the food and liquids we consume—which is known as postnatal Qi—and prenatal Qi, which we received from our parents. It warms us, protects us against exterior pathogens, holds our organs in place, promotes growth and development, and directs all our movements. Lao Zi, one of the earliest Daoist philosophers, noted in the *Dao De Jing* that Qi was difficult to grasp with the mind; it could only be felt.[30]

The therapeutic benefits of Tai Chi are likely to come from its emphasis on balance and harmony, continuous slow movements, rhythmic flexion of the lower limbs, extension of the upper body, the symmetrical arm motion, and the constant shifting of weight. Tai Chi appears to be a useful adjunctive therapy for patients with arthritis[31,32] and cardiovascular disease.[33] There is also evidence that Tai Chi may enhance physical fitness in older adults and improve postural stability.[34]

▶ QIGONG

Qigong (pronounced *chee-gong*) is part of the system of traditional Chinese medicine (TCM) that includes other therapies such as acupuncture and moxibustion, herbal medicine, acupressure massage, and nutrition. These therapies are discussed in detail in Chapter 9. In the practice of Qigong, the flow of Qi is regulated, and blockage of the flow of Qi is removed. Energy blocks or excess or deficient Qi may result from disease, injury, or stress.

Qigong is unique among TCM therapies because almost anyone can learn and practice it. However, it is best to study Qigong with a qualified teacher to maximize the benefits and avoid injury. An estimated 60 million people in China practice Qigong daily, primarily to maintain health and achieve long life.

Qigong is a combination of two ideas: Qi is the vital energy of the body, and Gong is the skill of working with the Qi. Medical Qigong for health and healing consists primarily of meditation, physical movements, and breathing exercises. Qigong practitioners develop an awareness of Qi sensations in their bodies and use their mind, or intention, to guide the Qi. The benefits of Qigong are said to extend be-

yond health and healing to enhance spiritual life and even special abilities such as psychic powers. Qigong is also used in martial arts to develop physical and mental powers for self-defense and healing.

Medical Qigong is divided into two parts: internal and external. Internal Qi is developed by individual practice of Qigong exercises. When Qigong practitioners become sufficiently skilled, they can use external Qi (*wai qi* or wei qi in Chinese) to "emit" Qi for the purpose of healing another person. This therapy has limited application on a large scale, because the number of skilled Qigong masters is limited. This chapter focuses on internal Qi, as almost everyone can learn Qigong exercises for maintaining health and for self-healing.

Medical Applications of Qigong

Between 1986 and 1996, 837 abstracts on medical uses of Qigong were published by Chinese researchers, more than half in English. These English-language abstracts have been entered into a database[35] and are readily accessible. The research on Qigong falls into two categories: first, the potential benefits of internal Qigong practice, and second, the effects of external or "emitted" Qi on humans, animals, cell cultures, and plants.[36,37] A number of examples from the research literature on Qigong follow.

Several groups in China have investigated the effects of Qigong on hypertension. Research on the short- and long-term effects of Qigong practice on hypertensive patients has been carried out at the Shanghai Institute of Hypertension by Wang et al.[38] Their research serves as a model of the effects of Qigong on many functions of the body. For these studies, the patients practiced "Yan Jing Yi Shen Gong" for 30 minutes twice a day. This Qigong exercise, claimed to be especially valuable for therapeutic purposes and delaying senility, consists of a combination of sitting meditation and gentle physical movements that emphasizes a calm mind, relaxed body, and regular respiration.

Stroke, Hypertension, and Mortality

In 1991, these researchers reported a 20-year controlled study of the anti-aging effects of Qigong on 204 hypertensive patients.[39] Recently, the researchers performed a 30-year follow-up study on 242 hypertensive patients who were divided randomly into a Qigong group (N = 122) and a control group (N = 120).[40] All patients were given drug therapy to control blood pressure, but only the experimental group practiced Qigong 30 minutes twice a day. The results show that the accumulated mortality rate was 25.4% in the Qigong group and 40.8% in the control group (P <.001). The incidence of stroke was 20.5% and 40.7% (P <.01), respectively, and the death rate as a consequence of stroke was 15.6% and 32.5%, respectively. The researchers also reported that over the 20-year period, blood pressure of the Qigong group stabilized, whereas that of the control group increased. During this period, the drug dosage for the Qigong group could be decreased and for 30% of the patients, could be eliminated. The drug dosage for the control group had to be increased.

Heart Function and Microcirculation

From a Chinese medicine perspective, older hypertensive patients usually have a deficiency of heart-energy, which can lead to a weakened function of the left ventricle and a disturbance of microcirculation. In a study of 120 male subjects 55 to 75 years of age, researchers evaluated the effects of Qigong by using echocardiography and indices of microcirculation.[41] The subjects were divided into three groups consisting of 46 hypertensive subjects with heart-energy deficiency, 34 without heart-energy deficiency, and 40 with normal blood pressure. Patients whose blood pressure measured more than 160/95 mm Hg were accepted as subjects after regulation with antihypertensive drugs for 4 weeks. The results showed that subjects with heart-energy deficiency experienced several im-

provements with Qigong practice: increases in cardiac output, ejection fraction, mitral valve diastolic closing velocity, and mean velocity of circumferential fiber shortening, while the total peripheral resistance decreased (P < .05–.01). Significant changes did not occur in the group without heart-energy deficiency.

Multiple quantitative evaluations of nail fold disturbance in the microcirculation were made on the above three groups by observing 9 indices of abnormal conditions: configuration of micrangium; micrangium tension; condition of blood flow; slowing of blood flow; thinner afferent limb; efferent and afferent limb ratio; color of blood; hemorrhage; and petechiae. At the beginning of the study, the incidence of microcirculation obstruction for the above three groups was 73.9%, 26.5%, and 17.5%, respectively. After practicing Qigong for 1 year, the group with heart-energy deficiency showed a decrease in nail fold microcirculation obstruction from 73.9% to 39.3% (P <.05). Significant changes did not occur in the group without heart-energy deficiency. The investigators emphasized that this study demonstrates the importance of selecting the type of Qigong exercise according to the patient's specific condition.

Bone Density

Aging may result in a decrease in bone density, especially in women. As a consequence, bones become more brittle and subject to fracture. Bone density was found to increase in male subjects who practiced Qigong for 1 year.[42] For 18 subjects 50 to 59 years of age, bone density increased from 0.627 ± 0.040 to 0.696 ± 0.069 g/cm^3. For 12 subjects aged 60 to 69 years, the bone density increase was somewhat less. However, for both age groups, the bone density increased to values exceeding those of normal men of the same age. It seems likely that Qigong therapy also would help restore the bone density of women. Further research on the applications of Qigong to osteoporosis is needed, both from prevention and treatment points of view.

Changes in Blood Chemistry in Hypertensive Patients

Auxiliary studies by Xu and coworkers[13] on the effects of Qigong exercise on the blood chemistry of hypertensive subjects show improvements in plasma coagulation fibrinolysis indices, blood viscosity, erythrocyte deformation index, plasma level of tissue-type plasminogen activator, plasminogen activator inhibitor, factor VIII–related antigen, and antithrombin III. In another study, the same researchers reported that Qigong exercise significantly and beneficially changed the activities of two messenger cyclic nucleotides (cyclic adenosine monophosphate and cyclic guanosine monophosphate).[14]

Cancer

Although the mechanisms remain elusive and difficult to understand from a Western perspective, research from China shows that emitted Qi from Qigong masters produced marked changes in cancer cell cultures from mice.[15, 16] In several studies, the effects of emitted Qi on tumors in animals have been reported. For example, emitted Qi was reported to inhibit the growth of implanted malignant tumors in mice but did not destroy the tumors. Encouraged by the results with animals, researchers have carried out clinical research on the effects of internal Qigong on human subjects with cancer. Detailed results are not available in English for all these clinical studies. In one study, patients with medically diagnosed malignant cancer were divided into a group of 97 patients who practiced Qigong and a control group of 30 patients. All patients received drugs, and the study group practiced Qigong for more than 2 hours a day over a period of 3 to 6 months. Both groups improved, but the study group showed improvement in

strength, appetite, freedom from diarrhea, and weight gain (3 kg [6.6 lb]) four to nine times greater than that of the control group. The phagocytic rate, one measure of the immune function, increased in the Qigong group, but decreased in the control group.[17]

Brain Waves

An extensive body of research has focused on the effects of Qigong on brain waves as measured by electroencephalography (EEG). During static, or sitting, meditation, alpha brain waves dominate beta waves and spread to the frontal areas of the brain.[18, 19] Kawano and Wang have found differences in the electroencephalograms of Zen Buddhist priests and Qigong masters. During almost all types of Qigong training, the frequency of the alpha waves increased from 0.6 to 1.0 Hz. During deep Zen meditation, the frequency decreased from -1.0 to -1.5 Hz, and sometimes theta waves appeared. Also, frontal and occipital alpha waves tended to synchronize with a phase difference that depended on the type of meditation. This phase difference became smaller with Qigong meditation (i.e., better synchronization) and larger with Zen meditation. These differences in brain function suggest that internal Qigong may be a semiconscious process that involves some awareness and activity, whereas Zen meditation may be a neutral process. Perhaps because of this difference, Qigong is considered a healing art, whereas Zen is generally not.

Blood Flow to the Brain

Rheoencephalography shows that Qigong exercise increases blood flow to the brain.[50] For 158 subjects with cerebral arteriosclerosis who practiced Qigong for 1 to 6 months, improvement was noted in symptoms such as memory loss, dizziness, insomnia, tinnitus, numbness of limbs, and vertigo headache. During these studies, a decrease in the plasma cholesterol level was also noted.

▶ MOVEMENT THERAPIES AS EXERCISE

In addition to mind–body or relaxation and centering practices, Hatha yoga, Tai Chi, and Qigong are also physical exercises that involve using the musculoskeletal system. There are many physical and mental benefits to exercise—improved fat metabolism, weight loss, and circulation. These benefits are discussed in detail in Chapter 13.

Bone density increases when reasonable mechanical stresses are placed on the bone over a period of time such as occurs with exercise. Exercise at the proper level can have the effect of increasing bone density, hence bone strength. Exercises such as yoga, Tai Chi and Qigong can be part of a regimen to counteract the effects of aging on bone such as osteoporosis and osteopenia. Exercise also improves coordination and may improve the balance of older persons, resulting in fewer falls and, hence, fewer fractures.

▶ FELDENKRAIS

Dr. Moshe Feldenkrais developed a system of movement and body awareness in Israel in the 1950s.[51,52] Although there is little research to document its effectiveness, this method is based on conventional neurological principles. It is based on the assumption that habitual movements and postures represent a disruption in the nervous system and that gentle movement and manipulation can replace old patterns of movement with new ones. The two main techniques used are a group process of "awareness through movement" and "functional integration," an individualized technique that uses movement and gentle manipulation.[53]

One exercise derived from Feldenkrais is an exercise where the spine is moved as if it were a chain. It is felt to be useful for relieving aches and pains, for reducing the effects of stress, and for helping people fall asleep. There are 26 moveable segments (vertebrae) in the spinal column starting with the tailbone (coccyx) and counting up to the base of the skull. Patients are taught to imagine that each of these segments is like a link in a chain, each capable of moving independently from the segment above and below it, but also, each attached to the segment above and below it. In one exercise, patients imagine that the tip of their tailbone (coccyx) is attached to a cable, which goes directly upward and is attached to a pulley on the ceiling, and that someone can pull the other end of the cable, which lifts their tailbone directly toward the ceiling. The spine, one segment at a time, is slowly lifted off the ground as if each vertebra were a link in a chain. This exercise requires very little muscular effort and is done in a relaxed manner, taking perhaps 30 seconds or more to lift the entire spine like a chain, and another 30 seconds to return to a neutral position.

▶ MASSAGE

Massage has been used for thousands of years in many different cultures for both prevention and treatment of a wide variety of conditions. Although it is less movement oriented than Hatha yoga, Tai Chi, or Qigong it involves the systematic and usually rhythmic stimulation of the soft tissues with pressure and stretching to elicit a therapeutic response. Massage therapy was introduced into the medical community in the United States after the Civil War and was rapidly accepted as part of most medical encounters until the early 1900s. Early in the twentieth century, therapeutic massage became more integrated into nursing practice, and then later into the practices of physical therapists and now licensed massage therapists.

Although there are many schools of massage that are not well known, massage as a complementary medical therapy is widely accepted as being beneficial, with a large body of research evidence to support its effectiveness.[54,55] Currently, massage now has the highest rate of physician referral in the United States of any of the complementary healing arts.[56] While not viewed as curative in and of itself for most medical problems, it can dramatically stimulate the self-healing response and speed recovery in a variety of clinical situations.

Therapeutic massage commonly will incorporate four basic techniques: friction, effleurage, pétrissage, and vibration/percussion. Friction is the process by which the therapist and the patient's skin and muscles move together. Friction is decreased with the use of massage oil. Effleurage refers to a series of long gliding strokes focusing on the superficial muscles. Pétrissage refers to the technique of kneading the muscles that is used to increase circulation to the muscle bed. Vibration and percussion are a series of fine or brisk movements that can be used to stimulate circulation and relaxation. There are many different types of massage that incorporate these and other techniques, including:

- Deep-tissue massage uses a variety of strokes to work both the superficial and deep muscles to release tension and increase relaxation.
- Sports massage emphasizes the use of massage to enhance athletic performance and increase the rate of recovery.
- Connective tissue massage works with light and deep massage of the superficial and deep connective tissue to stimulate the neural reflex arcs that connect the musculoskeletal system and the internal organs.
- Trigger-point massage and Shiatsu use deep finger pressure on trigger points or acupressure points.
- Reflexology is a type of foot massage based on the belief that zones and points on the feet correspond to other parts of the body and that the foot can be used a "map" of the body. Treatments are designed to open blocked nerve pathways and improve circulation in the foot in order to treat problems that may exist elsewhere in the body.
- Lymphatic drainage uses light strokes to stimulate the movement of lymphatic fluid, particularly in conditions where lymph flow may be compromised (edema, postmastectomy).
- Rolfing focuses on treatment of the connective-tissue fascia, a web throughout the body that responds to physical and emotional stress. Under stress, the fascia and connective tissue are felt to lose their elasticity, thereby restricting movement and motion from breathing patterns to actual movement. While Rolfing is often viewed as a form of massage therapy, it was begun with the intention of being a therapy complementary to orthopedic surgery. Rolfing traditionally begins with a 10-session series through which the connective tissue of the body is reset.

Touch is perceived through the circulatory and the nervous systems via the skin, the body's largest sensory organ. All of the forms of massage mentioned above share "laying on of the hands" as a common element. The physical contact of massage has the psychological effect of enhancing well-being and increasing relaxation as well as the physiological effects of increasing parasympathetic tone and reducing cortisol levels and sympathetic tone, and improving circulation.[57,58] Massage is generally contraindicated in any condition where there is active inflammation, particularly suspected bacterial infections. It should also be used with caution in patients with clotting disorders or pressure ulcers.

▶ CONCLUSION

Movement therapies take advantage of the fact that as living organisms we are all constantly in motion. From infancy to the end of life, we use movement and being touched or touching as a tool that shapes behavior and our interactions with the world. It is important when choosing a movement therapy for a patient that it be a joint decision based on the patient's interest, the practitioner's experience, and the availability of qualified movement practitioners. Some movement approaches involve complex series of movements where a trained instructor is critical, particularly for patients with medical conditions. Other movement approaches are easy to implement using self-instructional materials. Using movement as a tool to stimulate a therapeutic response is an essential part of the integrative medicine approach, reflecting our awareness that our ability to move is closely linked to our state of health.

REFERENCES

1. Johnson E. Anxiety, drug consumption, and personality correlates of yoga and progressive muscle relaxation. *Dissertation Abstr Int.* 1983;44: 1962.
2. Garfinkel M, Singhal A, Katz W, Allan D, Reshetar R, Schumacher H. Yoga-based intervention for carpal tunnel syndrome: a randomized trial. *JAMA.* 1998;280(18):1601–1603.
3. Haber D. Yoga as a preventive health care program for white and black elders: an exploratory study. *Int J Aging Hum Dev.* 1983;17(3):169–176.
4. Murugansan R, Govindarajulu N, Bera T. Effect of selected yogic practices on the management of hypertension. *Indian J Physiol Pharmacol.* 2000;44(2):207–210.
5. Patel C. Twelve-month follow-up of yoga and bio-feedback in the management of hypertension. *Lancet.* 1975;1(7898):62–64.
5a. Latha D. Efficacy of yoga theory in the management of headaches. *J Indian Psychol.* 1992;10: 41–47.
6. Nagarathna R. Yoga for bronchial asthma: a controlled study. *Br Med J.* 1985;(291):1077–1079.
7. Singh V, Britton J, Tattersfield A. Effect of yoga breathing exercises (pranayama) on airway reactivity in subjects with asthma. *Lancet.* 1990;335: 1381–1383.
8. Khanam A, Sachdeva U, Guleria R, Deepak K. Study of pulmonary and autonomic functions of asthma patients after yoga training. *Indian J Physiol Pharmacol.* 1996;40(4):318–324.

9. Raju P, Madhavi S, Prasad K, et al. Comparison of effects of yoga and physical exercise in athletes. *Indian J Med Res.* 1994;100:81–86.
10. Schmidt T, Wijga A, Von Zur Muhlen A, Brabant G, Wagner T. Changes in cardiovascular risk factors and hormones during a comprehensive residential three-month kriya yoga training and vegetarian nutrition. *Acta Physiol Scand Suppl.* 1997;640:158–162.
11. Shannahoff D, Beckett L. Clinical case reports: efficacy of yogic techniques in the treatment of obsessive compulsive disorders. *Int J Neurosci.* 1996;85(1–2):1–17.
12. Telles S, Reddy S, Nagendra H. Oxygen consumption and respiration following two yoga relaxation techniques. *Appl Psychophysiol Biofeedback.* 2000;25(4):221–227.
13. Schell F, Allolio B, Schonecke O. Physiological and psychological effects of Hatha-yoga exercise in healthy women. *Int J Psychosom.* 1994;41(1–4): 46–52.
14. Monro R, Coumar A, Nagarathna R, Dandona P. Yoga therapy for NIDDM: a controlled trial. *Complement Med Res.* 1992(6):66–68.
15. Schatz M. *Back Care Basics.* Berkeley, CA: Rodmell Press; 1992.
16. http://www.arthritisfoundation.org. Last access 2003.
17. Astin JA. Stress reduction through mindfulness meditation. Effects on psychological symptomatology, sense of control, and spiritual experiences. *Psychother Psychosom.* 1997;66:97–106.
18. Kabat-Zinn J, Wheeler E, Light T, et al. Influence of a mindfulness meditation-based stress reduction intervention on rates of skin clearing in patients with moderate to severe psoriasis undergoing phototherapy (UVB) and photochemotherapy (PUVA). *Psychosom Med.* 1998;60: 625–632.
19. Kabat-Zinn J, Lipworth L, Burney R. The clinical use of mindfulness meditation for the self-regulation of chronic pain. *J Behav Med.* 1985; 8(2):163–190.
20. Kaplan KH, Goldenberg DL, Galvin-Nadeau M. The impact of a meditation-based stress reduction program on fibromyalgia. *Gen Hosp Psychiatry.* 1993;15(5):284–289.
21. Sudsuang R, Chentanez V, Veluvan K. Effect of Buddhist meditation on serum cortisol and total protein levels, blood pressure, pulse rate, lung

volume, and reaction time. *Physiol Behav.* 1991; 50(3):543–548.

22. Swami Durgananda. *The Heart of Meditation.* South Fallsburg, NY: SYDA Foundation; 2002.

23. Wenneberg SR, Schneider RH, Walton KG, et al. A controlled study of the effects of the transcendental meditation program on cardiovascular reactivity and ambulatory blood pressure. *Int J Neurosci.* 1997;89:15–28.

24. Zamarra JW, Schneider RH, Besseghini I, et al. Usefulness of transcendental meditation program in the treatment of patients with coronary artery disease. *Am J Cardiol.* 1996;77(10):867–870.

25. Schneider RH, Staggers F, Alexander CN, et al. A randomized controlled trial of stress reduction for hypertension in older African Americans. *Hypertension.* 1995;26(5): 820–827.

26. Jevning R, Anand R, Biedebach M, et al. Effects on regional cerebral blood flow of transcendental meditation. *Physiol Behav.* 1996;59(3):399–402.

27. Barnes VA, Treiber FA, Turner JR, et al. Acute effects of transcendental meditation on hemodynamic function in middle-aged adults. *Psychosom Med.* 1999;61(4):525–531.

28. Jevning R, Wilson AF, Davidson JM. Adrenocortical activity during meditation. *Horm Behav.* 1978;10:54–60.

29. Cohen K. *The Way of Qigong: The Art and Science of Chinese Energy Healing.* New York: Ballantine Books; 1997.

30. Mitchell S. *Tao Ti Ching.* New York: Harper Collins; 1988.

31. Koh T. Tai Chi Chuan. *Am J Chinese Med.* 1981; 9:15–23.

32. Kirsteins AE, Dietz F, Hwang S. Evaluating the safety and potential use of a weight-bearing exercise, Tai Chi Chuan, for rheumatoid arthritis patients. *Am J Phys Med Rehabil.* 1991;70: 136–141.

33. Channer K, Barrow D, Barrow R, Osborne M, Ives G. Changes in hemodynamic parameters following Tai Chi Chuan and aerobic exercise in patients recovering from acute myocardial infarction. *Postgrad Med J.* 1996;72:349–351.

34. Tse S, Bailey D. Tai Chi and postural control in the well elderly. *Am J Occup Ther.* 1992;46: 295–300.

35. Qigong Database. Qigong Institute, 561 Berkeley Avenue, Menlo Park, CA 94025.

36. Sancier KM, Hu B. Medical applications of qigong and emitted qi on humans, animals, cell cultures,

and plants: review of selected scientific studies. *Am J Acupunct.* 1991;19(4):367–377.

37. Sancier KM. The effect of qigong on human body functions. Proceedings from the Fifth International Symposium on Qigong. Shanghai, China. 1994:179.

38. Wang C, Xu D, Qian Y. Medical and healthcare qigong. *J Tradit Chin Med.* 1991;11(4):296–301.

39. Kuang A, Wang C, Xu D, Qian Y. Research on the anti-aging effect of qigong. *J Tradit Chin Med.* 1991;11(2):153–158.

40. Wang C, Xu D, Qian Y, Shi W. Effects of qigong on preventing stroke and alleviating the multiple cerebro-cardiovascular risk factors: a follow-up report on 242 hypertensive cases over 30 years. Proceedings from the Second World Conference for Academic Exchange of Medical Qigong. Beijing, 1993:123–124.

41. Wang C, Xu D, Qian Y, Shi W, Bao Y, Kuang A. Beneficial effects of qigong on the ventricular function and micro circulation of deficiency in heart-energy hypertensive patients. Written communication, September 1993.

42. Xu D, Wang C. Clinical study of delaying effect on senility of hypertensive patients by practicing "Yang Jing Yi Shen Gong." Proceedings from the Fifth International Symposium on Qigong, Shanghai; 1994:109.

43. Ye M, Zhang R, Wu X, Wang Y, Shan J. Relationship among erythrocyte superoxide dismustase activity, plasma sexual hormones (T, E2), aging and qigong exercise [in English and Chinese]. Proceedings from the Third International Symposium on Qigong, Shanghai; 1990:28–32.

44. Kuang A, Wang C, Xu D, Qian Y. Research on "anti-aging" effect of qigong. *J Tradit Chin Med.* 1991;11(3):224–227.

45. Feng L. Effect of emitted qi on human carcinoma cells. Proceedings from the First World Conference for Academic Exchange of Medical Qigong. Beijing, 1988:1–4.

46. Feng L. Effect of emitted qi on the L 1210 cells of leukemia in mice. Proceedings from the First World Conference for Academic Exchange of Medical Qigong. Beijing, 1988:4–5.

47. Sun Q, Zhao L. Clinical observation of qigong as a therapeutic aid for advanced cancer patients. Proceedings from the First World Conference for Academic Exchange of Medical Qigong, Beijing; 1988:97–98.

48. Kawano K, Wang F. Difference between the EEG of Zen priests and internal qigong masters. *Soc Mind Body Sci.* 1994;3(1):99–104.

49. Machi Y. Various measurements of qigong masters for analyzing qigong mechanism. *Soc Mind Body Sci.* 1994;3(1):65–87.

50. Liu Y, He S, Xie S. Clinical observation on the treatment of 158 cases of cerebral arteriosclerosis by qigong. Proceedings from the Second World Conference on Academic Exchange of Medical Qigong. Beijing, 1993:125.

51. Feldenkrais M. *Awareness Through Movement: Health Exercises for Personal Growth.* San Francisco: Harper; 1991.

52. Feldenkrais M. *Body and Mature Behavior: A Study of Anxiety, Sex, Gravitation and Learning.* New York: International Universities Press; 1991.

53. Rywerant Y, Feldenkrais M. *The Feldenkrais Method.* New York: Keats Publishing, 1991.

54. Field T, Hernandez-Reif M, Seligman S. Juvenile rheumatoid arthritis: benefits from massage therapy. *J Pediatr Psychol.* 1977;22:607–617.

55. Field T, Sunshine W, Hernandez-Reif, et al. Chronic fatigue syndrome: massage therapy effects on depression and somatic symptoms in chronic fatigue. *J Chronic Fatigue Syndr.* 1997;3:43–51.

56. Astin J, Marie A, Pelletier K, et al. A review of the incorporation of complementary and alternative medicine by mainstream physicians. *Arch Intern Med.* 1998;79:1440–1447.

57. Hansen T, Kristensen J. Effects of massage, shortwave diathermy and ultrasound upon Xe disappearance rate from muscle and subcutaneous tissue in the human calf. *Scand J Rehabil Med.* 1973;5:179–182.

58. Cotton L, Roberts V. The prevention of deep vein thrombosis, with particular reference to mechanical methods of prevention. *Surgery.* 1977;81: 98–103.

CHAPTER 12

Homeopathy

EDWARD SHALTS

Homeopathy (from the Greek "omeos" [similar] and "pathos" [suffering]) is a system of medicine developed in the nineteenth century by the renowned German physician and chemist Samuel Hahnemann.[1,2] Hahnemann emphasized a holistic approach with the individualization of treatment, pioneering the concept of differential therapeutics. The approach he suggested represented a significant shift from the prevailing theoretical paradigm of the time—which was based on pathology and on the "theory of signatures"—to a holistic approach committed to addressing the entirety of psychosomatic changes characteristic to the illness in the particular individual. The theory of signatures, which Hahnemann rejected, stated that the therapeutic principles of a substance could be deduced from its physical appearance. For example, according to this theory, onion was beneficial in treatment of prostate problems because it looks like a prostate gland. From its inception, homeopathy sparked controversy, particularly because of Hahnemann's strong opposition to barbaric methods of treatment employed by mainstream medical practitioners of his time (blistering, phlebotomy, and purging) and to the polypharmacy that was prevalent at that time.

One of Hahnemann's great contributions to medicine at large was the notion of differential therapeutics. In acute trauma, for example, a victim with a combination of significant musculoskeletal pathology with the emphasis on bruising, swelling, and pain who does not feel that any kind of help is warranted despite objective severity of the trauma ("I am OK! I don't need any help") might need a homeopathic remedy *Arnica montana* (mountain arnica). Another person with the same severity of musculoskeletal pathology with the emphasis on bone trauma and a desire to lie absolutely still with severe discomfort and pain even at slight motion, might require *Bryonia,* a different remedy. A trauma victim with the main presentation of severe agitation and overwhelming fear of death might need yet another remedy, *Aconitum napellus* (monkshood). In essence, homeopathic pharmacology offers the differential therapeutics approach that is highly desired by any modern physician.[3–5]

▶ BASIC PRINCIPLES OF HOMEOPATHY

Principle of Similars

The main tenet of homeopathy is the principle of similars: a substance that can cause symptoms in a healthy person can stimulate self-healing in a person with a similar psychosomatic response to an illness. For example, a patient suffering from seasonal allergies with the main presentation of increased lacrimation; irritating, burning nasal discharge; pain at the route of the nose; and a general feeling of dullness and stupefaction, may benefit from a homeopathic preparation *Allium cepa* (onion), which causes a similar constellation of symptoms in healthy individuals. A different patient with seasonal allergic reactions characterized by irritating discharge from the eyes and bland, nonirritating nasal discharge, may benefit from a homeopathic preparation *Euphrasia* (eyebright), which tends to cause this constellation of symptoms in healthy volunteers.

The principle of similars can be restated in common biomedical terms as follows: a given concentration (or homeopathic dilution) of a substance may have opposite (not just different) effects if physiologic conditions are different (e.g., healthy versus ill organism). There also can be two different concentrations (or homeopathic dilutions) of a given substance that have opposite effects in a given physiologic state of a living system. A detailed analysis of this issue is presented in recent publications by Eskinazi[6] and Merrell and Shalts.[7]

Proving

In Hahnemann's time, the medicinal qualities of *China officinalis* (Peruvian bark), which was successfully employed in treatment of malaria, were attributed to its sour, astringent taste. Hahnemann's desire for a scientific, medical practice based on unbiased experimental data eventually led him to take significant doses of *C. officinalis* in an attempt to understand its mechanism of curative action in patients with malaria. After a few doses he developed symptoms similar to the symptoms that were characteristic for patients suffering from malaria. Subsequent to reproducing this experiment several times with consistently comparable results

and searching the medical literature available at the time unsuccessfully for a theoretical explanation for this phenomenon, Hahnemann adapted the principle of similars formulated by Hippocrates.[1] At the same time, he recognized the process of describing the medicinal characteristics of various substances by administering them to healthy volunteers as a valid method of creating homeopathic pharmacologic records. He named this process *Prüfung* (from "test," "experiment" in German). The English translation of this term is "proving." Further provings were performed by Hahnemann on himself, his family members, and students, and later on healthy volunteers *(provers)*. Eventually, a group of 50 doctors constituted the pool of provers that worked closely with Hahnemann and described the characteristics of approximately 100 substances of mineral, herbal, and animal origin.

Provings are essentially a phase I pharmacologic study, performed according to a strict protocol.[8] While conventional researchers are looking for physiologic tolerance in healthy individuals with a minimum of side effects, homeopaths pay attention to the opposite side of the coin, trying to see as many "side effects" they can possibly find. It is those "side effects" that they will use to prescribe upon as these are the qualities that characterize the distinct healing properties of that particular substance.

One could expect that different people will react to the same substance in a slightly different way. A medicine will theoretically tend to produce all symptoms in all provers, but in reality, when a proving is conducted properly, this does not happen. Depending on individual sensitivity, some subjects develop many symptoms, some develop significantly fewer symptoms, and others do not develop any symptoms at all. More often, some of the symptoms that are developed are common to many of the provers, while others are unique to certain individuals (Figure 12–1). Data collected from various provers represents "the picture" of the remedy.

The essence of the guidelines for proving a new substance is the administration of the test

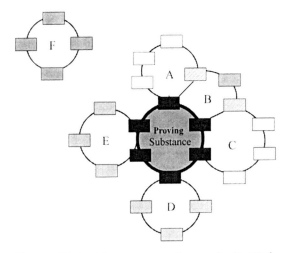

Figure 12-1. Here we see the cycle (a totality of possible symptoms) of adaptation for various provers A through F, as well as the cycle (all the symptoms possible) of the substance being proved. A number of segments (symptoms) represent the cycle. The boxes represent the segments of these cycles. It is clear that different subjects might experience some of the symptoms (A through E), all symptoms, or no symptoms at all (F). That depends on their individual sensitivity. A complete picture of the remedy is put together from the individual symptoms of sensitive provers. (*Reproduced with permission from Herscu P. Provings. Amherst, MA: The New England School of Homeopathy Press; 2002:33.*)

to subjects who are not taking other drugs, do not have serious illnesses, and are eating a simple diet.[2] A detailed protocol of provings is available.[8,9] The majority of provings carried out in the last 100–150 years were performed with substances diluted to 30c (10^{-60}) to ensure the safety of the volunteers. Despite the fact that it is almost 10^{10} times Avogadros number—and thus that the likelihood of any molecules of the original substance remaining in the tested dose is extremely small—authors report noticing a distinct effect in healthy individuals.[10–12] These symptoms elicited by diluted substances usually subside in a course of days or weeks.

Internet-based databases have been created to collect and systematize data received from ongoing provings (for example, www.nesh.com and www.dynamis.edu).

Provings were recently subjected to double-blind, placebo-controlled studies to ascertain the validity of the premise that biologically active substances in a homeopathic concentration of 30c (10^{-60}) can produce consistent symptoms that are clearly distinguished from placebo in healthy volunteers.[13–15] Interestingly, the reprovings of remedies that are well known in the homeopathic literature consistently show symptoms identical to descriptions in the original provings performed by Hahnemann and his team.[10,16]

Small Doses

Initially, Hahnemann prescribed remedies in the accepted (i.e., pharmacologic) dosages of the time. Many skeptics of homeopathy today incorrectly assume that Hahnemann and homeopathy were initially attacked for recommending doses of medicine too small to have any therapeutic benefit. However, for the first 20 years of his practice, Hahnemann primarily used medicinal doses that were only slightly diluted, commonly using the tincture of an herb or a 1:10 plant or mineral dose diluted two or three times. Hahnemann has never explained in writing why he diluted the remedies. One of the theories explaining his reason for dilutions suggests that he found that although patients improved in many cases, the drug often caused a severe initial aggravation of the symptoms. Such aggravation was to be expected because the drug itself was producing symptoms similar to those that had initially brought the patient to treatment. Still, it was understandably uncomfortable and alarming for the patients, and it precluded Hahnemann's ability to test (prove) some of the extremely toxic drugs in common use at that time, such as mercury and arsenic. He began reducing the doses by one-tenth and, as his patients continued to respond favorably even as their initial aggravations decreased in severity, Hahnemann continued to experiment with further 1:10 dilutions of previously diluted medicines. If there was a match within the framework of the principle of similars, the patient would be specifically sensitive to the remedy itself. As such, the doses necessary and sufficient to obtain a curative reaction were much lower than those needed to cause symptoms in healthy subjects. As he continued to strive for a subtler, less heroic healing action, Hahnemann further observed that progressive dilutions not only were less toxic but, paradoxically, more potent. According to another hypothesis, the early dilution procedures included vigorous shaking or "succussing" by hand in order to achieve complete homogenous dilution of the homeopathic medicine. Interestingly, contemporary experimental data suggest that succussion is an important step in the preservation of the biological activity of a highly diluted substance.[17,18]

The *Homeopathic Pharmacopeia of the United States*[19] is the official standard for the preparation of homeopathic medicines. Most are of plant origin, including flowers, leaves, roots, barks, and fruits. Although many are poisonous in their crude state, others are common medicinal herbs, foods, and spices. Homeopathy also uses preparations from minerals, venoms, secretions, milks, and hormones. Homeopathic medications have been incorporated in the Federal Food, Drug, and Cosmetic Act (FDCA) since 1938. Thus, homeopathic drug products are "drugs" as currently defined by US law. To date, close to 3,000 substances have been described in homeopathic literature.

The majority of homeopaths use two main types of dilutions: decimal (in increments 1:10) and centesimal (1:100). Each consecutive dilution is followed by vigorous shaking of the substance 20 to 40 times (vortex). This process is performed in modern homeopathic pharmacies that use sophisticated automated equipment. Table 12–1 explains the process of homeopathic dilutions.

Biological effects of high dilutions have been thoroughly investigated and described in numerous scientific publications. The most significant studies used the degranulation test on human basophils.[20–22] The first publications on the effect of high dilutions on basophils[23,24] reported that in vitro degranulation induced by various allergens was inhibited by high dilutions of bee venom (*Apis mellifica* 9c and 15c). Later studies[25,26] suggested as a possible mechanism of action the nonspecific blockade of immunoglobulin (Ig)E, the regulation of phospholipase activity, or the negative feedback of histamine on release. Results of a multicenter study under the guidance of Jacques Benveniste, conducted in collaboration with three laboratories in different countries, have indicated that human basophils are sensitive to infinitesimal doses of substances that are already known to have a stimulatory effect at ponderal doses, such as anti-IgE antibodies, calcium ionophores, and phospholipase A_2.[17] It was

▶ **TABLE 12–1** HOMEOPATHIC DILUTIONS

Centesimal		No. Succussions	Decimal	
Potency	Dilution		Potency	Dilution
1c	10^{-2}	100	1×	10^{-1}
2c	10^{-4}	200	2×	10^{-1}
3c	10^{-6}	300	3×	10^{-3}
6c	10^{-12}	600	6×	10^{-6}
12c	10^{-24}	1,200	24×	10^{-24}
30c	10^{-60}	3,000	30×	10^{-30}
200c	10^{-400}	20,000	200×	10^{-200}

also reported that to obtain maximum activity at the infinitesimal dilutions, the dilution process needed to be accompanied by vigorous succussion and that the stimulatory activity of the diluted and succussed antibody solutions persisted even after ultrafiltration. This study remains highly controversial, and the question of the biological mechanism of high dilutions remains unresolved. Bellavite and Signorini[18] recently summarized the in vitro research data on homeopathy, as well as data from animal models.

▶ THE HOMEOPATHIC EVALUATION

A homeopathic physician attempts to base a prescription on the unique characteristics of symptom patterns in a particular individual.[2,27,28] For example, two patients with tonsillitis might receive two different medications; one might have diffusely erythematous tonsils and an irritable mood, and the other might have a unilateral pustular presentation and an uncharacteristic sleepiness.

The homeopathic evaluation consists of the general medical examination with the standard organ/system review, but the complete evaluation moves significantly beyond these initial steps. The interview is structured to provide data necessary to match a unique symptomatologic picture of the patient with the characteristics of one of the remedies. The single most important factor in the evaluation is the chief complaint and the circumstances around it. Key points of the homeopathic interview are not dissimilar to a conventional history, but with much more detail. Key elements include:

1. *Mental/emotional* symptoms (i.e., mood, anxieties, and fears).
2. *Sensations* with concrete examples (e.g., burning as in hot or burning as in a chemical burn?)
3. *Location* of the symptom—The side of the body is also very important.

4. *Direction*—Does the symptom move or shift from one location to another?
5. *Concomitant symptoms*—What else is happening at the same time that the symptom is occurring? Underused in the majority of conventional medical approaches, this information is essential for a homeopath; it provides data that are unique to this particular individual.
6. *Modalities*—What makes the sensation occur, become worse or better? This can include temperature, position, food (or lack thereof), and time of day.
7. *Intensity*—Usually patients are asked to compare a present symptom to other symptoms they have had.
8. *Duration* of symptoms.
9. *Onset*—The actual date and time are very important. A symptom occurring late at night puts one in a different symptomatologic classification from one at 10 A.M.
10. *Sequence of events*—The circumstances before the patient experienced the symptom.

After taking the list of complaints as well as identifying important characteristics of the personality, lifestyle, and reactivity to emotional and physical events, the homeopath evaluates the case in its entirety. The homeopathic text on pharmacology, *Materia Medica,* is generally used to choose the appropriate remedy for the patient. This text[29–31] is based on the toxicology of the many substances in the homeopathic pharmacopeia elicited mainly in provings and descriptions of accidental poisoning. A cross-reference tool used for finding a group of remedies most closely corresponding to the symptomatologic complex presented by the patient is called a *repertory.*[32,33] Modern repertories are computerized and serve as a cross-reference tool allowing one to simultaneously search numerous databases.[34,35]

Frequently, the emerging clinical picture readily corresponds with the toxicologic picture of one of the common remedies (in homeopathic parlance they are called *polychrests*). However, such an "easy" match often is not immediately apparent. In that case, the homeopath *repertorizes* the case. Symptoms and physical findings are graded according to the level of importance and severity and are cross-referenced, using either print or computerized versions of the repertory. This analysis yields a list of remedies whose toxicologic picture closely corresponds to the case presented. A homeopath, using his or her knowledge of homeopathic toxicology, and sometimes after consulting one of numerous reference sources, then makes a final decision on the remedy to be prescribed.

Illustrative of the application of the method is the use of homeopathic preparations for treatment of fever. The "remedy-defining" qualities of each case are italicized in the following illustration. For example, the homeopathic remedy *Aconitum* (monkshood) is indicated when there is a *sudden* acute onset of fever or chills and fear with tremendous anxiety, agitation, restlessness, thirst, and *contracted pupils*. On the other hand, a patient who needs the homeopathic remedy *Belladonna* will present with the feeling of dry, burning heat without chills. The face and body will be warm to touch with icy cold extremities. The person may be delirious with hallucinations and photophobia, and sometimes will be experiencing twitching of the face and/or seizures. *The pupils are markedly dilated.* Importantly, both *Aconitum* and *Belladonna* can be applied in other clinical situations if the main presenting clinical picture is either of sudden severe panic, restlessness and fear (as in the use of *Aconitum* for a panic episode, especially caused by witnessing catastrophic events) or severe pain with redness, burning pain, and hot, red face with cold extremities (as in the use of *Belladonna* in case of acute otitis media).

► HOMEOPATHY TRAINING AND CERTIFICATION

Training

While in other countries homeopathic training and certification have been available for decades, the United States has not had full-time homeopathic schools or accredited professional education for more than 40 years. In the United States, homeopathy was taught in homeopathic medical schools beginning in the mid-nineteenth century. In 1900, there were 22 such schools, but by 1923—as a consequence of the Flexner report—there were only two.[6] The last homeopathic medical school in the United States (the homeopathic part of Hahnemann Medical School) was closed in 1949. Currently, there are general courses for consumers and professionals at various homeopathic schools in the United States that offer their own certificates. A number of these courses are reasonably comprehensive. However, there is currently no formal academic continuing medical education training in homeopathy in the United States.

Since homeopathy's inception, Europe has provided much of the impetus for homeopathy's research and use. Because of the public's interest, the European Parliament, in 1996, issued a mandate to the European Commission to examine whether homeopathy is beneficial. The subsequent report of the Commission's Homeopathy Medicine Research Group recommended that homeopathy be integrated into medical practice. Concordant with these recommendations, in January 1998, the French *Conseil National de l'Ordre des Medecins* (the equivalent of the American Medical Association) called for official recognition of homeopathy, accompanied by inclusion of homeopathy training in the undergraduate medical curriculum and the creation of a postgraduate degree.[36] Concurrently, a British commission, formed by the Prince of Wales to examine the possible integration of complementary health care into conventional medical practice, called for education and training in various complementary and alternative disciplines, including homeopathy, and for integrating their delivery into mainstream health care.[37] Prior to this, the Glasgow Homeopathic Hospital was already a part of the National Health Service of Great Britain.

Certification

Three states—Arizona, Nevada, and Connecticut—have implemented a process of certification of medical professionals practicing homeopathy. The American Board of Homeotherapeutics (ABH) has implemented a voluntary certification process that includes a written multiple-choice examination, an oral examination, a videotaped interview, and 10 case reports. A person can be admitted to examination only after completion of a required curriculum and clinical supervision. Physicians and osteopaths who meet the requirements of the ABH and the American Institute of Homeopathy (AIH) are awarded a title of Doctor of Homeopathy (DHt). As of this date, this certification process has not been recognized by US medical boards.

▶ CLINICAL OUTCOMES RESEARCH

Although there are many methodological challenges in research on the clinical effects of homeopathy—specifically the challenge of applying a randomized double-blind approach to a discipline that requires sophisticated individualized prescribing to be effective—there are a number of well-done studies of homeopathic interventions for specific conditions. Diagnoses studied to date include otitis media in children, allergic rhinitis, acute diarrheal syndromes, asthma, depression, and many others; where high-quality trials exist, they are included in the discussion of the specific conditions found elsewhere in this text.

To date, two meta-analyses of the clinical effects of homeopathy have been published.[38,39] A 1991 review by Kleinjnen at al. assessed 107 controlled trials in 96 published reports. Overall, of the 105 trials with interpretable results, 81 trials indicated positive results versus 24 trials in which no positive effects of homeopathy were found. In studies judged to have better research designs, 15 trials showed positive results, whereas in 7 trials, no positive results

could be detected. A more recent review by Linde at al.[39] assessed 186 double-blind and/or randomized trials, of which 119 met the inclusion criteria and 89 had adequate data for meta-analysis. The combined odds ratio was 2.45 in favor of homeopathy. The odds ratio for the 26 good-quality studies was 1.66, and when corrected for estimated publication bias, the ratio remained about the same (1.78). A detailed analysis of current research data can be found elsewhere.[7,18]

▶ PRACTICAL APPLICATIONS OF HOMEOPATHIC REMEDIES IN ACUTE CONDITIONS

Homeopathic pharmacotherapy offers the highly desirable advantage of differential therapeutics. Two different patients presenting within the same "conventional" diagnostic category may be prescribed two different homeopathic remedies based on the differences in their symptoms and various individual characteristics. Because of the complexity engendered by this individualized approach to prescribing, one needs to study homeopathy in depth for several years in order to apply homeopathic remedies effectively for treatment of most chronic conditions. According to homeopathic theory, effective treatment of a chronic illness requires sophisticated long-term treatment called "constitutional prescribing." It demands a high level of clinical and theoretical sophistication and requires extensive knowledge of homeopathic philosophy and pharmacology combined with clinical postgraduate training. Constitutional prescribing is outside of the scope of this chapter. On the other hand, prescribing for "true acutes" is more straightforward and may be learned in a significantly shorter format. This chapter introduces a few relatively simple homeopathic solutions for various acute conditions.

Homeopaths distinguish very clearly between acute and chronic illnesses. A so-called "true acute" is defined as a new, never experienced before, usually self-limiting condition.

For example, a person who suffered a traumatic injury will be considered presenting with an acute condition. On the other hand, a patient with history of repeated trauma may be approached as a person with a chronic condition. A single episode of otitis will be qualified as an acute condition. But if a child presents with frequent episodes of otitis media, (even if each of the episodes is accompanied by high fever and pain), the case will be treated as chronic. An acute exacerbation of eczema is still a part of the chronic illness according to homeopathic theory. I strongly advise against applying the data presented in this chapter for treatment of chronic conditions. Patients with chronic conditions should be referred to experienced homeopathic practitioners.

"Classical Homeopathy" versus Homeopathic Polypharmacy

Almost since the inception of homeopathy in the eighteenth century, a large group of physicians rooted in the conventional practice of polypharmacy and other "heroic" intrusive methods of treatment insisted on using combinations of various homeopathic remedies for treatment of particular diseases. The very same concept that Hahnemann fought in all his major writings was brought back under the flag of homeopathy. The term "classical homeopathy" was coined to distinguish Hahnemann's approach from the use of combination remedies and homeopathic polypharmacology. This polypharmacy approach, often called "homeopatherapeutics," is currently most popular in France. Both homeopathic "campuses" offer evidence-based research data to support the validity of their approach.[38–41]

Although this controversy between single remedies and combination approaches continues, there may be a role for both in practical homeopathic therapeutics. The combination homeopathic remedies are a result of an attempt to eliminate a need for a thorough homeopathic evaluation by combining the majority of

organ and pathology-specific remedies in one preparation. Some of these preparations can offer a substantial temporary relief for various self-limiting conditions. A number of the combination preparations have been studied in double-blind, placebo-controlled studies, with positive results reported for some indications.[40,41] The most popular and efficacious combination remedies are designed for the temporary relief of teething problems, baby colic, uncomplicated cough, vertigo, acute seasonal allergies, and uncomplicated cold/flu. Major reputable suppliers of combination and single homeopathic remedies in the United States can be found on various websites (e.g., www. HomeopathyHome.net).

The practitioner considering the use of a combination homeopathic must keep in mind one very important point. None of the combination remedies can provide a complete long-term alleviation of symptoms. This is especially true for treatment of chronic conditions. In fact, long-term (beyond 10–14 days) use of these preparations may cause a significant exacerbation of the illness. Many homeopathic practitioners feel that because of this potential for exacerbation, administration of combination remedies for chronic conditions, such as asthma or eczema—as opposed to acute conditions—is contraindicated.

Guidelines for Acute Prescribing

Basic Rules

Defining what is a "true acute" and what is an acute exacerbation of chronic illness is not a trivial issue in homeopathy. As outlined above, this distinction is critical, as the treatment approach to these two situations is very different. A *true acute* condition is usually characterized by prominent new symptoms. Usually the patient has never experienced these symptoms before. A very simple example of a true acute is an insect bite or acute trauma. An *acute exacerbation of chronic illness* characteristically contains old symptoms that are amplified as a result of various etiologic factors. For example, two patients may present with cough as a symptom. In one case, cough may be a part of the complex of symptoms of the acute exacerbation of asthma, in another it could be a part of the picture of croup or acute bronchitis. Another example is the distinction between a person presenting with habitual bruising—chronic condition—and one presenting with severe bruises as a consequence of plastic surgery or trauma. In some cases, the differences are not so obvious. For example, a true acute otitis and an acute exacerbation of chronic otitis media could be difficult to distinguish. The difference between true acutes and acute exacerbations must be considered prior to the initiation of homeopathic treatment.

Also important to consider in acute prescribing is the promptness of response to the homeopathic medication. Acute conditions respond to correctly prescribed homeopathic medication in minutes, sometimes hours. A child with fever of 103°F will feel better and will typically fall asleep in about 10–30 minutes after the administration of the correct homeopathic remedy. The lack of significant improvement of target symptoms shortly after the administration of the first dose of the homeopathic remedy usually indicates a need to reassess the patient in order to find another remedy. Chaotic administration of remedies without the sufficient data for the prescription should be avoided. A lack of improvement after a maximum of two to three various homeopathic remedies administered should indicate the need to abort any further attempts to treat with homeopathic remedies. Other means of treatment must be employed.

On the other hand, if the initial significant improvement of target symptoms is followed by the deterioration of the patient's condition a few hours after the administration of the first dose, the remedy should be repeated. A prompt improvement after an additional single dose of the homeopathic remedy ensues. The lack of a prompt response to the second dose of the remedy in this situation usually indicates a need to reassess the patient.

For acute prescribing in general, the use of remedies in 30c potency is recommended. Use of homeopathic remedies in higher potencies will be indicated for selected conditions/ remedies.

A final basic rule of both acute and chronic homeopathic prescribing is never to base the choice of a remedy on a *lack* of symptoms. If three or more very important symptoms requiring a particular remedy are present and the rest of the symptoms listed are not, it should not prevent a prescriber from choosing this remedy. For example, if a child has a very high fever and hot flushed face, glassy eyes with enlarged pupils, and seems to be delirious, but the extremities are also warm, *Belladonna* is most probably still indicated (for more details see a description of *Belladonna* in "Influenza and Colds" below). Presence of one of very characteristic symptoms (e.g., craving for lemonade, or glassy eyes, or face hot–extremities cold) confirms the prescription with other symptoms requiring the same remedy present.

SPECIFIC ACUTE CONDITIONS

Trauma and Surgery

Arnica montana (Mountain Arnica)
Arnica is the most important remedy for trauma and bruises. *Arnica* is frequently indicated in cases when trauma causes combined injury to skin, muscles, and bones. Blunt trauma, surgical trauma, traumatic tooth extraction, and birth trauma (to both mother and infant) are all appropriate indications. In severe trauma, for example, severe industrial accidents or serious motor vehicle accidents, *Arnica* 10M (a very high potency) should be given as soon as possible. In all other situations one dose of *Arnica* 200c is usually sufficient. External *Arnica* preparations (ointment, gel, and tincture) should never be used on nonintact skin.

Characteristic symptoms warranting use of *Arnica* include the following:

- Marked soreness, feeling as if bitten, tender to touch and pressure; bed feels too hard
- Worse: touch, pressure, slight movement
- Better: lying down with the head low, outstretched; sitting erect
- Emotional: frequently think they are fine and do not need any help; want solitude
- Mental and physical shock; restlessness after trauma

Specific conditions include the following:

- "Black eyes" from blows
- Loss of vision after injury, retinal hemorrhage, hyphemia
- Blows to the ear, posttraumatic nosebleeds
- Bruising after plastic surgery (e.g., rhinoplasty)
- Dental extractions with significant trauma and pronounced soreness
- Orthopedic surgery and other types of surgery where the trauma is significant
- Traumatic labor and delivery
- Muscular soreness after excessive exercise or exertion

BELLIS PERENNIS (COMMON DAISY OR LAWN DAISY)

Indicated for deep trauma and bruises, abdominal or pelvic trauma and surgery and deep muscle injuries.

Characteristic symptoms warranting use of *Bellis perennis* include the following:

- Frequently proximal lymphatic nodes become enlarged a few days after trauma
- Pain is better from cold applications

Specific conditions include the following:

- Blunt trauma to abdomen or pelvis with possible organ contusion
- Surgery with trauma to soft organs
- Traumatic arthritis

BRYONIA ALBA (WHITE BRYONY)

Indicated for any type of trauma to any type of tissue, but the most frequently encountered clinical situation is trauma to bone structures, including fracture.

Characteristic symptoms warranting use of *Bryonia* include the following:

- Severe exacerbation of pain after even a slightest movement
- Must lie still
- Better from firm pressure and from lying on the injured part

LEDUM (LABRADOR TEA)

Frequently indicated for large bruises or hematomas, such as in fractures.

Characteristic symptoms warranting use of *Ledum* include the following:

- Marked, pitting edema
- Injured areas are cold, at times icy cold, to touch
- Worse from heat or warm applications
- Better from ice or ice cold applications; the patient refuses to remove the cold
- Purplish, mottled discoloration remains long after the injury

RUTA (RUE)

Indicated for bruises to periosteum and areas where the bone structure is close to the surface, for injuries to joints or cartilage, and specifically for injuries of tendons.

Characteristic symptoms warranting use of *Ruta* include the following:

- Worse from lying on the painful side (compare to *Bryonia*)
- Worse from sitting or lying in general
- Better from continued motion, but worse on the first motion

OTHER REMEDIES FOR SELECTED TRAUMA-RELATED CONDITIONS

Millefolium (common yarrow)—specific remedy for falling from a height. Trauma resulting is hemorrhages—nose, lungs, rectum, etc. Pulmonary contusion and hemoptysis. Blunt trauma to the torso.

Aconitum (monkshood)—trauma accompanied by great fright or terror.

Cantharis (Spanish fly)—severe (second and third degree) burns. Useful in cases in which the burning seems to be much improved by cold applications. Patient categorically refuses to remove the cold pack even for a brief moment. Burns to mucous membranes, including chemical or electric burns.

Conium (poison hemlock)—injuries and contusions to glands such as the testes and breasts.

Hamamelis (witch hazel)—specific remedy for bleeding inside the eye after trauma.

Hypericum (St. John's wort)—injuries to areas with the high concentration of pain receptors, that is, the fingers, genitalia, and tongue. Crushing injuries to fingertips.

Sanguinaria (bloodroot)—specific remedy for pain in the top of the right shoulder, right-sided deltoid pain. Worse from motion. Much worse at night. Better from swinging the arm.

Strontium carbonicum (carbonate of strontia)—sprained ankle. Repeated twists and sprains of ankle.

Symphytum (comfrey)—specific remedy for blunt trauma to the eyeball (not the orbit). Nonunion of fractures.

Croup

ACONITUM (MONKSHOOD)

Useful in the first hours of the illness. If the patient is brought to the office on the second (or later) day of the illness, *Aconitum* is usually not indicated. Children and adults who require *Aconitum* are usually strong and healthy and develop strong reactions to infections with much heat and movement.

Characteristic symptoms warranting use of *Aconitum* include the following:

- Sudden onset that is frequently accompanied by fear and restlessness.

- Croup often begins after the exposure to cold, most frequently to a combination of dry cold and wind.
- The patient awakes from the first part of sleep with dry, barking cough.
- Stridor and suffocative cough accompanied by fear, terror. The child clings to parents.
- Symptoms worse on inspiration and after drinking (compare to *Spongia tosta*).
- No mucus present.

SPONGIA TOSTA (TOASTED SPONGE)

This is generally the most frequently indicated remedy in later stages (more than 24 hours) of croup.

Characteristic symptoms warranting use of *Spongia tosta* include the following:

- Dry, barking cough, like the sound of the saw going through wood. Some authors describe it as a "seal's bark."
- Stridor with noisy, whistling sounds.
- Worse at midnight, or immediately after. Much worse from cold air or cold drinks.
- Better with warm drinks or food, including nursing. Better when sitting upright or bent forward. Better with head bent forward (compare to *Hepar Sulphuris*).

HEPAR SULPHURIS

Hepar sulphuris calcareum is a complex preparation of potassium salts.

The patient is very irritable and cannot tolerate even minimal discomfort; often parents will report that child will scream at the slightest provocation.

Characteristic symptoms warranting use of *Hepar sulphuris* include the following:

- Croup comes on frequently between 2 and 4 A.M. or toward morning.
- Worse from being uncovered, or becoming even slightly cold.
- Better from throwing the head backward (compare to *Spongia tosta*).
- Thick, rattling mucus.

Influenza and Colds

Effective homeopathic treatment of flu and colds is possible but it is also complicated and requires skillful prescribing. A few frequently indicated remedies are described below. There are two generally indicated remedies for influenza and colds. The first is *Anas barbariae hepatis et cordis extractum 200c,* which is better known as *Oscillococcinum* (Boiron) or *Flu Solution* (Dolisos). It has been used for more than 65 years and has been evaluated in double-blind, placebo-controlled studies with positive outcome.[42] This remedy appears to be most efficacious in treatment of early stages of flu and common colds. A dose should be taken at the earliest onset of symptoms and repeated every 6 hours until symptoms resolve. The prophylactic value of this remedy is unclear. Many patients claim that taking a dose a day during the flu epidemic has been efficacious as a prophylactic measure.

The second remedy is *Influenzinum 9c.* Claims of a prophylactic value have been made for this remedy. In some countries, patients routinely take three to five pellets a day during the flu epidemic as a prophylactic measure. No research data is available.

The following are specific remedies for cold and flu.

ARSENICUM ALBUM (ARSENIC OXIDE)
Arsenicum Album is used to treat influenza or common cold accompanied by gastroenteritis, vomiting, and diarrhea. Unlike *Aconitum, Arsenicum Album* is indicated when there is a prodrome. Gastrointestinal complaints are usually prominent in the case.

Characteristic symptoms warranting use of *Arsenicum Album* include the following:

- High fever (up to 104°F) after a few days of prodrome. Fever may be followed by chill and rigors.
- Face is hot, and the patient craves open air and cold applications to the head and face yet the body is cold or chilled, and better from warmth.

- Thirsty for small sips of water (compare to *Bryonia*).
- Significant restlessness with weakness and a tendency to collapse.
- Significant anxiety with fear of dying from this illness (compare to *Aconitum*). Wants company at all times (compare to *Bryonia*).
- Worse around midnight or 1 A.M., or around noon or 1 P.M.

BRYONIA ALBA (WHITE BRYONY)
Muscular ache is an important symptom. Influenza tends to be slow in progressing. The key characteristic is desire to be absolutely still; patients tend to feel much worse from the slightest movement.

Characteristic symptoms warranting use of *Bryonia* include the following:

- Fever with the pronounced sensation of heat. Profuse perspiration.
- Chills begin distally (fingertips, toes, rarely the lips). Chills can be triggered by anger.
- Feel restless internally but cannot tolerate even the slightest motion.
- Very thirsty for large gulps of water at intervals (compare to *Arsenicum*).
- Severe frontal left-sided or occipital headaches.
- Generally symptoms are worse on the right side (except for the headache, which is left-sided).
- Irritable, averse to answering questions, and wants to be left alone (compare to *Arsenicum*).
- Worse generally around 9 P.M. Also worse from the slightest motion (as opposed to patients who need *Aconitum,* who have to move, and are generally restless).
- Patients are usually warm and feel worse in a warm room.

BELLADONNA
Any type of acute illness (including colds and flu) with rapid onset and extremely high (up to 105°F) fever, especially if accompanied by delirious state. A very commonly indicated rem-

edy for children with high fever. Compare to *Aconitum* (onset is also sudden, but the patient is very frightened and restless).

Key symptom is a flushed, red, face. Head is hot to touch, but hands and/or feet are cold. Combined with a few other characteristic symptoms, this symptom strongly confirms a need for *Belladonna*.

Characteristic symptoms warranting use of *Belladonna* include the following:

- Very high fevers.
- Delirium.
- Face is flushed, pupils are dilated (compare to *Aconitum* where the pupils are constricted).
- Craves lemons and, frequently, lemonade.
- Frequently severe right-sided headache (compare to *Bryonia* where the headache is left-sided).
- Headache is pounding; better in a dark, quiet room.
- Frequently right-sided sore throat or eye pain.
- Symptoms are frequently aggravated around 3 P.M.
- The patients may present with rapidly developing delirium or hallucinations (compare to *Baptisia tinctoria*).

BAPTISIA TINCTORIA (WILD INDIGO)

This is a relatively minor remedy. One of the very important symptoms is delirium with a sensation that the patient's body is broken into pieces or double. Advanced influenza with mental dullness or even stupor. Patient might fall asleep in the middle of the sentence. Tongue and pharynx are dry, can be suppurating with very offensive odor. Interestingly, they remain painless.

EUPATORIUM PERFOLIATUM (BONESET)

Frequently required in patients with severe, unbearable aching. The key symptom is terrible aching of bones; feels as if "the bones would break open."

Characteristic symptoms warranting use of *Eupatorium perfoliatum* include the following:

- Influenza with high fever (usually over 102°F) and severe, unbearable aching.
- Chills begin in the lumbar area and spread up the spine.
- Chills are worse after drinking.
- The patient is very chilly and sensitive to cold air.
- Thirst for cold drinks despite the chill (frequently during the chill).
- Desire cold food and ice cream.
- Restless from the pain, but motion does not ameliorate.
- Worse generally from 7 to 9 A.M.

GELSEMIUM (TRUMPET FLOWER)

Illness characterized by marked debility, weakness, and sleepiness. The onset of the fever is slow, over at least 24 hours to several days. The key symptom is pronounced weakness with trembling and heaviness of the extremities, eyelids, and head.

Characteristic symptoms warranting use of *Gelsemium* include the following:

- Chills running up and down the spine
- Chills that alternate with heat flushes
- Chills accompanied by fine tremors
- Minimal thirst
- Extreme sleepiness
- Head is very heavy
- Eyelids are half-shot or droopy
- Symptoms are aggravated around 10 A.M.
- The patient is somewhat depressed, feels dull

RHUS TOXICODENDRON (POISON IVY)

Influenza with aching and restlessness. The key symptoms are aches and pains that are ameliorated by constant movement. Aching of muscles and joints, which are worse with cold and better with heat.

Characteristic symptoms warranting use of *Rhus toxicodendron* include the following:

- Significant aching throughout the whole body.
- Very pronounced stiffness which makes the patient want to stretch.

- Chilly. Most of the complaints are much better from warm baths, applications, or drinks.
- Anxiety and restlessness in the patient with influenza.

Acute Otitis Media

Preliminary clinical research on use of homeopathy for otitis media seems to indicate that it can be effective in treatment of this condition.[43] Particularly given the current trend toward watchful waiting in treatment of otitis media, a familiarity with some of the commonly used homeopathics for this condition can be very helpful to the practitioner.

PULSATILLA (PASQUE FLOWER)
A frequently indicated remedy for this condition. The key symptoms are that the child is weepy, needs affection, and wants to be carried slowly and tenderly (compare with *Chamomilla*).

Characteristic symptoms warranting use of *Pulsatilla* include the following:

- Frequently high fever with pale face (compare to *Belladonna*).
- The illness begins with a "cold," frequently with thick green or yellow nasal discharge that develops into otitis media.
- Painful fullness or bursting sensation, usually in the left ear.
- Ear feels stopped with pulsating sensation or noises.
- Pain may extend to face and teeth.
- Changeable condition: one moment the child is very sick, the next moment playing, looks much improved.
- No thirst despite a very high fever.
- Worse with heat and at night.
- Better in the open and with cool air.
- The child is timid, weepy, whining pitifully (compare to *Chamomilla*), and wants attention and sympathy.

CHAMOMILLA (GERMAN CHAMOMILE)
Very frequently indicated in acute otitis in infants and toddlers. The key symptoms are that the child is unbearably irritable, screaming, and demanding, typically wanting to be carried at all times. Very disruptive in the waiting room (compare to *Pulsatilla*).

Characteristic symptoms warranting use of *Chamomilla* include the following:

- Exceptionally painful otitis; the patient is very sensitive to any pain.
- Frequently, one cheek is red and hot and the other is pale and cold.
- Inclined to arch backward.
- Worse from touching the ear; resists the ear examination.
- Better from being carried. Demands to be carried with the caregiver moving. Has a tantrum if put down (compare to *Pulsatilla*).

BELLADONNA
Sudden onset (compare to *Ferrum Phosphoricum*) of severe pulsating pain, especially on the right side. The key symptoms are a hot, flushed face with cold hands and/or feet.

Characteristic symptoms warranting use of *Belladonna* include the following:

- Very high (over 103°F) fever, glassy, glistening eyes, dilated pupils.
- Tympanic membrane is bright red, injected, and bulging.
- Worse at night, after midnight or at 3 P.M. Worse with even a slight jarring (compare to *Chamomilla*, in which patient wants to be carried all the time, and is worse when the caregiver stops).
- Better with warm wraps (compare to *Pulsatilla*, which is better from cold).
- Craves lemonade, but can be thirstless.
- The child is excited, frequently delirious with fever.

FERRUM PHOSPHORICUM (PHOSPHATE OF IRON)
Otitis media with a severe pain and high (usually over 103°F) fever. The key symptom is an acute situation that clearly requires treatment, but the patient presents no obvious modalities

and the illness sets in not as rapidly as in belladonna.

HEPAR SULPHURIS

Challenging to differentiate from *Chamomilla*. The key symptoms are that the patient is very sensitive to pain and screams from the pain, hates to be touched, and does not like to be moved or carried (compare to *Chamomilla*).

Characteristic symptoms warranting use of *Hepar sulphuris* include the following:

- Better from wrapping the ear, warmth.
- Must be well covered.
- Screams in pain even from a slightest attempt to uncover.

CONCLUSION

Homeopathy together with other modalities have been gaining a significant momentum among consumers in the United States. According to various sources, sales of homeopathic remedies double every year. On the other hand, the majority of medical professionals remain skeptical about homeopathy despite the growing body of scientific evidence of its efficacy. More well-designed large clinical studies and better education are the key to the future integration of homeopathy in the daily practice of physicians and other licensed professionals.

REFERENCES

1. Hahnemann S. Essay on a new principle for ascertaining the curative powers of drugs, and some examinations of the previous principles. *Hufeland J* 1796;2:391–439, 465–561.
2. Hahnemann S. *Organon of Medicine*. Kunzli J, Naude A, Pendleton P, trans. Blaine, Washington: Cooper Publishing; 1996:97–120.
3. Panos MB, Heimlich J. *Homeopathic Medicine at Home*. New York: Tarcher/Putnam; 1980.
4. Kruzel T. *The Homeopathic Emergency Guide*. Berkeley, CA: North Atlantic Books; 1992.
5. Morrison R. *Desktop Companion to Physical Pathology*. Nevada City, CA: Hahnemann Clinic Publishing; 1998.
6. Eskinazi D. Homeopathy re-revisited: is homeopathy compatible with biomedical observations? *Arch Intern Med.* 1999;159:1981–1987.
7. Merrell WC, Shalts E. Homeopathy. *Med Clin North Am.* 2002;86:47–62.
8. Herscu P, ed. *Provings*. Vol. I. *An Annotated Selection of Historic and Contemporary Writings*. Amherst, MA: New England School of Homeopathy Press; 2002.
9. Riley D, Seipt A, Zagon A. *Homeopathic Drug Proving Journal*. Santa Fe, NM: CTA Publishing; 1994.
10. Bellows HP. *The Test Drug Proving of the OO&L Society. A Reproving of Belladonna*. Boston: OO&L Society; 1906.
11. Sherr J. *Dinamic Provings*. Vol. 1. Malvern, Worcestern, England: Dynamis Books; 1997.
12. Herscu P. The proving of alcoholus. In: Herscu P, ed. *Provings*. Vol I. *An Annotated Selection of Historic and Contemporary Writings*. Amherst, MA: New England School of Homeopathy Press; 2002:143–320.
13. Shalts E. A double-blind placebo-controlled pilot study of the validity of provings as a method of finding pathogenic characteristics of homeopathic remedies. In: Herscu P, ed. *Provings*. Vol. II. *An Annotated Selection of Historic and Contemporary Writings*. Amherst, MA: New England School of Homeopathy Press; 2002:401–417.
14. Shalts E, Hoover TA, Herscu P. An investigation into the utility of placebo in provings. can a homeopath discern remedy from placebo? *Am J Homeopathic Med.* 2003;96(1):37–42.
15. Herscu P, Shalts E. Testing a novel experimental approach to proving studies. *Am J Homeopathic Med.* 2003;96(1):44–49.
16. Vieira GR. Clinical proving in Brasilia. *Eur J Classical Homeopathy.* 1996;2(7–8):35–42.
17. Davenas E, Beauvais F, Amara J, et al. Human basophil degranulation triggered by very dilute antiserum against IgE. *Nature.* 1988;333:816–818.
18. Bellavite P, Signorini A. *The Emerging Science of Homeopathy*. Berkeley, CA: North Atlantic Books; 2002.
19. *Homeopathic Pharmacopeia of the United States*. Washington, DC: American Institute of Homeopathy; 1979.
20. Benveniste J. The human basophil degranulation test as an in vitro method for the diagnosis of allergies. *Clin Allergy.* 1981;11:1.

21. Sainte-Laudy J. Standardisation of basophil degranulation for pharmacological studies. *J Immunol Methods*. 1987;98:279.

22. Cherruault Y, Guillez A, Sainte-Laudy J, Belon Ph. Etude mathematique et statistique des effets de dilutions successives de chlorhydrate d'histamine sur la réactivité des basophiles humains. *Biosciences*. 1989;7:63.

23. Poitevin B, Aubin M, Benveniste J. Effect d'Apis Mellifica sur la degranulation des basophiles humains in vitro. *Homéopathie Francaise*. 1985;73:193.

24. Poitevin B, Aubin M, Benveniste J. Approche d'une analyse quantitative de l'effet d'apis mellifica sur la degranulation des basophiles humains in vitro. *Innov Tech Biol Med*. 1986;7:64.

25. Poitevin B, Davenas E, Benveniste J. In vitro ommunological degranulation of human basophils is modulated by Lung histamine and Apis mellifica. *Br J Clin Pharmacol*. 1988;25:439.

26. ZDN (Zentrum zur Dokumentation für Naturheilverfahren). Poitevin B. Scientific bases of homeopathy. In: *Homeopathy in Focus*. Essen, Germany: VGM Verlag fur Ganzheitmedizin; 1990:42.

27. Vithoulkas G. *The Science of Homeopathy*. New York: Grove Press; 1980.

28. Rowe T. *Homeopathic Methodology*. Berkeley, CA: North Atlantic Books; 1998.

29. Kent JT. *Materia Medica of Homoeopathic Remedies*. London: Homoeopathic Book Service; 1989.

30. Boericke W. *Pocket Manual of Homoeopathic Materia Medica*. Santa Rosa, CA: Boericke & Tafel; 1927.

31. Vermeulen F. *Concordant Materia Medica*. Haarlem, The Netherlands: Emryss bv Publishers; 1997.

32. Kent JT. *Repertory of the Homoeopathic Materia Medica*. London: Homoeopathic Book Service; 1990.

33. Schroyens F, ed. *Synthesis. Repertorium Homeopathicum Syntheticum*. London: Homoeopathic Book Service; 1998.

34. *Radar*. Assesse, Belgium: Archibel SA.

35. *MacRepertory*. San Rafael, CA: Kent Homeopathic Associates.

36. Nau JY. Le Conseil de l'ordre des medecins reclame une reconnaissance officielle de l'homeopathie. *Le Monde*. February 13, 1998:10.

37. Foundation for Integrated Medicine (on behalf of the steering committee for the Prince of Wales's Initiative on Integrated Medicine, London, England: *Integrated Health Care: A Way Forward for the Next Five Years*). London: Foundation for Integrated Medicine; 1997.

38. Kleinjnen J, Knipschild P, ter Riet G. Clinical trials of homeopathy. *BMJ*. 1991; 302:316–23.

39. Linde K, Clausius N, Ramirez G, et al. Are the clinical effects of homeopathy placebo effects? A meta-analysis of placebo-controlled trials. *Lancet*. 1997;350:834–843.

40. Weiser M, Strosser W, Klein P. Homeopathic vs conventional treatment of vertigo: a randomized double-blind controlled clinical study. *Arch Otolaryngol Head Neck Surg*. 1998;124(8):879–885.

41. Oberbaum M, Yaniv I, Ben-Gal Y, et al. A randomized, controlled clinical trial of the homeopathic medication TRAUMEEL S in the treatment of chemotherapy-induced stomatitis in children undergoing stem cell transplantation. *Cancer*. 2001;92(3):684–690.

42. Vickers AJ, Smith C. Homoeopathic Oscillococcinum for preventing and treating influenza and influenza-like syndromes [review]. *Cochrane Database Syst Rev*. 2000;(2):CD001957.

43. Jacobs J, Springer DA, Crothers D. Homeopathic treatment of acute otitis media in children: a preliminary randomized placebo-controlled trial. *Pediatr Infect Dis J*. 2001;20(2):177–183.

CHAPTER 13

Physical Activity and Exercise

ROBERT B. LUTZ

All parts of the body that have a function, if used in moderation, and exercised in labors to which each is accustomed, become healthy and well developed and age slowly; but if unused and left idle, they become liable to disease, defective in growth and age quickly. This is especially so with joints and ligaments if one does not use them.

HIPPOCRATES

mens sano in corpore sano
(a sound mind in a sound body)

▶ INTRODUCTION

In spite of overwhelming evidence supporting the link between physical activity and health, Americans are becoming more sedentary. Statistics suggest that more than 60% of American adults currently fail to meet the US Surgeon General's recommendations.[1] It is stated that the single greatest contributor to this rise in inactivity is society itself; there is increasingly less need to be active as we focus on energy-saving devices in the home and the workplace, while built environments discourage walking and cycling in favor of the car.

Health promotion practices are fundamental to integrative medicine, as emphasis is placed upon living "healthy lifestyles." Physical activity is a component of such a style of living. In this regard, practitioners should seek to create opportunities for individuals to be "naturally active," in contrast to relying upon the formulaic exercise prescription that has historically served as the medical community's approach to exercise and physical activity. Research supports this shift in emphasis, as lifestyle-focused physical activity has been demonstrated to provide health benefits comparable to traditional exercise recommendations and, importantly, increases the likelihood of behavior change.

Health, and the determinants of this construct, are dynamic. They necessarily reflect the situations and context of the individual and change throughout an individual's life course. Consequently, discussion about "lifestyle" physical activity represents a dynamic process that seeks different approaches based upon an individual's stage in life (childhood, adulthood, senior) and the social context in which they reside.

▶ THE BURDEN OF PHYSICAL INACTIVITY

There are few things more natural than being active. From birth, activity is a natural part of our being. Yet as we age, activity becomes less natural. Rather, physical activity, for many of us, becomes a chore, something to check off on our "to-do list." With a focus on convenience and energy-saving devices, modernity has served to eliminate activity from our daily lives.

In some ways, "The major barrier to physical activity is the age in which we live. In the past, most activities of daily living involved significant expenditures of energy. In contrast, the overarching goal of modern technology has been to reduce this expenditure through the production of devices and services explicitly designed to obviate physical labor."[1] However, this comes at a cost. As seen in Table 13–1, convenience saving is activity lost.

Research, much of which dates back only to the 1980s, has identified the health-related benefits of physical activity. These benefits are undisputed. Much of this work has focused on the cardiovascular effects of aerobic exercise. Other identified benefits include improved muscular strength, flexibility and agility, increased bone density, improved lipid profiles, enhanced immune function, and improved insulin levels.[1] Physical activity reduces the risks for a number of chronic conditions, including cardiovascular disease, ischemic stroke, type 2 diabetes, colon cancer, osteoporosis, depression and anxiety, and fall-related injuries.[2] In 1996, *The Surgeon General's Report on Physical Activity and Health* summarized the findings to date and called for "commitment to healthy physical activity on all levels: personal, family, community, organizational, and national."

Every American should accumulate 30 minutes or more of moderate-intensity physical activity on most, preferably all, days of the week. . . . Adults who engage in moderate-intensity physical activity, i.e., enough to expend 200 Calories per day, can expect many of the health benefits described herein. . . . [O]ne way to meet this standard is to walk 2 miles briskly. . . . Most adults do not currently meet the standard described.[3]

▶ **TABLE 13–1** ENERGY EXPENDITURE FOR INACTIVE VERSUS ACTIVE LIVING

Inactive	kcal	Active	kcal
Using a garage door opener	<1	Lifting a garage door twice per day	2–3
Waiting for pizza delivery (30 minutes)	15	Cooking for 30 minutes	25
Using a leaf blower for 30 minutes	100	Raking leaves for 30 minutes	150
Using a lawn service	0	Gardening and mowing, each for 30 minutes per week	360
Putting the dog in the yard	2	Walking the dog for 30 minutes	125
Taking an elevator three flights	0.3	Walking up three flights of stairs	15
Parking as close as possible, 10-second walk	0.3	Parking in first spot, walk 2-minutes, 5 times per week	8
Shopping on line for 1 hour	30	Shopping at mall, walking for 1 hour	145–240
Paying for gas at the pump	0.6	Walking into the gas station to pay	5

Source: Adapted with permission from Blair SN, Nichaman MZ. The public health problem of increasing prevalence rates of obesity and what should be done about it. Mayo Clin Proc. 2002;77(2):109–113.

Despite these recommendations, Americans remain sedentary. Currently, 25% of adults report performing the recommended levels of physical activity; 29% report no leisure-time regular physical activity; and only 27% of high school students engage in the currently recommended levels of activity.[1] The increase in physical inactivity correlates with increases in many chronic diseases, including cardiovascular disease, stroke, type 2 diabetes mellitus, and some forms of cancer. Obesity, as a product of an imbalance of energy intake (diet) and energy expenditure (activity), is now recognized to be of "epidemic" proportions. The Surgeon General's *Call to Action to Prevent and Decrease Overweight and Obesity 2001* recognizes that an estimated 300,000 deaths per year might be attributable to obesity.[5,6]

In 1992, the American Heart Association identified physical inactivity as the fourth independent risk factor for cardiovascular disease. The World Health Organization notes that globally, physical inactivity accounts for an estimated 2 million deaths per year, making it one of the 10 leading causes of morbidity and mortality. Low levels of physical activity and fitness are associated with a twofold increase in all-cause mortality and cardiovascular mortality. This attributable risk is similar to or greater than that associated with hypercholesterolemia, diabetes mellitus, hypertension, and cigarette smoking.[7,8] The federal health initiative, Healthy People 2010, has identified physical activity as one of the 10 leading determinants of health.[9]

Research regarding the health-related benefits of physical activity has primarily focused on the physical/physiological component of health. As health has come to take on a more holistic definition, however, there has been a growing recognition that physical activity may provide more benefits than previously believed.

The World Health Organization (WHO), in its classic definition provided in 1948, stated that health was "a state of complete physical, social, and mental well-being, and not merely the absence of disease or infirmity." Subsequently, in the WHO Ottawa Charter on Health Promotion, a more functional approach was provided to this working definition: "Health is a resource for everyday life, not the object of living. It is a positive concept emphasizing social and personal resources as well as physical capabilities."[10]

Allowing for this broader definition, it is evident that physical activity can positively affect health at multiple levels. In physical activity research, a commonly used definition is, "Health is a human condition with physical, social, and psychological dimensions, each characterized on a continuum with positive and negative poles. Positive health is associated with a capacity to enjoy life and to withstand challenges; it is not merely the absence of disease. Negative health is associated with morbidity and in the extreme with premature mortality. . . . Wellness is a holistic concept describing a state of positive health in the individual and comprising physical, social, and psychological well-being."[11] Consistent with the guiding philosophy of integrative medicine that "engages the mind, spirit, and community as well as the body . . . to stimulate the body's innate healing,"[12] physical activity may serve as a fundamental component of any health-promoting recommendation.

▶ THE EVOLUTION OF PHYSICAL ACTIVITY RECOMMENDATIONS

A number of recommendations by expert panels and organizations concerning exercise and health were published in the 1960s and 1970s. These were based upon dose–response improvements identified with exercise training, especially aerobic exercise, and served to answer questions such as, "How much exercise is enough," and "What are the best exercises to improve fitness?" These recommendations used the training parameters of frequency, intensity, duration, and mode of exercise for answering these questions.

One of the earliest of these was "The Recommended Quantity and Quality of Exercise for Developing and Maintaining Fitness in Healthy Adults," released by the American College of Sports Medicine in 1978. It served as the guideline for public health recommendations provided to Americans, as well as serving as the framework for the development of the clinical exercise prescription.

Recognizing that this guideline addressed only cardiorespiratory fitness and body composition, it was updated in 1990 to include musculoskeletal fitness.[13] Additionally, it was acknowledged that the benefits of physical activity for overall health, independent of cardiovascular fitness, had been overlooked. Research suggested that health-related benefits could be achieved with lower levels of exercise training, reducing risks for chronic disease without necessarily affecting maximal oxygen consumption (VO_2max), the "gold standard" measure of cardiovascular fitness. Physically active adults developed higher levels of physical fitness that provided protection against many chronic diseases, such as cardiovascular disease, stroke, hypertension, and type 2 diabetes. A dose–response relationship was noted in most studies—low levels of physical activity and physical fitness were associated with increased all-cause mortality rates; conversely, increasing rates of activity and fitness demonstrated decreases in mortality rates. With this relationship, it was noted that regularly performed moderate-intensity activities (i.e., an additional 200 kcal/d or approximately 30 minutes per day) provided significant health benefits. "It has been pointed out that the quantity and quality of exercise needed to obtain health-related benefits may differ from what is recommended for fitness benefits. It is now clear that lower levels of physical activity than recommended by this position statement may reduce the risk for certain chronic degenerative diseases. . . ."[13] The most recent update of these recommendations has added the component of flexibility, although evidence supporting the benefit of this attribute is less robust.[14]

The physical activity objectives for Healthy People 2000 called for "an increase to at least 30% of the proportion of people aged 6 and older who engage regularly, preferably, daily, in light to moderate physical activity for at least 30 minutes per day." Data suggested, however, that Americans were falling short of these recommendations. A variety of reasons were cited with lack of time being the most common. Additionally, there was a concern that individuals may have believed that health benefits could only be derived from participation in continuous vigorous activity. This could have been perceived as a daunting challenge to overcome for individuals with low baseline activity levels. It was therefore essential to make people aware of the changing message.

In 1995, guidelines were released that focused on the public health impact of physical activity promotion.[3] They were based on research performed on individuals with lower cardiovascular functional capacity and demonstrated that more moderate levels of physical activity could produce significant benefits. Additionally, a dose–response relationship was identified. The stated objective of "encouraging increased participation in physical activity among Americans of all ages. . . . Every US adult should accumulate 30 minutes or more of moderate-intensity physical activity on most, preferably all, days of the week" has provided the overall framework for current efforts at getting the US population to become more active. These recommendations are based upon an energy expenditure of 3–4 kcal/kg/d, or approximately 1,000–2,000 kcal of extra energy expenditure per week. The amount of activity and therefore the caloric expenditure and the accumulated time spent in being active, rather than the manner in which this activity is performed, has become the emphasis of public health recommendations.

Three major differences exist as compared to previously mentioned recommendations: the intensity of exercise is *decreased* from 55–65% of maximum intensity to 50% for healthy adults (40% for individuals with very low initial fitness levels); the frequency is *increased* from 3 days per week to 5–7 days per week; and the opportunity of *accumulating* 30 minutes per day of activity in increments of 8–10 minutes is offered. These modifications are significant in that they provide increased opportunities to be physically active for individuals of low fitness levels, for those who are sedentary, and for those who claim insufficient time to exercise.

These health promotion-focused guidelines represent a point on a continuum of activity recommendations rather than a replacement for published guidelines. The dose–response relationship for physical activity and exercise is fairly consistent. The cardiorespiratory recommendations,[14] although adaptable to a significant percentage of American adults, are none-theless designed for those individuals who are interested in performing in the middle to high end of the physical activity/exercise continuum. Exercise intensity is inversely proportional to cardiovascular disease risk, irrespective of duration.[15] Given the current levels of activity/inactivity in America, 30 minutes of moderate activity on most days of the week represents a reasonable and obtainable goal for American adults and reflects a lower point on the physical activity/exercise continuum. Therefore, familiarization with these guidelines is essential for all health care providers. The challenge, however, is how to get individuals to follow through with these recommendations. Table 13–2 summarizes the various exercise recommendations described above.

▶ RECOMMENDATIONS FOR OTHER AGE GROUPS

Guidelines have been released for infants, toddlers, and preschool children.[16] These recommendations do not call for parents to start their children in exercise programs or enroll them in team sports. Rather, they recognize that children are naturally active from birth, but are often limited in their activities by such modern devices as strollers, playpens, and infant seats.

These may limit both physical and cognitive development and may set the stage for the development of sedentary behaviors, potentially leading to childhood, adolescent, and adult obesity. Whereas these devices are viewed by some as necessary for safety, many are actually used more out of convenience and may limit infants in their natural exploration of their environments. Children should be encouraged to be active from birth.

There are five guidelines for each age group. Their purpose is to provide information concerning age-appropriate activities, how environments should support activity, and identification of caregiver responsibilities to facilitate these activities.

Guidelines for Infants

Part of the infant's day should be spent with a caregiver or parent who provides systematic opportunities for planned physical activity. These experiences should incorporate a variety of baby games, such as peekaboo and pat-a-cake, and sessions in which the child is held, rocked, and carried to new environments.

Guideline 1. Infants should interact with parents and/or caregivers in daily physical activities that are dedicated to promoting the exploration of their environment.

Guideline 2. Infants should be placed in safe settings that facilitate physical activity and do not restrict movement for prolonged periods of time.

Guideline 3. Infants' physical activity should promote the development of movement skills.

Guideline 4. Infants should have an environment that meets or exceeds recommended safety standards for performing large-muscle activities.

Guideline 5. Individuals responsible for the well-being of infants should be aware of the importance of physical activity and facilitate the child's movement skills.

▶ **TABLE 13-2** PHYSICAL ACTIVITY AND EXERCISE RECOMMENDATIONS

Source	Objective	Mode	Intensity	Frequency	Duration	Resistance Training	Flexibility Training
ACSM (1978)	CV fitness Body composition	Endurance	70–85% HRmax	3–4 d/wk	20–60 min	n/a	n/a
ACSM (1990)	CV and musculoskeletal fitness Body composition	Endurance Strength	60–90% HRmax	3–5 d/wk	20–60 min	1 set, 8–12 reps 8–10 exercises 2 d/wk	n/a
CDC/ ACSM (1995)	Health promotion	Endurance accumulated in 8–10-min bouts	Moderate/hard	All/most days	≥30 min/d	n/a	n/a
ACSM (1998)	CV, musculoskeletal fitness, body composition, and flexibility	Endurance, strength, and flexibility	55/65–90% HRmax (minimum 10-min bouts accumulated per day)	3–5 d/wk	20–60 min/d	1 set, 8–12 reps 8–10 exercises 2–3 d/wk	2–3 d/wk

Abbreviations: ACSM = American College of Sports Medicine; CDC = Centers for Disease Control and Prevention; CV = cardiovascular; HRmax = maximum heart rate; n/a = not applicable; reps = repetitions.
Source: Adapted with permission from DHHS.[1]

Guidelines for Toddlers and Preschoolers

For toddlers, basic movement skills such as running, jumping, throwing, and kicking do not just appear because a child grows older, but emerge from an interaction between hereditary potential and movement experience. These behaviors promote physical and cognitive development and are influenced by the environment in which the child grows. For instance, a child who does not have access to stairs may be delayed in stair climbing; a child who is discouraged from bouncing and chasing balls may lag in hand–eye coordination.

Guideline 1. Toddlers should accumulate at least 30 minutes daily of structured physical activity; preschoolers at least 60 minutes.

Guideline 2. Toddlers and preschoolers should engage in at least 60 minutes and up to several hours per day of daily, unstructured physical activity and should not be sedentary for more than 60 minutes at a time except when sleeping.

Guideline 3. Toddlers should develop movement skills that are building blocks for more complex movement tasks; preschoolers should develop competence in movement skills that are building blocks for more complex movement tasks.

Guideline 4. Toddlers and preschoolers should have indoor and outdoor areas that meet or exceed recommended safety standards for performing large muscle activities.

Guideline 5. Individuals responsible for the well-being of toddlers and preschoolers should be aware of the importance of physical activity and facilitate the child's movement skills.

During the preschool years, children should be encouraged to practice movement skills in a variety of activities and settings. Instruction and positive reinforcement is critical during this time in order to ensure that children develop most of these skills before entering school.

Guidelines for Children and Adolescents

Children and adolescents are generally more active than adults. Unfortunately, available survey data suggest that a large percentage of youth fail to meet established guidelines for participating in physical activity. It is currently estimated that fewer than two-thirds of high school students participate in vigorous physical activity and less than half report performing stretching or strengthening exercises 3 or more days per week.[17] The decrease in activity that occurs with increasing age begins in early adolescence (boys at age 14 years and for girls at age 12 years)[18] and has been explained by a variety of reasons, including differing perceptions of the benefits of physical activity based upon gender, perceived competence and/or decreased level of fun, and perceived ability to be active (i.e., self-efficacy). Additionally, there is decreasing institutional support for activity, as schools have decreased time made available for physical education so as to increase time spent in classroom learning. Physical education is often taught by nonspecialists who have insufficient training to provide a well-rounded curriculum.[19] In such learning environments, a large amount of time is spent being inactive.[20] These facts have led to declines in cardiovascular fitness in school-aged youth over the past several decades.[21]

Physical activity provides many health-related benefits for young people. Improvements in cardiovascular and musculoskeletal fitness (e.g., aerobic fitness, blood pressure, muscular strength, bone mass), and metabolic parameters, such as blood lipids and glucose, have been noted.[1,22] Enhanced self-esteem and decreases in depression, anxiety, and stress, have likewise been identified.[23]

Much of the health-related rationale for emphasizing physical activity in youth is based upon the notion that behaviors developed in childhood may be maintained into later years. As the chronic diseases of adulthood are initiated many years before they manifest clinically, primary prevention is recommended. Data tracking physical activity across the life span are limited but suggest that this behavior tracks reasonably well from childhood into adulthood.[24] Conversely, childhood inactivity (and overweight/obesity) predicts adult inactivity. Given the evidence that cardiovascular disease begins early in life, and that disease risk factors[25–28] and physical activity behaviors[29–32] track over time, programs aimed at increasing activity in children could potentially prevent or delay the development of chronic diseases.[33]

Children (ages 5–12 years) are not little adults and therefore adult recommendations are not readily applicable. Children are naturally active, yet their activity occurs in short, vigorous intermittent bouts. They have relatively short attention spans and are relatively concrete thinkers. The current guidelines for childhood physical activity reflect these unique characteristics of childhood.[34]

Guideline 1. Elementary school children should accumulate at least 30–60 minutes of age-appropriate physical activity on all, or most, days of the week.

Guideline 2. An accumulation of more than 60 minutes and up to several hours per day of appropriate activities are encouraged for school-aged children.

Guideline 3. Some of the child's activity each day should be in periods lasting 10–15 minutes or more that includes moderate to vigorous activity. This activity will typically be intermittent in nature involving alternating moderate to vigorous activity with brief periods of rest and recovery.

Guideline 4. Extended periods of inactivity are discouraged for children.

Guideline 5. A variety of physical activities selected from the Physical Activity Pyramid is recommended.

Children and adolescents have also been provided with strength-training (resistance-training) guidelines.[35] Identified benefits include muscular strength and conditioning, improved sports performance, injury prevention and rehabilitation, and enhancement of long-term health. Participation in an appropriate strength-training program that focuses on technique is encouraged. Exercises performed without resistance should be learned, and upon mastery of appropriate skills, progressive resistance may be applied that permits 8–15 repetitions of an exercise. Appropriate warm up and cool down components should exist.

Recommendations for Seniors

Individuals older than age 65 years represent the fastest growing segment of the US population. They also represent the group with the greatest chronic disease burden and health care utilization, with an estimated 88% of individuals having at least one chronic disease.[36] Physical activity is essential to promote health and to prevent disability in seniors. Benefits have been demonstrated for cardiovascular disease; osteoarthritis and osteoporosis; type 2 diabetes mellitus; depression; cognition; postural stability and decreased risk of falls; musculoskeletal strength and fitness; and longevity.

> Participation in a regular exercise program is an effective intervention/modality to reduce/prevent a number of functional declines associated with aging. . . . Endurance training can help maintain and improve various aspects of cardiovascular function. . . . Strength training helps offset the loss in muscle mass and strength typically associated with normal aging. Additional benefits from regular exercise include improved postural stability, thereby reducing the risk of falling and associated injuries and fractures; and increased flexibility and range of motion. . . . [I]nvolvement in regular exercise can also provide a number of psychological benefits related to preserved cognitive function, alleviation of depression symptoms and behavior, and an improved concept of personal control and self-efficacy. . . . Thus, the benefits associated

with regular exercise and physical activity contribute to a more healthy, independent lifestyle, greatly improving the functional capacity and quality of life.[37]

Unfortunately, individuals older than age 50 years represent the most inactive segment of the US population.[1] Physical and physiological changes that accompany the aging process do not preclude individuals from being active, however, as physical activity is generally considered safe for healthy seniors. Although there are no established guidelines for this age group as there are with the other age groups, the above-mentioned adult guidelines provide a reference point that allows for adaptation, depending upon the unique status of the senior.

The American College of Sports Medicine currently recommends an exercise stress test for anyone older than age 50 years who is interested in beginning a vigorous exercise training program. This is probably unnecessary, however, for the majority of seniors who are interested in engaging in moderate intensity activity, such as walking or resistance training. Individuals should, however, be questioned to determine if any underlying risk factors (e.g., cardiovascular disease or diabetes) exist. For example, the PAR-Q (Physical Activity Readiness Questionnaire) is a commonly used instrument to assess whether further evaluation may be necessary[38]:

1. Has your doctor ever said you have heart trouble?
2. Do you frequently have pains in your heart and chest?
3. Do you often feel faint or have spells of severe dizziness?
4. Has a doctor ever said your blood pressure was too high?
5. Has your doctor ever told you that you have a bone or joint problem such as arthritis that has been aggravated by exercise, or might be made worse with exercise?
6. Is there a good physical reason not mentioned here why you should not follow an activity program even if you wanted to?

7. Are you over age 65 and not accustomed to vigorous exercise?

Although the physiological response to exercise is qualitatively, and often quantitatively, similar to that of younger adults, heart rate, stroke volume, and cardiac output performed at the same relative work rate are less in seniors. Conversely, peripheral resistance is generally higher. Cardiovascular adaptations and lessening of risk factors can occur for seniors when provided with the appropriate physiological stimulus.

Normal aging causes loss of muscle mass (sarcopenia) with changes identified as early as age 30 years. This is accompanied by a decrease in muscle strength by approximately 15% per decade between 50 and 70 years of age, and by about 30% thereafter. This loss of musculoskeletal fitness is a cause of significant morbidity and indirect mortality for seniors. Studies show, however, that these losses can be lessened through a program of resistance training that appropriately stresses the muscles.[39] Training programs should attend to the large muscle groups that are important for everyday functioning (e.g., shoulders and arms, spine, hips, knees, and ankles). Slowly performed repetitions that move the joint through the full functional range of motion should be performed. Although high-intensity programs of 8–12 repetitions with weight increases performed every 2–3 weeks based upon strength gains produce the greatest results in muscle strength, such programs are obviously not appropriate for everyone. Muscle endurance and smaller increases in muscle strength can be achieved by performing more repetitions of lesser weight. Individuals should follow appropriate breathing techniques (inhale before a lift, exhale during the lift, and inhale while lowering the weight) and avoid performing a Valsalva maneuver while lifting. Resistance training may also elicit positive changes in body composition by increasing energy requirements and decreasing body fat mass, has positive effects on bone health, and can significantly affect postural stability, thereby decreasing the risk of falls.

Flexibility training is the final component of current physical activity/exercise recommendations for seniors. Flexibility decreases with increasing age; maximum flexibility is seen in the mid to late twenties in both sexes. Flexibility programs provide for improvements in range of motion of many joints and mobility skills, such as ambulation, proprioception, and balance. Movement of the joint through the functional range of motion with recognition of current limitations is encouraged.

Seniors are encouraged to follow the current public health guidelines for accumulating a minimum of 30 minutes of moderate intensity activity on most days of the week. Identification of aerobic activities that are enjoyed, simple, and safe, based upon the individual's health status, should be performed. Resistance and flexibility training are likewise extremely important elements for a complete recommendation. Appropriate periods of warm up and cool down with stretching should be encouraged, and rapid changes in body temperature (e.g., immediately plunging into a pool after a workout) should be discouraged because of possible stress of the cardiovascular system. An algorithm (Figure 13–1) has been suggested that can provide a starting point for evaluation of a senior's current interest and past experience with physical activity and exercise.[40] Information obtained can then be used to tailor a program specific to individual needs and current health status. Programs should concurrently provide recommendations to increase physical activity while discouraging sedentary behaviors.

An important subset of the elderly population that benefits significantly from exercise programs is the frail elderly.[41] Such individuals are characterized by generalized weakness and an inability to perform the activities of daily living. Whereas in the past, frail elderly were seen as being beyond the assistance of exercise programs, research suggests the contrary, and frailty may be a direct result of physical

deconditioning combined with other factors (e.g., chronic disease and biological status). Therefore, it is important that physical activity and exercise be viewed as both a preventive and a treatment method for this population. Such exercise programs should include the three previously mentioned elements (cardiovascular, strength, and flexibility) and be specifically tailored to fit the limitations and the needs of the individual. Tai Chi, for example, provides all of these elements in an easily delivered program that provides significant benefits in decreasing morbidity in this population.[42]

▶ FROM DISEASE PREVENTION TO HEALTH PROMOTION

Historically, clinical medicine has concentrated upon the treatment of disease. Over the past few decades, growing recognition has developed concerning the role of behaviors in affecting disease initiation and progression. "Preventive medicine" has become a subspecialty within medicine, and the American Board of Preventive Medicine was incorporated under the laws of the State of Delaware on June 29, 1948, as "The American Board of Preventive Medicine and Public Health, Incorporated."

Three levels of prevention have been identified:

1. *Primary prevention:* actions and interventions that seek to identify risks and reduce susceptibility/exposure to health threats and disease incidence before disease onset.
2. *Secondary prevention:* detection and treatment of disease in its early stages to prevent progress or recurrence.
3. *Tertiary prevention:* intervention to lessen the effects of disease once it is already established.

Physical activity and exercise may function at all levels of prevention. Evidence suggests that regularly performed activity can successfully prevent the development of many chronic

Exercise in Older Patients

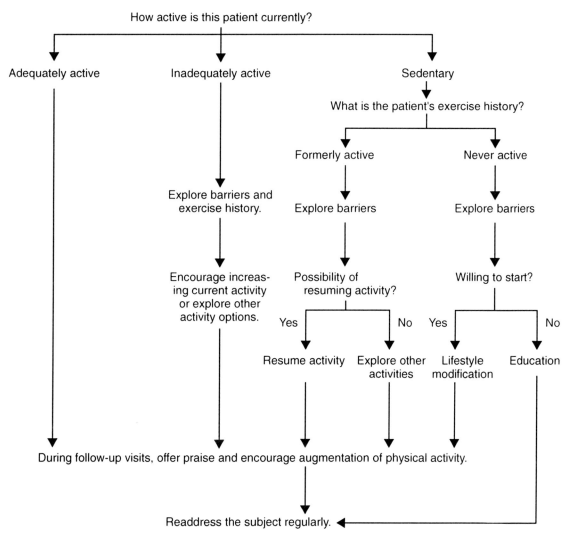

Figure 13–1. Exercise in older patients. *(Adapted with permission from Christmas and Andersen.[40])*

diseases. However, the optimal timing of physical activity interventions remains a research challenge. For example, it has been identified that enhanced dynamic weight-bearing exercise performed during the teen years may increase bone mass, an example of primary prevention.[13,41] This should theoretically lessen the risk of developing osteoporosis later in life.

The use of retrospective data to determine physical activity levels in youth is problematic, however, as it requires individuals to recall activity patterns that may have occurred decades before disease occurrence; conversely, longitudinal studies are expensive and difficult to perform. (Another example of primary prevention [Table 13–3] is how body mass index,

▶ TABLE 13–3 BODY MASS INDEX (BMI)

BMI	19	20	21	22	23	24	25	26	27	28	29	30	31	32	33	34	35
Height (inches)								Body Weight (pounds)									
58	91	96	100	105	110	115	119	124	129	134	138	143	148	153	158	162	167
59	94	99	104	109	114	119	124	128	133	138	143	148	153	158	163	168	173
60	97	102	107	112	118	123	128	133	138	143	148	153	158	163	168	174	179
61	100	106	111	116	122	127	132	137	143	148	153	158	164	169	174	180	185
62	104	109	115	120	126	131	136	142	147	153	158	164	169	175	180	186	191
63	107	113	118	124	130	135	141	146	152	158	163	169	175	180	186	191	197
64	110	116	122	128	134	140	145	151	157	163	169	174	180	186	192	197	204
65	114	120	126	132	138	144	150	156	162	168	174	180	186	192	198	204	210
66	118	124	130	136	142	148	155	161	167	173	179	186	192	198	204	210	216
67	121	127	134	140	146	153	159	166	172	178	185	191	198	204	211	217	223
68	125	131	138	144	151	158	164	171	177	184	190	197	203	210	216	223	230
69	128	135	142	149	155	162	169	176	182	189	196	203	209	216	223	230	236
70	132	139	146	153	160	167	174	181	188	195	202	209	216	222	229	236	243
71	136	143	150	157	165	172	179	186	193	200	208	215	222	229	236	243	250
72	140	147	154	162	169	177	184	191	199	206	213	221	228	235	242	250	258
73	144	151	159	166	174	182	189	197	204	212	219	227	235	242	250	257	265
74	148	155	163	171	179	186	194	202	210	218	225	233	241	249	256	264	272
75	152	160	168	176	184	192	200	208	216	224	232	240	248	256	264	272	279
76	156	164	172	180	189	197	205	213	221	230	238	246	254	263	271	279	287

Source: http://www.nhlbi.nih.gov/guidelines/obesity/bmi_tbl.htm

▶ TABLE 13–3 BODY MASS INDEX (BMI) (Continued)

BMI	36	37	38	39	40	41	42	43	44	45	46	47	48	49	50	51	52	53	54
Height (inches)									Body Weight (pounds)										
58	172	177	181	186	191	196	201	205	210	215	220	224	229	234	239	244	248	253	258
59	178	183	188	193	198	203	208	212	217	222	227	232	237	242	247	252	257	262	267
60	184	189	194	199	204	209	215	220	225	230	235	240	245	250	255	261	266	271	276
61	190	195	201	206	211	217	222	227	232	238	243	248	254	259	264	269	275	280	285
62	196	202	207	213	218	224	229	235	240	246	251	256	262	267	273	278	284	289	295
63	203	208	214	220	225	231	237	242	248	254	259	265	270	278	282	287	293	299	304
64	209	215	221	227	232	238	244	250	256	262	267	273	279	285	291	296	302	308	314
65	216	222	228	234	240	246	252	258	264	270	276	282	288	294	300	306	312	318	324
66	223	229	235	241	247	253	260	266	272	278	284	291	297	303	309	315	322	328	334
67	230	236	242	249	255	261	268	274	280	287	293	299	306	312	319	325	331	338	344
68	236	243	249	256	262	269	276	282	289	295	302	308	315	322	328	335	341	348	354
69	243	250	257	263	270	277	284	291	297	304	311	318	324	331	338	345	351	358	365
70	250	257	264	271	278	285	292	299	306	313	320	327	334	341	348	355	362	369	376
71	257	265	272	279	286	293	301	308	315	322	329	338	343	351	358	365	372	379	386
72	265	272	279	287	294	302	309	316	324	331	338	346	353	361	368	375	383	390	397
73	272	280	288	295	302	310	318	325	333	340	348	355	363	371	378	386	393	401	408
74	280	287	295	303	311	319	326	334	342	350	358	365	373	381	389	396	404	412	420
75	287	295	303	311	319	327	335	343	351	359	367	375	383	391	399	407	415	423	431
76	295	304	312	320	328	336	344	353	361	369	377	385	394	402	410	418	426	435	443

BMI, relates to risk of coronary artery disease, diabetes, and other health problems.) As secondary prevention, exercise programs initiated during the early stages of disease may demonstrate regression/delayed progression (e.g., weight-bearing exercise and osteopenia). Finally, upon disease diagnosis, an appropriately performed exercise program may improve disease status as seen with weight-bearing exercise and osteoporosis.[45]

Disease prevention often focuses upon "lifestyle" choices. Physical inactivity, nutrition, and tobacco usage are the leading contributors of preventable morbidity and mortality. Whereas addressing individual lifestyles holds great merit, this strategy, unfortunately, neglects to consider a fundamental issue of human behavior. Human behavior is dynamic and reflects the influence of many diverse factors, such as social and cultural norms, family and peer influence, economic status, and policies. Behaviors often change along an individual's life course. A focus solely upon individual behaviors and perceived ability to change behaviors may neglect to appreciate the context in which these behaviors are practiced.

How this is translated into an integrative approach for physical activity and exercise recommendations is important for consideration. Lifestyle choices reflect an individual's ability to take responsibility for their own lives, a proactive approach. In contrast, medicine has historically focused upon the treatment of disease in a reactive fashion. It is as important to provide appropriate recommendations for an individual as it is to understand the context in which the recommendations are being provided. Acknowledgment of the environment in which the person lives and plays provides opportunities for providing optimal recommendations that may be readily integrated into an individual's daily life. Failure to recognize these elements may find the most well-thought-out suggestions and well-meaning advice falling short of their desired outcomes.

Integrative medicine seeks to promote health as well as prevent disease. The World Health Organization (WHO) in 1947 provided a definition of health as "a state of complete physical, mental and social well-being, and not merely the absence of disease or infirmity." The World Health Organization convened the first International Conference on Health Promotion in Ottawa in 1986. A charter was drafted that has come to serve as the cornerstone of current promotion practices. It defined health promotion as "the process of enabling people to increase control over, and to improve, their health." Health was seen as "a resource for everyday life, not the objective of living. Health is a positive concept emphasizing social and personal resources, as well as physical capacities. Therefore, health promotion is not just the responsibility of the health sector, but goes beyond healthy lifestyles to well-being."[10] It is evident that health promotion requires a multilevel approach. As quoted by Breslow,[16] Henry E. Sigerist, the noted medical historian, stated "health is promoted by providing a decent standard of living, good labor conditions, education, physical culture, means of rest and recreation. . . . [H]ealth is not simply the absence of disease; it is something positive, a joyful attitude toward life and a cheerful acceptance of the responsibilities that life puts upon the individual."

Historically, the health-promoting effects of physical activity and exercise have been viewed and researched from a physiological/medical standpoint. Recommendations are viewed from the perspective of health and fitness objectives. Such an approach is limited. There is no context by which individuals and their "relationship" with activity and the environments in which they can be active are understood. What is the individual's past experience with exercise. What are the environmental barriers and supporters for engaging in this behavior? What medical conditions do they currently experience or are they at risk for developing? What do they hope to accomplish by becoming more active? These and other questions need to be entertained when attempting to encourage people to make active living a way of being.

Psychological and contextual elements play a significant role. Psychological elements include personal motivation for performance, effects upon mental well-being, outcome expectations (personal beliefs on activity/inactivity), and emotional attachment (positive emotions connected to an activity increase the likelihood of performance and maintenance). Contextual factors, such as location/physical environment, time (daily, seasonal, life course), and the sociocultural norms about activity may affect behavior. A complex and dynamic interplay of these factors affects the individual experience and response.[17] Therefore, attempts to move people to health-promoting behaviors must necessarily take into account all of these factors lest they fail to achieve their desired effects.

Structured Exercise versus Physical Activity

A "lifestyle" approach to physical activity recommendations has significant merit. Growing evidence supports the current recommendations of accumulating 30 minutes or more of moderate-intensity physical activity on most, preferably all, days of the week.[18,19] For many individuals, the health-related benefits of a lifestyle-focused activity program are appropriate starting points to incorporate lifetime physical activity. Additionally, acknowledging that for a significant percentage of Americans, "exercise" has been an intimidating concept, accumulating more daily activity is a nonthreatening means of improving health.

The intention of such recommendations, however, is not to discourage individuals from engaging in more vigorous forms of activity, but rather, to meet them where they feel most comfortable, and move them forward in a way that is health promoting, as well as possibly disease preventing. For some individuals, for example, those with chronic diseases, a structured, medically supervised format is necessary. Exercise, in addition to regularly performed physical activity, is an optimal situation.

For others, for example, those who find themselves sedentary but are interested in achieving the health-related benefits of being more active, simple daily living activities are a good starting point. And for those who consider themselves "healthy" and are not limited by chronic disease, moderate to vigorous exercise is an appropriate consideration.

The "exercise prescription" (see tinted box) has served as the foundation for physical activity and exercise recommendations. This formulaic approach is inadequate at many levels, however. For some, it is too regimented and structured. The instructions may be both intimidating as well as complicated and confusing. For others, the time commitment may be unrealistic for their busy lives. Therefore it becomes essential that health care providers who provide physical activity and exercise recommendations take a more reasonable approach: they must recognize the many factors that contribute to performance of behaviors and seek to partner with the individual, meeting them where they feel most comfortable and assisting them to achieve their goals and aspirations. Such an approach encourages individuals to take an active role in their own lives, while acknowledging the barriers and challenges that may exist to achieving behavior change.

Classically, the exercise prescription is defined by four components and remembered by the mnemonic FITT: Frequency, Intensity, Type, Tempo. The current recommendations define the amount and type of training necessary for developing and maintaining cardiorespiratory fitness, body composition, muscular fitness, and flexibility.[11] Recommendations usually call for engaging in certain activities, such as walking, bicycling, or swimming, for a defined duration at a given intensity for a specified number of times per week. Clinicians have been advised to provide these recommendations in a similar fashion to writing a medication prescription, using a prescription pad. It has been suggested that this may increase patient adherence. Empirical and clinical evidence, however, often finds exercise prescription failing for many individuals.

▶ THE EXERCISE PRESCRIPTION

Cardiorespiratory fitness and body composition

Frequency of training: 3–5 days per week.

Intensity of the exercise: 55/65–90% of maximum heart rate (HRmax) based upon the aerobic capacity goals and fitness level; lower intensity values are most applicable for less-fit individuals. (The prediction of HRmax using the equation "220 − age" was defined in the 1970s from a review of 10 studies in which the maximum age of individuals was <65 years, many of whom were either on medications or had cardiovascular risks that possibly affected calculations. A recent meta-analysis has determined that the equation "208 − 0.7 × age" more accurately predicts HRmax across a range of ages in adults.[51])

Light exercise: less than 60% of predicted HRmax.

Moderate exercise: 60–85% of predicted HRmax.

Vigorous exercise: greater than 85% of predicted HRmax.

Time spent: 20–60 minutes of continuous or intermittent (minimum of 10-minute bouts accumulated throughout the day) aerobic activity. The time is dependent upon the intensity—lower-intensity activities should be performed for longer periods of time (30 minutes or more); conversely, higher intensity training may be performed for 20 minutes or more. Because as total fitness is enhanced by training periods of longer duration and the risk of injury is increased with more intense training, moderate-intensity activities are recommended for adults.

Type of physical activity: any activity that uses large muscle groups that can be maintained continuously and is rhythmic in nature.

Musculoskeletal strength and endurance, body composition, and flexibility

Strength training: resistance training should be progressive, individualized, and work all major muscle groups. One set of 8–10 exercises, consisting of 8–12 repetitions that work the major muscle groups, performed through the full range of motion, should be performed 2–3 days per week. Multiple-set regimens may provide greater improvements.

Flexibility training: should be incorporated into the overall fitness program sufficient to develop and maintain range of motion. These exercises should stretch the major muscle groups and be performed a minimum of 2–3 days per week. Stretching should include appropriate static and/or dynamic techniques.

Progression: after an initial phase of 4–6 weeks of conditioning, activity levels can be slowly increased to the target range in most people; likewise, duration can be increased every 2–3 weeks. Most people reach an acceptable level of fitness within 6 months and enter the "maintenance" phase.

Maintenance: This can often be a challenging time for individuals as gains that may have come quickly and often early in their programs now seem few and far between. Encouragement and support from friends, family and clinicians can help people from regressing. Setting reasonable goals along the way of getting to this step can provide appropriate perspective as individuals may identify their accomplishments. The overall goal of this phase is to make activities a natural part of life.

Types of Physical Activity

Physical activity has been divided into work-related and leisure-time activity, with the latter further divided into exercise and sport.[50] An expanded version has been suggested for health promotion efforts that identifies five categories[47]: occupational activity; lifestyle activity; recreation activity; fitness activity; and sport activity. These categories are described below and summarized in Table 13–4.

Occupational activity relates to work performance. In current Western society, few occupations provide significant physical activity. The health benefits of occupational activity may be positive or negative, as some work requires vigorous physical activity while others place individuals at increased risk for injury or illness due to their sedentary nature or the potential exposure to toxins.

Lifestyle activities, because of their current focus, have been conceptualized in a number of ways. As currently defined within US research and recommendations, these are "self-selected activities, which include all leisure, occupational, or household activities that are at least moderate to vigorous in their intensity and could be planned or unplanned activities that are a part of everyday life."[52] They deemphasize the activity element in and of itself, focusing rather upon performing activities that are related to daily living. Many of these activities are performed routinely, such as climbing a set of stairs in the home, while others may require active intention to occur, such as bicycling to work rather than driving. An important element of this definition is that such activities are *selected* by the individual and can be performed consciously or by means of environmental modification, such as making stairs more accessible or posting signage to encourage use. When activities become an integral component of everyday living, they provide additional opportunities for accumulating physical activity and achieving the identified benefits of such performance.

Recreational activities are performed with an expectation of a positive outcome, often at an emotional level, such as pleasure, enjoyment or excitement. Secondary emphasis is placed upon the physical activity in and of itself. They are often identified as hobbies (note that lifestyle and recreational activities may demonstrate a significant degree of overlap).

Fitness activities are necessarily performed for health-related benefits. They have specific defined objectives and outcomes, and therefore may overlap with lifestyle and/or recreational activities when the outcome expectation is fitness (cardiovascular and/or musculoskeletal) related. The emotional component is often significant and may be viewed as either positive (e.g., working toward enhancing one's health) or negative (e.g., "needing" to exercise to decrease cardiovascular risk).

Sport activities are viewed as "competition-related" or are performed for their own sake. They may exist as hobbies, and therefore be considered recreational activities (e.g., pick-up basketball games) or when performed in a sense of competition or for their own sake, may emphasize the development or improvement of skills or achieving one's maximum performance. They have a significant emotional element that may, at times, allow performance when it is not in the best interest of the individual.

It is important to recognize that each category of activity is performed within a framework that extends beyond simply the physical and physiological. They exist within a specific spatial and temporal context and incorporate emotional and psychological elements into their performance. An individual's past and present experience with an activity and the development of self-efficacy around activity performance will significantly affect the likelihood of whether a given activity will be performed. Some activities, for example those that are work-related, are more directed at an outcome expectation, such as salary, and may have fewer emotional and psychological features. Conversely, other activities, such as those performed for recreation or for fitness and sport, have significant emotional and psychological elements that when positive, will serve to

▶ **TABLE 13-4** CATEGORIES OF ACTIVITIES

Category	Examples	Context	Psychological Meaning		Personal Choice	Health Benefits
			Outcome Expectations	Emotional Elements		
Occupational activity	Office work, construction work	Work	Productivity	Competence, boredom	0/min	0/min
Lifestyle activity	Commuting to work; climbing stairs	Daily living	Daily functioning	Competence, stimulation, fatigue	Mod	Mod
Recreational activity	Hiking, fishing, dancing	Leisure time	Recreation, social interaction, new experiences	Pleasure, enjoyment excitement	Max	Max
Fitness activity	Walking/running, bicycling, swimming	Leisure time	Fitness, health, well-being	Competence, exertion, stimulation	Max	Max
Sport activity		Leisure time	Skill development	Excitement, enjoyment		
Hobby	Skiing, Frisbee, ball games		Identifying personal limits, achieving results, well-being, enjoyment	Competence, self-expression, release	Max	Mod-Max
Competition	Above as competition				Mod	Mod-Max

Abbreviations: Max = maximum; Mod = moderate.
Source: Adapted from Marttila J, Leutakari J, Huppohen R, Miilunpalo S, Paronen O. The versatile nature of physical activity—on the psychological, behavioural and contextual characteristics of health-related physical activity. Patient Educ Couns. 1998;33:S29–S38.

strongly reinforce performance, and when negative, will discourage performance. Lifestyle-related activities, as an element of daily living, do not necessarily require a strong sense of motivation, but rather may become part of the "daily routine." As a means to increase activity in individuals who may not express interest in "exercising," incorporating such activities into their daily routine will indirectly serve to provide them with the identified health benefits associated with their performance. When physical activity recommendations are tailored for an individual in a manner that readily addresses the multiple considerations necessary to effectively promote behavioral change, the likelihood of success is enhanced.

► RECOMMENDATIONS FOR SUCCESSFUL EXERCISE COUNSELING: A WELLNESS-ORIENTED APPROACH TO PHYSICAL ACTIVITY

Although much is known about the benefits of physical activity and exercise, the challenge has been how best to translate this knowledge into practical application to promote behavior change. Numerous interventions, applied at levels from the individual and one-on-one counseling to group settings, and from the non-work/community to the work site, have demonstrated mixed success at increasing physical activity. Similar findings have been reported when looking at physical activity counseling in primary care health settings. Whereas many have demonstrated positive results in the short-term, few have found sustainable means to maintain positive behaviors.[1,53–55]

One possible explanation for this phenomenon is simply the approach that is often taken by those recommending physical activity and exercise. Formulaic recommendations, no matter how well meaning and biomedically appropriate, lack an appreciation of the context in which they are to be applied. It is easy to recommend to someone that based upon their cardiovascular risk profile, they should begin an exercise program that provides 30 minutes of aerobic exercise performed 3–5 times per week. But if this prescription is provided to someone who has historically hated exercise for varied reasons, it is unlikely that these recommendations will be followed.

Rather, it must be appreciated that physical activity behavior is not a simple act but rather a complex, often very demanding behavior that has become, because of current society, unnecessary for survival, and for the majority, unnecessary for livelihood. It therefore becomes an added element to everyday life that must be seen and experienced as worthwhile. Individuals who begin a program of activity or exercise may sometimes experience discomfort, a negative reinforcement for persistence. Environmental barriers both social (e.g., lack of support, busy schedules, and perceived insufficient time) and physical (e.g., lack of accessible facilities, absence of sidewalks, trails, and bicycle lanes) are many and are challenging to overcome. When physical activity is seen as part of the "to-do list" rather than as a function of daily living, there is a strong likelihood that other priorities will win out.

Another potential element for the lack of success in increasing physical activity is the focus of providing the recommendation itself. In clinical practice, the emphasis has been upon disease prevention. Patients have been given list of "not to dos" and "to dos" to ward off chronic disease. Certainly this has its merits where properly applied (e.g., preventive health screening). Recommending physical activity for preventing disease, although data support this relationship, requires a significant amount of active participation (i.e., exercise to enhance cardiovascular and/or musculoskeletal fitness) on the part of the individual that many find challenging. "Prevention" suggests that an outcome is inevitable unless efforts are taken. This is a very problem-focused approach.

In contrast, placing the emphasis upon health promotion creates a different perspective. Health should be viewed as multidimensional (personal, sociocultural, biological, spiritual, and psychological) and not seen as a goal in itself, but rather as a resource for everyday life. Having health allows an individual to potentially achieve their aspirations. This subtly shifts the frame of reference for receiving physical activity recommendations. Health now becomes a vital element for achieving "wellness," a multidimensional state of being describing the existence of positive health in an individual as exemplified by quality of life and a sense of well-being.[56] Such an approach is one that focuses upon potential. Taking a proactive role by engaging in those practices that support this objective allows for a sense of achievement as health and well-being are experienced. The knowledge that being active can enhance an individual's state of well-being and quality of life, even when experiencing disease, provides opportunities for individuals where previously few existed. It is this framework that serves as fundamental to recommending physical activity and exercise as such behaviors are "integrated" into an individual's state of being.

The US Preventive Services Task Force recommends that clinicians should counsel all patients on performing regular physical activities that are tailored to their health status and their personal lifestyle.[57] There is sufficient justification for this recommendation as moderate physical activity can serve as "first-line therapy and protection" against many chronic health conditions.[58] Currently, the provided message is insufficient in affecting significant behavioral change. Physicians' recommendations have significant impact on health-related habits of individuals, yet counseling for a variety of reasons is often omitted. Several barriers commonly cited by health care providers include lack of counseling skills, perceived ineffectiveness or confidence in counseling, and insufficient time, reimbursement, or support.[59]

Integrative medicine fundamentally asks health care providers to examine and explore their own lives, as speaking from experience greatly influences how physician messages are received. The incorporation of role modeling to demonstrate the personal value of physical activity increases patient willingness to follow through with the recommendations.[60]

Two elements provide the foundation for an integrative approach to physical activity and exercise recommendations—context and life course. Much has already been stated about the former, while the latter has been suggested through recognition of the importance of knowing the currently recommended guidelines for varying age groups. Behaviors that are introduced to children may significantly affect their performance in adulthood. Children who have negative physical activity experiences may grow up to be adults who perceive these experiences as aversive. Conversely, when activity is perceived as fun and becomes a natural part of everyday life for children, these positive experiences become fundamental to their way of life as they age. Physical activity and exercise can serve to address the multiple domains of health for individuals without being the focus—it becomes a resource for everyday living rather than an outcome. Thus, how these behaviors are introduced in childhood is a fundamental and necessary consideration.

Childhood and adolescence are times of life and development characterized by exploration and experiential learning. Providing youth with opportunities to appreciate how much fun being physically active can be is an important goal for parents and teachers alike. Children are naturally active and are the most physically active age group. Many, in spite of the growing statistics to the contrary, do achieve the current recommendations.[61] Activity levels drop off with increasing age, however, with adolescence demonstrating the most significant decrease, especially for girls and certain ethnic groups.[18]

Children are typically active in bouts or short bursts that accumulate throughout the day. A combination of factors that may be divided into physiological/developmental, environmental, and psychological, social and demographic, affect childhood physical activity behavior.[30] A child's physical health status, school physical education programs and community resources, parental and peer influence, self-efficacy, gender, age, and socioeconomic status, are but some of the numerous factors that correlate with activity levels. The challenge is to create environments and nurture children in a fashion whereby physical activity is a normative behavior, counteracting societal factors that encourage children to be inactive. Children currently spend more time in front of televisions, computers, and video games than with any other activity, other than sleeping. The average American child younger than 2 years of age watches an average of 1.6 hours of television per day, despite recommendations by the American Academy of Pediatrics that this age group not be exposed to television. Television becomes a baby-sitter for adults who themselves are often not achieving current recommendations for activity.

The challenge of increasing childhood activity may be approached by identifying leverage points that assist in creating opportunities to support physical activity as a way of life. Families that take an active, healthy, and appropriate interest in having their children experience the benefits of an active way of life, either through family-focused activities or through enrollment in school or after-school programs, provide opportunities for children to develop a sense of self-efficacy around an activity. Parents should serve as role-models as their influence is significant, especially for younger children. Advocating for strong physical education programs in schools and communities is essential, as children spend significant amounts of time in these environments. Advocating for parks and green spaces, and pedestrian and bike lanes, can serve to create policy decisions that support activity-promoting environments.

More commonly, clinicians find themselves providing recommendations to adults of varying ages. It is estimated that physical inactivity and poor nutrition combined account for approximately 14% of the annual adult US mortality and are second only to tobacco usage for causes of preventable morbidity and mortality.

Physical inactivity and poor nutrition account for more deaths than alcohol and drugs, firearms, and motor vehicle accidents combined.[62] These unhealthy behaviors significantly affect the quality of life for millions of individuals.

"Lifestyle modification" is a focus of health promotion and disease prevention efforts. It is suggested that appropriate behavioral change toward more healthy ways of living can significantly affect morbidity and mortality. Interventions are conceptually based on a number of theories and models that often target a single level of analysis, such as the individual, the "at-risk group," or the community. Given that the majority of these behavioral change theories/models were created by American psychologists and behavioral scientists, it is not surprising that the unit of analysis and change has been the individual and/or interpersonal.

More recently, broader approaches that seek to affect the environment and policy have been a subject of research efforts. These approaches attempt to target multiple levels concurrently and have been successfully implemented in tobacco cessaton programs. As physical activity behavior is complex and reflects an interaction of many elements, including personal, sociocultural, genetic, and environmental, it is likely that such multilevel approaches will be necessary to affect change. A number of theories (interrelated concepts, definitions, and propositions that present a *systematic* view of events or situations by specifying relations among variables, in order to *explain* and *predict* the events or situations) and models (generalized, hypothetical descriptions, often based on an analogy, and used to analyze or explain something) have been applied to the field of physical activity, and it is suggested that the success of activity counseling by primary care physicians is enhanced when this counseling is theoretically based.[59] Viewing recommendations from a contextual approach provides a broad-spectrum of opportunities for physical activity promotion. Commonly, aspects of the trans-theoretical model and social cognitive theory have been applied to recommending behavioral change in primary care. Identification of the individual's stage of change (i.e., precontemplation, contemplation, planning, action, and maintenance), providing the appropriate message for the stage, and acknowledgment of behavioral determinants that include predisposing factors (e.g., knowledge and attitudes), enabling factors (e.g., self-efficacy), and reinforcing factors (e.g., social support and internal/external rewards) provide a theoretical foundation.[63–78] Albeit, contextualizing all of this through seeking to understand an individual's past experience with this behavior, their goals and expectations, and environmental factors (physical, sociocultural, and socioeconomic) is essential to enhance successful change and maintenance. Recognition of the five levels of activity (work-related, lifestyle, recreation, fitness, and sports) creates an opportunity for providing recommendations that may be achieved at multiple levels, independently or interdependently.

A model proposed by Laitakari and Asikainen provides a structural framework for application of these contextual variables.[79] Five steps have been identified:

1. Assessment: there are four key subheadings under this stage.
   a. Quality-of-life concerns, goals, and expectations. This is potentially the most important consideration in the assessment stage as it defines the purpose for looking at initiating a behavioral change. It is necessary to identify and/or assist the individual in identifying their reasons for becoming (more) physically active (e.g., relaxation, vitality, and health-related benefits such as decreased disease risk, weight loss, feeling well, and preparation for an event).
   b. Health status/fitness status. An individual's current health and fitness status will affect recommendations and provide opportunities for seeing how this can be positively affected through activity.

   c. Health practices and attitudes. What does the person currently do and why? What new activities may be of interest? What are the skills and what is needed to go forward and/or to try something new? How do current practices, such as tobacco usage and dietary patterns, affect current health status, as well as affect the initiation of new behaviors?
   d. Life situation and environment. What is their current employment status? What type of work (e.g., amount of work-related physical activity) occurs? Is the current job primarily sedentary and if so, are there opportunities for adding activity to the work day? Are there hobbies that entail activity? Are there significant time constraints that will need to be addressed, and if so, how can potential solutions be identified? What does the individual's physical environment look like—urban versus suburban versus rural; access to trails, parks, and green spaces; proximity and access to recreation facilities; and weather considerations?
2. Target identification: Upon collecting information during the assessment, health care providers and the individual determine a realistic outcome for behavior initiation. This outcome must be prioritized, as it is easy to come up with many "targets" that individually may seem reasonable but when combined prove overwhelming. Likewise, the targeted outcome must be attainable and amenable to available resources. It may be the behavior itself, such as beginning a program of regular walking, or identification of an environmental consideration, for example, recognizing that a barrier to daily walking is the lack of available pedestrian pathways close to home. Therefore, the decision to drive a few miles to a community park is made. It is during this step that health care providers need to be aware of aspects of behavioral change theory as previously mentioned, because identification of the individual's stage of

readiness and providing the appropriate information and verbal support is important in providing assistance. Likewise, it is important to remember the five categories of physical activity that have been identified (see "Types of Physical Activity"). Consistent with an individual's desired outcome and their current condition, it is possible to provide activity recommendations that can be performed in a wide array of settings and situations. Ultimately, it is difficult to find a situation that is not amenable to some type of physical activity intervention—it may simply require creative "brainstorming" on the part of the health care provider and the individual to identify where the opportunities exist and how to best overcome perceived barriers.

3. Planning: This step combines elements of education, such as identification of objectives and determination of the optimal way of presenting information (written "exercise prescription" versus patient handouts versus verbal instruction), with an assessment of the determinants of behavioral change (predisposing, enabling, and reinforcing) to create a plan for behavior change. As noted with target identification, a determination of the individual's stage of behavior adoption is necessary to optimize the formulation of the action plan. Upon identification of how an individual currently fits within the categorization of physical activities, their goals and their expectations, and the context in which this behavior is to be initiated and maintained, consideration is given to what specific type(s) of activity will be performed. What is a reasonable starting point, including amount of time being spent and the frequency of performance? What venue will be chosen for this activity? Will it be done in an individual setting or with a group; if the latter, where does this group exist and how can the individual become connected? Are there seasonal considerations that need to

be factored into the program? What kind of support, if any, exists?

4. Implementation: This refers to the initiation of the plan. Fundamental to the success of this step, as well as those preceding it, is a strong relationship between the health care provider and the individual that is built upon mutual respect and consideration. It is far easier for counseling to occur when the former can relate and acknowledges the challenges that exist in changing behavior. Serving as a coach as well as a mentor can be a mutually rewarding experience.

5. Evaluation and Reformulation: The program should be periodically reevaluated, with acknowledgment of barriers and challenges that need to be overcome, and feedback and praise given for overcoming obstacles and achieving goals. Every visit should serve as an opportunity to check in and see how things are going. Assessment of an individual's stage of change should be performed, allowing determination of whether the program should be modified to reflect stage progression or regression. Monitoring of physical and health-related parameters, such as weight and blood pressure, can provide important reinforcement. Determination of how the program has affected an individual's perceived quality of life should be at the core of this step.

▶ THE ROLE OF PHYSICAL ACTIVITY AND EXERCISE IN SPECIFIC CONDITIONS

An integrative perspective incorporating physical activity specifically designed to address a medical condition might seem daunting to those who are attempting to bring this into their practice. The following examples of specific physical activity recommendations as they relate to disease states serve as a template for those interested in using depression, anxiety, and osteoporosis as case modules.

Depression and Anxiety

The prevalence of depression and anxiety is significant, with estimates ranging from 5–25% of the general population having symptoms consistent with the former and a lesser percentage with the latter. A large percentage of individuals presenting to primary care providers have symptoms suggestive of depression and it is likely that a significant number of people who have symptoms do not seek assistance. To date, the evidence is suggestive that physical activity and exercise may prevent depression and anxiety, as well as serve as a cornerstone of treatment.[80,81]

Depression

There appears to be an inverse relationship between physical activity, conditioning, and depression with depression being more common in individuals with lower levels of activity and higher levels of deconditioning. Epidemiological evidence suggests that those who become or are active are less likely to suffer from depressive symptoms. There also appears to be a dose–response relationship.[82,83] The majority of research has focused upon mild to moderate depression rather than severe depression, and has used a variety of measures. In clinically depressed individuals, physical activity appears to be as effective as other therapeutic modalities.[84,85] This effect is noted with both aerobic and resistance training/flexibility training forms of activity and is independent of fitness. There is evidence to suggest that continuous moderate intensity activity (30 minutes per day) is more beneficial than intermittent bouts (three 10-minute sessions per day).[86] The benefits have been identified in older adults,[87] as well as in adolescents.[88]

Anxiety

Anxiety, both acute (state) and chronic (trait), has been evaluated for effects of both acute (individual bout) and chronic (regular) exercise performance. The literature suggests that a moderate benefit exists for acute exercise and acute/state anxiety, with the majority of research looking at aerobic activity. Likewise, exercise programs of varying durations have a moderate effect upon both acute and chronic forms of anxiety. Meta-analysis looking at acute and chronic exercise has noted improvement in anxiety symptom scores. Aerobic activity demonstrates a larger effect than do resistance training/flexibility training programs. For improvement in chronic anxiety, a threshold duration was suggested of a minimum of 21 minutes per session, with maximal benefits achieved after 40 minutes.[89,90] The majority of research to date emphasizes that no causal relationship exists between anxiety and physical activity and exercise.

Historically, individuals with panic disorder have been discouraged from participating in exercise programs because of the belief that aerobic activity could trigger panic attacks. Exercise avoidance has been suggested to be an important element of panic disorder and may be a possible contributor to the pathophysiology.[91] Comparison of exercise programs with medications demonstrates efficacy superior to placebo. Although there has been minimal research in this area, evidence does suggest that exercise and physical activity improve the symptoms of panic disorder without necessarily triggering attacks.

The mechanism by which physical activity and exercise provide these mental health benefits is the subject of debate. It is probably multifactorial, with both psychological and physiological effects. Subjective feelings of well-being are enhanced. Psychological mechanisms, such as enhanced self-esteem and body image, self-efficacy, and mastery of skills and self-determination, have all been suggested as explanations for this observation. Overall, it appears that factors associated with the process of exercise are of significance.[81]

Similarly, increases in brain monoamines (norepinephrine, dopamine, and serotonin) have been identified with exercise, and the beta-endorphin hypothesis has long been used to explain the "runner's high." Irrespective of the exact mechanism, the benefits of physical activity and exercise are well acknowledged for individuals with mild to moderate depression and/or anxiety. The benefits are both direct and indirect, as subjective well-being and quality of life are enhanced through the knowledge that health benefits are being obtained. Additionally, evidence supports a preventive role. It is suggested that continuously performed moderate activity of any type provides the most benefits. Although there are no definitive exercise recommendations that appear to be uniformly appropriate, the evidence does suggest that the current public health recommendations of at least 30 minutes of moderate-intensity activity performed on most days of the week is an applicable message for individuals with depression and/or anxiety.

Osteoporosis

The morbidity and mortality associated with osteoporosis is significant. An estimated 30% of postmenopausal women meet the World Health Organization's diagnostic criteria for osteoporosis, while another 54% have osteopenia. Although men are less susceptible to osteoporosis than women because of their greater peak bone mass and larger bone size, they are not immune to osteoporotic fractures and demonstrate a higher mortality rate than women from pathologic hip fractures.[92] Bone remodeling is a normal physiological process, with relatively linear bone growth occurring during childhood and acceleration occurring with puberty. Approximately 95% of peak bone mass is experienced by the age of 17 years in girls and maybe 2–3 years later in boys. Individuals who do not achieve this peak bone mass by approximately age 20 years are at increased risk for developing osteoporosis later in life. Bone mass remains relatively uniform until approximately age 50 years at which time an imbalance occurs in the bone remodeling cycle that favors bone loss. The dynamic nature of bone is reflected by the phenomenon

of increased bone mass as a result of increased strain applied during weight loading. Conversely, lack of bone stress allows for rapid decreases in bone mass. Immobilization may result in up to 40% loss of original bone mass within 1 year, while those individuals subject to bed rest can significantly prevent bone loss by standing upright for as little as 30 minutes each day.[47]

Many factors affect bone mass. Genetics may affect up to 70% of the variation in bone mass.[47] Some factors are modifiable, however, to include medications and medical history (which have varying degrees of modifiability), nutrition, alcohol and tobacco usage, and physical activity (which can be significantly modified to affect prevention and treatment).

Evidence to support the effects of exercise and physical activity on bone mass is plentiful. Immobilization leads to significant loss of bone mass as a result of mechanical unloading. Conversely, skeletal loading has variable effects on bone mass, as demonstrated by weight lifters (increased bone mass) and chronic overexercise seen in women experiencing the female athlete triad (disordered eating, amenorrhea, and osteoporosis). Osteoporosis associated with this syndrome is a reflection of a complex interplay of nutritional deficits and hormonal changes that counteract the positive effects of mechanical stress.

Physical activity and exercise can serve as both prevention and treatment for osteoporosis. Ideally, physical activity should be looked upon as a preventive strategy. Data indicates that habitual physical activity performed in childhood and adolescence leads to increases in bone mineral density.[93,94] Likewise, site-specific increases in bone mineral density have been identified in premenopausal women and young adults with both endurance- and resistance-training programs.[95] Imposition of greater impact forces than what are commonly achieved by aerobic and resistance activities (e.g., jumping) demonstrate greater site-specific increases in bone mineral density,[96,97] as supported by observational studies in gymnasts. Findings in seniors are varied but do suggest that physical activity programs may decrease the rate of bone loss (rather than affecting gains in bone mass). The findings of some studies that demonstrate increases in bone mineral density greater than that achieved in younger individuals suggests a steeper dose–response curve reflecting their generally less-active lifestyles.

It is yet to be determined if exercise alone can prevent the bone loss that occurs during the postmenopausal years. Results are equivocal to date. The exercise-related increases in bone mass are usually only on the order of 1–3%, but this may be significant when combined with other modalities within an overall approach to prevention and management.

A few important points should be emphasized when providing physical activity and exercise recommendations. Musculoskeletal overload is essential. Weight-bearing activities, such as walking, are essential but in and of themselves insufficient to elicit significant changes in bone mass. Combining a walking routine with resistance training, and/or performing loaded walking (e.g., weighted vests) optimize the effects of this activity. Conversely, activities such as swimming that unload the skeleton do little to maintain bone mass (although other cardiovascular and musculoskeletal benefits are significant). Additionally, the responses to this overload are site specific—walking with a weighted vest most affects the pelvis, hips, and spine, but does nothing for the upper body. High-stress activities that are outside the normal physical stresses imposed, such as jumping or running, have the greatest effects upon bone mass. Changes that result from these types of activity require repetition as cessation demonstrates rapid declines in gains.

Therefore, a life course approach to providing physical activity and exercise recommendations is necessary. Keeping in mind the importance of a life course perspective, young women should be encouraged to be physically active to build a strong base. Appropriate nutritional choices should complement regularly performed dynamic and bone-stress-inducing activities that provide varying stresses to the musculoskeletal system. Rope jumping, running, and plyometrics are good examples of such activities. Upper body activities, such as structured resistance-training programs, should be a component of these recommendations. Adults of all ages should give consideration to the five categories of activity that were previously mentioned and identify how they can incorporate such recommendations into the framework of their daily lives. Older individuals with physical limitations can continue to benefit from structured exercise programs and should be encouraged to be regularly active as part of their daily routines. Gradual progression is important and encouraging individuals to listen to their bodies rather than working through pain and discomfort is necessary. Combining walking with resistance training and flexibility exercises can provide a stimulus to bone, as well as improve postural stability, thereby decreasing the risk of falls and potential pathologic fractures (e.g., quadricep- and ankle-strengthening exercises, combined with yoga asanas that increase flexibility of the hips and lumbar spine).

Conversely, not all exercises are good for individuals with osteoporosis. Care should be taken when recommending activity with the focus being upon improving functional capacity and quality of life. Programs should seek to minimize the potential for falls and avoidance of activities that increase the risk for fractures. For example, flexion of the lumbar spine creates significant anterior loading pressures upon the vertebral bodies, increasing the risk of compression fractures. Gradual progression of extension exercises for the spine produce less stress and can provide structural stability. Therefore, individuals should be cautioned about lifting with a flexed spine and encouraged to avoid forward flexion exercises. Resistance-training programs should be performed under close supervision to monitor technique and proper form. Subsequently, many simple exercises can be translated to the home environment, allowing for their incorporation into daily lifestyle activities.

► CONCLUSION

The process as presented may appear labor-intensive. Effectively delivering recommendations from this framework is not something that can be done in a short office visit. As the history of activity and exercise promotion has produced poor results to date,[98] a new model of physical activity promotion is necessary. Integrative medicine fundamentally provides an opportunity of exploring new models of behavior change, given its focus upon developing a partnership between provider and patient; the importance of self-awareness and role modeling on the part of the practitioner; and the importance of understanding an individual's life context and life trajectory. It is through a mutual commitment to exploration of possibilities that physical activity promotion within the context of an integrative medicine framework can identify the wealth of potential that can be obtained by creating a naturally active way of living.

REFERENCES

1. US Department of Health and Human Services. *Physical Activity and Health: A Report of the Surgeon General.* Atlanta, GA: US Department of Health and Human Services, Centers for Disease Control and Prevention, National Center for Chronic Disease Prevention and Health Promotion; 1996.
2. Task Force on Community Preventive Services. Recommendations to increase physical activity in communities. *Am J Prev Med.* 2002;22(4S):67–72.
3. Pate RR, Pratt M, Blair SN, et al. Physical activity and public health. *JAMA.* 1995;273:402–407.
4. Centers for Disease Control and Prevention. Physical activity trends—United States, 1990-1998. *MMWR Morb Mortal Wkly Rep.* 2001;50:166–169.
5. US Department of Health and Human Services. *The Surgeon General's Call to Action to Prevent and Decrease Overweight and Obesity.* Rockville, MD: US Department of Health and Human Services, Public Health Service, Office of the Surgeon General; 2001.
6. Allison DB, Fontaine KR, Manson JE, Stevens J, VanItallie TB. Annual deaths attributable to obesity in the United States. *JAMA.* 1999;282(16):1530–1538.
7. Kujala UM, Kaprio J, Sarna S, Koskenvuo M. Relationship of leisure-time physical activity and mortality: the Finnish twin cohort. *JAMA.* 1998;279:440–444.
8. Blair SN, Kampert JB, Kohl HW, et al. Influences of cardiorespiratory fitness and other precursors on cardiovascular disease and all-cause mortality in men and women. *JAMA.* 1996;276:205–210.
9. US Department of Health and Human Services. *Healthy People 2010.* 2nd ed. *With Understanding and Improving Health and Objectives for Improving Health.* Washington, DC: US Government Printing Office; 2000.
10. World Health Organization. *Ottawa Charter for Health Promotion.* Copenhagen, Denmark: World Health Organization, European Regional Office; 1986.
11. Bouchard C, Shephard RJ, Stephens T, Sutton JR, McPerson BD, eds. *Exercise, Fitness and Health: A Consensus of Current Knowledge.* Champaign, IL: Human Kinetics Books; 1990.
12. Gaudet TW. Integrative Medicine: the evolution of a new approach to medicine and to medical education. *Integr Med.* 1998;1(2):67–73.
13. ACSM position stand on the recommended quantity and quality of exercise for developing and maintaining cardiorespiratory and muscular fitness in healthy adults. *Med Sci Sports Exerc.* 1990;22:265–274.
14. Pollock ML, Gaesser GA, Butcher JD, et al. American College of Sports Medicine position stand: the recommended quantity and quality of exercise for developing and maintaining cardiorespiratory and muscular fitness, and flexibility in healthy adults. *Med Sci Sports Exerc.* 1998;30(6):975–991.
15. Tanesescu M, Leitzmann MF, Rimm EB, Willett WC, Stampfer MJ, Hu FB. Exercise type and intensity in relation to coronary heart disease in men. *JAMA.* 2002;288:1994–2000.
16. *ACTIVE START: A Statement of Physical Activity Guidelines for Children Birth to Five Years.* Reston, VA: National Association for Sport and Physical Education; 2002.

17. Kann L, Kinchen SA, Williams BI, et al. Youth risk behavior surveillance—United States, 1997. *MMWR Morb Mortal Wkly Rep.* 1998;47(SS-3):1–89.

18. Caspersen CJ, Pereira MA, Curran KM. Changes in physical activity patterns in the United States, by sex and cross-sectional age. *Med Sci Sports Exerc.* 2000;32(9):1601–1609.

19. Pate RR, Small ML, Ross JG, et al. School physical education. *J School Health* 1998;165(8):312–318.

20. Simons-Morton BG, Taylor WC, Snider SA, et al. Observed levels of elementary and middle school children's physical activity during physical education classes. *Prev Med.* 1994;23:437–441.

21. Kuntzleman CT, Reiff GG. The decline in American children's fitness levels. *Res Q Exerc Sport.* 1992;63:107–111.

22. Morrow JR, Freedson PS. Relationship between habitual physical activity and aerobic fitness in adolescents. *Pediatr Exerc Sci.* 1994;6:315–329.

23. Calfas KJ, Taylor WC. Effects of physical activity on psychological variables in adolescents. *Pediatr Exerc Sci.* 1994;6:406–423.

24. Malina RM. Tracking of physical activity across the lifespan. *President's Council on Physical Fitness and Sports Research Digest.* 2001;3(14);1–8.

25. Clarke WR, Schrott H, Leaverton P, Connor W, Lauer RM. Tracking of blood lipids and blood pressure in children: the Muscatine Study. *Circulation.* 1978;58:626–634.

26. Clarke WR, Lauer RM. Does obesity track in childhood? *Crit Rev Food Sci Nutr.* 1993;33:423–430.

27. Lauer RM, Anderson A, Beaglehole R, Burns T. Factors related to tracking of blood pressure in children: US National Center for Statistics Health Examination Survey Cycles II and III. *Hypertension.* 1984;6:307–314.

28. Webber L, Srinvanson S, Wattigney W, Berenson G. Tracking of serum lipids and lipoproteins from childhood to adulthood. *Am J Epidemiol.* 1991;133:884–899.

29. Kelder SH, Perry CL, Klepp KI, Lytle LL. Longitudinal tracking of adolescent smoking, physical activity, and food choice behavior. *Am J Public Health.* 1994;94:1121–1126.

30. Kohl WH, Hobbs KE. Development of physical activity behaviors among children and adolescents. *Pediatrics.* 1998;3:S549–S554.

31. Malina RM. Tracking of physical activity and physical fitness across the life span. *Res Q Exerc Sport.* 1996;57:48–57.

32. Nader P, Stone E, Lytle L, et al. Three-year maintenance of improved diet and physical activity: The CATCH cohort. *Arch Pediatr Adolesc Med.* 1999;153:695–704.

33. Berenson GS. *CV Risk Factors in Children: The Early Natural History of Atherosclerosis and Essential Hypertension.* New York: Oxford University Press; 1980.

34. Corbin CB, Pangrazi RP. *Physical Activity for Children: A Statement of Guidelines.* Reston, VA: NASPE Publications; 1998.

35. American Academy of Pediatrics Committee on Sports Medicine and Fitness. Strength training by children and adolescents. *Pediatrics.* 2001;107(6):1470–1471.

36. Hoffman C, Rice D, Sung H. Persons with chronic conditions: their prevalence and costs. *JAMA.* 1996;276:1478–1479.

37. ACSM position stand on exercise and physical activity for older adults. *Med Sci Sports Exerc.* 1998;30(6):992–1008.

38. Chisholm DM, Collis ML, Kulak LL, Davenport W, Gruber N. Physical activity readiness. *Br Columbia Med J.* 1975;17:375–378.

39. Evans WJ. Exercise training guidelines for the elderly. *Med Sci Sports Exerc.* 1999;31(1):12–17.

40. Christmas C, Andersen RA. Exercise and older patients: guidelines for the clinician. *J Am Geriatr Soc.* 2000;48:318–24.

41. Province M, Hadley E, Hornbrook M, et al. for the FICSIT Group. The effects of exercise on falls in elderly patients. *JAMA.* 1995;273(17):1341–1347.

42. Wolf SL, Barnhart HX, Kutner NG, et al. Reducing frailty and falls in older persons: an investigation of Tai Chi and computerized balance training. Atlanta FICSIT Group. Frailty and Injuries: Cooperative Studies of Intervention Techniques. *J Am Geriatr Soc.* 1996;44(5):489–97.

43. Bailey DA, Faulkner RA, McKay HA. Growth, physical activity, and bone mineral acquisition. *Exerc Sport Sci Rev.* 1996;24:233–265.

44. Bailey DA, McCulloch RG. Osteoporosis: are there childhood antecedents for an adult health problem. *Can J Pediatr.* 1992;5:130–134.

45. Marcus R. Role of exercise in preventing and treating osteoporosis. *Rheum Dis Clin North Am.* 2001;27(1):131–141.

46. Breslow L. From disease prevention to health promotion. *JAMA.* 1999;281(11):1030–1033.

47. Marttila J, Laitakari J, Nupponen R, et al. The ver-

satile nature of physical activity—on the psychological, behavioural and contextual characteristics of health-related physical activity. *Patient Educ Counsel.* 1998;33:S29–38.

48. Dunn AL, Marcus BH, Kampert JB, et al. Comparison of lifestyle and structured interventions to increase physical activity and cardiorespiratory fitness. *JAMA.* 1999;281(4):327–334.

49. Andersen RE, Wadden TA, Barlett SJ, et al. Effects of lifestyle activity vs. structure aerobic exercise in obese women: a randomized trial. *JAMA.* 1999;281(4):335–340.

50. Ainsworth BE, Montoye HJ, Leon AS. Methods of assessing physical activity during leisure and work. In: Bouchard C, Shephard RJ, Stephens T, eds. *Physical Activity, Fitness and Health: International Proceedings and Consensus Statement.* Champaign, IL: Human Kinetics; 1994:146–159.

51. Tanaka H, Monahan KD, Seals DR. Age-predicted maximal heart rate revised. *J Am Coll Cardiol.* 2001;37:153–156.

52. Dunn AL, Andersen RE, Jakicic JM. Lifestyle physical activity interventions: history, short- and long-term effects, and recommendations. *Am J Prev Med.* 1998;15(4):398–412.

53. Kalfas KJ, Long BJ, Sallis JF, et al. A controlled trial of physician counseling to promote the adoption of physical activity. *Prev Med.* 1996;25: 225–233.

54. Eakin EG, Glasgow RE, Riley KM. Review of primary care-based physical activity intervention studies. *J Fam Pract.* 2000;49:158–168.

55. The Writing Group for the Activity Counseling Trial Research Group. Effects of physical activity counseling in primary care: the Activity Counseling Trial: a randomized controlled trial. *JAMA.* 2001;286:677–687.

56. Corbin CB, Pangrazi RP. Toward a uniform definition of wellness: a commentary. *President's Council on Physical Fitness and Sports Research Digest.* 2001;3(15):1–8.

57. US Preventive Services Task Force. *Guide to Clinical Preventive Services.* 2nd ed. Baltimore, MD: Williams & Wilkins; 1996.

58. Chakravarthy MV, Joyner MJ, Booth FW. An obligation for primary care physicians to prescribe physical activity to sedentary patients to reduce the risk of chronic health conditions. *Mayo Clin Proc.* 2002;77:165–173.

59. Pinto BM, Goldstein MG, Marcus BH. Activity counseling by primary care physicians. *Prev Med.* 1998;27:506–513.

60. Harsha DM, Saywell RM, Thygerson S, Panozzo J. Physician factors affecting patient willingness to comply with exercise recommendations. *Clin J Sports Med.* 1996;6:112–118.

61. Sleap M, Tolfrey K. Do 9- to 12-year-old children meet existing physical activity recommendations for health? *Med Sci Sports Exerc.* 2001;33(4): 591–596.

62. McGinnis J, Foege W. Actual causes of death in the United States. *JAMA.* 1993;270:2207–2212.

63. Corbin CB, Prangrazi RP, Frank BD. Definitions: health, fitness, and physical activity. *Res Dig.* 2000;3(9):1–9.

64. Hochbaum GM. *Public Participation in Medical Screening Programs: A Sociopsychological Study.* Washington, DC: USPHS; 1958.

65. Rosenstock IM. The health belief model: explaining health behavior through expectancies. In: Glanz K, Rimer BK, Lewis FM, eds. *Health Behavior and Health Education. Theory, Research, and Practice.* San Francisco: Jossey-Bass; 1990.

66. Janz NK, Becker MH. The health belief model: a decade later. *Health Educ Q.* 1984;11(1):1–47.

67. Prochaska JO, DiClemente CC. *The Transtheoretical Approach: Crossing Traditional Boundaries of Change.* Homewood, IL: Dorsey Press; 1984.

68. Prochaska JO, DiClemente CC, Norcross JC. In search of how people change. *Am Psychol.* 1992;47(9):1102–1114.

69. Bandura A. *Social Foundations of Thought and Action: A Social-Cognitive Theory.* Englewood Cliffs, NJ: Prentice-Hall; 1986.

70. Bandura A. Health promotion from the perspective of social cognitive theory. *Psychol Health.* 1998;13:623–649.

71. Fishbein M, Ajzen I. Belief, attitude, intention, and behavior: an introduction to theory and research. Boston, MA: Addison-Wesley, 1975.

72. Ajzen I, Fishbein M. *Understanding Attitudes and Predicting Social Behavior.* Englewood Cliffs, NJ: Prentice-Hall; 1980.

73. Ajzen I. *Attitudes, Personality and Behavior.* Homewood, IL: Dorsey Press; 1998.

74. Stokols D. Establishing and maintaining healthy environments: toward a social ecology of health promotion. *Am Psychol.* 1992;47:6–22.

75. McLeroy KR, Bibeau D, Steckler A, Glanz K. An ecological perspective on health promotion programs. *Health Educ Q.* 1988;15(4):351–377.

76. Sallis JF, Owen N. Ecological models of health behavior. In: Glanz K, Rimer BK, Lewis FM, eds. *Health Behavior and Health Education*. 3rd ed. San Francisco: Jossey-Bass; 2002.

77. *Theory at a Glance. A Guide for Health Promotion Practice*. Available at: http://oc.nci.nih.gov/services/Theory_at_glance/HOME.html. Accessed 8/25/03.

78. Glanz K, Rimer BK, Lewis FM, eds. *Health Behavior and Health Education*. 3rd ed. San Francisco: Jossey-Bass; 2002.

79. Laitakari J, Asikainen TM. How to promote physical activity through individual counseling—a proposal for a practical model of counseling on health-related physical activity. *Patient Educ Counsel*. 1998;33:S13–S24.

80. Paluska SA, Schwenk TL. Physical activity and mental health current concepts. *Sports Med*. 2000;29(3):167–180.

81. Fox KR. The influence of physical activity on mental well-being. *Public Health Nutr*. 1999;2(3a):411–418.

82. Paffenbarger RS, Lee I-M, Leung R. Physical activity and personal characteristics associated with depression and suicide in American college men. *Acta Psychiatr Scand*. 1994;89(S377):16–22.

83. Farmer ME, Locke BZ, Moscicki EK, et al. Physical activity and depressive symptoms: The NHANES I epidemiological follow-up study. *Am J Epidemiol*. 1988;128:1340–1351.

84. Shepard RJ. Physical activity, health and well-being at different life stages. *Res Q Exerc Sport*. 1995;66(4):298–302.

85. Craft LL, Landers DM. The effect of exercise on clinical depression and depression resulting from mental illness: a meta-analysis. *J Sport Exerc Psychol*. 1998;20(4):339–357.

86. Osei-Tutu KEK, Campagna PD. Psychological benefits of continuous vs. intermittent moderate intensity exercise. *Med Sci Sports Exerc*. 1998;30(suppl 15):S117.

87. King AC, Taylor CB, Haskell WL. Effects of differing intensities and formats of 12 months of exercise training on psychological outcomes in older adults. *Health Psychol*. 1993;12(4):292–300.

88. Steptoe A, Butler N. Sports participation and emotional well-being in adolescents. *Lancet*. 1996;347:1789–1792.

89. Calfas KJ, Taylor WC. Effects of physical activity on psychological variables in adolescents. *Pediatr Exerc Sci*. 1994;6(4):406–423.

90. Petruzzello SJ, Landers DM, Hatfield BD, et al. A meta-analysis of the anxiety-reducing effects of acute and chronic exercise. *Sports Med*. 1991;11(3):143–182.

91. Zimetbaum P, Josephson ME. Evaluation of patients with palpitations. *N Engl J Med*. 1998;338(19):1369–1373.

92. Poor G, Atkinson EJ, Lewallen DG, et al. Age-related hip fractures in men: clinical spectrum and short-term outcomes. *Osteoporos Int*. 1995;5(6):419–426.

93. Bailey D, McKay HA, Mirwald RL, et al. A six-year longitudinal study of the relationship of physical activity to bone mineral accrual in growing children: the University of Saskatchewan Bone Mineral Accrual Study. *J Bone Miner Res*. 1999;14:1672–1679.

94. Bradney M, Pearce G, Naughton G, et al. Moderate exercise during growth in prepubertal boys: changes in bone mass, size, volumetric density, and bones strength: a controlled prospective study. *J Bone Miner Res*. 1998;13(12):1814–1821.

95. Friedlander AL, Genant HK, Sadowsky S, et al. A two-year program of aerobics and weight-training enhances BMD of young women. *J Bone Miner Res*. 1995;10(4):574–585.

96. Bassey EJ, Rothwell MC, Little JJ, et al. Pre- and postmenopausal women have different bone mineral density responses to the same high impact exercise. *J Bone Miner Res*. 1998;13:1805–1813.

97. Arnett MG, Lutz B. The effects of rope jump training on the os calcis stiffness index of postpubescent girls. *Med Sci Sports Exerc*. 2002;34(12):1913–1919.

98. Laitakari J, Miilunpalo S. How can physical activity be changed: basic concepts and general principles in the promotion of health-related physical activity. *Patient Educ Counsel*. 1998;33(Suppl):S47–S59.

CHAPTER 14

Spirituality and Health

VICTOR S. SIERPINA AND MICHELLE SIERPINA

Substantial data exists demonstrating the impact of spiritual and religious practices on health outcomes. This chapter summarizes the clinical and epidemiological literature relating to spirituality and health, and briefly describes the phenomenon known as nonlocal healing. It offers suggested techniques for sensitively discussing spiritual matters with patients, and describes several published models for taking a spiritual history.

Healers in traditional societies have always interwoven their healing and spiritual practices. Examples of such traditional blending of the healing of body and spirit include Aesculapian temple dreamworkers, Navajo sandpainting practices, the ritual Lakotah use of the medicine wheel (Figure 14–1), and the shamanic tradition shared by many cultures of a healing journey to "retrieve the ill person's soul." The tribal medicine man or woman is both healer and spiritual leader. The Lakotah medicine man saw healing as occurring through the continuity between man and nature. The miraculous healings attributed to Jesus in the *Bible* are another example of the traditional connection[1] between spiritual practice and healing. Traditional Chinese medicine does not differentiate spiritual and mental healing from physical healing; nor does Ayurveda or the traditional indigenous healing systems of Africa. Rather, all of these traditions consider spiritual practices an integral part of a holistic healing continuum.

Almost all traditional healing systems have held that man is inextricably connected both to nature and to others in the society. Individual health involves balance in the interconnectedness between humankind and the earth, between humans and other humans, and between the individual and the spiritual powers. This balance is maintained through an interchange of energy between the earth and the people through healthy social interactions, and through regular spiritual practice.

With the advent of Cartesian thinking and the "scientific method" in the seventeenth century in Western civilization, a separation between the realms of material body and spirit developed: morality and spirituality became the exclusive domain of the church, while the scientists were left to explore the material world and the physical functions of the human body. The benefit of the Cartesian split of mind–body and spirit was that it relieved, for a time, the tension that blamed all illness on personal misconduct or sin. Science was freed from explaining existential and philosophical issues beyond its experimental and observational processes.

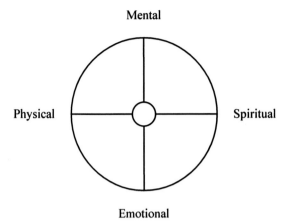

Mental

Physical   Spiritual

Emotional

Figure 14–1. Medicine wheel. The medicine wheel, permeated with spirit, was a symbol of all of life, not a mere pantheistic icon. Spirit coincides with values leading to mental thoughts, which initiate physical actions. The emotional reactions cycle back to inform and compare to the spiritual values. The medicine wheel symbolized the belief that spirit animates all living beings and even inanimate ones: stone, sky, weather, water, and fire.

Over time, however, contemporary man's quest for knowledge and the scientific explanation of the world has failed to address the disconnection between the mind–body and human spirituality. Although the mechanism remains unknown, scientific studies reveal an association between health care outcomes and prayer, religious practices, beliefs, and spiritual orientation toward life. The development of quantum theory has also supported the existence of an inextricable relationship between all aspects of the universe: physical, psychical, and spiritual.

Viktor Frankl eloquently defined man's "search for meaning" as the ultimate quest in our species, a quest that addresses life's core issues—health, illness, suffering, death, and the understanding and acceptance of our humanness.[2] An examination of the connection between this "search for meaning" and the human experience of health and illness—and a commitment to explore this connection with our patients—constitutes an important piece of the integrative medicine approach.

▶ DEFINITIONS OF SPIRITUALITY AND RELIGION

The distinction between "spirituality" and "religion" is not always clear to those entering into an exploration of this field. One can define spirituality broadly and intrapersonally as *an inherent aspect of every human being that relates to the Absolute—that domain where values and meaning exist.* Religion is more external and interpersonal, *a body of beliefs and practices defined by a community or society to which its adherents mutually subscribe.* While these definitions are not mutually exclusive, it is important to note that one can be religious without being spiritual and spiritual without being religious, or one can, of course, be both. The social dimensions and manifestations of one's values represent the intersection of one's religious or spiritual practices with other individuals and with society. One helpful way to more easily understand this boundary is by examining the distinctions between one's own personal spirituality and the organized religion or religious practices to which one may have been exposed.

Spirituality is ineffable, constituting "one's relationship to the Absolute."[3] Most health and religion studies have addressed religious practice using attendance at religious services as a measurable variable. Although imprecise, this approach has at least provided a means to begin to describe the association between health care and personal beliefs in the realm of spirituality and religion. The impact of a personal spirituality practiced outside of the context of organized religion is not adequately characterized by this approach, and neither are the transpersonal aspects of prayer or how intentionality and nonlocal healing affect clinical or basic science outcomes.

▶ TAKING A SPIRITUAL HISTORY

Cultural competency—the ability to understand patients' beliefs and attitudes as a manifestation of their cultural and ethnic background—is critical to the effective practice of patient-centered or relationship-centered medicine. The spiritual history is an important part of understanding this cultural context for each patient and will help the health care provider recognize the impact religious practices and spiritual beliefs have on patients' health and their health-related choices.

The practitioner who obtains vital information about a patient's belief system may better understand why the patient makes certain choices while not selecting other seemingly rational ones. It would be inappropriate and perhaps even insensitive to query every patient about spiritual beliefs on the first visit. In a lon-gitudinal therapeutic relationship, however, these issues will emerge, often spontaneously and organically. Spiritual matters may seem to have little relevance to minor, self-limiting illnesses like colds and flu. On the other hand, even minor illnesses may bring messages from the body or the psychospiritual dimension. They may signal imbalance, that the immune system is under stress, or that a conflict in one's life values and one's actions is resulting in illness.

It may be easier for health care providers to recognize the importance of addressing patients' spiritual needs during major illness, hospitalization, surgery, and terminal disease. A skilled clinician may use Maslow's hierarchy of needs to guide assessing patient readiness and the appropriateness of discussing spiritual matters.[4] The case history that follows illustrates the importance of an awareness of the role of spirituality in a patient's life.

▶ Case Example: Ophelia B.

In teaching medical students and house staff about the importance of spirituality in the clinical care setting, perhaps nothing is as effective as an experience with a patient for whom their religious and spiritual beliefs are intrinsic to their world view and directly impact their medical care.

One busy afternoon, I (Dr. VSS) was working with Dr. SG, a third year-resident, and we were admitting Ophelia B, an elderly African American woman with a new diagnosis of multiple myeloma. When Dr. SG and I entered the patient's room, we found it filled with family members, friends, and an impressive 6'7" gentleman who identified himself as Ophelia's minister.

We greeted and shook hands as I introduced my resident and myself as the attending physician. We asked if we could have some time alone with the patient to perform her history and physical.

"Actually, Doc," said the gigantic minister, "we were just about to pray together. Could you come back in a little while?"

Looking way up at the minister, I restrained a flicker of impatience as I quickly realized how essential this moment was for the patient.

Rather than leaving, expressing annoyance, or trying to assert some kind of medical authority, I politely asked, "Do you mind if we join you in the prayer?"

The patient was clearly pleased, as was the minister.

"Of course, doctor. We'd be pleased to have you join us," said the minister with a smile.

We joined hands in a circle of care and prayer around the patient's bed. I glanced over at my resident who was wide eyed with this development, clearly a novel experience for her.

The minister, a daughter, and a son each said a few words of prayer. I took the opportunity to compose a short prayer of my own in the spirit of the moment. The patient closed with a short prayer for her family and for the medical team.

Throughout the rest of her hospitalization, the patient and her family members used every opportunity to express hope, gratitude, and optimism based on the fact that her medical team was connected with her on a spiritual level. As standard chemotherapy protocol was implemented, the enrollment of the patient's faith, her minister, and her joy that the medical team supported the importance of her faith system in her healing process all helped Ophelia and her family adjust to a difficult problem.

While we never took a formal spiritual history as described below (we didn't need to in this case), our willingness to engage with the patient around the importance of *her* belief system was instrumental in enhancing the therapeutic relationship. By providing not only conventional medical care but empowering her by affirming the value of her beliefs in the healing process, the quality of the patient's experience with a serious illness was substantially improved. It was clearly important to her that not only her minister and family enjoin her spiritual beliefs but that her medical team did as well. This fit with the belief of many religious African Americans that the doctor is "God's mechanic"; the closer we can align ourselves with this belief system, the more patient rapport we can establish.[5]

Dr. SG expressed appreciation at the opportunity to expand her range of clinical behaviors to include a higher degree of sensitivity and direct support to patients regarding their spiritual belief system. Simply joining hands in a circle of prayer in that hospital room provided a connection for Ophelia that could most likely not have happened in any other way.

Approaches to Spiritual History-Taking

There are a number of published models for how to take a sensitive but thorough spiritual history. These are not inflexible templates or formulaic approaches. Rather, they provide students and clinicians with vocabulary and techniques that reassure both patient and clinician. The challenge of taking a spiritual history can be likened to the difficulties or even the embarrassment of inquiring about domestic violence, sexual practices, or substance abuse. Like these, it represents an important part of the biopsychosocial history, which should not be omitted simply because of the physician's discomfort with the topic. Table 14–1 presents four useful models for taking a spiritual history.[4]

▶ EPIDEMIOLOGY OF RELIGION AND HEALTH

Almost every major disease or condition, whether physical or mental, has been shown to be positively affected by a patient's religious practice.[3] More than 1,600 studies have shown religious involvement, attendance, and social support from a religious community to have substantive health benefits. This remains true even when lifestyle factors such as smoking, alcohol consumption, marital status, and other expected confounders are factored out. An in-depth review of the epidemiology of religion and of the impact of religion and prayer on specific health conditions is beyond the scope of this chapter; consequently, we provide the reader with information on where to find such a review, and with a few examples

▶ **TABLE 14-1** FOUR MODELS OF TAKING A SPIRITUAL HISTORY

Three Questions[6]	FICA[7]
1. What helps you get through tough times?	Faith
2. Who do you turn to when you need support?	Impact
3. What meaning does this experience have for you?	Community
	Assist

Hope[4]	Spiritual History[8]
Hope—sources of	Spiritual belief system
Organized religion	Personal spirituality
Personal spirituality or practice	Integration with spiritual community
Effects on medical care and End of life Issues	Ritualized practices and restrictions
	Implications for medical care
	Terminal event planning

of studies that demonstrate particularly important points.

Dale Matthews and colleagues from the National Institute for Healthcare Research have developed an extensive bibliography of clinical research related to spiritual topics documenting the scope of evolving scientific inquiry. This appears in four volumes entitled *The Faith Factor.*[10–13] A second invaluable resource in this area is *Handbook of Religion and Health,*[14] which systematically catalogues and critically reviews more than 1,600 studies.

One question that is often raised is whether religious practice or attendance is simply a proxy for social support, and that the benefits attributed to religion are in fact not distinct from those known to derive from any social network. A study done by Oxman and colleagues[15] found that cardiac patients who reported religious beliefs or social support and social network recovered faster and survived longer than did patients who did not. This study examined religious participation and social support separately and found that these were additive variables. Each alone was a positive predictor of improved health, but taken together the outcomes increased. Religion, as defined above, adds to the individual's social support network.

An early study at Duke University reported similar findings. In the Duke Longitudinal Study of Aging,[16] 252 men were followed for 25 years. Religious affiliation was negatively associated with mortality. A rigorous longitudinal study examined the relationship between religious attendance and all-cause mortality over a 28-year period and found that attending services once per week was associated with a 36% reduction in mortality during the follow up period.[17] Of interest is that in this report, frequent church attendees were more likely, rather than less likely, to have impaired mobility. This offsets a common criticism of church attendance-type studies in which the critics assert that attendance statistics create a selection bias for a healthier population. The logic is that the less mobile and already sick are less likely to attend services. The opposite was found to be the case here. Many studies also show positive relationships between religious involvement and improved mental health or decreased experiences of depression and medical interventions related to mental illness.[18–20]

In addition to their demonstrable effects on mortality, for many people their religious practices offer them substantial coping behaviors with end-of-life issues, the loss of function and pain that may accompany aging and illness, and the loss of loved ones. These coping mechanisms can help to relieve stress, define meaning, and further personal and spiritual growth when facing life's greatest challenges. End-of-life choices regarding resuscitation and terminal care are often informed by a patient's and their family's belief system. One religious group might opt for every possible medical intervention no matter how complex or costly. Another might peacefully accept an end-of-life transition with minimal medical intervention and appropriate comfort care and pain relief. While inquiring about end-of-life choices, such as code/no code status, it is vital that health care practitioners be sensitive to the patient's predominant belief system, as well as to the patient's personal and community sources of support and comfort.

► PRAYER AND NONLOCAL HEALING

Another body of literature examines the direct effects of prayer, positive intentionality, and directed thought on people, animals, and microbes, and even on random events. In *Spiritual Healing, Scientific Validation of a Healing Revolution*,[21] psychiatrist Daniel Benor concisely reviews 124 controlled scientific studies of "spiritual healing." He defines spiritual healing as "a systematic, purposeful intervention by one or more persons aiming to help another living being (person, animal, plant, or other living system) by means of focused intention, hand contact, or *passes* to improve their condition."[22]

In a landmark study, cardiologist Randolph C. Byrd followed nearly 400 coronary care unit patients in a San Francisco hospital.[23] Byrd's rigidly designed, double-blind, randomized study found that patients who were prayed for required fewer antibiotics than did those in the control group, and needed no intubations or mechanical ventilators, while many in the control group did. Mortality was lower among the prayed-for group, although the difference was not statistically significant.

A second double-blind, randomized, controlled study by William Harris and his colleagues on coronary care unit patients in Kansas City, Missouri, included nearly 1,000 patients.[24] This work showed that distant intercessory prayer was associated with positive medical outcomes in coronary patients in the range of 10–11%.

AIDS patients received positive distant intentionality in a study done by Sicher, Targ, and their colleagues.[25] This randomized, double-blind study showed that those who were the focus of distant healing had statistically significantly fewer AIDS-related health problems after 6 months. Nonlocal intentionality also has been studied in other life forms and in inanimate objects.

► CONTROVERSIES IN SPIRITUALITY AND MEDICINE

The current confluence of spirituality and medicine is controversial. Many studies support the beneficial effect of religion and religious practice on health. Others examine patient beliefs and expectations for spiritual support from physicians and the effects of distant prayer or nonlocal healing. Critics cite methodological flaws and believe several significant ethical issues remain unresolved. In one succinct overview of this subject, VandeCreek, a chaplain, challenges physicians' professionalism and ethical standard when providing spiritual care, as well as the notion of any physician advocacy for religious aspects of patient care.[26] He outlines these concerns:

1. Patients' religious diversity is a problem area. Plurality and heterogeneity of religious beliefs make it difficult to initiate religious discussions or to pray with patients. Physicians may not be well trained to manage this diversity. However, the author does, nevertheless, agree that taking a spiritual history is important.

2. Religious faith and practice are a source of conflict, guilt, and family and intercultural discord for some patients. Advocates of addressing spirituality in clinical care emphasize the comfort and meaning patients derive from their beliefs. The author challenges physicians initiating dialogue about such complex and sensitive matters in the health care setting.
3. Physicians may not possess the requisite interpersonal and intrapersonal skills to facilitate religious conversations. Skills learned in chaplaincy and psychotherapy training are essential. No published research has examined what physician skills are necessary for this area, nor how they might be taught.
4. Physicians might proselytize about their own deeply held religious beliefs. This is an inappropriate use of medical authority.
5. Physicians who include religious issues in the medical context risk crossing boundaries and diminishing religion to a mere medical "intervention." Is medicine's focus on health and illness appropriately merged with religious discussion and recommendations about spiritual practices? He argues that this alliance can trivialize religion by subsuming it to medical treatment.

VandeCreek concludes that religion and spirituality cannot be totally separated from medical practice. Patients may raise religious concerns with their physicians and some adequately trained physicians may well participate in these discussions. He suggests that much additional research and discussion are necessary before this area becomes a standard part of medical practice.

Other authors argue that the science underlying the association of religion and health is flawed; that church attendance and health outcomes data should be viewed cautiously; and that only clinical trials rather than epidemiologic studies on church attendance are likely to be definitive.[27] They further argue that many studies fail to control for confounders,

such as behavioral and genetic differences, and stratification variables, such as age, sex, education, ethnicity, socioeconomic status, and health status. They state that many epidemiology of religion studies report conflicting findings.[28] These authors are concerned that mixing physician authority and religious issues can be dangerously coercive. They question whether results are generalizable to gravely ill patients, non-Protestants, and tertiary surgical patients, for example.

In essence, such authors argue that the association between religion, spirituality, and health is weak, making it premature to promote faith and religion as adjunctive to medical treatments. They feel that patients who draw upon religious faith may be supported, but that prayer, religious activity, or attendance should not be prescribed.

Countering these arguments, Dossey takes the position that physicians and nurses cannot ignore sensitive issues just because they are uncomfortable with them.[29–31] This area provides an opportunity, Dossey contends, to remove the labels of modern medicine as "too remote, too technical, and too uncaring." In the same vein, the family medicine literature on spirituality suggests that taking a thorough spiritual history can greatly improve the physician's understanding of his or her patients, especially in the palliative care or end-of-life setting.[7] Studies from both primary care settings and inpatient populations consistently find that many patients are interested in discussing spiritual matters with their physicians.[32–34] A survey of family physicians reports that 79% describe themselves as having a strong religious or spiritual orientation.[35] Furthermore, a majority of family physicians believe that spiritual well-being is an important factor in health.[36] The physician with proper training in this area can use his or her own philosophical and spiritual beliefs in a sensitive manner to enhance the healing relationship without imposing these particular beliefs on or prescribing these particular beliefs for the patient. Unfortunately, most studies show that, lacking time and adequate training, physicians tend to discuss spiritual matters infrequently with their patients and make few referrals of hospitalized patient to chaplains.[36]

The controversy regarding the proper place for spiritual interventions in the clinical setting is paralleled by a similar controversy regarding how—and even whether—prayer and other spiritual practices can or should be studied. A balanced discussion about the controversy of academic health centers studying the efficacy of intercessory prayer notes the arguments in favor of conducting such research[37]:

1. The academic medical center should seek new knowledge concerning therapeutics, irrespective of the source of the original hypotheses.
2. Medical research has an obligation to respond to the demand of the body politic in selecting topics for research.
3. Clinical trials of intercessory prayer take no position on the existence of God.

The same authors go on to outline the major criticisms of academic prayer research:

1. It is impossible to design a controlled trial of the efficacy of prayer.
2. An academic medical center conducting a clinical trial of intercessory prayer is offensive to religion.
3. Clinical trials of the efficacy of prayer are an attempt to prove the existence of God.

Potential problems in prayer research are many, including denominationalism, placebo effect, "dosage," causality, and informed consent. Nonetheless, promoting further research among those in the academic community is one way to diminish the existing controversy.

Although complete consensus among all participants in this area of investigation is not likely, Table 14–2 outlines a number of points that seem to be widely agreed upon by many experts in this area at this point.

▶ RECOMMENDATIONS FOR CLINICIANS

Although there are certainly challenges and significant barriers to effective communication

---

▶ **TABLE 14-2** CONSENSUS POINTS IN THE DEBATE ABOUT RELIGION, SPIRITUALITY, AND HEALTH

1. Health care, spirituality, and religion have interrelationships.
2. Prescribing or proselytizing religious or spiritual practices by health care providers is inappropriate.
3. Prayer with patients can be appropriate if patient initiated.
4. Taking a spiritual history is a matter of cultural competency to be considered in certain, though not all, medical encounters.
5. Further research on both the epidemiology of religion and the efficacy of prayer are indicated by previous research and necessary to define spirituality's place in health care.
6. Communicating about spiritual matters with patients is a delicate matter, similar to communicating about domestic violence, sexual orientation or practice, substance abuse, and other difficult subjects. Training of health care providers in this skill is an educational challenge.
7. Closer collaboration with and referrals to trained clergy or chaplains is an important part of managing the issue of spirituality in health care.
8. The role of spirituality and religion in the health care setting is decided among the individual patient, the family, and the health care provider.
9. Potential problems of ethical issues, power issues, and blurring of scientific and religious boundaries are all challenges.

in this area, the clinician who believes that the spiritual component is valid, relevant, and helpful to patient care will discover effective ways to introduce it. This may require a change in practice habits and the learning of new ways of being with patients, and also may elicit concerns about the clinician's own beliefs.

The issue of plurality and heterogeneity of beliefs is a real one. The health care provider who starts from a patient-centered position, respecting patients' beliefs and choices whatever they may be, will demonstrate good communication, compassion, and caring. While it is inappropriate to impose one's own view of religion or spirituality (or other topics for that matter) on patients, there may be times when the patient asks about the clinician's views and values.

Fully understanding one's own belief system and knowing how it gives life meaning and purpose is essential to effectiveness in this area. The beliefs of the patient and of the health care provider may not coincide. To answer patient's questions, one will have to have examined certain existential questions that occur in medical practice, for example, the death of a child, a life-threatening illness, and how to make end-of-life choices. Furthermore, a solid grounding in one's own belief system can prevent the all-too-frequent physician burnout that occurs when values and the reality of medical care seem to clash. Medicine is not a "value-free" zone or profession. Medical choices are value laden. The health care provider's spiritual position is intrinsic to how choices are made.

The physician must make choices: whether to pray with patients, how to create a healing environment in the office, how to address unanswerable questions, and how to find meaning for patients, their families, and the physician, even in pain and suffering. In the context of a clear but evolving personal belief system, these dilemmas become easier, although never truly simple.

REFERENCES

1. *Holy Bible.* "Matthew 7:16." New International Version. Grand Rapids, MI: Zondervan; 1994.

2. Frankl V. *Man's Search for Meaning.* New York: Simon & Schuster; 1984.

3. Dossey L. The future of medicine: the role of spirituality and meaning. International Wellness Conference. Galveston, TX. January 18, 2002.

4. Anandarajah G, Hight E. Spirituality and medical practice using the HOPE questions as a practical tool for spiritual assessment. *Am Fam Physician.* 2001;63:81–89.

5. Mansfield CJ, Mitchell J, King DE. The doctor as God's mechanic? Beliefs in the southeastern United States. *Social Sci Med.* 2002;54(3):399–409.

6. Kinney C. Three questions. Galveston, TX: The University of Texas Medical Branch at Galveston, School of Nursing; 1999.

7. Puchalski C, Romer A. Taking a spiritual history allows clinicians to understand patients more fully. *J Palliat Med.* 2000;3:129–137.

8. Maugans T. The spiritual history. *Arch Fam Med.* 1990;5:11–16.

9. Sierpina V. Mind, body, and now . . . spirit. In: *Integrative Health Care: Complementary and Alternative Therapies for the Whole Person.* Philadelphia: FA Davis; 2001:48–55.

10. Matthews D, Larson D, Barry C. The faith factor. In: *An Annotated Bibliography of Clinical Research on Spiritual Subjects.* Vol. 1. Rockville, MD: National Institute for Healthcare Research; 1993.

11. Matthews D, Larson D, Barry C. The faith factor. In: *An Annotated Bibliography of Clinical Research on Spiritual Subjects.* Vol. 2. Rockville, MD: National Institute for Healthcare Research; 1993.

12. Matthews D, Larson D, Barry C. The faith factor. In: *An Annotated Bibliography of Clinical Research on Spiritual Subjects.* Vol. 3. Rockville, MD: National Institute for Healthcare Research; 1995.

13. Matthews D, Larson D, Barry C, et al. The faith factor. In: *An Annotated Bibliography of Clinical Research on Spiritual Subjects: Prevention and Treatment of Illness, Addictions, and Delinquency.* Vol 4. Rockville, MD: National Institute for Healthcare Research; 1997.

14. Koenig H, McCoullough M, Larson D. *Handbook of Religion and Health.* New York: Oxford University Press; 2001:53–382.

15. Oxman T. Lack of social participation or religious strength and comfort as risk factors after cardiac surgery in the elderly. *Psychosom Med.* 1995;57:5–15.

16. Palmore E. Predictors of the longevity difference: a 25-year follow-up. *Gerontology*. 1982;22:513–518.

17. Strawbridge W, Cohen R, Shema S, et al. Frequent attendance at religious services and mortality over 28 years. *Am J Public Health*. 1997;87:957–961.

18. Koenig H, Cohen H, Blazer D, et al. Religious coping and depression among elderly, hospitalized medically ill men. *Am J Psychiatry*. 1992;149:1693–1700.

19. Koenig H, George L, Peterson B. Religiosity and remission of depression in medically ill older patients. *Am J Psychiatry*. 1998;155:536–542.

20. Levin J, Markides K, Ray L. Religious attendance and psychological well-being in Mexican Americans: a panel analysis of three-generations of data. *Gerontologist*. 1996;36:454–463.

21. Benor D. *Spiritual Healing, Scientific Validation of a Healing Revolution*. Southfield, MI: Vision Publications; 2001.

22. Benor D. *Spiritual Healing, Scientific Validation of a Healing Revolution*. Southfield, MI: Vision Publications; 2001:4.

23. Byrd R. Positive therapeutic effects of intercessory prayer in a coronary care unit population. *South Med J*. 1988;81:826–829.

24. Harris W, Gowda M, Kolb J, et al. A randomized, controlled trial of the effects of remote, intercessory prayer on outcomes in patients admitted to the coronary care unit. *Arch Intern Med*. 1999;159:2273–2278.

25. Sicher F, Targ E, Moore D. A randomized double-blind study of the effect of distant healing in a population with advanced AIDS. Report of a small scale study. *West J Med*. 1998;169:356–363.

26. VandeCreek L. Physicians providing spiritual care: professional and ethical challenges. *The Park Ridge Center Bulletin;* 2000:7–8.

27. Sloan R, Bagiella E, VandeCreek L. Should physicians prescribe religious activities? *N Engl J Med*. 2000;342:1913–1916.

28. Sloan R, Bagiella E, Powell T. Religion, spirituality, and medicine. *Lancet*. 1999;353:664–667.

29. Dossey L. *Healing Words: The Power of Prayer and the Practice of Medicine*. San Francisco: Harper Collins; 1993.

30. Dossey L. *Be Careful What You Pray For . . . You Just Might Get It*. San Francisco: Harper Collins; 1997.

31. Dossey L. Do religion and spirituality matter in health? A response to the recent article in the Lancet. *Altern Ther Health Med*. 1999;5:16–18.

32. King D, Bushwick B. Beliefs and attitudes of hospital inpatients about faith healing and prayer. *J Fam Pract*. 1994;39:349–352.

33. Maugans T, Wadland W. Religion and family medicine: a survey of physicians and patients. *J Fam Pract*. 1991;32:210–213.

34. Ehman J, Ott B, Short T, et al. Do patients want physicians to inquire about their spiritual or religious beliefs if they become gravely ill? *Arch Intern Med*. 1999;159:1803–1806.

35. Daaleman T, Frey B. Spiritual and religious beliefs and practices of family physicians—a national survey. *J Fam Pract*. 1999;48:98–104.

36. Ellis M, Vinson D, Ewigman B. Addressing spiritual concerns of patients: family physicians' attitudes and practices. *J Fam Pract*. 1999;48:105–109.

37. Halperin E. Should academic medical centers conduct clinical trials of the efficacy of intercessory prayer? *Acad Med*. 2001;76:791–797.

CHAPTER 15

Informatics and Integrative Medicine

Over the past 20 years, physicians have witnessed a publication revolution, with an ever-increasing number of new medical journals emerging. With this information explosion, keeping up-to-date with the scientific literature by reading selected journals is no longer possible. This is as true for the field of integrative medicine as for general medicine. Students and clinicians are now increasingly dependent upon electronic literature searching to identify and retrieve relevant, current, and worthwhile clinical and scientific information. Thus, it is critical to know where to look for high-quality information and how to search effectively.

To access the literature on integrative medical practice, including clinical studies, two types of searches need to be performed: (1) conventional medical topics in standard biomedical databases and (2) complementary and alternative medicine (CAM) practices in a wider variety of bibliographic and informational databases such as herbal *materia medicas,* specialized databases, and organizational, academic, and government websites.

Because integrative medicine encompasses a large area of study and many therapeutic practices, it is necessary to think broadly when conducting a literature search. In searching one

must be prepared to use the separate disciplines as foci of the search. To do this effectively, it is advisable to become familiar with the concepts and terminology that comprise each field of study. This is discussed in detail in "How to Search" below. Areas to consider when searching include the following:

- Herbal medicine/botanicals
- Nutrition/supplementation
- Mind–body medicine, including hypnosis, imagery, biofeedback, and meditation/relaxation
- Spirituality
- Traditional and indigenous systems of medicine
- Homeopathy
- Manipulative and manual medicine
- Movement therapies
- Environmental medicine
- Energy approaches
- Anthropological/cultural medicine

▶ DATABASE COVERAGE

Because of the broad nature of CAM practices, effective searching requires the use of MEDLINE, additional databases, and specific search strategies to ensure quality retrieval of information.

MEDLINE

The number of randomized controlled trials in CAM has approximately doubled every 5 years.[1] In 1996 approximately 1,500 articles on CAM were added to MEDLINE,[2] while in 2001 3,650 were added. When searching MEDLINE under the term *complementary therapies* approximately 83,000 citations are retrieved (as of January 2003), a 120% increase over the number of articles retrieved in 1999.[3] Yet, while a good starting point, searching MEDLINE alone will not yield an adequate retrieval on CAM topics. In general, MEDLINE searching retrieves approximately 50% of all known randomized controlled trials on a given topic. In CAM, as a result of several factors, a MEDLINE search will frequently yield far less than 50%.

The number of CAM journals indexed by MEDLINE is not comprehensive. As of 1998, MEDLINE indexed approximately 23% of the world's medical journals and only 10% of CAM journals.[4] Thus of approximately 695 CAM journals worldwide, 69 were indexed in MEDLINE. While MEDLINE currently indexes approximately 600 CAM journals, there is still a significant amount of CAM literature not covered by this database. Thus, MEDLINE searching must be supplemented by other databases that index additional CAM journals, particularly for certain topics such as manual medicine, herbal medicine, and traditional and indigenous medicine.

The number of MEDLINE search terms (MeSH [MEDLINE Subject Headings]) in CAM is also limited. MeSH headings are a restricted thesaurus of standard medical terms that help to organize and bring together articles by concept. While these are being continually revised and expanded by the National Library of Medicine, there is still inadequate indexing of CAM concepts. Although the MeSH heading "complementary therapies" includes more terms than the previous heading "alternative medicine," many important topics are still omitted. Thus a more comprehensive search strategy is required, including the addition of other MeSH

headings as well as keyword or text word searching (see "How to Search" below).

In addition, many CAM studies exist that have never been fully published in any journal. These include randomized controlled trials that appear in conference proceedings, dissertations, and US patent records. Others sources are needed to access these materials.

Other Databases

Various biomedical databases are available that, when used in conjunction with MEDLINE, will provide more complete information on a CAM topic. Some databases cover specific areas of practice such as nutrition, dietary supplements or herbal medicine. Others index the international literature more extensively. Because CAM practices have been more thoroughly studied and integrated into medical practice in Europe, for example, access to this literature yields a more robust retrieval. In addition, information on traditional and indigenous medical practices requires access to a variety of information sources from international publications that are not readily accessible to the Western researcher.[1–7] Each of the websites noted below was accessed on 8/13/03.

ACULARS (ACUPUNCTURE LITERATURE ANALYSIS AND RETRIEVAL SYSTEM)

Produced by the Beijing Institute of Information and Library of the Academy of Traditional Chinese Medicine in Beijing, the database contains more than 40,000 references on acupuncture and moxibustion from more than 500 biomedical journals and conference proceedings from China and abroad. Searches are available for a fee in English and Chinese through the Retrieval Section, Institute of Information on Traditional Chinese Medicine, China Academy of Traditional Chinese Medicine, 18 Beixincang, Dongzhimen Nei, Beijiing, 100700, P.R. China. Tel: (10)4032167, (10)4014411-3232; Fax: (10)4032167; e-mail wulc@sun.ihep.ac.cn.

AMED (ALLIED AND COMPLEMENTARY MEDICINE)

AMED is produced by the Health Care Information Service of the British Library. It references more than 500 CAM journals, mostly European titles in English. It provides broad coverage of complementary medicine focusing on clinical data and research studies. Searching AMED extends coverage of CAM topics, as MEDLINE indexes about half the CAM journals indexed by AMED. It is searchable by MeSH terms, as well as by AMED key words. AMED is available through online vendors such as OVID, Dialog, SilverPlatter, and Ebsco through your medical library or by subscription.

AMERICAN JOURNAL OF CLINICAL NUTRITION (WWW.AJCN.ORG/SEARCH.DTL)

This is a searchable free database of *The American Journal of Clinical Nutrition* (full text from 1999 to present; abstracts from 1975 to 1998) as well as the capability of searching approximately 300 other journals by clicking on the button "search across multiple journals."

CAM CITATION INDEX (WWW.NLM.NIH.GOV/NCCAM/ CAMONPUBMED.HTML#)

Produced by the National Center of Complementary and Alternative Medicine of NIH, the CAM Citation Index contains more than 180,000 bibliographic citations from the MEDLINE database from 1963 to the present, covering all aspects of complementary medicine. Access is free.

ARCAM (ARTHRITIS AND COMPLEMENTARY MEDICINE DATABASE) AND CAMPAIN (COMPLEMENTARY AND ALTERNATIVE MEDICINE AND PAIN DATABASE) (WWW.CAMPAIN.UMM.EDU/RIS/RISWEB.ISA)

This database was developed by the Complementary Medicine Program at the University of Maryland, a leading international center for research, patient care, education, and training in the integration of evidenced-based complementary medical approaches for patient care.

The database lists 10,000 references, including 3,000 controlled clinical trials, from 14 databases on the use of CAM for acute and chronic pain. Access is free.

CARDS (COMPUTER ACCESS TO RESEARCH ON DIETARY SUPPLEMENTS) (HTTP://ODS.OD.NIH.GOV/)

This database of federally funded research projects on dietary supplements was developed by the National Institutes of Health Office of Dietary Supplements in order to provide helpful information for researchers, health care providers, industry, and the general public. The database can be searched by researcher, dietary supplement, health condition or funding institution.

CINAHL (CUMULATIVE INDEX TO NURSING AND ALLIED HEALTH LITERATURE) (WWW.CINAHL.COM)

CINAHL provides coverage of English language journals, books, audiovisual materials, selected conference proceedings, and dissertations in all areas of nursing, allied health, health education, and transcultural nursing. It offers substantial coverage of CAM topics in the nursing, physical therapy, and occupational therapy literature, especially manual, mind–body and energy approaches. Available through OVID, Ebsco, DataStar, and Silver Platter through your medical library or by subscription or directly through CINAHL Information Systems.

CISCOM (CENTRALIZED INFORMATION SERVICE FOR COMPLEMENTARY MEDICINE) (WWW.RCCM.ORG.UK/CISCOM/CISCOM_ INTRO.ASP)

Developed by the Research Council for Complementary Medicine, London, this database contains more than 5,000 randomized trials and 80,000 references combining information from MEDLINE, AMED, and other European specialty databases. There is no direct access to the database, but individual searches can be ordered through the Research Council on their website.

COCHRANE LIBRARY (WWW.COCHRANE.ORG)

Developed by an independent international group of medical researchers and physicians who prepare systematic reviews of controlled clinical trials in all areas of medicine, the Cochrane database is available through many academic institutions or through individual subscription via the Internet or on CD-ROM. A subscription can be purchased for either the complete database or for selected parts. A complementary medicine field was added in 1996; it has issued more than 60 systematic reviews, including acupuncture, massage, homeopathy, and herbal medicine. In addition, the Cochrane Controlled Trials Registry on CAM extensively covers the international scientific research literature, and includes trials from many sources that are not indexed in MEDLINE. To search phrases use quotation marks, for example, "integrative medicine." Wild cards can also be used, for example, migraine* for migraine, migraines, migraine-like.

EMBASE (WWW.EMBASE.COM)

This European database covers the biomedical literature, indexing more than 3,500 international journals. It includes many CAM journals that are not indexed in MEDLINE, and is especially thorough in the areas of pharmaceuticals and herbal medicine. It is an expensive fee-based database with access provided by major database vendors such as OVID, Dialog, SilverPlatter, and DataStar, or directly through the publisher, Elsevier Science Publishing.

HEALTHSTAR (WWW.NCBI.NLM.NIH.GOV/PUBMED)

Articles in HealthStar focus on the economic and administrative aspects of health care delivery, including health services research, planning and policy, technology assessment, administration, and research. Topics include the evaluation of patient outcomes; effectiveness of procedures, programs, products, services and processes; administration and planning of health facilities and services; health insurance; health policy; financial management; health services research; laws and regulation; personnel administration; quality assurance; licensure and accreditation; and medical legal issues. HealthStar has been incorporated into MEDLINE. It is available as a separate file through OVID.

HOMINFORM (WWW.HOM-INFORM.ORG)

Produced by the British Homeopathic Library at Glasgow Homeopathic Hospital, this database contains approximately 20,000 references dating back to 1911. Searching is free; copies of articles can be ordered.

IBIDS (INTERNATIONAL BIBLIOGRAPHIC INFORMATION ON DIETARY SUPPLEMENTS DATABASE) (HTTP://ODS.OD.NIH.GOV)

Produced by the Office of Dietary Supplements of the National Institutes of Health and the National Agricultural Library, this bibliographic database covers the worldwide scientific literature on dietary supplements (vitamins, minerals, herbal, and botanical supplements) from 1986 to the present. Information includes their use in human nutrition, role in disease, chemical composition, biochemical roles, antioxidant activity, food fortification, population use, and more. The database can be searched in two ways: the complete database or peer-reviewed citations only. A pop-up window keyword list of dietary supplements and herbal terminology is available online. Simple searches can be done by typing in keywords. An advanced search mode is also available to search combined terms for greater specificity. Truncation symbols and wild cards can also be used to locate variant forms of a keyword.

MANTIS (MANUAL, ALTERNATIVE AND NATURAL THERAPY INDEX SYSTEM) (WWW.HEALTHINDEX.COM)

MANTIS, formerly Chirolars database, thoroughly covers the peer-reviewed chiropractic, osteopathic, and manual medical literature. Most of the fully indexed journals are not indexed in MEDLINE. In addition, MANTIS provides some coverage of herbal medicine, homeopathy, naturopathy, physical therapy, and traditional Chinese medicine. The database contains more than 40,000 records dating from 1880 to the present, and is updated monthly. It is searchable by MeSH heading since 1999, and by its own specialized controlled vocabulary. MANTIS is available via OVID and Dialog. An affordable option is to subscribe directly from the manufacturer, Action Potential.

NAPRALERT (NATURAL PRODUCTS ALERT) (WWW.INFO.CAS.ORG/ONLINE/DBSS/ NAPRALERTS.HTML)

Maintained by the Program for Collaborative Research in the Pharmaceutical Sciences, College of Pharmacy, University of Illinois at Chicago, the NAPRALERT subscription database contains extracted information from more than 150,000 scientific research articles from 1650 to the present on natural products (pharmacology, biologic activity, ethnomedicine, and plant chemistry). It contains abstracts from journals, patents, and meeting abstracts. Data from NAPRALERT searches rank-order organisms as to their probability of having a specific biological activity. NAPRALERT is a fee-based resource available directly on the Internet.

PsycINFO (WWW.APA.ORG/PSYCINFO/PRODUCTS)

Produced by the American Psychological Association (APA), this is a good source of information on mind-body and other CAM therapies relevant to stress and psychological issues. PsycINFO provides worldwide coverage of more than 1,300 professional and academic journals, books, dissertations, and conference proceedings in psychology and related disciplines. It is available through the APA and through database vendors such as OVID, Dialog, DataStar, Ebsco, and SilverPlatter.

USDA NATIONAL NUTRIENT DATABASE FOR STANDARD REFERENCE (WWW.NAL.USDA.GOV/FNIC/FOODCOMP/)

Prepared by the Agricultural Research Service's Nutrient Data Laboratory, food composition products datasets can be searched or downloaded. Datasets include a nutrient database, isoflavones (214 foods), carotenoids (215 foods), *trans*-fatty acids (214 foods), and more.

Newspapers

Many newspapers offer free searching of the most recent 7–14 days with full text retrieval. Older articles are archived. While there is often no fee to search the archives, a fee may be charged to retrieve the full text of any archived article. Some papers require a subscription in order to access both current and archived material. The following sites are good sources for U.S. and international newspapers.

ONLINE NEWSPAPERS (*www.onlinenewspapers.com*)

This web site provides broad coverage of local and national publications that can be searched by region (North America, South America, UK, Europe, Asia, Middle East, Africa), country, and state.

THE INTERNET PUBLIC LIBRARY (*www.ipl.org/div/news/*)

The Internet Public Library is a public service organization of the University of Michigan School of Information. It covers online newspapers from around the world organized by country, state, city, and title.

YAHOO (*http://d5.dir.dcn.yahoo.com/news_and_media/ newspapers/*)

The newspaper directory is organized by region and categories such as alternative newsweeklies, publishers and organizations.

▶ HOW TO SEARCH

Basic training in search techniques by a medical librarian is highly advised. This will greatly improve search technique in terms of the amount of information retrieved and the relevance of that information. Learning how to think about and construct a search will be useful for any topic you are investigating or whichever database you are searching. In addition, it is essential to become familiar with the vocabulary of integrative medicine, both in order to select useful search terms and to explore a topic thoroughly.[8]

Searching MEDLINE

MeSH Headings

If there is a MeSH heading for your topic of interest it should be used. If there are subtopics to your term, it is usually advisable to use them all by "exploding" your term. This is important because MEDLINE indexes articles by using the most specific MeSH term that applies. Thus, if you type in "complementary therapies" you will only retrieve general articles on the topic of CAM. Unless you "explode" your term, you will not retrieve articles on the subtopics included under the hierarchical term "complementary therapies," thus missing articles indexed under particular CAM therapies such as acupuncture, homeopathy, and massage. Unless your search is highly specific it is a good idea to select as many synonyms or related concepts as possible. For example, when searching for the role of spirituality in medicine various search terms should be used, including *religion, spirituality,* and *faith healing,* among others.

While you will certainly become increasingly familiar with MeSH headings in integrative medicine the more frequently you search, it is difficult to know all the headings that may apply to any given search. That is why many database systems, such as OVID, include a feature called *mapping.* Typing a word into the search box that is not a MeSH term provides related terms that are generated by the system. You can then choose the terms that most closely match your concept. If no appropriate terms appear, then search your term as a keyword

(see "Text Word or Keyword Searching" below). If you retrieve any articles that are relevant, select them and identify which MeSH headings were used to index them. Then search under those MeSH terms. Another way to find related concepts in the OVID system is to type in your term, go to the screen where it is mapped, and then click *Scope.* This will provide information on the usage of the term, its history as a MeSH heading, and related terms to search.

Text Word or Keyword Searching

Searching by keyword may seem like a simple and direct strategy, but you will be ignoring the work done by indexers who have pulled together many articles on each topic in MeSH headings that are a conceptual match, even if the specific keyword you choose does not appear in the form you have used. On the whole, keyword searching should be saved for those topics that do not have MeSH headings or when your search using MeSH headings has produced an inadequate retrieval, and should be done in a specific way (see below). Searching by text word can also supplement a search by MeSH headings, as there is a possibility that an article was either misclassified or not fully classified.

A text word search looks for the presence of the specific word or words you typed in the any listing in the database, including in the title, abstract, authors' names, and the institution where the research was done. The program identifies the word(s) exactly as typed. For example, if you type in the word *herb* you will not retrieve articles where the word appears as *herbal, herbalist,* or *herbalism,* and you may miss many potentially useful articles. Because of this it is important to use a search technique called "truncation" or a "wildcard" when doing keyword searches in order to retrieve all variant forms of a word. Different databases use different truncation symbols. For example, databases provided through OVID use the *$* to indicate retrieval of an unlimited number of letters after the word you enter. In other words, if you type in *herb$* you will retrieve articles with the words *herb, herbs, herbal, herbalist,* or *herbalism.* The use of the *?* will retrieve the word you have typed with one or zero characters added. So *herb?* will retrieve *herb* or *herbs* only. As you can see, this will make a significant difference in the number of articles you retrieve.

Subheadings

Subheadings classify articles on a particular MeSH topic into smaller categories, such as adverse effects, psychology, epidemiology, physiopathology, rehabilitation, complications, and so on (e.g., diabetes/diet therapy). Thus, they are best used when you are looking for a very specific aspect of your topic. They are also useful when many articles have been retrieved, as they are a good way to more closely focus your search. However, if you begin your search by limiting by subheading, it is very possible that you will miss relevant articles, as indexing by subheadings is often inadequate or incorrectly classified. If you have used subheadings and your retrieval is small, try searching again without attaching any subheadings to your MeSH terms.

Combining Search Terms

To create a flexible search, it is helpful to search each term separately, establishing a separate set for each term. These can then be combined with the Boolean operators *AND, OR,* and *NOT.*

AND will find citations in which both terms are applied, thus limiting a search. *OR* will find citations that contain either or both terms, thus expanding a search. *NOT* will exclude citations containing the selected term. *NOT* should be used with caution, as articles will be eliminated that contain that term but which might also contain information on topics you are interested in. An example of such a strategy follows.

Sample Search Strategy

SEARCH STRATEGIES

When you type in a search term you create a "set" consisting of the articles you retrieve. For example, if you were to search for articles on the use of biofeedback or hypnosis in the treatment of migraine you would type in:

Set 1   Explode *hypnosis*
Set 2   Explode *biofeedback*
Set 3   Explode *migraine*
Set 4   (1 or 2) and 3

Your retrieval in set 4 represents those articles that discuss either the use of hypnosis or biofeedback or both for migraines.

In searching databases it is advisable to use the *Help* feature to become familiar with the structure of that database and the commands, fields and limits available for use. They will differ in each database. Even though the MEDLINE database is the same no matter which company is providing access to it, the commands will differ according to the software. This is especially true for the wildcard symbols and command searching (the use of specific commands rather than clicking on menu options to search a database). For instance, in OVID, command searching for biofeedback in the title field will be entered as *biofeedback.ti.* In PubMed (the free US government version of MEDLINE), the entry will be *biofeedback[ti].*

Other Search Limits

Some databases provide a variety of ways to limit and thereby more closely target your search. Common limits include *language, age, species, male* or *female, year* or *range of years,* and publication type such as *review, multicenter study, randomized controlled clinical trial,* or *guidelines.*

Other Types of Searches

In addition to searching by subject, you can also search by author or by journal. These types of searches will usually be provided as a menu option that will guide you in the proper

way to enter the appropriate information in that database.

Sample Search Terms

Table 15–1 includes some sample search terms on specific broad topics in CAM that will help to familiarize you with the vocabulary in the field. If you are using a system that allows you to save searches, these search strategies can be saved individually and can serve as a tem-

▶ **TABLE 15–1** CAM SEARCH TERMS

CM Approaches	
Explode *Complementary Therapies*	Exploding this term will retrieve general articles on CM and specific articles on the modalities that are subtopics of the term *complementary therapies.* Coverage is broad but not inclusive of all CM topics Or search *integrative medicine* or *alternative medicine* using the keyword search option.
Major categories under this heading include:	
Acupuncture Therapy	
Homeopathy	
Massage	
Medicine, Traditional	
Mind–Body and Relaxation Techniques	
Musculoskeletal Manipulations	
Phytotherapy	
Psychoneuroimmunology	
Sensory Art Therapies	
Spiritual Therapies	
Aromatherapy	
Aromatherapy	Or search *essential oils* as a keyword term or use the name of particular oils as keywords.
Explode *Oils, Volatile*	
Environmental Medicine	
Explode *Environmental and Public Health*	
Explode *Environmental Health*	
Explode *Preventive Medicine*	
Explode *Public Health*	
Air Pollution	
Environmental Exposure	
Water Pollution	
Food Contamination	

▶ **TABLE 15–1** CAM SEARCH TERMS *(Continued)*

Exercise and Movement Approaches
  Dance Therapy
  Exercise
  Exercise Therapy
  TaiJi
  Yoga

Or use keyword searching for other approaches such as *Qi gong* or *Qigong* or *Chi kung* (variant spellings) or *Feldenkrais, Trager, Alexander Technique,* or *Rolfing,* among others.

Energy Medicine
  Therapeutic Touch
  Explode *Electromagnetics*
  Explode *Phototherapy*
  Magnets
  Color therapy
  Sound

Use keyword searching for *Reiki, energy medicine, magnets, magnet therapy, or biomagnetic.*

Herbal Medicine
  Explode *Medicine, Herbal*
  Explode *Phytotherapy*
  Explode *Plant Extracts*
  Explode *Drugs, Chinese Herbal*
  Explode *Plants, Medicinal*
  Explode *Plant Oils*

Or search names of specific herbs. Some herbs have MeSH headings indexed under the universal scientific plant name rather than the common name. The scientific name can be found in an herbal medicine print resource or online at www.herbmed.com. Other herbs must be searched as key words.

Many articles are indexed according to plant constituents rather than by plant name, as much research is conducted on the constituents of the plant and not on the whole plant. These include *alkaloids, flavones, glycosides, resins, and tannins,* among others, and they are MeSH headings. For instance, much of the research on soy is indexed under its constituents *genistein* and *daidzen.* A good search strategy would use all these terms: *soybeans* or *genistein* or *daidzen.*

Manual Medicine
  Explode *Musculoskeletal Manipulations*

Or use keyword searching for other techniques such as *myofascial release, tui na,* or *tuina* (variant spellings).

  Explode *Manipulation, Chiropractic*
  Explode *Manipulation, Osteopathic*
  Explode *Manipulation, Spinal*
  Massage
  Kinesiology, Applied
  Reflexology

Mind–Body Approaches
  Biofeedback
  Explode *Hypnosis*
  Imagery
  Meditation
  Psychophysiology
  Relaxation
  Relaxation Techniques

Continued

▶ **TABLE 15–1** CAM SEARCH TERMS *(Continued)*

Nutritional Approaches	
Explode *Nutrition*	Or search specific vitamins, minerals, or
Explode *Dietary Supplements*	supplements
Explode *Antioxidants*	
Explode *Vitamins*	
Explode *Minerals*	
Explode *Fatty Acids*	
Explode *Diet*	
Explode *Dietary Therapy*	
Explode *Carotene*	
Explode *Retinoids*	
Explode *Fish Oils*	
Explode *Health Food*	
Explode *Vegetarianism*	
Explode *Diet, Macrobiotic*	
Spirituality	
Explode *Religion*	Or search keywords *prayer* or *spiritual healing*
Religion and Psychology	
Religion and Medicine	
Pastoral Care	
Spirituality	
Spiritual Therapies	
Faith Healing	
Shamanism	
Traditional and Indigenous Systems of Medicine	
Explode *Medicine, Traditional*	Use key word searching for *Tibetan Medicine,*
Medicine, African Traditional	*Native American Medicine,* or any other
Medicine, Arabic	traditional healing system that does not have
Medicine, Ayurvedic	its own MeSH heading
Medicine, Kampo	
Medicine, Oriental Traditional	
Explode *Acupuncture*	
Explode *Acupuncture Therapy*	
Explode *Drugs, Chinese Herbal*	

plate to be combined in any way for future searches.

Getting the Full-Text Article

Some databases have the complete article available for downloading. Those that are not online can be ordered through an academic or hospital library that you are affiliated with or through commercial services such as Ingenta (www.ingenta.com) or DocDeliver (www. docdeliver.com).

Ordering a Professional Information Search

If you are unable to do your own search, you can contact the medical librarian at your institution or order a search from a professional researcher. The Association of Independent Information Professionals (1–888–544–2447 or www.aiip.org) offers a referral program in which they will try to match your search needs with up to three AIIP members who have expertise in that subject area. There is no fee for this referral service. Fees for an information search, however, will be negotiated with each information professional. Most referrals are made within 2 business days.

Subscription Services

While the databases described above are predominantly collections of bibliographic citations, subscription services usually offer full text information on the topics they cover. These often include drug and herbal monographs and detailed information on health conditions and treatments. They are geared to the individual practitioner in scope and pricing, although institutional access is also available.

AcuBase 2.003 (www.trigram.com)
AcuBase 2.003 software (available on CD-ROM) is a practice management suite of services for traditional Chinese medicine. It consists of a Reference Library of acupoints, herbs, formulas, patent formulas, review topics, and herb/drug information, as well as a Practice Management component for billing, vendors, inventory, electronic billing, etc. It is produced by Trigram products and is sold by various distributors listed on their website.

AltMeDex (www.micromedex.com)
Produced by Thomson MICROMEDEX, AltMeDex contains 110 US Pharmacopoeia herbal monographs, which are updated quarterly. It covers herbal, vitamin, mineral, and other dietary supplements in clinically focused, evidence-based monographs covering administration, dosing, warnings, precautions, contraindications, and interactions. AltMeDex is available on disk.

IBIS (The Interactive Body/Mind Information System) (www.ibismedical.com/ibis.html)
Produced by Integrative Medical Arts, IBIS covers 282 medical conditions and provides treatment information from more than 12 systems of natural medicine and CAM therapies including nutrition, acupuncture, botanical medicine, Chinese medicine, and homeopathy. It also includes an extensive materia medica of more than 2,400 individual foods, herbs, and remedies. It is available on CD-ROM for PC and Macintosh. An Internet version is in development.

Integrative Medicine (www.onemedicine.com)
This suite of services was created by Integrative Medicine Communications and includes information on health conditions and treatments, including herbs, supplements, and conventional remedies, cross-referenced with interactions and practice guidelines where appropriate. Also includes a monthly news services covering evidenced-based information on alternative therapies and botanical medicines, and a weekly news service covering current research, new products, regulatory activities, reports on toxicity and adverse events, and integrative medicine business. Information is peer reviewed by an advisory board of leaders in the field of integrative medicine.

Natural Medicines Comprehensive Database (www.naturaldatabase.com)
This affordable subscription database is produced by the *Pharmacist's Letter* and the *Prescriber's Letter*. It is a comprehensive, referenced, and up-to-date database that covers clinical information on herbs and dietary supplements, including interactions. The information is ordered by the level of scientific evidence currently available.

Natural Standard (www.naturalstandard.com)
Developed by clinicians and researchers from over 50 academic institutions, this evidenced-based information resource covers herbs and

supplements and a wide variety of health conditions. It provides extensive, referenced, and evaluated scientific information designed to help clinicians and patients in the decision making process. Individual and institutional subscriptions are available at an affordable price.

QIGONG DATABASE (WWW.QIGONGINSTITUTE.ORG/ DATABASE.HTML)

Developed by the Qigong Institute, this database covers clinical trials and experimental research on medical Qigong from China and other countries. It contains approximately 1,600 references from 1994 to 1999 and uses keyword searching. Citations include a substantial number of English-language abstracts with data tables and statistical analysis. The database is available only on CD-ROM and can be ordered directly from the Qigong Institute.

TRADITIONAL CHINESE MEDICINE DATABASE SYSTEM (WWW.CINTCM.COM/INDEX.HTM)

Two databases are available from the Institute of Information on Traditional Chinese Medicine, Chinese Academy of Traditional Chinese Medicine. The first database, TCMLARS, contains approximately 73,275 references on traditional Chinese medicine published since 1984, including Chinese herbal medicine, acupuncture, moxibustion, Qigong, and Chinese massage. The second database, the Traditional Chinese Drug Database, is a 545-drug Chinese *materia medica*.

▶ INTERNET WEBSITES

The Internet is a huge repository of information that lacks consistent peer review, editorial systems, or safeguards. Because the quality of information varies so widely, it is imperative to learn how to evaluate websites, particularly those that provide medical information.

How to Evaluate Websites

The most important factor in evaluating a website is the site's credibility because this impacts any assessment of the quality of the information provided. Various criteria can help in this process.

1. Publisher—It is essential to identify who is publishing the material. Look for well-known sources such as journals, universities, research centers, libraries, government agencies, and professional organizations. Other credible organizations include consumer advocacy groups, voluntary health-related organizations, and organizations of providers. Websites can also be published by commercial sponsors and by professional and lay individuals. While these may seem to be potentially biased sources, the addition of the following evaluative criteria will help to distinguish those that are reliable from those that are unreliable.

2. Authority (expertise in the field)—Look for clearly identified authorship and/or source including the qualifications and credentials of their own and cited authors. All references to other publications, especially clinical studies, should be identified with the correct bibliographic citation so that the user can obtain the original source material for further reading and independent verification. In addition, editorial practices and reviewers should be identified. The website should provide the opportunity for feedback and interactivity through e-mail. The choice of links to other sites should meet the same criteria as the website content.

3. Trustworthiness (assessment of bias)—The site should include disclosure of potential conflicts of interest, disclosure of the mission, purpose and standards for posting information, and clear indication on the use of information gathered about users. Be aware of claims that appear to be unreal-

istic. Appropriate disclaimers that address a site's limitations, scope, and purpose should be posted as well.

4. Content quality—Assessment of quality includes the currency of the information, as indicated by posting of the date of website updates and policies regarding updating. While the accuracy of information is difficult to evaluate, the substance and depth of content may help to determine this. In addition, the site should be well organized so that information is presented in a logical format. The content should be understandable relative to its intended users.

5. Design quality—The technology used should facilitate the location of information, not complicate it. The organization of the site should serve to locate information quickly and provide ease of use. Links between sites should match the original site's audience, allow free movement between sites, and should be selective. The aesthetics of the site, color coordination, lack of clutter, unobtrusive backgrounds, and legibility of text should also contribute to comfort and ease of use. Use of a variety of text, audio, and visual formats can enhance preferences and learning styles.

6. Rating System: HONCode (Health on the Net Foundation)—This self-governing body was developed to promote ethical standards for online health information. Websites are evaluated according to eight specific criteria and the HONCode logo is issued to sites that meet these criteria. To date, this is the most widespread attempt to apply a code of conduct to online health information, although there is great overall interest in ways to increase the authority and safety of health information on the Internet.

How to Perform a Web Search

Search techniques can vary from search engine to search engine. As a general rule, however, there are several search strategies that can generally be used to improve the quality and limit the quantity of information retrieval.

- Keywords—Once you have decided on your search question, select the relevant keywords and enter them individually. For example, to search for the use of biofeedback or hypnotherapy in the treatment of migraines, you would enter *biofeedback hypnotherapy migraine* in the search box.

- Searching phrases—When searching a particular phrase, such as "integrative medicine," it is helpful to put the phrase in quotation marks so that each word is not searched separately. This will improve the relevancy of your retrieval.

- Plus or minus signs—To increase search precision you can put a plus sign before a word that must appear in your search results. For instance to search the use of valerian for insomnia you would enter *+valerian +insomnia +sleep* in the search box. The use of a minus sign would indicate that you are excluding that word from your search results. For instance to search herbs other than St. John's wort that are used in depression, you would enter *+herbs +depression − st john's wort*.

Recommended Websites

Websites offer a variety of useful information to those interested in CAM practice.[9-16] The selected websites in this section begin with those offering general CAM information and are then categorized by therapeutic approach. Specialized sites that address specific areas of health, as well as evidenced-based medicine sites, are described separately under "Special Areas" and "Evidence-Based Medicine." An overview of all information resources for each field of CAM practice can be found in Table 15-2.

▶ **TABLE 15-2** CHART OVERVIEW OF INFORMATION RESOURCES

	Databases	Websites	Subscription Databases

General	AMED
	CINAHL
	CISCOM
	Cochrane
	EMBASE
	MEDLINE
		American Holistic Medical Association
		American Holistic Nurses Association
		Center for Health and Healing
		National Center for Complementary and
		  Alternative Medicine
		National Foundation for Alternative Medicine
		Physicians Committee for Responsible
		  Medicine
		Rosenthal Center for Complementary and
		  Alternative Medicine
			IBIS
			Integrative medicine

Acupuncture	ACULARS
	AMED
	Cochrane
	EMBASE
	MANTIS
	MEDLINE
		Acupuncture.com
		Acupuncture Consensus Statement
			Traditional Chinese
			  Medicine
			  Database
			Acubase

Cross-cultural medicine	AMED CINAHL MEDLINE PsycINFO		IBIS
Energy medicine	AMED CINAHL CISCOM Cochrane EMBASE MEDLINE PsycINFO	International Association of Reiki Professionals Nurse-Healers Professional Association	
Environmental medicine	EMBASE MEDLINE	Environmental Protection Agency Healthcare Without Harm Natural Resources Defense Council Sustainable Hospitals Project	

Herbal	Cochrane
	MEDLINE
	EMBASE
	NAPRALERT
		American Botanical Council
		HerbMed
		Herb Research Foundation
			AltMedEx
			IBIS
			Integrative
			  Medicine
			Natural Medicines
			  Comprehensive
			  Database
			Natural Standard

Homeopathy	Cochrane CISCOM EMBASE HomInform MEDLINE	Homeopathic Educational Services Homeopathic Trust National Center for Homeopathy	

▶ **TABLE 15-2** CHART OVERVIEW OF INFORMATION RESOURCES *(Continued)*

	Databases	Websites	Subscription Databases
Manual	CINAHL	American Chiropractic Association	IBIS
	Cochrane	American Massage Therapy Association	Integrative Medicine
	EMBASE	American Osteopathic Association	
	MANTIS	Associated Body Work and Massage	
	MEDLINE	Professionals	
		ChiroWeb	
		National Certified Board for Therapeutic	
		Massage & Bodywork	
		Touch Research Institute	
		Upledger Institute	
Mind–Body	AMED	Academy for Guided Imagery	IBIS
	CINAHL	American Society of Clinical Hypnosis	Integrative Medicine
	CISCOM	Association of Applied Psychophysiology &	
	Cochrane	Biofeedback	
	EMBASE	Biofeedback Certification Institute of America	
	MEDLINE	Center for Mindfulness in Medicine, Health	
	PsycINFO	Care & Society	
		Health Journeys	
		Institute for Integrative Aromatherapy	
		International Medical & Dental Hypnotherapy	
		Association	
		Mind/Body Medical Institute	
		National Association of Holistic	
		Aromatherapy	
		Society of Clinical & Experimental Hypnosis	
		The Milton Erickson Foundation	
		Transcendental Meditation	
Movement therapies	AMED	Alexander Technique International	
	CIHAHL	American Society for the Alexander Technique	
	Cochrane	American Yoga Association	
	EMBASE	Feldenkrais Guild	
	MANTIS	Qigong Institute	
	MEDLINE	Rolf Institute	
		Trager Approach	
		Yoga Research & Education	
Nutrition	American	ConsumeberLab.com	Natural Medicines
	Journal of	FNIC	Comprehensive
	Clinical	FoodFind	Database
	Nutrition	Supplement Watch	
	CARDS		
	database		
	CINAHL		
	Cochrane		

Continued

► **TABLE 15–2** CHART OVERVIEW OF INFORMATION RESOURCES *(Continued)*

	Databases	Websites	Subscription Databases

Nutrition (cont.)	EMBASE
	IBIDS
	  database
	MEDLINE
	USDA
	  Nutrient
	  Database		

Sensory therapies	CINAHL MEDLINE PsycINFO	American Art Therapy Association American Art Therapy Research Web Site American Dance Therapy Institute American Music Therapy Association Institute for Music Research	

Spirituality	AMED
	CINAHL
	Cochrane
	EMBASE
	MEDLINE
	PsycINFO
		Center for the Study of Science & Religion
		  at Columbia University
		Center for Study of Religion, Spirituality,
		  & Health
		Fetzer Institute
		John Templeton Foundation
		Spirituality and Health	

Traditional and indigenous	ACULARS CISCOM Cochrane EMBASE MANTIS MEDLINE	American Institute of Vedic Studies Ayurvedic Institute National Institute of Ayurvedic Medicine	TCM database Qigong database Acubase 2003

Sites have been selected based on the following criteria: the contribution of the organization to the field of integrative medicine, the depth and quality of information provided, and the provision of specific types of information including *materia medicas,* legislative and regulatory updates, research databases, informational databases, ongoing research projects, resource reviews and recommendations, practitioner locators, funding information, and educational information including schools, boards, accrediting bodies, training programs, and licensing and certification information.

General CAM Information

AMERICAN HOLISTIC MEDICAL ASSOCIATION (WWW.HOLISTICMEDICINE.ORG)
The website of this professional association for medical doctors, doctors of osteopathy, and medical students covers consumer information, conferences, the American Holistic Medical Association newsletter online, and a browseable physician membership directory.

AMERICAN HOLISTIC NURSES ASSOCIATION (WWW.AHNA.ORG)
AHNA is a nonprofit membership of organizations of nurses that supports research, education,

and the promotion of holistic health care. Its website covers conference information, the organization's holistic nursing certification program, and a list of other certificate programs endorsed by the American Holistic Nurses Association.

CONTINUUM CENTER FOR HEALTH AND HEALING (WWW.HEALTHANDHEALINGNY.ORG)

This educational and evidence-based website is an initiative of the Continuum Center for Health and Healing, an integrative medical center that is part of Beth Israel Medical Center in New York City. Extensive information is provided on 30 CAM, traditional, and indigenous therapeutic approaches, research and guidelines on these approaches, a professional education section for fellowships, courses and conferences, a resource section covering organizations, books, journals, audiotapes, videotapes, and databases on each topic, and a Health A to Z section, annotating recent high-quality research on 66 health conditions.

NATIONAL CENTER FOR COMPLEMENTARY AND ALTERNATIVE MEDICINE (WWW.NCCAM.NIH.GOV)

The National Center for Complementary and Alternative Medicine is one of the 27 institutes and centers that make up the National Institutes of Health. Its website contains information about CAM, classification of CAM practices, fact sheets, news and events, consensus reports, clinical trial awards data, current and completed research projects, funding opportunities and priorities, and more.

NATIONAL FOUNDATION FOR ALTERNATIVE MEDICINE (WWW.NFAM.ORG)

This not-for-profit organization was formed to identify effective CAM treatments available outside the United States, to evaluate the protocols and treatment outcomes, and to report the findings to the public. The foundation serves as an international CAM clearinghouse, providing comprehensive, research-based information on CAM treatments for degenerative diseases. Its website covers research initiatives,

reviews of international clinics treating degenerative diseases, and information on wellness, prevention, and treatment.

PHYSICIANS COMMITTEE FOR RESPONSIBLE MEDICINE (WWW.PCRM.ORG)

Founded in 1985, this nonprofit organization promotes preventive medicine and nutrition and conducts clinical research. Its website provides information on the organization's research projects, research controversies and issues, an online magazine called *Good Medicine,* resources, physician referral, recent medical news, and the work of the organization's initiative, The Cancer Project.

THE RICHARD AND HINDA ROSENTHAL CENTER FOR COMPLEMENTARY AND ALTERNATIVE MEDICINE, COLUMBIA UNIVERSITY (WWW.ROSENTHAL.HS.COLUMBIA.EDU)

The Center's objectives are to conduct rigorous scientific research into the effectiveness, safety, and mechanisms of action of CAM remedies and practices, to develop professional training and educational programs, and to serve as a respected source of information about CAM. Its website includes information about Center projects, CAM courses and events, including a guide to CAM courses taught at medical schools, women's health resources, botanical medicine, and CAM research and information resources, including a directory of databases. Also discussed is the Center's role as one of 16 specialty research centers funded by the National Center for Complementary and Alternative Medicine at the NIH and the Center for Complementary and Alternative Medicine Research in Women's Health.

Acupuncture

ACUPUNCTURE.COM (WWW.ACUPUNCTURE.COM)

This site provides a referral database by geographical area; traditional Chinese medicine resources including books, music, videotapes, software, quality herbs, and medical supplies;

extensive links; and articles and research about acupuncture and traditional Chinese medicine.

ACUPUNCTURE CONSENSUS STATEMENT, NATIONAL INSTITUTES OF HEALTH CONSENSUS DEVELOPMENT CONFERENCE STATEMENT (HTTP://ODP.OD.NIH.GOV/CONSENSUS/CONS/ 107/107_INTRO.HTM)

This site presents the full 1997 consensus statement on acupuncture based on the findings of a nonfederal, nonadvocate, 12-member panel of experts in the fields of acupuncture, pain, psychology, psychiatry, physical medicine and rehabilitation, drug abuse, family practice, internal medicine, health policy, and epidemiology, among others. The NIH organized this 2.5-day conference to evaluate the scientific and medical data on the uses, risks, and benefits of acupuncture procedures for a variety of conditions.

Energy Approaches

REIKI: INTERNATIONAL ASSOCIATION OF REIKI PROFESSIONALS (WWW.IARP.ORG/)

The International Association of Reiki Professionals' website provides general information on Reiki, a search service for locating Reiki practitioners and teachers, and a database of Reiki articles.

THERAPEUTIC TOUCH: NURSE HEALERS– PROFESSIONAL ASSOCIATES INTERNATIONAL (WWW.THERAPEUTIC-TOUCH.ORG/ DEFAULT.ASP)

The official organization for therapeutic touch, its website provides information on therapeutic touch, a geographic listing of teachers, and recommended resources including books, audiotapes, and videotapes, conference information, position statements, and more.

Environmental Medicine

ENVIRONMENTAL PROTECTION AGENCY (WWW.EPA.GOV)

The website of this government agency provides information and educational resources on pollutants, pesticides, wastes, ecosystems, cleanup, water, air, human health, and more.

HEALTH CARE WITHOUT HARM (WWW.NOHARM.ORG)

Founded in 1996, this coalition of 360 organizations in 40 countries is designed to reform the environmental practices of the health care industry. This includes supporting the development and use of environmentally safe materials, technology, and products, and educating health care institutions and all affected constituencies about the environmental and public health impact of the health care industry. Its website provides resources, news, organizations, events, and a searchable library by topic and type of document including fact sheets, government information, newspaper and magazine articles, and press releases.

NATIONAL RESOURCES DEFENSE COUNCIL (WWW.NRDC.ORG)

This large membership organization is dedicated to protecting the planet's wildlife and natural resources and to ensuring a safe and healthy environment. Its website covers such topics as clean air and energy, toxic chemicals and health, clean water and oceans, global warming, cities and green living, and environmental legislation.

SUSTAINABLE HOSPITALS PROJECT (WWW.SUSTAINABLEHOSPITALS.ORG/)

A project of the Lowell Center for Sustainable Production of the University of Massachusetts Lowell, this website covers ways to reduce occupational and environmental hazards in hospitals including latex, mercury, needles, polyvinyl chloride, alternative products, better practices, and resources.

Herbal Medicine

AMERICAN BOTANICAL COUNCIL (WWW.HERBALGRAM.ORG)

The American Botanical Council is a leading nonprofit educational and research organization in phytomedicine. Membership includes

15 online herbal monographs, as well as access to Herbclip online, an herbal medicine database of 1,500 critical reviews of important current journal articles that is updated quarterly. Extensive links include medicinal herbal education programs, regulatory/government resources, safety/toxicology information, and statistical information.

HERBMED (WWW.HERBMED.ORG)

This interactive herbal database is a project of the Alternative Medicine Foundation. Information on more than 100 herbs is hyperlinked to the scientific articles in MEDLINE, providing an evidence-based information resource for health professionals and the general public. Six categories of information are provided for each herb: evidence for activity, warnings, preparations, mixtures, mechanisms of action, and other.

HERB RESEARCH FOUNDATION (WWW.HERBS.ORG)

The website of this well-respected nonprofit educational and research organization features herbal news, fact sheets, recommended herbal books, a "hotline service" for calls on herbal questions, custom herbal research service, and information packets on common herbs for sale.

Homeopathy

HOMEOPATHIC EDUCATIONAL SERVICES (WWW.HOMEOPATHIC.COM)

This leading US center for homeopathic resources, established by Dana Ullman, covers selected books, tapes, research, medicines, medicine kits, software for the general public and the health professional, and correspondence courses. More than 40 specific ailments and their homeopathic treatments are described. This site also has a research section that describes developments in the field.

HOMEOPATHIC TRUST (WWW.TRUSTHOMEOPATHY.ORG)

The website of the British Homeopathic Association and Homeopathic Trust provides accurate, research-based information on homeopathy.

NATIONAL CENTER FOR HOMEOPATHY (WWW.HOMEOPATHIC.ORG)

A leading homeopathic organization in the United States, its website includes a research section with abstracts of journal articles and a resource section of professional societies, associations, schools, and products and services.

Manual Medicine

AMERICAN CHIROPRACTIC ASSOCIATION (WWW.AMERCHIRO.ORG)

The main professional chiropractic organization website provides information on chiropractic, a reference section on AHCPR guidelines, new research, grants, legislative updates, and a listing of chiropractic councils, state delegates, and state associations.

AMERICAN MASSAGE THERAPY ASSOCIATION (WWW.AMTAMASSAGE.ORG)

The web site of this major association of massage therapists offers information on massage therapy, massage school listings by state with school profiles, national certification, a massage therapist locator by state, and the last five issues of *Massage Therapy Journal* online.

AMERICAN OSTEOPATHIC ASSOCIATION (WWW.AOA-NET.ORG)

The American Osteopathic Association (AOA) is a national professional association of osteopathy that accredits colleges of osteopathic medicine, osteopathic internships and residency programs, and health care facilities. Its website offers general information on osteopathic medicine, links to AOA programs, a selection of full-text articles from the *Journal of the American Osteopathic Association*, a list of US osteopathic colleges, information for postdoctoral physicians, and information on research and grants.

ASSOCIATED BODYWORK AND MASSAGE PROFESSIONALS (WWW.ABMP.COM)

This professional membership association provides professionals and consumers with information and services on massage, body-work, and somatic therapies including benefits of these therapies, print resources on massage therapy, a practitioner finder by geographical location and type of massage practice, massage boards and requirements, and a list of accredited schools searchable by state.

CHIROWEB (WWW.CHIROWEB.COM)

This site offers more than 7,000 articles and research reviews, a chiropractor referral directory and other chiropractic news, government reports, and general information on chiropractic.

NATIONAL CERTIFICATION BOARD FOR THERAPEUTIC MASSAGE AND BODYWORK (WWW.NCBTMB.COM)

The National Certification Board for Therapeutic Massage and Bodywork website offers information on national certification including eligibility requirements, application fees, scheduling, and recertification. It also covers continuing education and a nationally certified practitioner search by geographical area.

TOUCH RESEARCH INSTITUTE (WWW.MIAMI.EDU/TOUCH-RESEARCH/INDEX.HTML)

The Touch Research Institute at the University of Miami is the first academic center devoted solely to the study of touch and its applications in science and medicine to promote health and to treat disease. Research at the center began in 1982. Its website covers research at the Institute, including published studies and reviews, journal articles, studies in review, and ongoing studies.

UPLEDGER INSTITUTE (WWW.UPLEDGER.COM)

The Institute was founded by an osteopathic physician to support craniosacral therapy through education programs, clinical research, and therapeutic services. The website covers the Institute's educational programs, as well as articles, citations, books, and a practitioner locator.

Mind–Body Medicine
AROMATHERAPY
INSTITUTE OF INTEGRATIVE AROMATHERAPY (WWW.AROMA-RN.COM)

The Institute has a five-part diploma program in aromatherapy approved for 156 contact hours of continuing education credits through the American Holistic Nurses Association. The website covers course information, book reviews, fact sheets, workshops, and conferences.

NATIONAL ASSOCIATION FOR HOLISTIC AROMATHERAPY (WWW.NAHA.ORG)

The National Association for Holistic Aromatherapy (NAHA) is a nonprofit association involved in setting national standards and guidelines for aromatherapy education and certification in the United States. The website covers its educational guidelines, a directory of schools and educators in compliance with NAHA guidelines, and NAHA's quarterly journal with online access available.

BIOFEEDBACK
ASSOCIATION FOR APPLIED PSYCHOPHYSIOLOGY AND BIOFEEDBACK (WWW.AAPB.ORG)

The website of this nonprofit organization, which is composed of clinicians, researchers, and educators in biofeedback and related disciplines, provides an introduction to biofeedback and appropriate conditions for biofeedback treatment, current research, information on meetings and workshops, and links to its publications and to related websites.

BIOFEEDBACK CERTIFICATION INSTITUTE OF AMERICA (WWW.BCIA.ORG)

The Biofeedback Certification Institute of America is an educational organization that was founded in 1981. Its website offers information on biofeedback, general biofeedback, and electroencephalogram biofeedback training programs, and the certification process.

HYPNOSIS

AMERICAN SOCIETY OF CLINICAL HYPNOSIS (WWW.ASCH.NET)

Founded by Milton Erickson in 1957, the American Society of Clinical Hypnosis is the largest US organization for health and mental health care professionals who use clinical hypnosis. Its website provides practitioner referral by geographic area, certification information, clinical hypnosis workshop schedules, and conference information.

INTERNATIONAL MEDICAL AND DENTAL HYPNOTHERAPY ASSOCIATION (WWW.INFINITYINST.COM)

The website provides a list of hypnosis schools approved by the organization, a speaker service and referral service, book and videotape reviews, articles, and specialty certification information.

THE MILTON H. ERICKSON FOUNDATION (WWW.ERICKSON-FOUNDATION.ORG)

The website provides training information, publications, and links to other professional hypnosis and psychological organizations, publishers, and Milton H. Erickson Institutes around the world.

SOCIETY FOR CLINICAL AND EXPERIMENTAL HYPNOSIS (HTTP://IJECH.EDUC.WSU.EDU/SCEH/SCEHMAIN.HTM)

This website provides free access to an interactive database with 11,725 references to hypnosis, related material in scholarly journals and books, presentations from professional meetings, and article abstracts from the *International Journal of Clinical and Experimental Hypnosis* from 1997 to the present.

IMAGERY

ACADEMY FOR GUIDED IMAGERY (WWW.HEALTY.NET/AGI)

Directed by Martin L. Rossman and David E. Bresler, the Academy for Guided Imagery (AGI) is an educational organization providing accredited postgraduate training for health care professionals in interactive guided imagery. The AGI website lists the organization's professional training programs, a professional e-mail broadcast service, and information on its books and audiotapes.

HEALTH JOURNEYS (WWW.HEALTHJOURNEYS.COM)

Developed by Belleruth Naparstek, LISW, a pioneer in the field of imagery and health, this website provides research information on guided imagery, a collection of resources on wellness, diseases, disorders, and chronic illness, an explanation of the imagery process, practice tips, and a discussion forum.

MEDITATION/RELAXATION

CENTER FOR MINDFULNESS IN MEDICINE, HEALTH CARE AND SOCIETY AT THE UNIVERSITY OF MASSACHUSETTS MEDICAL CENTER (WWW.UMASSMED.EDU/CFM/)

The Center was established to further the practice and integration of mindfulness on an individual, institutional, and societal level. It sponsors a wide range of clinical, research, education, and outreach initiatives in the public and private sectors. This includes the well-known Stress Reduction Program, the oldest and largest academic medical center–based stress reduction program in the United States, developed by Jon Kabat-Zinn, PhD, and Saki Santorelli, EdD, as well as a range of professional training programs and corporate workshops, courses, and retreats. The website covers the history of the Center, its stress reduction program, conference information, professional education, workplace programs, research, outreach, a bibliography, and selected guided meditation tapes.

MIND/BODY MEDICAL INSTITUTE (WWW.MBMI.ORG/DEFAULT.ASP)

The Institute was founded in 1988 as a nonprofit scientific and educational organization based on the work of Herbert Benson at Harvard Medical School on the "relaxation response." The website covers research, education, training, clinical programs, books, videotapes, audiotapes, and more.

TRANSCENDENTAL MEDITATION (WWW.TM.ORG)

As the official US website of the transcendental meditation (TM) program, it describes the program and covers scientific research on TM, places to study, news articles and books, and a discussion of the uses of TM to enhance function and treat a variety of conditions.

Movement Therapies

ALEXANDER TECHNIQUE INTERNATIONAL (WWW.ATI-NET.COM)

The Alexander Technique International (ATI) is a worldwide professional organization for the Alexander Technique. Its website offers general information on the technique, an up-to-date international listing of ATI teachers, training, and upcoming workshops and events, articles on learning and teaching the technique, and a resource section of books, journals, audiotapes, videotapes, and articles.

AMERICAN SOCIETY FOR THE ALEXANDER TECHNIQUE (WWW.ALEXANDERTECH.COM)

The American Society of the Alexander Technique is the largest professional association of Alexander teachers in the United States. Its website provides a listing of certified teachers and information on teacher training and board certification, workshops, classes, and events, and a search service for related books and online articles.

AMERICAN YOGA ASSOCIATION (WWW.AMERICANYOGAASSOCIATION.ORG)

This not-for-profit educational organization focuses on high-quality yoga instruction. Its website describes the organization's varied educational programs, books, and instructional videotapes, and includes a section on self-help topics such as yoga and arthritis.

FELDENKRAIS GUILD OF NORTH AMERICA (WWW.FELDENKRAIS.COM)

As the professional organization of practitioners and teachers, the Guild works to promote and enforce the correct practice of the Feldenkrais Method. Only those personally trained by Dr. Feldenkrais or who have graduated from a Guild-accredited training program are eligible to be certified and become members. The website contains extensive information on the theory and practice of the method, sample exercises, articles of interest, where to find practitioners and training, book and tape resources, and links to additional sites.

QIGONG INSTITUTE (WWW.QIGONGINSTITUTE.ORG)

The Institute works to incorporate Qigong into traditional Western medical practices via education, research, and clinical studies. Its Qi newsletter includes lectures and information on events. The Institute's website includes articles contributed to scientific journals and magazines, a directory of teachers and therapists, information on lectures and workshops, books and videotapes, and a database of citations from original sources for clinical and experimental research on Qigong.

ROLF INSTITUTE ® OF STRUCTURAL INTEGRATION (WWW.ROLF.ORG)

The official Rolfing site provides extensive information on Ida Rolf's theory and practice of Structural Integration. As the only certifying body for Rolfers, it provides curriculum for basic and advanced training, and promotes research and education relating to the practice and effectiveness of this modality. There are online resources for books, tapes, and articles of interest, as well as research information, a practitioner locator, and answers to commonly asked questions.

THE TRAGER APPROACH (WWW.TRAGER-US.ORG)

The United States Trager Association is a member of Trager International and represents the Trager Approach in the United States. Its website covers information on the Trager Approach, professional trainings, classes and workshops, online articles, and practitioner locators by geographic area.

Yoga Research and Education Center (www.yrec.org)

Established by Georg Feuerstein, the Yoga Research and Education Center is an international network of yoga researchers, educators, and practitioners. The website provides guidance on finding a yoga teacher, school, or class, and offers recommended audiotapes and videotapes, information on the different types of yoga, articles and reviews, and affiliated institutions and organizations.

Nutrition/Supplementation

ConsumerLab.com (www.consumerlab.com)

This website provides independent test results on vitamins, herbs, minerals, dietary supplements, and functional foods, and on testing for identity, potency, standardization, purity, bioavailability, and consistency. Part of the information is free access. The full database requires a small subscription fee.

Food and Nutrition Information Center (www.nal.usda.gov/fnic)

This website, produced by the National Agricultural Library, has compiled a broad range of information including a Food and Nutrition Information Center resource list that provides links to major organizations, databases, and FDA guidelines, reports, and studies, and a searchable A–Z health topic section consisting of substantial links to a wide variety of authoritative sources of health information. Food composition databases include carotenoid database, isoflavone database, trans fatty acid database, and others.

Food Find (http://nutrition.about.com/library/foodfind/blfoodfind.htm)

Provides the nutrient composition of individual foods in six categories: fruits, vegetables, breads/grains, dairy, nut/seed, and fast food.

Supplement Watch (www.supplementwatch.com)

A self-funded corporation of scientists, physiologists, nutritionists, and other health care professionals who provide timely, evidence-based advice on dietary supplements. Categories include Supplements A to Z, summarizing all relevant data on a particular supplement, searchable by supplement or category; Product Reviews and Brand Recommendations, which rates each branded supplement that is evaluated; Nutrition Counselor which is an interactive module providing a lifestyle survey and report; Articles; and Ask the Experts.

Sensory Art Therapies
ART THERAPY
American Art Therapy Association (www.arttherapy.org)

The American Art Therapy Association is a national organization that sets the standards for the education and practice of art therapy. Their website provides information regarding professional credentialing, legislation, licensure, educational programs, and issues pertaining to the practice of art therapy.

American Art Therapy Research (www.arttherapy.org/resources/research/art_therapy_research.htm)

The research branch of the American Art Therapy Association (see above), its website covers research resources, research articles and books, online articles, outcomes bibliography, statistical resources, and information on conducting and publishing research.

DANCE THERAPY
American Dance Therapy Institute (www.adta.org)

The American Dance Therapy Institute works to establish and maintain the highest levels of competency and education in the field of dance therapy. It publishes *The American Journal of Dance Therapy*, provides a list of therapists who have met their standards, publishes monographs, and monitors graduate programs for those pursuing credentials. Its website contains information on the mission of the organization, credentialing, education, and research.

MUSIC THERAPY

AMERICAN MUSIC THERAPY ASSOCIATION (WWW.MUSICTHERAPY.ORG)

Founded in 1998, the American Music Therapy Association sets the standard for training and certification in music therapy. It publishes several journals and newsletters, including the *Journal of Music Therapy, Music Therapy Perspectives,* and *Music Therapy Matters.* The website provides fact sheets on the use of music therapy with different groups, a Music Therapy Listserv providing a discussion forum, and Music Therapy E-News, an electronic newsletter. There is also information on how to find a practitioner or to obtain training in the field, as well as products, conferences, and other resources.

INSTITUTE FOR MUSIC RESEARCH (HTTP://IMR.UTSA.EDU)

An initiative of the University of Texas at San Antonio, the Institute for Music Research was established to promote research into music psychology and technology. It provides a number of resources, including an online computer database called CAIRSS (Computer-Assisted Information Retrieval Service System), which contains thousands of articles on music research. It also sponsors conferences and research projects, while faculty members give presentations worldwide. A number of audiotapes, multimedia software, and books are also available through the Institute.

Spirituality

CENTER FOR THE STUDY OF SCIENCE AND RELIGION AT COLUMBIA UNIVERSITY (WWW.COLUMBIA.EDU/CU/CSSR/)

Founded in 1999, the Center is an interdisciplinary, interschool, collaborative forum for the examination of issues lying at the boundary of the scientific and religious ways of comprehending the world and our place in it. The Center sponsors educational initiatives, including undergraduate and other course work, a research fellowship, and a calendar of events open to the public.

THE CENTER FOR THE STUDY OF RELIGION/SPIRITUALITY AND HEALTH (WWW.DUKESPIRITUALITYANDHEALTH.ORG)

The purpose of the Center is to conduct multidisciplinary research on the effects of religion or spirituality on physical and mental health. The website describes the Center's postdoctoral fellowship program and includes annotated research reports, recommended books on various aspects of spirituality and health and a calendar of events.

THE FETZER INSTITUTE (WWW.FETZER.ORG)

This nonprofit educational organization supports mind/body/spirit health care approaches through education and research. Its website provides information on the organization's philosophy, programs, reports, articles, and recommended resources.

JOHN TEMPLETON FOUNDATION (WWW.TEMPLETON.ORG)

The Foundation supports more than 150 projects, studies, awards programs and publications worldwide. The website provides information on funding guidelines and initiatives, spirituality and health programs (including highlights from the medical literature and an annotated bibliography under "Spirituality and Healing in Medicine" course), a science and religion section, an online newsletter *Progress in Theology,* the Templeton Foundation University lecture series, and more.

SPIRITUALITY AND HEALTH (WWW.SPIRITUALITYHEALTH.COM)

This website was developed by the Publishing Group of Trinity Church of New York City with an advisory group of theologians, philosophers, researchers, teachers, and writers in order to explore spirituality and healing. The site includes a news section, articles on spiritual issues and practice, essays, a database of more than 15,000 reviews of current books, audiotapes, films, and videotapes with online purchase available, a discussion forum, and interactive self-tests on spirituality and health.

Ayurvedic Medicine
AMERICAN INSTITUTE OF VEDIC STUDIES (WWW.VEDANET.COM)
Founded by Dr. David Frawley, the Institute is an educational center teaching the system of Vedic and yogic knowledge. The website offers information on schools and programs, a list of courses and calendar of events, and a listing of online books and articles.

AYURVEDIC INSTITUTE (WWW.AYURVEDA.COM)
The Institute is one of the world's leading Ayurvedic schools and is headed by medical director Dr. Vasant Lad. The Institute is developing an information center that will include an Ayurveda herbal *materia medica,* an online database of Ayurvedic herbs, including botanical, Sanskrit, and common names, pharmacologic action, indications, contraindications, constituents, and more.

THE NATIONAL INSTITUTE OF AYURVEDIC MEDICINE (WWW.NIAM.COM)
Founded by Scott Gerson, MD, The National Institute of Ayurvedic Medicine (NIAM) is an educational center, a collaborative research facility, and a Panchakarma Retreat Center. The NIAM Research Library has one of the largest collections of Ayurvedic literature in the United States. The Institute's website offers information on the basic principles of Ayurveda; current research; an Ayurvedic medicinal plant chart (some with full monographs); educational programs and correspondence courses; and a schedule for Panchakarma retreats and other events.

Special Areas

Pain
PAIN LINKS
(WWW.PAINLINKS.ORG/CHRONIC.PAIN.HTML)
This well-selected directory of websites provides a variety of information on chronic pain (divided into links, organizations, and information).

PAIN RESEARCH AT OXFORD
(WWW.JR2.OX.AC.UK/BANDOLIER/PAINRES/PRINTRO.HTML)
A resource for systematic reviews on pain and anesthesia including acute pain, chronic pain, arthritis, migraine and headache, and safety issues.

Cancer
COMMONWEAL CANCER PROJECT
(WWW.COMMONWEAL.ORG)
Commonweal is a 25-year-old health and environmental research institute that focuses on helping people with cancer find and assess treatment options and work toward physical, mental, emotional, and spiritual healing.

Other programs include a children and young adults program to help those with learning, social, or emotional difficulties; training for childcare and juvenile justice professionals; training for physicians and professionals who work with people with life-threatening illnesses; and support for local, national, and international initiatives that contribute to environmental health.

CYBERBOTANICA: PLANTS AND CANCER TREATMENTS
(HTTP://BIOTECH.ICMB.UTEXAS.EDU/BOTANY)
Part of the Indiana University Biotech Project, this website provides information on botanical compounds currently used in cancer treatment.

OFFICE OF CANCER COMPLEMENTARY AND ALTERNATIVE MEDICINE
(HTTP://OCCAM.NCI.NIH.GOV)
Presents Best Case Series and pilot clinical trials using CAM modalities, CAM cancer treatment trials, CAM information from the PDQ cancer database, MD Anderson Cancer Center, and more.

THE CANCER PROJECT
(WWW.CANCERPROJECT.ORG)
This special project of the Physicians Committee for Responsible Medicine is dedicated to advancing new approaches to cancer prevention

and survival through nutrition education and research. The website covers Committee's research initiatives, cancer prevention and survival information, cancer commentaries, news, a food-as-medicine section, and an "ask the dietitian" feature.

THE SIMONTON CANCER CENTER (WWW.SIMONTONCENTER.COM)

This website provides information on the Simonton approach (a comprehensive cognitive-behavioral self-help therapy for patients with cancer and their support persons), online programs on imagery and visualization, training programs in cancer counseling, and tape and book resources.

Immunology

CENTER FOR COMPLEMENTARY AND ALTERNATIVE MEDICINE RESEARCH IN ASTHMA, ALLERGY, AND IMMUNOLOGY (WWW_CAMRA.UCDAVIS.EDU/)

A National Center for Complementary and Alternative Medicine (NCCAM) research center (University of California at Davis), the Center promotes research into the use of CAM therapies for asthma and allergies. Select Current Studies, then Botanicals, to view information on current research studies involving immune boosting herbs.

Women's Health

NORTH AMERICAN MENOPAUSE SOCIETY (WWW.MENOPAUSE.ORG)

This scientific nonprofit organization addresses the impact of menopause on women's health during midlife and beyond. The website has information for health care professionals and consumers, including recently published studies with expert commentary, information on a menopause practitioner competency examination, educational materials, conference information, and reports on the state of the knowledge about menopause and related therapies.

ROSENTHAL CENTER FOR COMPLEMENTARY AND ALTERNATIVE MEDICINE—WOMEN'S HEALTH INFORMATION RESOURCES (WWW.ROSENTHAL.HS.COLUMBIA.EDU/ WOMEN.HTML)

This website includes an annotated listing of women's health resources on the Internet by category, including academic centers; government sites; electronic journals; women's health issues such as fertility, osteoporosis, and heart disease; and other research resources. These include general conventional medicine sites as well as complementary medicine sites.

SusanLoveMD.org (WWW.SUSANLOVEMD.COM)

The Susan Love MD Breast Cancer Foundation provides advice and information on breast cancer, including significant resources on women and wellness and complementary approaches to self-care. The website includes information on decision making, clinical trial information, a list of recommended scientific articles and conference information.

Evidence-Based Medicine

BANDOLIER EVIDENCE-BASED HEALTHCARE (WWW.JR2.OX.AC.UK/BANDOLIER/BOOTH/ BOOTHS/ALTMED.HTML)

Produced by Oxford University, Oxford, UK, Bandolier is a print and Internet journal covering systematic reviews and meta-analyses of CAM therapies, particularly herbs and supplements, acupuncture, homeopathy, massage, and safety issues. Other topics include cognitive-behavioral therapy, biofeedback, music therapy, exercise, prayer, relaxation, therapeutic touch, and yoga.

DARE: DATABASE OF ABSTRACTS OF REVIEWS OF EFFECTIVENESS (UNIVERSITY OF YORK) (HTTP://NHSCRD.YORK.AC.UK/DAREHP.HTM)

This database of quality assessed reviews is produced by the British National Health Service. These systematic reviews of the research evidence evaluate and synthesize results, providing a comprehensive summary of the available evidence on a given topic.

SUM Search (University of Texas/SGIM)
(http://sumsearch.uthscsa.edu/)

Selects the best websites to search, organizing results from the broadest level of information to the narrowest. Includes textbooks, review articles, practice guidelines, systematic reviews, and original research.

TRIP Database (Centre for Research Support) (www.tripdatabase.com)

An amalgamation of hyperlinks from evidence-based sites available on the Internet from around the world. There are more than 29,000 links from more than 75 sites of high-quality medical information on evidence-based topics. The database now includes links to peer-reviewed journals and "eTextbooks," and is updated monthly.

REFERENCES

1. Vickers A. Recent Advances: complementary medicine. *BMJ*. 2000;321:683–686.
2. Barnes J, Abbot NC, Harkness E, et al. Articles on complementary medicine in the mainstream medical literature: an investigation of MEDLINE, 1966 through 1996. *Arch Intern Med*. 1999; 159(15):1721–1725.
3. Allais G, Voghera D, De Lorenzo C, et al. Access to databases in complementary medicine. *J Altern Complement Med*. 2000;6(3):265–74.
4. Ezzo J, Berman BM, Vickers AJ, et al. Complementary medicine and the Cochrane collaboration. *JAMA*. 1998;280(18):1628–1630.
5. Rupert RL. Searching chiropractic literature: a comparison of three computerized databases. *J Manip Physiol Ther*. 1997;20(4):285–288.
6. Tomasulo P. MANTIS—manual, alternative, and natural therapy index system database. *Med Ref Serv Q*. 2001;20(3):45–55.
7. Tomasulo P. A new source of herbal information on the web: the IBIDS Database. *Med Ref Serv Q*. 2000;19(1):53–57.
8. Bastyr University: Library: Resources: Using CAM MEDLINE. Available online at www.bastyr.edu/library/resources/researchguide/cammedline.asp. Last accessed 8/13/03.
9. Cassileth BR. Resources for alternative and complementary cancer therapies. *Cancer Pract*. 1998; 6(5):299–301.
10. Cline RJW, Haynes KM. Consumer health information seeking on the Internet: the state of the art. *Health Educ Res*. 2001;16(6):671–692.
11. Friedman Y. Navigating the world of alternative medicine. Worthwhile websites. *Am J Nurs*. 2001; 101(3):87–9.
12. He M, Yan X, Zhou J, et al. Traditional Chinese medicine database and application on the web. *J Chem Inf Comput Sci*. 2001;41(2):273–277.
13. Huang MB. Internet resources for Tibetan medicine. *Med Ref Serv Q*. 2001;29(1):61–67.
14. Owen DJ. Herbal resources on the Internet. *Med Ref Serv Q*. 1999;18(4):39–56.
15. Stone VI, Fishman DL, Frese DB. Searching online and web-based resources for information on natural products used as drugs. *Bull Med Libr Assoc*. 1998;86(4): 523–527.
16. Thomson T. Web resources for CAM researchers. *Complement Ther Med*. 2000;8:216–217.
17. Wootton JC. Web watch. Alternative and complementary therapies. *AIDS Patient Care Stds*. 1998;12(10):811–13.

CHAPTER 16

Selected Issues in Environmental Medicine

ANDREA GIRMAN, LAUREN VIGNA, AND ROBERTA LEE

Environmental medicine—the examination of the impact of environmental factors on health and illness—is an enormous field, worthy of an entire textbook. It is also a vital component of the integrative medicine approach, as seeing the patient in the context of his or her environment, and the influences of that environment on the patient's health, is critical to the "whole person" approach, which is at the core of integrative medicine. Traditionally, other than in the case of asthma or specific allergic illness, physicians have not typically done environmental assessment as part of ongoing care.

Various topics from the field of environmental medicine are touched on throughout this text including multiple chemical sensitivity syndromes in Chapter 17 and food sensitivities in Chapters 7 and 21. Choices regarding organic versus nonorganic foods, and the challenges posed by dioxins, polychlorinated biphenyls (PCBs), and mercury in the food chain are discussed in Chapter 30. Other important aspects of this field which are not covered in this text involve occupational exposures to toxic chemicals and/or radiation, and the pressing questions regarding the long-term safety of genetically engineered and/or irradiated foods.

This chapter addresses three specific topics in environmental medicine: the influence of drinking water on health and on illness, the impact of air pollution, and the phenomenon known as sick building syndrome. Although a comprehensive discussion of environmental influences on health is beyond the scope of this text, we hope that the subjects introduced here and elsewhere will raise awareness regarding the importance of environmental assessment as a part of integrative medicine's approach to the patient.

▶ WATER AND HEALTH

Eighty percent of the surface of the Earth is covered by water. Despite this abundance, only a tiny fraction of freshwater (1%) is available for human consumption. Nearly 97% of the Earth's water supply exists as seawater, and another 2% is frozen in ice caps and glaciers. Water continuously circulates between the Earth's surface and atmosphere in what is known as the hydrological cycle. Freshwater—water that has a relatively low amount of total dissolved solids as measured in parts per million—is present in the atmosphere, but it also exists as surface water and groundwater. Surface water represents all water that exists in a state that is open to the atmosphere (streams, rivers, reservoirs, lakes, and oceans). Groundwater is freshwater that filters into the ground, and is held in soil and rock formations known as aquifers. These aquifers are a precious resource, heavily used for both consumer (wells and springs) and agricultural (irrigation) needs.

As a vital nutrient, water plays a critical role in a myriad of physiological processes. More than 60% of the weight of the human body is water, and while a human being can live more than a month without food, a person could only live as long as 1 week without water.

Access to Clean and Safe Water

Compared to a majority of the global community, most Americans today have access to relatively reliable and safe drinking water. This unparalleled access comes as a result of a series of regulatory reforms and technological advances over the past century. Public awareness and concern for controlling water pollution in the United States was heightened in June 1969, after the Cuyahoga River in Cleveland, Ohio, caught fire and burned for 4 days. Outrage over the burning river eventually led to enactment of the Federal Water Pollution Control Act Amendments of 1972, commonly known as the Clean Water Act (CWA) after its amendment in 1977. The CWA established the basic structure for regulating discharges of pollutants into US waters, and gave the United States Environmental Protection Agency (EPA) authority to implement pollution control programs. Under the CWA, the EPA set water-quality standards for all contaminants in *surface* waters, as well as wastewater standards for industry, made it unlawful for any person to discharge any pollutant from a "point" source (municipal sewage plants and industrial facilities) into navigable waters, and funded the construction of sewage treatment plants.[1] More recent attention has been given to "nonpoint" source pollution created when rainwater runs off from sources such as streets, construction sites, and farms.

Similar concern for the state of the nation's public drinking water supply and its impact on public health led Congress to pass the Safe Drinking Water Act (SDWA) in 1974, and to first amend it in 1986. Under this Act, the EPA is mandated to set and enforce two national health-based quality standards for naturally occurring and synthetic contaminants found in tap water, to regulate discharges made to groundwater sources, and to monitor the patency of public water systems infrastructure.[2] Pollutant standards for tap water include the maximum contaminant goal level and the maximum contaminant level. The maximum contaminant goal level is the level of contaminant that is not expected to cause adverse health effects over a lifetime of exposure; this standard includes a safety margin and acts as a standard guideline without penalty for violation. The maximum contaminant level is an enforceable standard that is set as close to the maximum contaminant goal level as possible, and is the maximum permissible level of contaminant allowed in tap water. Additional significant amendments to the SDWA were made in 1996, enhancing the law in a number of ways, including by recognizing source water protection, establishing a fund for water system improvements, increasing public access to information about drinking water, and creating more stringent guidelines for both microbial contaminants and the by-products of chemical disinfection.

Despite enactment of the CWA, the SDWA, and several other laws designed to protect US water resources, a recent review in *Environmental Health Perspectives* suggests that the nation will continue to face significant challenges to providing safe drinking water. Areas of concern are systemic (the deteriorating US water system infrastructure, increasing consumer and industrial demand, and increasing foreign ownership of US water systems); regulatory (nonenforcement of and persistent noncompliance of public water systems with current EPA regulatory standards); environmental (depletion of surface water and groundwater sources faster than they can be replenished, global climate effects, acid rain, and urban sprawl); technological (resistance of pathogens to standard disinfection approaches); and biomedical (the impact of disinfection by-products and chemical contaminants on human health; and the emergence of new waterborne pathogens) in nature.[3] Subsequent to the attacks of September 11, 2001, attention is also being directed at the vulnerability of national water resources to acts of terrorism.[1]

The scope of the aforementioned water issues is clearly quite broad, yet warrants investigation by any health care provider interested in the environmental issues encompassed by an integrative approach to health. This is particularly relevant given rising consumer interest in water quality and safety, SDWA requirements that water utilities provide Consumer Confidence Reports—detailed annual reports of a community's water source, contaminants, and possible health effects—to all customers, and the perception that health care providers are trusted information sources on these issues.[5]

Water and Human Health

Although water is generally considered a critical biophysical nutrient, research documenting its impact on health is lacking overall. The limited numbers of studies that exist indicate some benefit of optimal hydration in decreasing the relative risk of fatal coronary heart disease in men and women,[6] and a possible protective association between zinc and magnesium content in domestic drinking water and type 1 diabetes.[7] One animal study suggests that water quality may impact the severity of neuropathology in Alzheimer's disease, but its relevance in human patients is unknown.[8] Other research has focused on the mineral content of water—from both tap and bottled sources—and the effect that constituents such as calcium, sodium, and magnesium might have on disease states such as osteoporosis, hypertension, and the risk of sudden death.[9,10]

Total-body dehydration has been reported to result in a significant decrease in forced expiratory volume at 1 second in young adults with exercise-induced asthma,[11] and has been described as a common finding in severe acute childhood asthma.[12] Fluid hydration has been mentioned as appropriate supportive care in both adults and children with underlying pulmonary disease.[13–15] However, little research has focused on the potential preventive or acute therapeutic effects of optimal hydration in individuals with acute or chronic pulmonary (or other) disease.

Water and Human Disease

The true magnitude of water-associated disease in the United States is not known. While the American Society for Microbiology has estimated that up to 900,000 individuals become ill and up to 900 individuals die annually in the United States from waterborne infectious agents,[16] no such estimate exists for the health burden of waterborne chemical contaminants. In a recent survey of 2,000 adults conducted by the National Environmental Education and Training Foundation, 75% of participants indicated concern for the quality and safety of their drinking water, and nearly 25% reported avoiding tap water for health or aesthetic concerns.[17] A growing body of evidence suggests that these concerns are justified.

Waterborne Infectious Disease

Numerous surveys demonstrate contamination of both US surface water and groundwaters by a variety of pathogens.[18–20] Although the Centers for Disease Control and Prevention (CDC) routinely collect information on the occurrences of waterborne infectious illness,[21–25] this data is generally thought to grossly underrepresent actual incidence.[26] Many waterborne infectious illnesses are never reported, and at least one study estimates that as much as 35% of gastrointestinal illnesses may be attributable to the consumption of drinking water that meets current federal water quality standards.[27]

Enteric bacterial agents such as *Shigella* spp. and *Campylobacter* spp. are predominantly responsible for drinking-water disease outbreaks, while illness associated with recreational water contamination is primarily caused by *Pseudomonas* spp., *Shigella* (shigellosis), and *Legionella*. Enteric viruses such as Norwalk virus, rotavirus, caliciviruses, adenoviruses, and hepatitis A have all been transmitted by water,[28] but little is known about their occurrence in water or their endemic rates of infection. The enteric protozoa *Cryptosporidium parvum* and *Giardia lamblia* are the organisms most responsible for waterborne disease outbreaks. One study found *Cryptosporidium* oocysts in 80% of US surface water samples[29]; another study reported a drinking water-associated cryptosporidiosis outbreak despite state-of-the-art water treatment.[30] The highly infectious nature of *Cryptosporidium,* its resistance to chlorine disinfection and its filter-escaping small size make it a pathogen not only of significant threat to the US water supply but also with significant public health implications, especially for immunocompromised individuals.[31]

In its most recent analysis, the CDC reported an increase of drinking water outbreaks associated with both surface water and groundwater contamination by infectious agents,[32] and noted that the majority of groundwater outbreaks were associated with private or non-community wells not regulated by the EPA. This is an important finding, given that up to half of the population of some states in the United States receive their drinking water from private or household wells.[33] The CDC also reported that recreational water outbreaks involving gastroenteritis doubled from the previous survey period, and were most frequently associated with *Cryptosporidium parvum* in treated water (swimming pools or interactive fountains) and with *Escherichia coli O157:H7* in freshwater. *E. coli O157:H7* is an emerging pathogen of concern, a pathogen newly linked to waterborne illness or recently recognized. Other members of this class include *Mycobacterium avium* complex, *Legionella pneu-*

mophila, Helicobacter pylori, Vibrio cholera O139, hepatitis E, and *Cyanobacteria* (blue-green algae).[34–37]

Compounding the issue of waterborne illnesses caused by existing and emerging pathogens is another marked clinical concern: the public health threat represented by waterborne pathogen resistance to multiple antibiotics.[38,39] This may be the result of source-water contamination by antibiotic and bioactive chemicals used in the human population,[40] by unregulated and massive use of antibiotics in agriculture and aqualculture,[41] and by gene exchange of antibiotic resistance and virulence factors on biofilms forming on the inner surface of water system structures such as pipes and holding tanks.[42]

Waterborne Chemical Contaminants

Chlorine was first used in the United States to sterilize city water in 1908, and continues to be the most common and important drinking water disinfectant. However, mounting evidence suggests carcinogenic and possibly other health effects associated with disinfection by-products, compounds formed by the interaction of chlorine and organic molecules in water. While dozens of disinfection by-products exist, the trihalomethanes are the most studied and the only by-product to have a drinking water standard.[43] Epidemiological studies link disinfection by-products to increased cancer risks of the bladder, rectum, esophagus, and breast.[44,45] Links have also been suggested between disinfection by-products (trihalomethanes) and an increased risk of adverse reproductive outcomes, including spontaneous abortion and neural tube defects.[46–50] Significant clinical concern is also being raised about the impact of synthetic organic compounds on human and ecological health.[51,52] These contaminants result from the production, use, and disposal of numerous industrial, agricultural, medical, and household chemicals. They include industrial by-products (dioxin, polychlorinated biphenyls, perchloroethylene, and methyl-*tert*-butyl ether); pesticides (dichlorodiphenyltrichloroethane [DDT], aldrin, endrin, chlordane, and heptachlor); herbicides; over-the-counter, prescription, and veterinary pharmaceuticals; hormones; household cleaners; and personal care products.[53] Epidemiologic studies have found associations between perchloroethylene-contaminated public drinking water and lung cancer, and possibly colorectal cancer.[54,55] Methyl-*tert*-butyl ether (MTBE), a common gasoline additive, is linked to carcinogenesis in animals[56] and is known to contaminate groundwater sources via leaking fuel tanks.[57,58] The endocrine disrupter dioxin is also associated with increased prevalence and severity of endometriosis in nonhuman primates, and is implicated in the pathobiology of the disease in humans as well.[59]

As discussed above many organic wastewater contaminants are ubiquitous, persistent and potent toxins capable of reaching groundwater supplies. A recent US Geological Survey found organic wastewater contaminants in 80% of streams sampled downstream from a wide range of areas at high risk for human, industrial, and agricultural impact—a clear indication that they are neither removed by wastewater treatment nor biodegraded.[60] Seventy-five percent of streams sampled had more than one organic wastewater contaminant; the median was seven. Compounds most frequently detected included coprostanol (fecal steroid), *N,N*-diethyltoluamide (insect repellant), caffeine (stimulant), and triclosan (antimicrobial disinfectant).

The US Geological Survey raises a number of critical issues related to water contamination by organic compounds. The individual or additive (either synergistic or antagonistic) health effects of chronic organic water contaminant exposure on humans, animals, and plants are not known. Many organic wastewater contaminants lack drinking-water guidelines or advisories; of the estimated 75,000 chemicals in use, the EPA currently has drinking water standards for only 54 organic chemicals or chemical groups.[61] For example, organic water contaminants such as MTBE and the disinfection by-product *N*-nitrosodimethyl-amine (*N*-NDMA) have an

ubiquitous environmental presence and raise concerns about human toxicity at low levels. Despite this, no federal standards exist for these compounds in drinking (tap or bottled) water.

Ultimately, the number of new and different contaminants released into the national water system has grown faster than the ability of federal regulatory agencies to classify, regulate, and monitor them. Alarmingly, drinking water standards for even the small number of monitored chemicals are routinely violated. According to the EPA, nearly 30 million Americans drink water each year from systems reporting violations of health-based standards.[62]

Other water contaminants of health concern include heavy metals such as arsenic, cadmium, lead, and mercury; nitrates resulting from fertilizer application and septic tank seepage; and radon. Fluoride is also a water constituent of considerable controversy. Although fluoride may enter water from natural deposits, it is most frequently added during water-treatment processes in order to prevent dental caries. Nonnatural sources of fluoride used as additives in water treatment come from the industrial by-products of phosphate fertilizer production and aluminum smelting. The upper intake level for fluoride is 10 mg/d for US adults and children no longer at risk for dental fluorosis (>8 years of age). Intakes slightly in excess of this level for 10 or more years increase the risk of preclinical (stage 1) skeletal fluorosis; intakes less than 10 mg/d have not been shown to cause adverse health effects, although some uncertainty remains with respect to bone strength, cancer, and reproductive effects.[63]

Water Solutions

Given the ubiquitous presence of contaminants in national water sources including drinking water, total avoidance of either infectious or chemical agents seems impossible. Integrative medical interventions should be tailored to address the specific health issues that definitively (or theoretically) are associated with ingestion of waterborne contaminants. Despite this, any intervention must begin with an investigation of each patient's unique susceptibility and his or her risk of microbial and chemical exposure. For healthy patients desiring to optimize their wellness, the best therapeutic interventions may be education, prevention, and tailoring a lifestyle that minimizes overall body toxicologic burden.

Given the clinical implications, physicians and patients must begin to educate themselves about the health risks involved by using any water source—whether tap or bottled—on a daily basis. Three basic questions provide the most critical information: Where does the water come from? What is in the water? How is the water handled and treated?

Who's at Risk?

By virtue of living on Earth at this time in history, we have all been and will all continue to be exposed to environmental contaminants to varying degrees. However, some groups of individuals are particularly vulnerable to the toxic effects of waterborne infectious pathogens and chemical compounds (Table 16–1).

Numerous studies detail the significant morbidity and mortality associated with waterborne infectious agents in immunocompromised individuals.[61–66] Similarly, the higher risk from waterborne microbial pathogens seen in the elderly may be related to reduced immunity, as well as to diminished resilience from underlying malnutrition or chronic disease states and a greater exposure to institutional environments.[67,68] Associations between trihalomethane exposure and miscarriages in pregnant women were previously discussed.

Children of all ages comprise one of the most vulnerable populations to environmental pollutants. A report recently compiled by Greater Boston Physicians for Social Responsibility (in conjunction with the Clean Water Fund) examined the contribution of toxic chemicals to the epidemic of neurodevelopmental, learning, and behavioral disabilities in children.[69] The report provides a comprehensive scientific review of the impact that exposure to heavy metals such as lead and mercury, dioxins, and PCBs, pesticides, and organic solvents has on the developing fetal, neonatal, and childhood nervous system.

Because dioxins in a mother's body are mobilized from fatty tissue stores and concentrated in breast milk, the dioxin exposure of breastfeeding neonates is estimated to be 50

▶ **TABLE 16–1** SELECTED PATIENT SUSCEPTIBILITIES

Contaminant	Neonates	Infants–Children	Pregnant Women*	Immuno-compromised	Elderly
Lead	XXX	XXX	XXX		
Nitrates	XXX		XX		
DBPs			X?		
E. coli O157:H7		XXX			XX
Enteroviruses	XXX				
Cryptosporidia				XXX	XX
Hepatitis E			XXX		
Adenovirus				XXX	
MAC				XXX	XX

*With the exception of hepatitis E, all of the susceptibilities listed are for the fetus.
Abbreviations: DBPs = dibutylphthalates; MAC = *Mycobacterium avium*-intracellular complex.
Note: Summary table of categories of patients at higher risk than the general population for specific exposures. The number of X's is a qualitative judgment by the authors of the relative degree of susceptibility, weighing both frequency and severity of adverse health effects.
Source: Physicians for Social Responsibility. Drinking Water and Disease. *Washington, DC: Physicians for Social Responsibility; 2000.*

times that of adults.[70,71] Formula-fed infants may be exposed to increased levels of lead and nitrates (concentrated by boiling tap water for formula preparation) as well as the xeno-estrogen bisphenol-A (released by microwaving baby bottles containing a plastic monomer inner coating).[72] Other studies have found statistically significant associations between perchlorate exposure and elevated newborn thyroid-stimulating hormone levels,[73] as well as an increased prevalence of infectious disease in childhood resulting from immunotoxic exposures during pregnancy and breast-feeding.[74]

Older children may be at higher risk for waterborne infectious disease outbreaks related to recreational exposure. At least one study documented measurable levels of enterovirus in 100% of wading pools sampled.[75] Drinking fountains in schools also represent potential sources of waterborne contaminants. One recent study found lead levels above federal standards in 222 of New York City's 990 elementary schools.[76] In addition, associations between childhood exposure to volatile organic compounds in drinking water and cancer continue to be investigated.[77,78] Limitations clearly exist in estimating the true impact of waterborne toxins on all populations, yet this may be especially true for children. The EPA's maximum contaminant levels have been extrapolated from animal studies and are based on an adult male's body weight and water consumption.[79]

Not a Drop to Drink?

Educating health conscious patients as well as those in more vulnerable health states is of paramount importance for physicians, given the ubiquitous nature of the water issues addressed here. In general, any steps that individuals make to inform themselves about the condition of their drinking water, or about measures that can be taken to reduce exposure to waterborne contaminants in both drinking and non-drinking sources, will be beneficial. Numerous resources exist that are dedicated to educating

both professionals and the public about water safety.

Water Disinfected by Heat

Two methods of disinfecting water are boiling and distilling. Boiling water for 1 minute is a convenient way to kill most harmful microbes present in water. However, it does not remove harmful chemical contaminants, and boiling for longer than 1 minute concentrates levels of contaminants such as lead and nitrates that are present in water. Survey studies also raise concerns about contaminants resulting from the distillation process.[80]

Bottled Water

Americans' increasing concern over the quality of their drinking water continues to spur the growth of the bottled water industry—a market worth an estimated $7 billion in 2002. Consumer surveys indicate that individuals most often choose bottled water for heath and taste reasons. Although often perceived as a more healthy alternative to drinking tap water, studies suggest that the quality and contents of bottled waters can differ significantly.[81,82] A recent investigation by the National Resources Defense Council sampled 1,000 bottles of water from 103 different brands, and found that 33% of the brands had at least one bottle that violated state or industry standards for contaminants.[83] Contaminants included pathogenic bacteria as well as synthetic organic (trihalomethanes and plastic-derived chemicals) and inorganic (arsenic) compounds.

Because many states lack stringent bottled water regulatory programs, individuals should be encouraged to purchase bottled waters that are qualified as interstate (not intrastate) commerce or are nationally distributed. Bottled waters distributed across state lines are subject to a much higher degree of regulatory standards, including federal standards for maximum contaminant levels and good manufacturing practices. In addition, bottled water manufacturers who are members of the International Bottled Water Association adhere to the most

---

▶ **WATER INFORMATION RESOURCES**

The following sources provide comprehensive information on a wide variety of useful water-related topics—from regulatory policy and home water testing, to toxic body burden effects, and preventive health strategies.

Books

Ingram C. *The Drinking Water Book.* Berkeley, CA: Ten Speed Press; 1991.

Kupua A'o LK. *Don't Drink the Water.* Pagosa Springs, CO: Kali Press; 1998.

Physicians for Social Responsibility. *Drinking Water and Disease: What Health Care Providers Should Know.* Washington, DC: PSR; 2000.

Water Quality Testing

NSF International (www.nsf.org)

Websites

American Water Works Association (www. awwa.org)

Centers for Disease Control and Prevention (www.cdc.gov/ncidod/diseases/water/drinking.htm)

Clean Water Action (www.cleanwateraction. org)

Clean Water Fund (www.cleanwater.org)

Environmental Working Group (www.ewg.org/reports/bodyburden/index.php)

National Resources Defense Council (www.igc.org/nrdc)

Physicians for Social Responsibility (www. psr.org)

United States Environmental Protection Agency (www.epa.gov/safewater)

United States Geological Survey (www. water.usgs.gov)

---

stringent accepted standards. Waters sold interstate are legally required by the FDA to annually provide a full analysis of all bottled water contents such as minerals, infectious agents, radioactive materials, and organic and inorganic contaminants. Individuals may also request content information on the water source used for bottling, and should be encouraged to discontinue using brands from manufacturers who are reluctant to respond to requests on either bottled water contents or source information.

Finally, the filtration and other disinfection processes used by many manufacturers to purify bottled water products can be limited in their ability to remove all contaminants. As discussed previously, there are increasing concerns regarding toxic compounds that are byproducts of water management methods. These include the carcinogenic trihalomethanes and *N*-nitrosodimethylamine,[84,85] as well as byproducts of ozone treatment, the most com-

monly employed method of disinfecting bottled waters and an increasingly used process in municipal water systems.[86,87]

Water Filters

Patients interested in using home water filtration products to improve tap water quality should be aware that no home filtering system will remove every contaminant of concern. Before purchasing a water purifying unit—from either inexpensive portable systems to expensive full home reverse-osmosis systems—patients should be encouraged to contact their local municipal water system for an analysis of contaminants. A filtration unit providing a content removal that best matches contaminants present in the municipal system should be selected.

NSF International provides water filter certification based on standards developed by the American National Standards Institute, and provides consumer assurance that claims made by the water filter manufacturer are valid. Individuals should also be instructed to care for their water filtration systems as instructed by the manufacturer, as replacing water filters and/or providing regular maintenance appropriately will guarantee the best level of protection.

▶ AIR AND HEALTH

In this section we discuss air pollution and its effects on health. An optimally functioning respiratory system is essential for good health. Each day, we provide our bodies with 24,000 breaths, which equals approximately 2 gallons of air per minute, or 3,000 gallons per day. Because breathing is essential to life, we must ensure that the quality of the air we inhale each day is optimal. This section reviews the common air pollutants, as well as diseases linked with contaminated air. We also discuss methods of achieving cleaner air and the role antioxidants may play in protecting from air pollutants.

What Contaminants Are in the Air?

The Clean Air Act of 1970 authorized the EPA to set standards for six different outdoor air contaminants including ground level ozone, particulate matter, carbon monoxide, nitrogen oxide, sulfur dioxide, and lead. These exposure standards are referred to as the National Ambient Air Quality Standards and consist of a concentration and averaging time that attempts to account for weather changes. Air pollution is also measured by the Pollutant Standard Index, which ranges from 0 to 500, measuring the above-mentioned pollutants except lead and nitrogen dioxide. A Pollutant Standard Index rating of 100 or greater indicates a federal standard has been exceeded for one of the four toxins. Other indoor air pollutants include environmental tobacco smoke, mold spores, and mercury vapor.

Ground-level ozone is a gas composed of three oxygen atoms, and is created by a chemical reaction between oxides of nitrogen and any volatile organic compounds (VOCs). Ozone can be "good " or "bad" depending on its position in the atmosphere. "Good" ozone occurs naturally high in the earth's stratosphere and protects the earth from ultraviolet sun rays. In the lower atmosphere, ozone is considered "bad," and is usually created by motor vehicle exhaust, gasoline vapors, and industrial solvents. Peak ozone levels occur in hot, dry summertime weather that is stagnant and muggy, and can be carried hundreds of miles, creating air pollution far from its original source.

Particulate matter includes particles in the air, such as dust, soot, liquid droplets, and smoke. Particles can come from a variety of sources, including motor vehicles, unpaved roads, industrial sites, and wood burning. Particle formation can also occur by chemical reactions from combustible fuels. Particulate matter can be especially damaging to the environment as well as to public health, because the particles can change chemical and nutrient balances in water and soil, thereby destroying natural ecosystem balance.

Carbon monoxide (CO) is formed when carbon molecules in fuel are not completely combusted. Motor vehicle exhaust accounts for approximately 56% of CO emissions nationwide. As CO is colorless and odorless, it is difficult to assess unless specifically measured using a CO detector. Other sources of CO include cigarette smoke, industrial processing, woodstoves, and natural sources such as forest fires.

Nitrogen oxides form during high-temperature combustion processes, such as those involved in industry, motor vehicles, and electrical utilities. Many of the nitrogen oxides are also colorless and odorless like CO, and can be carried over many miles by wind, creating regional, as well as local, pollution. Nitrogen oxides contribute to the formation of acid rain, and can also change the nutrient and chemical balance in soil and water. They are the only emission monitored by the EPA that has *increased* by 10% since 1970.

Sulfur dioxide is a gas that is readily formed by the extraction of gasoline from oil, metals extracted from ore, or by the burning of coal and oil. Over half of the sulfur dioxide in the air comes from coal-burning electrical utilities, other sources being petroleum refineries, metal processing utilities, and cement plants. Like nitrogen oxides, sulfur dioxide also contributes to acid rain, and particles can be carried by winds over long distances. Asthmatics are particularly affected by high levels of sulfur dioxides.

Lead is a naturally occurring compound found today mostly in metal processing plants and smelters. Motor vehicles were another primary source of lead pollution prior to the disuse of leaded gasoline by most passenger vehicles. Children and infants are at greatest risk, not only through air contamination, but also through soil, water, and lead paint chips.

Air and Disease

Many diseases are associated with air pollution, including heart disease,[88] lung cancer,[89] stroke,[90] rhinoconjunctivitis in children,[91] asthma development,[92] and asthma-related mortality.[93]

One study done in The Netherlands examined daily variations in air pollution and mortality during the period from 1986 to 1994. The study's conclusions showed that "specific cardiovascular causes of death, heart failure in particular, are more strongly associated with air pollution than total cardiovascular mortality."[94]

Another study[90] recently looked at stroke and air pollution in Seoul, Korea, and measured daily stroke deaths and daily air pollution data taken from 20 sites, correlating these with measures of particulate matter, sulfur dioxide, nitrogen dioxide, ozone, and carbon monoxide. This study's conclusions revealed a statistically significant association between ischemic stroke mortality and level of air pollution. According to this study, the increase in relative risk of dying from ischemic stroke with increased air pollution is 3–6%, depending on the pollutant examined. The study did not examine the mechanism of how air pollution

might cause stroke, but it is speculated that an increase in free radicals produced by the pollution causes an increase in the inflammatory response and enhanced blood coagulation, therefore adding to the risk for stroke.

Multiple studies show that asthma and allergies have an association with air pollution. One study examined exposure to indoor molds[91] and allergic sensitization. The results revealed children exposed to high levels of mold spores were more likely to suffer from rhinoconjunctivitis and allergic sensitization; the children most affected were those who still lived in their home of birth. A study in France examined the short-term effects of air pollution in mild-to-moderate asthmatic children who were followed for 3 months,[95] and showed statistically significant associations between ozone and an increase in asthma attacks and respiratory infections. Increases in nitrogen dioxide were also associated with nocturnal cough and respiratory infections.

A study performed with adults in Germany[96] also showed an association with ambient air particulate matter and an increase in asthma symptoms and inhaler use. Other studies[97] have examined nitrogen dioxide and ozone and have shown both to be linked with exacerbating severe asthma and even a related cause of death in asthmatic individuals.

Lung cancer is also linked to both indoor and outdoor air pollution. A study done in China[98] looked at females with new diagnoses of primary lung adenocarcinoma and indoor air pollutants, such as cooking fumes, as well as other sources of indoor/outdoor air pollution and other demographic data. The results showed a statistically significant increase with lung cancer and exposure to indoor cooking fumes. A California study[99] examined more than 6,000 nonsmokers during the period 1977–1992 for incidence of new lung cancers in relation to ambient air pollutants. The results showed an increased relative risk of 3.56 for males exposed to a defined level of ozone and a relative risk of 5.21 associated with particulate matter exposure. Females had increase in relative risk (2.14) with increased sulfur dioxide exposure, as well as increased relative risk (1.25) with particulate matter exposure.

Long-term exposure to pollutants was also studied by Pope and Burnett,[89] using the American Cancer Prevention Study II statistics. Of the 1.2 million participants, they were able to study those in metropolitan areas for which air pollution data was available. As expected, cigarette smoking was associated with a significant higher all-cause mortality rate. Also noted was an 8% increase in lung cancer mortality related to increased particulate matter ambient concentrations. Of note, much research still needs to be done in order to completely assess the effect air pollution has on health. Critics argue that there are limitations in the current studies, and that air pollution alone is a difficult risk factor to isolate. This being said, there nevertheless are some actions that can be taken to promote better air and better respiratory health.

Clean Air Solutions

The most effective treatment for air pollution is prevention. In July 2002, the Bush Administration announced its plans for Clear Skies legislation, which will set strict mandatory emissions caps on sulfur dioxide, nitrogen oxides, and mercury. The EPA projects that by 2020 public health benefits will include prevention of 12,000 premature deaths and total $93 billion saved per year, far outweighing the cost of the project at $6.5 billion.

Air cleaners are another way some harmful toxins can be removed. Three types of air cleaners exist: mechanical filters, ion generators, and electronic air cleaners. Mechanical filters clean by forcing air through fibers that may contain an adhesive or electrical charge for particles to stick to. They usually consist of flat or pleated material to allow for greater surface area. HEPA (high-efficiency particulate air) filters are of the mechanical type.

Ion generators come in portable units only, and clean air by generating static charges to remove particles. Some types of ion generators may produce ozone, which, as discussed earlier, is an outdoor air toxin. Electronic air cleaners work by trapping charged particles in an electric field, on a series of flat plates or on fibers. This type can be portable or connected to central heating or air conditioning systems. Other newer systems on the market are referred to as hybrid devices, and combine two or more of the methods of air cleaning described.

Air cleaning serves as an addition to two other important methods for reducing pollutants in indoor air. These include most importantly, source control, or prevention, such as smoking cessation and emissions control. Source control can be difficult when not all pollutants are easily identifiable, such as carbon monoxide. Ventilation reduces indoor air pollutants by bringing outside air indoors. Some systems use mechanical ventilation with exhaust fans or air exchangers, but opening windows and doors can also aid in ventilation. One must keep in mind, however, that outdoor air itself may contain high levels of contaminants, and ventilation and air cleaning should remain balanced.

The role of antioxidants in protecting from the health effects of air pollution recently gained attention because of their ability to scavenge free radicals. We know that excessive exposure to reactive oxygen and nitrogen species is what causes oxidative stress and leads to damage of DNA proteins as well as lipids. Tobacco smoke, as well as air pollution, contain reactive oxygen and nitrogen, and thus can lead to DNA damage. The body uses antioxidants to ward off this damage, hence the idea exists that supplemental antioxidants may help decrease the oxidative stress caused by air pollution.[100] Grievink et al.[101] examined adults with chronic respiratory conditions and their dietary intake or serum concentration of vitamin C and beta-carotene. The results showed that "serum beta-carotene, and to a lesser extent dietary vitamin C and beta-carotene, may attenuate peak expiratory flow decreases due to air pollution in subjects with chronic respiratory symptoms." Two other studies by Grievink examined acute effects of ozone on lung function and the ability of antioxidants to modulate these effects.[102] Lung function was measured in Dutch cyclists, and results suggest that daily intake of 100 mg of vitamin E and 500 mg of vitamin C was statistically significant in showing partial protection against the effects of ozone on lung function in cyclists. Other research examined the relation between lung function and beta-carotene and alpha-tocopherol.[103] The results showed *no* relation between plasma alpha-tocopherol and lung function. A trend but no statistical significance in lung function improvement was seen in patients with higher beta-carotene levels.

▶ SICK BUILDING SYNDROME

The clearest way into the universe is through a forest wilderness.

JOHN MUIR

Shelters and building structures have protected humans since the beginning of recorded history. For the most part, buildings have been viewed as a means of providing shelter and a safe environment that can prevent exposure to the elements. The idea of a building as a potential cause of illness seems foreign and was not recognized until the early 1970s.[104] The phenomenon is thought to have developed as building structures were deliberately "tightened" to conserve energy in response to the Middle East oil embargo.[105] The term "sick building syndrome" (SBS), first officially reported in 1984,[106] is now a commonly recognized term used to describe symptoms related to indoor air quality such as off-gassing in the environment. The syndrome has been difficult to define, and multiple causes have been proposed for its etiology. In 1984, a World Health Organization Committee report suggested that up to 30% of new and remodeled buildings worldwide had reports related to SBS.[107]

Sick Building Syndrome and Building-Related Illness Defined

The term sick building syndrome is used to describe a situation in a building where more people than normal have various symptoms or feel ill and the etiology is not attributable to live agents, bacteria, or molds. The symptoms may be reported in association with a specific room or zone or may be spread throughout an entire building.[108] The term "building-related illness" (BRI), in contrast, is used when symptoms of diagnosable illness (such as asthma or allergic rhinitis) are identified and can be attributed directly to airborne building contaminants.

The complaints commonly reported with SBS are often similar to those found in many common illnesses and allergies (see Table 16–2). In many cases, the symptoms are so vague that most sufferers will not see a physician and may not take time off work.[109] An important diagnostic clue, however, is that most patients with SBS report relief after leaving the building. In contrast, the symptoms related to BRI—although often similar to those of SBS—may require prolonged recovery times after leaving the building. Risk factors for SBS are known to include female sex, atopy, a low-paying job category, frequent tasks involving the handling of paper, use of a video display terminal, a history of airway hyperrreactivity, and preexisting respiratory or dermatologic disease.[110]

▶ **TABLE 16–2** SYMPTOMS ASSOCIATED WITH SICK BUILDING SYNDROME

Eyes	Itching, dry, watering
Nose	Irritated, itching, runny, dry
Throat	Sore, dry mouth
Head	Headache, lethargy, irritability, difficulty concentrating
Skin	Dryness, itching, irritation
Lung	Dry cough, chest tightness
General	Nausea, fatigue, low grade fever

Source: Adapted from Appleby P. ABC of work-related disorders: building-related illnesses. BMJ. 1996; 313(7058):674–677.

Frequently, both SBS and BRI are a result of poor building operation or inconsistent maintenance in accordance with its original design. At other times SBS or BRI will be a problem resulting from poor design alone. Unfortunately, in the early 1990s, when sick building syndrome was first reported in the literature, the lack of a clear conceptual framework for defining these illnesses made it easy to ascribe this syndrome to mass psychogenic illness or mass hysteria.[111] However, subsequent studies that evaluated respiratory impairments discredited psychogenic illness theories, as the syndrome was more thoroughly evaluated and more reports of chronic symptoms and dysfunction continued to emerge.[112]

Environmental Factors in SBS

While there has been no single cause of SBS identified to date, a number of factors have been identified that contribute to the symptoms. Environmental factors that make SBS more likely include high concentrations of particulate matter, extremes in thermal comfort, reduced humidity, insufficient fresh air supply, excessive air movement, poor lighting, microbial contamination, and volatile organic compounds and noise. Table 16–3 provides a more complete list.[113–117]

The data suggesting an association between particulate matter and increased SBS symptoms in the workplace has been mostly observational. Intervention studies on the effect of reducing surface contaminants have had mixed results.[118] However, residential studies have extensively documented adverse health outcomes of airborne particles and benefits from removal.[119] Particles that have been implicated include animal dander, molds, dust mites, and bacterial agents.

Biological air pollutants can be found to some degree in every home, school, and workplace. Sources include outdoor air, as well as

▶ **TABLE 16–3** RISK FACTORS FOR SICK BUILDING SYNDROME

Characteristics of work and building
Sedentary occupation, clerical work
More than half of occupants using display screen equipment >5 hours
Maintenance problems identified
Low ceilings (<2.4 m [7.9 feet])
Many movements of furniture
Large area of open shelving and exposed paper
Sealed building and city centre location
Large size—typically an occupied floor area >2,000 m² (6,561.7 square feet)
Centralized control of environmental conditions (no local control of heating, etc.)
Building more than 15 years old
Large areas of soft furnishings, carpets, and fabrics
Environmental factors
Low room humidity
Low supply rate of outdoor air
Smoking permitted in work areas
Damp areas and visible mold growth
Dust, solvents, and ozone emissions from printers and copiers
Low-frequency fluorescent lamps creating subliminal flicker
High room temperature
Excess supply rate of outdoor air
Dusty atmosphere
Gaseous emissions (volatile organic compounds) from building materials
Low-frequency noise

Source: Reproduced with permission from Appleby PH. ABC of work-related disorders: building-related illnesses. BMJ. 1996;313(7058):674–677.

human and animal occupants who can act as vectors for viruses, bacteria, and insect-borne illnesses. Water reservoirs and other damp indoor surfaces can serve as breeding grounds for fungi and bacteria. High humidity (greater than 50%) is particularly important, as this generally encourages dust mite proliferation and increased fungal growth on damp surfaces.[120] A number of steps can be taken to reduce concentrations of particulate matter, including (1) providing adequate ventilation to reduce aerosolized particles, (2) keeping equipment water reservoirs clean and avoiding areas of standing water; (3) repairing leaks and seepage quickly and replacing carpets within 24 hours of damage; (4) controlling humidity to keep levels between 30% and 50%; (6) cleaning carpets and furniture regularly; (7) covering mattresses and washing toys at temperatures above 54.4°C (130°F) to kill dust mites; and (8) considering a HEPA filtration system. The merits of removing particulate matter and specifics of different filtration systems are discussed earlier in this chapter.

Another potential contributing factor to SBS is the presence of VOCs, including formaldehyde, pesticides, solvents, and cleaning agents. Formaldehyde, which has been classified by the EPA as a probable human carcinogen, is one of the few indoor air pollutants that can be readily measured; home testing kits are readily available. Until the early 1980s, urea-formaldehyde foam insulation was used as a major insulation source for homes. It is now seldom used, and most experts feel that most homes insulated with this foam are now considered safe because the off-gassing has ceased.[121] However, formaldehyde-based resins are still found in many plywood finishes, paneling, fiberboard, and particleboard materials, and are used frequently in mobile and conventional home construction as subflooring and paneling, as well as in commercial buildings.[122]

At room temperature, VOCs, including formaldehyde, are emitted as gases from certain solids or liquids. One source notes that formaldehyde off-gasses are in substantial quantities only when the humidity level is higher than 50%.[123] Airborne formaldehyde acts as an irritant to the conjunctiva and lower respiratory tract. Symptoms of formaldehyde exposure include tingling or burning of the eyes, nose, and throat, chest tightness, and wheezing. Some patients will experience an acute reaction to formaldehyde vapor, which can be associated with hypersensitivity. Approximately 10–20% of those experiencing formaldehyde reactions may have hyperreactive airways, predisposing them to the effects of formaldehyde vapors.[124] One study of residential exposure compared neurobehavioral and respiratory parameters in individuals who were living in manufactured homes and in renovated buildings to those in subjects with known formaldehyde exposure at work, and found similar adverse effects in both groups. The authors of this study found that "exposure to indoor air produced abnormal simple and choice reaction time, abnormal balance with eyes open and with the eyes closed, abnormalities of color confusion, reduced verbal recall and elevated abnormal moods";[125] the authors suggest that these findings point to formaldehyde as having a major role in health problems related to indoor air.

Benzene and perchloroethylene are other common VOCs; these, as well as a wide array of other VOCs, are emitted by products that are used in the home, office, and school, and in crafts or in hobby activities. These products, of which there are thousands in common use, include hair sprays, rug and oven cleaners, paints and lacquers, dry-cleaning fluids, office copiers and printers, glues and adhesives, and permanent markers (Table 16–4). It is estimated that there may be over 70, 000 industrial chemicals in use that have the potential to create effects attributable to environmental or chemical exposure.[126] Ventilation at 10 liters per second per person appears to reduce the incidence of symptoms related to SBS, including those from exposure to VOCs.[127] Because of this fact, the installation of new carpeting or other materials known to be high in VOCs should be done in a well-ventilated area to minimize concentrations of the potentially harmful off-gasses.

Carbon monoxide (CO) is a non-VOC gas that is commonly noted as a potential hazard.

▶ **TABLE 16–4** COMMON INDOOR AIR POLLUTANTS AND THEIR SOURCES

Tobacco smoke

Ozone from photocopiers and printers

Dust from outdoor air, skin, paper, printer and photocopier toner

Carbon monoxide from traffic and tobacco smoking

Oxides of nitrogen from traffic, gas cookers

Isocyanates: toluene, diphenylmethane, hexamethylene

   Typical indoor concentrations: $50–10^3$ µg/m^3 (trace)

   Sources: adhesives, sealants, tobacco smoke, wall and floor coverings, paint, and moth crystals

Formaldehyde

   Typical indoor concentration: 1–0.06 parts per million (0–0.03 parts per million outdoors)

   Sources: urea foam insulate, fabrics, carpets, floor and wall coverings, plywood, lacquer, gypsum
     board, disinfectants

Source: Adapted from Appleby PH. ABC of work-related disorders: building-related illnesses. BMJ. 1996;313(7058): 674–677.

Carboxyhemoglobin levels of 2.0–3.5% have been measured in nonsmokers in indoor environments where the CO concentration has been 4–10 parts per million. It has been reported that heavy cigarette smoking or intake of exhaust fumes from exogenous sources can create carboxyhemoglobin concentrations of 5–10%.[128] At this level, cognitive dysfunction, decreased alertness, dizziness, and headache have been reported, representing an occult form of carbon monoxide poisoning.[129]

Other environmental factors contributing to SBS include light and noise. Low-frequency noise seems to be one of the nonspecific factors commonly present in SBS environments, whereas high-frequency noise does not seem to have deleterious effects. The importance of noise in the etiology of SBS and its potential negative effects remains somewhat unclear in the literature.[130,131] Low-frequency fluorescent lamps creating subliminal flicker have also been reported as contributory.[132] Eye strain and headache are often reported, especially with conventional white fluorescent lighting.[133] It has been suggested that to minimize effects from fluorescent lighting, incandescent or natural lighting should be used whenever possible.

Building-related illnesses have specific causes and are not discussed in this section. However, for a comprehensive summary of all illnesses with related symptoms and suggested ways to address these illnesses, the reader is referred to the websites of the Environmental Protection Agency at www.epa.gov and the National Center for Environmental Health at www.cdc.gov/nceh/airpollution/mold/moldfacts.htm.

Taking an Environmental History

Environmental contaminants in general are increasingly coming to the attention of the public; sick building syndrome and its effects represent only one of a growing number of concerns related to this area. Frequently, the presentation of SBS is very vague: a headache, myalgia, rash, respiratory difficulty, or other symptom seeming to have no attributable etiology in the immediate history. Rarely is the consideration of an environmental factor entertained. In one study reviewing 2,922 histories taken by 137 third-year medical students, 91% of the cases documented smoking status and 70% documented occupation, but specific occupational exposures were documented in only 8.4% of cases. Patients younger than 40 years of age and women were less likely than older patients or men to have occupation and industry noted.[134] It appears that in the area of environmental health, physicians are lagging behind the public in awareness regarding these exposures.[135] Furthermore, the histories for SBS require identifying clusters of illness; physicians typically are trained to interview individuals for

Exposure History

COMMUNITY

For each of the items listed below:	Do you presently live nearby				If you ever lived nearby, please write the years.
Heavy traffic	☐ No	☐ Yes *(please specify)*	○ highway	○ busy street	_____
Vehicle idling area	☐ No	☐ Yes *(please specify)*	○ auto	○ bus / truck	_____
Dump site	☐ No	☐ Yes *(please specify type)* _____			_____
Farm(s)	☐ No	☐ Yes *(please specify type)* _____			_____
Industrial plant(s)	☐ No	☐ Yes *(please specify type)* _____			_____
Polluted lake / stream	☐ No	☐ Yes *(please specify type)* _____			_____
Nuclear power plant	☐ No	☐ Yes			_____
Hydro towers	☐ No	☐ Yes			_____
Other potential hazards	☐ No	☐ Yes *(please specify type)* _____			_____

Do you protect yourself from excess sun exposure? ☐ rarely ☐ occasionally ☐ often ☐ always

HOME & HOBBY

How long have you lived in your present residence? _____ **How old is it?** _____

What type of dwelling is your residence? ☐ house ☐ mobile home
☐ apartment → ○ basement ○ above store ○ highrise → *floor* _____

Ownership? ☐ owner occupied ☐ rental ☐ public housing

How is your home heated? ☐ forced air ☐ hot water radiators ☐ space heater ☐ baseboard heaters

What type of fuel is used for heating? ☐ natural gas ☐ oil ☐ wood ☐ electricity ☐ propane

Do you use: ☐ central vacuum? ☐ HEPA filter vacuum? ☐ other vacuum? _____

Have you done any renovating? ☐ No ☐ Yes → When? _____
What? _____

Do you own / lease a car? ☐ No ☐ Yes → Age? _____ **Smoking permitted inside?** ○ No ○ Yes

Do you use pesticides or herbicides (bug or weed killers, flea / tick sprays, collars, powders, pellets, etc.):

① **in your home?** ☐ No ☐ Yes *(please specify type)* _____

② **on your pets?** ☐ No ☐ Yes *(please specify type)* _____

③ **on your lawn or garden?** ☐ No ☐ Yes *(please specify type)* _____

What is your water source for bathing? ☐ city ☐ well ☐ other *(please specify* _____)

Environmental Health Clinic, Sunnybrook & Women's College Health Sciences Centre
Ontario College of Family Physicians

compiled by Dr. L. M. Marshall
print design by Helen Kwan

Figure 16–1. An excerpt from the Ontario College of Family Physicians' environmental history form.

For each of the items listed below:	Do you presently have in your <u>HOME</u>?	If you ever had, please write the years.
Damp, musty basement or crawl space	☐ No ☐ Yes → ○ slight ○ severe	_____
Wet windows or outside closet walls (condensation)	☐ No ☐ Yes → ○ slight ○ severe	_____
Water leaks	☐ No ☐ Yes → ○ slight ○ severe	_____
Visible mould	☐ No ☐ Yes → ○ slight ○ severe	_____
Crumbling pipe insulation	☐ No ☐ Yes → ○ slight ○ severe	_____
Flaking paint	☐ No ☐ Yes → ○ slight ○ severe	_____
Stagnant stuffy air	☐ No ☐ Yes → ○ slight ○ severe	_____
Gas or propane stove	☐ No ☐ Yes	
Other gas appliances	☐ No ☐ Yes *(please specify)* _____	_____
Wood stove or fireplace	☐ No ☐ Yes	_____
Carbon monoxide detector(s)	☐ No ☐ Yes	_____
Air conditioning	☐ No ☐ Yes → ○ central ○ individual rooms	_____
Electrostatic air cleaner	☐ No ☐ Yes	_____
Other air cleaner(s)	☐ No ☐ Yes *(please specify)* _____	_____
Carpets	☐ No ☐ Yes → Where? _____ How old? _____	_____
Old vinyl linoleum	☐ No ☐ Yes	_____
Photocopier / fax machine / printer	☐ No ☐ Yes → Type? _____	_____
Garage	☐ No ☐ Yes → ○ attached ○ underground	_____
Smoker(s)	☐ No ☐ Yes → Who? _____	_____
Pets	☐ No ☐ Yes *(please specify)* _____	_____
Indoor plants	☐ No ☐ Yes → How many? _____	_____

Do you use an electric blanket?   ☐ No   ☐ Yes → Years _____

Do you use dust mite-proof: Pillow cover(s)?   ☐ No   ☐ Yes   **Mattress cover(s)?**   ☐ No   ☐ Yes

What product(s) do you usually use: *(please specify brands)*

bathroom cleanser _____   floor / wall cleanser _____

laundry detergent _____   fabric softener _____

What hobbies do you have? _____

What hobbies do members of your household have? _____

Have you ever personally done any of the following:

☐ furniture stripping / refinishing   Years: _____

☐ home renovating   Years: _____   *(please specify type)* _____

☐ art work (e.g. painting, ceramics, stained glass, leather work, etc.)   Years: _____   *(please specify type)* _____

☐ other non-occupational activities with exposure to toxic chemicals
   Years: _____   *(please specify type)* _____

Environmental Health Clinic, Sunnybrook & Women's College Health Sciences Centre
Ontario College of Family Physicians

compiled by Dr. L. M. Marshall
print design by Helen Kwan

OCCUPATION

1. **Do you presently do volunteer work and/or work for pay?**

   ☐ Volunteer work → *Number of hours per week:* _____ *Type:* _____

   ☐ Work for pay → *Number of hours per week:* _____

   ☐ Unable to work for pay due to health problems → *Date stopped work:* _____
   Reason(s): _____

   ☐ On disability benefits → *Type:* _____

2. **Starting with your present or most recent job, please list all of the paying jobs you have ever had.**
   Please use the back of this page if necessary.

Company Name & Work Location	From Mth / Yr	To Mth / Yr	Job Title & Description	Exposures*	Protective Measures / Equipment **
1.	/	/			
2.	/	/			
3.	/	/			
4.	/	/			

* Please list the significant chemicals, dusts, fibres, fumes, radiation, biologic agents (e.g. bacteria, moulds, viruses) and physical agents (e.g. extreme heat, cold, vibration, noise) that you were exposed to at this job.

** Please list any protective measures taken (e.g. showering at work, laundering clothes at work, etc.) or protective equipment used (e.g. gloves, apron, mask, respirator, hearing protectors, etc.).

3. **The following questions are about your present or most recent work environment:**

   Age of Building: _____ Number of Floors: _____ Approximate number of occupants: _____

   Neighbourhood: ☐ rural ☐ commercial ☐ industrial

   Which of the following are / were on the same floor as your work station in your present or most recent work environment?

   ☐ bank of computers ☐ partitions or room dividers ☐ unvented copy machines

   ☐ unvented smoking areas ☐ carpets → *How old?*_____

   ☐ central air conditioning ☐ windows that open

   Can / could you smell odours from the following in your present or most recent work environment?

   ☐ laboratory ☐ cafeteria ☐ manufacturing area ☐ parking garage in or near the building

   Have any of the following occurred in your work environment over the past 12 months or the last 12 months you worked in your most recent job?

   ☐ use of pesticides → ○ indoors ○ outdoors ☐ fire, smoke ☐ flood, water leaks ☐ carpet cleaning

   ☐ new flooring, furniture, etc. *(please specify)* _____ ☐ construction ☐ renovation

   ☐ painting ☐ chemical spill, leak *(please specify)* _____ ☐ accidents ☐ stress

   On average, how would you describe your present or most recent work environment?

Lighting	☐ too much glare	☐ satisfactory	☐ too dim	
Temperature	☐ too hot	☐ satisfactory	☐ too cold	☐ too variable
Air Movement	☐ too stuffy	☐ satisfactory	☐ too drafty	
Humidity	☐ too dry	☐ satisfactory	☐ too humid	
Odour	☐ none ☐ moderate	☐ strong	*Specify:* _____	
Noise	☐ little ☐ moderate	☐ a lot		
Your Comfort Overall	☐ unsatisfactory	☐ somewhat satisfactory	☐ satisfactory	
Co-workers' Comfort Overall	☐ unsatisfactory	☐ somewhat satisfactory	☐ satisfactory	

Environmental Health Clinic, Sunnybrook & Women's College Health Sciences Centre
Ontario College of Family Physicians

compiled by Dr. L. M. Marshall
print design by Helen Kwan

Figure 16–1. An excerpt from the Ontario College of Family Physicians' environmental history form. *(Continued)*

SCHOOL (if applicable)

How old is your or your child's school? _____   Number of floors: _____   Number of occupants: _____

Have additions been made to the original building?   ❑ No   ❑ Yes → When? _____

Number of portable classrooms in use: _____

Hours per day you or your child spends in a portable classroom: _____

School neighbourhood: ❑ rural   ❑ suburban   ❑ urban

Is your or your child's school located near any of the following:

Heavy traffic   ❑ No   ❑ Yes *(please specify)*   ○ highway   ○ busy street

Vehicle idling area   ❑ No   ❑ Yes *(please specify)*   ○ auto   ○ bus / truck

Dump site   ❑ No   ❑ Yes *(please specify type)* _____

Farm(s)   ❑ No   ❑ Yes *(please specify type)* _____

Industrial plant(s)   ❑ No   ❑ Yes *(please specify type)* _____

Polluted lake / stream ❑ No   ❑ Yes *(please specify type)* _____

Nuclear power plant   ❑ No   ❑ Yes

Hydro towers   ❑ No   ❑ Yes

Other potential hazards ❑ No   ❑ Yes *(please specify type)* _____

Which of the following does your or your child's school have? *(Please check all that apply)*

❑ carpeted classrooms   ❑ central air conditioning   ❑ art room – exhaust hood?   ○ No ○ Yes
❑ unvented copy machine(s)   ❑ windows that open   ❑ laboratory – exhaust hood? ○ No ○ Yes
❑ flaking paints   ❑ mouldy smell   ❑ workshop – exhaust hood?   ○ No ○ Yes

Have any of the following occurred in your or your child's school during the current or last school year?
(Please check all that apply)

❑ carpet cleaning   ❑ construction   ❑ renovation   ❑ painting
❑ new flooring or furniture *(please specify)* _____   ❑ flood, water leaks
❑ roof tarring   ❑ use of pesticides / herbicides → ○ indoors ○ outdoors

Are the following products used in your or your child's school during the school year?
(Please check all that apply)

❑ deodorizer strips   ❑ furniture wax or polish   ❑ odourous cleaning products
❑ floor wax   ❑ scented washroom soap   ❑ spray paints
❑ permanent markers   ❑ strong-smelling art supplies

Does your or your child's school have a policy regarding the use of personal scented products by staff and students?

❑ No   ❑ Yes *(please specify)* → ○ prohibition of scented products   ○ encouragement of unscented products

Environmental Health Clinic, Sunnybrook & Women's College Health Sciences Centre
Ontario College of Family Physicians

compiled by Dr L. M. Marshall
print design by Helen Kwan

Exposure History

PERSONAL

Natural Inhalant Allergies

Do you think you are allergic to any seasonal pollens, animal danders, dust, mites, or moulds?

❏ No   ❏ Yes *(please specify)* _____

Have you ever had allergy tests?   ❏ No   ❏ Yes

If YES, please specify:

Age	Year	Type of Test	Results	Treatments (e.g. avoidance, shots, medications)	Improvement 0 = worse 1 = none 2 = a little 3 = some 4 = a lot

Synthetic Chemicals

Have you ever had symptoms you linked with exposure to any synthetic (man-made) chemical at a level that did not seem to bother most people (e.g. paints, perfumes, cosmetics, diesel exhaust, jet fuel, tar, etc.)?

❏ No   ❏ Yes

(*'Linked'* means that the symptom started or worsened within 48 hours after you were exposed to something, or the symptom improved or disappeared after you were no longer exposed to it.
'Exposure' means being near, touching, smelling, breathing in, eating, drinking, swallowing or injecting something.)

If YES, please specify chemical(s) and symptom(s):

Man-made Chemical	Symptoms Linked with Low Level Exposure	Presently Affected? 1 = a little 2 = somewhat 3 = a lot	In the Past 1 = a little 2 = somewhat 3 = a lot

How often do you use SCENTED personal products? *(please check)*

Scented Products	Soap	Lotion	Cosmetics	Hair permanent	Hair tint	Perfume/aftershave	Other(s) *(please specify)*
Never	❏	❏	❏	❏	❏	❏	❏ _____
Occasionally	❏	❏	❏	❏	❏	❏	❏ _____
Daily	❏	❏	❏	❏	❏	❏	❏ _____

Artificial Materials

How many metal dental fillings / caps do you currently have? silver / mercury _____ gold _____

Have you had silver / mercury fillings removed? ❏ No ❏ Yes → Number removed: _____ Year(s): _____

Do you have other artificial materials in your body (e.g. pins, screws, plates, meshes, valves, implants, etc.)?

❏ No   ❏ Yes *(please specify)* _____

Smoking History

Do you currently use tobacco (daily or almost every day)?

❏ No   ❏ Yes *(please specify)* → ○ cigarettes ○ cigars ○ snuff ○ chewing tobacco

• If **YES**, average number per day: _____ Number of years: _____

• If **NO**, have you ever used tobacco (daily or almost every day)?   ○ No   ○ Yes

· If YES, number of years you used tobacco: _____ Average number per day: _____

· Date you last used tobacco regularly: Year _____

Have you ever experimented with "recreational drugs"?   ❏ No   ❏ Yes

Environmental Health Clinic, Sunnybrook & Women's College Health Sciences Centre
Ontario College of Family Physicians

compiled by Dr. L. M. Marshall
print design by Helen Kwan

Figure 16–1. An excerpt from the Ontario College of Family Physicians' environmental history form. *(Continued)*

Travel Illnesses

Have you ever experienced significant symptoms when travelling?   ☐ No   ☐ Yes

If YES, please specify:

Age	Year	Location	Symptoms

Blood Transfusion

Have you had blood transfusion(s)?   ☐ No   ☐ Yes → Year(s) _____

Living Situation / Supports

Who lives at home with you? _____

Are you: ☐ single   ☐ married / cohabitating   ☐ separated   ☐ divorced   ☐ widowed

Do you have spiritual beliefs / practices which help you cope?
☐ No   ☐ Yes *(please comment)* _____

Are you part of a religious community which helps you cope?
☐ No   ☐ Yes *(please estimate the number of contacts in the last 12 months)* _____

Who backs you up best with your present health problems? _____

What other supports do you have? _____

Stresses

Type of Stress	Ever had it?	When? *Please specify Year(s)*	Comments
Loss of someone close	☐ No ☐ Yes		
Illness in someone close	☐ No ☐ Yes		
Loss of job	☐ No ☐ Yes		
Change of job	☐ No ☐ Yes		
Change of workplace	☐ No ☐ Yes		
A move	☐ No ☐ Yes		
Marriage	☐ No ☐ Yes		
Separation	☐ No ☐ Yes		
Divorce	☐ No ☐ Yes		
Pregnancy	☐ No ☐ Yes		
Alcohol / drug addiction	☐ No ☐ Yes		
Alcohol / drug addiction in someone close	☐ No ☐ Yes		
Physical abuse	☐ No ☐ Yes		
Emotional abuse (being put down, called names)	☐ No ☐ Yes		
Sexual abuse	☐ No ☐ Yes		
Other *(please specify)*	☐ No ☐ Yes		

Environmental Health Clinic, Sunnybrook & Women's College Health Sciences Centre
Ontario College of Family Physicians

compiled by Dr. L. M. Marshall
print design by Helen Kwan

DIET & DRUG

1. **Who grocery shops for you?** _____

   Where? ☐ chain grocery store   ☐ health food store   ☐ market   ☐ others *(please specify)* _____

2. **Who cooks for you?** _____

3. **Please indicate foods and beverages most typically consumed for each of the following meals and the times at which they are most typically eaten.**

Foods / Snacks	Please Specify	Time	Beverage(s)	Please Specify	Time
Breakfast			Breakfast		
Mid-Morning			Mid-Morning		
Lunch			Lunch		
Mid-Afternoon			Mid-Afternoon		
Dinner			Dinner		
Evening			Evening		

4. **How much of the following beverages do you consume regularly and have you linked any symptoms with drinking them?**

   ☐ **water** → Number of 8 oz glasses per 24 hours _____ ○ city ○ charcoal-filtered ○ distilled ○ reverse osmosis
   ○ bottled (glass) ○ bottled (plastic)   Any symptoms linked? _____

   ☐ **beer, ale** → Number of 12 oz bottles per week _____ Any symptoms linked? _____

   ☐ **wine** → Number of 6 oz glasses per week _____ Any symptoms linked? _____

   ☐ **spirits** (e.g. whisky, rum) → Number of 1½ oz drinks per week _____ Any symptoms linked? _____

   ☐ **coffee** → Number of 8 oz cups per 24 hours _____ Any symptoms linked? _____

   ☐ **tea** → Number of 8 oz cups per 24 hours _____ Any symptoms linked? _____

   ☐ **cola** → Number of 12 oz drinks per 24 hours _____ ○ regular ○ diet Any symptoms linked? _____

   ☐ **other(s)** *(please specify)* _____ Any symptoms linked? _____

5. **Do you eat fish?**   ☐ No   ☐ Yes → On average, how many days per week? _____ How many times per day? _____
   Type(s) of fish eaten (e.g. tuna, salmon, etc.): _____

6. **Please list foods / beverages that do not agree with you** (e.g. stuffy runny nose, heartburn, bloating, diarrhea, sleepiness, difficulty thinking or concentrating, etc.) **or cause allergic reactions** (e.g. hives, rashes, shortness of breath, wheezing, anaphylaxis, etc.)**:**

List foods / beverages that are a problem	What problem(s) do they give you?	Approximately how often do you eat / drink them?			
		Never	Occasionally	Daily	More than once a day

7. **Please list any foods / beverages that you crave or that help you to feel better and the time(s) the craving usually occurs:**

List foods / beverages that you crave or that help you to feel better	Time(s) of craving	What problem(s), if any, do they give you?	Approximately how often do you eat / drink them?		
			Never	Occasionally	Daily

Environmental Health Clinic, Sunnybrook & Women's College Health Sciences Centre
Ontario College of Family Physicians

compiled by Dr. L. M. Marshall
print design by Helen Kwan

Figure 16–1. An excerpt from the Ontario College of Family Physicians' environmental history form. *(Continued)*

8. **Please list all PRESCRIPTION medications you currently take on a regular basis, including birth control pills and allergy injections: ***

Name of prescription medication	Dose (e.g. mg, ml, IU)	How often do you take it?	How long have you taken it?	If you have side effects, please specify

* Use additional paper if necessary.

9. **Please list all NON-PRESCRIPTION medications you currently take on a regular basis, including vitamins, minerals, herbs, remedies, etc.: ***

Name and brand of non-prescription medication	Dose (e.g. mg, ml, IU)	How often do you take it?	How long have you taken it?	If you have side effects, please specify

* Use additional paper if necessary.

10. **Drug Adverse Reactions: Please list ANY medication / anesthetics / immunizations you have had to stop taking because of side effects or allergic reactions:**

Name of medication / immunization	Type of side effects or allergic reaction that caused you to stop it	Age	Year

11. **Have you EVER had an emergency injection of adrenaline (epinephrine) for a reaction to any medication, food, insect sting, or other substance?**

❑ No   ❑ Yes → What year(s)? _____

To what? _____

specific medical diagnosis, not necessarily informed by the perspective of a group of people with similar symptoms of concern. This lack of a "public health" perspective can be a major hurdle in making the appropriate diagnosis of SBS or any other environmental/occupational exposure.

Because there are so many chemicals in the environment with potentially deleterious effects on health—an estimated 70,000 or more—running through a checklist of possible exposures as part of standard history taking is impractical. An organized approach in history taking has been proposed using the CH2OPD2 mnemonic: community, home, hobbies, occupation, personal habits, diet, and drugs. A complete environmental history questionnaire is available via the Ontario College of Family Physicians website at www.ocfp.ca/English/OCFP/Communications/Publications, compiled by Dr. L. Marshall[136]; an excerpt from this history form is provided in Figure 16–1.

▶ CONCLUSION

It is clear that many more studies are needed to shed light on the particular effects of environmental exposures in SBS, and on the more subtle effects on health of VOCs and other chemicals, both in the workplace and at home. Nonetheless, even lacking this specific data, an integrative practitioner can take a thorough environmental history. With the increased index of suspicion for environmental illness we are proposing here, and with attention to the appearance of clusters of similarly inexplicable symptoms in the community, we may be able to identify causes of illness—including SBS—previously overlooked with use of the conventional approach. By logical extension, this awareness of the impact of environmental factors can also enhance our understanding at a most fundamental level of the delicate interconnections between nature, the individual, and the community.

For a successful technology, reality must take precedence over public relations, for Nature cannot be fooled.

RICHARD P. FEYNMAN

REFERENCES

1. United States Environmental Protection Agency Laws and Regulations. Available at: www.epa.gov/region5/water/cwa.htm.
2. United States Environmental Protection Agency Office of Groundwater and Drinking Water. Available at: www.epa.gov/safewater/.
3. Levin RB, Epstein PR, Ford TE, et al. US drinking water challenges in the twenty-first century. *Environ Health Perspect.* 2002;10(1):43.
4. United States Environmental Protection Agency Chemical Emergency Preparedness and Prevention. Available at: http://yosemite.epa.gov/oswer/ceppoweb.nsf/content/ct-epro.htm.
5. National Environmental Education and Training Foundation (NEETF) and Roper Starch Worldwide. *The National Report Card on Safe Drinking Water: Knowledge, Attitudes and Behaviors.* Washington, DC: NEETF; 1999.
6. Chan J, Knutsen SF, Blix GG, et al. Water, other fluids, and fatal coronary heart disease: the Adventist Health Study. *Am J Epidemiol.* 2002; 155(9):827.
7. Zhao HX, Mold MD, Stenhouse EA, et al. Drinking water composition and childhood-onset type 1 diabetes mellitus in Devon and Cornwall, England. *Diabet Med.* 2001;18(9):709.
8. Sparks DL, Lochhead J, Horstman D, et al. Water quality has a pronounced effect on cholesterol-induced accumulation of Alzheimer amyloid beta (Abeta) in rabbit brain. *J Alzheimers Dis.* 2002;4(6):519.
9. Azoulay A, Garzon P, Eisenberg MJ. Comparison of mineral content of tap water and bottled waters. *J Gen Intern Med.* 2001;16(3):168.
10. Garzon P, Eisenberg MJ. Variation in the mineral content of commercially available bottled waters: implications for health and disease. *Am J Med.* 1998;105(2):125.
11. Maxwell P, Cerney F, Ohtake P, Leddy J. Dehydration and exercise—induced bronchospasm.

Report to the American College of Sports Medicine. American College of Sports Medicine Annual Meeting; June 3, 1999; Seattle, WA.

12. Potter PC, Klein M, Weinberg EG. Hydration in severe acute asthma. *Arch Dis Child.* 1991; 66(2):216.

13. Jeng MJ, Lemen RJ. Respiratory syncytial virus bronchiolitis. *Am Fam Physician.* 1997;55(4):1139.

14. Lemen RJ. Respiratory syncytial virus and bronchiolitis. *Zhonghua Min Guo Xiao Er Ke Yi Xue Hui Za Zhi.* 1995;36(2):78.

15. Gross NJ. Chronic obstructive pulmonary disease: current concepts and therapeutic approaches *Chest.* 1990;97(suppl 2):19S.

16. American Society for Microbiology. *Microbial Pollutants in our Nation's Water.* Washington, DC: American Society for Microbiology; 1999.

17. National Environmental Education and Training Foundation (NEETF) and Roper Starch Worldwide. *The National Report Card on Safe Drinking Water: Knowledge, Attitudes and Behaviors.* Washington, DC: NEETF; 1999.

18. Harvey S, Greenwood JR, Picket MJ, et al. Recovery of *Yersinia enterocolitica* from streams and lakes of California. *Appl Environ Microbiol.* 1976;32(3):352.

19. Rose JB, Gerba CP, Jacobowaki W. Survey of potable water supplies for *Cryptosporidium* and *Giardia. Environ Sci Technol.* 1991;25:1393.

20. LeChevalier MW, Norton WD, Lee RG. Occurrence of *Giardia* and *Cryptosporidium* spp. in surface water supplies. *Appl Environ Microbiol.* 1991;57(9):2610.

21. Lee SH, Levy DA, Craun GF, et al. Centers for Disease Control and Prevention. Surveillance for waterborne-disease outbreaks—United States, 1999–2000. *MMWR Morb Mortal Wkly Rep.* 2002; 51(8):1.

22. Barwick RS, Levy DA, Craun GF, et al. Surveillance for waterborne-disease outbreaks—United States, 1997–1998. *MMWR Morb Mortal Wkly Rep.* 2000;49:1.

23. Levy DA, Bens MS, Craun GF, et al. Surveillance for waterborne-disease outbreaks—United States, 1995–1996. *MMWR Morb Mortal Wkly Rep.* 1998; 47(5):1.

24. Kramer MH, Herwaldt BL, Craun GF, et al. Surveillance for waterborne-disease outbreaks—United States, 1993–1994. *MMWR Morb Mortal Wkly Rep.* 1996;45(1):1.

25. Moore AC, Herwaldt BL, Craun GF, et al. Surveillance for waterborne disease outbreaks—United States, 1991–1992. *MMWR Morb Mortal Wkly Rep.* 1993;42(5):1.

26. Ford TE. Microbiological safety of drinking water: United States and global perspectives. *Environ Health Perspect.* 1999;107(suppl 1):191.

27. Payment P, Richardson L, Siemiatycki J, et al. A randomized trial to evaluate the risk of gastrointestinal disease due to consumption of drinking water meeting current microbiological standards. *Am J Public Health.* 1991;81(6):703.

28. Griffin DW, Donaldson KA, Paul JH, et al. Pathogenic human viruses in coastal waters. *Clin Microbiol Rev.* 2003;16(1):129.

29. LeChevalier MW, Norton WD. Giardia and cryptosporidium in raw and finished water. *J Am Water Works Assoc.* 1995;87:54.

30. Goldstein ST, Juranek DD, Ravenholt O, et al. Cryptosporidiosis: an outbreak associated with drinking water despite state-of-the-art water treatment. *Ann Intern Med.* 1996;125(2):158.

31. Rose JB. Environmental ecology of *Cryptosporidium* and public health implications. *Annu Rev Public Health.* 1997;18:135.

32. Lee SH, Levy DA, Craun GF, et al. Centers for Disease Control and Prevention. Surveillance for waterborne-disease outbreaks—United States, 1999–2000. *MMWR Morb Mortal Wkly Rep.* 2002; 51(8):1.

33. Barron G, Buchanan S, Hase D. New approaches to safe drinking water. *J Law Med Ethics.* 2002; 30(suppl 3):158.

34. Hegarty JP, Dowd MT, Baker KH. Occurrence of *Helicobacter pylori* in surface water in the United States. *J Appl Microbiol.* 1999;87(5):697.

35. Goodman KJ, Correa P, Tengana Aux HJ, et al. *Helicobacter pylori* infection in the Colombian Andes: a population-based study of transmission pathways. *Am J Epidemiol.* 1996;144(3):290.

36. Klein PD, Graham DY, Gaillour A, et al. Water source as risk factor for *Helicobacter pylori* infection in Peruvian children. Gastrointestinal Physiology Working Group. *Lancet.* 1991;337(8756):1503.

37. Rustin PA, Rose JB, Haas CN, et al. Risk assessment of opportunistic bacterial pathogens in drinking water. *Rev Environ Contam Toxicol.* 1997;152:57.

38. Gaudreau C, Gilbert H. Antimicrobial resistance of clinical strains of *Campylobacter jejuni* subsp.

jejuni isolated from 1985–1997 in Quebec, Canada. *Antimicrob Agents Chemother.* 1998;42:2106.

39. Weber JT, Mintz ED, Canizares R, et al. Epidemic cholera in Ecuador: multidrug-resistance and transmission by water and seafood. *Epidemiol Infect.* 1994;112(1):1.

40. Halling-Sorensen B, Nors Nielsen S, Lanzky PF, et al. Occurrence, fate and effects of pharmaceutical substances in the environment—a review. *Chemosphere.* 1998;36(2):357.

41. Levy RB. Multidrug resistance—a sign of the times. *N Engl J Med.* 1998;338(19):1376.

42. Doolittle MM, Cooney JJ, Caldwell DE. Tracing the interaction of bacteriophage with bacterial biofilms using fluorescent and chromogenic probes. *J Ind Microbiol Biotechnol.* 1996;16(6):331.

43. Physicians for Social Responsibility. *Drinking Water and Disease: What Health Care Providers Should Know.* Washington, DC: Physicians for Social Responsibility; 2000.

44. Koivusalo M, Pukkala E, Vartianinen T. Drinking water chlorination and cancer—a historical cohort study in Finland. *Cancer Causes Control.* 1997;8(2):192.

45. Morris RD, Audet AM, Angelillo IF, et al. Chlorination, chlorination by-products, and cancer: a meta-analysis. *Am J Public Health.* 1992;82(7):955.

46. Deane M, Swan SH, Harris JA, et al. Adverse pregnancy outcomes in relation to water consumption: a re-analysis of data from the original Santa Clara County Study, California, 1980–1981. *Epidemiology.* 1992;3(2):94.

47. Savitz DA, Andrews KW, Pastore LM. Drinking water and pregnancy outcome in central North Carolina: source, amount, and trihalomethane levels. *Environ Health Perspect.* 1995;103(6):592.

48. Waller K, Swan SH, DeLorenze G, et al. Trihalomethanes in drinking water and spontaneous abortion. *Epidemiology.* 1998;9(2):134.

49. Swan SH, Waller K, Hopkins B, et al. A prospective study of spontaneous abortion: relation to amount and source of drinking water consumed in early pregnancy. *Epidemiology.* 1998;9(2):126.

50. Klotz JB, Pyrch LA. Neural tube defects and drinking water disinfection by-products. *Epidemiology.* 1999;10(4):383.

51. Environmental Working Group. *Consider the Source: Farm Runoff, Chlorination Byproducts, and Human Health.* Washington, DC: Environmental Working Group; 2001.

52. Conacher D. *Troubled Waters on Tap: Organic Chemicals in Public Drinking Water Systems and the Failure of Regulation.* Washington, DC: Center for the Study of Responsive Law; 1988.

53. Daughton CG, Ternes TA. Pharmaceuticals and personal care products in the environment: agents of subtle change? *Environ Health Perspect.* 1999;107(suppl 6):907.

54. Paulu C, Aschengrau A, Ozonoff D. Tetrachloroethylene-contaminated drinking water in Massachusetts and the risk of colon-rectum, lung, and other cancers. *Environ Health Perspect.* 1999;107(4):265.

55. Williams P, Benton L, Warmerdam J, et al. Comparative risk analysis of six volatile organic compounds in California drinking water. *Environ Sci Technol.* 2002;36(22):4721.

56. Ahmed FE. Toxicology and human health effects following exposure to oxygenated or reformulated gasoline. *Toxicol Lett.* 2001;123(2–3):89.

57. Fayolle F, Vandecasteele JP, Monot F. Microbial degradation and fate in the environment of methyl tert-butyl ether and related fuel oxygenates. *Appl Microbiol Technol.* 2001;56(3–4):339.

58. Lince DP, Wilson LR, Carlson GA, et al. Effects of gasoline formulation on methyl-*tert*-butyl ether (MTBE) contamination in private wells near gasoline stations. *Environ Sci Technol.* 2001;35(6):1050.

59. Rier S, Foster WG. Environmental dioxins and endometriosis. *Toxicol Sci.* 2002;70(2):161.

60. Kolpin DW, Furlong ET, Meyer MT, et al. Pharmaceuticals, hormones, and other organic wastewater contaminants in US streams, 1999–2000: a national reconnaissance. *Environ Sci Technol.* 2002;36:1202.

61. Physicians for Social Responsibility. *Drinking Water and Disease: What HealthCare Providers Should Know.* Washington, DC: Physicians for Social Responsibility; 2000.

62. EPA. *National Public Water System Annual Compliance Report and Update on Implementation of the 1996 Safe Water Drinking Act Amendments.* Washington, DC: Environmental Protection Agency; 2000.

63. Whitford GM. The metabolism and toxicity of fluoride. In: *Monographs in Oral Science.* Vol. 16. New York: Karger Press; 1996.

64. Hoxie NJ, Davis JP, Vergeront JM, et al. Cryptosporidiosis-associated mortality following a massive waterborne outbreak in Milwaukee, Wisconsin. *Am J Public Health.* 1997;87(12):2032.

65. Goldstein ST, Juranek DD, Ravenholt O, et al. Cryptosporidiosis: an outbreak associated with drinking water despite state-of-the-art water treatment. *Ann Intern Med*. 1996;125(2):158.

66. Dillingham RA, Lima AA, Guerrant RL. Cryptosporidiosis: epidemiology and impact. *Microbes Infect*. 2002;4(10):1059.

67. Physicians for Social Responsibility. *Drinking Water and Disease: What Health Care Providers Should Know*. Washington, DC: Physicians for Social Responsibility; 2000.

68. Bannister P, Mountford RA. Cryptosporidium in the elderly: a cause of life-threatening diarrhea. *Am J Med*. 1989;86(4):507.

69. Greater Boston Physicians for Social Responsibility. *In Harm's Way: Toxic Threats to Child Development. A Report by Greater Boston Physicians for Social Responsibility Prepared for a Joint Project with Clean Water Fund*. Cambridge, MA; 2000.

70. Greater Boston Physicians for Social Responsibility. *In Harm's Way: Toxic Threats to Child Development. A Report by Greater Boston Physicians for Social Responsibility Prepared for a Joint Project with Clean Water Fund*. Cambridge, MA; 2000.

71. Environmental Working Group. *MOM's . . . and POPS: Persistent Organic Pollutants in the Diets of Pregnant and Nursing Women*. Washington, DC: Environmental Working Group; 2000.

72. Brotons JA, Olea-Serrano MF, Villalobos M, et al. Xenoestrogens released from lacquer coatings in food cans. *Environ Health Perspect*. 608;103(6, 1995.

73. Brechner RJ, Parkhurst GD, Humble WO, et al. Ammonium perchlorate contamination of Colorado River drinking water is associated with abnormal thyroid function in newborns in Arizona. *J Occup Environ Med*. 2000;42(8):777.

74. Richter-Reihhelm HB, Althoff J, Schulte A, et al. Workshop report. Children as a special subpopulation: focus on immunotoxicity. Federal Institute for Health Protection of Consumers and Veterinary Medicine (BgVV), 15–16 November 2001, Berlin Germany. *Arch Toxicol*. 2002;76(7):377.

75. Keswick BH, Gerba CP, Goyal SM. Occurrence of enteroviruses in community swimming pools. *Am J Public Health*. 1981;71(9):1026.

76. The Hall Water Report. Lead Found in Tap Water in 20% of NYC Elementary Schools. *Hall Water Rep*. 2002;16(21):7.

77. Massey-Stokes M, Lanning B. Childhood cancer and environmental toxins: the debate continues. *Family Community Health*. 2002 ;24(4):27.

78. Davies SM, Ross JA. Childhood cancer etiology: recent reports. *Med Pediatr Oncol*. 2003;40(1):35.

79. The Hall Water Report. *Cancer kids vs polluted drinking water: is it a matter of society's priorities? Hall Water Rep*. October 1999.

80. Dabeka RW, Conacher HB, Lawrence JF, et al. Survey of bottled drinking waters sold in Canada for chlorate, bromide, bromate, lead, cadmium and other trace elements. *Food Addit Contam*. 2002;19(8):721.

81. Ikem A, Odueyungbo S, Egiebor NO, et al. Chemical quality of bottled waters from three cities in eastern Alabama. *Sci Total Environ*. 2002; 285(1–3):165.

82. Azoulay A, Garzon P, Eisenberg MJ. Comparison of mineral content of tap water and bottled waters. *J Gen Intern Med*. 2001;16(3):168.

83. The National Resources Defense Council. *Bottled Water: Pure Drink or Pure Hype?* New York: The National Resources Defense Council; 1999.

84. Barret S, Hwang C, Guo Y. Occurrence of NDMA in drinking water: a North American survey 2001–2002 [abstract]. American Water Works Annual Conference; June 15–18, 2003; Anaheim, CA.

85. Kohut KD, Andrews SA. N-nitrosodimethylamine formation in drinking water due to amine-based polyelectrolytes. Proceedings from the Water Quality Technology Conference and Exhibition; November 10–14, 2002; Seattle, WA.

86. Shang NC, Yu YH, Ma HW. Variation of toxicity during the ozonation of monochlorophenolic solutions. *J Environ Sci Health Part A Tox Hazard Subst Environ Eng*. 2002;37(2):261.

87. Paraskeva P, Graham NJ. Ozonation of municipal wastewater effluents. *Water Environ Res*. 2002;74(6):569.

88. Hoek G, Brunekreef B, Fischer P, van Wijnen J. The association between air pollution and heart failure, arrhythmia, embolism, thrombosis, and other cardiovascular causes of death in a time series study. *Epidemiology*. 2001;12(3):355–357.

89. Pope CA III, Burnett RT, et al. Lung cancer, cardiopulmonary mortality, and long-term exposure to fine particulate air pollution. *JAMA*. 2002;287(9): 1132–1141.

90. Hong YC, Lee JT, Kim H, Kwan HJ. Air pollution: a new risk factor in ischemic stroke mortality. *Stroke* 2002;33(9):2165–2169.

91. Jacob B, Ritz B, Gehring U, et al. Indoor exposure to molds and allergic sensitization. *Environ Health Perspect.* 2002;110(7):647–653.

92. Ponsonby AL, Dwyer T, Kemp A, Couper D, Cochrane J, Carmichael A. A prospective study of the association between home gas appliance use during infancy and subsequent dust mite sensitization and lung function in childhood. *Clin Exp Allergy.* 2001;31(10):1544–1552.

93. Stevenson LA, Gergen PJ, Hoover DR, Rosenstreich D, Mannino DM, Matte TD. Sociodemographic correlates of indoor allergen sensitivity among United States children. *J Allergy Clin Immunol.* 2001;108(5):747–752.

94. Hoek G, Brunekreef B, Fischer P, van Wijnen J. The association between air pollution and heart failure, arrhythmia, embolism, thrombosis, and other cardiovascular causes of death in a time series study. *Epidemiology.* 2001;12(3): 355–357.

95. Just J, Segala C, Sahraoui F, Priol G, Grimfeld A, Neukirch F. Short-term health effects of particulate and photochemical air pollution in asthmatic children. *Eur Respir J.* 2002;20(4):899–906.

96. Klot S, Wolke G, Tuch T, Heinrich J, et al. Increased asthma medication use in association with ambient fine and ultrafine particles. *Eur Respir J.* 2002;20(3):691–702.

97. Sunyer J, Basagana X, Belmonte J, Anto JM. Effect of nitrogen dioxide and ozone on the risk of dying in patients with severe asthma. *Thorax.* 2002;57(8):687–693.

98. Zhou BS, Wang TJ, Guan P, Wu JM. Indoor air pollution and pulmonary adenocarcinoma among females: a case-control study in Shenyang, China. *Oncol Rep.* 2002;7(6):1253–1259.

99. Beeson WL, Abbey DE, Knutsen SF. Long-term concentrations of ambient air pollutants and incident lung cancer in California adults: results from the AHSMOG study. *Environ Health Perspect.* 1998;106(12):813–823.

100. Bowler RP, Crapo JD. Oxidative stress in allergic respiratory diseases. *J Allergy Clin Immunol.* 2002;110(3):349–356.

101. Grievink L, van der Zee SC, Hoek G, Boezen HM, van't Veer P, Brunekreef B. Modulation of the acute respiratory effects of winter air pollution by serum and dietary antioxidants: a panel study. *Eur Respir J.* 1999;13(6):1439–1446.

102. Grievink L, Zijlstra AG, Ke X, Brunekreef B. Double-blind intervention trial on modulation of ozone effects on pulmonary function by antioxidant supplements. *Am J Epidemiol.* 149(4): 306–314, 1999.

103. Grievink L, Smit HA, Veer P, Brunekreef B, Kromhout D. Plasma concentrations of the antioxidants beta-carotene and alpha-tocopherol in relation to lung function. *Eur J Clin Nutr.* 1999;53(10):813–817.

104. Hodgson M. Field studies on the sick building syndrome. *Ann N Y Acad Sci.* 1992;641:21–36.

105. World Health Organization. *Indoor Air Quality Research. Euro Reports and Studies. Report No. 103.* Copenhagen: WHO; 1984.

106. Finnigan MS, Pickering CAC, Burge PS. The sick building syndrome: prevalence studies. *Br Med J.* 1984;289:1573–1575.

107. Indoor air facts no. 4 (revised): Sick Building Syndrome (SBS). Available at: http://www.epa.gov/iag/pubs/sbs.html. Accessed October 8, 2002.

108. Indoor air facts no. 4 (revised): Sick Building Syndrome (SBS). Available at: http://www.epa.gov/iag/pubs/sbs.html. Accessed October 8, 2002.

109. Appleby P. ABC of work-related disorders: building-related illnesses. *BMJ.* 1996;313(7058):674–677.

110. Marshall L, Weir E, Abelsohn A, et al. Identifying and managing adverse environmental health effects: 1. Taking an exposure history. *CAMJ.* 2002; 166(8)1049–1055.

111. Kreiss K. The sick building syndrome: where is the epidemiological basis? *Am J Public Health.* 1990;80:1172–1173.

112. Kilburn K. Indoor effects after building renovation and in manufactured homes. *Am J Med Sci.* 2000;320(4):249–254.

113. Niven RM, Fletcher AM, Pickering CA, et al. *Occup Environ Med.* 2000;57(9):627–634.

114. Harrison J, Pickering CAC, Fargher EB, et al. An investigation of the relationship between microbial and particulate indoor air pollution and the sick building syndrome. *Respir Med.* 1992;86: 225–235.

115. Dietert RR, Hedge A. Toxicological considerations in evaluating indoor air quality and human health impact of new carpet emissions. *Crit Rev Toxicol.* 1996;26:633–707.

116. Teeuw KB, Vandenbroucke-Grauls CM, Verhoef J. Airborne gram-negative bacteria and endotoxin in sick building syndrome. A study of Dutch governmental office buildings. *Arch Intern Med.* 1994;154:2339–2345.

117. Persson Waye K, Rylander R, Benton S, et al. Ef-

fects on performance and work quality due to low-frequency ventilation noise. *J Sound Vibration.* 1997;205:467–474.

118. Mendell M, Fisk W, Petersen M, et al. Indoor particles and symptoms among office workers: results from a double-blind cross-over study. *Epidemiology.* 2002;13(3):296–304.

119. Institute of Medicine, Committee on the Assessment of Asthma and Indoor Air. Impact of ventilation and air cleaning on asthma. In: *Clearing the Air: Asthma and Indoor Air Exposure.* Washington, DC: National Academy Press; 2000:327–393.

120. Indoor air pollution: an introduction for health professionals. Available at: http://www.epa.gov/iaq/pubs/hpguide.html. Accessed September 26, 2002.

121. May J. *My House is Killing Me.* Baltimore, MD: John Hopkins University Press; 2001:247.

122. Indoor air pollution: an introduction for health professionals. Available at: http://www.epa.gov/iaq/pubs/hpguide.html. Accessed September 26, 2002.

123. May J. *My House is Killing Me.* Baltimore, MD: John Hopkins University Press; 2001:247.

124. Indoor air pollution: an introduction for health professionals. Available at: http://www.epa.gov/iaq/pubs/hpguide.html. Accessed September 26, 2002.

125. Kilburn K. Indoor air effects after building renovation and in manufactured homes. *Am J Med Sci.* 2000;320(4):249–254.

126. Marshall L, Weir E, Abelsohn A et al. Identifying and managing adverse environmental health effects: 1.Taking an exposure history. *CAMJ JAMC.* 2002;166(8)1049–1055.

127. Menzies D , Bourbeau J. Current concepts: Building related illnesses. *N Engl J Med.* 1997;337(21): 1524–1531.

128. Horvath SM, Dahms TE, O'Hanlon JF. Carbon monoxide and human vigilance: a deleterious effect of present urban concentration. *Arch Environ Health.* 1971;23:343–347.

129. Heckerling PS, Leikin JB, Maturen A, et al. Predictors of occult carbon monoxide poisoning in patients with headache and dizziness. *Ann Intern Med.* 1987;107:174–176.

130. Appleby P. ABC of work-related disorders: building-related illnesses. *BMJ.* 1996;313(7058): 674–677.

131. London Hazards Center, Interchange Studios, Hampstead Town Hall Center, London: Sick building syndrome: causes, effects and control. 1990. Available at: http://www.lhc.org.uk/members/pubs/books/sbs/sb-toc.htm. Accessed March 2, 2002.

132. Appleby P. ABC of work-related disorders: building-related illnesses. *BMJ.* 1996;313(7058): 674–677.

133. London Hazards Center, Interchange Studios, Hampstead Town Hall Center, London: Sick building syndrome: causes, effects and control. 1990. Available at: http://www.lhc.org.uk/members/ pubs/books/sbs/sb-toc.htm. Accessed March 2, 2002.

134. McCurdy SA, Morrin LA, Memmott MM. Occupational history collection by third-year medical students during internal medicine and surgery inpatient clerkships. *J Occup Environ Med.* 1998; 40(8):680–684.

135. Merret EF. Human health and the environment. Are physician educators lagging behind? *JAMA.* 1999;281:1661.

136. Marshall L, Weir E, Abelsohn A, et al. Identifying and managing adverse environmental health effects: 1.Taking an exposure history. *CAMJ JAMC.* 2002;166(8)1049–1055.

PART III

Integrative Approaches to Specific Conditions

CHAPTER 17

Integrative Approach to Allergy

RANDY J. HORWITZ AND ROBERT Y. LIN

We understand much of the pathophysiologic origin of many allergic diseases, including allergic rhinitis, allergic conjunctivitis, contact dermatitis, asthma, and venom allergy. The central role of inflammation in allergic respiratory disease and in eczema has also been elucidated and appreciated. Other forms of hypersensitivity, however, are still poorly understood. The traditional allopathic concept of allergy implies a known and reproducible mechanism of patient reactivity (such as allergen-specific immunoglobulin IgE). This is in contrast to the more widely used lay concept of allergy as a reactivity that recurs in any given patient, sometimes with different manifestations, regardless of mechanism. Broadening of the definition of allergy to include idiosyncratic reactions and/or a tendency to reactivities with different stimuli is probably useful when encountering patients and trying to evaluate their concerns as well as their actual current symptoms. This construct gives importance not only to whether the patient has an "allergic disease" but also to whether they are "atopic"; in other words, whether they have a tendency towards allergic or hypersensitivity phenomena. The allopathic physician tends to treat each disease state separately. An integra-

tive approach might additionally consider measures to diminish an "atopic" predisposition.

This chapter focuses on a limited number of allergic diseases, some of which typify the ambiguity of the term "allergic." For chronic urticaria, a known mechanism does not exist for most patients, whereas it is well-defined for allergic conjunctivitis. For food allergy, immediate reactions may or may not have an allergen-specific IgE mechanism, whereas delayed reactions never do. Environmental hypersensitivity is a controversial area, which has been the focus of an entire medical subspecialty (clinical ecology), albeit one not officially recognized by the American Medical Association.

▶ CHRONIC URTICARIA

Chronic urticaria is a common disorder for which an underlying cause often cannot be identified. However, it is usually a benign disorder that frequently resolves spontaneously. The typical urticarial lesion consists of a wheal, or plaque, whose borders expand and may include a central, undisturbed area. Urticarial lesions can vary in size from less than 1 cm (0.4 inches) to more than 30 cm (11.8 inches) in diameter (giant urticaria). There may be a region of erythema (flare) around each individual lesion, and lesions often coalesce to form irregular shapes. When treated with antihistamines, the urticarial lesions may be barely raised and only manifest with round or serpiginous macules, often with central clearing. Symptoms associated with chronic urticaria include pruritus or burning, but may include angioedema, a diffuse swelling that may involve the eyes, lips, hands, or feet. In some patients, angioedema may predominate and typical urticarial lesions are absent.

Pathophysiology

The pathophysiology of chronic urticaria is not well understood, although mast cell-derived histamine plays a major role. In some cases, physical stimuli, such as cold temperature or pressure (dermographism) initiates the urticaria.[1] While such triggers are readily identifiable, they often begin suddenly and with no prior history of intolerance to the stimuli.

The urticarias are conventionally classified by their frequency, duration, and associated symptoms. Chronic idiopathic urticaria (CIU) is defined as daily (or near daily) urticaria, persisting for at least 6 weeks, for which no cause is identified.[2] It is characterized by spontaneously occurring pruritic wheals that individually last less than 24–36 hours. Accompanying angioedema, which tends to be more long-lived and nonpruritic, is frequently observed in CIU patients. A similar disorder, chronic recurrent urticaria has an intermittent course. Acute urticaria may persist for several weeks after an infection or drug hypersensitivity reaction, but usually lasts less than 6 weeks. In patients who present only with angioedema, without associated urticaria, one must consider the possibility of C1-esterase inhibitor deficiency. Such a reaction can also manifest after exposure to an angiotensin-converting enzyme inhibitor.

Chronic idiopathic urticaria typically presents without constitutional symptoms (such as fever, arthralgia, or weight loss) or any laboratory markers of inflammation. The histopathology of a skin biopsy, usually unnecessary in CIU, shows only perivascular mononuclear cells. It is important to differentiate the urticarial diseases from urticarial vasculitis, which has a different course and treatment.[3] Vasculitic lesions tend to be more persistent, without a waxing and waning course. In addition, the patient will frequently present with systemic symptoms, an increased erythrocyte sedimentation rate, and, occasionally, a decrease in serum C4 levels (hypocomplementemic urticarial vasculitis).

Chronic idiopathic urticaria is associated with thyroid autoantibodies in as many as 30–40% of patients.[1] The presence of these autoantibodies may have some therapeutic implications. In some CIU patients who fail to respond to conventional therapy (including corticosteroids), the addition of thyroxine has improved symptoms, even in the presence of normal thyroid function tests.[1]

Although chronic urticaria seems to be an atopic disorder, most studies fail to show an association of CIU with other more "classical" atopic diseases, such as asthma, allergic rhinitis, and eczema. Furthermore, although allergy tests are commonly employed in the evaluation of patients with chronic urticaria, few studies show an association between CIU and the presence of IgE to either aeroallergens or ingestants. One possible exception to this rule is in the case of mite hypersensitivity, which some studies implicate as a cause of chronic urticaria in certain patients.[5,6] Non-IgE exacerbations of chronic urticaria have been demonstrated for aspirin, other nonsteroidal antiinflammatory drugs, and for certain pseudoallergens. The pseudoallergen category, which includes food preservatives and food additives, is favored by certain European investigators as a causative factor in urticaria,[7] but is generally regarded as a minor contributor to the disease.[1,2] Of note is that these compounds cannot be detected through any form of allergy testing. Chronic idiopathic urticaria is usually not associated with high-grade eosinophilia, which, if observed, mandates a search for parasites as an etiologic agent.[8] Low-grade eosinophilia is sometimes observed in chronic urticaria patients who have coexisting atopic disease.

There are many forms of physical urticaria. These include solar, aquagenic, vibratory, pressure, cholinergic, and cold urticarias. The cholinergic and cold forms are the most common of these. Cholinergic urticaria occurs frequently in younger patients, and may be associated with atopic diseases such as allergic rhinitis and asthma. Typically, eruptions of small pruritic papules occur after exposure to heat or exercise or even stress. This is in contrast to the typical large wheals seen in CIU. Occasionally, the patient with cholinergic urticaria will have bronchospasm and other signs of systemic histamine release following exer-

cise or rises in body temperature. This scenario is similar to that observed with exercise-induced anaphylaxis, which may be difficult to distinguish from cholinergic urticaria with extracutaneous manifestations.[9] Cold urticaria consists of wheals that develop after cold exposure. An ice cube application for 5 minutes may induce a wheal in the shape of the applied cube after 5–10 minutes (Figure 17–1). Some patients only develop hives with total-body exposure to cold. Cold urticaria is sometimes associated with a cryoprotein, so a complete work-up should include cold agglutinins, cryoglobulins, and syphilis tests to exclude these secondary causes. Another physical urticaria is dermographia, also called dermatographia. Some authors also refer to it as factitious urticaria.[1] Dermographia consists of

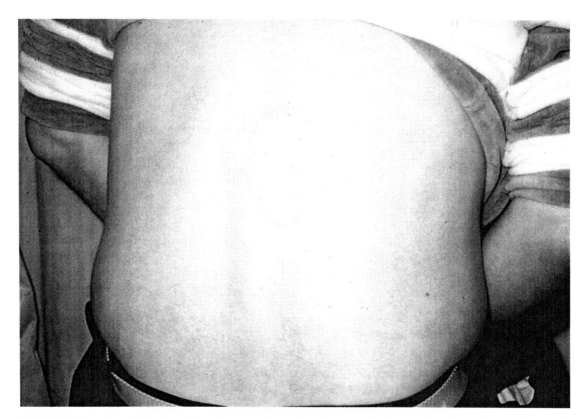

Figure 17–1.   Example of cold urticaria induced by the application of an ice cube to the back for 5 minutes.

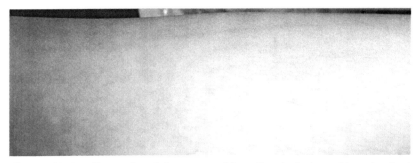

Figure 17–2. Example of dermographic urticaria induced by physical stroking.

urticaria induced by physical stroking (Figure 17–2). Patients often complain of itching and hives that occur at bra strap or belt contact areas. These pruritic lesions tend to be brief in duration but are recurrent. Delayed pressure urticaria, unlike dermographism, occurs several hours after direct pressure to the skin, and may be associated with arthralgias.[10] Lesions tend to be long-lived, with many persisting for longer than 24 hours.[10]

▶ Case Example 1: Urticaria

A 56-year-old retired man presented to the clinic with pruritus and hives for 3 years. He initially had hives only during the summer months, but recently they continued into the fall. He believed that there was an association of the hives with swimming and cold exposure. He was treated successfully with cetirizine, but still developed recurrences whenever a dose was missed. The physical examination revealed vitiligo over much of the skin, but no active lesions. Laboratory testing revealed a normal erythrocyte sedimentation rate of 4 mm/h, and normal thyroid function. No eosinophilia was observed on the complete blood cell count, and the office spirometry was normal. The patient was continued on cetirizine but began to have hives despite regular administration, and montelukast was added to his regimen. On a subsequent visit, hives were noted on the patient's wrist and leg. The patient continued to have breakthrough hives despite taking the medications regularly. A burst of prednisone was prescribed, which provided temporary relief. Despite the addition of famotidine to his regimen, the patient required another prednisone burst 6 months later. The patient then decided to consult an integrative medicine specialist.

Conventional Approach

Because of the presumptive association of mast cells with histamine release, it is not surprising that H_1-receptor blockade is a cornerstone of conventional therapy for urticaria. Nonsedating antihistamines, such as cetirizine, fexofenadine, and loratadine, are efficacious in CIU. As the chronic urticarias may persist for years, it is desirable to use the safest medication possible, especially in children and women of childbearing age. Although the older, first-generation antihistamines (such as chlorpheniramine and diphenhydramine) have a longer track record for safety in pregnancy, the sedating qualities of these medications, along with their short serum half-lives, make them undesirable for long-term treatment. Still, in pregnancy, the first-generation antihistamines are preferred, especially if required in the first or second trimester. Some patients with CIU have remission of their disease during pregnancy, in a manner similar to rheumatoid arthritis, where endogenous steroid production has been postulated to play a role.

In studies of chronic urticaria, the conventional treatments decrease hive numbers and associated symptoms, but complete resolution often does not occur. It is useful to quantify the frequency of hive occurrence, the associated symptoms and the overall impact on the patient's daily life. Several scoring systems exist for such purposes, and are based upon the number of wheals on the body, the relative pruritic intensity, and the patient-determined quality-of-life index.[1] The location of the lesions and the presence of angioedema may be more troublesome to some patients than simply the number of hives or itching severity. This should be taken into account when planning a treatment regimen. Patients may prefer to have a few hives and take little or no medication.

Physical urticarias are treated with medication and avoidance of the stimulus if possible. Cold urticaria is problematic and potentially lethal with swimming.[11] Anxiolytic medication may be considered for cholinergic urticaria in addition to H_1-receptor antagonists.[1]

If H_1-receptor blockade with newer, nonsedating antihistamines is ineffective in treating chronic urticaria, other medications should be considered. The older, first-generation antihistamines may have additional, nonhistamine-mediated, effects on the allergic response,[2] and thus may be added to a nonsedating antihistamine regimen. For example, hydroxyzine or diphenhydramine may be used in a patient already taking a daily nonsedating H_1 blocker. In addition, concomitant administration of H_2 receptor antagonists with H_1-receptor antagonists

has been useful in some patients with chronic urticaria or dermographism.[12–14]

There are other, less-studied agents used for the control of chronic urticaria. Leu-kotriene antagonists also show efficacy in patients with acetylsalicylic acid or food additive-associated chronic urticaria.[15] It is unclear whether leukotriene antagonists have a significant effect in those patients for whom histamine receptor blockade has failed.[16] Some authors believe that doxepin, a sedating tricyclic antidepressant with both H_1-and H_2-blocking effects, is helpful in patients who do not respond to H_1-receptor blockade. Caution must be exercised when using tricyclic medications, because these drugs can cause cardiovascular abnormalities. Ketotifen, a prescription mast cell-stabilizing drug not yet available in the United States shows efficacy in chronic urticaria, and is used frequently by Canadian specialists treating chronic urticaria.[17]

Oral corticosteroids have been used for the treatment of chronic urticaria, with mixed results. Although long-term corticosteroid use may be effective, the risk-to-benefit ratio is less than desirable, even with alternate-day dosing regimens.[2] Topical cortico-steroids are often prescribed for chronic urticaria, but the variable location and evanescent nature of the lesions make this approach "hit or miss." Other, less common, treatments that are effective in small studies of "refractory patients" include nifedipine,[18] cyclosporine,[19] plasmapheresis,[20] intravenous immunoglobulin,[21] and stanozolol.[22]

Avoidance of aspirin and related nonsteroidal antiinflammatory drugs (NSAIDs) is often recommended. An alternative to traditional NSAIDs is the cyclooxygenase (COX)-2 antagonists, which are effective and well-tolerated, even among aspirin-sensitive patients.[23] Botanical antiinflammatories, containing extracts of ginger *(Zingiber officinale)*, turmeric *(Curcuma longa)*, or boswellia, are an integrative option to the traditional NSAIDs.

Patients with urticarial vasculitis should be examined for underlying infections, such as hepatitis B or C, and autoimmune diseases, such as systemic lupus erythematosus. Clinical responses to rheumatologic medications have been observed for some patients with urticarial vasculitis.[3,24,25] These medications include dapsone, hydroxychloroquine, sulfasalazine, colchicine, and corticosteroids.

Integrative Medicine Approach

For many patients, identifying the cause of their chronic urticaria takes precedence over symptom control. The search for exogenous agents that cause CIU exacerbations typically centers around foods, food additives, or microbial products. Limited, anecdotal reports show an association between dust mite and candidal hypersensitivity and chronic urticaria. This has led some clinicians to prescribe antifungals, yeast-free diets, and mite avoidance measures in selected patients. However, the evidence of efficacy for these approaches is weak.

Nutritional Approaches

Dietary causes of chronic urticaria are supported by a number of controlled challenge studies showing that both food and food additives can induce hives. Volatile aromatic compounds in certain vegetables and spices (such as tomatoes and parsley) have been demonstrated as causing exacerbations of CIU. Food dyes and preservatives (Table 17–1) and natural salicylates (such as dried fruits, plums, and licorice) have also been implicated. To explore food-related chronic urticaria, an elimination diet is a reasonable first step. Specific diet therapy proposed by Zuberbier and colleagues[7,26] is based not only on avoidance of food additives, fruits, seafood, and packaged food, but also involves avoidance of certain vegetables, which presumably contain "volatile" aromatic compounds. The elimination diet is prescribed for 2–3 weeks, and patients who respond are then "challenged" with various categories of "pseudoallergens" in order to further ascertain the offending agent(s). Other elimination and rotational diets have been proposed,[27] including a rice and lamb hypoallergenic food-elimination diet. These diets have not been studied in depth, but have proven useful for many patients.

There are many anecdotal reports of successful vitamin remedies for chronic hives. These include vitamin B_{12} injections, quercetin (citrus bioflavonoid), and vitamin C. None of these compounds has been studied in placebo-controlled trials. Quercetin, a plant flavonoid that stabilizes mast cells,[28] is often used in the treatment of chronic urticaria. Quercetin treatment has reportedly had better results treating allergic rhinitis than treating chronic urticaria,[29] but its safety profile and efficacy in some individuals make it an attractive option.

Botanical Approaches

Bromelain, a proteolytic enzyme from pineapples, has also been suggested for use in patients with urticaria. The known actions of bromelain include interference with malignant cell growth, inhibition of platelet aggregation, fibrinolytic activity, and antiinflammatory action.[30] Bromelain also lowers kininogen and bradykinin serum and tissue levels, and has an influence on prostaglandin synthesis. These effects have direct relevance to allergic disease. The usual dose of bromelain is variable and sometimes based on enzymatic activity, but doses between 300 and 1500 mg daily have been used. Some precaution is warranted with the use of bromelain, because it can be allergenic and can cause clinical hypersensitivity reactions by itself. In fact, bromelain-reactive individuals often have false-positive pollen ra-

▶ **TABLE 17–1** COMMON ALLERGENIC FOOD ADDITIVES

Chemical Compound	Type
Azorubine	Food dye
Benzoic acid	Food preservative
Sodium bisulphite	Food preservative
Sulphur dioxide	Food preservative
Sunset yellow	Food dye
Tartrazine	Food dye

dioallergosorbent tests (RASTs), because of cross-reacting carbohydrate determinants.[31] Bromelain is commonly combined with quercetin in the treatment of urticaria.

Stinging nettle is another herbal that is commonly prescribed for urticaria, although it has not been as well studied for this as it has been for other allergic conditions.

Mind–Body Approaches

Stress is often purported to be a factor in chronic urticaria, but whether it precedes the diagnosis or manifests as a result of the rash is unclear. This is particularly true for cholinergic urticaria, where cholinergic blockade abolishes the lesions.[1] Stress reduction would thus appear to be a logical adjunct in treating certain chronic urticaria patients. Guided imagery and visualization techniques are very helpful in such cases. While well-controlled studies involving stress-

reduction therapy are difficult to design, there is no risk with these modalities, and the potential benefits to the patient warrant the liberal and enthusiastic recommendation of such techniques.

Other Therapies

The discovery that ultraviolet therapy can be beneficial in many cases of chronic urticaria[32] has led some naturopathic specialists to recommend sun or tanning salon exposure. This is logical, but not well-studied. Inherent risks of solar radiation may also limit such global recommendations.

Acupuncture[33] has also been reported to be useful in the treatment of chronic urticaria, but controlled studies are lacking. Additionally, no one has examined the ability of the complete traditional Chinese medicine approach to urticaria, as opposed to simply the acupuncture component.

▶ Case Example 1: Urticaria Conclusion

The man with the 3-year history of chronic idiopathic urticaria seen in our clinic was treated first with nutritional counseling. We recommended a modified elimination diet. He avoided dairy products (including eggs, milk, and any products containing casein hydrolysates), chicken, fruits, nuts, and food additives. In addition, we recommended that he restrict his protein ingestion to 10–15% of his total caloric intake, because most allergic reactions are the result of protein allergens. He started taking quercetin, as well as vitamins B_{12} and C. In addition, he began a program of daily journaling to report symptoms, as well as

to explore sources of inner stress in his life. He underwent two sessions of guided imagery, which focused on symptomatic control of the pruritus associated with his hives. Within a period of 5 weeks, he noted a modest decrease in the frequency of his eruptions. More importantly, when he did have an exacerbation, his symptoms were quite mild, and the duration of his hives was markedly reduced. As a result of the dietary modifications, the patient lost 25 pounds. Encouraged by the weight loss, he began an exercise program that still continues. Eighteen months after his initial visit, his urticaria went into remission.

▶ ALLERGIC CONJUNCTIVITIS

Allergic conjunctivitis is a fairly common disorder, frequently accompanied by allergic rhinitis, thus giving rise to its usual designation, allergic

rhinoconjunctivitis. Allergic conjunctivitis manifests with symptoms of ocular pruritus, although other symptoms such as tearing, irritation, stinging, and burning may also be present. Corneal symptoms, such as photophobia and blurred vision, may occur with more severe cases. Ocular secretions may be somewhat thickened, and both palpebral and bulbar conjunctival injection is often observed. Chemosis, or swelling of the conjunctiva, can also be seen.

Pathophysiology

Allergic conjunctivitis is more often seasonal than perennial, with spring symptoms predominating largely as a result of grass and tree pollenosis. The indoor allergens, such as cat dander and dust mites, are usually associated with perennial symptoms. Specific IgE to suspected aeroallergens are not always identified, but conjunctival IgE levels are usually elevated in allergic conjunctivitis. The author (RYL) has observed several Chinese immigrant patients who have spring allergic conjunctivitis symptoms but manifest with delayed type hypersensitivity skin reactions to tree and grass pollens.[34] No pollen-specific IgE was noted in these patients when they presented.

There are two other forms of allergic conjunctivitis that have distinct clinical features: vernal conjunctivitis and giant papillary conjunctivitis. Vernal conjunctivitis is a chronic, bilateral disease that often occurs in atopic individuals beginning in childhood or in young adulthood. It often begins in the spring, thus giving rise to the term vernal. Along with pruritus, there is often a foreign-body sensation in the eye, and the upper tarsal conjunctiva shows cobblestoning from papillary hypertrophy. Vernal conjunctivitis may be difficult to manage, but usually remits by the third decade of life. Giant papillary conjunctivitis is linked to the use of contact lenses and manifests with ocular burning, itching, and tearing. Like vernal conjunctivitis, upper tarsal cobblestoning is observed. Both giant papillary conjunctivitis and vernal conjunctivitis are characterized by increased eosinophils in the involved tissues.

▶ Case Example 2: Conjunctivitis

A 32-year-old man from North Dakota was referred to an allergist for seasonal allergies since the age of 25. His allergic symptoms are seasonal—March through June—and began as nasal congestion with rhinorrhea, but recently evolved into predominantly ocular complaints. His symptoms consist of ocular itching and a "grainy" feeling in the eyes, often associated with mucoid secretions. He had been treated with oral antihistamines and nasal corticosteroids in the past, without relief. At the time of our evaluation, he was using olopatadine, cetirizine, and fluti-casone nasal spray. He denies any other atopic diseases except skin sensitivity to PABA (para-aminobenzoic acid). Physical examination revealed bulbar conjunctival injection and mild edema of the inferior turbinates.

Fluorometholone and nedocromil ophthalmic drops were added to his regimen. RASTs were strongly reactive to several tree pollens. The patient returned in 2 weeks and reported little relief. He did not want to use "steroids" and thus did not use the fluorometholone prescription.

Conventional Medicine Approach

Drug therapy is the cornerstone of conventional therapy of perennial allergic conjunctivitis, unless there is a clearly defined allergen for which avoidance is an alternative. Because allergic conjunctivitis is often accompanied by allergic rhinitis, initial therapies typically employ systemic antihistamines. Nonspecific vasoconstrictors, such as naphazoline, methylcellulose tears, and saline drops, are also helpful in mild cases. For patients not responding to these initial measures, a broad range of prescription ocular medications are available. The mechanism of action of such medications include antiinflammatory, mast cell-stabilizing, H_1-receptor blocking, or a combination of these. Mast cell-stabilizing ophthalmics include pemirolast, nedocromil, lodoxamide, ketotifen, and cromolyn. Ocular antihistamines include emedastine, levocabastine, and azelastine. Olopatadine is an antiallergic ophthalmic preparation that has both histamine-receptor blocking and mast cell-stabilizing effects. Nedocromil and lodoxamide have both H_1-receptor blocking and mast cell-stabilizing effects. Several nonsteroidal antiinflammatory medications are also available in ophthalmic preparations, including diclofenac and ketorolac.

Ketorolac is FDA approved for treatment of allergic conjunctivitis. However, it is associated with ocular stinging and, in practice, have been replaced by the histamine receptor/mast cell stabilizing ophthalmics in the treatment of allergic ocular disease. The addition of systemic antihistamines is not usually effective in those patients who do not respond to nonsteroid antiallergic ophthalmics.

Corticosteroid ophthalmics are essential for patients with allergic conjunctivitis who do not respond to other medications. Prior to initiating treatment with an ocular steroid preparation, care must be exercised to be sure of the correct diagnosis, because many conditions may be worsened by the drug. All corticosteroid preparations can potentially raise intraocular pressure in susceptible individuals, but this rise is usually transient. Fluorometholone 0.1% eye drops is a useful treatment for ocular allergies. This steroid penetrates the cornea well, but is inactivated in the anterior chamber, which may theoretically result in a lower incidence of glaucoma and cataract formation than with prednisolone or dexamethasone. Loteprednol is a steroidal ophthalmic preparation that is approved for treating iritis, postsurgical ocular inflammation, and

allergic conjunctivitis; it has also been used to treat giant papillary conjunctivitis.[35,36] The dangers associated with use of ocular corticosteroids for extended periods include the long-term risk of cataract formation and the potential for elevated intraocular pressure. Thus, most physicians limit the use of such medications to 10 days or less, a difficult proposition when treating perennial symptoms.

Immunotherapy with pollen extracts is commonly used to treat allergic rhinoconjunctivitis, particularly when the disease has not responded to conventional pharmacologic modalities. Immunotherapy using pollen extracts is generally more effective than immunotherapy with non-pollen extracts, and because allergic conjunctivitis is most frequently seasonal (and pollen related), immunotherapy has particular potential for successful treatment in this disorder. Unfortunately, most studies do not differentiate between rhinitis and conjunctivitis symptom scores when evaluating the efficacy of immunotherapy. The main disadvantages of immunotherapy are the potential for serious systemic reactions and the long time required to build up and maintain an efficacious dosing regimen. There is considerable interest in the prospect of monoclonal anti-IgE treatment in the near future. One product, olizumab (a humanized, monoclonal anti-IgE antibody preparation), has recently received FDA approval for the treatment of allergic asthma. It has demonstrated efficacy in allergic rhinitis and asthma, and is expected to be given as a regular subcutaneous injection, possibly through self-injection.

Systemic reactions are not a problem with this medication. It is likely that patients with allergic conjunctivitis will also benefit from this medication.[37]

Integrative Medicine Approach

BOTANICAL MEDICINES

Although there is little evidence-based literature regarding the treatment of allergic conjunctivitis using complementary therapies, several approaches may be useful. Herbal and vitamin therapies, as outlined for the treatment of chronic urticaria, are also recommended for allergic rhinoconjunctivitis. External ocular compresses and eye washes made from natural substances are quite popular. Typically, gauze pads or cotton balls are soaked in the specified solution and then applied over the eyes. Eyebright *(Euphrasia officinalis)*, chamomile *(Matricaria recutita)*, fennel seed *(Foeniculum vulgare)*, marigold *(Calendula officinalis)*, plantain *(Plantago lanceolata)*, and flax *(Linum usitatissimum)* are recommended as compresses for ocular infection, irritation, and inflammation. The first five herbs are made into a tea (1 teaspoon herb in 1 cup hot water), which is cooled and used with compresses three to four times daily. Flax is usually used as a poultice (1 oz bruised flax seed steeped in 4 oz water for 15 minutes, with subsequent wrapping in cheesecloth for each application). Eye washes with goldenseal *(Hydrastis canadensis)* and boric acid are also recommended. These preparations are available commercially, or can be prepared by adding 10 drops of a goldenseal tincture and 1 teaspoon of boric acid to 1 cup of distilled water. Eye washes may be administered with an eye cup or a sterile dropper. Combination Ayurvedic and Chinese herbal ophthalmics are also commercially available, such as Opthacare.[38]

HOMEOPATHY

Homeopathic ophthalmics may be purchased as prepared solutions. One popular brand is the Similasin line (#1, #2, and #3). Combination and individual remedies containing Apis, Euphrasia, and/or Sabadilla are also purported to be effective for allergic conjunctivitis. Various dilutions are used, 12x to 30c every 1–4 hours. One uncontrolled study of a homeopathic preparation of Euphrasia found it to be both safe and effective, but the dilution was not fixed.[39]

Finally, acupuncture is occasionally used to treat allergic conjunctivitis. While no controlled studies have been published describing clinical efficacy for this condition, many of our patients have found relief from ocular pain and congestion from this treatment modality.

▶ Case Example 2: Conjunctivitis Conclusion

The patient with allergic conjunctivitis and the desire to avoid ocular steroid medications was seen in clinic and desired a botanical treatment. We recommended topical eye drops made from eyebright *(Euphrasia officinalis)*, a plant long used to treat mucous membrane inflammation and ocular conjunctivitis. He used it seasonally, and titrated the dose to achieve symptom control. No side effects were experienced. In addition, we recommended that he experiment with stinging nettle and quercetin for his nasal symptoms. He began using stinging nettle *(Urtica dioica)*, but at last follow-up he revealed that he restarted oral loratadine, which he said provided adequate symptom control.

▶ FOOD ALLERGIES

Food allergies are an increasingly common problem in the primary care setting. There is little difficulty in recognizing an acute, anaphylactic hypersensitivity reaction, and the allergist typically has little trouble in identifying the causative agent, using a complete dietary history along with skin tests and in vitro blood tests. The recognition and identification of a putative food allergen in a patient with vague gastrointestinal complaints, however, presents a more difficult clinical challenge. At least part of the difficulty arises from the lack of clarity in conventional terminology used by both the public and the medical community.

Although the general public uses the term allergy loosely when describing untoward physiological reactions, the allergist employs a more precise and distinct terminology. An adverse food reaction is one in which any abnormal reaction occurs following the ingestion of a specific food or food additive. This broad category is often subdivided for clarity into toxic and nontoxic reactions. Toxic reactions, such as bacterial food poisoning, are generalized to the population, and affect most individuals in a similar fashion, provided an equivalent dose is ingested. These are not discussed here. There are two types of nontoxic food reactions that are described: true food allergies and food intolerance. True food allergies are those reactions caused by a distinct immunological reaction, such as an IgE-mediated anaphylactic reaction to peanuts in sensitive individuals. The other category of nontoxic food reaction is food intolerance, and is far more common in general practice. An intolerance is a reproducible adverse reaction to a specific food or group of foods without a clearly identifiable immune mechanism. It is a broad category, and may be as clear as abdominal discomfort related to a lactose intolerance to dairy products, or as vague as a worsening of arthritic symptoms in response to wheat-containing foods. Often, only a heightened awareness and a clinical suspicion will guide the practitioner to consider the possibility of a food intolerance mitigating a patient's symptoms. The precise classification of adverse food reactions can be useful in predicting the risk of a dangerous anaphylactic reaction or determining appropriate adjunct therapy, but in and of itself, does little to ameliorate the symptoms of the patient.

Pathophysiology

The gastrointestinal tract has evolved to absorb, extract, and use energy from ingested food. The immune mechanisms of the gut are responsible for differentiating potential pathogens (such as bacteria, viruses, and parasites) from inert food proteins and glycoproteins. A series of sophisticated physical and immunological barriers has evolved to accomplish this, including a resilient mucosal layer, gastrointestinal enzymes, and antigen-specific IgA molecules in the lymphoid tissue of the gut.

In classical food allergy syndromes, intact foods are mechanically and enzymatically cleaved into small peptides, a small fraction of which is absorbed into the bloodstream. Some of these food antigens may be presented to T lymphocytes and may trigger gastrointestinal symptoms. Alternatively, the food antigen may encounter sensitized mast cells bearing specific IgE antibody. This interaction triggers the release of potent biochemical mediators of allergy, including histamine, prostaglandins, and leukotrienes. In addition to anaphylaxis, many severe, nongastrointestinal symptoms, such as urticaria (hives) or respiratory symptoms (wheezing), may occur. Oral allergy syndrome is a fairly common contact urticarial reaction occurring in the oropharynx that results in pruritus and angioedema of the lips, tongue, and throat following ingestion of certain fruits ands vegetables. Certain of these foods, such as apples, melons, or bananas, cross-react with tree pollens (ragweed, birch), and can be problematic in people with those plant allergies (Table 17–2). Cooking these foods greatly reduces their allergenicity.

The pathophysiology of the nonclassical adverse food reactions is more complex and ill-defined. This broad and heterogeneous group of symptoms constitutes the majority of dietary reactions seen in an integrative medicine practice. The difficulty in identifying such food reactions is largely a result of the diverse constellation of symptoms that are provoked by dietary causes.

Pathophysiological explanations are elusive, although an exaggerated reaction to a digestive product of a particular food, an impairment of the intestinal barrier function,[10] or a generalized inflammatory reaction[11] have all been proposed. Patients may present with diverse and seemingly unrelated symptoms, such as

▶ **TABLE 17-2** COMMON PATTERNS OF CROSS-REACTIVITY BETWEEN ALLERGENS

Allergenic Pollen	Cross-Reacting Foods
Alder	Carrots, celery, cherries, hazelnuts, peaches
Birch	Apples, raw potatoes, carrots, celery, hazelnuts
Grass	Melons, tomatoes, cereal grains
Latex	Avocados, bananas, papaya, kiwi
Mugwort	Celery, apples, kiwi, peanuts
Ragweed	Apples, bananas, cantaloupe, honeydew, watermelon

▶ **TABLE 17-3** FOOD ALLERGY SYMPTOMS

Abdominal pain (cramping, bloating)
Diarrhea
Gastroesophageal reflux
Oral allergy syndrome
Respiratory symptoms (cough, hoarseness)
Urticaria, angioedema
Vomiting

headaches, fatigue, irritable bowel symptoms (cramping, bloating, and diarrhea), or arthralgias[42,43] (Table 17-3). Among the other disease entities that must be excluded are celiac disease (wheat gluten enteropathy), lactose intolerance, and inflammatory bowel disease.

Prevalence

The prevalence of classical food allergy is highest during the first few years of life. Nearly one-third of newborns followed prospectively for 3 years demonstrated an adverse food reaction.[44] Fortunately, most children outgrow their sensitivity within 5 years, with the exception of the peanut and tree nut allergies. Food allergies that begin in late childhood or adulthood will persist unless complete avoidance of the offending allergen from the diet is achieved. Tolerance to the allergen will usually occur within 2 years of an appropriate elimination diet.[45,46]

Surprisingly few foods are responsible for most documented food reactions. In children, these include milk, eggs, peanuts, fish, soybeans, wheat, and tree nuts. In adults, the most commonly implicated foods are peanuts, tree nuts, shellfish, and fish. Of these allergens, peanuts, tree nuts, and shellfish are the longest-lasting and most resistant to tolerance.

▶ Case Example 3: Food Intolerance

AM is a 37-year-old female with a history of mild asthma and allergic rhinitis since childhood, who presented to clinic with abdominal bloating and cramping for the past 2 years. She denied nausea, vomiting, fevers, or weight loss. Lately, her symptoms have been increasing in both frequency and severity. She has been seen in the emergency room on three separate occasions, with no formal diagnosis made. Her outpatient work-up has consisted of a several abdominal ultrasonographs, abdominal computerized tomography scans, colonoscopy, stool analyses, and blood tests. Gastroenterology consultation resulted in a presumptive diagnosis of irritable bowel syndrome, and the patient achieves slight relief from the antispasmodic Bentyl (dicyclomine hydrochloride). Allergy consultation was obtained, and screening skin test and RAST food panels were negative. The patient has begun to decrease her oral intake in order to continue to maintain a busy work schedule and her social activities. Her present attitude toward food is anxious.

Conventional Medicine Approach

The conventional approach to classical food allergy is relatively straightforward, but often depends upon the astute clinician associating the symptomology with a particular dietary practice. An anaphylactic, respiratory, or urticarial reaction immediately after eating peanuts, or a peanut-containing product is a straightforward diagnosis. More commonly, the putative allergen is masked amidst a myriad of food and food additives present in the modern diet. The appropriate starting point is a complete food recall diary of the previous 24–48 hours (with emphasis upon foods consumed in the immediate 90-minute period prior to an hypersensitivity reaction). Anaphylaxis is most common among patients allergic to peanuts, shellfish, or tree nuts, so these ingredients are always suspect.[47]

There are several diagnostic tests that are routinely performed by the allergist. The skin test, preferably using fresh foods, is a common starting point. It is important to remember, however, that a positive skin test only confirms the presence of allergen-specific IgE in the bloodstream—it never confirms a food allergy. Only 40% of individuals with a positive skin test to a food allergen will actually manifest a symptom when that food is ingested.[48,49] The remainder have a clinically insignificant skin test reaction. A positive skin test to a food that is typically well-tolerated does not mandate further investigation. The true value of the skin test is to exclude the presence of an IgE-mediated allergy, as seen in a negative skin test. In cases where a patient has a skin condition that precludes extensive skin testing (such as eczema), or in infants that do not tolerate the procedure, a RAST may be substituted. Here, levels of allergen-specific IgE in the blood are measured. Again, such tests merely indicate the presence of the antibody, and caution should be exercised to prevent the incorrect identification of a causative agent. Like the skin test, a negative RAST is useful in excluding a presumed allergen.

Finally, the gold standard of food sensitivity tests is the double-blind, placebo-controlled, food challenge. The basic design of a food challenge involves feeding gradually increasing doses of the suspected food at predetermined time intervals until either symptoms occur, or a normal portion of the food ingested openly is tolerated. The suspected food (or additive) is usually freeze-dried, encapsulated, and given to the patient in a blinded fashion in order to eliminate both patient and observer bias. A food challenge is completed when the patient has an obvious reaction to the food, or when a normal portion of the food has been ingested openly without symptoms. The length of time a patient is observed in between doses and after completion of the challenge depends upon several factors including the timing and severity of previous reactions. In severe reactions, a "late-phase," or delayed reaction, may occur many hours later, and must be considered.

There are no adequate pharmacologic therapies for controlling food allergies. Strict avoidance of identifiable food allergens is essential, with care to check food labels with respect to "hidden" ingredients. Also, in severe allergies, it is necessary to be aware of food handling and preparation techniques, to avoid inadvertently cross-contaminated food products. In addition, many individuals should carry an epinephrine self-injector (such as EpiPen) to use in the event of accidental exposure. Antihistamines offer some level of relief for mild food allergies, such as mild urticarial reactions. A compound that has been used with mixed success in the past is oral cromolyn sodium, marketed as Gastrocrom.[50] Although the drug has been used successfully for eosinophilic gastroenteritis, the efficacy in classical IgE-mediated food allergy is equivocal.[51]

Integrative Medicine Approach

Integrative approaches to the diagnosis of adverse food reactions requires the practitioner to be aware of a possible dietary link with the physical or somatic complaint. Often, a lifelong dietary practice will suddenly present with an idiosyncratic reaction. Indeed, the medical literature is replete with reports of diet-associated (or exacerbated) conditions. Autoimmune disorders, constipation, gastroesophageal reflux disease, and even nephropathy are associated with ingestion of cow's milk in susceptible individuals.[52–54] Interestingly, in a majority of cases, patients had been ingesting dairy products for years with no overt symptoms. Food-induced symptoms have also been reported in up to 50% of patients with irritable bowel disease.[55–57] The integrative practitioner will not usually order diagnostic allergy tests, but rather will use a trial of an elimination diet as a diagnostic as well as therapeutic tool. The most commonly used elimination diets in the integrative practice are wheat and dairy restricted (see "Nutritional Approaches"). The glycoproteins in these foods are commonly involved in a myriad of symptoms.

There are numerous untested methods of diagnosis that are used by a minority of practitioners. Many of these methods are purported to accurately identify those foods that are responsible for a myriad of symptoms. Among the more popular alternative diagnostic techniques are applied kinesiology,[58] where muscle strength (either the practitioner's or the patient's) is monitored in response to a putative allergen; allergen-specific serum IgG levels (IgG RAST), which some practitioners believe corresponds to gut immune status; and food immune complex assays, which reportedly measure circulating antibody–food complexes in the bloodstream. These methods are used by a subpopulation of complementary and alternative care medicine practitioners, and there are presently no adequately controlled trials to support their widespread use.

Nutritional Approaches

The nutritional approach to food sensitivity requires a thoughtful and logical approach to discern the causal relationship of symptoms to a particular food item. Food diaries are often helpful in this regard. Haphazard guessing and random elimination of individual foods is ill-advised. A better approach is a trial of a modified elimination diet. This diet consists of "hypoallergenic foods" including lamb, chicken, potatoes, rice, banana, apple, and cruciferous vegetables (such as cabbage, brussels sprouts, and broccoli). In the event of an oral allergy syndrome, the banana and apple may be withheld. Careful avoidance of dairy products and wheat-containing foods should be maintained. All cow's milk products should be avoided, including skim milk, cheese, yogurt, sour cream, whey, casein, sodium caseinate, calcium caseinate, and all foods containing these ingredients. Typically, soy or rice milk is allowed, with the caveat that some people may be sensitive to these foods. In our experience, however, a combined sensitivity to milk, soy, and rice is extremely rare. The elimination diet is continued for at least 8–10 days. If there is a food sensitivity that is contributing to the patient's symptoms, an improvement should be seen (typically by day 5 or 6 of the diet). After completing the initial 10 days, a new food item may be introduced every 2 days with a vigilant watch for a recurrence of symptoms. If the symptoms are related to an adverse food reaction, they will usually recur more dramatically within 48 hours of ingestion.

A different method used by some practitioners is the more drastic water fast. In this model, symptoms usually resolve by the fifth day, after which the reintroduction of single foods begins, with monitoring for recurrence of symptoms. This method is extreme, and should only be employed under medical supervision. The effects of fasting on the immune system are well described.[59,60] Fasting decreases mitogen- and antigen-induced lymphocyte proliferative responses,[61] suppresses interleukin (IL)-2 production,[62] and may cause a transient immunosuppression.[63]

The use of probiotics has emerged as a significant intervention for gastrointestinal immune-mediated illness. The theory behind this practice is that the diet and the microflora composition of the intestine may have a significant effect on inflammation and other immune functions. Introduction of probiotics, or specific strains of healthy gut microflora, promotes gut permeability barrier functions and lessens inflammation. Studies show that probiotic bacterial strains can regulate intestinal immunity and perhaps improve oral tolerance to innocuous environmental antigens.[61–66] The most common strains of bacteria that are used in practice are *Lactobacillus* and *Bifidobacterium* spp.

Botanical Medicines

Certain botanical preparations are used to calm the symptoms of adverse food reactions. In the case of upper respiratory symptoms, quercetin, a bioflavonoid obtained from buckwheat and citrus fruit, has been used prophylactically. In addition, extracts of stinging nettles *(Urtica dioica)* possess antihistaminic properties. Specific gastrointestinal reactions to foods may be managed expectantly. Enteric-coated capsules of peppermint oil can be helpful for abdominal pain related to bowel spasms,[68] but may exacerbate gastroesophageal reflux. Teas prepared from chamomile or ginger root have long been regarded as effective "stomach pain" relievers, even for children..[67] Licorice root preparations (preferably deglycyrrhizinated) reportedly promote mucosal healing in the gastrointestinal tract.[69] Licorice has antispasmodic, antiinflammatory, expectorant, laxative, and soothing properties.[70] Triphala is a mixture of three ayurvedic herbs and has long been used to regulate bowel function. It also exerts a mild laxative effect.

Manipulative Approaches

Hands-on techniques have proven efficacy in musculoskeletal conditions, such as back pain, but also can be useful in patients with gastrointestinal symptoms (abdominal pain, cramping, and diarrhea). The thought is that following ingestion of a reactive food, the presence of a somatovisceral reflex can perpetuate symptoms. Manual manipulation of the abdominal muscles is used to decrease pain as well other symptoms.

Mind–Body Approaches

There are strong links between the mind and the body, and seminal studies by Ader and Cohen led to the development of psychoneuroimmunology as a distinct field of study.[71–73] There are numerous clinical studies demonstrating the impact of psychological state upon allergic diseases. Asthma has long been known to be influenced by stress and anxiety.[74] In addition, anxiety and depression are noted to be common comorbid conditions among those individuals with gastrointestinal manifestations of their food sensitivities, as well as irritable bowel syndrome. The use of mind–body modalities such as hypnosis, meditation, and biofeedback, is a safe and effective way of modulating the response of the autonomic nervous system to food intolerances by controlling underlying stress conditions.[75] Meditation is a useful practice for many, varied medical conditions. There are numerous practice styles, and we often suggest several possibilities for each patient. Although no studies have focused exclusively on the control of allergic disease processes, there is ample evidence to support efficacy in cases of many diverse chronic diseases, including gastrointestinal disorders.[76–78]

Journaling is another useful technique to lessen stress and improve somatic symptoms. We advise patients to express their feelings about events in their lives that were traumatic or stressful by using words or pictures. The efficacy of this powerful technique has been demonstrated in several diseases, including asthma and rheumatoid arthritis.[79]

▶ Case Example 3: Food Intolerance Conclusion

AM, our anxious woman with presumptive irritable bowel syndrome, was seen in our clinic, and several mind–body and nutritional recommendations were made. She began a meditation practice daily and underwent several sessions with a clinical hypnotist. She became adept at self-hypnosis and was now able to calm her gastrointesti-nal symptoms when they first arose. In addition, she instituted a strict wheat- and dairy-elimination diet, which reduced the frequency of her symptoms by more than 90% per her report. She is slowly adding back foods and gradually expanding her dietary repertoire. We also ordered a celiac antibody panel, which was negative.

▶ ENVIRONMENTAL ALLERGIES

Few topics in allergy promote more divisiveness than the subject of environmental sensitivities. This broad category encompasses a diverse array of clinical entities such as multiple chemical sensitivities, sick building syndrome, and even the Gulf War syndrome (Table 17–4). As a group, these disorders are often termed "functional somatic syndromes," and their very existence is a matter of debate. Barsky and Borus[80] established a definition for this syndrome that has been embraced by the conventional medical establishment:

> Functional somatic syndrome refers to several related syndromes that are characterized more by symptoms, suffering, and disability, than by disease-specific, demonstrable abnormalities of structure or function.

The conventional medical community regards the majority of these disorders as psychosomatization disorders, and notes an association of various psychological disorders (e.g., depres-sion, anxiety) in patients with environmental sensitivity. On the opposite end of the spectrum are the "clinical ecologists," a growing population of practitioners that seek to diagnose and treat these patients with uncommon laboratory tests and treatment regimens. There are no studies demonstrating their effectiveness, so we have no objective way to evaluate these doctors' claims. In view of the lack of adequate pathophysiological explanations and definitive therapies for these syndromes, it becomes the role of the integrative physician to examine both approaches, and to focus on treatment modalities that will ultimately benefit the patient and the patient's symptoms. Respect and compassion for the patient, as well as for the patient's perceptions of disease, are mandatory.

Pathophysiology

The large number and diversity of potential etiologies and physical manifestations reported precludes a unified pathophysiological explanation for this condition. There are a few characteristics that most of the environmental sensitivities share, including multiple subjective symptoms, often unrelated; sensitivity to extremely low doses of common chemicals; large numbers of substances that elicit symptoms; lack of demonstrable abnormalities in accepted laboratory or diagnostic tests; symptom duration of greater than 6 months; and many unrelated organ systems affected. Although the triggers may differ, most of these conditions produce similar symptoms.

▶ **TABLE 17–4** ENVIRONMENTAL SENSITIVITIES

Candida hypersensitivity
Electromagnetic field effects
Multiple chemical sensitivities or idiopathic environmental intolerance
Sick building syndrome
Silicone Implant reactivities
Video display terminal intolerance

Multiple chemical sensitivity (MCS; also called idiopathic environmental intolerance) is a prototypical environmental sensitivity condition. There are no scientifically accepted diagnostic criteria for MCS, nor even an accepted definition of MCS. The list of chemical exposures that have been reported is immense, and includes perfumes, gasoline, diesel fumes, cleaning solvents, and even amalgams in dental fillings. Offending substances are usually identified by a characteristic odor. The symptoms reported typically bear no relationship to the established toxicities of the compounds, nor do they occur at toxic concentrations. Patients with MCS, as a group, have a higher-than-normal history of abuse during childhood. as well as higher-than-normal family histories of substance abuse and cardiovascular and respiratory diseases.[81] In addition, in a small study population of people with MCS followed for 8 years, a majority met *Diagnostic and Statistical Manual of Mental Disorders,* 4th ed., criteria for mood, anxiety, or somatoform disorders.[82] As is the case with chronic fatigue syndrome, it is difficult to determine whether the psychological symptoms reported are the cause or the effect of the MCS symptoms. Some experts believe that MCS (as well as other intolerances to environmental chemicals) is a complex but real phenomenon that can be elicited by both stress and chemicals.[83] Immunologic, toxicologic, sociologic, and psychogenic models have been proposed to explain these phenomena,[84–86] but none are widely accepted.

A subcategory of MCS is the "sick building syndrome," also termed nonspecific building-related illnesses. The condition has been appreciated for nearly 25 years, and seeks to explain symptoms occurring in susceptible individuals in a particular indoor environment. Typically, affected people report headache, mucosal irritation (nose and throat), eye irritation, and confusion after variable exposures to the "toxic" locale. There are many hypotheses suggested to explain the syndrome, including exposure to volatile organic compounds (VOCs) and bioaerosols. It has been suggested that low levels of exposure in areas with poor ventilation and humidification may affect a small percentage of the population.[87,88]

Another common environmental sensitivity that has been reported is the "*Candida* hypersensitivity syndrome." This condition is often self-diagnosed by patients presenting to an integrative medicine clinic, usually based upon information gleaned from popular magazines and books geared to the lay audience. It is not to be confused with the conventional diagnoses of local or systemic candidiasis. Thus, the appearance of *Candida* in the oropharynx of those using inhaled steroid preparations (thrush), or in the bloodstream of patients undergoing chemotherapy, is unrelated to candidal hypersensitivity. Rather, this condition is thought to occur in certain people who develop a sensitivity to candidal toxins released from the *Candida albicans* that normally exists in the gastrointestinal and vaginal tracts.[89,90] Although this toxin has never been identified, it has been reported to act as an immunosuppressant.

► Case Example 4: Environmental Sensitivity

BW is a 44-year-old woman who presents to clinic with a list of 25 environmental triggers for a myriad of physical symptoms. Factors such as strong odors, food dyes, electromagnetic fields from household appliances, and the building in which she previously worked all elicited a somatic symptom. These complaints included nausea, headache, vertigo, joint pains, and heart palpitations. Her symptoms have grown in intensity and frequency over the past several years. All conventional test results have been negative. The patient is divorced and lost her administrative job last year as a consequence of excessive absences. She has filed a lawsuit against her previous employer for building-related illnesses and unfair dismissal.

Conventional Medicine Approaches

Conventional medical approaches differ depending upon the practitioner. There are no set protocols for evaluation and treatment of the patient with environmental sensitivity. The prudent approach, however, mandates a careful evaluation to exclude potentially serious and treatable conditions. Often the patient has both a symptom to report as well as a proposed etiology that may seem far-fetched to the practitioner. However, the symptom must be evaluated in its own right, and an open-minded approach is essential to develop a rational work-up plan. Only after excluding treatable conditions can the health care provider explore interventions that may be beneficial.

Typically, the conventional physician will order a number of laboratory or imaging studies to screen for physiological disease. When negative results are obtained, the patient may recommend alternative or unproven diagnostic techniques to provide an explanation for the symptoms. Usually, the patient will need to obtain these tests at their own expense, and with a risk of losing credibility and a relationship with their physician. Should the patient desire to use an unproven therapeutic modality, further alienation and compromise of the doctor–patient relationship may result.

The attitudes of mainstream medicine to these environmental conditions are best illustrated by the statements of recognized medical organizations. The American College of Physicians questions the existence of an environmental illness ". . . because of a lack of clinical definition."[91] It also noted there was "inadequate support" for the basic beliefs of clinical ecology, and that "the diagnoses and treat-ments involve procedures of no proven efficacy." This view is also supported by the American College of Occupational Medicine.[92] The American Academy of Allergy[93] has stated: "The idea that the environment is responsible for a multitude of human health problems is most appealing. However, to present such ideas as facts, conclusions, or even likely mechanisms without adequate support, is poor medical practice."

Some conventional practitioners recognize the association of various comorbid psychological conditions with the presence of environmental sensitivities, and initiate referrals for psychological interventions or prescribe psychotropic medications. This can be useful; however, there can often be a lack of validation or empathy for the patient's perceived symptoms. A harsh dismissal of the patient's concerns, by words or deeds, on the part of the physician does little to help treat this complex entity.

Integrative Medicine Approach

The integrative approach to these environmental sensitivities does not stress definitive diagnoses. Instead, attention is focused upon a suitable holistic treatment regimen that can be individualized to deal with specific symptoms. In the case of MCS, for example, precise diagnosis of causative agents from a large, unrelated list is usually futile, and avoidance is generally impossible. Rather than attempting to define those specific chemicals that are causing somatic complaints, integrative practitioners suggest modalities that ameliorate symptoms and let the patient regain control of his or her life. Typical approaches include nutritional support, modest environmental control measures, mind–body techniques, and homeopathy. An individualized combination of these interventions often serves the sensitive patient well.

Nutritional Approaches

Integrative physicians typically recommend an antiinflammatory/antioxidant diet based upon the supposition that there could be mediators of inflammation or allergy that are involved in the environmental sensitivity syndrome. These dietary modifications are beneficial to a wide range of patients with environmental sensitivities and are quite safe. Even without a clearly defined pathophysiologic mechanism, the stressors felt by these patients likely has a detrimental physiological effect, and the use of antioxidants in foods and as supplements may ameliorate some of these conditions.

Table 17–5 summarizes our standard recommendations. Briefly, these recommendations are designed to lower the exposure to potential allergenic proteins and glycoproteins, increase the intake of natural antioxidants, and decrease the exposure to compounds that may contribute to inflammatory mediator production (i.e., lower exposure to proinflammatory compounds). The dietary guidelines are generally easy to integrate into a daily routine, and thus far have been very effective in mitigating the putative effects of environmental sensitivities. Perhaps the most attractive feature of these dietary guidelines is the overall beneficial effect that is reported by patients, with no adverse consequences.

Some practitioners have developed specific nutritional regimens for particular sensitivities. For example, in patients with presumed *Candida* hypersensitivity, a diet low in sugars, dietary yeast, and "moldy" foods (such as some aged cheeses) is frequently prescribed. There are no well-controlled studies documenting efficacy of this "yeast-free" approach in patients with "candidal sensitivity," and we often prefer generic modified elimination diets to delineate food provocateurs of the symptoms that patients ascribe to candidal hypersensitivity.

Homeopathy

Homeopathy has helped individuals with a wide variety of disorders, and we find it particularly well-suited for hypersensitive individuals, because the healing compounds, called "remedies," are present in highly dilute concentrations. In fact, most are so dilute that no active molecules remain—simply the "memory" of the active compound in the water diluent. Thus, unlike many herbal or nutritional treatments, the likelihood of adverse effects to the sensitive individual from the treatment is very low. Symptom improvement in individuals with a variety of sensitivities is possible, and the technique is well-tolerated.

Environmental Control Measures

Most patients will go to any extreme in an effort to reduce debilitating symptoms. Patients should be warned that many "clinical ecologists"

▶ **TABLE 17–5** ANTIINFLAMMATORY DIETARY CONSIDERATIONS

- Decrease total dietary protein to 10–15% of your daily caloric intake
- Use plant proteins in place of animal-derived proteins
- Eliminate milk and dairy products
- Increase your supply of natural antioxidants by dramatically increasing fruit and vegetable intake
- Eat organic foods whenever possible
- Eliminate polyunsaturated vegetable oils, margarine, vegetable shortening, all partially hydrogenated oils, and all foods that might contain *trans*-fatty acids (i.e., deep-fried foods)
- Increase your intake of omega-3 essential fatty acids

may recommend relocation to other parts of the country, or even to rebuild a home in order to lessen their environmental exposures. These interventions are expensive, and have never been clearly shown to reduce symptoms. Although there is no "elimination diet" counterpart for the ill-defined triggers of somatic disorders, there are some measures that are useful. Patients are advised to consult with an allergist for skin testing, particularly for the detection of dust mite and common mold allergens. In general, *Alternaria* and *Cladosporium* spp. are the allergenic molds most commonly found (both indoors and outdoors) throughout the United States, although *Aspergillus* and *Penicillium* spp. are also common. If tests are positive for either allergen, then a trial of humidity control, as well as removal of mite breeding areas, is indicated. This may include carpet removal in the sleeping areas, regular hot water washing of bed linens, and regular vacuuming (with a mask).

Mind–Body Approaches

As with food allergies, patients with functional sensitization disorders are well-served by the introduction of self-hypnosis, guided imagery, or journaling. These techniques are useful in inducing a state of relaxation, as well as allowing the patient to visualize their healing. For example, a patient may be able to visualize themselves in a building where they experience their symptoms, or tasting a "forbidden" food. As long as the risk for anaphylaxis and true immediate hypersensitivity has been removed, such mind–body techniques are safe and usually effective. Furthermore, the ability to self-induce a trance relaxation state is particularly useful for those patients who are reluctant to leave their homes for fear of a "toxic" reaction. It is a proven stress-reducing modality that affords the patient a level of symptom control that they can regulate.

Meditation is also beneficial in dealing with symptoms of chronic pain or somatic complaints resulting from putative environmental irritants. We find that patients who meditate regularly are able to tolerate gradually increasing levels of their putative triggers without symptoms. In addition, the frequency and intensity of breakthrough symptoms seems to be diminished. As with food intolerances, there are no published trials of this modality for environmental sensitivities.

Finally, many patients have reported success using eye movement desensitization and reprocessing (EMDR), a controversial psychotherapeutic technique that combines elements of the standard modalities (e.g., psychodynamic, behavioral, and cognitive) with eye movements. The technique has been used for a variety of conditions, ranging from posttraumatic stress disorder to depression.

Botanical Medicines

There are no studies to support the use of herbal compounds specifically for environmental sensitivities, but much has been written about their role in allergic disease in general. These include stinging nettles *(Urtica dioica)*[94] and licorice root (Glycyrrhiza glabra),[95] which exhibit antiinflammatory activities. In addition, there are tonifying herbs and herb blends, also called tonics, that are used to restore strength and vigor, and typically are taken for an extended period of time. While these compounds have no specific role in environmental sensitivity, they often restore a sense of well-being in the patient.

▶ CONCLUSION

Allergic diseases have been plaguing mankind for centuries. They are often described as inappropriate or exaggerated responses to environmental compounds, an evolutionary remnant of a formerly useful biological defense or even one of nature's mistakes. Perhaps the real mistake is our assumption that we actually understand the mechanism and purpose behind the allergic response. The interactions between the immune system and the mind, for exam-

▶ Case Example 4: Environmental Sensitivity Conclusion

Patient BW was evaluated in clinic, and found to be mildly depressed, perhaps because of situational circumstances. She had a difficult childhood, with vivid memories of physical and psychological abuse as a child. These episodes were never properly addressed, and the memories have plagued her since their occurrence. We recommended that these issues be validated and addressed formally by using a psychodynamic intervention. She began receiving psychotherapy, along with a series of guided imagery sessions designed to allow her to mentally prepare for the inevitable exposures that she feared in public life. In addition, she altered her diet (per the recommendations described above), and lost 15 pounds over the course of several months. She also began an exercise program, with regular walking. Since initiating these changes, she feels better, claims to have improved self-esteem, and is exploring a return to the workforce (part-time) in the near future.

ple, transcend anything that would have been imagined as recently as three decades ago.

Integrative medicine respects these voids in our knowledge, and operates under the assumption that the human body possesses immense healing potential in and of itself. It is our challenge, as practitioners, to find the individual key that will unlock the healing force in our patients. Implicit in such an approach, however, is a healthy respect for the advances in modern pharmaceuticals and therapeutics. No complementary or alternative modalities have yet been described that work as well as epinephrine and intravenous fluid replacement to reverse the effects of anaphylaxis. Integrative medicine offers the unique opportunity to blend these seemingly disparate approaches to patient care in an open-minded and flexible manner.

REFERENCES

1. Greaves M. Chronic urticaria. *J Allergy Clin Immunol.* 2000;105(4):664–672.
2. Kaplan AP. Clinical practice. Chronic urticaria and angioedema. *N Engl J Med.* 2002;346(3): 175–179.
3. Mehregan DR, Hall MJ, Gibson LE. Urticarial vasculitis: a histopathologic and clinical review of 72 cases. *J Am Acad Dermatol.* 1992;26(3 pt 2): 441–448.
4. Zauli D, Deleonardi G, Foderaro S, et al. Thyroid autoimmunity in chronic urticaria. *Allergy Asthma Proc.* 2001;22(2):93–95.
5. Numata T, Yamamoto S, Yamura T. The role of mite allergen in chronic urticaria. *Ann Allergy.* 1979;43(6):356–358.
6. Lodi A, Di Berardino L, Chiarelli G, et al. [Chronic urticaria and allergy to Acari. Experience with a specific desensitization therapy.] *G Ital Dermatol Venereol.* 1990;125(5):187–189.
7. Zuberbier T, Pfrommer C, Specht K, et al. Aromatic components of food as novel eliciting factors of pseudoallergic reactions in chronic urticaria. *J Allergy Clin Immunol.* 2002;109(2): 343–348.
8. Van Dellum RG, Maddox DE, Dutta EJ. Masqueraders of angioedema and urticaria. *Ann Allergy Asthma Immunol.* 2002;88(1):10–14.
9. Casale TB, Keahey TM, Kaliner M. Exercise-induced anaphylactic syndromes. Insights into diagnostic and pathophysiologic features. *J Amer Med Assn.* 1986;255(15):2049–2053.
10. Dover JS, Black AK, Ward AM, Greaves MW. Delayed pressure urticaria. Clinical features, laboratory investigations, and response to therapy of 44 patients. *J Am Acad Dermatol.* 1988;18(6): 1289–1298.

11. Brandes K. [Cold urticaria and swimmer's death.] *Z Allgemeinmed.* 1970;46(24):1219–1220.

12. Kaur S, Greaves M, Eftekhari N. Factitious urticaria (dermographism): treatment by cimetidine and chlorpheniramine in a randomized double-blind study. *Br J Dermatol.* 1981;104(2):185–190.

13. Phanuphak P, Schocket A, Kohler PF. Treatment of chronic idiopathic urticaria with combined H_1 and H_2 blockers. *Clin Allergy.* 1978;8(5):429–433.

14. Harvey RP, Wegs J, Schocket AL. A controlled trial of therapy in chronic urticaria. *J Allergy Clin Immunol.* 1981;68(4):262–266.

15. Pacor ML, Di Lorenzo G, Corrocher R. Efficacy of leukotriene receptor antagonist in chronic urticaria. A double-blind, placebo-controlled comparison of treatment with montelukast and cetirizine in patients with chronic urticaria with intolerance to food additive and/or acetylsalicylic acid. *Clin Exp Allergy.* 2001;31(10):1607–1614.

16. Ellis MH. Successful treatment of chronic urticaria with leukotriene antagonists. *J Allergy Clin Immunol.* 1998;102(5):876–877.

17. Grant SM, Goa KL, Fitton A, et al. Ketotifen: a review of its pharmacodynamic and pharmacokinetic properties, and therapeutic use in asthma and allergic disorders. *Drugs.* 1990;40:412.

18. Bressler RB, Sowell K, Huston DP. Therapy of chronic idiopathic urticaria with nifedipine: demonstration of beneficial effect in a double-blinded, placebo-controlled, crossover trial. *J Allergy Clin Immunol.* 1989;83(4):756–763.

19. Grattan CE, O'Donnell BF, Francis DM, et al. Randomized double-blind study of cyclosporin in chronic "idiopathic" urticaria. *Br J Dermatol.* 2000;143(2):365–372.

20. Grattan CE, Francis DM, Slater NG, Barlow RJ, Greaves MW. Plasmapheresis for severe, unremitting, chronic urticaria. *Lancet.* 1992;339(8801):1078–1080.

21. O'Donnell BF, Barr RM, Black AK, et al. Intravenous immunoglobulin in autoimmune chronic urticaria. *Br J Dermatol.* 1998;138(1):101–106.

22. Brestel EP, Thrush LB. The treatment of glucocorticosteroid-dependent chronic urticaria with stanozolol. *J Allergy Clin Immunol.* 1988;82(2):265–269.

23. Nettis E, Di PR, Ferrannini A, Tursi A. Tolerability of rofecoxib in patients with cutaneous adverse reactions to nonsteroidal anti-inflammatory drugs. *Ann Allergy Asthma Immunol.* 2002;88(3):331–334.

24. Lopez LR, Davis KC, Kohler PF, Schocket AL. The hypocomplementemic urticarial-vasculitis syndrome: therapeutic response to hydroxychloroquine. *J Allergy Clin Immunol.* 1984;73(5 pt 1):600–603.

25. O'Loughlin S, Schroeter Al, Jordan RE. Chronic urticaria-like lesions in systemic lupus erythematosus. *Arch Dermatol.* 1978;114(6):879–883.

26. Zuberbier T, Chantraine-Hess S, Hartmann K, Czarnetzki BM. Pseudoallergen-free diet in the treatment of chronic urticaria. A prospective study. *Acta Derm Venereol.* 1995;75(6):484–487.

27. Murray MT, Pizzorno JE Jr. Urticaria. In: Pizzorno JE Jr, ed. *Textbook of Natural Medicine.* 2nd ed. Edinburgh: Churchill-Livingstone; 1999:1561–1571.

28. Johri RK, Zutshi U, Kameshwaran L, Atal CK. Effect of quercetin and Albizzia saponins on rat mast cell. *Indian J Physiol Pharmacol.* 1985;29(1):43–46.

29. Thornhill SM, Kelly AM. Natural treatment of perennial allergic rhinitis. *Altern Med Rev.* 2000;5(5):448–454.

30. Murray MT, Pizzorno JE Jr. Urticaria. In: Pizzorno JE Jr, ed. *Textbook of Natural Medicine.* 2nd ed. Edinburgh: Churchill-Livingstone; 1999:619–627.

31. Gailhofer G, Wilders-Truschnig M, Smolle J, Ludvan M. Asthma caused by bromelain: an occupational allergy. *Clin Allergy.* 1988;18(5):445–450.

32. Olafsson JH, Larko O, Roupe G, Granerus G, Bengtsson U. Treatment of chronic urticaria with PUVA or UVA plus placebo: a double-blind study. *Arch Dermatol Res.* 1986;278(3):228–231.

33. Chen CJ, Yu HS. Acupuncture treatment of urticaria. *Arch Dermatol.* 1998;134(11):1397–1399.

34. Lin RY. Delayed hypersensitivity to pollen skin prick tests and seasonal rhinitis. *J Allergy Clin Immunol.* 1995;95:911–912.

35. Asbell P, Howes J. A double-masked, placebo-controlled evaluation of the efficacy and safety of loteprednol etabonate in the treatment of giant papillary conjunctivitis. *CLAO J.* 1997;23(1):31–36.

36. Howes JF. Loteprednol etabonate: a review of ophthalmic clinical studies. *Pharmazie.* 2000;55(3):178–183.

37. Casale TB, Condemi J, LaForce C, et al. Effect of omalizumab on symptoms of seasonal allergic

rhinitis: a randomized controlled trial. *JAMA.* 2001;286(23):2956–2967.

38. Biswas NR, Gupta SK, Das GK, et al. Evaluation of Opthacare eye drops—a herbal formulation in the management of various ophthalmic disorders. *Phytother Res.* 2001;15(7):618–620.

39. Stoss M, Michels C, Peter E, Beutke R, Gorter RW. Prospective cohort trial of Euphrasia single-dose eye drops in conjunctivitis. *J Altern Complement Med.* 2000;6(6):499–508.

40. Sanderson IR, Walker WA. Uptake and transport of macromolecules by the intestine: possible role in clinical disorders (an update). *Gastroenterology.* 1993;104:622–639.

41. Carol M, Lambrechts A, Van Gossum A, Libin M, Goldman M, Mascarte-Lemone E. Spontaneous secretion of interferon gamma and interleukin 4 by human intraepithelial and lamina propria gut lymphocytes. *Gut.* 1998;42:643–649.

42. Pacor ML, Lunardi C, Di Lorenzo G, et al. Food allergy and seronegative arthritis: report of two cases. *Clin Rheumatol.* 2001;20(4):279–281.

43. Mansfield LE, Vaughan TR, Waller SF, et al. Food allergy and adult migraine: double-blind and mediator confirmation of an allergic etiology. *Ann Allergy.* 1985;55:126–129.

44. Bock SA. Prospective appraisal of complaints of adverse reactions to foods in children during the first three years of life. *Pediatrics.* 1987;79:683–688.

45. Pastorello E, Stochi L, Pravetonni V, et al. Role of the elimination diet in adults with food allergy. *J Allergy Clin Immunol.* 1989;84:475–483.

46. Sampson HA, Scanlon SM. Natural history of food hypersensitivity in children with atopic dermatitis. *J Pediatr.* 1989;115:23–27.

47. Sampson HA. Food allergy: from biology toward therapy. *Hosp Pract.* 2000;35(5):67–83.

48. Bock A, Buckley J, Holst A, et al. Proper use of skin tests with food extracts in the diagnosis food hypersensitivity. *Clin Allergy.* 1978;8:559–564.

49. Atkins FM, Steinberg SS, Metcalf DD. Evaluation of immediate adverse reactions to foods in adult patients. I. Correlation of demographic, laboratory, and prick skin test data with response to controlled oral food challenges. *J Allergy Clin Immunol.* 1985;75:646–651.

50. Edwards AM. Oral sodium cromoglycate: its use in the management of food allergy. *Clin Exp Allergy.* 1995;25(suppl 1):31–33.

51. Burks W, Sampson HA. Double-blind placebo-controlled trial of oral cromolyn in children with atopic dermatitis and documented food hypersensitivity. *J Allergy Clin Immunol.* 1988;81:417–423.

52. Sandberg DH, McIntosh RM, Bernstein CW, et al. Severe steroid-responsive nephrosis associated with hypersensitivity. *Lancet.* 1977;1:388–391.

53. Lagrue G, Laurent J, Rostoker G, Lang P. Food allergy in idiopathic nephrotic syndrome. *Lancet.* 1987;2:277.

54. Howanietz H, Lubec G. Idiopathic nephrotic syndrome, treated with steroids for five years, found to be allergic reaction to pork. *Lancet.* 1985;2:450.

55. Svedlund J, Sjodin I, Dotevall G, Gillberg R. Upper gastrointestinal and mental symptoms in the irritable bowel syndrome. *Scand J Gastroenterol.* 1985;20:595–601.

56. Young E, Stoneham MD, Petruckevitch A, et al. A population study of food intolerance. *Lancet.* 1994;343:1127–1130.

57. Nanda R, James R, Smith H, et al. Food intolerance and the irritable bowel syndrome. *Gut.* 1989;30:1099–1104.

58. Garrow JS. Kinesiology and food allergy. *BMJ.* 1988;296:1573.

59. Goldhamer A, Lisle D, Parpia B, et al. Medically supervised water-only fasting in the treatment of hypertension. *J Manipulative Physiol Ther.* 2001;24(50):335–9.

60. Kjeldsen-Kragh J, Haugen M, Borchgrevink CF, et al. Controlled trial of fasting and one-year vegetarian diet in rheumatoid arthritis. *Lancet.* 1991;338:899–902.

61. Holm G, Palmblad J. Acute energy deprivation in man: effect on cell-mediated immunological reactions. *Clin Exp Immunol.* 1976;25:207–211.

62. Savendahl L, Underwood L. Decreased interleukin-2 production from cultured peripheral blood mononuclear cells in human acute starvation. *J Clin Endocrinol Metab.* 1997;82:1177–1180.

63. Fraser DA, Thoen J, Reseland J, et al. Decreased CD-4+ lymphocyte activation and increased IL-4 production in peripheral blood of rheumatoid arthritis patients after acute starvation. *Clin Rheumatol.* 1999;18(5):394–401.

64. Majamaa H, Isollauri E. Probiotics: a novel approach in the management of food allergies. *J Allergy Clin Immunol.* 1997;99:179–186.

65. Pelto L, Isolaurie E, Lillius EM, Nuutila J, Salminen S. Probiotic bacteria downregulate the milk-induced inflammatory response in milk-hypersensitive subjects but have a immunostimulatory effect in healthy subjects. *Clin Exp Allergy*. 1998;28:1474–1479.

66. Isolaurie E. Probiotics in the prevention and treatment of allergic disease. *Pediatr Allergy Immunol*. 2001;12(14):56–59.

67. Blumenthal M, ed. *Herbal Medicine: Expanded Commission E Monographs*. Newton. MA: Integrative Medicine Communications; 2000.

68. Kline RM, Kline JJ, Di Palma J, Barbero GJ. Enteric-coated, pH-dependent peppermint oil capsules for the treatment of irritable bowel syndrome in children. *J Pediatrics*. 2001;138(1):125–128.

69. Gaby AR. Deglycyrrhizinated licorice treatment of peptic ulcer. *Townsend Lett*. 1988;60:306–311.

70. Newall CA, Anderson LA, Philpson JD. *Herbal Medicine: A Guide for Healthcare Professionals*. London, UK: The Pharmaceutical Press; 1996.

71. Ader R, Cohen N. Behaviorally conditioned immunosuppression and murine systemic lupus erythematosus. *Science*. 982;215:1534–1536.

72. Ader R, Cohen N. CNS-immune system interactions: conditioning phenomena. *Behav Brain Sci*. 1985;8:379–395.

73. Ader R, Grota LJ, Cohen N. Conditioning phenomena and immune function. *Ann N Y Acad Sci*. 1987;496:532–544.

74. Rietveld S, Everaerd JW, Creer TL. Stress-induced asthma: a review of research and potential mechanisms. *Clin Exp Allergy*. 2000;30:1058–1066.

75. Gonsalkorale WM, Houghton LA, Whorwell PG. Hypnotherapy in irritable bowel syndrome: a large-scale audit of a clinical service with examination of factors influencing responsiveness. *Am J Gastroenterol*. 2002;97(4):954–961.

76. Kabat-Zinn J, Lipworth L, Burney R, et al. Four-year follow-up of a meditation-based program for the self-regulation of chronic pain: treatment outcomes and compliance. *Clin J Pain*. 1987;2:159–173.

77. Kabat-Zinn J, Wheeler E, Light T, et al. Influence of a mindfulness meditation-based stress reduction intervention on rates of skin clearing in patients with moderate to severe psoriasis undergoing phototherapy (UVB) and photochemotherapy (PUVA). *Psychosom Med*. 1998;60: 625–632.

78. Keefer L, Blanchard EB. A one-year follow-up of relaxation response meditation as a treatment for irritable bowel syndrome. *Behav Res Ther*. 2002;40(5):541–546.

79. Smyth JM, Stone AA, Hurewitz A. Effects of writing about stressful experiences on symptom reduction in patients with asthma or rheumatoid arthritis: a randomized trial. *JAMA*. 1999;281:1304–1309.

80. Barsky AJ, Borus JF. Functional somatic syndromes. *Ann Intern Med*. 1999;130:910–921.

81. Bell IR. Early life stress, negative paternal relationships, and chemical intolerance in middle-aged women: support for a neural sensitization model. *J Womens Health*. 1998;7(9):1135–1147.

82. Black DW, Okiishi C, Schlosser S. The Iowa follow-up of chemically sensitive persons. *Ann N Y Acad Sci*. 2001;933:48–56.

83. Bell IR, Baldwin JC, Schwartz GE. Sensitization studies in chemically intolerant individuals: implications for individual difference research. *Ann N Y Acad Sci*. 2001;933:38–47.

84. Sparks PJ, Daniell W, Black DW, et al. Multiple chemical sensitivity syndrome: a clinical perspective. I. Case definition, theories of pathogenesis, and research needs. *J Occup Med*. 1994;36:718–730.

85. Cotterill JA. Total allergy syndrome. *Lancet*. 1982;1:628–629.

86. Green MA. "Allergic to everything": 20th century syndrome. *JAMA*. 1985;253:842.

87. Marks PJ, Daniel EB. The sick building syndrome. *Immunol Allergy Clin North Am*. 1994;14:521–535.

88. Brooks SM, Weiss MA, Bernstein IL. Reactive airways dysfunction syndrome. Case reports of persistent airways hyperreactivity following high-level irritant exposures. *Am Rev Respir Dis*. 1985;27:473–476.

89. Truss CO. Tissue injury induced by Candida albicans: mental and neurological manifestations. *J Orthomol Psych*. 1978;7:17.

90. Truss CO. Restoration of immunologic competence to *Candida albicans*. *J Orthomol Psych*. 1980;9:287.

91. Terr AI. Clinical ecology. *Ann Intern Med*. 1989;111:168–178.

92. American College of Occupational and Environmental Medicine. *Position Statement: Multiple Chemical Sensitivities*. April 27, 1993.

93. American Academy of Allergy and Clinical Immunology Executive Committee. Position statement on clinical ecology. *J Allergy Clin Immunol.* 1986;78:269–270.

94. Riehemann K. Plant extracts from stinging nettle *(Urtica dioica),* an antirheumatic remedy, inhibit the proinflammatory transcription factor NF-kappaB. *FEBS Lett.* 1999;442(1): 89–94.

95. Okimasu E, Moromizato Y, Watanabe S, et al. Inhibition of phospholipase A_2 and platelet aggregation by glycyrrhizin, an antiinflammatory drug. *Acta Med Okayama.* 1983;37: 385–391.

CHAPTER 18

Integrative Approach to Cardiovascular Health

Steven F. Horowitz

Cardiovascular disease remains the leading cause of death in Western countries; in the United States, there are more than 700,000 cardiac deaths annually. It is estimated that by the year 2020 cardiovascular disease will become the number one killer worldwide. The full extent of suffering from atherosclerosis is hard to estimate, as stroke, kidney dysfunction, and loss of limbs and eyesight from vascular disease are not included in these estimates, yet are part of the same systemic illness. Tremendous progress has been made in understanding the molecular biology and physiology of atherosclerosis, and advancements in surgical and pharmacologic treatments have markedly improved outcomes in both acute coronary syndromes and chronic disease.

Numerous genetic markers of increased coronary disease risk have been identified in the areas of lipid metabolism, diabetes mellitus, and hypertension. However, while diseases that are predominantly or exclusively genetically determined, such as muscular dystrophy, have little variation in incidence rates around the world, coronary artery disease mortality is remarkably variable, suggesting a strong influence of acquired or environmental factors on disease occurrence. This is not surprising, considering the five major cardiovascular risk factors are substantially influenced by lifestyle choices[1]: abnormal blood lipids, obesity, diabetes mellitus, cigarette smoking, and sedentary lifestyle.

Death rates from coronary artery disease have traditionally been higher in the United States than in France and Japan. Even within the United States, there is a wide variation in disease occurrence, with less coronary disease along the West Coast and more in the East. Further evidence of the impact of environment on risk factors and coronary disease incidence comes from epidemiologic studies of native populations that migrate from regions of low disease risk to high-risk countries. For instance, Japanese citizens who move from Japan to Hawaii develop higher cholesterol levels and coronary disease incidence rates. Native-born Japanese who move to the US mainland develop even higher serum cholesterol and coronary disease rates that are nearly 50% higher than those who move to Hawaii.[2,3] Similarly, people from the Punjab in India who move to West London, England, develop not only a cardiovascular risk profile that is higher than that in India, but a cardiovascular disease mortality that is higher than that among white West

Londoners in the same environment.[4] This finding suggests that adverse environmental factors may not only increase risk, but may interact with previously dormant genetic predispositions such as abnormal lipoprotein patterns, to create a higher risk of cardiovascular-related death.

Thus, many epidemiologic studies suggest that acquired cardiovascular risk is of great importance in determining whether (or when) genetic predisposition to coronary artery disease becomes clinically manifest. Some researchers estimate that only approximately 10% of coronary disease is truly genetically unavoidable, with the rest of the at-risk population developing disease because of the interaction between genetic, environmental, cultural, and behavioral factors. In the United States, death rates have progressively dropped over the last three decades, while in other areas of the world, such as Southeast Asia and the former Soviet Union, there is evidence of alarming mortality rate increases. Even in the United States there is evidence of a recent increase in key cardiovascular risk factors, such as cigarette smoking, sedentary lifestyle, obesity, and diabetes mellitus, suggesting the potential for future increases in disease incidence. This and other data provide compelling support for the concept that coronary disease development and progression can be substantially addressed through nonallopathic means, predominantly involving diet and life-style interventions.

▶ APPROACH TO THE PATIENT

It has become progressively more difficult to apply the labels of alternative, complementary, and even integrative medicine to the practice of cardiology. Supplementation with high-dose vitamins and neutraceuticals has long been considered the domain of "alternative" practitioners, yet niacin, a vitamin, is a mainstay of allopathic lipid therapy when administered at 50 to 100 times the normal daily requirements. Similarly, moderate exercise, diet, and weight loss have long been advocated by physicians for prevention and treatment of coronary disease, yet more extreme approaches may be considered radical or "alternative" by many physicians, despite evidence in the literature supporting their value over moderate recommendations.

Currently, the lines between therapeutic strategies are blurring, with tradition, culture, economics and bias often determining whether an approach is considered mainstream or unorthodox, regardless of the evidence. As Dr. Dean Ornish has stated, "if you cut open a patient's chest and implant veins from his legs it is considered standard, acceptable medical treatment, while if you treat the patient with diet, exercise, and relaxation therapy it's considered radical."[5] It is evident that full integration of evidence-based therapeutic strategies in cardiology is uncommon. Too often the commitment of individual health care providers is to specific therapies rather than to the patient, regardless of whether the provider comes from an allopathic or alternative background.

Interventions aimed at lifestyle change represent a mainstay of primary and secondary coronary disease prevention. When chronic coronary disease is known to be present, these techniques are valuable adjunctive therapies used together with pharmaceuticals as necessary. However, lifestyle changes, diet, and vitamin supplementation have no role in the care of the acutely ill patient with an unstable coronary syndrome, and may in fact delay lifesaving interventions or surgical therapy in patients who lose time searching for noninvasive alternatives. This chapter focuses on the evidence accumulated in the literature to support the use of nonallopathic therapies as primary or adjunctive treatments for chronic heart disease.

▶ LIFESTYLE

For most people, lifestyle choice represents the most important factor that influences their risk of developing coronary artery disease. For example, a cigarette smoker destined to sustain a myocardial infarction will have it on average a decade earlier than a nonsmoker. Other lifestyle-related risk factors of importance for the development of coronary artery disease include lack of exercise, obesity, diabetes mellitus and, most controversial of all, choice of diet.

Diet

Although a growing body of literature has provided evidence-based direction for cardiovascular health through nutrition, significant controversies remain. These controversies are fueled in the lay press, as seemingly discordant diets gain equal publicity and vocal advocacy. Hippocrates wrote, "Thy food shall be thy cure," but the question of which food remains unanswered. Nonetheless, some basic nutritional concepts are well documented and supported in the literature.

First, there appears to be a strong epidemiologic link between saturated animal fat consumption, serum cholesterol levels in adulthood, and atherosclerotic death in most parts of the world. Total dietary fat intake appears to be less-well linked to the risk of cardiovascular disease. More specific observational data shows favorable cardiovascular outcomes with consumption of foods rich in monounsaturated fat such as olive oil and some tree nuts (almonds and walnuts). Unfortunately, there remains a significant volume of conflicting data, even in some instances surrounding the consumption of saturated fats. Avocados, for example, have been avoided in many diets because of their high fat content. Studies, however, show lowering of cholesterol with avocados, which are rich in monounsaturated fat.

Alluding to information from epidemiologic studies without benefit of prospective trial outcome data may produce layers of assumptions based more on extrapolation than on solid research. Most prospective diet intervention trials are invariably too small or too short to demon-strate differences in outcome, although several show improvement in risk factors, well-being, coronary angiograms, myocardial perfusion measured by positron emission tomography scans, and coronary event rates. Some of these trials are marred by manipulation of multiple variables simultaneously. For instance, in the St. Thomas' Atherosclerotic Regression Study (STARS), standard care was compared with two arms involving dietary intervention that included low fat, high fiber, and high omega-3 intake (one group also included cholestyramine).[6] Although event-free survival and angiograms were improved, it is not clear which of the multiple dietary interventions was responsible for the improvement.

Low-fat diets have produced uneven results regarding cholesterol lowering and improvement in cardiovascular outcome. Some studies, such as the Oslo Diet Heart study, show significant cholesterol lowering and fewer cardiac-related deaths but no change in overall mortality after 11 years of follow-up.[7] The American Heart Association has promoted diets containing up to 30% of calories as fat and 200 to 300 mg/d of cholesterol, with up to 10% saturated fat allowed. Despite the popularity of the American Heart Association Step I and Step II diets, there is little or no evidence that low-density lipoprotein-cholesterol (LDL-C) is significantly altered, and there is no data supporting outcome improvement.[8,9] In the Lifestyle Heart Trial,[10] more extreme fat restrictions (less than 10% of total calories) in a small group of highly motivated patients resulted in marked improvement in angina, slight but significant coronary disease regression as demonstrated by serial angiography, and improvement in myocardial perfusion assessed by positron emission tomography imaging. The diet was essentially vegan except for small amounts of nonfat dairy products, and total cholesterol intake was under 15 mg/d. The trial included three other lifestyle changes: yoga, moderate aerobic exercise, and group support. Evidence of improvement occurred despite a slight increase in triglycerides and a fall in high-density lipoprotein-cholesterol (HDL-C). Total cholesterol and LDL-C fell significantly (37%). There was a direct relationship between progression or regression of coronary disease and adherence to the full program in this small group of patients. Although patients undergoing this combined lifestyle approach continued to show improvement, as measured by both symptoms and laboratory tests at 5 years, no conclusions concerning outcomes could be reached. Additionally, because multiple interventions were used, it was not possible to know whether all components were necessary to obtain coronary disease regression or stabilization. Nonetheless, the trial produced valuable laboratory-based data about the potential for engineering sustained "healing" of coronary lesions without medications and with lifestyle changes only.

An observational study by Sdringola et al.[11] addressed the issue of a very-low-fat diet combined with cholesterol-lowering medication. Patients were classified as undergoing poor, moderate, or maximal treatment, the latter category consisting of a combination of a very-low-fat diet, regular exercise, and statin medication. Follow-up at 5 years demonstrated an event rate of only 6.6% in the maximal treatment group, as compared with 20.3% and 30.6% in the moderate and poor treatment groups. Of note, improved positron emission tomography imaging correlated with a better long-term clinical outcome. Although the study participants were not randomized, and multiple "healthful" behaviors may have skewed the results, the study does suggest the potential for additional benefit from the combined use of modalities thought to have value individually. Of note, the maximal treatment group had the lowest LDL via lifestyle and statin medication. It is possible that more aggressive therapy with statins alone may have achieved the same benefit without the need for lifestyle change. At the very least, however, as in the Lifestyle Trial, intense changes in diet and exercise may offer the potential to reduce the need for some medical and interventional therapies.

The Lyon Diet heart study sought to explain the Cretan paradox: a low incidence of coronary artery disease on the isle of Crete despite relatively high cholesterol levels. The authors compared a Mediterranean diet with a prudent Western diet and randomized 605 post-myocardial infarction patients. The Mediterranean diet consists of little meat or saturated fats, but a great deal of vegetables, fruit, bread, cereals, and wine, with some cheese. It also contains other dietary items like purslane, a dandelion-like plant used in salads and high in vitamin E. The diet also contains olive oil, rich in antioxidants and monounsaturated fatty acid, and walnuts, rich in fiber and alpha-linolenic acid. In addition, the intervention group was given a canola oil-based margarine to ensure a high intake of alpha-linolenic acid. The study was planned for 4 years but was stopped early because of the power of the results. There was a 70% reduction in cardiac events, including death, and the effect was seen within 2 months of starting the study. Despite the change in diet and beneficial outcome in the intervention group, there was no difference in LDL-C cholesterol levels, and other standard risk factors remained independently predictive of coronary events.[12,13]

Although the study was stopped early, follow-up at 4 years demonstrated retained benefit, as the intervention group easily maintained a Mediterranean style diet.[11] The ability of the intervention group to continue on a cardiac-event-lowering diet after the trial had ended is of considerable interest because of the difficulty many patients have in following more restrictive, and perhaps less palatable, recommendations. The study was later criticized because participants knew their groups prior to consenting for the study, and the intervention group received canola oil margarine as a supplement.[15] Nonetheless, in an accompanying editorial by Leaf, it was noted that "relatively simple dietary changes achieved greater reductions in risk of all cause and coronary heart disease mortality than any of the cholesterol-lowering studies to date."[16]

Considering the magnitude of the benefit in the Lyon Trial, the intrinsic difficulty in performing this type of dietary intervention study, and the fact that the dietary changes are unlikely to be harmful, it appears reasonable to direct cardiac patients toward a Mediterranean-style diet. Because cholesterol levels remained a risk factor despite marked outcome improvement with a Mediterranean diet, it is logical to assume further cholesterol lowering would provide incremental benefit. It is likely that the addition of statin medication would have added value considering the mean LDL-C level was 161 mg/dL in the interventional group. Whether additional nutritional interventions aimed specifically at cholesterol lowering without diminishing the dietary omega-3 monounsaturated fat or alpha-linolenic acid content of the Mediterranean diet would provide improved outcomes remains speculative, but has support in the literature.[17]

The importance of omega-3 fatty acids and linolenic acid in cardiovascular disease prevention has been bolstered by basic research demonstrating stabilization of cell membranes and prevention of fatal ventricular arrhythmias in animal models of ischemic heart disease. The impact of fish oil on clotting was presaged by Viking tales of Greenlanders bleeding easily in combat. Despite a diet rich in mammal meat, Eskimos had little coronary disease prior to the introduction of Western diets. Unlike land-based mammals, those mammals eaten by Eskimos stood atop the arctic food chain, deriving fat from deep sea fish and plankton rich in omega-3 fatty acids. Deep sea fish, although rich in omega-3 fatty acids, is not the only source of this essential fatty acid. Two ounces of salmon provides the recommended daily dose of slightly more than 1 g of omega-3 fatty acids, but the same amount can be found in half a teaspoon of flaxseed oil, three-quarters of a teaspoon of canola oil, 6 oz of tofu or 0.5 oz of walnuts. Other foods, such as broccoli and kale, contain omega-3 fatty acids, but would require 5 to 8 cups per day to exceed 1 g.

Usually large, randomized, well-controlled clinical trials offer more definitive information about treatment strategies than do epidemiologic studies and often clarify relationships only suggested by small randomized trials. However, the advantage of randomized trials may be somewhat attenuated when applied to the very difficult task of outpatient dietary interventions. For example, several epidemiologic studies suggest lower cardiovascular morbidity and mortality in populations subsisting on plant-based diets. Seventh Day Adventists who adhere to a vegetarian diet, for example, have a third of the cardiovascular risk found in nonvegetarian Adventists.[18] Although these nonrandomized observational studies may be hampered by confounding variables (e.g., vegan Seventh Day Adventists may demonstrate other healthful behaviors), it is also likely that religious members will adhere to a strict vegetarian diet than will randomized subjects in a controlled trial. Thus, patient nutrition may be one key factor in cardiovascular health that is not easily modified nor well suited for study in randomized trials.

The paucity of outcome data in prospective, controlled nutritional trials has allowed for criticism of general recommendations by some members of the scientific community, as well as continued advocacy of unproven diets by nonscientists, physicians, and others. As is true of most medical recommendations, it is still necessary for physicians to make them based on the data that is available, incomplete as that may be. To do so, the concept of *principio non nocarum* (first do no harm) must be adhered to in order to avoid recommendations that include well-known risks pitted against hypothetical gains.

Diets rich in fruits, vegetables, omega-3 fatty acids, almonds, walnuts, whole grains, and monounsaturated fatty acids are likely to be cardiovascular friendly with little or no downside. Similarly, avoidance or limitation of refined white flour and sugar, saturated animal fat, *trans*-fatty acids, and partially hydrogenated vegetable oils is likely to be valuable. Diets used for weight loss that omit or severely limit all carbohydrates and allow for unlimited saturated fat and animal protein intake have neither an epidemiologic nor a strong observational study-based rationale and should be avoided pending more definitive research. Weight loss appears to be short term only. Whether this dietary approach proves to be an alternative to gastrointestinal surgical procedures for patients with intractable obesity and carbohydrate addiction remains to be evaluated. In general, avoidance of obesity through caloric restriction coupled with exercise is likely to promote cardiovascular health and is a reasonable recommendation. Diets rich in fruits and vegetables and low in sodium are recommended for patients with hypertension, although long-term impact on outcome is unknown despite a demonstrated favorable impact on blood pressure.[19]

Regardless of the diet recommendation, serial monitoring of lipids, triglycerides, and weight is critical, as long-term noncompliance is, unfortunately, the rule, rather than the exception. Individual substrate and metabolic differences between patients as well as nutritional recommendation misinterpretations commonly require additional diet modifications and education. For instance, patients on very-low-fat diets may need to learn about vegetarian protein sources and avoidance of high-glycemic-index foods. Reliance on simple rather than complex carbohydrates may result in weight gain and hypertriglyceridemia; in addition, vegans may require B_{12} and L-carnitine supplementation.

Exercise

An active lifestyle provides significant protection from coronary artery disease. It is estimated that 200,000 deaths in the United States are attributable to a sedentary lifestyle.[20] Exercise capacity, when initially recorded on a treadmill, is inversely related to the future risk of death in patients with known coronary disease. Remarkably, there is evidence that duration on a treadmill provides similar, compelling prognostic information for noncardiac subjects as well. Thus, a person without heart disease but with limited exercise capacity is at the same

high risk of dying as a patient with coronary disease and limited exercise capacity.[21] Conversely, people with an excellent exercise capacity have similar benign outcomes, whether or not the stress test is positive.

There are multiple physiologic effects of exercise that relate to overall improvement in cardiovascular risk. For instance, exercise is intimately related to maintenance of ideal body weight. It is rare for overweight and obese patients to maintain weight loss with dieting alone.[22] Exercise diminishes blood pressure, favorably affects clotting, lightens depression, and is usually associated with other positive lifestyle changes. Although there is some controversy over the effect of exercise on LDL-C, chronic exercise does elevate HDL, although usually to a minimal degree. Other favorable metabolic changes include a shorter postprandial clearance time for atherogenic particles, less central obesity, and lower plasma insulin levels.[23]

The positive impact of exercise on atherosclerosis may transcend its effect on risk factors. Beneficial effects of exercise on coagulation, vascular function, autonomic tone, and inflammation have been reported.[24] In a study involving more than 72,000 women, the risk of coronary events was inversely related to weekly energy expenditure.[25] The benefits of exercise occur in minimally active subjects when compared with sedentary individuals, but there is additional gain from vigorous exercise. In a meta-analysis of 27 studies of exercise and coronary disease prevention, there was a clear association of sedentary lifestyle with increased risk, estimated at 1.8:1. In addition, a "dose-response" relationship existed between amount of exercise and additional benefit.[26] The risk of death from any cause in patients who could not exercise past 5 metabolic equivalents (METS) was approximately double the risk of death in people who could exercise more than 8 METS.[27]

In the Harvard Alumni Study, there was a 20% reduction in coronary disease risk associated with moderate activity levels.[28] Moderate exercise was defined as more than 4,200 kcal per week of walking, cycling, swimming, or yard workout. Exercise exceeding 4,200 kcal/wk is valuable in diminishing the incidence of fatal coronary artery disease in both men and women,[29] and multiple short exercise sessions are just as good as a single long session for diminishing cardiovascular risk.[30] Although the risk of death is reduced in people who exercise regularly, there is a slightly higher risk of death during exercise. This risk is small, and further diminished in people who are accustomed to regular, vigorous exercise.[31] Although numerous studies document the incremental value of higher levels of aerobic exercise, there is a disproportionate increase in survival with minimal exercise when compared to a sedentary lifestyle.[32] Thus, benefits accrue from the metabolic effects of low grade, chronic exercise as well as from more vigorous aerobic training. Regular, low-grade exercise alters carbohydrate and lipid metabolism and is more likely to result in sustained weight loss over time.[33] Small increases in HDL occur within weeks of regular aerobic training, but also occur with low-grade exercise at 6 to 24 months. Other metabolic benefits include favorable changes in LDL particle size and composition, although no change in total LDL occurs. Over time, plasma insulin levels and central obesity also improve.[34]

Explaining the relationship between obesity, fasting glucose and triglyceride determinations and coronary artery disease, St. Pierre et al. noted coronary risk to be significantly higher when abnormal fasting glucose, hypertriglyceridemia, and central obesity were present.[35] The phenomenon of central obesity and high triglycerides has been referred to as the "hypertriglyceridemic waist" phenotype and is associated with the atherogenic, metabolic triad 80% of the time. This triad consists of hyperinsulinemia, hyperapolipoproteinemia B, and small, dense LDL particle production, and is associated with an increased risk of type 2 diabetes and coronary artery disease.[36] While the predisposition to develop this condition may be genetically determined, the clinical manifestations of this syndrome are heavily dependent on lifestyle, especially diet and exercise. As discussed above, numerous studies document change in cardiovascular risk as populations move from one culture to another, usually, but not exclusively, involving moves from an Oriental to Western environment. Of note, low HDL may not be a significant risk factor unless associated with an elevated LDL or the metabolic syndrome.[37] The metabolic syndrome, now involving more than 40% of middle-aged Americans, consists of increased abdominal fat, hypertriglyceridemia, hypertension, low HDL, and insulin resistance. Causes include obesity and sedentary lifestyle acting in concert with genetic predisposition. The metabolic syndrome increases coronary disease risk independently of cholesterol and LDL levels, and is increasing in frequency in the general population.[38]

There is substantial evidence that cardiovascular risk and mortality are favorably influenced by a change in activity level, even in middle age and older persons. Cardiac rehabilitation is also useful in the elderly. General improvement in well being, obesity, exercise capacity, and HDL have been reported with exercise in the elderly, as well as improvement in heart rate variability, a powerful marker of outcome.[39–41] Blair estimated enhanced survival as the result of exercise, stating that "reductions in death rates of 9% to 15.3% could be expected if all nonfit people became fit."[42–43] Unfortunately, maintenance of a long-term exercise program is difficult. Only a small minority of cardiac patients who join rehabilitation programs will continue exercising. It appears sedentary lifestyle, like morbid obesity and many addictions, is essentially an intractable "disease."

Alcohol and Heart Disease

Alcohol is unique among dietary components because of its well-documented cardiovascular benefits as well as its toxicity.[44] Observational and epidemiologic studies demonstrate a strong relationship between alcohol intake and decreased coronary artery disease mortality.[45] The French paradox—relatively less cardiovascular disease than would be predicted based on dietary fat content—has long been attributed to the French penchant for red wine. The validity of this relationship was questioned by Artaud-Wild et al., who found no evidence of a French paradox when coronary disease incidence was compared specifically to dairy fat intake.[46] In general, however, most studies support an inverse relationship between alcohol consumption and coronary artery disease incidence, although the specific advantage of red wine over other alcoholic beverages remains unclear.

Wine intake has been reported to confer 25–35% more coronary disease protection than beer or hard liquor consumption, but other confounding variables may mitigate these findings. Wine drinkers in general appear to have healthier diets and smoke less than beer and hard liquor drinkers.[47] A more recent, comprehensive comparison of the protective value of red wine, white wine, beer, and liquor in more than 38,000 male health care professionals revealed no advantage to any specific type of drink when beverages were normalized for grams of alcohol.[48] These results differed from a report of 129,000 patients receiving benefit only from moderate wine intake (red or white) and not beer or hard liquor.[49] What is clear is that there is a U-shaped curve of cardiovascular (and all-cause) mortality associated with frequency of alcohol intake. Regarding dietary alcohol, it appears that "teetotalers" and heavy drinkers are both at increased risk of dying.

Explanations for alcohol's cardiovascular benefit include diminished clotting capacity and platelet aggregation, higher HDL, diminished inflammation, improved endothelial function, and enhanced antioxidant activity from flavonoids and other substances found in grape juice, skin, and seeds.[50,51] Similar polyphenol antioxidants may be found in green tea and chocolate.

There are many uncontrolled variables in existing epidemiologic studies and sufficient remaining uncertainty to prohibit sweeping recommendations about alcohol use in the general population. This is especially true of a substance with substantial short- and long-term toxicity and potential for abuse and addiction. Alcohol remains a common cofactor in a large percentage of fatal automobile accidents, homicides, and suicides. Long-term use is associated with a host of potentially fatal health conditions, including pancreatitis, liver cirrhosis, encephalopathy, and (possibly) some types of cancer.[52] Even cardiovascular deaths are more frequent with heavy alcohol intake, and derive from cardiomyopathy, hypertension, and hemorrhagic stroke; acute myocardial infarction may be associated with binge drinking. More than two drinks per day is associated with hypertension; cessation of heavy drinking will lower blood pressure even in nonhypertensive subjects.[53] Any recommendations must take into account the fact that as much as 10% of the US population may encounter difficulty controlling alcohol intake at some time in their adult lives. Thus, patients with personal or family histories of alcohol abuse may not be well served by general recommendations to "drink moderately."

It is not yet clear whether there are identifiable subgroups of the population that would most benefit from adding or increasing dietary alcohol.[54] For example, a study by Zairis et al. suggests a long-term benefit of moderate alcohol consumption only for coronary disease patients with elevated C-reactive protein, a marker for intravascular inflammation and a predictor of future coronary events.[55] In the study by Artaud-Wild et al., alcohol use was evaluated, along with saturated fat and dairy intake, for its potential impact on cardiovascular death in a study involving nutritional data from 40 countries.[56] Alcohol may have actually increased the risk of death in countries with the healthiest diets and lowest intrinsic cardiovascular risk. Because elevated C-reactive protein is influenced by diet and other standard risk factors, it is possible that the risk:benefit ratio of alcohol becomes favorable only with high states of oxidative burden. More research is needed to answer the question of whether thin, athletic vegans should abstain from alcohol, while those who regularly eat cheeseburgers are best served by washing them down with an alcoholic beverage.

Despite limited data, Ecker and Klatsky[56a] attempted to address this pragmatically with an algorithm, suggesting that one to three drinks per week for nondrinkers at risk of coronary disease, increasing to one drink per day in people who are older, are at higher risk, or who already drink occasionally. Their suggestion that heavy drinkers limit their intake to two drinks per day may be unrealistic, and abstention with tighter control of risk factors may represent a safer alternative. To date, clarification of the U-shaped curve of overall survival for subgroups of coronary disease patients as well as the general population at risk for coronary disease (and alcoholism) needs to be more thoroughly mapped out before precise recommendations can be made.

Personality and Heart Disease

A number of personality types are associated with an increased incidence of coronary artery disease. The original descriptions of type A personality included a sense of time urgency and aggressive behavior. Friedman and Ulner hypothesized that hyperaggressiveness and free-floating hostility result from an inadequate self-esteem, leading to emotional exhaustion, lack of personal caretaking, abnormal physiology, and, ultimately, coronary events.[57] Although somewhat controversial, most studies have suggested a doubling of cardiovascular risk with type A behavior. So-called type D behavior combines depression, worry, and social isolation, and may increase coronary disease deaths fourfold. Multiple studies have identified social isolation as a risk for increased all-cause mortality. Anxiety by itself may increase sudden death in coronary disease patients, and

major depression may be responsible for a fourfold increase in incidence of cardiac deaths. In a study of 218 patients followed for 18 months after a myocardial infarction, nearly half were found to have moderate or severe depression.[58] Of the 21 deaths occurring in the follow-up period, 18 were among the depressed patients. A number of physiologic changes may occur with anxiety, anger, and depression, including arrhythmias, vasoconstriction, hypertension, platelet aggregation, and plaque rupture. It seems logical, therefore, to aggressively treat anxious or depressed patients at risk for coronary disease, even though there is insufficient evidence that this approach prevents the excess mortality associated with these conditions.

Dietary Supplements and Herbs

There are many allopathic pharmaceuticals used for the treatment of cardiovascular disease that are originally derived from plants.[59] Digoxin, for example, a drug in continuous use for more than 150 years, was originally employed as a tea made from the leaves of the foxglove, or digitalis, plant. This drug has largely been replaced by angiotensin-converting enzyme inhibitors (ACEIs) for the treatment of heart failure, because ACEIs prolong life as well as relieve symptoms. Digoxin still has a role, in combination with ACEIs, in diminishing symptoms and maintaining the patient's improved clinical status. Digoxin is also used for regulating heart rate in atrial fibrillation.

Lovastatin, the first of the "statin" medications that are now the mainstays of pharmaceutical cholesterol lowering, derives from the fungus *Aspergillus terreus*. Lovastatin can also be found naturally in preparations of red rice yeast, an over-the-counter supplement with cholesterol-lowering properties. The statin medications have demonstrated a 20–30% improvement in outcome in both primary and secondary coronary artery disease prevention.

Many common components of plant-based diets have antioxidant or antiinflammatory properties with potential benefit for cardiovascular health. Oxidation of LDL and the inflammatory response to endothelial injury are thought to be major components of the atherosclerotic process. The Mediterranean diet, for example, is commonly thought of as consisting primarily of olive oil, red wine, and fish. In fact, there are many differences between the Mediterranean and Western diets. Purslane (family Portulacaceae), for example, is a dandelion-like vegetable grown in the Middle East. It is a common ingredient in salads, high in vitamin E, and isolated for use as a medicinal herb. In laboratory studies of the sativa variety of *Portulaca oleracea,* significant analgesic and antiinflammatory properties have been identified. This is in addition to studies describing the value of purslane as an anti-spasmodic affecting both skeletal and smooth muscle.[60]

Garlic has been promoted as a valuable food additive for maintenance of cardiovascular health, although its purported ability to lower serum cholesterol has come under question in more recent trials.[61,62] However, there are several other antiatherosclerotic properties that have been documented in a laboratory setting that may have clinical relevance. Several studies show diminished LDL oxidation, lowered plasma fibrinogen, and increased fibrinolytic activity in patients taking garlic supplements.[63,64] Campbell et al. demonstrated the ability to reduce atherosclerosis by more than 64% in a rabbit model, despite the fact that induced hypercholesterolemia did not improve. Using aged garlic extract, both the area of endothelial lipid infiltration and neointimal carotid artery thickening were diminished in the group of hypercholesterolemic rabbits receiving garlic.[65] Despite these promising laboratory findings, there is still controversy based on the clinical studies involving humans regarding the health benefits of garlic.

Among nonnutritive plant components, tea has maintained its special position as a healthful drink dating back to the ancient Far East. Brewed leaves from the *Camellia* species of tea tree are high in polyphenol compounds,

containing large quantities of active flavonoids. Polyphenol compounds are plant-derived substances with a variety of antioxidant and antiinflammatory properties. Prominent among this large group of compounds are the flavonoids, which consist of flavanones, flavones, isoflavones, flavonols, anthrocyanidines and proanthrocyanidines. Included within these subgroupings are catechins and quercetins. Polyphenols counter inflammation through several intracellular mechanisms, including inhibition of leukotrienes, thromboxane A_2, and prostaglandin formation. Additional beneficial effects involve diminished histamine production and reduced platelet activating factor. Because polyphenols are commonly found in many plant-based foods, vegetarianism invariably involves a large polyphenol intake.

Although there are many active components shared equally between green and black tea such as methylxanthines and flavonoids, green tea contains three times more catechins than black tea.[66] Although tea is an abundant source of catechins, they are also found in apples, chocolate, purple grapes, and red wine.[67,68] There are in vitro and animal studies supporting the value of the components of tea for prevention of LDL oxidation, improvement of endothelial function, and as an aid for reducing glucose concentration in diabetes. However, human studies are less clear, and prospective outcome studies do not exist. Based on promising laboratory studies and a low likelihood of harm, it is reasonable to consider tea as a valuable nonnutritive plant source of antioxidants that may have a wide range of health benefits.

A member of the Rosaceae family, hawthorn (*Crataegus oxyacantha*) has been used for a variety of cardiovascular ailments, including mild heart failure, angina, and hypertension.[69] There is supporting laboratory data suggesting hawthorn berries are rich in flavonoids and crataegus acid, and suggesting improved coronary blood flow and inotropism in animals. Beneficial impact on ischemic myocardium is thought to occur because of scavenging of free oxygen radicals.[70] There is some supporting laboratory data suggesting that hawthorn may be valuable as an antiarrhythmic and lipid-lowering agent, but solid human studies are lacking. Several studies in the German literature, including placebo-controlled, double-blinded tests, support the use of hawthorn as effective in the treatment of mildly symptomatic congestive heart failure.[71,72] One study, using a randomized, double-blind, placebo-controlled format, failed to demonstrate benefit in patients with mild symptoms.[73] However, most other studies, virtually all appearing in the German literature, support the use of hawthorn as effective for New York Heart Association (NYHA) class II heart failure. A number of mild adverse side effects have been described (e.g., dizziness and agitation), but hawthorn is generally well tolerated at therapeutic doses.

An additional nonnutritional herb in widespread use is ginkgo biloba. A number of studies have suggested value for ginkgo as a treatment for leg claudication secondary to peripheral vascular disease. The impact on walking time is minimal,[74,75] however, and does not compare favorably with regular exercise. Ginkgo may be useful as an adjunct to exercise in the treatment of claudication, but should not be seen as a substitute for exercise as the mainstay of therapy.

Among supplements, beta-carotene initially held the most promise as a potentially important treatment for the prevention of coronary artery disease. Like vitamins E and C, serum beta-carotene levels were found to be higher in subjects without coronary disease when compared with the serum of coronary artery disease patients. This led to the widespread assumption that supplementing vitamins C, E, and beta-carotene would be useful for both primary and secondary coronary disease prevention. Two randomized trials of beta-carotene supplementation in high-risk patients found no benefit at all. One trial, in fact, found harm from beta-carotene supplementation when given daily. After an average 4 years of follow-up of 18,000 smokers, former smokers, and workers previously exposed to asbestos,

the group randomized to beta-carotene 30 mg/d (and 25,000 IU of vitamin A) had a higher death rate from both lung cancer and cardiovascular disease.[76,77] It has been postulated that daily supplementation with beta-carotene might have the paradoxical effect of producing a relative carotene deficiency by interfering with the absorption of dozens of other naturally occurring carotenoids.[78] Similar studies with vitamin C and E supplementation have failed to show value in prevention of coronary disease despite initially optimistic reports.[79]

Coenzyme Q10 (CoQ10), also known as ubiquinone, is a lipophilic antioxidant and key component of the mitochondrial respiratory chain. Coenzyme Q10 has been proposed as potentially useful in angina, congestive heart failure, hypertension, and hyperlipidemia, and for preservation of myocardial function during heart surgery.

There is some controversy over purported decreases in coenzyme Q10 with the use of statin medications (beta-hydroxy-beta-methylglutaryl [HMG]-coenzyme A reduction inhibitors). More recently, Bleske et al. showed no diminution of CoQ10 as the result of either pravastatin or atorvastatin therapy.[80] Perhaps the most clinically relevant application of CoQ10 is in the area of preservation of myocardial function in the operating room. The myocardium of patients undergoing open-heart surgery who are treated with CoQ10 appear to maintain their aerobic efficiency during reperfusion, have higher adenosine triphosphate levels, and are protected from creatine kinase oxidative inactivation.[81]

The widespread use of CoQ10 for congestive heart failure is logically based on findings of diminished coenzyme in the failing myocardium. Multiple studies appear to support CoQ10 supplementation, but many deficiencies were present in small or scientifically weak publications. To address the lack of solid data, Khatta et al.[82] studied 46 patients in a randomized, double-blind, controlled trial and found no evidence of improved exercise tolerance, aerobic capacity, or left ventricular function with CoQ10 200 mg/d. Although the possibility exists the study dose of 200 mg/d was inadequate, most of the prior studies showing benefit occurred at lower doses. At present, although CoQ10 is a necessary component of healthy cell metabolism, there is little quality evidence suggesting supplementation is a valuable treatment for heart failure, and nothing to suggest outcomes are improved. This is an area that could benefit from additional well-done research studies, perhaps at higher doses of CoQ10.

Folic acid, in combination with vitamins B_6 and B_{12}, has emerged as a potentially valuable compound for the prevention and treatment of atherosclerosis.[83] Folic acid appears to be important for the regulation of homocysteine, an amino acid associated with thrombosis and atherosclerosis.[84] Previously, only very high levels of homocysteine were thought to be related to coronary disease. More recent data suggests levels as low as 12 μmol/L may increase the risk of vascular disease. In addition to vitamin B_6, B_{12}, and folic acid deficiencies, a number of conditions may contribute to hyperhomocystinemia, including inherited metabolic disorders, renal failure, hypothyroidism, and psoriasis.[84] Of interest, cholestyramine, niacin, and fibric acid derivatives, commonly used to treat high cholesterol, can also cause hyperhomocystinemia. Homocystinemia levels increase with age and are higher in men and postmenopausal women. Smoking and coffee intake are both associated with higher homocysteine levels.

Although there appears to be a continuous (rather than threshold) relationship between homocysteine levels and vascular disease, some authors have questioned whether high homocysteine levels are simply associated with vascular disease and represent a disease marker only. A number of other compounds may lower homocysteine levels, including betaine, choline, and penicillamine. The American Heart Association has stated that there is insufficient outcome data to recommend routine homocysteine testing and treatment, except in very-high-risk patients. However, treatment with B

vitamins and folate supplementation is relatively benign and fairly inexpensive, and can be covered adequately with a standard multivitamin pill. While this course of supplementation may yet be proven unnecessary after more definitive studies are completed, it is unlikely to be proven harmful, and is a reasonable recommendation for patients at risk.

Vitamin E supplementation has long been advocated for cardiovascular health. Initial observational studies appeared to confirm the value of this antioxidant vitamin both in men and women.[85,86] However, prospective, randomized trials failed to demonstrate diminished cardiovascular or all-cause mortality,[87] or improvement in atherosclerosis assessed by serial carotid ultrasonograph studies. At present, while there is laboratory evidence of the potential importance of vitamin E as an antioxidant, the current status of clinical studies does not support its use as a supplement.

Despite the continued, passionate advocacy of supplements for cardiovascular disease treatment and prevention, Willett and Stampfer[88] recommend only a daily multivitamin that does not exceed FDA dosage limitations. It is clear that much good outcomes research has yet to be done to clarify observational studies and initial, encouraging laboratory reports about many supplements and neutraceuticals. Unfortunately, numerous epidemiologic and observational studies are "contaminated" by multiple simultaneous healthful lifestyle changes that frequently appear together in patients who do not have coronary artery disease. As with the evaluation of any drug or intervention, the concept of *principio non nocarum* should govern patient recommendations.

Although not commonly viewed as an herb or a supplement, *theobroma cacao* contains a number of cardiovascular relevant compounds worthy of exploration. Theobroma translates to "food of the Gods," an apt name for chocolate, originally used by priests and royalty in Aztec Mesoamerica. The cacao bean contains a number of polyphenol antioxidants and other compounds active against reactive oxygen species.

The polyphenols present in chocolate are similar to those in red wine and tea, and are more concentrated in dark chocolate. Forty grams of chocolate is estimated to contain the equivalent antioxidant content of 10 servings of fruit and vegetables. Among the 300 or so compounds found in chocolate are substances that inhibit platelet aggregation, stimulate endorphin release, elevate serotonin levels, and improve mood. Whether these benefits outweigh the downsides of high saturated fat and high calorie content plus sugar and milk additives remains to be determined.[89,90]

The Healthy Mindset: Effective Implementation of Lifestyle Change

When applied to cardiovascular disease, preventive medicine in Western society is a concept most people accept, few people practice, and almost no one pays for. Despite the fact that coronary disease can often be detected years or even decades before the onset of symptoms, most of the $200 billion annual price tag is spent on the treatment of symptomatic disease and end-organ failure, with little resources allotted to screening and prevention.

Unfortunately, the reliance on therapeutic rather than preventive strategies fosters a "magic bullet" mentality in the West. For example, many patients believe taking statin medication obviates the need for careful nutrition and caloric reduction. Patients may not alter sedentary lifestyle or diet, but simply add medications, fiber, alcohol, olive oil, duck pâté, or a host of supplements in the mistaken belief that they are now completely protected regardless of lifestyle choices. It is clear that no single strategy, medication, or intervention provides a guarantee for the complete avoidance of negative cardiac events. The combination of multiple preventive strategies probably affords the best primary and secondary preventions of coronary disease.

In a survey of nearly 85,000 female nurses, initially free of cardiovascular disease, the risk of developing type 2 diabetes mellitus was assessed prospectively.[91] A low-risk group of women was identified who did not smoke, had a body mass index less than 25, performed 30 minutes of moderate to vigorous exercise daily, consumed a diet high in fiber and polyunsaturated fat and low in *trans*-fatty acids and high glycemic index foods, and averaged half an alcoholic drink per day. This "ideal" group had only a fifth of the cardiovascular disease that developed in the rest of the nurses; however, fewer than 1 in 20 nurses qualified for the "ideal" group. Body mass index was most closely related to the development of diabetes, a major risk factor for cardiovascular disease, with nearly a 40-fold increased incidence among the most obese subjects. Although more research data is needed in this area, it appears likely that those patient who embrace the full spectrum of lifestyle changes are most likely to have less morbidity and mortality in the long run.

Hennekens[92] has suggested the potential benefit of modifying risk factors on cardiovascular outcome includes a 20–30% improvement with cholesterol lowering, 15–20% improvement with blood pressure control, 50–70% with cessation of cigarette smoking, 35–55% with normalization of obesity, and 35–55% with increased physical activity. Thus, patients who develop a healthy mindset that encompasses control of all modifiable cardiovascular risk factors and compliance with antihypertensive and cholesterol-lowering medications have an excellent chance of radically altering their outcome. For most stable coronary disease patients, these estimates of improved outcomes cannot be currently matched (or even approached) by invasive techniques or medications alone.

It appears that a healthy mindset and the ability to permanently modify behavior is relatively uncommon yet exceedingly important. At present enormous sums of money are being spent to conquer a largely behavioral disease using pharmacology, surgery, catheterization-based interventions, and genetic engineering.

This paradox is brought home by Jonas and Eaton who estimated that if just 10% of adults started a regular walking program, $5.6 billion would be saved annually.[93]

▶ SUMMARY OF RECOMMENDATIONS

Acute coronary syndromes should be evaluated urgently, preferably in an emergency room. These syndromes are manifested by a change in frequency or duration of angina, the occurrence of new angina or chest pain at rest, and unexplained shortness of breath, syncope, or diaphoresis in a patient at risk. Those patients with suspected unstable angina or acute myocardial infarction should undergo coronary angiography (unless there are mitigating circumstances) with an eye toward stenting or coronary artery bypass grafting as indicated. Misguided searches for dietary, supplemental, or alternative therapeutic options in the acute setting may cost valuable time and myocardium.

Patients with stable chronic coronary artery disease should be evaluated with laboratory and noninvasive testing to stratify risk and understand the need for further invasive testing. Coronary disease patients, even those with severe three vessel or left main obstruction, may have minimal symptoms despite evidence of severe and extensive myocardial ischemia on stress testing. Prognosis correlates well with laboratory evidence of severe ischemia, even in the absence of symptoms. Laboratory evidence of severe disease suggests the need for coronary angiography even without chest pain. This is especially important in patients with minimal discomfort, as coronary disease is frequently silent, and patients, unfortunately, present with myocardial infarction and death as the first symptom in an alarmingly high percentage of cases.

Patients with chronic coronary disease but without evidence of severe ischemia should be treated with lifestyle modification and medication. To date, catheter-based coronary interventions, including elective stenting, in patients with stable coronary syndromes, do not favorably change outcome in this group of patients. The algorithm of therapy might change with the introduction of coated stents.

▶ **TABLE 18-1** INTERVENTIONS WITH GOOD EVIDENCE FOR IMPROVED OUTCOME

Angiotensin-converting enzyme inhibitors and beta-blockers for secondary prevention
Avoidance of saturated fat derived from animal and dairy products
Avoidance of *trans*-fatty acids and partially hydrogenated vegetable oils
Beta blockers
Control of hypertension
Coronary artery bypass surgery (selected patients)
Inclusion of foods rich in omega-3 fatty acids in diet
Inclusion of fruits, vegetables, and legumes in diet
Low-dose aspirin for secondary prevention or as primary prevention for moderate to high risk
   patients
Regular aerobic exercise
Regular low-grade exercise
Smoking cessation
Statin medications and other lipid-lowering drugs for primary and secondary prevention
   (e.g., high-dose niacin)
Weight loss in overweight and obese patients

▶ **TABLE 18–2** INTERVENTIONS THAT ARE LIKELY TO BE VALUABLE
AND PROBABLY IMPACT OUTCOME

Alcohol intake (½ to 2 drinks/day)
Coated intracoronary stents
Enhanced external counterpulsation (EECP)
Folic acid, B_6, B_{12} supplements for the treatment of hyperhomocysteinemia
Increased fruits and vegetables
Low salt diet for hypertension
Medical therapy of depression and anxiety (e.g., selective serotonin reuptake inhibitors)
Multiple, simultaneous lifestyle interventions (vegetarianism, very-low-fat diet, relaxation therapy,
 and measures aimed at improving social isolation and depression)
Treatment of psychologic risk factors with cognitive therapy, group support, relaxation therapy
Vegetarianism
Vitamin E supplementation

People at risk of developing cardiovascular disease, which includes most people in the United States, should embrace a lifestyle that is likely to delay or avoid the development of atherosclerosis. Medications for high blood pressure and high cholesterol should be added if the patient does not succeed using lifestyle modification. Medications should be a first-line choice if blood pressure and cholesterol are very elevated. It is understood that new research will add to existing recommendations and replace others with outcome based data. Tables 18–1, 18–2, and 18–3 summarize the available interventions for prevention and treatment of stable coronary heart disease.

▶ **TABLE 18–3** TREATMENTS THAT MAY
(OR MAY NOT) IMPACT ON OUTCOME

Chocolate
Heart failure supplements (hawthorn,
 coenzyme Q10)
Supplementation with L-carnitine, L-arginine
Supplementation with magnesium, garlic,
 lecithin, phosphatidyl choline, other
 phytonutrient supplementation
 (isoflavones, polyphenols)

REFERENCES

1. Myers J. Exercise and cardiovascular health. *Circulation*. 2003;107(1):e2–e5.
2. Robertson TL, Katz H, Rhoeds GG, et al. Epidemiologic studies of coronary heart disease and stroke in Japanese men living in Japan, Hawaii, and California. Incidence of myocardial infarction and death from coronary heart disease. *Am J Cardiol*. 1977;39:239–249.
3. Worth RM, Katz H, Rhoads GG, Kagan K, Syme SL. Epidemiologic studies of coronary heart disease and stroke in Japanese men living in Japan, Hawaii and California: mortality. *Am J Epidemiol*. 1975;102(6):481–490.
4. Williams B. Westernized Asians and cardiovascular disease: nature or nurture? *Lancet*. 1995;345(8947):401–402.
5. Ornish Dean. Personal communication.
6. Watts GF, Lewis B, Brunt JN, et al. Effects on coronary artery disease of lipid-lowering diet, or diet plus cholestyramine, in the St. Thomas' Atherosclerosis Regression Study (STARS). *Lancet* 1992;339:563–569.
7. Leren P. The Oslo diet-heart study: eleven-year report. *Circulation*. 1870;42:935–942.
8. Hunninghake DB, Stein EA, Dujovne CA, et al. The efficiency of intensive dietary therapy alone or combined with lovastatin in outpatients with hypercholesterolemia. *N Engl J Med*. 1993;328:1213–1219.
9. Stefanick ML, Mackey S, Sheehan M, et al. Effects of diet and exercise in men and postmenopausal

women with low levels of HDL cholesterol and levels of LDL cholesterol. *N Engl J Med.* 1998; 339:12–20.

10. Ornish D, Brown SE, Schwerwitz LW, et al. Can lifestyle changes reverse coronary heart disease? The Lifestyle Heart Trial. *Lancet.* 1990;336: 129–133.

11. Sdringola S, Nakagawa K, Nakagawa Y, et al. Combined intense lifestyles and pharmacologic lipid treatment further reduce coronary events and myocardial perfusion abnormalities compared to usual care cholesterol lowering drugs in coronary artery disease. *J Am Coll Cardiol.* 2003;41(2):263.

12. de Lorgeril M, Renaud S, Mamelle N, et al. Mediterranean alpha-linolenic acid-rich diet in secondary prevention of coronary heart disease. *Lancet.* 1994;343:145–149.

13. de Lorgeril M, Salen P, Monjand I, Delaye J. The diet heart hypothesis in secondary prevention of coronary heart disease. *Eur Heart J.* 1997;18: 14–18.

14. de Lorgeril M, Salen P, Martin JL, Monjand I, Delaye J, Mamelle N. Mediterranean diet traditional risk factors and the rate of cardiovascular complications after myocardial infarctions. Final report of the Lyon Diet Heart Study. *Circulation.* 1999;99:779–785.

15. Yancy WS, Westinar EC, French PA. Califf run diets and clinical coronary events—the truth is out there. *Circulation.* 2003;107:10–16.

16. Leaf A. Dietary prevention of coronary heart disease–the Lyon Diet Heart Study. *Circulation.* 1999;99:733–735.

17. Ornish D, Scherwitz LW, Billings JH, et al. Intensive lifestyle changes for reversal of coronary heart disease. *JAMA.* 1998;280:2001–2007.

18. Phillips RL, Lemon FR, Beeson WL, Kuzma JW. Coronary heart disease mortality among Seventh-Day Adventists with differing dietary habits: a preliminary report. *Am J Clin Nutr.* 1978;10 suppl: 5191–5198.

19. Sacks FM, Svetkey LP, Vollmar WM, et al. Effects on blood pressure of reduced dietary sodium and the dietary approaches to stop hypertension (DASH) diet. *N Engl J Med.* 2001;344:3–10.

20. Paffenberger RS, Hyde RT, Wing AL, et al. The association of changes in physical activity level and other lifestyle characteristics with mortality among men. *N Engl J Med.* 1993;328:538–545.

21. Myers J, Prakash M, Froelicher V, et al. Exercise capacity and mortality among men referred for exercise testing. *N Engl J Med.* 2002;346(11): 793–801.

22. Byers T. Body weight and mortality. *N Engl J Med.* 1995;333:723–724.

23. Manson JE, Hu FB, Rich-Edwards JW, et al. A prospective study of walking as compared with vigorous exercise in the prevention of coronary heart disease in women. *N Engl J Med.* 1999;341: 650–658.

24. Balady GJ. Survival of the fittest—more evidence. *N Engl J Med.* 2002;346:832–833.

25. Hu FB, Stampfer MJ, Manson JE, et al. Trends in the incidence of coronary heart disease and changes in diet and lifestyle in women. *N Engl J Med.* 2000;343:530–537.

26. Berlin JA, Colditz GA. A meta-analysis of physical activity in the prevention of coronary heart disease. *Am J Epidemiol.* 1990;132:612–628.

27. Blair SN, Kohl HW 3rd, Paffenbarger RS Jr, et al. Physical fitness and all-cause mortality. A prospective study in healthy men and women. *JAMA.* 1989;262(17):2395–2401.

28. Sesso HD, Paffenberger RS, Lee I. Physical activity and coronary heart disease in men: the Harvard Alumni Health Study. *Circulation.* 2000; 102(9):975–980.

29. Oguma Y, Sesso HD, Paffenberger RS JR, Lee I. Physical activity and all cause mortality in women. *Br J Sports Med.* 2002;36(3):162–172.

30. Lee I, Sessio HD, Paffenberger RS. Physical activity and coronary heart disease risk in men: does the duration of exercise episodes predict risk? *Circulation.* 2000;102(9):981–986.

31. US Public Health Service, Office of the Surgeon General. *Physical Activity and Health: A Report of the Surgeon General.* Atlanta, GA: US Department of Health and Human Services, Centers for Disease Control and Prevention, National Center for Chronic Disease Prevention and Health Promotion; 1996.

32. Berlin JA, Colditz GA. A meta-analysis of physical activity in the prevention of coronary heart disease. *Am J Epidemiol.* 1990;132:612–628.

33. Fletcher GF, Balady, Amsterdam EA, et al. Exercise standards for testing and training: a statement for healthcare professionals from the American Heart Association. *Circulation.* 2001;104: 1694–1740.

34. Fletcher GF, Balady GJ, Amsterdam EA, et al. Exercise standards for testing and training: a state-

ment for healthcare professionals from the American Heart Association. *Circulation*. 2001;104:1694–1740.

35. St-Pierre J, Lemieux I, Vohl MC, et al. Contribution of abnormal obesity and hypertriglyceridemia to impaired fasting glucose and coronary artery disease. *Am J Cardiol*. 2002;90(1):15–18.

36. Lamarch B, Tehernof A, Moorjani S, et al. Small, dense low-density lipoprotein particles as a predictor of the risk of ischemic heart disease in men. Prospective results from the Quebec Cardiovascular Study. *Circulation*. 1997;95:69–75.

37. Lemieux I, Despres JP, Cantin B, et al. Low HDL-cholesterol without the metabolic risk is not predictive of an increased CHD risk? Evidence from the Quebec Cardiovascular Study. *Diabetes*. 2002;51 (suppl 2):A9.

38. Expert panel on Detection, Evaluation and Treatment of High Blood Cholesterol in Adults. Executive Summary of the Third Report of The National Cholesterol Education Program (NCEP). Expert Panel on Detection, Evaluation, and Treatment of High Blood Cholesterol in Adults (Adult Treatment Panel III). *JAMA*. 2001;285:2486–2497.

39. Lavie CJ, Milani RV, Littman AB. Benefits of cardiac rehabilitation and exercise training in secondary coronary prevention in the elderly. *J Am Coll Cardiol*. 1993;22:678–683.

40. Stable A, Mattsson E, Ryder L, et al. Improved physical fitness and quality of life training of elderly patients after acute coronary events—a one-year followup randomized controlled study. *Eur Heart J*. 1999;20:1475–1484.

41. Stahle A, Nordlander R, Bergfeldt L. Aerobic group training improves exercise capacity and heart rate variability in elderly patients with a recent coronary event. A randomized controlled study. *Eur Heart J*. 1999;20:1638–1646.

42. Blair SN, Kohl HW 3rd, Barlow CE, et al. Changes in physical fitness and all-cause mortality. A prospective study of healthy and unhealthy men. *JAMA*. 1995;123:52–53.

43. Blair SN, Kampert JB, Kohl HW 3rd, et al. Influences of cardiorespiratory fitness and other precursors on cardiovascular disease and all-cause mortality in men and women. *JAMA*. 1996;276:205–210.

44. Renaud S, de Lorgeril M. Wine, alcohol, platelets and the French paradox for coronary heart disease. *Lancet*. 1992;339:1523–1526.

45. Klatsky A, Friedman GD, Siegelaub AB. Alcohol consumption before myocardial infarction. Results from the Kaiser-Permanente epidemiologic study of myocardial infarction. *Ann Intern Med*. 1974;81(3):294–301.

46. Artaud-Wild SM, Conner SL, Sexton G, Conner WE. Differences in coronary mortality can be explained by differences in cholesterol and saturated fat intakes in 40 countries but not in France or England. *Circulation*. 1993;88(6):2771–2779.

47. Klatsky A. Drink to your health? *Sci Am*. 2003;288(2):74–81.

48. Mukamal K, Conigrave K, Mittleman M, et al. Roles of drinking pattern and type of alcohol consumed in coronary heart disease in men. *N Engl J Med*. 2003;348(2):109–118.

49. Klatsky A, Friedman G, Armstrong MA, Kipp H. Wine, liquor, beer and coronary heart disease mortality. *Circulation*. 2002;supp. A3602:106–119.

50. Goldberg IJ, Mosca L, Piano MR, Fisher EA. Wine and your heart: a science advisory for healthcare professionals from the Nutrition Committee, Council on Epidemiology and Prevention, and Council on Cardiovascular Nursing of the American Heart Association. *Circulation*. 2001;103:472–475.

51. Friedman JE, Parker C III, Li L, et al. Select flavonoids and whole juice from purple grapes inhibit platelet function and enhance nitric acid release. *Circulation*. 2001;103:2792–2798.

52. Klatsky A. Drink to your health? *Sci Am*. 2003;288(2):74–81.

53. Muntwyler J, Hennekens CH, Buring JE, Gaziano JM. Mortality and light to moderate alcohol consumption after myocardial infarction (Physicians Health Study). *Lancet*. 1998;352:1882–1885.

54. Goldberg IJ. To drink or not to drink? *N Engl J Med*. 2003;348(2):163–164.

55. Zairis MN, Papadaki O, Lyras A, et al. Inflammatory status and moderate alcohol consumption, results from the GENERATION study. *Circulation*. 2002;106:19.

56. Artaud-Wild SM, Conner SL, Sexton G, Conner WE. Differences in coronary mortality can be explained by differences in cholesterol and saturated fat intakes in 40 countries but not in France or England. *Circulation*. 1993;88(6):2771–2779.

56a. Ecker RR, Klatsky AL. Doctor, should I have a drink? An algorithm for health professionals. *Ann NY Acad Sci*. 2002;957:317–320.

57. Price VA, Friedman M, Ghandour G, Fleisch-mann N. Relationship between insecurity and Type A behavior. *Am Heart J.* 1995;129(3): 488–491.

58. Frasure-Smith N, Lesperance F, Talajic M. Coronary heart disease/myocardial infarction: Depression and 18 month prognosis after myocardial infarction. *Circulation.* 1995;91:999–1005.

59. DeSinet PAGM. The role of plant-devised drugs and herbal medicine in healthcare. *Drugs.* 1997; 54(6):802–840.

60. Chan K, Islam MW, Karmil M, et al. The analgesic and anti-inflammatory effects of *Portulaca oleracea* L. subsp. *Satriva* (Haw.) *Calak.* *J Ethnopharmacol.* 2000;73:445–451.

61. Neil HAW, Silegy CA, Lancaster T, et al. Garlic powder in the treatment of moderate hyperlipidaemia: a controlled trial and meta analysis. *J R Coll Physicians Lond.* 1996;30:329–334.

62. Simons LA, Balasubramaniam S, Von Konigsmar KM, et al. On the effect of garlic on plasma lipids and lipoproteins in mild hypercholesterolemia atherosclerosis. 1995;113:219–225.

63. Bordia AH, Jostii HK, Sanadhya YK, Bhu N. Effect of essential oil of garlic on serum fibrinolytic activity in patients with coronary artery disease. *Atherosclerosis.* 1977;28:155–159.

64. Campbell JH, Campbell GR. Heparin-sulfate degrading enzymes induce modulation of smooth muscle phenotype. *Exp Cell Res.* 1992;200: 156–167.

65. Campbell JH, Efendyr JL, Smith NJ, Campbell GR. Molecular basis by which garlic suppresses atherosclerosis. *J Nutr.* 2001;131:10065–10095.

66. Difresne CJ, Farnworth ER. A review of latest research findings on the health promotion properties of tea. *J Nutr Biochem.* 2001;12:404–421.

67. Arts IC, Hollman PCH, Kromhout D. Chocolate as a source of tea flavonoids. *Lancet.* 1999; 354(9177):488.

68. Hollman PCH, Hertog MGL, Katan MB. Analysis and health effects of flavonoids. *Food Chem.* 1996;57:43–46.

69. Miller AL. Botanical influences on cardiovascular disease. *Altern Med Rev.* 1998;3:432–441.

70. Rigelsky JM. Hawthorn: pharmacology and therapeutic uses. *Am J Health Syst Pharm.* 2000;59(5): 417–422.

71. Schmidt U, Kuhn U, Ploch M, et al. Efficacy of the hawthorn abstract LI 132 (600 mg/d) during eight weeks' treatment [German]. *Munch Med Wocensehr.* 1994;132:513–519.

72. Weikl VA, Assimus KD, Neukum-Schmidt A, et al. Objective confirmation of the efficacy of a special Crataegus WS 1442 in patients with cardiac insufficiency (NYHA II) [German]. *Fortschr Med.* 1996;114:291–296.

73. Bodigheimer K, Chase D. Effectiveness of hawthorn extract at a dosage of 3 × 100 mgs per day. Multicentre double-blind trial with 85 NYHA stage II heart failure patients [German]. *Munch Med Wochenschr.* 1994;136:51–61.

74. Kleignen J, Knipschild P. Ginkgo biloba. *Lancet.* 1992;340:1136–1139.

75. Ernst E. Ginkgo biloba in der Behandlung der Claudicatio intermittens cine systematische Recherche anhand Kontroliester Studien in der Literatur. *Fortschr Med.* 1996;114:85–87.

76. Omenn GS, Goodman GE, Thornquist MD, et al. Effects of a combination of beta carotene and vitamin A on lung cancer and cardiovascular disease. *N Engl J Med.* 1996;334(18): 1150–1155.

77. Hennekens, CH, Buring JE, Manson JE, et al. Lack of effect of long-term supplementation with beta carotene on the incidence of malignant neoplasms and cardiovascular disease. *N Engl J Med.* 1996;334(18):1145–1149.

78. DeSinet PAGM. Current health status of beta carotene supplementation. *Int Pharm J.* 1996;10: 213–214.

79. Yusuf S, Dagenais G, Pogue J, et al. Vitamin E supplementation and cardiovascular events in high-risk patients. The Heart Outcomes Prevention Evaluation Study Investigators. *N Engl J Med.* 2000;342:154–160.

80. Bleske BE, Willis RA, Anthony M, et al. The effect of pravastatin and atorvastatin on coenzyme Q10. *Am Heart J.* 2001;142(2):E2.

81. Crestanello JA, Kamelgard J, Lingle DM, Mortenson SA, Rhode M, Whitman GJR. Elucidation of a tripartite mechanism underlying the improvement in cardiac tolerance to ischemia by coenzyme Q10 pretreatment. *J Thorac Cardiovasc Surg.* 1996;111(2):443–450.

82. Khatta M, Alexander BS, Krichten CM, et al. The effect of coenzyme Q10 in patients with congestive heart failure. *Ann Intern Med.* 2000;132(8): 636–640.

83. Topol EJ. *Textbook of Cardiovascular Medicine.*

2nd ed. Baltimore, MD: Lippincott Williams and Wilkins; 2002:200–204.

84. Leshadri N, Robinson K. Homocysteine, B vitamins, and coronary artery disease. *Med Clin North Am.* 2000;84:215–237.

85. Stampfer MJ, Hennekens GH, Manson JE, et al. Vitamin E consumption and the risk of coronary disease in women. *N Engl J Med.* 1993;328: 1444–1449.

86. Rimm EB, Stampfer MJ, Ascherio A, et al. Vitamin E consumption and the risk of coronary heart disease in men. *N Engl J Med.* 1993;328: 145–156.

87. Yusef S, Dagenais G, Pogue J, et al. Vitamin E supplementation and cardiovascular events in high-risk patients. The Heart Outcomes Prevention Evaluation Study Investigators. *N Engl J Med.* 2000;342:154–160.

88. Willett WC, Stampfer MJ. Clinical Practice. What vitamins should I be taking doctor? *N Engl J Med.* 2001;345:1819–1824.

89. Weisburger JH Chemopreventive effects of cocoa polyphenols on chronic diseases. *Exp Biol Med.* 2001;226(10):891–897.

90. Lee R, Balick MJ. Chocolate: healing "food of the Gods?" *Alternat Ther Health Med.* 2001;7(5): 120–122.

91. Hu FB, Stampfer MJ, Manson JE, et al. Trends in the incidence of coronary heart disease and changes in diet and lifestyle in women. *N Engl J Med.* 2000;343:530–537.

92. Hennikens CH. Antioxidant vitamins and cardiovascular disease: Current and future directions. Presentation. Alternative Medicine: Implications for clinical practice. Harvard Medical School Department of Continuing Medical Education. 1999, Boston, MA.

93. Jonas TF, Eaton CB. Cost-benefit analysis of walking to prevent coronary heart disease. *Arch Fam Med.* 1994;3:703–710.

CHAPTER 19

Integrative Approach to Chronic Fatigue Syndrome

BETSY B. SINGH, SIVARAMA P. VINJAMURY, AND VIJAY J. SINGH

Chronic fatigue syndrome (CFS) refers to a pattern of symptoms not attributable to other diseases or illnesses. Onset of CFS is generally reported as insidious and is characterized by a severe fog-like fatigue that may be reported to "come and go" or may begin and not end for months at a time.[1] The fatigue factor of CFS is not relieved by rest or sleep and results in reduction of occupational, social, or personal activities. To make the diagnosis of CFS, symptoms must have been persistent for 6 months or more, be of recent onset, and not secondary to environmental stressors.[2] The diagnosis of CFS is made primarily via history and clinical examination and requires the presence of four or more of the following symptoms: impaired short-term memory; sore throat; tender cervical or axillary lymph nodes; muscle pain; multijoint pain; headaches of a new type, pattern, or severity; nonrefreshing sleep; or malaise lasting more than 24 hours poststrenuous exertion.[3]

While there is a specific range of symptoms related to the syndrome, there is no clear etiological basis for the disorder. No abnormal neurological or physical findings are generally reported. Thus, CFS is a diagnosis of exclusion. It is also a subjective and relativistic diagnosis

in the sense that the symptoms presented suggest an ongoing illness without the presence of readily identifiable disease-related factors.

▶ PATHOPHYSIOLOGY

A definitive understanding of the cause or causes of CFS has not yet been established.[1] Likewise, epidemiological studies have not consistently identified common presentation factors or patterns. However, a variety of potential causal links have been investigated, including viral or bacterial infection, immune dysregulation, dysautonomia, and neuroendocrine dysfunction. Many CFS researchers now suspect that this condition may ultimately be caused by multiple triggers in genetically, environmentally, or otherwise susceptible individuals.[5,6] The major factors implicated to date in the pathogenesis of CFS are outlined below.

Infection

Direct and indirect evidence points to the involvement of active viral (Epstein-Barr virus and/or human herpesvirus 6) or bacterial infections *(Chlamydia pneumoniae)* in the development of CFS. For quite some time, Epstein-Barr virus in particular was believed to play a causative role; however, a single agent has not yet been found in all CFS patients that can be recognized as a marker.[7,8] This suggests that infection may be a contributing trigger but not a definitive cause per se. The usefulness of testing for the presence of these infectious agents in CFS patients has not been established.

Immune Dysregulation

A number of abnormalities are often found in immune function in patients with CFS, including increased natural killer cell activity, increased number of activated T cells, decreased lymphocyte stimulation, and increased production of some proinflammatory cytokines.[8] The presence of these abnormalities is not diagnostic, and the exact role of these changes in the pathophysiology of CFS remains unclear; some authors speculate that CFS represents a state in which the immune system is in a chronic state of upregulation, but not functioning effectively, and that the increase in inflammatory mediators resulting from this activation is the cause of many of the symptoms of the condition.

Another intriguing area of recent research into pathophysiology is the potential role of ribonuclease (RNase) L levels in pathogenesis. RNase L fights infection by degrading viral RNA. Because CFS patients have been found to have a new low molecular weight (37 kDa) form of this enzyme and low levels of normal RNase L (80 kDa), it has been proposed that dysfunction in the 2–5A synthetase RNase L antiviral pathway may be a predisposing factor in CFS. The presence of this abnormal enzyme in other diseases and whether it can serve as a marker for CFS are currently being studied.[9]

Dysautonomia

Studies at Johns Hopkins University show that a low blood volume, abnormal sympathetic tone, and neurological dysfunction cause orthostatic intolerance (hypotension with change of posture associated with nausea and giddiness) in CFS patients. Further research is underway to understand the role of autonomic nervous system dysfunction in CFS.[10,11]

Neuroendocrine Dysfunction

Abnormalities evident on single-photon emission computed tomography (SPECT) scans of the brain show perfusion deficiencies in the lateral frontal and temporal regions in many patients with CFS. This may be an important finding because the latest evidence seems to indicate that the memory and concentration deficits are independent of any depression experienced by CFS patients, and thus may represent a discrete manifestation of neurological dysfunction. A study that examined the serotonergic activation of the hypothalamic–pituitary–adrenal (HPA) axis also found a possibly deficient function in this area in CFS patients.[12] One additional study of neurotransmitter function found an increased prolactin response to buspirone in CFS patients; this finding may indicate abnormal function in the dopaminergic system.[13] As implied by the serotonin study,[12] many investigators now feel that there may be a dysfunction of the HPA stress axis in patients with CFS and fibromyalgia syndrome.[14] Low circulating cortisol levels have been found in some patients with CFS, and in some patients may be linked to abnormally small adrenal glands.[12] As in the studies examining the relationship between CFS and depression, it is difficult to determine whether the adrenal dysfunction present in some patients is the cause of CFS or the result of a chronic illness.

Genetic Disorders

The isolation and discovery in patients with CFS of autoantibodies to lamin B-1—a component of the cellular structure—has created more interest in an autoimmune explanation of CFS.[15] Further research is needed on the role of autoimmunity in the pathogenesis of CFS.

▶ PREVALENCE AND NATURAL HISTORY

The reported prevalence of CFS is influenced by the case definitions used, the patient's self-report of symptoms, physician assessment, population demographics, and the relationship of the symptoms to other more common disorders. Currently, data does not support a socioeconomic explanation of the presentation of CFS; patients come from all socioeconomic strata. CFS generally occurs in young adults, with a peak onset between 20 and 40 years of age, and is found more commonly in women.[16] The prevalence of CFS in the general community is roughly 0.2–0.7%; the prevalence in the primary care setting is 0.5–2.5%, depending on the case definition used. There are multiple case definitions found in the published literature: CDC 1988, Australia 1990, Oxford 1991, and CDC 1994. The CDC 1994 definition is the most widely used; however, different studies have used different definitions, making the distinctions between the definitions of some importance.[3,17–20] Table 19–1 outlines these definitions.

The condition known as myalgic encephalomyelitis (ME), which was given a specific case definition only 12 years ago,[21] shares much of the symptom profile of CFS. Before this case definition became available to help distinguish ME from CFS, it is likely that persons with either condition were considered to have the same syndrome. Factors common to both ME and CFS, which contributed to the initial difficulty in differential diagnosis, were similar fatigue presentations and presence of neurological and cognitive problems. However, ME is more likely to be precipitated by a respiratory or gastrointestinal infection; symptoms may be more dramatic if onset follows a neurological, cardiac, or endocrine problem presentation. Uses of differential case definitions and confusion with other disease entities contribute to the wide range of data reported on prevalence, etiology, and pathophysiology of CFS.[22]

It is important to note that despite the developing science in this area, there remain many skeptics in the medical community who continue to believe that CFS, ME, and other similar syndromes are not physiologic in origin, but are a result of utilization of poor coping strategies by patients. One psychiatrist has compared CFS to neurasthenia, a psychiatric diagnosis of the late nineteenth century.[23] However, in a recent in-depth study of 15 females with CFS, investigators found that the coping mechanisms that were employed by patients were similar to those of patients with other chronic illnesses. The implication of this finding is that the psychological symptoms that frequently accompany CFS may be an effect of the illness, rather than its cause, as is often suggested. Rather than finding dysthymia or panic disorder, which are associated with CFS by some, the investigators found obsessional and healthy neurotic defense levels operating and an improvement in symptoms with increased social support. Physician validation was considered important along with maintenance of relationships with family, friends, and participation in spiritual activities in order to maintain hope for continued improvement.[24] Thus skeptical physicians can do harm to patients who are doing their best to cope with the symptoms of CFS.

A number of other studies have examined the link between CFS and psychiatric conditions. In a prospective study of concurrent psychiatric conditions in 405 patients who came to an academic medical center with CFS,

▶ **TABLE 19–1** CRITERIA FOR CASE DEFINITIONS OF CFS

Case Definitions of CFS	Criteria
US Centers for Disease Control (CDC) 1988	6 months of devastating persistent and relapsing fatigue Functional activity—50% decrease in activity 6 or 8 symptoms required; physical signs sometimes required Neuropsychiatric symptoms may be present New onset required Exclusions: any preexisting organic or psychiatric disease, bipolar disorder, and substance abuse
US Centers for Disease Control and Prevention (CDC) 1994	6 months' duration of persisting fatigue Substantial reduction of previous levels of occupational, social, or personal activities 4 or more of the following symptoms required and have persisted for at least 6 months; impairment in memory, pharyngitis, painful cervical and axillary lymph nodes, muscle weakness and joint pain without inflammation, sleep disturbances Exclusions: hypothyroidism, chronic hepatitis B or C, tumors, certain depression, substance abuse, bipolar disorder, psychosis, eating disorders, and obesity
Australia 1990	6 months' duration of persisting fatigue Substantial functional impairment—commotion of daily activities Postphysical exertion fatigue No symptoms specified Cognitive or neuropsychiatric symptoms required New onset not required Exclusions: known physical causes, psychosis, bipolar disorder, substance abuse, eating disorders
United Kingdom 1991 "Oxford Criteria"	6 months' duration of persisting fatigue Functional impairment—affects physical and mental normal functioning No symptoms specified Cognitive or neuropsychiatric symptoms may be present Definite onset required Exclusions: known physical causes, psychosis, bipolar disorder, eating disorder, organic brain disease, substance abuse Other psychiatric disorders (depressive illness, anxiety disorders) are not reasons for exclusion

depression was the most common psychiatric disorder (58%), with panic disorder diagnosed in an additional 14%. Somatization disorder was diagnosed in 10% of the patients. Sleep disorders were found in 2% of the patients. Seventy-eight percent of the CFS patients in total received a psychiatric diagnosis. The investigators concluded that patients meeting the criteria for CFS are likely to have mood, anxiety, or somatoform disorders.[25] The challenge as always is to determine to what degree the psychiatric condition is a result of the chronic illness of CFS, and to what degree it is the primary explanation for the symptoms. This distinction is often impossible to make clearly in clinical practice.

▶ Case Example: Chronic Fatigue Syndrome

A 45-year-old woman presented with symptoms of tiredness, fatigue, nonrefreshing sleep, poor concentration and loss of memory, and musculoskeletal pain for more than 6 months. She said her symptoms did not improve after rest and often her fatigue exacerbated with relatively minor physical or mental activity. She tried over-the-counter painkillers and sleep aids in addition to multivitamins, but nothing helped her. These symptoms resulted in substantial reduction in her day-to-day activities, both at home and at work. On examination, no abnormal physical or mental findings were found clinically. Laboratory investigations such as complete blood cell count, thyroid function tests, liver function tests, erythrocytic sedimentation rate, serum electrolytes, and routine urinalysis were done to exclude other disorders before diagnosing the condition as CFS. She seemed frustrated with her fatigue and its impact on her life but did not exhibit signs of clinical depression, hence a referral for a psychological work-up seemed premature.

Conventional Treatment

Appropriate conventional treatment includes medical, psychological, and social support. To date, no pharmacologic agent has been discovered that provides a "cure" for CFS or a period of time when the patient is completely symptom free. As many persons with CFS report drug sensitivities similar to patients with fibromyalgia, pharmacological interventions can often produce additional problems as a consequence of side effects. Nevertheless, conventional drug therapies can be helpful to some patients with CFS.

Even though clinical trials do not show consistent benefit from antidepressant therapy, in practice some patients do benefit from their use. Selective serotonin reuptake inhibitors, tricyclic antidepressants, and nefazodone have all been used for treatment of CFS-associated depression, for muscle and joint pain, and for the sleep problems that often accompany CFS.[26,27] In one antidepressant trial, overall improvement was noted for participants receiving antidepressant therapy with phenelzine, along with improved vigor.[28] Some patients report improvement in subjective perception of energy and functional ability through the use of moclobemide.[29] Nonsteroidal antiinflammatory drugs and other over-the-counter analgesics are often self-prescribed by CFS patients, and physicians should be aware of the potential for gastrointestinal complications related to these medications if they are overused.

A number of other conventional medications have been studied for treatment of CFS, although none are currently in widespread use. Glucocorticoid therapy[30] helps to reduce reported fatigue in certain CFS patients. A clinical study of the relationship between CFS and 5-HT$_3$ receptor antagonists found pronounced improvement for patients treated with tropisetron (Navoban [Novartis]).[31]

Ampligen is a synthetic nucleic acid product that stimulates the production of interferons, and appears to be a biological response modifier with both antiviral and immuno-modulatory activity. Preliminary studies show moderate benefit in physical performance and cognition in three separate clinical trials without any evidence of significant toxicities. The Food and Drug Administration (FDA) to date has not approved Ampligen for widespread use, and its administration in CFS patients is currently investigational/experimental.[32]

Conventional treatment also includes referral to local social service agencies when inability to work and the consequent lifestyle changes that occur impact the patient and family. Patients may also have high school or college studies disrupted. In a trial comparing social support using a buddy system versus a wait-list control, participants in the social support group experienced significantly greater improvement than did those who did not receive support.[33]

The role of exercise in CFS is controversial. Some researchers report that exercise can be potentially damaging,[34] leading to increased impairment in cognitive functions, delayed recovery from exercise, and shortened endurance time. Other studies have found exercise, particularly mild and carefully graded exercise, to be beneficial for patients with CFS.[35,36]

A variety of exercise interventions, some graded, have been tested against a variety of comparison groups such as flexibility/relaxation, standard care, or placebo groupings. In general, the graded exercise studies found significant improvement on overall improvement measures and fatigue. At least one study indicated greater improvement on wellness scores in the exercise-intervention group than in the comparison group.[36]

Normal exercise programs may sometimes provoke a relapse in CFS patients,[37] so activity must be very carefully graded, extremely gentle, and aimed toward improving function. There is also some evidence that excessive rest can be detrimental to CFS patients; thus, it is important to address this question of how to incorporate exercise to prevent the deterioration that apparently can accompany a completely sedentary lifestyle in the patient with CFS.[38]

Integrative Strategies

Research into complementary/alternative treatment strategies for CFS to date is limited and is generally insufficient for a consensus. Because of this, clinical decision-making in this area is challenging and must incorporate a number of factors in addition to the available published evidence, including success of therapies used by the patient previously, patient preferences, and physician knowledge and experience in treating CFS. Although it has not been adequately studied to date, the role of a supportive, open-minded physician willing to consider a wide variety of treatment options for CFS is considered by many patients a critical factor in their recovery. Many CFS patients have a history of very negative experiences with the conventional health care system. In one study, CFS patients reported receiving insufficient information about their disorder and inadequate emotional support from physicians. Many reported turning to alternative or complementary forms of treatment as a result. The most commonly reported difficulties in communication with physicians were regarding etiology and treatment options for CFS.[39] The most widely used complementary and alternative care medicine therapies for CFS are summarized below.

Manipulative Medicine

Although data on manipulative approaches to CFS are somewhat limited, in clinical practice these approaches can be invaluable. There is some preliminary data for several approaches worth mentioning. A study comparing massage therapy to a sham transcutaneous electrical nerve stimulation treatment for CFS showed significant improvement in fatigue, sleep, and myalgia in patients receiving massage therapy.[40] Another study of 80 patients compared osteopathic manipulation to routine care for CFS and found that overall improvement scores were significantly higher for persons receiving osteopathic treatment.[41] The relevance of these findings is limited by the fact that this trial was not randomized or blinded and that the dropout rate was quite high (28%).

Chiropractic approaches to CFS have not been extensively studied. Farinelli reported promising results in a pilot study of patients receiving a program of nutritional and herbal supplements in conjunction with a specific protocol of adjustments at C1-C2. The author reports that this group of patients had reported complete relief of symptoms even after 6 months.[42] Similar studies on the effect of chiropractic care on patients diagnosed with CFS are underway at other centers.[43] The hypothesis informing the use of manipulation in CFS is that somatovisceral reflexes involving the cervical spine, in particular, may play a role in the autonomic dysfunction often seen in CFS; consequently, adjustment of the spine can play a role in alleviating CFS symptoms. It should be stressed that research on manipulative approaches to CFS is very preliminary and hypothesis-generating only at this point.

Mind–Body Therapies

Mind–body interventions, which include cognitive behavior therapy (CBT) and relaxation or meditation practices, show a great deal of promise in CFS. Although many of these studies have been conducted in combination with other interventions, making it more difficult to determine the source of change, CBT appears to be the most promising approach. In general, CBT as a primary investigative therapy has reduced fatigue and improved overall quality of life in a number of studies.[44] One randomized controlled trial (RCT) ($n = 278$) of CBT versus no treatment and CBT versus guided support, found improvement in physical function and measures of impairment and mental health for those in the CBT group over the 8-month period of the trial.[45] A second, nonblinded RCT comparing CBT to counseling ($n = 45$), found no differences.[46] A third study, an RCT ($n = 60$) comparing CBT to relaxation, found no difference in depression scores, but the CBT group was significantly improved on the factors of physical functioning, impairment/impact, social functioning, and occupational functioning.[47]

In a combined study of CBT and medical care versus medical care only, the combination showed significant improvement in activity level, impairment/impact, and depression, but did not show any difference in anxiety levels.[48]

Research to date has not delineated a specific number of sessions or duration of CBT treatment to recommend to CFS patients.[44] The goal of CBT is not quick relief of symptoms; maximization of capacity to problem solve in daily life and live as functionally as possible is the goal of the treatment approach. Attitudes, beliefs, and behaviors that may have inhibited recovery or optimum function are identified. Then, physical, medical, and behavioral changes may be begun at an individualized pace that will keep the patient moving forward toward maximization of quality of life. As the patient begins to grapple with the changes required for living a fuller life, recognizing each progressive step as a victory born of their cognitive and behavioral efforts, the patient will begin to live at a higher level of function than believed possible before CBT was begun. It is important to remember that learning how to think and behave differently are therapeutic changes that a patient can carry with them at all times and continue to grow in their use even after formal CBT has been terminated.

Homeopathy

At least one randomized trial comparing individually selected homeopathic remedies to placebo has been conducted. Each group had 32 patients; the trial was double-blind and had a 5% dropout rate. The homeopathic remedies were selected based on the symptoms of the patients. Findings indicate a significant improvement in patients receiving the active product.[49] Geraghty described three case studies on chronic fatigue syndrome following a viral infection in young people in which patients were treated with Cobaltum Phosphoricum, Calcium Phosphoricum, and Cadmium Phosphoricum.[50] All three fully recovered following this treatment.

Nutritional Support

Deficiencies of many common vitamins and essential nutrients are common in CFS patients. In addition, some investigators believe that patients with CFS may have a defect in cellular energy production and/or a risk of decreased vitamin utilization. Studies reveal that vitamins B_6, B_{12}, C, and E, Coenzyme Q10, essential fatty acids, L-carnitine, L-glutamine, magnesium, zinc, and folic acid are deficient in most CFS patients.[51]

Essential Fatty Acid Supplementation

It has been widely believed that dysfunctional changes in essential fatty acid metabolism are a major cause for hyper- and hyporesponsiveness in immune function in CFS. However, a recent trial conducted by Warren[52] calls this belief into question. In this study, 50 patients who fulfilled the Oxford Criteria for CFS were randomly allocated to treatment with either Efamol Marine (an omega-3 essential fatty acid supplement) or placebo for 3 months. At the end of 3 months, investigators reported that although the symptoms of CFS generally improved with time, this improvement was not significant, and there were no significant differences between the treatment and placebo groups. This finding is in sharp contrast to an earlier, often-quoted study of fish oil supplementation[53] in which 85% of patients had a clinically significant improvement of symptoms.

Magnesium

Although the role of magnesium in the pathogenesis of CFS is controversial, at least one study has shown magnesium supplementation to be beneficial for patients with CFS. This could be because of an increased oxidative stress in severe magnesium deficiency causing exacerbation of the chronic inflammatory state in patients with CFS. Studies are underway to understand the mechanism and role of magnesium in CFS.[54]

Coenzyme Q10

Coenzyme Q10 (CoQ10) plays a critical role in cellular respiration and has been found to be deficient in many CFS patients.[55,56] A study by Judy et al.[57] reported that 90% of clinical symptoms disappeared after CoQ10 100 mg daily was given for 3 months. Interestingly, this study reported that 85% of patients on CoQ10 had decreased postexercise fatigue.

L-Carnitine

L-Carnitine deficiency can be associated with impaired mitochondrial function.[58] Studies indicate that a decrease in free serum carnitine level is common in CFS patients and can be correlated with symptom severity. However the results in clinical trials are equivocal; only one-third of these patients responded dramatically to 3–4 g of oral supplementation per day.[59]

Folic Acid

Folic acid supplementation has been tried with the assumption that serum folic acid deficiency in CFS patients could cause cerebrospinal fluid folate deficiency that may contribute to fatigue, mental depression, and immunosuppression in these patients. However, small dosages (800 μg) for a short duration (1 week) resulted in no positive effects in a double-blind crossover trial conducted in a small sample.[60] In another study, large doses as high as 10,000 μg of folate produced satisfactory results in a group of patients after 2–3 months of folate supplementation.[61] More research is needed to determine the exact dose and role of folic acid in CFS

Vitamin B_{12}

As with folic acid, there is insufficient scientific data to substantiate the efficacy of vitamin B_{12} in CFS patients.[62] Some informal observations made by Lapp and Cheney while treating their patients indicate a mixed response in 2,000 patients when vitamin B_{12} 2,500–5,000 μg was given every 2 or 3 days for 2–3 weeks. In clinical practice, regular B_{12} supplementation remains a widely used treatment; many CFS patients report a short-lived, but substantial, improvement in energy level with regular B$_{12}$ injections.[63]

Other Nutrients

Brailey and Lord[64] report that 75% of chronic fatigue symptoms resolved when 15 g/d of a wide range of free-form amino acids was given to CFS patients for 3 months.

Nicotinamide adenine dinucleotide (reduced form) appears potentially helpful as well, with at least one trial demonstrating a better overall symptom improvement score in subjects supplemented with 10 mg daily than in controls.[65]

L-Tryptophan, zinc, sodium, and vitamin C are other commonly used nutrients that some clinicians believe are helpful in reducing CFS symptoms for some patients. Further research is needed on these nutrients and their role in CFS.[66]

Dietary Manipulation

Dietary manipulation is often used as an approach to CFS symptoms. One survey to analyze the dietary intake and selected nutrient concentrations in patients with chronic fatigue syndrome reported that 54% of a sample of CFS patients attempted unspecified dietary changes on their own and that 73% of these people found that the dietary changes reduced their fatigue.[67] Meydani reported that the release of inflammatory cytokines might be reduced by eliminating food intolerances through dietary modifications.[68]

Wheat and milk and preservatives such as benzoates, nitrites, nitrates, food colorings, and other additives have caused food intolerance in CFS patients and studies show that their elimination results in a reported decrease in the severity of symptoms.[69] Organically grown dietary fruits and vegetables are preferable so as to avoid unnecessary exposure to pesticides, which may cause food intolerance and might also potentially tax the body's detoxification systems, which may already be abnormally stressed in patients with CFS. Despite lack of

direct evidence, alcohol, sugars, and caffeine are believed to cause exacerbation of CFS symptoms,[70] and patients are often advised to avoid these substances because of their possibly deleterious effects on immune function and on the HPA axis.

Botanical/Herbal Treatments

Herbal approaches to CFS have not been extensively studied to date. Evening primrose oil, *Echinacea*, ginkgo biloba, ginseng, St. John's wort, licorice, and blueberries are commonly used substances and might be beneficial in alleviating the CFS symptoms. To date, however, none of these has been adequately studied for a specific role in treatment of CFS.

Ginkgo biloba is a powerful antioxidant and has the capacity to improve cerebral blood flow, memory, and cognition deficits caused by cerebral insufficiency.[71,72] Blueberries have the highest oxygen radical absorbance capacity among many fruits and vegetables; because of this, some clinicians believe that blueberries may have a significant role in treating the symptoms of CFS through antioxidant activity. Panax ginseng is a tonic and adaptogenic herbal that stimulates hypothalamic output and adrenocorticotrophic hormone and hence adrenal cortex function, thereby increasing stamina.[73,74] *Echinacea angustifolia* and *Echinacea purpurea* are used to enhance phagocytic activity in order to improve antigen recognition, which may lead to better immune responsiveness.[75] *Cordyceps sinensis, Rhodeola rosea,* and Siberian ginseng (*Eleuthero senticosus*) are botanicals with adaptogenic qualities and are often used as supportive treatment in CFS as well.

Hypericum perforatum (St. John's wort) is used in CFS for its dual role of antiviral and antidepressant effects.[76] This herb improves cognitive function for some patients who are depressed,[77] and may be helpful with the concentration and "brain fog" symptoms characteristic of CFS. Nevertheless, to date, studies assessing the specific role of St. John's wort in CFS are not available.

Licorice supplementation on a regular basis has been shown to help CFS sufferers, particularly those with orthostatic intolerance. This benefit is probably mediated by the effect of licorice on blood pressure and fluid retention.[78,79]

Acupuncture/Chinese Medicine

There is not enough scientific literature to definitively support the role of traditional Chinese medicine (TCM) in CFS. Traditionally, CFS is treated as a liver and Qi stagnation and spleen and Qi deficiency in TCM. Cheung et al.,[80] in a case series, observed that the combination of acupuncture and TCM formulas was beneficial in reducing many of the symptoms of CFS. The study reports a 100% reduction in symptoms such as fatigue, insomnia, and headache at the end of 1 month. These researchers used CDC 1994 criteria for diagnosis and selection of cases and compared them with TCM diagnosis liver and Qi stagnation and spleen and Qi deficiency. The researchers in this case series used Gui Pi Tang as the base formula and added other herbs to the combination based on the symptom profile of each patient. For sore throat, Huang qin and Jie geng were added; for depression, Chai hu was added; for headache, Bai zhi was added; and for joint aches, Du huo and Fang feng were added. The herbal prescription was taken three times per day. Acupuncture was administered three times per week, and three sets of acupoints were used alternately. The total duration of the trial was 4 weeks.

Ayurveda

Chronic fatigue syndrome is treated in Ayurveda, traditional Indian medicine, as predominantly an imbalance of *vata* with some minor changes in the *pitta* levels. Ashwagandha* *(Withania somnifera),* which has been studied for its adaptogenic and immunomodulatory action, is often recommended for patients with CFS. In one study, using a mouse model of chronic fatigue, herbal preparations found effective were *Withania somnifera* root extract, BR-16A® (an ayurvedic formula made up of Brahmi, Ashwagandha, Bach, Giloe, Amla, Shankhapushpi), and Siotone® granules (another ayurvedic formula containing Ashwagandha, Kapikachchhu, Gokshura, Shatavari, and Silajit). All the three preparations were found to be "compared favorably" to conventional anti-depressant drugs such as imipramine, desipramine, tranylcypromine, alprazolam, mianserin, idazoxan, and fluoxetine in their effectiveness.[81] An interesting case study conducted at the Raj Medical Center in Iowa, described total remission of CFS symptoms after a combination of internal cleansing, external oil, and herbal treatments.[82]

Yoga

Yoga postures, pranayama, relaxation, and meditation are powerful tools for helping CFS patients. It is believed that yoga's gentle, restorative poses increase circulation and oxygen flow, soothing the mind without irritating the body. One survey of a group of 150 patients with chronic fatigue asked them to list all of the interventions they were using for their fatigue—from the alternative to the conventional, including physical activity and pharmaceuticals.[83] Two years later, the same patients were asked to name the treatment that had helped them most. The preliminary findings indicated that yoga appeared to help the CFS patients more than any other treatment. Although there are no well-designed research studies on the effect of yoga in CFS, anecdotal evidence indicates a role for yoga in CFS.

---

*Ashwagandha is the Sanskrit name for *Withania somnifera* in Latin. Sanskrit is the language used in the Ayurvedic system

▶ Case Example: Chronic Fatigue Syndrome Conclusions

It is important for the physician caring for a patient with CFS to make an attempt to build a relationship with the patient based on an understanding of the impact of the diagnosis on the patient and a willingness to assist the patient in problem-solving in day-to-day life. Management of pain and management of covarying symptoms, such as gastrointestinal problems and unrestful sleep, must be pursued over the long term to give the patient the best quality of life. It is also very important for physicians to help patients develop realistic expectations for their outcome. As "cure" is not what is anticipated, the physician should discuss with patients what their current expectation is for normal function, and determine if it is realistic in the short term or whether it might be more appropriate as a goal to work toward. The ideal physician will partner with patients to reach these goals, making referrals to other practitioners when necessary.

An integrative strategy, a blending of conventional and alternative options, seems the most efficient way to manage this patient's physical and mental fatigue. She has had this health problem less than a year and has not tried many prescription drugs. However, her suffering has caused significant frustration, and lack of motivation and interest in her activities. The line of treatment must focus on reducing her physical fatigue, as well as assisting her with coping strategies, while she realigns her personal activity expectations with her current levels of function. At first, a symptomatic treatment with antidepressants or analgesics must be considered. Later, emphasis on nutritional deficiencies and diet must be given a priority because she may have been neglecting proper food intake because of her pain, fatigue, and altered mood state secondary to her condition. Prescription drugs, over-the-counter preparations, and lifestyle support must be offered to optimize outcome.

Both the patient and the family should receive support in making a transition to a lifestyle that will allow the patient to maximize his or her contributions to family and society without making the patient feel guilty or depressed over slowed or temporarily disrupted progress toward previously established goals. Both personal and family psychological support may be required to create an atmosphere in which the patient can adjust goals without a feeling of failure or disappointment. Where available, a support group for the patient and for the family may assist both in reaching a better understanding of the syndrome and in learning coping skills from others who have experienced the same struggles.

REFERENCES

1. Holmes GP. Defining the chronic fatigue syndrome. *Rev Infect Dis.* 1991;13(suppl 1):S53–S55.
2. Fukuda K, Straus S, Hickie I, et al. The chronic fatigue syndrome: a comprehensive approach to its definition and study. International Chronic Fatigue Syndrome Study Group. *Ann Intern Med.* 1994;121(12):953–959.
3. Sharpe MC, Archard LC, Banatvala JE, et al. Chronic fatigue syndrome: guidelines for research. *J R Soc Med.* 1991;84:118–121.
4. Komaroff AL, Buchwald DS. Chronic fatigue syndrome: an update. *Annu Rev Med.* 1998;49:1–13.
5. Farrar DJ, Locke SE, Kantrowitz FG. Chronic fatigue syndrome. 1: Etiology and pathogenesis. *Behav Med.* 1995;21(1):5–16.
6. Evengard B, Klimas N. Chronic fatigue syndrome:

probable pathogenesis and possible treatments. *Drugs.* 2002;62(17):2433–2446.

7. Yamanishi K. Chronic fatigue syndrome and virus infection: human herpesvirus 6 (HHV-6) infection. *Nippon Rinsho.* 1992;50(11):2612–2616.

8. Hassan IS, Bannister BA, Akbar A, Weir W, Bofill M. A study of the immunology of the chronic fatigue syndrome: correlation of immunologic parameters to health dysfunction. *Clin Immunol Immunopathol.* 1998;87(1):60–67.

9. Suhadolnik RJ, Reichenbach NL, Hitzges P, et al. Changes in the 2-5A synthetase/RNase L antiviral pathway in a controlled clinical trial with poly(I)-poly(C12U) in chronic fatigue syndrome. *In Vivo.* 1994;8(4):599–604.

10. Bou-Holaigah I, Rowe PC, Kan J, Calkins H. The relationship between neurally mediated hypotension and the chronic fatigue syndrome. *JAMA.* 1995;274:961–967.

11. Streeten DH, Thomas D, Bell DS. The roles of orthostatic hypotension, orthostatic tachycardia, and subnormal erythrocyte volume in the pathogenesis of the chronic fatigue syndrome. *Am J Med Sci.* 2000;320(1):1–8.

12. Parker AJ, Wessely S, Cleare AJ. The neuroendocrinology of chronic fatigue syndrome and fibromyalgia. *Psychol Med.* 2001;31(8):1331–1345.

13. Sharpe M, Clements A, Hawton K, Young AH, Sargent P, Cowen PJ. Increased prolactin response to buspirone in chronic fatigue syndrome. *J Affect Disord.* 1996;41(1):71–76.

14. Gaab J, Huster D, Peisen R, et al. Hypothalamic–pituitary–adrenal axis reactivity in chronic fatigue syndrome and health under psychological, physiological, and pharmacological stimulation. *Psychosom Med.* 2002;64(6):951–962.

15. Konstantinov K, von Mikecz A, Buchwald D, Jones J, Gerace L, Tan EM. Autoantibodies to nuclear envelope antigens in chronic fatigue syndrome. *J Clin Invest.* 1996;98(8):1888–1896.

16. Salztein BJ, Wyshak G, Hubbuch JT, Perry JC. A naturalistic study of the chronic fatigue syndrome among women in primary care. *Gen Hosp Psychiatry.* 1998;20(5):307–316.

17. Manu P, Lane TJ, Matthews DA. Chronic fatigue and chronic fatigue syndrome: clinical epidemiology and aetiological classification. *Ciba Found Symp.* 1993;173:23–31(discussion 31–42).

18. Holmes GP, Kaplan JE, Gantz NM, et al. Chronic fatigue syndrome: a working case definition. *Ann Intern Med.* 1988;108:387–389.

19. Fukuda K, Straus SE, Hickie I, et al. The Chronic fatigue syndrome: a comprehensive approach to its definition and study. *Ann Intern Med.* 1999; 121(12):953–959.

20. Lloyd AR, Hickie I, Boughton CR, Spencer O, Wakefield D. Prevalence of chronic fatigue syndrome in an Australian population. *Med J Aust.* 1990;153:522–528.

21. Dowsett EG, Goudsmit E, Macintyre A, Shepherd C, et al., London criteria for M.E. In: *Report from The National Task Force on Chronic Fatigue Syndrome (CFS), Post Viral Fatigue Syndrome (PVFS), Myalgic Encephalomyelitis (ME).* Bristol, UK: Westcare; 1994:96–98.

22. Dowsett EG, Ramsay AM, McCartney RA, Bell EJ. Myalgic encephalomyelitis (M.E.)—a persistent enteroviral infection? *Postgrad Med J.* 1990;66: 526–530.

23. Deale A. Neurasthenia in young women. *Am J Obstet.* 1894;29:190–195 (cited in Wessely S, Hotopf M, Sharpe M. *Chronic Fatigue and Its Syndromes.* Oxford: Oxford University Press; 1999:105).

24. Wessely S, Chalder T, Hirsch S, Wallace P, Wright D. The prevalence and morbidity of chronic fatigue and chronic fatigue syndrome: a prospective primary care study. *Am J Public Health.* 1997; 87:1449–1455.

25. Wessely S, Nimnuan C, Sharpe M. Functional somatic syndromes: one or many? *Lancet.* 1999, 354(9182):936–939.

26. Goodnick PJ, Sandoval R. Psychotropic treatment of chronic fatigue syndrome and related disorders. *J Clin Psychiatry.* 1993;54:13–20.

27. Hickie I. Nefazodone for patients with chronic fatigue syndrome. *Aust N Z J Psychiatry.* 1999; 33(2):278–280.

28. Natelson BH, Cheu J, Pareja J, Ellis SP, Policastro T, Findley TW. Randomized, double-blind, controlled placebo-phase in trial of low-dose phenelzine in the chronic fatigue syndrome. *Psychopharmacol (Berl).* 1996;124:226–30.

29. Hickie IB, Wilson AJ, Wright JM, Bennett BK, Wakefield D, Lloyd AR. A randomized, double-blind placebo-controlled trial of moclobemide in

patients with chronic fatigue syndrome. *J Clin Psychiatry.* 2000;61(9):643–648.

30. McKenzie R, O'Fallon A, Dale J, et al. Low-dose hydrocortisone for treatment of chronic fatigue syndrome: a randomized controlled trial. *JAMA.* 1998;280(12):1061–1066.

31. Spath M, Welzel D, Farber L. Treatment of chronic fatigue syndrome with 5-HT$_3$ receptor antagonists—preliminary results. *Scand J Rheumatol Suppl.* 2000;113:72–77.

32. Strayer DR, Carter WA, Brodsky I, et al. A controlled clinical trial with a specifically configured RNA drug, poly(I).poly(C12U), in chronic fatigue syndrome. *Clin Infect Dis.* 1994;18(suppl 1): S88–S95.

33. Shlaes JL, Jason LA. A buddy/mentor program for PWCs. *CFIDS Chronicle.* 1996;Winter:21–25.

34. Paul L, Wood L, Behan WM, Maclaren WM. Demonstration of delayed recovery from fatiguing exercise in chronic fatigue syndrome. *Eur J Neurol.* 1999;6(1):63–69.

35. Fulcher KY, White PD. Randomized controlled trial of graded exercise in patients with the chronic fatigue syndrome. *BMJ.* 1997;314(7095): 1647–1652.

36. Powell P, Bentall RP, Nye FJ, Edwards RH. Randomised controlled trial of patient education to encourage graded exercise in chronic fatigue syndrome. *BMJ.* 2001;322(7283):387–390.

37. Ohashi K, Yamamoto Y, Natelson BH. Activity rhythm degrades after strenuous exercise in chronic fatigue syndrome. *Physiol Behav.* 2002;77(1):39–44.

38. Silver A, Haeney M, Vijayadurai P, Wilks D, Pattrick M, Main CJ. The role of fear of physical movement and activity in chronic fatigue syndrome. *J Psychosom Res.* 2002;52(6): 485–493.

39. Deale A, Wessely S. Patients' perceptions of medical care in chronic fatigue syndrome. *Soc Sci Med.* 2001;52(12):1859–1864.

40. Field TM, Sunshine W, Hernandez-Reif M, et al. Massage therapy effects on depression and somatic symptoms in chronic fatigue syndrome. *J Chronic Fatigue Syndr.* 1997;3:43–51.

41. Perrin RN, Edwards J, Hartley P. An evaluation of the effectiveness of osteopathic treatment on symptoms associated with myalgic encephalomyelitis. A preliminary report. *J Med Eng Technol.* 1998;22:1–13.

42. Farinelli E. Effective treatment for chronic fatigue syndrome case studies of 70 patients. Proceedings of the International Conference on Spinal Manipulation; March, 1989:259–263.

43. Gerow G, Poierier MB, Alt R. Chronic fatigue syndrome. *J Manipulative Physiol Ther.* 1992;15(8): 529–535.

44. Price JR, Couper J. Cognitive behaviour therapy for adults with chronic fatigue syndrome. *Cochrane Database Syst Rev.* 2000(2):CD001027.

45. Prins JB, Bleijenberg G, Bazelmans E, et al. Cognitive behaviour therapy for chronic fatigue syndrome: a multicentre randomised controlled trial. *Lancet.* 2001;357(9259):841–847.

46. Ridsdale L, Godfrey E, Chalder T, et al. Chronic fatigue in general practice: is counselling as good as cognitive behaviour therapy? A UK randomised trial. *Br J Gen Pract.* 2001;51(462):19–24.

47. Deale A, Chalder T, Marks I, Wessely S. Cognitive-behavior therapy for chronic fatigue syndrome: a randomized controlled trial. *Am J Psychiatry.* 1997;154(3):408–414.

48. Sharpe M, Hawton K, Simkin S, et al. Cognitive behaviour therapy for the chronic fatigue syndrome: a randomized controlled trial. *BMJ.* 1996;312(7022):22–26.

49. Awdry R. Homeopathy and chronic fatigue—the search for proof. *Int J Altern Complement Med.* 1996;14:12–16.

50. Geraghty J. Homeopathic treatment of chronic fatigue syndrome: three case studies using Jan Scholten's methodology. *Homeopathy.* 2002;91(2): 99–105.

51. Werbach MR. Nutritional strategies for treating chronic fatigue syndrome. *Altern Med Rev.* 2000; 5(2):93–108.

52. Warren G, McKendrick M, Peet M. The role of essential fatty acids in chronic fatigue syndrome. A case-controlled study of red-cell membrane essential fatty acids (EFA) and a placebo-controlled treatment study with high dose of EFA. *Acta Neurol Scand.* 1999;99(2):112–116.

53. Behan PO, Behan WM, Horrobin D. Effect of high doses of essential fatty acids on the postviral fatigue syndrome. *Acta Neurol Scand.* 1990; 82(3):209–216.

54. Haward JM, Davies S, Hunisett A. Magnesium and chronic fatigue syndrome. *Lancet.* 1992; 340:426.

55. Kwong LK, Kamzalov S, Rebrin I, et al. Effects

of coenzyme Q(10) administration on its tissue concentrations, mitochondrial oxidant generation, and oxidative stress in the rat. *Free Radic Biol Med.* 2002;33(5):627–638.

56. Lapp CW. Chronic fatigue syndrome is a real disease. *N C Fam Physician.* 1992;43(1):6–11.

57. Judy W. Southeastern Institute of Biomedical Research, Bradenton, Florida; Presentation to the 37th Annual Meeting, American College of Nutrition; October 13, 1996. In: Werbach MR. Nutritional strategies for treating chronic fatigue syndrome. *Altern Med Rev* 2000 Apr;5(2):93–108.

58. Plioplys AV, Plioplys S. Serum levels of carnitine in chronic fatigue syndrome: clinical correlates. *Neuropsychobiology.* 1995;32(3):132–138.

59. Plioplys AV, Plioplys S. Amantadine and L-carnitine treatment of chronic fatigue syndrome. *Neuropsychobiology.* 1997;35(1):16–23.

60. Kaslow JE, Rucker L, Onishi R. Liver extract-folic acid-cyanocobalamin vs placebo for chronic fatigue syndrome. *Arch Intern Med.* 1989;149(11):2501–2503.

61. Botez MI, Botez T, Leveille J, et al. Neuropsychological correlates of folic acid deficiency: facts and hypotheses. In: Botes MI, Reynolds EH, eds. *Folic Acid in Neurology, Psychiatry, and Internal Medicine.* New York: Raven Press; 1979:435–461.

62. Heap LC, Peters TJ, Wessely S. Vitamin B status in patients with chronic fatigue syndrome. *J R Soc Med.* 1999;92(4):183–185.

63. Lapp CW, Cheney PR. The rationale for using high-dose cobalamin (vitamin B_{12}). *CFIDS Chronicle Physicians Forum.* 1993;Fall:19–20.

64. Brailey JA, Lord RS. Treatment of chronic fatigue syndrome with specific amino acid supplementation. *J Appl Nutr.* 1994;46:4–8.

65. Forsyth LM, Preuss HG, MacDowell AL, Chiazze L Jr, Birkmayer GD, Bellanti JA. Therapeutic effects of oral NADH on the symptoms of patients with chronic fatigue syndrome. *Ann Allergy Asthma Immunol.* 1999;82(2):185–191.

66. Vassallo CM, Feldman E, Peto T, Castell L, Sharpley AL, Cowen PJ. Decreased tryptophan availability but normal postsynaptic 5-HT2c receptor sensitivity in chronic fatigue syndrome. *Psychol Med.* 2001;31(4):585–591.

67. Nisenbaum R, Jones A, Jones J, Reeves W. Longitudinal analysis of symptoms reported by patients with chronic fatigue syndrome. *Ann Epidemiol.* 2000;10(7):458.

68. Meydani SN. Dietary modulation of cytokine production and biologic functions. *Nutr Rev.* 1990; 48(10):361–369.

69. Manu P, Matthews DA, Lane TJ. Food intolerance in patients with chronic fatigue. *Int J Eat Disord.* 1993;13:203–209.

70. Emms TM, Robers TK, Butt HL, et al. Food intolerance in chronic fatigue syndrome. Presented at the American Association for Chronic Fatigue Syndrome Conference [abstract no. 15]. January 2001; Seattle, WA.

71. Rigney S, Kimber S, Hindmarch I. The effect of acute doses of standardized ginkgo biloba extract on memory and psychomotor performance in volunteers. *Phytotherapy Res.* 1999;13:408–415.

72. Solomon PR, Adams F, Silver A, Zimmer J, DeVeaux R. Ginkgo for memory enhancement: a randomized control trial. *JAMA.* 2002;288(7):835–840.

73. Nocerino E, Amato M, Izzo AA. The aphrodisiac and adaptogenic properties of ginseng. *Fitoterapia.* 2000;71(suppl 1):S1–S5.

74. Filaretov AA, Bogdanova TS, Mitiushov MI, Podgovina TT, Srailova GT. Effect adaptogens on the activity of the pituitary-adrenocortical system in rats. *Biull Eksp Biol Med.* 1986;101(5):573–574.

75. Percival SS. Use of echinacea in medicine [review]. *Biochem Pharmacol.* 2000;60(2):155–158.

76. Schulz V. Clinical trials with hypericum extracts in patients with depression—results, comparisons, conclusions for therapy with anti-depressant drugs. *Phytomedicine.* 2002;9(5):468–474.

77. Siepmann M, Krause S, Jorashchky P, Muck-Weymann M, Kirch W. The effects of St. Johns's wort extract on heart rate variability, cognitive function and quantitative EEG: a comparison with amitriptyline and placebo in healthy men. *Br J Clin Pharmacol.* 2002;54(3):277–282.

78. Baschetti R. Chronic fatigue syndrome and licorice. *N Z Med J.* 1995;108:156–157.

79. Bou-Holaigah I, Rowe PC, Kan J, Calkins H. The relationship between neurally mediated hypotension and the chronic fatigue syndrome. *JAMA.* 1995;274:961–967.

80. Cheung CKT, Cheung FCW, Cheung JCP. Treatment of ten cases of chronic fatigue syndrome with Chinese herbs, acupuncture and diet precautions. *W J Acupunct Moxibustion.* 2000;10(1):1–6.

81. Kaur G, Kulkarni SK. A Comparative study of antidepressants and herbal psychotropic drugs in a

mouse model of chronic fatigue. *J Chronic Fatigue Syndr.* 2000;6(2):23–36.

82. Lansdorf N. A natural treatment approach to chronic fatigue syndrome—a case study. The Maharishi Vedic Medicine approach to chronic fatigue syndrome. Available at: http:// www.theraj.com/cfs/index.html. Accessed January 23, 2003.

83. Kelly AL. Rest for the weary. *Yoga J.* March/Apr 2001. Available at: http://www.yogajournal.com/health/124_1.cfm. Accessed January 23, 2003.

CHAPTER 20

Integrative Approach to Endocrinology

Tieraona Low Dog

▶ DIABETES MELLITUS

Pathophysiology

Diabetes is a metabolic disorder that is most commonly diagnosed by the presence of an abnormal glucose metabolism that usually presents as an abnormally elevated plasma glucose. In this illness, the body is unable to properly produce and use insulin. Chronic elevation of blood glucose is associated with long-term damage, dysfunction, and failure of various organs, especially the eyes, kidneys, nerves, heart, and blood vessels. Diabetes is the leading cause of blindness, end-stage kidney failure, and circulatory problems leading to amputation.[1]

Although there are many factors that help to regulate fuel metabolism, insulin and its antagonist glucagon are the primary hormones involved in diabetes. Insulin increases the transportation of glucose (and amino acids) and concomitantly stimulates glycogen and fat formation. Glucagon, on the other hand, stimulates the formation of glucose and the breakdown of fat and glycogen. An abnormal balance between these two hormones and an inability

to perform their normal functions is a hallmark of diabetes.

After eating a meal, particularly a meal of carbohydrate and protein, the beta cells of the pancreas secrete insulin. As the ratio of insulin to glucagon increases, the liver begins to increase glycogen synthesis and inhibit gluconeogenesis in order to store excess fuel. The muscle cells use glucose for their energy needs, as well.

When fasting, there are low levels of insulin and increased levels of glucagon. If fasting continues, cyclic adenosine monophosphate (cAMP) will begin to break down fat to release free fatty acids for fuel to be used by the liver and muscles, reserving the scarce supplies of glucose for the brain and central nervous system. Acetate, resulting from the use of free fatty acids by the liver, is converted to ketoacids that can be used by the brain if necessary to meet its energy needs. The American Diabetes Association and the World Health Organization use a fasting plasma glucose (FPG) concentration of 126 mg/dL (7.0 mmol/L) as the primary diagnostic criteria for the presence of diabetes.[2,3] Random glucose over 200 with symptoms or an abnormal GTT (glucose tolerance test) is also diagnostic.

Type 1 versus Type 2 Diabetes

Type 1, or juvenile-onset, diabetes has the primary problem of not producing enough insulin. This type accounts for less than 10% of all diabetics. This form of diabetes results from a cellular-mediated autoimmune destruction of the insulin secreting, or islet, cells of the pancreas. One or more of these autoantibodies are noted in 85–90% of individuals when fasting hyperglycemia is initially detected. In this form of diabetes, the rate of islet cell destruction can be variable, being rapid in some individuals and slow in others.[4] Autoimmune destruction of islet cells can be the result of a genetic predisposition, environmental factors, or, in some cases, unknown causes. Individuals with type 1 diabetes are at risk for the development of other autoimmune disorders such as Graves disease and pernicious anemia.

Type 2 diabetes, once referred to as non–insulin-dependent or age-onset diabetes, accounts for the vast majority of patients with diabetes. These individuals do not have antibodies to their islet cells but become resistant to using the insulin they produce. At least initially, these individuals do not need insulin treatment. More than 75% of type 2 diabetics are obese. Obesity itself can cause insulin resistance; even those who are not obese but who have an increased percentage of body fat in the abdominal region arc at risk.[5] Recent research suggests that fat cells produce a hormone that interferes with the action of insulin.

Type 2 diabetes may develop gradually over time and frequently goes undiagnosed for many years, as symptoms in the early stages are often not severe enough for patients to notice. Symptoms such as lethargy, irritability, weight loss, blurred vision, cuts that are slow to heal (particularly in the extremities), and numbness in the hands or feet are often subtle. Type 2 diabetes is most commonly controlled with oral drugs and lifestyle modifications, including healthy eating, weight loss, and exercise. Despite this, more than 35% of patients with this form of diabetes need insulin injections to maintain adequate control of blood glucose levels.

The complications of diabetes can stem from either type 1 or type 2 disease. Diabetes is the leading cause of blindness in people older than age 20 years and is associated with almost half of the cases of end-stage renal disease. The circulatory problems associated with diabetes in combination with nerve damage may cause diabetic neuropathy leading to amputation, a four- to fivefold increased risk of heart disease, and impotence.

Gestational Diabetes

Risk assessment for gestational diabetes mellitus (GDM) should be undertaken at the first prenatal visit. Women who are at risk for GDM should be screened at the first prenatal visit and again between 24 and 28 weeks.[6] Table 20–1 outlines the risk factors for gestational diabetes.

GDM complicates roughly 4% of all pregnancies in the United States.[7] Pregnant women with GDM have an increased incidence of pregnancy-induced hypertension, polyhydramnios, and cesarean section. There is an increased incidence of fetal macrosomia, shoulder dystocia, and metabolic problems in the newborn. Long-term, these infants may be at increased risk for obesity and type 2 diabetes. Clinical recognition of GDM is important because treatment and antepartum fetal surveillance can reduce perinatal morbidity and mortality.[8]

Epidemiology/Prevalence

Diabetes has become an epidemic in the United States and is closely associated with the rise in obesity, a decrease in physical activity, and changes in food consumption habits. Over the past 30 years the incidence of diabetes has risen from around 1 or 2% of the population to more than 7%. The actual number of diabetics is undoubtedly higher because many

▶ **TABLE 20-1** RISK FACTORS FOR GESTATIONAL DIABETES

- Those with a history of GDM
- History of recurrent spontaneous abortions or unexplained intrauterine fetal death
- History of recurrent preeclampsia
- Family history of diabetes mellitus in first-degree relatives
- Previous macrosomic infant (>4,000 g)
- Excessive weight gain (>18.1 kg [40 lb] during pregnancy)
- Maternal age over 30 years
- Fasting plasma glucose >105 mg/dL on two separate occasions
- Marked obesity
- Member of an ethnic group at high risk for diabetes (e.g., Native American)

GDM, gestational diabetes mellitus.

people have the disease for a long period before it is diagnosed or even before they have symptoms that cause them to seek medical attention. It is currently estimated that there are more than 15 million diabetics in the United States and that more than 5 million persons with diabetes are not aware that they have the disease.

Throughout the world, the prevalence of type 2 diabetes mellitus has increased dramatically during the past two decades.[9] More alarming is the recent steady demographic shift in type 2 diabetes to younger populations. This type of diabetes used to be associated with the elderly, and those with the disease would often die before the complications associated with diabetes set in. According to a recent estimate from the Centers for Disease Control and Prevention (CDC), the incidence of diabetes has increased almost 40% for those younger than age 50 years and almost 70% for those younger than age 40 years. Decreased physical activity, increasing obesity, and changes in food consumption are implicated in this epidemic.[10]

Genetics plays a role in diabetes, although rather than directly inheriting the disease, it seems some people inherit a susceptibility to the disease. This underscores the important role that obesity plays in the appearance of the disease. The familial nature of diabetes has been known for centuries, and as we further

define the human genome, new therapeutic strategies will undoubtedly emerge.

Conventional Medical Therapy

Prevention

Diabetes, particularly type 2, can be prevented if particular attention is paid to the risk factors for diabetes, which include obesity, lack of physical activity, poor diet (fat, refined carbohydrate, and fiber intake), and cigarette smoking.[11] These are factors under the control of patients and should be addressed at every possible opportunity for those at risk. There is good data suggesting that reduction in weight and increase in physical activity will reduce the risk of diabetes (as well as that of other diseases). Although there is less-conclusive evidence for specific dietary factors, it is reasonable to address these issues. If patients modify the risk factors under their control, the expression of the disease, even in susceptible individuals, will be reduced. Although widely touted, beta-carotene, taken as a dietary supplement, has not been shown to reduce the risk for type 2 diabetes.[12]

Treatment Options

For new-onset diabetes that is not insulin requiring, a trial of dietary modification, weight loss, and exercise alone is indicated. Treatment approaches for type 2 diabetes should consider the individual's increased risk of altered lipid levels, hypertension, obesity, and vascular damage. Hyperglycemia increases the risk of cardiovascular disease, making hyperlipidemia a disorder of concern that requires aggressive treatment.[13]

Conventional pharmaceutical therapy falls into several categories. All are designed to improve glycemic control as measured by the plasma glucose levels and hemoglobin (Hb) A1c. The 1998 United Kingdom Prospective Diabetes Study (UKPDS) demonstrated fairly convincingly that a modest reduction in HbA1c (less than 1%) in patients with type 2 diabetes is associated with improvement in long-term outcomes, particularly in prevention of microvascular complications. Oral hypoglycemic medications fall into several categories, according to their mechanism of action, and may be used alone or in combination with insulin therapy.

The sulfonylureas are designed to stimulate insulin production by the pancreas. They work via a complex mechanism that ultimately results in portal hyperinsulinemia and reduced hepatic glucose production. Factors that predict a good response to this group of drugs include recent diagnoses, mild- to-moderate fasting blood sugar (220 to 240 mg/dL), high fasting C-peptide level, no history of insulin therapy, and absence of islet cell or glutamic acid decarboxylase antibodies.[14]

Metformin (Glucophage), a biguanide, stimulates glucose uptake and storage by the liver in order to control blood sugar levels. This agent enhances the sensitivity of both liver and muscle tissue to insulin and inhibits hepatic gluconeogenesis.[15] Clinical trials demonstrate that metformin decreases the fasting plasma glucose level by 60 to 70 mg/dL and the HbA1c value by 1.5 to 2.0 percentage points in patients with poorly controlled diabetes. In addition to lowering plasma glucose levels, metformin also reduces plasma triglyceride and low-density lipoprotein (LDL) levels.[16] It is the only oral agent that reduces some of the vas-

cular complications when used alone, and is increasingly being used as the primary monotherapy in newly diagnosed type 2 diabetics.

Acarbose (Precose and Glyset), a glucosidase inhibitor, inhibits starch digestion by competitively inhibiting the ability of enzymes (maltase, isomaltase, sucrase, and glucoamylase) in the small intestinal brush border to break down oligosaccharides and disaccharides into monosaccharides.[17] By slowing the process of digestion and absorption, these drugs slow the entry of glucose into the systemic circulation, thereby allowing the pancreas extra time to increase insulin secretion in response to the slowed increase in plasma glucose level. For these reasons it is obviously most effective in patients who have postprandial hyperglycemia.

The thiazolidinediones (TZDs) are medications that act directly on peripheral tissues to increase the uptake of glucose. Troglitazone maleate (Rezulin) was associated with severe hepatotoxicity, which led to its withdrawal from the US market in March 2000. Two TZDs are currently available: pioglitazone (Actos) and rosiglitazone (Avandia). One advantage of this class of medications is their beneficial effects on lipids and possibly other cardiovascular parameters (i.e., hypertension and inhibiting progression of early atherosclerotic lesions), making them valuable in patients with metabolic syndrome.[18] Pioglitazone and rosiglitazone have not been associated with liver toxicity in pre- and postmarketing studies; nonetheless, until long-term research is available, the FDA recommends monitoring liver enzymes regularly. A disadvantage of the TZDs worth noting is their cost—prices typically run around $150 per month.

Oral agents are often prescribed in combination for enhanced glucose control. The most common combination therapy of conventional oral hypoglycemic agents is metformin plus a sulfonylurea.[19] One benefit of this prescribing strategy is the additional glucose and lipid-lowering effects of the combination approach. If a combination regime of metformin and sulfonylurea fails to produce acceptable blood glucose control, other options include the addition of a bedtime (neutral protamine Hagedorn [NPH]) insulin dose or institution of a regimen of insulin injections as needed.

Insulin Therapy

For type 1 diabetes, and for type 2 diabetes uncontrolled by diet and oral agents, insulin is currently the treatment of choice. Insulin comes in a variety of different forms, primarily distinguished by the length of action. Combinations of long- and short-acting insulins are typically used in a given patient. Insulin is also now often delivered with a pump that can be programmed to deliver a specific dose of a specific type of insulin when needed.

Integrative Medicine Approaches

There are more than 200 different combinations of medications, insulin, and lifestyle modifications in use today for the treatment of diabetes. Modification of risk factors through lifestyle interventions is essential for successful treatment of diabetes. Lifestyle interventions should include diet, exercise, smoking cessation, and stress management. Exercise strategies are covered in depth in Chapter 13, and will not be extensively discussed here. Clearly, any treatment plan should include a regular exercise program that is tailored to the individual. Individuals without significant complications should engage in both aerobic and weight-bearing activities to improve muscle strength, manage weight, improve insulin sensitivity, and to reduce the risk of cardiovascular disease.[20]

A large government survey (The Medical Expenditure Panel Survey) looked at the use of complementary and alternative medicine (CAM) by more than 21,000 people.[21] CAM was defined as "approaches to health care that are different from those typically practiced by medical doctors in the United States." Respondents were presented with a list that included practices such as acupuncture, nontraditional nutri-

tion advice or lifestyle diets, massage therapy, herbal remedies, biofeedback, meditation, and imagery or relaxation techniques. Of those surveyed, 825 people had diabetes. Eight percent of the people with diabetes reported using CAM, compared with only 5% of their counterparts without diabetes. The most common types of CAM used were nutrition advice and lifestyle diets—naturopathic or homeopathic nutrition/diets, megadoses of vitamins, and the Atkins diet—followed by spiritual healing, herbal remedies, massage therapy, and meditation training.

Nutritional Approaches

Fiber/Whole Grains

Fiber decreases postprandial glucose and insulin concentrations in those with diabetes and in those with normal glucose levels.[22] Epidemiologic studies have also reported inverse associations between dietary fiber and serum insulin.[23] Although both soluble and insoluble fiber appear beneficial, researchers report a stronger association between insoluble fiber and diabetes risk. The Nurses' Health Study found that the combination of a high glycemic load and a low cereal fiber intake increased the risk of diabetes (relative risk [RR] = 2.50; 95% confidence interval [CI], 1.14–5.51) when compared with a low glycemic load and high cereal-fiber intake. This study also suggests that grains should be consumed in a minimally refined form to reduce the incidence of diabetes.[24] Almost identical findings were noted in the Health Professionals' Follow-up Study.[25] These findings were reaffirmed recently by the Iowa Women's Health Study. This prospective study of postmenopausal women found strong inverse associations between incidence of diabetes and intakes of total grains, whole grains, dietary fiber, cereal fiber, and dietary magnesium after multivariate adjustments for several risk factors for diabetes were done.[26] It should be noted that whole grains contain substantially more dietary fiber and magnesium than refined grains and that grains consumed in an intact form may have a more dramatic effect on glycemic response than refined grains with a smaller particle size.[27]

Psyllium is a viscous water-soluble fiber that has long been used as a bulk laxative with a good safety record. Soluble fibers improve glycemic control in type 2 diabetes. Psyllium reduced postprandial glucose levels in one study,[28] while another study reported a reduction in fasting blood glucose.[29] A crossover study of the effects of psyllium taken immediately before breakfast and dinner compared with the effects of cellulose placebo supplementation in individuals with type 2 diabetes, found that postprandial serum glucose values were 14% lower after breakfast, 31% lower after lunch, and 20% lower after dinner when psyllium was taken before the morning and evening meal.[30] A more recent study of patients with type 2 diabetes found similar results.[31] Given the safety of psyllium and its beneficial effects upon glucose and lipids, the addition of this fiber to individuals with diabetes seems sensible.

Magnesium

Magnesium is the fourth most abundant cation in the body and affects many cellular functions, including transport of potassium and calcium ions. In addition, magnesium modulates signal transduction, energy metabolism and cell proliferation. Magnesium deficiency is not uncommon among the general population and its intake has steadily decreased over the years, especially in the Western world.[32] Certain populations may be particularly vulnerable to magnesium deficiency as one study in urban African American women found.[33] Hypomagnesemia is a common characteristic of diabetes mellitus. Fiber-rich cereal products decrease diabetes risk (see "Fiber/Whole Grains"). The superior magnesium content of these foods may account for a substantial part of this benefit. High-magnesium diets have preventive activity in certain rodent models of diabetes, while mag-

nesium depletion is associated with insulin resistance.[34] Research has found that alterations in glucose levels influence magnesium homeostasis independently of insulin levels in type 1 diabetic patients. This is thought to be a result of increased renal magnesium clearance during periods of hyperglycemia.[35]

The relationship between hypomagnesemia and diabetic neuropathy is intriguing. Circulating ionized magnesium levels were found to decrease with increases of plasma HbA1c and triglycerides in type 2 diabetic patients with incipient or overt nephropathy, after adjusting for age, sex, body mass index, diabetes duration, systolic and diastolic blood pressure, hypoglycemic therapy, plasma creatinine, creatinine clearance, plasma cholesterol, and fasting glucose.[36] Similar results were seen in individuals with type 1 diabetes. Patients with type 1 diabetes, disturbed nerve conduction velocity and low erythrocyte magnesium levels (<2.3 mmol/L) were given oral magnesium supplements for 1 year. When compared to controls, this study found that under unchanged metabolic control, supplementation with magnesium improved nerve conduction, especially in younger patients with a shorter duration of diabetes.[37]

Magnesium supplementation may also be important when considering the vasoconstrictive effects of hypomagnesemia and the magnitude of vascular disorders seen in those with diabetes.[38] Patients with diabetes, and those with significant risk factors for the disorder, should be encouraged to limit refined grains and to acquire their energy from whole grain products rich in magnesium. Supplementation with magnesium may be necessary in those who have low dietary intake of these substances. Only 1% of the total body magnesium pool is extracellular, and simply checking total serum magnesium may obscure true deficiencies of magnesium in patients with arrhythmia and diabetes mellitus.[39] One note of caution: patients with renal disease may have hypermagnesemia, making supplementation unnecessary and unwise.

Vitamin E

Diabetics have been noted to have an abnormally large amount of free radicals triggered by hyperglycemia. Vitamin E theoretically should arrest some of the harmful effects of free radicals through its antioxidant activity. Researchers have noted that plasma levels of lipid hydroperoxidases are higher in insulin-resistant individuals when compared to those who are insulin sensitive. This suggests increased lipid peroxidation, reduced clearance, or both. These findings are associated with significantly lower plasma concentrations of carotenoids and tocopherols. Although studies have not been able to determine a cause and effect relationship, an integrated analysis of the available literature strongly suggests that tocopherols, and perhaps carotenoids, should be added to the growing list of environmental factors known to modulate insulin effects.[40] Vitamin E also appears to increase intracellular magnesium levels when given at doses of 600 IU/d.[41] Given the potential benefit of antioxidants for the prevention of other diseases and the difficulty in obtaining enough from the diet, supplementation with vitamin E may be wise for diabetics. The usual dosage is 400 IU/d.

Vitamin C

Some studies show that diabetics have at least 30% lower levels of circulating vitamin C than do those persons without the disorder. Scientists question whether the increased oxidative stress seen in diabetes ultimately depletes antioxidant reserves. While vitamin C supplementation lowers cellular sorbitol concentrations and reduces capillary fragility, it shows little impact on blood glucose concentration.[42] The question of whether diabetes decreases vitamin C levels or increases the demand for this nutrient was recently addressed. A study of newly diagnosed diabetics and controls failed to find any statistically significant association between diabetes and vitamin C concentration after a multivariate adjustment was performed that included total vitamin C consumption, body mass index, educational level, cigarette smoking, and other factors.[43] Individuals should follow the recommendations set forth with the new food pyramid guidelines that encourage five to seven servings of fruits and vegetables every day. Diabetics who do not smoke and who follow this guideline should be able to obtain adequate levels of vitamin C in their diet. If not, a supplement containing 500 mg of vitamin C should be taken one to two times per day.

Vanadium

Vanadium is a transitional element capable of existing in different oxidation states and forming complex ions. Numerous investigations have demonstrated the beneficial effect of vanadium salts on diabetes in streptozotocin (STZ)-diabetic rats, in rodents with genetically determined diabetes, and in human subjects. Vanadyl sulfate ($VOSO_4$), an oxidative form of vanadium, reduces hyperglycemia and insulin resistance in animal models. Small clinical studies of short duration in type 2 diabetes have shown beneficial effects, primarily a reduction in fasting plasma glucose and HbA1c without changes in plasma insulin levels.[44] A recent study of 11 type 2 diabetics given $VOSO_4$ 150 mg/d for 6 weeks found improved hepatic and muscle insulin sensitivity.[45] Although the exact cellular mechanisms via which vanadium works are not currently known, preliminary data suggest that the effects of vanadium may be mediated by a synergy between several postreceptor events in the insulin-signaling cascade in target tissues.[46]

The few studies available for review used a dosage range of 100–150 mg/d of vanadyl sulfate or sodium metavanadate. While the preliminary data is certainly promising, concerns have arisen about the long-term safety of inorganic vanadium salts. Treatment of diabetic animals has been associated with side effects, including gastrointestinal discomfort and decreased body weight. In addition, vanadium salts have been reported to exert toxic effects on the liver and kidney. Concerns have been cited of possible accumulation of vanadium in the spleen and testes when used long-term leading to immunotoxicity and possible reproductive toxicity. Because of potential developmental toxicity, there is a serious question about the safety of vanadium supplementation during pregnancy and while breast-feeding.[47] Recently, it was suggested that organic vanadium compounds are much safer than inorganic vanadium salts and are not associated with any gastrointestinal discomfort or hepatic or renal toxicity.[48] Clearly, this is an area of needed research given the potential benefit of vanadium in diabetes but also the potential harm of a substance that would have to be used long-term for the management of a chronic disorder.

Chromium

Chromium is an essential trace element for mammals and is required for maintenance of proper carbohydrate and lipid metabolism. This element improves the glucose–insulin system in individuals with diabetes with no detectable effects on control subjects. Chromium improves insulin binding, insulin receptor number, and beta-cell sensitivity, and increases insulin sensitivity in target tissues. While the mechanism of action on a molecular level has been elusive, recent research indicates that the chromium-binding oligopeptide chromodulin may play a unique role in the autoamplification of insulin signaling.[49] Supplementation of 162 diabetic patients (48 with type 1 and 114 with type 2 diabetes) with chromium picolinate 200 μg/d enabled 118 patients to reduce their daily dose of insulin, sulfonylurea, or metformin. The success rate was slightly greater in patients with type 2 diabetes (74%) than in patients with type 1 diabetes (71.6%). Placebo administration was ineffective and no significant differences between genders were noted.[50]

One hundred eighty Chinese patients with type 2 diabetes, age 35–65 years, were divided into three groups of 60 and supplemented with placebo or chromium picolinate 100 or 500 μg

2 times per day for 4 months. Improvements in the glucose–insulin system were highly significant in the subjects receiving 500 μg twice per day with less or no significant improvements in the subjects receiving 100 μg twice per day after 2 and 4 months. Limitations of this study included concurrent diabetic treatments (hypoglycemic medications, insulin, traditional Chinese medicines, and diet). The dose of 1,000 μg/d is much larger than what is normally used; however, there were no reports of toxicity in the study.[51] Interestingly, the 200 μg/d did not produce significant results and this is the dose most commonly recommended for glucose intolerance.

Not all studies have shown a favorable effect on blood glucose. A randomized placebo-controlled study of 76 patients with established atherosclerotic disease (25 had type 2 diabetes) given 250 μg chromium or placebo for up to 16 months (mean duration was 11.1 months) failed to find any statistically significant change between groups in fasting glucose, total cholesterol, or low-density lipoprotein. An increase in high-density lipoprotein was noted in the chromium group ($p < 0.005$), along with a decrease in serum triglycerides ($p < 0.02$). In the diabetic subgroup, 12 received placebo and 13 were treated with chromium. Although mean serum chromium levels significantly increased in the treatment group after 3 months of supplementation, there was no significant change in mean fasting glucose concentration. In fact, there was a small increase in mean fasting serum glucose in diabetics receiving chromium, but these changes were not statistically significant.[52] It is questionable, however, whether the chromium salt used in this trial (chromium chloride) provided an adequate amount of bioavailable chromium. When chromium is bound to picolinate it forms an organic complex that facilitates its absorption. One must also wonder if chromium is beneficial for diabetics who are not deficient in the element.

The evidence for chromium should be considered preliminary for the treatment of diabetes. Adverse effects appear to be minimal, however, excessive dietary chromium inhibits the absorption of zinc and iron. There is also no convincing evidence that chromium is beneficial for weight loss.

Fish Oil

Fish oil improves nerve conduction velocity and increases Na-K-ATPase activity in diabetic animals. Studies also suggest that fish oil may be effective in the prevention of diabetic neuropathy.[53] Fish oil also reduces triglycerides by roughly 45% without significant change in LDL in type 2 diabetics with hypertriglycedemia.[54]

Botanical Medicines

Insulin resistance remains a major therapeutic problem that is treated primarily with dietary management and/or pharmaceutical agents. The use of botanicals to address diabetes is popular in many countries and is growing in the United States. World ethnobotanical information indicates that approximately 800 plants are used for the control of diabetes mellitus, with almost 150 of these found in Mexico.[55] Although most lack scientific studies, there is preliminary data available for some. Patients may use nutritional supplements and herbs to lower blood sugar, reduce the risk of diabetic retinopathy, ease neuropathic pain, and enhance their overall vitality. The following is a brief list of the most commonly used and/or promising antidiabetic agents.

Bitter Melon (Momordica charantia)

Bitter melon unripe fruit and seeds are used in Australia, South America, and Asia (especially India) for the treatment of diabetes. The "active" principles are not known. Researchers have found a galactose-binding lectin with insulin-like activity from the seeds; others believe that the hypoglycemic activity is a result of the presence of another compound in the seed (2,6-diaminopyrimidinol-5-D-glucopyranoside); yet others maintain that a nonnitrogenous neutral substance (charantin) is the active

ingredient.[56] Charantin appears to be best extracted in alcohol.

Studies provide conflicting data and are primarily limited to animal research using experimentally induced diabetic rats. Of the two open trials in non–insulin-dependent diabetes mellitus (NIDDM) patients, one noted improved glucose tolerance in 73% of type 2 diabetics given 2 ounces of juice,[57] while the other found both fasting and postprandial serum glucose levels were reduced (p<0.001) in 86% of patients (n = 100) using Karolla (bitter melon fruit).[58] A study using an alcoholic extract of the pulp was conducted in normal glucose primed rats and STZ (streptozocin)-induced diabetic rats. This study noted improved glucose tolerance resulting in a 26% reduction in plasma glucose at 3.5 hours, as compared to a 40–50% reduction at 1, 2, and 3.5 hours in STZ-rats treated with metformin. Bitter melon was found to have roughly 25% the efficacy of tolbutamide in reducing blood sugar in normal glucose-primed rats. Although there was no increase in insulin secretion, a dramatic increase in the rate of glycogen synthesis was noted.[59] A more recent study found that STZ-induced diabetic rats orally fed bitter melon fruit juice increased their number of beta cells as compared to untreated diabetic rats (p<0.004); however, the absolute number was still significantly less than found in normal rats.[60] Only one study was found that failed to show any hypoglycemic activity with the use of bitter melon. Wistar rats rendered hyperglycemic by STZ and then fed a diet containing freeze-dried bitter gourd powder at 0.5% level for 6 weeks failed to experience a reduction in blood glucose levels.[61] It should be noted, however, that the preparation used in this trial differed from those used in other studies, as it did not contain the seed and was freeze-dried.

Fenugreek (Trigonella foenum-graecum)

Fenugreek is found primarily in the Middle East, India, and Mediterranean countries. The seeds are commonly used as a food spice and are employed in medicine for their nutritive, hypocholesterolemic, and hypoglycemic effects. Researchers believe that the appetite-stimulating and lipid-lowering activities of fenugreek are a result of high fiber content and steroid saponins,[62] while the antidiabetic activity is a result of the high fiber content[63] of the seeds and the presence of 4-hydroxyisoleucine (stimulates insulin secretion).[64] The hypoglycemic effects of fenugreek have been demonstrated in experimentally induced diabetic rats, dogs, mice, healthy volunteers,[65] and in insulin-dependent diabetes mellitus (IDDM) and NIDDM patients.[66] Preliminary data suggest glucose levels fall an average of 13.2–23.09% with higher doses. Studies also suggest that disrupted free radical metabolism in diabetic animals are normalized with the addition of fenugreek seed into the diet.[67] Raw fenugreek seeds reduce total serum cholesterol, LDL/VLDL cholesterol and triglyceride levels in experimental animal[68] and human studies.[69] The lipid-lowering, antioxidant, hypoglycemic activity of this fiber may prove a useful addition to the diet of diabetics.

Ginseng (Panax quinquefolius and P. ginseng)

Ginseng remains one of the most popular herbal supplements sold on the American market. Two species dominate the trade: Asian ginseng *(Panax ginseng)* and American ginseng *(Panax quinquefolius)*. There have been two trials conducted to determine if American ginseng has hypoglycemic activity. One randomized, double-blind, placebo-controlled study (n = 19; 10 nondiabetic adults and 9 adults with NIDDM) found that 3 g of powdered ginseng reduced postprandial glycemia when taken 40 minutes before glucose challenge in both groups.[70] A recent crossover study (n = 12) found that doses of 1–3 g were equally effective in reducing postprandial glycemia in nondiabetics when given 40 minutes before a 25-g glucose challenge but not at 20, 10, or 0 minutes.[71] (Crude ginseng root was used in this study.) The

authors concluded that reduction in postprandial glycemia is time dependent but not dose dependent. A double-blind, placebo-controlled randomized study of 36 NIDDM patients found a reduction in fasting blood glucose and body weight, and improved mood with both 100 and 200 mg doses of ginseng but a reduction in hemoglobin A1c and improved physical activity was noted only with the 200 mg dose. (The composition of ginseng product was not stated in the study.) This data should be considered promising but preliminary.

Gymnema (Gymnema sylvestre)

Gymnema has been used for the treatment of diabetes in India for 26 centuries. It is used as tea and in encapsulated form. In vitro and animal studies show that gymnema has hypoglycemic activity. Studies in STZ-induced diabetic rats found that when given GS4 (a water-soluble standardized gymnema extract) orally for 20 days, pancreatic beta cells were doubled, while fasting blood glucose returned to near-normal levels. Researchers speculate that this herbal therapy helps repair/regenerate the endocrine pancreas.[72] An open trial of 22 NIDDM patients on conventional oral hypoglycemic agents were provided GS4 400 mg/d for 12–18 months as an adjunctive therapy. All participants experienced a significant reduction in blood glucose, glycosylated hemoglobin, and glycosylated proteins. Many were able to reduce the dose of their prescription medication, while five were able to completely discontinue their medication. Increased insulin levels were noted after GS4 supplementation in this study.[73] Another study was conducted to determine the effect of GS4 in 27 patients with IDDM. Patients were given 400 mg/d of GS4 in addition to their insulin for 10–12 months. Patients were noted to have a reduction in fasting blood glucose, glycosylated hemoglobin, and glycosylated plasma protein levels when compared to those receiving insulin only. Interestingly, serum lipids returned to near-normal levels in those receiving GS4.[74]

Gymnema appears to be a promising herb with a relatively good safety profile and may be of benefit as an adjunctive therapy in patients with IDDM or NIDDM.

Stevia (Stevia rebaudiana)

Stevia is a perennial shrub indigenous to South America. For centuries the leaves have been used as a sweetener and medicine. The constituents responsible for its sweetness were identified in 1931; stevioside, a glycoside, was found to be approximately 100 times sweeter than sucrose at a 10% sucrose concentration. Japan is the largest consumer of stevia leaf and extract, where it is used as a multipurpose sweetener. Although stevia is approved as a food additive in a number of countries (e.g., Japan, Brazil) it is sold as a dietary supplement in the United States. (Interestingly, the FDA ruled that stevia is safe as a dietary supplement but not as a food additive!) Stevia has no calories, no carbohydrates, and does not elevate blood glucose—all beneficial for diabetics. Stevia is used as a folk treatment for diabetes in Paraguay and Brazil. In vitro studies suggest that stevioside stimulates insulin release via a direct action on beta cells.[75] In preliminary studies, stevioside reduced systolic and diastolic blood pressure in hypertensive adults when given 250 mg TID for 3 months.[76] It was also determined that stevia is not cariogenic.[77]

Stevia appears to be a safe and effective sweetener for diabetics that may also have hypoglycemic and antihypertensive activity. It is currently available at a number of health food stores and over the Internet. Most products are standardized to stevioside and rebaudioside content.

Evening Primrose Oil (Oenothera biennis)

Evening primrose is an indigenous North American plant that has been used in Native American medicine for the treatment of skin diseases and arthritis. In contemporary therapeutics, evening primrose seed oil is recommended for a variety of conditions including atopic dermatitis, mastalgia, premenstrual syndrome, and diabetic neuropathy. Evening primrose seed oil is a rich source of essential fatty acids, particularly gamma-linolenic acid. Two double-blind, placebo-controlled randomized studies have found evening primrose seed oil of benefit in patients with diabetic neuropathy. A 1993 study (n = 111) found that evening primrose seed oil was significantly more effective than placebo in relieving 13 of 16 parameters (standard tests including sensation, hot and cold thresholds, and tendon reflexes). Conduction and neurological values were improved over placebo. Although sex, age, and diabetes type did not influence the results, those with relatively well-controlled diabetes fared better than did those with poorly controlled diabetes. The dose was evening primrose seed oil 6,000 mg/d, providing 480 mg/d of gamma-linolenic acid.[78] Another study (n = 22) found a statistically significant increase in median and peroneal nerve conduction and improvement in neuropathic symptoms (numbness, pain, paresthesias).[79] A study in diabetic rats found that dietary administration of gamma-linolenic acid can prevent the deficit in nerve conduction velocity induced by diabetes. There was no significant association between this prevention of the nerve conduction velocity deficit with nerve fatty acid composition, changes in neuronal sugar and polyol contents, Na^+-K^+-exchanging adenosine triphosphatase (ATPase) activity, or ouabain binding. This is supportive of the hypothesis that gamma-linolenic acid acts through indirect mechanisms, probably by improving neuronal blood supply and/or conceivably involving a shift in prostanoid metabolism.[80] Additional studies in animals suggest that gamma-linolenic acid is of most benefit in early deficits in peripheral nerve conduction, with little likelihood of reversing late deficits.[81] There may be additional therapeutic benefit when gamma-linolenic acid is combined with alpha-lipoic acid.[82]

Capsicum (Capsicum spp)

Capsicum (chili) peppers are widely used as a warming, pungent spice and are also available, in various forms, as dietary supplements and pharmaceutical preparations. The oleoresin and capsaicin (the major capsaicinoid in the fruit) are used in topical preparations for the relief of postherpetic neuralgia, rheumatoid arthritis, osteoarthritis, and painful diabetic neuropathy. Capsaicin causes a local depletion of substance P, an endogenous neuropeptide involved in the transmission of pain impulses from peripheral nerves to the spinal column.[83] This occurs as the result of capsaicinoids binding to VR1, a fatty acid receptor present only on C fibers, which leads to desensitization or degeneration of the sensory afferent.[84] When first applied, capsaicin intensely activates primary sensory neurons, resulting in local reddening and increased pain sensation. With repeated application, analgesia occurs, although it may take up to 72 hours for substance P to be completely depleted. Capsaicin must be repeatedly applied to the painful area to achieve the desensitization of the sensory neurons.[85] Four double-blind, placebo-controlled trials found capsaicin effective for the treatment of diabetic neuropathy.

Pure capsaicin preparations are available in strengths of 0.025% and 0.075%. The cream, or ointment, must be applied four times per day for at least 8–12 weeks and then can often be used two to three times per day to maintain analgesia.

Bilberry (Vaccinium myrtillus)

Bilberry fruit is rich in anthocyanosides that have been shown to act as powerful antioxidants. These substances support connective tissue via stabilization of collagen[86] and reduce capillary fragility.[87] Two small, double-blind, placebo-controlled studies showed improved ophthalmoscopic patterns in patients with diabetic retinopathy[88] and/or hypertensive retinopathy.[89] Two open trials showed reduction in hemorrhages[90] and vascular permeability.[91] Retinal protection may result from the inhibition of retinal phosphoglucomutase and glucose-6-phosphatase.[92] Although the data should be considered preliminary, there is enough to suggest that bilberry fruit extract may be beneficial for the prevention/treatment of diabetic retinopathy given its antioxidant and vascular stabilizing activity. Clinical trials have all been conducted on preparations standardized to contain 25% anthocyanidins. The dosage range is usually 360–600 mg/d, depending upon the condition being treated. Therapeutic benefits normally take 4–8 weeks to appear and so the product should be taken for at least 2 months.

Homeopathy

Homeopathy as a medical therapy has no controlled clinical trials available for the treatment of diabetes or its complications. *Syzygium jambolanum*, an Indian plant of which the seeds are used to make a homeopathic remedy, has been reported to be useful in the treatment of diabetes, particularly for treatment of diabetic ulcers. However, there are only case reports in the homeopathic medical literature.

Mind–Body Medicine

There is limited research available for review to determine the effectiveness of mind–body medicine for improving glucose control or reducing the complications of diabetes. One study of 552 diabetics found that those who regularly attended religious services had a lower level of C-reactive protein than did diabetics who did not regularly attend services, indicating a possible cardio-protecting effect. After adjusting for demographic variables, health status, smoking, social support, mobility, and body mass index, the association between religious attendance and C-reactive protein remained significant for respondents with diabetes (RR = 1.90; 95% CI, 1.03–3.51).[93]

There may be a role for Tai chi in elderly diabetic patients, especially for those with early peripheral neuropathy. Recent investigations have found that Tai chi is beneficial to cardiorespiratory function, strength, balance, flexibility, microcirculation, and psychological profile, and can reduce the risk of falls in elderly individuals.[91]

► HYPOTHYROIDISM

Pathophysiology

Primary hypothyroidism is caused by a decreased production of thyroid hormones by the thyroid gland. This leads to a generalized slowdown in metabolic function. Hypothyroidism is a relatively common disorder that, in adults, is usually caused from primary thyroid failure. This may be a result of autoimmune disease or therapies that ablate the thyroid (radioactive iodine or radiation to the neck). In adults living in the United States, chronic autoimmune (Hashimoto's) thyroiditis is a common cause. Sometimes the disorder can be the result of iodine deficiency or excess, or from a genetic defect that prevents the appropriate synthesis of thyroid hormone. Medications such as lithium and amiodarone can inhibit thyroid hormone synthesis, although, amiodarone can also cause hyperthyroidism.[95] Lithium causes hypothyroidism in 5–15% of patients, and goiter in up to 37% of patients. Thyroid function tests should be performed prior to initiating lithium therapy, and at 6-month intervals thereafter.[96]

Secondary and tertiary syndromes are rare causes of hypothyroidism. Pituitary dysfunction leads to insufficient quantities of thyroid-stimulating hormone (TSH) being produced. This can be the result of pituitary insufficiency, pituitary tumors, and a consequence of pituitary surgery. Tertiary hypothyroidism indicates that the problem lies in the hypothalamus.

Conventional Treatment Approach

There are several brands of thyroid hormone replacement available in the United States. Most contain T_4, assuming that most individuals will be able to convert this into the active form of T_3 in the peripheral tissue. Some T_3 preparations are also available. Desiccated thyroid extract is available, but it is not routinely used by most practitioners because of batch-to-batch variability in potency. The conventional approach is to use a thyroid replacement product containing T_4 only and titrate the dose to attain normal serum TSH.

Integrative Treatment Strategies

Thyroid Hormone Replacement

Popular texts directed at the lay public advocate the use of products containing both triiodothyronine (T_3) and thyroxine (T_4) extracts as being potentially more effective in treating symptoms of hypothyroidism than the T_4-alone products. These combination medications are available both from animal sources (pig thyroid in Armour thyroid) and from synthetic sources (Thyrolar). Even in some conventional endocrinology circles, more attention is currently being paid to using combinations of T_4 and T_3 for the treatment of hypothyroidism based on the premise that not all tissues are equally able to convert T_4 to T_3 and that some patients do not respond well to treatment with T_4 alone. One study has reported improved mood with combination hormones in patients with hypothyroidism.[97] More research is needed to determine the true benefit or need for administering both T_4 and T_3; however, in patients with low T_3 levels, this may be the preferred treatment, if selenium deficiency is not present.

Another area of some controversy is the treatment of what has been incorrectly called in the alternative medicine world "subclinical hypothyroidism." This term has been used to describe a state in which TSH and other laboratory measures of thyroid function are within normal limits but the patient still reports symptoms of fatigue, weight gain, cold sensitivity, dry skin, and constipation, which are potentially attributable to hypothyroidism. This condition, which would more properly be named "symptomatic euthyroid state," is often diagnosed by alternative or integrative physicians, even in patients who have never been formally hypothyroid by laboratory values. When these patients are treated with low levels of thyroid hormone, there is often a substantial improvement in symptoms.

Nutritional Supplements

SELENIUM

Selenium is a cofactor of the antioxidant enzyme glutathione peroxidase and of the thyroid hormone-converting enzyme iodothyronine 5'-deiodinase. There is evidence that selenium deficiency can lead to hypothyroidism. Iodothyronine 5'-deiodinase is a selenium-containing enzyme responsible for ensuring the conversion of thyroxine (T_4) into 3,5,3'-triiodothyronine (T_3) in the thyroid and peripheral tissues. Regulation of this enzyme depends, in part, on selenium and iodine status.[98] Selenium deficiency significantly decreased tissue T_3 concentrations in the hippocampus, hypothalamus, and striatum in rats, whereas no significant changes were found in the cerebellum, cerebral cortex, and brain stem. Tissue T_4 concentrations were only marginally affected, with the exception of a 35% increase in the cerebral cortex. This study suggests that certain tissues may be more vulnerable to selenium deficiency than other tissues.[99] A study of patients with phenylketonuria or milder hyperphenylalaninemias on protein-restricted diets at risk for selenium deficiency found that free thyroxine and reverse triiodothyronine (rT_3) levels were inversely correlated with selenium. Reduced conversion of T_4 and rT_3 was likely a result of the lower levels of selenium found in this group of patients.[100] Although most individuals in the United States are not iodine deficient, if iodine deficiency is present, iodine should be replaced first followed by selenium supplementation.[101] The dose for selenium supplementation should not exceed 200 μg/d. Toxicity has been reported in association with intakes of >700 μg/d.[102]

Botanical Medicines

KELP (LAMINARIA SPP)

Kelp is recommended by many herbalists for the treatment of hypothyroidism, given that it is a rich source of iodine, a substance essential for the synthesis of thyroid hormones. This seaweed was a powerful treatment for hypothyroidism in areas where the diet was deficient in iodine and goiter was endemic. However, since the introduction of iodized salt, iodine deficiency is relatively rare in Western countries. Paradoxically, too much iodine can actually lead to a reversible type of hypothyroidism. Iodine-induced hypothyroidism permits a persistent Wolff-Chaikoff effect. One study of 22 patients with spontaneously occurring primary hypothyroidism found that 12 (54.5%) became euthyroid after restricting iodine intake for 3 weeks.[103] Another study of 1,061 Japanese adults living in coastal Japan found that the prevalence of autoantibody-negative hypothyroidism is more prevalent and marked in those consuming higher amounts of iodine. The researchers stressed that excessive iodine intake be considered in cases of hypothyroidism.[104] Even more interesting was the case of a young woman who developed iodine-induced hypothyroidism because of excessive transcutaneous absorption of iodine in sea-bath salts. She had been using iodized sea-bath salts for 3 months in a hot-water bath as a slimming technique. Her thyroid function returned to normal after discontinuation of the salts.

Kelp and other seaweeds can certainly be added to the diet for their flavor and abundant minerals; however, these substances are probably only minimally useful for the treatment of hypothyroidism in those who consume dairy, seafood, processed food, or who use table salt. Patients with mild hypothyroidism who want to try kelp should have their thyroid function rechecked in 8–12 weeks. If no improvement is noted, appropriate replacement should be implemented. And bear in mind, some individuals will actually experience a worsening of hypothyroidism with the addition of kelp, bladderwrack, or other iodine-containing herbs, if their diet already contains sufficient amounts of this substance.

► HYPERTHYROIDISM

Pathophysiology

Hyperthyroidism, also referred to as thyrotoxicosis, is defined as any condition in which elevated levels of thyroid hormones are present. While both T_4 and T_3 are elevated in hyperthyroidism, T_3—the more metabolically active of the two—is usually elevated to a greater degree. The most common cause of hyperthyroidism is the autoimmune condition Graves' disease (toxic diffuse goiter). Other causes include toxic adenoma, toxic multinodular goiter, silent thyroiditis, subacute thyroiditis, and postpartum thyroiditis. Hyperthyroidism can also be caused from excessive iodine intake and in patients taking too much thyroid medication. Graves' disease is an autoimmune condition, the trigger for which is unknown. Immunoglobulins that stimulate thyroid activity are the hallmark of the disorder. Studies being done on genetic markers in Graves' disease indicate that a gene mutation/inherited defect is implicated in the development of the disease. Individuals with other autoimmune disorders (e.g., diabetes and lupus) are at risk for developing this disorder.

Toxic adenoma refers to a solitary nodule within the thyroid gland that produces excessive amounts of thyroid hormones. Toxic multinodular goiter occurs in middle-aged and elderly individuals with a long-standing history of goiter. This condition almost always occurs in iodine-deficient areas of the world, where goiter is often endemic.

Hyperthyroidism is approximately seven times more likely to occur in women than in men, and most cases are reported in the third and fourth decades of life. In rare instances, patients with hyperthyroidism can develop a life-threatening condition called thyrotoxic crisis, or thyroid storm. This can occur as the result of a serious stressor (surgery, infection, trauma) in a poorly managed patient. Approximately 25% of patients will die, even with appropriate medical attention.

Conventional Treatment

The major treatments used in conventional medicine are designed to limit the amount of thyroid hormones being produced by the gland. This can be achieved via a number of different strategies. Oral antithyroid medications interrupt hormone synthesis by preventing the organification of iodide in the thyroid. Thionamides (methimazole, carbimazole, and propylthiouracil) are the most popular pharmacologic agents currently used in the management of hyperthyroidism. Roughly 25% of patients with Graves disease will experience remission after 3–18 months of treatment.

If hyperthyroidism recurs, patients are usually given radioiodine therapy. Ablation of the thyroid tissue can also be accomplished with the administration of radioactive iodine. Radioactive iodine therapy (^{131}I) is often the second choice for treatment, after the thionamides. Radioactive iodine takes the place of iodine in the organification process in the thyroid gland, leading to destruction of the thyroid cells. The goal of treatment is to deliver a dose that destroys enough of the gland to eliminate the hyperthyroidism, while leaving enough intact tissue to prevent hypothyroidism. Unfortunately, a considerable number of patients will become hypothyroid and need hormone replacement.

Subtotal thyroidectomy by an experienced surgeon can be performed to remove enough thyroid tissue to eliminate the hyperthyroidism, while preserving enough tissue to prevent hypothyroidism. Surgical complications include damage to the recurrent laryngeal nerve leading to vocal cord paralysis. Postoperative complications include hypoparathyroidism, hemorrhage, and hypothyroidism. A skilled surgeon is essential, as up to 40% of patients will experience recurrence of hyperthyroidism because of insufficient removal of tissue.[105]

In cases of mild hyperthyroidism, beta-blockers are often prescribed. These drugs provide symptomatic relief of adrenergic symptoms such as tremor, arrhythmia, tachycardia, and anxiety. They also provide some inhibition of peripheral conversion of T_4 to T_3, thus providing additional protection from thyrotoxic effects. It should be noted, however, that these drugs have no effect on the production or release of thyroid hormones and so are usually used as an adjunctive therapy alongside anti-thyroid medications, radioactive iodine, or in preparation for surgery.

Integrative Approaches

Nutritional Supplements
ANTIOXIDANTS
Patients with hyperthyroidism experience an increase in oxidative stress and damage. It is believed that these oxidative processes play a role in the genesis of hyperthyroidism-induced damage. Vitamins C and E and selenium levels are decreased in hyperthyroid patients as compared to controls, leading a number of researchers to recommend dietary supplementation with antioxidants.[106] A group of 24 patients with hyperthyroidism taking propylthiouracil were noted to have reduced antioxidant function when compared to 15 healthy controls. One thousand milligrams of ascorbic acid was given to both groups for 30 days. Both groups showed significant improvement in antioxidant status and reduction of oxidative stress by the end of the study.[107] Vitamin E supplementation was shown to significantly reduce oxidative stress in hyperthyroid rat models by decreasing glutathione peroxidase activity, while increasing glutathione activity.[108] Animal studies show that supplementation with vitamin E and/or C protects apolipoproteins from the in-creased oxidation that occurs during hyperthyroid states.[109] A study in patients with mild to moderately severe Graves' ophthalmopathy found that 9 of 11 patients (82%) treated with oral antioxidants showed improvement as compared to 3 of 11 (27%) in the placebo group (p < 0.05). Reduction in soft-tissue inflammation was the disease component that responded most dramatically to treatment.[110]

Practitioners should consider supplementation with ascorbic acid and vitamin E in patients with hyperthyroidism. The dose for vitamin C is 1–2 g/d; for vitamin E, 400–600 IU. Many flavonoid-rich plants, such as bilberry, *Ginkgo biloba*, and hawthorn, also possess potent antioxidant activity.

Botanical Medicines
BUGLEWEED (*LYCOPUS EUROPAEUS* OR *L. VIRGINICUS*)
Herbalists have used bugleweed as a remedy for palpitations, fever, menorrhagia, nosebleeds, and anxiety since ancient times. Research has found that this herb can be beneficial for treating the symptoms of mild hyperthyroidism. In vitro studies of freeze-dried aqueous extracts of *L. europaeus* and *L. virginicus*, as well as *Melissa officinalis* and *Lithospermum officinale*, found that these substances interacted with important components of Graves' disease–immunoglobulin (IgG), inhibiting their ability to bind to the TSH receptor and activate the thyroid, although this effect was more pronounced with *Lithospermum* and *Melissa* than with *Lycopus*.[111] The active inhibitory constituents are thought to be rosmarinic acid, ellagic acid, and luteolin-7-beta-glucoside. These substances also appear to inhibit peripheral T_4-5'-deiodination to T_3.[112] While most experimental research was done with parenteral administration in animals, oral administration in rats noted only a reduction in T_3, likely caused by reduced peripheral conversion. TSH and T_4 levels were reduced only when the ethanolic extract of *Lycopus* was administered intraperitoneally. Interestingly, luteinizing hormone was also reduced with intraperitoneal

administration.[113] *Lycopus* lowers serum pro-lactin levels[114] and has also been noted to have significant antioxidant effect in vitro.[115] This may also be an additional benefit in Graves' disease as a recent study presented encouraging results in the treatment of mild-to-moderate Graves' ophthalmopathy with antioxidant agents.[116] No therapeutic trials of *Lycopus* have been conducted in humans, which is somewhat surprising. The German Commission E recognizes the following uses of *Lycopus* based upon pharmacological data only: "mild hyperthyroid conditions with neuroanatomic dysfunction, also breast tension and tenderness (mastodynia)." Rare cases of thyroid enlargement have been reported with long-term use of this herb. Dose recommendations range from 0.2–2 g/d of crude drug or equivalent.[117]

A patient with very mild hyperthyroidism may benefit from a trial of *Lycopus* for 8–12 weeks. Laboratory and symptom evaluation should be closely monitored. Herbalists often recommend that motherwort *(Leonurus cardiaca)* and/or hawthorn *(Crataegus* spp) be taken in addition to bugleweed for additional quieting effects upon the heart. This herb is not appropriate for moderate-to-severe cases of hyperthyroidism. Because of the antigonadotropic and antithyrotropic effects of this herb, it should not be used during pregnancy.

GROMWELL *(LITHOSPERMUM OFFICINALE)*
Although this herb is not used to the extent bugleweed is for the treatment of mild hyperthyroidism, it has been just as well studied. When freeze-dried extracts of *Lithospermum* were injected into animals, it was found to lower TSH, T_4, and T_3 levels. At the level of the pituitary, it blocks the activity of TSH, by interfering with TSH binding at the thyroid gland.[118] It also appears to suppress the iodide pump and block the release of thyroid hormones from the thyroid gland. Outside the thyroid gland, *Lithospermum* inhibits the liver enzyme I-iodothyronine deiodinase, decreasing peripheral conversion of T_4 to T_3.[119] An in vitro study found the freeze-dried extract decreased the ability of the antibodies to bind to thyroid tissue in Graves' disease.[120] There have been no human clinical trials to evaluate the effectiveness of *Lithospermum* in cases of hyperthyroidism.

The same cautions and contraindications for bugleweed should be considered with gromwell. The dose is variable, however, *King's* recommends that a strong infusion of the dried root, 1 ounce to 1 pint water be given every 3 hours in tablespoonful doses.[121] It should be noted that the Eclectics used *L. officinale* primarily for its diuretic effect and the treatment of acute and chronic cystitis.

LEMON BALM *(MELISSA OFFICINALIS)*
Lemon balm has been revered as a calmative, antispasmodic and antiseptic since ancient Greece. Lemon balm has similar antithyroid activity to *Lithospermum*. In vitro studies found that freeze-dried aqueous extracts of lemon balm were able to block the binding of bovine TSH to human thyroid membranes and binding of Graves autoantibodies.[122] There are no human clinical trials evaluating the effectiveness of lemon balm for hyperthyroidism. The calmative effects of lemon balm would also be beneficial for relieving some of the symptoms associated with hyperthyroidism. Lemon balm is quite safe when used appropriately. The dose for tincture (1:5) is generally 3–5 mL BID–TID.

MOTHERWORT *(LEONURUS CARDIACA)*
Motherwort has been used in many parts of the world as a "heart tonic" for palpitations and tachycardia. Alkaloids in the herb, such as leonurine, have sedative and hypotensive activity. Studies in animals demonstrate hypotensive, antiarrhythmic, antispasmodic, anxiolytic, and sedative effects. The German Commission E recognized motherwort for the treatment of cardiac disorders associated with anxiety and for symptomatic relief in hyperthyroidism.[123] The dose of tincture (1:5) is generally 2–4 mL BID–TID. Given the uncertain effects upon the uterus, motherwort should not be used during pregnancy.

Lifestyle Recommendations

Smoking significantly increases the risk for more severe Graves' ophthalmopathy and increases oxidative damage. Patients should be counseled and encouraged to stop smoking. Antioxidant supplementation should be considered.

Eating a diet rich in cruciferous vegetables may help reduce thyroid activity. Rutabagas, Brussels sprouts, turnips, and red cabbage are thought to have the greatest antithyroid potential. Soy isoflavones have also exhibited antithyroid activity. These foods, therefore, can be a useful dietary recommendation for hyperthyroid patients.

REFERENCES

1. DeFronzo R. Pharmacologic therapy for type 2 diabetes mellitus. *Ann Intern Med.* 1999;131: 281–303.
2. Expert Committee on the Diagnosis and Classification of Diabetes Mellitus. Report of the expert committee on the diagnosis and classification of diabetes mellitus. *Diabetes Care.* 1997;20: 1183–1197.
3. Alberti K, Zimmer P. Definition, diagnosis and classification of diabetes mellitus and its complications, part 1: diagnosis and classification of diabetes mellitus, provisional report of a World Health Organization consultation. *Diabet Med.* 1998;15:539–553.
4. Zimmet PZ, Tuomi T, Mackay R, et al. Latent autoimmune diabetes mellitus in adults (LADA): the role of antibodies to glutamic acid decarboxylase in diagnosis and prediction of insulin dependency. *Diabet Med.*1994;11:299–303.
5. Kissebah AH, Vydelingum N, Murray R, et al. Relationship of body fat distribution to metabolic complications of obesity. *J Clin Endocrinol Metab.* 1982;54:254–260.
6. Singh S. Gestational diabetes mellitus. In: Frederickson HL, Wilkins-Haug L, eds. *OB/GYN Secrets.* Philadelphia: Hanley & Belfus; 1991.
7. Engelgau MM, Herman WH, Smith PJ, German RR, Aubert RE. The epidemiology of diabetes and pregnancy in the US, 1988. *Diabetes Care.* 1995;18:1029–1033.
8. Langer O, Rodriguez DA, Xenakis EMJ, McFarland MB, Berkus MD, Arrendondo F. Intensified versus conventional management of gestational diabetes. *Am J Obstet Gynecol.* 1994;170: 1036–1047.
9. Harris MI, Flegal KM, Cowie CC, et al. Prevalence of diabetes, impaired fasting glucose, and impaired glucose tolerance in US adults. The Third National Health and Nutrition Examination Survey, 1988–1994. *Diabetes Care.* 1998;21: 518–526.
10. Stern MP, Gonzalez C, Mitchell BD, Villalpando E, Haffner SM, Hazuda HP. Genetic and environmental determination of type II diabetes in Mexico City and San Antonio. *Diabetes.* 1992;41:484–492.
11. Manson JE, Spelsberg A. Primary prevention of non–insulin-dependent diabetes mellitus. *Am J Prev Med.* 1994;10(3):172–184.
12. Liu S, Ajani U, Chase C, et al. Long-term carotene supplementation and risk of type 2 diabetes mellitus. *JAMA.* 1999;282:1073–1075.
13. Lehto S, Ronnemaa T, Haffner SM, et al. Dyslipidemia and hyperglycemia predict coronary heart disease events in middle-aged patients with NIDDM. *Diabetes.* 1997;46:1354–1359.
14. Blaum CS, Velez L, Hiss RG, Halter JB. Characteristics related to poor glycemic control in NIDDM patients in community practice. *Diabetes Care.* 1997;20:7–11.
15. Stumvoll N, Nurjhan N, Perriello G, et al. Metabolic effects of metformin in non–insulin-dependent diabetes mellitus. *N Engl J Med.* 1995;333: 550–554.
16. Jeppesen J, Zhou MY, Chen YD, Reaven GM. Effect of metformin on postprandial lipemia in patients with fairly to poorly controlled NIDDM. *Diabetes Care.* 1994;17:1093–1099.
17. Lebovitz HE. A new oral therapy for diabetes management: alpha-glucosidase inhibition with acarbose. *Clin Diabetes.* 1995;13:99–103.
18. Inzucchi SE. Oral antihyperglycemic therapy for type 2 diabetes. *JAMA.* 2002;287:360–372.
19. Lebovitz HE. Stepwise and combination drug therapy for the treatment of NIDDM. *Diabetes Care.* 1994;17:1542–1544.
20. American College of Sports Medicine. Position stand: exercise and type 2 diabetes. *Med Sci Sports Exerc.* 2000;32(7):1345–1360.
21. Egede L, Zheng D, Ye X, et al. The prevalence and pattern of complementary and alternative medicine use in individuals with diabetes. *Diabetes Care.* 2002;25:324–329.

22. Anderson JW. Fiber and health: an overview. *Am J Gastroenterol.* 1986;81:892–897.

23. Vitelli LL, Folsom AR, Shahar E, et al. Association of dietary composition with fasting serum insulin level: the ARIC Study. *Nutr Metab Cardiovasc Dis.* 1996;6:194–202.

24. Salmerón J, Manson JE, Stampfer MJ, et al. Dietary fiber, glycemic load, and risk of non–insulin-dependent diabetes mellitus in women. *JAMA.* 1997;277:472–477.

25. Salmeron J, Ascherio A, Rimm EB, et al. Dietary fiber, glycemic load, and risk of NIDDM in men. *Diabetes Care.* 1997;20(4):545–550.

26. Meyer KA, Kushi LH, Jacobs DR Jr, et al. Carbohydrates, dietary fiber, and incident type 2 diabetes in older women. *Am J Clin Nutr.* 2000; 71:921–930.

27. Jenkins EJA, Wesson V, Wolever TM, et al. Wholemeal versus wholegrain breads: proportion of whole or cracked grain and the glycaemic response. *BMJ.* 1988;297:958–960.

28. Florholmen J, Arvidsson-Lenner R, Jorde R, Burhol PG. The effect of Metamucil on postprandial blood glucose and plasma gastric inhibitory peptide in insulin-dependent diabetics. *Acta Med Scand.* 1982;212:237–239.

29. Fagerberg SE. The effects of a bulk laxative (Metamucil) on fasting blood glucose, serum lipids and other variables in constipated patients with non–insulin dependent adult diabetes. *Curr Ther Res.* 1982;31:166–172.

30. Pastors JG, Blaisdell PW, Balm TK, Asplin CM, Pohl SL. Psyllium fiber reduces rise in postprandial glucose and insulin concentrations in patients with non–insulin-dependent diabetes. *Am J Clin Nutr.* 1991;53:1431–1435.

31. Anderson JW, Allgood LD, Turner J, et al. Effects of psyllium on glucose and serum lipid responses in men with type 2 diabetes and hypercholesterolemia. *Am J Clin Nutr.* 1999;70:466–473.

32. Saris NE, Mervaala E, Karppanen H, et al. Magnesium. An update on physiological, clinical and analytical aspects. *Clin Chim Acta.* 2000;294(1–2): 1–26.

33. Fox CH, Ramsoomair D, Mahoney MC, et al. An investigation of hypomagnesemia among ambulatory urban African Americans. *J Fam Pract* 1999;48(8):636–639.

34. McCarty MF. Toward practical prevention of type 2 diabetes. *Med Hypotheses.* 2000;54(5):786–793.

35. Djurhuus MS, Skott P, Vaag A, et al. Hyperglycaemia enhances renal magnesium excretion in type 1 diabetic patients. *Scand J Clin Lab Invest.* 2000;60(5):403–409.

36. Corsonello A, Ientile R, Buemi M, et al. Serum ionized magnesium levels in type 2 diabetic patients with microalbuminuria or clinical proteinuria. *Am J Nephrol.* 2000;20(3):187–192.

37. Engelen W, Bouten A, De Leeuw I, De Block C. Are low magnesium levels in type 1 diabetes associated with electromyographical signs of polyneuropathy? *Magnes Res.* 2000;13(3): 197–203.

38. Whang R, Sims G. Magnesium and potassium supplementation in the prevention of diabetic vascular disease. *Med Hypotheses.* 2000;55(3): 263–265.

39. Sasaki S, Oshima T, Matsuura H, et al. Abnormal magnesium status in patients with cardiovascular diseases. *Clin Sci.* 2000;98(2):175–181.

40. Facchini FS, Humphreys MH, DoNascimento CA, et al. Relation between insulin resistance and plasma concentrations of lipid hydroperoxides, carotenoids, and tocopherols *Am J Clin Nutr.* 2000;72:776–779.

41. Paolisso G, Tagliamonte MR, Barbieri M, et al. Chronic vitamin E administration improves brachial reactivity and increases intracellular magnesium concentration in type II diabetic patients. *J Clin Endocrinol Metab.* 2000;85(1):109–115.

42. Will JC, Byers T. Does diabetes mellitus increase the requirement for vitamin C? *Nutr Rev.* 1996;54(7):193–202.

43. Will JC, Ford ES, Bowman BA. Serum vitamin C concentrations and diabetes: findings from the third National Health and Nutrition Examination Survey, 1988–1994. *Am J Clin Nutr.* 1999;70: 49–52.

44. Cohen N, Halberstam M, Shlimovich P, et al. Oral vanadyl sulfate improves hepatic and peripheral insulin sensitivity in patients with non–insulin-dependent diabetes mellitus. *J Clin Invest.* 1995;95:2501–2509.

45. Cusi K, Cukier S, DeFronzo RA, et al. Vanadyl sulfate improves hepatic and muscle insulin sensitivity in type 2 diabetes. *J Clin Endocrinol Metab.* 2001;86(3):1410–1417.

46. Poucheret P, Subodh V, Grynpas MD, McNeill JH. Vanadium and diabetes. *Mol Cell Biochem.* 1998;188:73–80.

47. Domingo JL. Vanadium and diabetes. What about vanadium toxicity? *Mol Cell Biochem.* 2000;203: 185–187.

48. Srivastava AK. Anti-diabetic and toxic effects of vanadium compounds. *Mol Cell Biochem.* 2000;206(1–2):177–182.

49. Vincent JB. Elucidating a biological role for chromium at a molecular level. *Acc Chem Res.* 2000;33(7):503–510.

50. Ravina A, Slezak L, Rubal A, Mirsky N. Clinical use of the trace element chromium (III) in the treatment of diabetes mellitus. *J Trace Elements Exp Med.* 1995;8(3):183–190.

51. Anderson RA, Cheng N, Bryden NA, et al. Elevated intakes of supplemental chromium improve glucose and insulin variables in individuals with type 2 diabetes. *Diabetes.* 1997;46: 1786–1791.

52. Abraham AS, Brooks BA, Eylath U. The effects of chromium supplementation on serum glucose and lipids in patients with and without non–insulin-dependent diabetes. *Metabolism.* 1992;41(7): 768–771.

53. Gerbi A, Maixent JM, Ansaldi JL, et al. Fish oil supplementation prevents diabetes induced nerve conduction velocity and neuroanatomical changes in rats. *J Nutr.* 1999;129:207–213.

54. Patti L, Maffettone A, Lovine C, et al. Long-term effects of fish oil on lipoprotein subfractions and low-density lipoprotein size in non–insulin-dependent diabetic patients with hypertriglycidemia. *Atherosclerosis.* 1999;146:361–367.

55. Alarcon-Aguilara FJ, Roman-Ramos R, Perex-Gutierrez S, et al. Study of the anti-hyperglycemic effect of plants used as antidiabetics. *J Ethnopharmacol.* 1998;61:101–110.

56. Kalpana P, Srinivasan K. Effect of dietary intake of freeze-dried bitter gourd *(Momordica charantia)* in streptozotocin induced diabetic rats. *Die Nahrung.* 1995;39(4):262–268.

57. Welihinda J, Karunanayake EH, Sheriff MH, Jayasinghe KS. Effect of *Momordica charantia* on the glucose tolerance in maturity-onset diabetes. *J Ethnopharmacol.* 1986;17(3):277–282.

58. Ahmad N, Hassan MR, Halder H, Bennoor KS. Effect of *Momordica charantia* (Karolla) extracts on fasting and postprandial serum glucose levels in NIDDM patients. *Bangladesh Med Res Counc Bull.* 1999;25(1):11–13.

59. Sarkar S, Pranava M, Marita R. Demonstration of the hypoglycemic action of *Momordica charantia* in a validated animal model of diabetes. *Pharmacol Res.* 1996;33(1):1–4.

60. Ahmed I, Adeghate E, Sharma AK, et al. Effects of *Momordica charantia* fruit juice on islet mor-phology in the pancreas of streptozotocin-diabetic rat. *Diabetes Res Clin Pract.* 1998;40(3): 145–151.

61. Kalpana P, Srinivasan K. Effect of dietary intake of freeze-dried bitter gourd *(Momordica charantia)* in streptozotocin induced diabetic rats. *Die Nahrung.* 1995;39(4):262–268.

62. Sauvaire Y, Baissac Y, Leconte O, et al. Steroid saponins from fenugreek and some of their biological properties. In: Waller G, Yamasaki K, eds. *Saponins Used in Food and Agriculture.* New York: Plenum Press; 1996.

63. Ribes G, Sauvaire C, Da Costa JC, et al. Antidiabetic effects of subfractions from fenugreek seeds in diabetic dogs. *Proc Soc Exp Biol Med.* 1986;182:159.

64. Sauvaire Y, Baissac Y, Leconte O, et al. Steroid saponins from fenugreek and some of their biological properties. In: Waller G, Yamasaki K, eds. *Saponins Used in Food and Agriculture.* New York: Plenum Press; 1996.

65. Khosla P, Gupta DD, Nagpal RK. Effect of *Trigonella foenum graecum* (fenugreek) on blood glucose in normal and diabetic rats. *Indian J Physiol Pharmacol.* 1995;39(2):173–174.

66. Raghuram TC, Sharma RD, Sivakumar B, Sahay BK. Effect of fenugreek seeds on intravenous glucose disposition in non–insulin-dependent diabetic patients. *Phytother Res.* 1994;8:83–86.

67. Ravikumar P, Anuradha CV. Effect of fenugreek seeds on blood lipid peroxidation and antioxidants in diabetic rats. *Phytother Res.* 1999;13(3): 197–201.

68. Udayasekhara Rao P, Sesikeran B, Srinivasa Rao P, et al. Short term nutritional and safety evaluation of fenugreek. *Nutr Res.* 1996;16(9):1495–1505.

69. Praveen KB, Dasgupta DJ, Prashar BS, Kaushal SS. Preliminary report: effective reduction of LDL cholesterol by indigenous plant products. *Curr Sci.* 1987;56(12):80–81.

70. Vuksan V, Sievenpiper JL, Koo VY, et al. American ginseng (*Panax quinquefolius* L.) reduces postprandial glycemia in nondiabetic subjects and subjects with type 2 diabetes mellitus. *Arch Intern Med.* 2000;160(7):1009–1013.

71. Vuksan V, Sievenpiper JL, Wong J, et al. American ginseng (*Panax quinquefolius* L.) attenuates postprandial glycemia in a time-dependent but not dose-dependent manner in healthy individuals. *Am J Clin Nutr.* 2001;73(4):753–758.

72. Shanmugasundaram ER, Gopinath KL, Radha

Shanmugasundaram K, Rajendran VM. Possible regeneration of the islets of Langerhans in streptozotocin-diabetic rats given Gymnema sylvestre leaf extracts. *J Ethnopharmacol.* 1990;30(3): 265–279.

73. Baskaran K, Kizar Ahamath B, Radha Shanmugasundaram K, Shanmugasundaram ER. Antidiabetic effect of a leaf extract from *Gymnema sylvestre* in non–insulin-dependent diabetes mellitus patients. *J Ethnopharmacol.* 1990;30(3): 295–300.

74. Shanmugasundaram ER, Rajeswari G, Baskaran K, et al. Use of *Gymnema sylvestre* leaf extract in the control of blood glucose in insulin-dependent diabetes mellitus. *J Ethnopharmacol.* 1990;30(3):281–294.

75. Jeppesen PB, Gregersen S, Poulsen CR, Hermansen K. Stevioside acts directly on pancreatic beta cells to secrete insulin: actions independent of cyclic adenosine monophosphate and adenosine triphosphate-sensitive K+ channel activity. *Metabolism.* 2000;49(2):208–214.

76. Chan P, Tomlinson B, Chen YJ, et al. A double-blind, placebo-controlled study of the effectiveness and tolerability of oral stevioside in human hypertension. *Br J Clin Pharmacol.* 2000;50(3): 215–220.

77. Das S, Das AK, Murphy RA, et al. Evaluation of the cariogenic potential of the intense natural sweeteners stevioside and rebaudioside A. *Caries Res.* 1992;26(5):363–366.

78. Keen H, Payan J, Allawi J, et al. Treatment of diabetic neuropathy with gamma-linolenic acid. The gamma-linolenic acid multicentre trial group. *Diabetes Care.* 1993;16(1):8–15.

79. Jamal GA, Carmichael H. The effect of gamma-linolenic acid on human diabetic peripheral neuropathy: a double-blind, placebo-controlled trial. *Diabet Med.* 1990;7:319–323.

80. Head RJ, McLennan PL, Raederstorff D, Muggli R, Burnard SL, McMurchie EJ. Prevention of nerve conduction deficit in diabetic rats by polyunsaturated fatty acids *Am J Clin Nutr.* 2000;71: 386S–392S.

81. Biessels GJ, Smale S, Duis SE, et al. The effect of gamma-linolenic acid-alpha-lipoic acid on functional deficits in the peripheral and central nervous system of streptozotocin-diabetic rats. *J Neurol Sci.* 2001;182(2):99–106.

82. Cameron NE, Cotter MA. Effects of antioxidants on nerve and vascular dysfunction in experimental diabetes. *Diabetes Res Clin Pract.* 1999; 45(2–3):137–146.

83. Guzzo CA, Lazarus GS, Werth VP. Dermatological pharmacology. In: Gilman AG, Goodman LS, Rall TW, et al., eds. *Goodman & Gilman's The Pharmacological Basis of Therapeutics.* 9th ed. New York: McGraw-Hill; 1996:1612.

84. Robbins W. Clinical applications of capsaicinoids. *Clin J Pain.* 2000;16(2):S86–S89.

85. Fusco BM, Giacovazzo M. Peppers and pain. The promise of capsaicin. *Drugs.* 1997;53(6): 909–914.

86. Mian E, Curri SB, Lietti A, Bombardelli E. Anthocyanosides and the walls of the microvessels: further aspects of the mechanism of action of their protective effect in syndromes due to abnormal capillary fragility [translated from Italian]. *Minerva Med.* 1977;68:3565–3581.

87. Cohen-Boulakia F, Valensi PE, Bonlahdour H, et al. In vivo sequential study of skeletal muscle capillary permeability in diabetic rats: effect of anthocyanosides. *Metabolism.* 2000;49(7):880–885.

88. Perossini M, Guidi G, Chiellini S, Stravo D. Diabetic and hypertensive retinopathy therapy with *Vaccinium myrtillus* anthocyanosides (Tegens). Double-blind, placebo-controlled trial. *Ann Oftalmol Clin Ocul.* 1987;113:1173–1190.

89. Repossi P, Malagola R, De Cadilhac C. The role of anthocyanosides on vascular permeability in diabetic retinopathy. *Ann Oftalmol Clin Ocul.* 1987;113:357.

90. Orsucci PL, Rossi M, Sabbatini G, et al. Treatment of diabetic retinopathy with anthocyanosides: a preliminary report. *Clin Ocul.* 1983;4:377.

91. Scharrer A, Ober M. Anthocyanosides in the treatment of retinopathies [translated from German]. *Klin Monatsbl Augenheilkd.* 1981;178:386–389.

92. Leung AY, Foster S. *Encyclopedia of Common Ingredients Used in Foods, Drugs, and Cosmetics.* 2nd ed. New York: Wiley & Sons; 1996.

93. King DE, Mainous AG 3rd, Pearson WS. C-reactive protein, diabetes, and attendance at religious services. *Diabetes Care.* 2002;25(7):1172–1176.

94. Lan C, Lai JS, Chen SY. Tai Chi Chuan: an ancient wisdom on exercise and health promotion. *Sports Med.* 2002;32(4):217–224.

95. Khanderia U, Jaffe CA, Theisen V. Amiodarone-induced thyroid dysfunction. *Clin Pharm.* 1993;12(10):774–779.

96. Gittoes NJ, Franklyn JA. Drug-induced thyroid disorders. *Drug Saf.* 1995;13:46–65.

97. Bunevicius R, Kazanavicius G, Zalinkevicius R, Prange AJ Jr. Effects of thyroxine as compared with thyroxine plus triiodothyronine in patients with hypothyroidism. *N Engl J Med.* 1999;340: 424–429.

98. Bouvier N, Millart H. Relationships between selenium deficiency and 3,5,3'-triiodothyronine (T3) synthesis. *Ann Endocrinol.* 1997;58(4):310–315.

99. Campos-Barros A, Meinhold H, Walzog B, Behne D. Effects of selenium and iodine deficiency on thyroid hormone concentrations in the central nervous system of the rat. *Eur J Endocrinol.* 1997; 136(3):316–323.

100. van Bakel MME, Printzen G, Wermuth B, Wiesmann UN. Antioxidant and thyroid hormone status in selenium-deficient phenylketonuric and hyperphenylalaninemic patients. *Am J Clin Nutr.* 2000;72:976–981.

101. Kohrle J. Thyroid hormone deiodination in target tissues-a regulatory role for the trace element selenium? *Exp Clin Endocrinol.* 1994;102(2): 63–89.

102. Civil ID, McDonald MJ. Acute selenium poisoning: case report. *N Z Med J.* 1978;87:354–356.

103. Tajiri J, Higashi K, Morita M, et al. Studies of hypothyroidism in patients with high iodine intake. *J Clin Endocrinol Metab.* 1986;63(2):412–417.

104. Konno N, Makita H, Yuri K, et al. Association between dietary iodine intake and prevalence of subclinical hypothyroidism in the coastal regions of Japan. *J Clin Endocrinol Metab.* 1994;78(2): 393–397.

105. Wilson JD, Foster DW, Kronenberg HM, Larsen PR. *Williams Textbook of Endocrinology.* 9th ed. Philadelphia: WB Saunders; 1997:425–515.

106. Aliciguzel Y, Ozdem SN, Ozdem SS, et al. Erythrocyte, plasma, and serum antioxidant activities in untreated toxic multinodular goiter patients. *Free Radic Biol Med.* 2001;30(60);665–670.

107. Seven A, Tasan E, Inci F, et al. Biochemical evaluation of oxidative stress in propylthiouracil treated hyperthyroid patients. Effects of vitamin C supplementation. *Clin Chem Lab Med.* 1998; 36(10): 767–770.

108. Seven A, Seymen O, Hatemi S, et al: Antioxidant status in experimental hyperthyroidism: effect of vitamin E supplementation. *Clin Chim Acta.* 1996;256(1):65–74.

109. Dirican M, Tas S. Effects of vitamin E and vitamin C supplementation on plasma lipid peroxidation an on oxidation of apolipoprotein B-containing lipoproteins in experimental hyperthyroidism. *J Med Invest.* 1999;46(1):29–33.

110. Bouzas EA, Karadimas P, Mastorakos G, Koutras DA. Antioxidant agents in the treatment of Graves' ophthalmopathy. *Am J Ophthalmol.* 2000; 129(5):618–622.

111. Auf'mkolk M, Ingbar JC, Kubota K, et al. Extracts and auto-oxidized constituents of certain plants inhibit the receptor-binding and the biological activity of Graves' immunoglobulins. *Endocrinology.* 1985;116(5):1687–1693.

112. Auf'mkolk M, Kohrle J, Gumbinger H, et al. Antihormonal effects of plant extracts: iodothyronine deiodinase of rat liver is inhibited by extracts and secondary metabolites of plants. *Horm Metab Res.* 1984;16(4):188–192.

113. Winterhoff H, Gumbinger HG, Vahlensieck U, et al. Endocrine effects of *Lycopus europaeus* L. following oral application. *Arzneimittelforschung.* 1994;44(1):41–45.

114. Sourgens H, Winterhoff H, Gumbinger HG, Kemper FH. Antihormonal effects of plant extracts. TSH and prolactin suppressing properties of *Lithospermum officinale* and other plants. *Planta Med.* 1982;45:78–86.

115. Lamaison JL, Petitjean-Freytet C, Carnat A. Medicinal *Lamiaceae* with antioxidant properties, a potential source of rosmarinic acid. *Pharm Acta Helv.* 1991;66(7):185–188.

116. Bouzas EA, Karadimas P, Mastorakos G, Koutras DA. Antioxidant agents in the treatment of Graves' ophthalmopathy. *Am J Ophthalmol.* 2000; 129(5):618–622.

117. Schulz V, Hansel R, Tyler VE. *Rational Phytotherapy: A Physicians' Guide to Herbal Medicine.* 3rd ed. Berlin: Springer-Verlag; 1998:245.

118. Brinker F. Inhibition of endocrine function by botanical agents. 1. *Boraginacea* and *Labiatae.* *J Nat Med.* 1990;1:10–18.

119. Auf-mkolk M, Kohrle J, Gumbinger H, et al. Antihormonal effects of plant extracts: iodothyronine deiodinase of rat liver is inhibited by extracts and secondary metabolites of plants. *Horm Metab Res.* 1984;16(4):188–192.

120. Auf'mkolk M, Ingbar JC, Kubota K, et al. Extracts and auto-oxidized constituents of certain plants inhibit the receptor-binding and the biological activity of Graves' immunoglobulins. *Endocrinology.* 1985;116(5):1687–1693.

121. Felter HW, Lloyd JU. *King's American Dispen-*

satory. 18th ed. Sandy, OR: Eclectic Medical Publications; 1983:1198–1199.

122. Aufmkolk M, Ingbar JC, Kubota K, et al. Extracts and auto-oxidized constituents of certain plants inhibit the receptor-binding and the biological ac-

tivity of Graves' immunoglobulins. *Endocrinology.* 1985;116(5):1687–1693.

123. Blumenthal M, Busse WR, Goldberg A, et al: *The Complete German Commission E Monographs.* Austin, TX: American Botanical Council; 1998.

CHAPTER 21

Integrative Approach to the Gastrointestinal System

Leo Galland

The most critical function of the gastrointestinal (GI) tract is the digestion of food and the absorption of nutrients. The GI tract also serves the entire body as an organ of immune surveillance and response, detoxification, and neuroendocrine regulation. Digestive functions are supported physically by mastication, peristalsis, enzymes, and secretions that enhance enzyme activity. Absorptive functions are facilitated by the immense surface area of the small intestine, with its villi and microvilli, and the transmucosal, energy-driven processes of active transport and facilitated diffusion that occur along the entire length of the small and large intestines. From the perspective of pathology, the barrier function of the alimentary canal is as important as its absorptive function. In effect, the mucosal surface is an external surface that has been internalized, but which remains continuous with the external environment. From the buccal mucosa to the anal sphincter, every centimeter of the GI tract is colonized by bacteria, with the colon bearing the greatest load. Every meal bathes this surface with antigens, organisms, and pharmacologically active substances derived from food and drink.

The serosal side of the GI mucosa is a site of active surveillance. Two-thirds of the body's lymphocytes reside here, concentrated in Peyer patches or scattered as intraepithelial lymphocytes, making the small intestine the largest immunologic organ of the human body.[1] Intestinal lymphocytes recognize soluble and insoluble antigens that cross the mucosal barrier by passive diffusion or endocytosis. This normal physiologic process, called *gut antigen sampling*, may be greatly altered during states of inflammation. A complex neurologic network regulates intestinal motility and interacts with the intestinal immune system. This network produces and uses every neurotransmitter found in the central nervous system (CNS). Although the gut nervous system interacts continuously with the CNS, it is complete enough to function in isolation, and has been dubbed "the second brain."[2]

GI disorders are not merely "digestive disorders." Most gastrointestinal diseases result from dysfunction among the complex regulatory relationships mentioned above, and their effects are not limited to the gastrointestinal tract. Integrated therapies for GI disorders, as presented in this chapter, extend beyond the substitution of a "natural treatment" for a drug (e.g., the use of peppermint oil instead of vagolytics for relieving intestinal cramps[3]). They derive from applying the principles of patient-centered diagnosis (described in Chapter 4) to the integrated physiology of the GI tract. Two concepts that are often neglected in conventional teaching play a central role in this application: dysbiosis and permeability.

▶ DYSBIOSIS AND THE NORMAL GI FLORA

Symbiosis is Greek for living together. We live together with about 100 trillion microbes, most of them residing in the colonic lumen, where there are as many colony-forming units (CFUs) as there are cells in the adult human body. More than 500 species of bacteria live in the healthy human alimentary canal; in the average adult, they weigh about 1 kg (2.2 lb).[4] Table 21–1 describes the predominant organisms at different sites.

Table 21–2 shows the typical composition of stool flora. In health, the relationship is either beneficial (eu-symbiosis, or mutualism) or neutral in its effects (commensalism). The normal colonic microflora ferment soluble fiber to yield short-chain fatty acids that supply 5–10% of human energy requirements.[4] Endogenous flora synthesize at least seven essential nutrients, supplementing dietary intake: folic acid, biotin, pantothenic acid, riboflavin, pyridoxine, cobalamin, and vitamin K.[4] They participate in the metabolism of drugs, hormones, and carcinogens, including digoxin,[5] sulfasalazine, and estrogens.[6] By demethylating methylmercury, gut flora protect mice from mercury toxicity.[7] They prevent potential pathogens from estab-

▶ **TABLE 21–1** MUCOSAL BACTERIA OF THE GI TRACT

- Colon: anaerobic spirochetes, fusiform bacteria
- Ileum: coccobacilli
- Oral: anaerobes (*Corynebacterium, Actinomyces, Bacteroides, Spirochaetas, Fusobacterium*), and aerobes (*Streptococcus* and *Lactobacillus*)
- Stomach: lactobacilli, yeasts

▶ **TABLE 21–2** COMPOSITION OF NORMAL STOOL FLORA

Eubacterium, 26 spp	25.5%
Bacteroides, 20 spp	22.6%
Bifidobacterium, 8 spp	11.5%
Peptostreptoccus	8.9%
Fusobacterium, 5 spp	7.7%
Ruminoccus, 11 spp	4.5%
Lactobacillus, 7 spp	2.4%
Streptococcus	1.6%
Clostridium	0.6%
Enterobacter	0.5%

lishing infection by numerous mechanisms, including production of short-chain fatty acids and bacteriocin (an endogenous antibiotic); induction of a low oxidation-reduction potential; competition for nutrients; deconjugation of bile acids (which renders them bacteriostatic); blockade of adherence receptors; and degradation of bacterial toxins.[8]

Germ-free animals have moderate defects in immune function when compared to control animals. These include lower levels of natural antibodies, hyporesponsive macrophages and neutrophils, defective production of colony-stimulating factors, leukopenia, lymphoid hypoplasia, subnormal interferon levels, and weak delayed hypersensitivity responses. They are more susceptible to infection with intracellular parasites such as *Listeria, Mycobacterium,* and *Nocardia,* but are not more susceptible to viral infection.[4] The immunologic effects of normal gut flora are in part caused by antigenic stimulation and in part by the bacterial origin of specific immune activators, such as endotoxin lipopolysaccharide and muramyl dipeptides.[4,9] The gut flora of healthy individuals is quite stable; largely because of interbacterial inhibition.[10] Alteration in the level of normal flora by antibiotics has long been known to allow secondary infection by pathogenic bacteria and yeasts.[11]

Dysbiosis, or dys-symbiosis, occurs when the relationship between gut flora and the human host becomes injurious to the host (parasitism). In dysbiosis, organisms of relatively low intrinsic virulence—organisms that usually exist in a state of mutualism or commensalism with their hosts—promote illness. This differs from infection, in which a highly virulent organism attaches to the mucosal lining and either invades the mucosa (like *Shigella flexneri*) or secretes a potent toxin (like *Vibrio cholerae*). The normal indigenous flora protect against pathogens; dysbiosis, however, may predispose to infection. Recent use of ampicillin, for example, increased the risk of diarrhea following exposure to food-borne *Salmonella*, presumably because ampicillin pretreatment depleted indigenous organisms.[12] Conversely, administration of *Lactobacillus* GG (*L. casei* var *rhamnosus,* strain GG) prevents development of traveler's diarrhea, which is usually caused by food-borne pathogens.[13] The pathogenicity of *Entamoeba histolytica* depends upon the colonic bacterial milieu. When invasive strains of *E. histolytica* are grown in culture, their zymodeme patterns change to those of nonpathogenic strains if they are cocultured with colonic flora obtained from healthy individuals. When nonpathogenic strains are incubated with the bacterial flora obtained from patients with amebic dysentery, the reverse happens: they assume the zymodeme patterns of invasive organisms. Consequently, amebic pathogenicity is influenced by the indigenous colonic flora of the host.[14]

At least five mechanisms of disease associated with dysbiosis have been described:

1. As already mentioned, the loss of beneficial microbes may cause disease by removal of the protective effects of the normal gut flora. Antibiotic-induced diarrhea not only involves the overgrowth of toxin-producing bacterial species, such as *Clostridium difficile,* but the loss of the neutralizing effect of the normal colonic flora on clostridial toxins.[15]

2. Microbial enzymes may modify selected intraluminal substrates, producing noxious substances. Microbial alteration of bile acids

is thought to play a pathogenic role in cholelithiasis and colon cancer. The primary bile acids, cholate and chenodeoxycholate, are synthesized in the liver. Deoxycholic acid (DCA), a secondary bile acid, is produced from cholate by colonic bacteria. In the colon, DCA is a tumor promoter, and fecal DCA concentrations are directly proportional to the rate of colon cancer in populations studied.[16] DCA that is absorbed from the colon enters the portal circulation and reaches the liver, from which it is excreted in bile. DCA in bile increases its saturation with cholesterol. In patients with cholelithiasis, the degree of bile cholesterol supersaturation (the main reason for stone formation) correlates directly with DCA concentration.[17] Colonic dysbiosis thereby contributes to cholelithiasis.

3. Microbial antigens may cross-react with mammalian antigens, stimulating autoimmunity. Ankylosing spondylitis, for example, occurs almost exclusively in human leukocyte antigen (HLA)-B27–positive individuals. Immunologic cross-reactivity has been shown for HLA-B27 antigen expressed on the host cell membrane and antigens present in *Klebsiella pneumoniae, S. flexneri,* and *Yersinia enterocolitica,* suggesting molecular mimicry in the pathogenesis of this disease.[18] Workers in Australia have demonstrated bacteria with cross-reactive antigenic determinants in bowel flora of B27-positive ankylosing spondylitis patients; these bacteria are almost never found in B27-positive controls without ankylosing spondylitis.[19]

4. Components of the microbial cell wall may stimulate nonspecific, dysfunctional immune responses that produce local or systemic inflammation. Intestinal lymphocytes from patients with Crohn's disease, but not controls, show a mitogenic response to *Enterobacter* and *Candida albicans,* both normally present in the small intestine.[20] Bacterial endotoxemia has been described in patients with psoriasis[21] and cystic

acne.[22] Activation of the alternative complement pathway by gut-derived endotoxin may play a role in the pathogenesis of these disorders.

5. Bacterial enzymes may destroy host enzymes or components of the host's biological response system. In small bowel bacterial overgrowth, for example, destruction of pancreatic and brush-border enzymes by bacterial proteases may cause maldigestion and malabsorption.[23] *Pseudomonas* species colonizing the gut can inactivate interferon gamma.[24]

In addition to its role in antibiotic-induced diarrhea and small bowel bacterial overgrowth, intestinal dysbiosis may contribute to the pathogenesis of ulcerative colitis, Crohn's disease, irritable bowel syndrome (IBS), peptic ulcer disease, gastroesophageal reflux disease (GERD), gastric cancer, and colon cancer.[25,26] Integrated therapies for patients with these disorders should include treatments that restore normal alimentary tract symbiosis.

▶ REGULATION OF GI FLORA

The principal factors that regulate the composition and distribution of the GI flora are diet, motility, the nature of GI secretions, immune function, and the ingestion of antibiotic or probiotic substances.

Dietary Factors

Carbohydrates, including fiber, serve as substrates for bacterial and fungal growth and fermentation. Table 21–3 lists products of bacterial fermentation. Simple carbohydrates tend to increase both growth and fermentation by microbes in the mouth, stomach, and upper small intestine.[27,28] Complex carbohydrates increase these activities in the ileum,[29] and soluble fiber (found in fruit, legumes, and some whole grains) normally exerts its effects in the cecum

▶ **TABLE 21-3** PRODUCTS OF MICROBIAL FERMENTATION IN GUT

- Acetaldehyde
- Acetic acid
- Acetone
- Butanol
- Butylene glycol
- Butyric acid
- CO_2
- Ethanol
- Formic acid
- Hydrogen
- D-Lactic acid
- Propionic acid

and colon.[30] Feeding soluble fiber to rodents increases the bacterial biomass and enzyme concentration in the cecum. Insoluble fiber, found in many vegetables and in wheat bran, by contrast, decreases the cecal biomass and enzyme concentrations, mostly by dilution, and perhaps also by inhibition.[31] In patients with gallstones whose bile is supersaturated with cholesterol, wheat bran added to the diet lowers cholesterol saturation and DCA concentration in bile, probably by interfering with colonic bacterial enzyme activity.

Products of gut microbial fermentation, especially short-chain fatty acids like butyrate, nourish colonic epithelial cells and lower stool pH. A slightly acidic stool is associated with protection against colon cancer.[32] In the small bowel, fermentation products may act as irritants. Lactic acid, for example, is a major factor in producing the symptoms of lactose intolerance.

Protein induces intestinal bacteria to synthesize enzymes involved in peptide, amino acid, and amine catabolism, including peptidases, ureases, and tryptophanases.[33] The putrefactive odor of stool is largely caused by this enzyme activity, as is the production of ammonia. Tryptophanase not only contributes to putrefaction, but also yields carcinogenic indoles and skatoles, which may contribute to the epidemiologic association between high-protein diets and colon cancer.[34] The diamino acid, glutamine, in contrast, nourishes the small intestinal epithelium and the lymphocytes of the gut-associated lymphoid tissue.

The effects of dietary fat on GI microflora are complex. Free fatty acids are bacteriostatic; the presence of these in milk confers protection against intestinal infection with bacteria and protozoa. Increased bile flow, induced by fat ingestion, is also bacteriostatic. The protozoan *Giardia lamblia*, however, thrives in the presence of bile. High rates of biliary secretion produce an increase in fecal bile acid concentration and at the same time increase fecal pH. Both these features are associated with an increase in the rate of colon cancer in humans and animals.[35]

Among micronutrients, iron appears to have the greatest impact on gut flora, because all microbes, except lactobacilli and bifidobacteria, depend upon iron for growth and metabolism. Feeding iron to patients with bowel disease, especially when concentrated in pill form, can induce the overgrowth of pathogenic species. Lactoferrins are iron-binding proteins found in colostrum and in leukocytes. Lactoferrins aid with intestinal iron absorption and inhibit bacterial, fungal, and protozoan growth. Lactoferrins in breast milk help to prevent diarrheal disease in infancy.[36]

Motility

Peristalsis moves the gut contents distally and helps to maintain the bacterial concentration gradient from stomach to anus. Altered motility may allow small bowel bacterial overgrowth and may increase mucosal exposure to irritants.[37] Motility, in turn, is influenced by diet, neuroendocrine factors, and consumption of drugs and herbs. As a general rule, dopaminergic neurons inhibit and serotoninergic neurons enhance motility, although different receptor subtypes are active at different sites in the enteric nervous system.[38] High-fiber diets tend to stimulate motility and decrease intesti-

nal transit time. Simple sugars have a bifold effect. They shorten small bowel transit but inhibit large bowel transit. This effect appears to be mediated by the vagus nerve, which is stimulated by the ingestion of sweet food, regardless of its glucose content. A potential effect of this phenomenon is to increase the delivery of unabsorbed nutrients into the cecum and to permit greater bacterial metabolism of those nutrients in the colon.

Herbs and spices have numerous pharmacologic effects. Ginger and capsicum, in particular, increase GI motility.[39]

GI motility is also influenced by emotional distress, which may either stimulate or inhibit motility of the bowel and gallbladder and the secretion of gastric acid and duodenal bicarbonate. Changes in GI flora resulting from stress effects on motility are subtle, but may be significant. Russian cosmonauts experienced a decrease in stool concentrations of lactobacilli and bifidobacteria before space missions (dietary changes were not described)[40]; anger and hostility have been accompanied by an increase in the levels of tryptophanase-producing bacteria in stool. The activity of these might increase colonic putrefactive activity and the production of carcinogens from high-protein foods. GI flora, in turn, may have considerable influence on gut motility; this is discussed in "Functional Digestive Disorders."

Secretions

Gastric HCl has the most significant influence of all GI secretions. HCl is not only the first line of biological defense against the acquisition of enteric infections, it helps to maintain relatively low concentrations of bacteria and fungi in the stomach, despite the high nutrient density that occurs postprandially.[11] Hypochlorhydria, whether resulting from pathology or drugs, increases susceptibility to infection with enteric pathogens and also permits increased gastric colonization with bacteria and yeasts.[12] Bacterial enzymes may convert dietary nitrates or nitrites to carcinogenic nitrosamines (one link between hypochlorhydria and gastric cancer).[43] The gastric microbial overgrowth resulting from strong acid suppression or the hypochlorhydria of aging causes vitamin B_{12} malabsorption and gastric synthesis of ethanol following carbohydrate consumption.[44]

The other secretory products with significant influence on GI flora are secretory immunoglobulin A (sIgA) and mucins. Both impair bacterial attachment to mucosal epithelium, interfering with mechanisms of pathogenicity.

Immunity

The immune regulatory network in the gut is composed of antigen-presenting cells, effector cells, and the cytokines they produce, and antibodies, primarily sIgA. The most intense activity occurs in the jejunum and ileum. Intestinal columnar epithelium, which consists of normal enterocytes, functions as antigen-presenting cells, ingesting soluble antigen by endocytosis, transporting it to the serosal surface of the epithelium and presenting antigens to intraepithelial lymphocytes. Most intraepithelial lymphocytes have a CD-8 (cytotoxic/suppressor) phenotype and generate an immune response that is largely immune suppressive. Normal immune tolerance for dietary antigens appears to depend upon this enterocyte-mediated immune activity. Intraepithelial lymphocyte activity, however, is not always immune suppressive. The cytokines produced by intraepithelial lymphocytes may stimulate macrophages to produce inflammatory cytokines, which contribute to the pathogenesis of inflammatory bowel disease (IBD) (see "Inflammatory Bowel Disease").

The small bowel epithelium is punctuated by squat, noncolumnar epithelial cells called M cells, which have a large indentation on the serosal side in which macrophages reside. M cells ingest and transport particulate or insoluble antigens and deliver them to their associated macrophages, which then travel to Peyer's patches and present the antigen to Peyer's patch lymphocytes. The predominant phenotype of Peyer's patch lymphocyte is CD-4 (helper); their activation leads to an increase in IgA specific to the antigen presented. Impaired small bowel immunity, whether acquired or congenital, permits colonization by pathogens and can also permit small bowel bacterial overgrowth. Pathologically heightened immunity (sensitization) to components of the normal flora occurs during the course of IBD.

Intestinal immune function, like systemic immunity, can be strongly influenced by diet and nutritional status. Protein-calorie malnutrition, by impairing cell-mediated immunity and secretion of IgA, may cause small bowel bacterial overgrowth.[45] Deficiencies of specific nutrients have demonstrated effects on systemic immunity, which may predispose to GI disease. Low blood levels of zinc,[46] iron,[47] vitamin A,[48] and selenium[49] are associated with increased susceptibility to mucosal yeast infection. These deficiencies, and others, are common among patients with chronic gastrointestinal disorders, especially IBD.[50–53] They may occur because of self-imposed dietary restrictions, maldigestion, malabsorption, excessive loss through GI secretions, or the effects of therapeutic drugs. Sulfasalazine and its derivatives, for example, impair folic acid transport.[54] Proton pump inhibitors may permit gastric bacterial overgrowth with secondary deficiencies of vitamin B_{12} and malabsorption of fat-soluble nutrients.[55] Correction of nutritional deficiency is important for maintenance or restoration of normal intestinal immune function. Dietary fats have important immune-modulating effects in the intestinal tract. The antiinflammatory effects of omega-3 essential fatty acids have been used in the treatment of patients with IBD (discussed in "Crohn's Disease").

Antibiotics and Probiotics

Traditional cuisines from many cultures contain foods with natural antibiotic or probiotic activity. Many spices have these intrinsic antimicrobial components; most are heat labile, destroyed by heating at 90°C (194°F) for 20 minutes.[56] Spices appear to have initially been added to food as preservatives. Human ingestion of these, uncooked or lightly cooked, may protect against enteric infection or microbial overgrowth in the upper bowel. Ginger, for example, contains more than 400 biologically active components that provide antiinflammatory, antiulcer, and antiparasitic effects; it has long been used for the treatment of digestive complaints.[57] Garlic is mentioned in the earliest Vedic medical texts. Its antimicrobial activity was first demonstrated by Pasteur, and Schweitzer employed it for the treatment of amebic dysentery at his clinic in Africa. The dose needed to obtain significant benefit is at least 10 g (about three small cloves) per day.[58,59] Onion, another member of the *Allium* family, has similar antimicrobial benefits but requires larger doses.[60,61] Turmeric may relieve flatulence by reducing the concentration of fermentative bacteria; it also has antifungal activity and antiinflammatory activity. The effective dose is about 1 g/d.[62,63] Cinnamon has antifungal activity.[64] Sage and rosemary contain the essential oil eucalyptol, which kills *C. albicans,* helminths, and many bacterial species.[65] Oregano contains more than 30 biologically active ingredients of which 12 have antibiotic, antiviral, antiparasitic, or antifungal effects.[66] Thyme was used as a vermifuge in ancient Egypt.[67]

Fermented foods, such as sauerkraut or yogurt, contain lactic acid bacteria such as *L. plantarum* or *L. bulgaricus,* respectively, that can successfully colonize the small and large intestines. Daily consumption of yogurt decreased the frequency of monilial vaginitis in a controlled study, but only if the yogurt contained viable organisms.[68] Numerous probiotic supplements are commercially available in the United States. The most intensively studied are *Lactobacillus* GG (a strain of *L. casei* var. *rhamnosus*),[69] *L. plantarum* (which naturally grows on plant surfaces and is found in cultured plant foods), and *Saccharomyces*

boulardii (a yeast similar to baker's yeast that was originally cultured from lichee nuts in French Indochina during the 1920s).[70] *Lactobacillus* GG and *S. boulardii* protect against antibiotic-induced and traveler's diarrhea. Administration of *L. plantarum* to patients undergoing major abdominal surgery decreased the incidence and severity of postoperative infection.[71] Unlike the lactobacilli, *S. boulardii* is not part of the normal flora and is only found in the gut if it is ingested. It stimulates production of sIgA and can neutralize *Clostridium difficile* toxin A. *S. boulardii* helps prevent recurrent pseudo-membranous colitis caused by *C. difficile*. New preparations of probiotics are being tested for therapeutic benefits in IBD (see "Ulcerative Colitis").

▶ INTESTINAL PERMEABILITY AND GUT BARRIER FUNCTION

The intestinal epithelium is the site of vectorial transport of solvents, solute, and macromolecules between the intestinal lumen and the circulation. The net effect is regulated by the tightness or leakiness of the barrier. Transport and barrier functions are physiologically regulated and may be significantly altered under conditions of disease.[72] Two routes for transport are possible: transcellular or intercellular (paracellular). The regulation of each is separate and specific. Transcellular transport may occur by passive or facilitated diffusion (e.g., water and magnesium), by active transport (e.g., glucose and most vitamins and minerals), or by endocytosis (particulate matter and macromolecules) (see Tables 21–4, 21–5,

▶ **TABLE 21–4** NUTRIENTS ABSORBED BY ACTIVE TRANSPORT

- Amino acids, peptides
- Monosaccharides
- Sodium, zinc, copper, iron, calcium
- Vitamins

▶ **TABLE 21–5** NUTRIENTS ABSORBED
BY DIFFUSION

- Free fatty acids
- Magnesium
- Monoglycerides, lysolecithin

▶ **TABLE 21–6** SMALL INTESTINAL
ENDOCYTOSIS

- Antigens
- Macromolecules
- Micelles
- Microbes

and 21–6, and Figure 21–1). The transport of macromolecules, including intact dietary protein, across the small intestinal epithelium is a normal physiologic process that occurs after each meal.[73] Intact enzymes, such as urokinase, can be absorbed.[74] Dietary macromolecules normally enter the systemic circulation postprandially, in immunocompetent healthy volunteers.

Bacterial translocation, sometimes producing septicemia, is a pathological process usually resulting from impairment of mucosal immunity, induced by hypoxia or starvation.[75] Cardiopulmonary bypass[76] and hypovolemic shock[77] induce splanchnic hypoxia and are associated with bacteremia by this mechanism. Total parenteral nutrition starves the intestinal mucosa and may be complicated by septicemia,

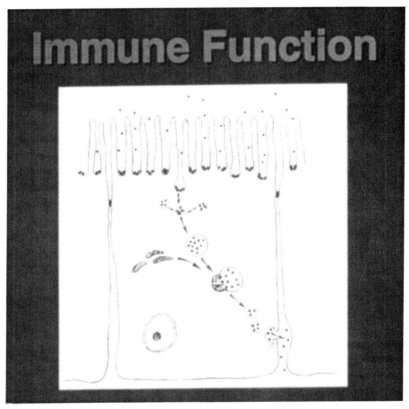

Figure 21–1. Endocytosis as a mechanism of transepithelial transport of macromolecules.

also by this mechanism.[78] The bacteria causing sepsis in patients receiving total parenteral nutrition enter the circulation from the GI tract, not usually from the intravenous catheter.

The other conditions in which normal gut barrier function involving transcellular permeability is excessively increased are genetic. In hemochromatosis and in idiopathic hypercalciuria, excessive absorption of iron or calcium, respectively, results from enhancement of enzyme-driven active transport resulting from gene mutations.

Nutritional deficiency has complex effects on transcellular mucosal permeability. For minerals like calcium, iron, or zinc, which require specific transport proteins for absorption, deficiency causes a compensatory, physiologic increase in the activity of the transport protein. It is possible that nutritional deficiencies that impair cellular energy metabolism may cause malabsorption by hampering active mucosal transport. In vitamin B_3 deficiency, for example, small intestinal function is impaired even though the villous architecture remains normal, perhaps because some active transport processes are specifically dependent upon the B_3-containing cofactors nicotinamide adenine dinucleotide or nicotinamide adenine dinucleotide phosphate.[79–81] Evidence for similar effects caused by other nutritional deficiencies is lacking.

The most common increases in intestinal permeability follow the paracellular route. Paracellular transport is always passive and is normally limited by cellular adhesion molecules that make up the tight junctions, adherens junctions, and desmosomes that knit adjacent cells together (Figure 21–2). Contraction of the epithelial cell cytoskeleton opens adherens junctions, transiently increasing paracellular permeability. This may be stimulated by high intraluminal concentrations of glucose or by excessive cholinergic stimulation in the small intestine.[82] Experiments with rodents that are genetically bred to produce a cholinergic response to stress (characterized by low frequency of avoidance behaviors) indicate that immersion stress and cold stress in these animals produce a measurable increase in paracellular permeability that can be blocked by anticholinergic agents and that does not occur in animals bred differently.[83] Similar effects appear to occur in humans, but definitive studies have not been performed. The healthy first-degree relatives of patients with Crohn's disease represent a human population with a statistically significant increase in intestinal permeability,[84] which is probably constitutional. Increased permeability may play an etiologic role in Crohn's disease, allowing abnormal entry of microbial antigens into the gut wall.[85] Cholinergic neural pathways may play a contributory role.

Another physiologic influence on paracellular permeability is an endogenous peptide called Zot (zona occludens toxin), which transiently loosens tight junctions. Infectious agents such as *Vibrio cholerae*, the cause of cholera, produce Zot analogues that irreversibly open tight junctions, causing a leaky gut.[86] The leaky gut of cholera is a separate phenomenon from the diarrhea associated with cholera, which is caused by toxic stimulation of mucosal adenylate cyclase. Prostaglandin E, on the other hand, helps to maintain normal paracellular permeability.[87] Exposure to cyclooxygenase inhibitors, like aspirin and nonsteroidal anti-inflammatory drugs (NSAIDs) causes a transient increase in paracellular permeability that may be blocked by administration of the prostaglandin E analogue misoprostol.[88] Exposure to high doses of NSAIDs for about 2 weeks renders this increase in permeability resistant to misoprostol but reversible with the antibiotic metronidazole.[89] A sustained increase in small bowel permeability, as induced during the treatment of rheumatoid arthritis with NSAIDs, results in sensitization to gut microbial antigens and microscopic enteritis.[90] Reduction of mucosal antigen exposure and the gut inflammatory response with metronidazole is needed for reversal of hyperpermeability in these circumstances. This mechanism may explain the benefits of antibiotic therapy in the treatment of patients with IBD and rheumatoid

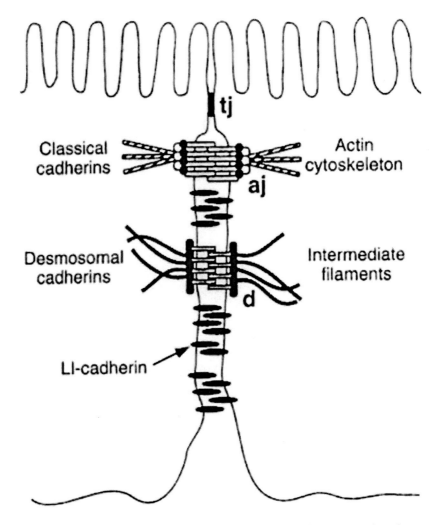

Figure 21-2. Representation of adhesive cell-cell contacts by classical cadherins, desmosomal cadherins, and LI-cadherin in the intestinal mucosa. aj = Adherens junction; d = desmosomes; tj = tight junctions.

arthritis.[91] Antibiotics not only alleviate symptoms in these patients but also behave like disease-modifying agents.[92]

Other factors that may produce a pathological increase in paracellular permeability include infectious agents (viral, bacterial, and protozoan),[93,94] ethanol,[95] exposure to cytotoxic drugs such as methotrexate,[96] and ingestion of foods that provoke an allergic or inflammatory response.[97] Following exposure to allergenic foods, permeability sharply increases.[98] Most of this increase can be averted by pretreatment with sodium cromoglycate,[99] indicating that release from mast cells of atopic mediators like histamine and serotonin is responsible for the increase in permeability.

Claude André, a leading French research worker in gut permeability, has proposed that measurement of gut permeability is a sensitive and practical screening test for the presence of food allergy and for following response to treatment. In Andre's protocol, patients with suspected food allergy ingest 5 g each of the innocuous sugars lactulose and mannitol. These sugars are not metabolized by humans, and the amount absorbed is fully excreted in the urine within 6 hours. Mannitol, a monosaccharide, is passively transported through intestinal epithelial cells; mean absorption is 14% of the administered dose (range: 5–25%). In contrast, the intestinal tract is impermeable to lactulose, a disaccharide; less than 1% of the administered dose is normally absorbed. The differential excretion of lactulose and mannitol in urine is then measured. The normal ratio of lactulose/mannitol recovered in urine is less than 0.03. A higher ratio signifies excessive lactulose absorption caused by excessive paracellular permeability. The lactulose/mannitol challenge test is performed fasting and again after ingestion of a test meal. At the Hôpital St. Vincent de Paul in Paris, permeability testing has been effectively used with allergic infants to determine which dietary modifications their mothers needed to make while breast-feeding and which of the "hypoallergenic" infant formulas they needed to avoid in order to relieve their symptoms.[100]

Increased intestinal permeability may contribute to illness by permitting excessive exposure to luminal antigens derived from microbes or food.[101] Increased permeability stimulates classic hypersensitivity responses to foods and to components of the normal gut flora; bacterial endotoxins, cell wall polymers, and dietary gluten may cause "nonspecific" activation of inflammatory pathways mediated by complement and cytokines.[102] In experimental animals, chronic low-grade endotoxemia causes the appearance of autoimmune disorders.[103]

Leaky gut syndromes are clinical disorders associated with increased intestinal permeability. They include inflammatory and infectious bowel diseases[104]; chronic inflammatory arthritides[105]; cryptogenic skin conditions such as acne,[106] psoriasis,[107] and dermatitis herpetiformis[108]; eczema[109]; irritable bowel syndrome[110]; AIDS[111]; chronic fatigue syndromes; and cystic fibrosis.[112] Hyperpermeability may play a primary etiologic role in the evolution of each disease, or may be a secondary consequence of it. Unless specifically investigated, the role of altered intestinal permeability in patients with leaky gut syndromes often goes unrecognized. The availability of safe, noninvasive, and inexpensive methods for measuring small intestinal permeability makes it possible for clinicians to look for the presence of altered intestinal permeability in their patients and to objectively assess the efficacy of treatments.

Treatment of hyperpermeability states has two phases:

1. *Remove the cause.* This includes the treatment of an intestinal infection, avoidance of enterotoxic drugs (primarily NSAIDs and ethanol), and elimination of food allergens from the diet. Diagnostic methods for food allergy are controversial and a discussion of the merits and pitfalls of each method is beyond the scope of this chapter. Andre's method (described above) uses an increase in permeability to diagnose food allergy and is therefore specific to the role of food in creating hyperpermeability.

2. *Nourish the gut.* Under normal conditions, intestinal epithelium has the fastest rate of mitosis of any tissue in the body; old cells slough and a new epithelium is generated every 3–6 days.[113] The metabolic demands of this normally rapid cell turnover must be met if healing of damaged epithelium is to occur. When these are not met, hyperpermeability is exacerbated.[114] To maintain its integrity, this epithelium requires all the nutrients needed for cellular growth and repair: protein, calories, vitamins, minerals, and essential fatty acids. Glutamine, among

all the amino acids, appears to have a special role in restoring normal small bowel permeability and immune function.[115] Patients with intestinal mucosal injury secondary to chemotherapy or radiation benefit from glutamine supplementation with less villous atrophy, increased mucosal healing, and decreased passage of endotoxin through the gut wall.[116] At a dose of 1,600 mg daily, glutamine use was associated with the rapid radiographic healing of peptic ulcers, prior to the advent of H_2 blockers.[117] Glutamine does not appear to play a trophic role in the colon, however. In the large bowel, this role is played by butyric acid, which is generated by the fermentation of soluble fiber. Supplementing the diet with glutamine at intakes of 5–30 g/d decreases small intestinal hyperpermeability in severely ill individuals. Feeding butyrate by mouth is unlikely to have any effect on the large bowel, because it is readily absorbed in the jejunum. Butyrate enemas, however, have been used to nourish colonic segments that are surgically isolated from the fecal stream.[118]

Prostaglandins play a key role in the maintenance of normal paracellular permeability, although the specific prostaglandin balance for optimal permeability is unknown. In experimental animals, fish oil feeding ameliorates the intestinal mucosal injury produced by methotrexate and, additionally, blunts the systemic circulatory response to endotoxin.[119] In tissue culture, both n-3 and n-6 essential fatty acids stimulate wound healing of intestinal epithelial cells.[120] Consumption of large amounts of vegetable oils, on the other hand, tends to increase the free radical content of bile and to exacerbate the effects of endotoxin.[121]

Other trophic factors that may be helpful in improving enteric epithelial hyperpermeability include:

1. *Lactobacilli.* The ability of *Lactobacillus acidophilus* preparations to improve altered permeability has not been directly tested, but is suggested by the ability of live cultures of *L. acidophilus* to diminish radiation-induced diarrhea,[122] a condition directly produced by the loss of mucosal integrity. *Lactobacillus* GG limits diarrhea caused by rotaviral infection in children, and improves the hyperpermeability associated with rotaviral infection.[123]

2. *Epidermal growth factor,* a polypeptide that stimulates growth and repair of epithelial tissue, is widely distributed in the body, with high concentrations being detectable in salivary and prostate glands and in the duodenum. Saliva can be a rich source of epidermal growth factor, especially the saliva of certain nonpoisonous snakes. The use of serpents in healing rituals may reflect the value of ophidian saliva in promoting the healing of wounds. Thorough mastication of food may nourish the gut by providing it with salivary epidermal growth factor. Purified epidermal growth factor heals ulceration of the small intestine.[124]

3. *Gamma oryzanol,* a complex mixture of ferulic acid esters of phytosterols and other triterpene alcohols derived from rice bran, has been extensively researched in Japan for its healing effects in the treatment of gastric and duodenal ulceration, which are thought to be secondary to its potent antioxidant activity.[125]

Although epithelial integrity is the main factor maintaining normal permeability, it is not the only factor. Secretory IgA plays a supportive role. Levels may be boosted by administration of the nonpathogenic yeast, *S. boulardii.* Clinical trials have demonstrated the effectiveness of *S. boulardii* in the treatment or prevention of traveler's diarrhea,[126] *C. difficile* diarrhea,[127] and antibiotic diarrhea.[128] Experimental data suggest that the yeast owes its effect to stimulation of sIgA secretion[129] and macrophage activation.[130] Passive elevation of gut immunoglobulin levels can be produced by feeding bovine colostrum or egg yolk extracts[131] that are rich in IgA and IgG. Feeding IgG and IgA orally is effective in preventing infantile necrotizing enterocolitis,[132] a disorder thought to be caused by the hyperpermeability of the infantile gut. Bovine colostrum, 125 mL three times a day, fed to healthy human volunteers was shown to prevent the increase in intestinal permeability produced by indomethacin administration.[133]

Severely ill patients are often treated with "bowel rest," clear-liquid diets, or total parenteral nutrition. Alternative practitioners sometimes use juice fasts for "cleansing." Whatever the therapeutic value of these methods, they carry with them the risk of inducing hyperpermeability of the small intestine. Patients fasted or fed only liquids develop intestinal villous atrophy, depletion of sIgA, and translocation of bacteria from the gut lumen to the systemic circulation.[134] Feeding glutamine reverses all these abnormalities. The only demonstrated exception to this has been patients with rheumatoid arthritis. Fasting decreases intestinal permeability in patients with rheumatoid arthritis, possibly because fasting in these patients is accompanied by discontinuation of NSAIDs, avoidance of food allergens, and decreased activation of enteric lymphocytes.[135]

Fiber supplements have complex effects on gut permeability and bacterial composition. Low-fiber diets increase permeability. Dietary supplementation with insoluble fiber, such as pure cellulose, decreases permeability.[136] Dietary supplementation with highly soluble fiber sources, such as fruit pectin or guar gum, has a biphasic effect. At low levels, it reverses the hyperpermeability of low-residue diets, probably by a mechanical bulking effect that stimulates synthesis of mucosal growth factors. At high levels of supplementation, it produces hyperpermeability, probably by inducing synthesis of bacterial enzymes that degrade intestinal

mucins.[137,138] For maximum benefit with regard to intestinal permeability, dietary fiber supplementation should contain a predominance of insoluble fiber.

Repairing abnormal permeability, restoring healthy gut flora, and improving intestinal immune function are essential goals in the integrative treatment of gastrointestinal disorders. The achievement of these goals is supported by specific dietary therapies, nutritional supplements, probiotic flora, and herbs. Herbs with antibiotic, antiinflammatory, and antispasmodic activity have been used for millennia in many different cultures for problems such as abdominal pain, diarrhea, and constipation.[139,140] Contemporary studies often show that herbal therapies employed for intestinal disorders demonstrate antimicrobial activity against common intestinal pathogens,[141–151] although clinical research may show them to have less activity than modern antibiotics.[152] Antimicrobial herbs readily available in the United States include the leaves of *Artemisia annua* (sweet sagewort or qinghao), a plant that yields the lactone artemisinin (qinghaosu), which is the basis for a new class of antimalarial compounds widely used in Asia and Africa[153]; the roots of *Berberis aquifolium* (Oregon grape or barberry), *Hydrastis canadensis* (goldenseal), and *Coptis chinensis* (goldthread), which yield the alkaloid berberine[154–157]; the bulb of *Allium sativum* (garlic); and the fruit of *Juglans nigra* (black walnut).[158–160] Along with probiotics, their use may aid the establishment of desirable changes in the gut flora.[161]

Other modalities that have shown benefit for treatment of chronic gastrointestinal disorders include mind–body therapies[162] and acupuncture.[163] Specific information about multicomponent, integrative, evidence-based approaches to patients with inflammatory bowel disease, irritable bowel syndromes, and acid-peptic disorders is presented below. The potential role of these therapies in preventing cancers of the gastrointestinal tract is mentioned, where data exist.

▶ INFLAMMATORY BOWEL DISEASE

Both dysbiosis and hyperpermeability play central roles in the immunopathology of the inflammatory bowel diseases, which are "thought to result from inappropriate and ongoing activation of the mucosal immune system driven by the presence of normal luminal flora . . . facilitated by defects in both barrier function and the mucosal immune response. Accumulating evidence suggests that the luminal flora is a requisite and perhaps central factor in the development of inflammatory bowel disease."[164] Although Crohn's disease and ulcerative colitis show important differences, especially in response to integrative therapies, and are discussed separately, the two conditions also share a great deal. Both show genetic and environmental influences, may be aggravated by nonsteroidal anti-inflammatory drugs,[165] and are sometimes improved by antibiotics,[166,167] although antibiotic therapy is more consistently effective for active Crohn's colitis than for ileitis or ulcerative colitis. In both types of IBD, an increased number of surface-adherent and intracellular bacteria have been observed in mucosal biopsies.[168,169] Mucosal immune responses provoked by these bacteria, however, are distinctly different in the two disorders. The predominant response in Crohn's disease involves lymphocytes with a type 1 T-helper cell (Th1) response, whereas ulcerative colitis appears to feature lymphocytes with an atypical type 2 T-helper cell (Th2) response.[170] Th1 responses are mediated by interferon gamma (IFN-γ) and interleukin-12 (IL-12), whereas Th2 responses are mediated by interleukin-5 (IL-5) and transforming growth factor-β. Inflammation in both types of IBD involves stimulation of macrophages, which produce interleukin-1 (IL-1) and tumor necrosis factor-α (TNF-α), and activation of the multifunctional regulator, nuclear factor-$\kappa\beta$.[164] The antiinflammatory cytokine, IL-1 receptor antagonist, is decreased in both diseases.[171] Inflammation in IBD is associated with an increase in markers of oxidative stress and decreased levels of antioxidants. Zinc and copper or the zinc- and copper-dependent enzyme, superoxide dismutase, are reduced in mucosal biopsies from patients with both types of IBD.[172] Oxidative stress caused by inflammation produces a loss of 73% of reduced ascorbate in the bowel epithelium of IBD patients.[173] Plasma levels of vitamins A and E are lower and plasma levels of the oxidative stress marker, 8-hydroxy-deoxyguanosine, are higher in IBD patients than in controls.[174]

Patients with Crohn's disease and ulcerative colitis may also share some dietary and psychological risk factors. Small studies from northern Europe found a greater than average premorbid intake of sugar and bread among patients with both types of IBD[175]; self-reported intolerance of specific foods was over four times more common for patients with each type of IBD than for controls.[176] Two-thirds of food-intolerant patients reported sensitivity to one or two foods and one-third experienced symptom provocation with multiple foods; the most commonly reported problem foods were onions, cabbage, apples, strawberries, citrus fruit, and beef.

Several studies have looked at anxiety, depression, perceived stress, and stressful life events as related to disease activity among patients with IBD, and a few have evaluated the role of psychotherapy in the treatment of patients with IBD. Of 80 patients in a British study, most believed there was a close link between personality, stress, and disease activity; 42 thought a stressful life event or a "nervous personality" had initiated the disease.[177] A German study, however, found no relationship between stressful life events, feelings of pressure or conflict, or fear of separation and symptomatic exacerbations of Crohn's disease or ulcerative colitis.[178] Italian researchers studied the relationship of perceived stress with endoscopic appearance of the rectal mucosa in 46 asymptomatic outpatients with ulcerative colitis. The level of perceived stress over the previous 2 years was higher in the 11 patients with mucosal abnormalities than in the 35 patients with a normal rectal mucosa ($P = .004$). The authors believed their findings represented a "true link between psychological factors and ulcerative colitis activity."[179] Intriguing research from Germany describes an "uncoupling" of the adrenal steroid and autonomic nervous system responses to stress in patients with IBD. Among healthy controls, stress responses activate the adrenal cortex and the autonomic nervous system together, so that levels of neuropeptide Y and plasma cortisol vary together. Among IBD patients, levels of neuropeptide Y and cortisol are inversely related, so that autonomic nervous system activation does not evoke the immune-modulating effects of cortisol. Some of this disparity may be caused by prior use of adrenal steroids. The relative insufficiency of adrenal function present among IBD patients, which is suggested by this research, may explain stress-induced exacerbations of disease.[180]

The quality of life of patients with IBD is inversely proportional to both psychosocial distress and disease activity, as might be expected; however, psychosocial function and coping may be better predictors of quality of life than disease activity itself.[181] Adaptive adjustment to IBD has been conceptualized as a process involving the interaction of three challenges: illness uncertainty, loss and change, and suffering.[182] Enhancement of adaptive adjustment and prevention of psychosocial distress should play an important role in the treatment of patients with IBD. Interventions of potential value include enhancing problem-solving and coping skills, enhancing the positive appraisal of uncertainty, increasing personal control, and increasing social support.[183]

Three prospective studies of different types of psychotherapy for patients with IBD have failed to show any improvement in medical outcome compared with standard medical care.[184–186] An effective, "patient-centered" intervention was designed by a team at the University of Manchester. During a 15–30-minute consultation, physicians designed personalized self-management strategies for each patient.

The goal was to ensure that patients could recognize relapse and that patients and physicians could agree on a mutually acceptable treatment protocol for the patient to initiate at onset of a relapse. Physicians specifically asked patients about the symptoms they had experienced during past relapses and reviewed past and current treatments that had been used to control symptoms, emphasizing the specific effectiveness of each and its acceptability to the patient. Compared to a control group that received customary care, the intervention group required one-third as many doctor visits and one-third as many hospitalizations. The difference in outcome was not related to specific treatments employed but rather to the empowerment of patients to be actively involved in managing their own care.[187] This self-management approach effectively addressed the adaptive challenges described above, with significant benefit to patients.

► CROHN'S DISEASE

Small intestinal permeability is increased in noninflamed tissue[188] of patients with Crohn's disease and in healthy first-degree relatives of patients with Crohn's disease, suggesting that a predisposition to hyperpermeability may be a risk factor for its development.[189] Aspirin causes an exaggerated increase in intestinal permeability in first-degree relatives of patients with Crohn's disease, as compared to controls.[190] The rate of relapse among Crohn's disease patients who have entered remission is directly related to the measurement of small intestinal permeability using the lactulose/mannitol probe described above[191] (Figure 21–3). Hyperpermeability may be the result of microscopic inflammation, but it also increases exposure of the intestinal immune system to luminal antigens. The intraepithelial lymphocytes of patients with Crohn's disease are abnormally sensitive to antigens derived from indigenous bowel bacteria and yeast.[20] Small bowel bacterial overgrowth may aggravate

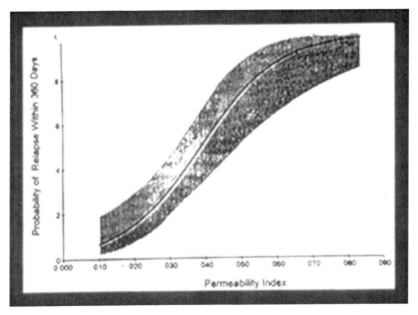

Figure 21-3. Probability of a Crohn's disease relapse within 1 year.

inflammation in patients with Crohn's disease, and has been identified in 30% of hospitalized patients in one study.[50] The immune response underlying the pathology of Crohn's disease, as in other granulomatous diseases, is driven by Th1 lymphocytes and their cytokine, IL-12. These Th1 products promote a self-sustaining cycle of activation with macrophages that includes IL-2, which further increases Th1 activity, and IL-1, IL-6, IFN-γ, and TNF-α, which promote a broader inflammatory response. Inflammation increases oxidative stress in the bowel mucosa.[192] A growing body of research indicates that the normal intestinal microflora is essential for provoking inflammation in Crohn's disease, and one study has shown adherent strains of *Escherichia coli* bound to the ileal mucosa.

Using the language of patient-centered diagnosis, the predominant theory of Crohn's disease holds that the key mediators (IL-12, IFN-γ, TNF-α, and reactive oxygen intermediates) are activated by exposure to triggers derived from the normal gut flora, and that the usual antecedents are genetic predisposition and/or the occurrence of a precipitating event that damages intestinal mucosal integrity, such as acute enteritis. High sucrose intake predisposes to Crohn's disease.[193,196] The control of Crohn's disease is enhanced by dietary avoidance of sucrose and other refined carbohydrates,[197] suggesting that the sugar/disease relationship may be significant, not coincidental.

The hygiene hypothesis has been invoked to explain the increasing prevalence of Crohn's disease during the past century. The most intriguing incarnation of this theory attributes the increase to lack of exposure to helminths. Helminth infestation was virtually universal among humans until the late nineteenth century; its prevalence has declined substantially at the same time and with the same demographics as the increased incidence of IBD. Helminth infestation provokes an immune response that is Th2 mediated, with the main cytokines being IL-4, IL-5, and IL-11. Th2 activity naturally downregulates Th1 activity. Furthermore, IL-11 is immune suppressive and antiinflammatory; its synthesis may explain the low levels of clinical allergy in children with heavy parasitic infestation. Researchers at the University of Iowa have induced remission in patients with refractory Crohn's disease by administering the eggs of a nonpathogenic pork roundworm.[198]

Various studies have identified other triggers for patients with Crohn's disease.[199] Although feelings of "being under pressure" are associated with the activity of Crohn's disease, to date there has been no validation for the notion that stressful life events can trigger exacerbation.[200] Food presents numerous triggers. Patients with Crohn's disease often show immunologic hypersensitivity to a component of *Saccharomyces cerevisiae* (baker's and brewer's yeast).[201] Feeding a suspension of *S. cerevisiae* may provoke symptoms in asymptomatic patients.[202] The East Anglican Multicentre Controlled Trial, conducted under the auspices of Cambridge University, evaluated the value of diet in the treatment of patient's with active Crohn's disease.[203] The first phase consisted of 2 weeks of a defined elemental diet, during which 84% of the patients achieved clinical remission accompanied by a significant decrease in erythrocyte sedimentation rate and C-reactive protein and an increase in serum albumin. Patients were then randomized to receive treatment with prednisolone or treatment with a specific food exclusion diet. To determine which foods each patient needed to avoid, a structured series of dietary challenges was conducted. At 6 months, 70% of patients treated with diet were still in remission as compared with 34% of patients being treated with prednisolone. After 2 years, 38% of patients treated with specific food exclusion were still in remission as compared with 21% of steroid-treated patients. Patients who did not comply with their diets were regarded as being treat-

ment failures, even if they remained in complete remission. In previous uncontrolled studies, some of the same authors had used a diet consisting of one or two meats (usually lamb or chicken), one starch (usually rice or potatoes), one fruit, and one vegetable instead of the elemental diet in order to induce remission. Compliance with the specific food elimination diet was associated with a rate of relapse of less than 10% per year.[204] Table 21–7 lists the individual foods found to provoke symptoms in this study. Most patients reacted adversely to more than one food.

Help with maintenance of remission has also been demonstrated in a randomized blinded trial, using an enteric-coated fish oil extract that supplied eicosapentaenoic acid (EPA) 1,800 mg/d and docosahexaenoic (DHA) 900 mg/d.[205] Based upon clinical symptoms and laboratory indices of inflammation, 59% of those receiving fish oil remained in remission at 1 year as compared to 26% of those receiving placebo. The main side effect of fish oil was reversible diarrhea, which occurred in 10%. The effect of fish oils in Crohn's disease patients may involve more than pharmacologic

▶ **TABLE 21–7** FOODS PROVOKING CROHN'S ACTIVITY IN TOTAL OF 64 PATIENTS

• Wheat	28
• Dairy	28
• *Brassica* vegs	16
• Corn	12
• Yeast	11
• Tomatoes	11
• Citrus fruits	10
• Eggs	10
• Tap water	8
• Coffee	8
• Banana	8
• Potatoes	7
• Lamb	7
• Pork	7
• Beef	5
• Rice	5

suppression of inflammation. Biochemical studies indicate that 25% of patients with IBD show evidence of essential fatty acid deficiency.[206] The leukocytes of patients with Crohn's disease have abnormalities in the uptake and metabolism of essential fatty acids, which correlates with low levels of zinc.[207] Zinc deficiency is common among patients with Crohn's disease, as is selenium deficiency, another mineral important for normal essential fatty acid metabolism. Zinc and selenium supplementation may offer additional benefits to patients with Crohn's disease. Zinc is important for growth and repair. Zinc-deficient adolescents with Crohn's disease grow and mature more normally when zinc deficiency is treated; as would be expected. Anecdotally, correction of zinc deficiency as a specific intervention has been associated with global clinical improvement, suggesting that zinc replacement may have beneficial effects on disease activity.[208] Both zinc and selenium are cofactors for inducible enzymes with antioxidant effects (superoxide dismutase and glutathione peroxidase, respectively). Oxidant stress is characteristic of inflammation in the mucosa of patients with IBD; correction of zinc or selenium deficiency may help to alleviate inflammation by supporting antioxidant responses.

The author has used the clinical science just reviewed to develop a practical, individualized approach for treatment of patients with Crohn's disease, which was associated in a case series with induction of complete clinical remission with discontinuation of all medication in 30% and varying degrees of improvement in symptom scores (range: 40–90%; mean: 65% improvement) and laboratory parameters in the remainder. There were no patients whose condition deteriorated or who did not experience some improvement in symptoms.[209] This approach is divided into three phases.

Phase One: Initial Exclusion Diet. Although the few foods elimination diet of the Cambridge researchers may be used, a broader and easier initial nutritional intervention is a modified Paleolithic diet that is free of cereal grains, milk and soy products, and potatoes, and very low in disaccharides such as sucrose. This diet is described in a book, *Breaking the Vicious Cycle*[210] and referred to as the specific carbohydrate diet (SCD; for more information go to www.scd.org). In the author's experience, this diet alone has improved symptoms in 55% of patients, being most effective in those with ileitis. (Of note, the diet permits the use of certain cultured dairy products. It also does not eliminate some of the vegetables or fruits found to provoke symptoms in published studies.)

Phase Two: Modified Exclusion Diet. In those patients responding with a 50% or greater reduction in symptoms over 30 days when using SCD, a slight expansion of the initial diet is permitted, within the guidelines detailed in *Breaking the Vicious Cycle*. In those patients who do not show a 50% reduction in symptoms, further dietary changes are made on an individual basis. The most common changes are (1) elimination of all milk-derived products; (2) reduction in dietary yeast and monosaccharides by eliminating honey, fruit, vinegar, and any fermented foods; (3) substitution of rice and potatoes for nut flours (the major source of complex carbohydrate in the SCD).

Phase Three: Nutritional Supplementation. Delayed-release fish oil capsules supplying 2,700 mg of n-3 fatty acids a day and a multivitamin and mineral supplying folic acid 800 μg, zinc 25 mg, selenium 200 μg, and vitamin E 400 mg. Vitamin E is used for its antioxidant effects, although controlled studies of its use have not been conducted. For those with ileitis, glutamine 3,000–6000 mg/d is also used, usually in a formulation that includes either gamma-oryzanol 300 mg/d or epidermal growth factor derived from a glandular extract.

Probiotics and prebiotics must be used with caution in patients with Crohn's disease, because their effects are highly unpredictable. Although occasional small studies have shown benefits from administration of nonpathogenic bacteria,[211] induction of remission by an elemental diet has been associated with a reduction in fecal *Lactobacillus* concentrations,[212] and all bacteria, even friendly flora, may activate Th1 responses.

Various antibiotic regimens are used in conventional therapy for Crohn's disease, either to treat acute exacerbations or induce remission of chronic disease. Their use is compatible with the strategy outlined above, with one exception. Some patients experience an exacerbation of symptoms when taking antibiotics, perhaps as a result of the yeast sensitivity which is common among patients with Crohn's disease. These patients may require antifungal therapy instead of or in addition to antibiotics.

▶ Case Example 1: Crohn's Disease Responsive to Fluconazole

A 21-year-old woman experienced the sudden onset of severe right-lower-quadrant abdominal pain and diarrhea following a trip to France. Radiologic evaluation revealed an ileocolic fistula and a diagnosis of Crohn's disease was made. Stool examination showed cysts of *Entamoeba histolytica*. Her gastroenterologist began treatment with ciprofloxacin and her abdominal pain steadily increased, so she sought an alternative therapy to antibiotics for the treatment of her condition. During her initial interview, she revealed that she had suffered a respiratory infection while traveling and had received an antibiotic from a French physician. The onset of symptoms following one antibiotic and the aggravation of symptoms while taking another, suggested that the antibiotics were the triggers for her

symptoms, perhaps by encouraging the overgrowth of antibiotic-resistant organisms. *Clostridium difficile* was not found in stool, but there was a high level of yeast seen in stool. Ciprofloxacin therapy was immediately discontinued and fluconazole (Diflucan) 200 mg/d was started. A low-sugar, low-yeast diet was recommended. Within 4 days she was pain free. She continued to follow a yeast-elimination diet for a period of 2 years, observing a transient return of abdominal pain upon consumption of bread or beer. She continued to use Diflucan intermittently for several months for control of symptoms, with no other medication. As of 2003, she has been in complete clinical and laboratory remission for 3 years. She has not been compliant with the use of nutritional supplements.

▶ ULCERATIVE COLITIS

Compared to Crohn's disease, the immunopathology of ulcerative colitis is not as clearly understood and the role of intestinal permeability is less certain, because colonic permeability is extremely difficult to measure. Microbial triggers appear to be equally as important, however, with effector cells thought to

be atypical Th2 lymphocytes, which produce transforming growth factor-β and IL-5. Circumstantial evidence associating abnormal strains of *E. coli* to inflammation in ulcerative colitis led to a therapeutic protocol in which treatment with 1 week of oral gentamicin, followed by the administration of a nonpathogenic, standardized *E. coli* strain, was superior to mesalazine for maintenance of remission.[213]

Other probiotic therapies have not been tested in controlled trials, although pouchitis (post-colectomy inflammation of the ileal pouch) has been shown to respond to very high doses (450 billion CFUs per day or more) of a mixture of lactic acid and bifidobacteria.[211] This preparation is now being tested as an aid to maintenance of remission in patients with ulcerative colitis.[215] Several natural products have shown promise as aids to inducing remission in ulcerative colitis. Fish oils, supplying approximately 3,200 mg of EPA and 2,000 mg of DHA per day, decrease symptoms and lower the levels of leukotriene B4 in stool, with improvement demonstrated after 12 weeks of therapy.[216] Lower doses, as used in other trials, do not appear to be effective and fish oil therapy has not been associated with maintenance of remission in ulcerative colitis, as it has been in Crohn's disease.[205] The Ayurvedic herb boswellia, 300 mg three times a day, was as effective as the 5-ASA (5-aminosalicyclic acid) derivative mesalamine in reducing symptoms of active ulcerative colitis.[217] An extract of aloe vera, concentrated to a mucopolysaccharide concentration of 30% of solid weight, was demonstrated to reduce symptoms and indices of inflammation in controlled studies.[218] Butyric acid nourishes the colonic epithelium, encouraging differentiation of cells. Butyrate enemas are beneficial for healing distal ulcerative colitis and postsurgical diversion colitis.[118] Wheat grass juice, 100 cc taken twice daily for 1 month, tested in a small placebo-controlled trial of patients with distal ulcerative colitis,[219] produced a significant reduction in rectal bleeding, abdominal pain and disease activity as measured by sigmoidoscopy. A germinated barley foodstuff containing glutamine-rich protein and hemicellulose-rich fiber was given to patients with mild to moderate active ulcerative colitis who had been unresponsive to or intolerant of standard treatment in a nonrandomized, open-label study. At a dose of 20–30 g/d this treatment resulted in significant clinical and endoscopic improvement, associated with an increase in stool butyrate concentrations.

Previous work by this group had demonstrated that stool butyrate production by enteric bacteria suppressed binding of the inflammatory gene regulator nuclear factor kappa B.[220]

Compared to patients with Crohn's disease, patients with ulcerative colitis are less likely to have specific food intolerance and more likely to harbor intestinal protozoa. Controlled studies of diet for ulcerative colitis have not been performed, but observers who have published uncontrolled studies have estimated that 15–20% of patients with ulcerative colitis have food allergy or specific food intolerance, with cow's milk protein being the leading offender.[221] Because hydrogen sulfide produced by enteric flora inhibits the epithelial effects of butyrate,[222] a low-sulfur diet has been advocated for maintenance of remission in ulcerative colitis. This diet, which is markedly different from the SCD used for treatment of Crohn's disease, eliminates eggs, cheese, whole milk, ice cream, mayonnaise, soy milk, mineral water, nuts, cruciferous vegetables, beef, pork, and sulfited alcoholic beverages. A preliminary study following four patients after an acute exacerbation of chronic ulcerative colitis found no relapses or adverse nutritional effects over a 5-year period.[223]

Colitis caused by *Entameba histolytica*, and occasionally other protozoa, may be confused with ulcerative colitis.[224] Protozoan infection is more likely in patients with recent onset, onset after the age of 30 years, or poor response to conventional antiinflammatory medication. The boundary between infectious and "idiopathic" colitis is very fuzzy, however. Acute gastrointestinal infection often precedes the development of IBD,[225] and patients with ulcerative colitis are at greater risk of intercurrent colonic infection than controls, possibly because the inflammation already present increases susceptibility. Spontaneous overgrowth of *C. difficile* without antecedent antibiotic exposure is not unusual in patients with ulcerative colitis and may be a cause for a sudden onset of rectal bleeding.[226] Stool testing for protozoan infestation is more likely to be accurate when performed by a laboratory that specializes in tropical medicine or parasitology than when performed by a general laboratory.[227] The presence of protozoa in stool of a patient with long-standing, stable, mild to moderate ulcerative colitis is most likely to be significant if the patient has experienced a recent exacerbation.[228] Charcot-Leyden crystals in stool, sometimes used as a sign of amebic or helminthic infection, are not reliable indices of infection in patients with IBD, because eosinophil degranulation (the source of Charcot-Leyden crystals) is a component of disease activity.

In the author's previously unpublished case series of patients seeking integrative treatment of ulcerative colitis, over 30% of patients were infested with an organism, the majority harboring *E. histolytica*. In 14% of all patients, eradication of the organism produced a long-term clinical and pathologic remission, indicating that these patients may indeed have been suffering from an infectious colitis. In 18% of all patients, eradication of the organism ended the acute exacerbation and returned the patient to his or her previous state of stable ulcerative colitis. The following questions are most useful in gauging the likelihood that a patient may respond to specific antimicrobial therapy.

1. How long ago was a diagnosis of ulcerative colitis made?
2. How long have you been experiencing gastrointestinal symptoms?
3. Was the onset of your symptoms preceded by any of the following: foreign travel, acute gastroenteritis, the use of antibiotics, or intimate contact with a person suffering from gastrointestinal symptoms?
4. Since the onset of your gastrointestinal symptoms, have you been treated with antibiotics for any reason? Which ones? Did your gastrointestinal symptoms change during or after antibiotic use; if so, how?

More recent onset of symptoms, or recent exacerbation, onset associated with high-risk sit-uations for acquiring enteric or colonic infection, and improvement of symptoms when using antibiotics all increase the likelihood of a specific microbial trigger. Exacerbation of symptoms associated with antibiotic use suggests the presence of *C. difficile* toxicity or a fungal trigger for inflammation (as described in the case report above in a patient with Crohn's disease).

After the identification and treatment of specific microbial triggers and control of possible dietary triggers, administration of probiotics, fish oils, aloe mucopolysaccharides, and Boswellia may be helpful for patients with chronic disease, in addition to or sometimes in place of conventional therapies. Acupuncture and moxibustion are commonly employed by practitioners of Chinese medicine for treatment of ulcerative colitis. Uncontrolled studies from China claim excellent results.[229,230] One small study of moxibustion found evidence of enhanced cellular immunity and decreased antibody production associated with improvement of diarrhea in patients with ulcerative colitis,[231] suggesting downregulation of the Th2 response network. A review of studies from both Chinese and Western literature supports the efficacy of acupuncture in the regulation of gastrointestinal motor activity and secretion through opioid and other neural pathways.[232] Controlled clinical trials with ulcerative colitis patients have not yet been conducted.

▶ "FUNCTIONAL" DIGESTIVE DISORDERS

Conditions such as IBS, nonulcer dyspepsia, and biliary dyskinesis are often grouped together as functional bowel disorders with a high mutual comorbidity and frequent association with other painful conditions such as fibromyalgia, migraine headache, and vulvar pain syndromes.[233] Various explanations have been put forward to explain the association. In France and Germany, what knits these conditions together is often thought of as "latent tetany" or "spasmophilia," a condition that involves calcium or magnesium deficiency and the effects of stress. In the United States and the United Kingdom, the concept evoked is one of visceral hypersensitivity. Most contemporary research attempts to understand the role of neurotransmitters and other biochemical mediators in functional bowel disorders, so that agonist and antagonist drugs may be developed.[234,235] Although the role of serotonin and its receptors has received considerable attention lately,[236] numerous nonserotonergic mechanisms of pain and altered motility are likely to be involved.[237,238] A recent review in *Lancet* emphasizes the inadequacy of all concepts about the nature of these disorders and of the "functional" label applied to them.[239] Many patients with IBS have evidence of inflammation on colonoscopy, many dyspeptic patients show mild to moderate gastritis on endoscopy, and sphincter of Oddi dysfunction, which is part of the construct of biliary dyskinesia, may be associated with severe cholecystitis and/or pancreatitis. One problem with basing a diagnostic system upon observed pathology is that histology may lack sensitivity in assessing the role of inflammation as an illness mediator. In all hospitals, for example, some percentage of appendices removed because of suspected appendicitis will be histologically normal. A research team in Ireland found that a third of these contained elevated concentrations of inflammatory cytokines, indicating that inflammation was occurring without its characteristic microscopic changes.[240]

The fuzzy border between "functional" and "organic" bowel disease reveals itself in the similar responses to nutritional therapies. The Cambridge group employs the same dietary strategies to treat patients with IBS as with Crohn's disease (described in "Crohn's Disease"). In their hands, specific food intolerance is present in almost 50% of patients with diarrhea-predominant IBS and the majority of these patients can achieve complete control of IBS symptoms by adhering to a diet that eliminates their triggers.[241] The most common food triggers for patients with IBS are similar to the food triggers for patients with Crohn's disease: wheat, corn, cow's milk, and yeast are high on the list, with most patients having more than one food trigger. They have found that patients with diarrhea-predominant IBS have increased concentrations of prostaglandin E_2 in stool, a presumed mediator of diarrhea and intestinal cramping in these patients. They believe that food intolerance in IBS results from altered gut microbial ecology (dysbiosis). Patients with food-intolerant IBS have marked instability of the fecal flora with an increased aerobe:anaerobe ratio and excessive colonic fermentation.[242] Employing a whole-body chamber for measuring hydrogen and methane production, they observed that patients with IBS produced more hydrogen and methane than controls. The exclusion diet they employed reduced hydrogen and methane production of IBS patients to normal but had no effect on the hydrogen and methane production of the control group.[243] The mechanism for the relationship among specific food intolerance, excessive prostaglandin E_2 production, and abnormal colonic fermentation has not been clearly explained, but treatment of the condition with a permanent exclusion diet has remained a mainstay of treatment.

Others have suggested that food intolerance in IBS has an immunologic basis and may represent food allergy, although laboratory tests and skin testing do not have a high predictive value in determining which foods need to be avoided.[244] More than 20% of British patients referred to specialists with a diagnosis of IBS had antigliadin or antiendomysial antibodies, and almost 5% had histologic evidence of celiac disease.[245] One percent of the total population had occult celiac disease without the presence of endomysial antibodies. As another example, Type I hypersensitivity to *C. albicans* has been described in a group of patients with IBS.[246] Ingestion of an extract of *C. albicans* produced cramps and diarrhea in these patients during a double-blind challenge. Most *Candida*-allergic patients were also hypersensitive to food yeasts contained in bread, beer, wine, vinegar, fruit juices, and dried fruits. A yeast-elimination diet cleared IBS in 40% of *Candida*-allergic patients; an additional 40% needed additional treatment with oral nystatin to eliminate symptoms.

Not only have multiple types of food intolerance been described in patients with IBS, varied types of abnormal gut fermentation have also been described. A team at Cedars-Sinai Medical Center used breath testing for hydrogen and methane to identify the presence of small bowel bacterial overgrowth in patients who met the Rome criteria for IBS (described in Table 21–8). In their patient population, 78% had breath tests suggesting small bowel bacterial overgrowth and were treated with antibiotics; repeat testing indicated that small bowel bacterial overgrowth was no longer present in slightly more than half of those treated.[247] Antibiotic therapy improved diarrhea and abdominal pain in these patients; 48% of patients who responded to treatment no longer met criteria for IBS by the end of the study.

British researchers have used blood ethanol concentration in response to oral glucose loading as a way to measure abnormal gut fermentation.[248] Although they have not studied this phenomenon in relationship to IBS specifically, many of the polysymptomatic patients studied have chronic gastrointestinal symptoms, including abdominal pain and distension and alterations of bowel function. In their study populations, most patients respond better to antifungal drugs than to antibiotics, indicating that fungal dysbiosis may be as likely to cause symptoms of IBS as bacterial dysbiosis.

Other frequently described triggers for IBS include parasitic infection, exposure to environmental chemicals, and psychological distress. *Giardia lamblia*[249] and *Blastocystis hominis*[250] have been identified in stool specimens of 15–40% of patients diagnosed with IBS. Antiprotozoan therapy improved symptoms of the majority of patients treated for giardiasis; carriers of *E. histolytica* cysts, however, do not show improvement in IBS after treatment.

A correlation between emotional distress and symptoms of IBS has long been noted by patients and practitioners.[251] The neuroendocrine response to minor stressors differs between individuals with and without IBS, although the anomalies described do not directly explain the clinical syndrome. Somatostatin levels, for example, are significantly higher in patients with IBS than in controls and correlate with the presence of intestinal symptoms,[252] but this may represent a secondary or compensatory response, because somatostatin is an endogenous visceral analgesic. Various psychotherapeutic techniques have been employed in an effort to diminish symptoms of patients with IBS. In one study, relaxation

▶ **TABLE 21–8** ROME II DIAGNOSTIC CRITERIA FOR IBS

- At least 12 weeks of abdominal pain or discomfort with 2 of the following:
  Relief with defecation
  Onset associated with a change in stool frequency
  Onset associated with a change in appearance of stool
- Supportive symptoms:
  Fewer than 3 bowel movements a week
  More than 3 bowel movements a day
  Stool quality: hard/lumpy or watery/mushy
  Straining at defecation
  Urgent bowel movements
  Feeling of incomplete defecation
  Passing mucus with bowel movements
  Abdominal distension or fullness

response meditation was tested in matched pairs of 16 adults randomized to 6 weeks of meditation training or 6 weeks of symptom monitoring. Meditation was superior to control for reduction of flatulence ($P = .03$) and belching ($P = .02$) only. At 3-month follow-up, these improvements had been maintained and a significant improvement was also noted for diarrhea, but not for constipation.[253] In a larger, randomized study (120 patients) that combined relaxation training with psychotherapy, significant improvement was found for diarrhea and intermittent, stress-induced abdominal pain but not for constipation or constant abdominal pain.[254]

Several studies have examined the effect of cognitive behavior therapy (CBT) on symptoms of IBS. Although the protocols used differ in their details, most employ the following standard components: IBS information and education; relaxation techniques (which may include progressive muscle relaxation, electromyelogram-assisted muscle relaxation or thermal biofeedback); and training in coping with illness, problem-solving, and/or assertiveness. Control groups vary. Most consist of patients receiving standard medical care, with or without assignment to symptom-monitoring waiting lists. Few studies control for the increased attention and contact with therapists given to those receiving CBT. A British study compared 12 weeks of individual psychotherapy with supportive listening and found that psychotherapy improved both physical and emotional symptoms, but the effect was significant for women only. Treatment effects persisted for 1 year after therapy ended.[255] Research at the State University of New York at Albany, where almost all published US studies of CBT for IBS have been done, found insignificant improvement for CBT when compared to a control protocol of "pseudo-meditation and EEG alpha-lowering biofeedback."[256] This same group found that the presence of an Axis-1 psychiatric disorder significantly lowered the likelihood that a patient with IBS would improve with CBT.[257] Almost

all other studies, including those from the Albany group, show improvement in psychological measures with CBT: a decrease in distress, disability, and avoidance behaviors and an increase in quality of life and feelings of control. In some studies, psychological improvement is not associated with a significant improvement in GI symptoms, even though severity of physical and emotional distress covaries.[258,259] When GI symptoms appear to be improved by CBT, improvement in somatic symptoms is closely related to improvement in psychological functioning[260,261] and may be sustained for 2 years after the end of treatment.[262] One study that showed benefits of CBT for GI symptoms found a self-help support group to offer no advantage over the waiting list control.[263] A cognitive-behavioral family intervention was superior to standard pediatric care for children with recurrent abdominal pain,[264] producing a higher rate of complete elimination of pain, lower levels of relapse at 6- and 12-month follow-up, and lower levels of interference with their activities as a result of pain.

Hypnotherapy using gut-directed guided imagery for patients with severe, refractory IBS was compared to psychotherapy in a landmark British study and found to be dramatically more effective.[265] Benefits of hypnosis were sustained 18 months after cessation of treatment.[266] Hypnotherapy also improved the patients' quality of life and reduced absenteeism from work.[267] Positive effects of hypnosis for IBS patients have been confirmed in reports from the Netherlands[268] and the United States,[269] with pain and flatulence showing the greatest symptom improvement. In the US study, which involved only 12 patients, state and trait anxiety scores were also seen to decrease significantly, and results at the 2-month follow-up point indicated good maintenance of treatment gains. It is noteworthy that no significant correlation was found between initial susceptibility to hypnosis and treatment gain. Moreover, a positive relationship was found between the presence of psychiatric diagnoses and overall level of improvement, the opposite of the effect seen with CBT. It is likely that the bene-fits of hypnotherapy extend beyond stress man-agement. A single session of self-hypnosis dra-matically reduced recurrent abdominal pain in children within 3 weeks in an uncontrolled study.[270] Direct suggestion influences auto-nomic function; 5 minutes of preoperative sug-gestion was associated with faster recovery of normal bowel motility and earlier hospital dis-charge in patients undergoing major abdominal surgery.[271] Hypnotherapy produces a change in measured rectal sensitivity of patients with IBS,[272] an effect not seen with CBT even when GI symptoms improve.[273]

Biofeedback uses instruction and operant conditioning rather than suggestion in an effort to improve self-regulation of autonomic and skeletal muscle function. Combined with pelvic floor muscle exercise, it has shown consistent benefits for the treatment of fecal incontinence in adults[274–276] but not children[277]; the quality of this research, however, has been questioned.[278] Biofeedback demonstrates variable and limited effectiveness for control of constipation or ab-dominal pain, perhaps because the techniques employed do not address the underlying mech-anisms. Anal canal sphincterometry alone did not help overcome constipation,[279] but small case studies that combined sphincterometric feedback with general biofeedback-assisted re-laxation have claimed substantial improvement of severe chronic constipation in patients with slow transit[280] or excessive anal sphincter tone.[281] Biofeedback was not helpful in the treatment of chronic constipation among chil-dren,[282] but showed some benefit when added to a high-fiber diet for children with recurrent abdominal pain.[283]

Acupuncture effects autonomic nervous sys-tem function and GI motility and has repeat-edly been shown to relieve postoperative nau-sea and vomiting,[284] an effect blocked by local anesthesia, indicating that it is mediated by neural circuits.[285] Acupuncture has also been reported to reduce abdominal pain associated with numerous different disorders,[286–288] in-cluding cancer.[289,290] IBS as an entity does not exist in traditional Chinese medicine, so the use of acupuncture to treat IBS in China, where most studies of acupuncture are done, can only be assessed by using surrogate concepts that may not fulfill Western criteria for IBS. An un-controlled pilot study from England reports sig-nificant symptomatic improvement of patients with IBS receiving acupuncture,[291] but a Ger-man study found no benefit in treatment of adults with chronic constipation,[292] and a trial comparing real and sham acupuncture found inconsistent results. There was a significant re-sponse to the first true acupuncture treatment, but it was not maintained with continued acupuncture therapy.[293]

▶ INTEGRATIVE THERAPIES FOR IBS

An integrated approach to the problem of IBS is much like an integrated approach to the problem of IBD and requires answering a se-ries of questions:

Are There Microbial Triggers?

Parasites
Examination of stool for ova and parasites by a lab that specializes in parasitology will pro-duce a positive response rate of 7–48%, de-pending upon the laboratory, the selection of patients, and the time of year. Parasitic infec-tion is most likely to be important in patients with a distinct onset of altered bowel habits at onset. Long duration of symptoms and the pres-ence of chronic constipation do *not* exclude protozoan infection. Chronic giardiasis, re-sponsive to antimicrobial therapy, is as often characterized by constipation as by diarrhea.[291] The author has encountered patients in whom severe gastrointestinal symptoms present for as long as 20 years have totally cleared upon treat-ment of giardiasis. Initial treatment options in-clude a number of antiprotozoan drugs and herbs and *S. boulardii*, which stimulates sIgA secretion.

Yeasts

Patients who have developed IBS after exposure to antibiotics, or whose IBS is exacerbated by antibiotics, are likely to have dysbiosis as a trigger. Yeast overgrowth, sometimes associated with yeast hypersensitivity, depletion of normal flora or, occasionally, clostridial overgrowth, are possible. Examination of stool for *C. difficile* toxin and microscopic stool examination for yeast can be helpful. Several studies have described intestinal candidiasis as a cause of chronic diarrhea, with diarrhea responding to antifungal medication.[295,296] In one interesting study, the yeasts seen on microscopic stool exam failed to grow on culture and were described as "dead fecal yeasts."[297] This observation is consistent with unpublished observations by the author when using rectal swabs. The growth of yeast from culture of a rectal swab was a poor predictor of symptomatic response to antifungal drugs. Patients who showed abundant yeast on microscopic examination but who had negative cultures, were highly likely to report symptomatic improvement with antifungal drug therapy. Rectal mucus from these patients was capable of inhibiting the growth of a standardized culture of *C. albicans* on nutritive agar. This research has two implications: (1) Stool cultures for fungus are unreliable tests for predicting which patients with chronic GI symptoms will respond to antiyeast therapy. (2) Pathogenesis of yeast-associated intestinal disorders involves a vigorous or hyperactive host response, such that rectal mucus contains antifungal factors not present in patients without yeast-associated illness. In addition to antifungal drugs or herbs, dietary restriction of simple carbohydrates and administration of lactobacilli and other probiotics may be helpful.

Bacterial Overgrowth

Patients whose IBS symptoms improve when taking antibiotics may be suffering from bacterial overgrowth. Timed breath analysis for hydrogen and methane after a glucose or lactulose challenge may be helpful in confirming this diagnosis, if available, and if precautions are taken to avoid the many causes of false readings. Foods and herbs with antimicrobial activity are potentially useful as adjuncts to treatment. These include uncooked oils of garlic, oregano, thyme, and rosemary.

Achlorhydria is a potential contributor to small bowel bacterial overgrowth, allowing bacteria and yeast to grow in the stomach and duodenum. The most common causes of achlorhydria are prolonged use of proton pump inhibitors and chronic atrophic gastritis, a complication of infection with *Helicobacter pylori* and possibly a result of normal aging. Alternatives to the use of proton pump inhibitors and strategies for *H. pylori* eradication are discussed in "Acid Peptic Disease." If normal gastric pH cannot be restored, there may be value in administration of hydrochloric acid supplements to aid in control of small bowel bacterial overgrowth. Because bacterial proteases can destroy brush-border and pancreatic enzymes, symptoms associated with bacterial dysbiosis may also be relieved by the administration of supplemental digestive enzymes.

Are There Dietary Triggers?

Food may influence IBS in two ways; to apply either, a thorough dietary history should be taken.

First, specific food intolerance may provoke symptoms. This intolerance may be pharmacologic (e.g., caffeine or other alkaloids in coffee increasing gut motility), digestive (e.g., lactose intolerance), immunologic (e.g., gluten intolerance), or allergic. A few foods exclusion diet of the type employed by the Cambridge group (described for Crohn's disease) may be of value.

Second, the physical/chemical composition of food may alter GI function by increasing bile flow (fats and oils), increasing microbial growth (carbohydrates), or stimulating intestinal baroreceptors (fiber). Increasing dietary fiber can be helpful for chronic constipation but has no consistent effect in IBS, probably because IBS is not a single entity. There is no single diet for IBS.

A practical strategy begins with an analysis of the patient's eating habits. Patients whose habits reflect the lowest common denominator among US adults or children (high fat and sugar, low fiber, fast food eaten quickly) should be counseled about a healthier dietary pattern of a type that has been shown to prevent chronic disease: decreased sugar, fat, and refined carbohydrates, increased consumption of vegetables, fruit and whole grains, substitution of water for coffee and alcohol, and more leisurely meals, eaten with friends and family. For many patients, these simple and obvious changes will reduce symptoms markedly. Patients who become worse with such changes should be asked what foods they are eating more. If more complex carbohydrate and fiber are associated with worsening of symptoms, a lower carbohydrate diet or the SCD should be considered. Patients who do not benefit from a healthier dietary pattern may be candidates for an exclusion diet.

What Are the Sources of Stress in This Person's Life?

People often know what these are when asked directly. The response to a few simple, open-ended questions, such as those that follow, may reveal other sources of stress.

Were there any associated emotional events at the onset of symptoms?

How are things going for you at work/in school/at home?

How well do you get along with your spouse/parents/children/close friends/coworkers?

Are you satisfied with work, family life/social life?

Are there people you can confide in or trust?

Do you feel financially secure?

What are your main sources of stress and of pleasure?

Identifying major life stressors may allow appropriate interventions that dissipate the impact of stress. Knowing the patient in this way also enables the doctor to treat the patient empathically, which enhances the quality of the interaction. A strong and trusting relationship between doctor and patient has a significant impact on the long-term management of IBS, independent of any specific treatments employed.

Are There Other Disorders Present That Might Be Contributing to Chronic GI Symptoms?

By definition, chronic GI symptoms caused by a systemic illness, such as hypothyroidism, are not IBS. The latent tetany syndrome (LTS), however, bears discussion, because it is not recognized in North America. LTS is a state of neuromuscular hyperexcitability characterized by clearly defined electromyographic abnormalities and symptoms caused by spastic contraction of skeletal or smooth muscle. Although LTS can be produced by calcium deficiency, alkalosis, and hyperventilation, most individuals with LTS do not show these features. As a group, individuals with LTS have lower levels of serum or erythrocyte magnesium than a control population and abnormal responses to parenteral magnesium challenge suggesting magnesium deficiency.[298] LTS is associated with IBS, fibromyalgia, and migraine headache, and administration of physiologic doses of magnesium improves symptoms in most cases.[299] The administration of magnesium to a patient with IBS can be difficult; patients with diarrhea may be sensitive to the cathartic effect of magnesium. On the other hand, patients with constipation and abdominal pain, who show other manifestations of LTS, such as anxiety, skeletal muscle spasms, fatigue, and delayed sleep onset, may benefit from recommended daily allowance doses of magnesium (300–400 mg/d).

The combination of digestive complaints with symptoms of reactive airways disease has been termed reactive intestinal dysfunction syndrome.[300] Table 21–9 lists the environmental chemical exposures that precipitate reactive intestinal dysfunction syndrome. Once the condition has been established, symptoms are triggered by exposure to low levels of multiple volatile substances, including perfumes and carpet fumes. Symptoms of reactive intestinal dysfunction syndrome are abdominal distension, abdominal pain, diarrhea, vomiting, and constipation. The researchers who described this syndrome speculate that activation of neurotransmitters in the lung and the GI tract by the offending chemicals is the mechanism. Although many physicians are likely to attribute reactive intestinal dysfunction syndrome to psychological distress or "just IBS," attempts to treat chemical sensitivities of this type with dismissal or with psychotherapy are usually unsatisfactory to doctors and a source of frustration and anger to patients. It is the author's experience that outcome is better and the doctor–patient relationship stronger if the patient's observations are taken seriously. Patients should be encouraged to examine and test their attributions with the cooperation of the physician. Patients with environmental chemical sensitivities are often sensitive to drugs or herbs

▶ **TABLE 21–9** CHEMICAL TRIGGERS PROVOKING SYMPTOMS OF REACTIVE INTESTINAL DYSFUNCTION SYNDROME

- Anesthetics
- Carbonless copy paper
- Diazinon
- Dursban
- Epoxy
- Herbicides
- Isocyanates
- Lacquer
- Methylene chloride
- Paint
- Paraffin
- Toluene
- Trichloroethylene
- Triphenylmethane

ingested orally, but environmental modification can be very helpful for symptom control.

Once these four questions have been answered and appropriate treatments implemented, there remain numerous therapeutic options for control of symptoms. Hypnotherapy, guided imagery and other mind–body approaches should be encouraged. Peppermint oil can relieve abdominal cramping, possibly working as a calcium channel blocker in the gut.[301] Recommended doses are 0.2–0.4 mL (374–748 mg) for adults and half that dose for children. Probiotic therapy using *Lactobacillus plantarum* has demonstrated superiority to placebo in improving pain, regulating bowel habits, and decreasing flatulence.[302] Aloe vera and psyllium may be helpful in the treatment of constipation.[303,304] Fructooligosaccharides, a mixture of complex fermentable carbohydrates from various vegetable sources, especially chicory, relieves constipation and enhances the growth of bifidobacteria.[305] Other natural products that may help with chronic constipation include ginger, which enhances motility, and triphala, a mixture of herbs used in Ayurveda.[306] Side effects of these are minimal, but both peppermint oil and ginger extracts may aggravate esophageal reflux. Enteric coated, pH-dependent capsules decrease the likelihood of heartburn. *Atractyloides lancea* rhizome, a component of many traditional Chinese medicines, is another motility enhancer.[307]

An intriguing study published in *Journal of the American Medical Association* demonstrated that a mixture of herbs employed in traditional Chinese medicine could effectively relieve symptoms of IBS. The study design permitted a striking observation. Patients with IBS were evaluated by a practitioner of traditional Chinese medicine, who wrote each of them an individual prescription based upon the tenets of Chinese diagnosis. Treatment was randomized and blinded. One-third received the specific herbal formula prescribed, one-third received a standard herbal formula that the group of practitioners had agreed in advance would relieve symptoms of most patients with IBS, and one-third received placebo. During the 6 months of the study, the two groups receiving herbal therapies showed a comparable and significant relief of symptoms as compared to the placebo group. After the herbs were discontinued, the group receiving the standardized formula slowly relapsed, so that 6 months later they were as symptomatic as the placebo group. The group receiving individualized therapies, however, did not relapse after treatment was discontinued.[308] The unheralded implication of this study is that traditional Chinese medicine, when practiced according to its own principles, does not merely relieve symptoms of IBS, but enables a change in the individual being treated.[309]

The principles of evaluation and treatment for IBS may be successfully applied to other "functional" GI disturbances, as illustrated in the following case report.

▶ Case Example 2: Severe Refractory Constipation in an Infant

A second opinion was sought by the parents of a 2-year-old girl who suffered from severe constipation and abdominal pain. The infant had always seemed to have some difficulty with bowel movements, but the problem was accentuated after her first birthday and had become progressively worse. Stool was scanty and dry, bowel movements were infrequent, and stooling was slow and associated with crying. The pediatrician suggested milk of magnesia and fruit juice, which helped for about two weeks, and then prescribed a polyethylene glycol laxative and a stool softener, which relieved symptoms for a month, after which all treatments became ineffective. A pediatric gastroenterologist rendered a diagnosis of redundant, atonic colon and prescribed senna along with polyethylene glycol. His rationale was that the child had to move her bowels painlessly every day or the situation would worsen. The parents were told that she would need to continue this regimen indefinitely.

The first step in reevaluating the problem was to take a chronological feeding history. She had been nursed for 2 months and fed a cow's milk formula until age 12 months. Solid food had been slowly introduced beginning at age 5 months and cow's milk had become a dietary staple when formula was discontinued, which was about the same time as constipation became problematic. Cow's milk hypersensitivity is an established cause of childhood constipation. The parents reluctantly eliminated cow's milk from the child's diet, but were afraid to discontinue senna because the specialist had warned them against doing so. Fructooligosaccharides and *Lactobacillus* GG were added as supplements. When her stool became loose, senna and then polyethylene glycol were slowly discontinued. After 2 months of milk avoidance, fructooligosaccharides, and lactobacillus, the child had daily, soft, painless bowel movements and required no further medication.

▶ ACID–PEPTIC DISEASE

Hydrochloric acid produces much of the cellular damage and symptomatology of peptic ulcer disease, gastritis, and GERD. The major etiologic factor in duodenal ulceration now appears to be *H. pylori* infection, which destroys somatostatin-producing antral cells that downregulate HCl production.[310] Cigarette smoking contributes to duodenal ulceration by impairing duodenal bicarbonate secretion.[311] Additional potential triggers are those that increase gastric acid secretion by neurogenic or histaminergic mechanisms: emotional distress,[312] alcohol use,[313] and exposure to food allergens.[314] NSAIDs and aspirin are the most common causes of gastritis and gastric ulceration in the industrial world. Even low-dose aspirin therapy, as used for prevention of cardiovascular events, triples a person's risk of hospitalization for GI bleeding.[315] The presumed mechanism is inhibition of prostaglandin production, which increases mucosal sensitivity to acid-induced damage.

The relationship between *H. pylori* and gastric disease is complex. It causes gastric inflammation by stimulating Th1 lymphocytes and provoking release of several inflammatory cytokines, in particular interleukin-8 (IL-8), a potent neutrophil activator expressed by gastric epithelial cells.[316] In addition to peptic ulcer disease, *H. pylori* may cause or contribute to antral gastritis, atrophic gastritis, hypertrophic gastritis, gastric adenocarcinoma, gastric lymphoma,[316] and NSAID gastropathy.[317] The varied diseases provoked by the single trigger reflect the variety of physiological responses evoked by its presence. Eradication of *H. pylori* with antibiotics and proton pump inhibitors has revolutionized conventional treatment of these conditions. In dyspeptic patients infected with *H. pylori,* the use of proton pump inhibitors alone, without eradication of *H. pylori,* actually increases the incidence of atrophic gastritis.[318]

Several natural products have been advanced as alternatives to antibiotics for treatment of *H. pylori* infection. Garlic and garlic extracts inhibit growth of *H. pylori* in culture at concentrations that can be obtained from consumption of raw garlic or garlic oil capsules.[319,320] The minimal inhibitory concentration (MIC) for aqueous garlic extract to produce 90% inhibition of all *H. pylori* strains tested was 5 mg/mL.[321] Fresh garlic was four times more effective than boiled garlic. The proton pump inhibitor omeprazole was synergistic with aqueous garlic extract for 47% of strains tested. The MIC for one garlic-derived compound, thiosulfinate, was 40 μg/mL.[322] A study

from China revealed that garlic consumption was inversely associated with risk of acquiring *H. pylori* infection or developing aggressive precancerous gastric lesions.[323] High consumption of raw or cooked garlic is associated with decreased incidence of gastric cancer, one complication of *H. pylori* infection.[324,325] Use of garlic capsules, however, conferred no protection against gastric cancer in a retrospective Dutch study that coincidentally found an inverse association between gastric cancer and consumption of onions.[326] No clinical trials using aqueous garlic extract or garlic oil for treatment of *H. pylori* infection have been conducted. Sulforaphane, a sulfur-containing phytochemical that contributes to the distinctive odor of cabbage, has also demonstrated bacteriostatic and bacteriocidal activity against reference strains and clinical isolates of *H. pylori*. Its MIC was less than 4 μg/mL, even against antibiotic-resistant organisms.[327]

In China, patients with chronic gastritis usually have *H. pylori* infection and may have signs of "damp heat" or "blood stasis." Herbal remedies used in traditional Chinese medicine for clearing heat and removing blood stasis, such as Coptis Root Decoction for Purging Stomach Fire, inhibit the growth of *H. pylori* at therapeutic concentrations.[328] Evodia fruit (the raw, dried fruit of *Evodia rutaecarpa*) has been used in traditional Chinese medicine for 2,000 years for treatment of GI disorders and pain, as part of remedies thought to improve blood circulation and dispel stagnant cold.[329] Among its alkaloids are unique quinolones with MIC against *H. pylori* of less than 0.05 μg/mL, which is similar to the MIC of amoxicillin and clarithromycin, antibiotics that are used worldwide for the eradication of *H. pylori*. Of interest, the antimicrobial activity of these quinolone alkaloids was highly selective against *H. pylori*, showing almost no activity against other intestinal bacteria.[330] *Pistacia lentiscus* resin, or mastic gum, which is used as a food component in the Mediterranean and as treatment for gastric disorders by traditional healers, kills *H. pylori* in vitro at concentrations equivalent to administration of 1,000 mg twice a day. In the author's unpublished personal series, mastic gum was effective in eradication of *H. pylori,* using the stool antigen test, in 75% of cases; the cure rate with conventional therapy at present is 96%. Egg yolk anti-*H. pylori* antibody inhibited serum anti-*H. pylori* IgG production and the incidence of acute gastritis in *H. pylori*-infected Mongolian gerbils. In human volunteers infected with *H. pylori,* urea breath testing showed decreased urease activity after antibody ingestion.[331]

Other herbal products traditionally used for the treatment of dyspepsia have antiulcerogenic activities that are independent of antibiotic effect. Licorice, aloe gel, and capsicum (chili) have been used extensively for treatment of dyspeptic symptoms, and their clinical efficacy has been documented. Botanical compounds with antiulcer activity include flavonoids (quercetin, naringin, silymarin, and anthocyanosides), saponins (from *Panax japonicus* and Kochia scoparia), gums, and mucilages (i.e., gum guar and myrrh).[332] Removal of glycyrrhizin from licorice increases safety without compromising antiulcer efficacy.[333,334] Cabbage juice[335] and artichoke leaf[336] extracts have both been used traditionally in Europe for treatment of dyspeptic symptoms, but scientific studies of effectiveness and mechanism of action are lacking. These therapies are worth exploring in patients with nonulcer dyspepsia as an alternative to the chronic use of antisecretory therapies.

Although bland diets are traditionally used for treatment of peptic ulcer disease in Western societies, Asian studies show that turmeric is useful in symptomatic relief of gastric ulcers,[337] and that chili protects against aspirin-induced gastritis in humans.[338] A retrospective Chinese study concluded that high intake of chili was associated with a decreased risk of peptic ulcer disease,[339] although a similar study from India found an increased risk of gastric cancer associated with high intake of chili.[340] Traditional Japanese (Kampo) herbal formulas used for treating ulcers have strong antioxidant activity, scavenging superoxide radicals and in-

hibiting the generation of hydroxyl radicals.[341] One Kampo medicine (TJ43) also enhanced gastric emptying, an effect that few drugs have.[342] Gamma-oryzanol, a group of antioxidants derived from rice bran oil and useful in the treatment of small bowel hyperpermeability, has antiulcer properties in animals.[343]

Before *H. pylori* infection was established as a major risk factor for duodenal ulcer disease, its primary trigger was considered to be emotional distress. Today, psychotherapeutic approaches to duodenal ulcer disease are infrequently researched. However, a study of the rate of ulcer healing in Korea found that patients entered into an integrative stress management program healed better than a control group who were given a relaxation tape.[344] A Norwegian study, however, found that short-term cognitive therapy had no effect on the 1-year recurrence rate of duodenal ulcer disease.[345]

Acupuncture has been used for the treatment of epigastric pain independent of diagnosis[346,347] and for chronic gastritis[348] in uncontrolled studies. Electroacupuncture was found to improve gastric emptying in diabetic patients.[349]

With the decline in gastric disease caused by *H. pylori* has come a substantial increase in GERD and esophageal adenocarcinoma.[350] Like the more common squamous cell carcinoma of the esophagus, the incidence of adenocarcinoma is inversely related to consumption of folic acid, beta-carotene, and vitamins E and C.[351] Some researchers believe that certain strains of *H. pylori* actually work to prevent GERD[352]; others that the association is coincidental. GERD results from esophageal exposure to gastric contents, including HCl, pepsin, and bile, and it may be complicated by esophageal metaplasia (Barrett esophagus), dysplasia, and carcinoma. Proton pump inhibitors reduce symptoms and cure esophagitis in up to 90% of cases, but do not diminish reflux.[353] They appear to replace acid reflux with nonacid reflux. Reflux itself is caused by transient relaxation of the lower esophageal sphincter not related to swallowing. These are motor reflexes preprogrammed in the brain stem in response to gastric vagal mechanoreceptors. Postprandial gastric distension is an important trigger for lower esophageal sphincter relaxation by this mechanism. A more physiological mechanism for reducing reflux is to reduce postprandial gastric distension by consumption of small meals eaten slowly in a relaxed fashion. Calcium ions increase contraction of the lower esophageal sphincter (LES),[354] so calcium salts in powdered, chewable, or liquid form with meals may also prevent reflux. Calcium used this way is not functioning as an antacid but as a tonifying agent. High-fat meals delay gastric emptying and may aggravate reflux, although in individuals with gastric fermentation caused by bacterial or yeast overgrowth, fat may be less provocative than carbohydrate, which increases postprandial gastric distension through fermentation. There are numerous uncontrolled anecdotal reports of supplementation with hydrochloric acid (betaine HCl) and/or digestive enzymes reducing symptoms of GERD. These may achieve their effect through enhanced gastric emptying, which decreases gastric distension. Reflux symptoms have also been relieved by capsules of red-pepper powder, 2.5 g/d, taken before meals for 5 weeks, in a placebo-controlled trial.[355] Liquid sodium alginate, which is derived from seaweed, was shown to decrease the frequency but not the duration of reflux episodes in a small clinical trial.[356]

▶ CONCLUSION

The chief functions of the GI tract—digestion, absorption, elimination, and immune surveillance—are strongly influenced by the interplay of the autonomic nervous system, permeability/vectorial transport and the microbial milieu. GI function determines, and to a large extent is determined by, nutritional status. Alterations in intestinal permeability, microbial flora, and neuroendocrine regulation are key factors in the pathophysiology of most of the common GI diseases. Some of the most frequently used drugs have detrimental effects on GI function.

NSAIDs increase permeability, causing inflammation and blood loss. Proton pump inhibitors and antibiotics each contribute to microbial dysbiosis. Alternative or complementary therapies for chronic GI disorders are therefore highly desirable. Their successful application depends upon a patient-centered approach: an understanding of the antecedents, triggers and mediators likely to be operative in each patient and the influence that each of these has on GI function and microecology. Therapeutic attention should focus on dietary composition, micronutrient sufficiency, the regulation of GI motility and secretions, antibiotic and probiotic substances, and central nervous system modulation of autonomic function.

REFERENCES

1. Targan RS, Kagnoff FM, Brogan MD, Shanahan F. Immunologic mechanisms in intestinal disease. *Ann Intern Med.* 1987;106:854–870.
2. Gershon MD. The enteric nervous system: a second brain. *Hosp Pract.* 1999;34(7):31–32, 35–38, 41–42 passim.
3. Pittler MH, Ernst E. Peppermint oil for irritable bowel syndrome: a critical review and metaanalysis. *Am J Gastroenterol.* 1998;93(7):1131–1135.
4. Mackowiak PA. The normal microbial flora. *N Engl J Med.* 1982;307:83–93.
5. Lindenbaum J, Rund DG, Butler VP Jr. Inactivation of digoxin by gut flora: reversal by antibiotic therapy. *N Engl J Med.* 1981;305:789–794.
6. Gorbach S. The role of intestinal flora in the metabolism of drugs, hormones and carcinogens. *Infect Dis.* 1982;12:4–30.
7. Rowland IR, Robinson RD, Doherty RA. Effects of diet on mercury metabolism and excretion in mice given methylmercury: role of gut flora. *Arch Environ Health.* 1984;39:401–408.
8. Savage DC. Colonization by and survival of pathogenic bacteria on intestinal mucosal surfaces. In: Britton G, Marshall K, eds. *Adsorption of Microorganisms to Surfaces.* New York: Wiley; 1980:175–206.
9. Stokes CR. Induction and control of intestinal immune response. In: Newby TJ, Stokes CR, eds. *Local Immune Responses of the Gut.* Boca Raton, FL: CRC Press; 1984:97–142.

10. Sprunt K, Redman W. Evidence suggesting importance of role of interbacterial inhibition in maintaining balance of normal flora. *Ann Intern Med.* 1968;68:579–590.

11. Seelig MS. O Mechanisms by which antibiotics increase the incidence and severity of candidiasis and alter the immunological defenses. *Bacteriol Rev.* 1966;30:442–459.

12. Sun M. In search of Salmonella's smoking gun. *Science.* 1984;226:30–32.

13. Oksanen PJ, et al. Prevention of travellers' diarrhoea by *Lactobacillus* GG. *Ann Med.* 1990;22(1): 53–56.

14. Mirelman D. O Effect of culture condition and bacterial associates on the zymodemes of *Entamoeba histolytica*. *Parasitol Today.* 1987;3:37–40.

15. Torres JF, Camorlinga M, Munoz O. Neutralization of cytotoxic activity of *Clostridium difficile* with fecal flora. *Arch Invest Med (Mex).* 1987;18(4):315–317.

16. Hill MJ, Drasar BS, Williams REO. Faecal bile-acids and clostridia in patients with cancer of the large bowel. *Lancet.* 1975;325:535–539.

17. Low-Beer TS. How the colon begets gallstones. *Lancet.* 1998;351:612–613.

18. Yu DTY, Choo SY, Schaack T. Molecular mimicry in HLA-B27–related arthritis. *Ann Intern Med.* 1989;111:581–591.

19. McGuignan LE, Prendergast JK, Geczy AF, Edmonds JP, Bashi HV. Significance of non-pathogenic cross reactive bowel flora in patients with ankylosing spondylitis. *Ann Rheum Dis.* 1986;45: 566–571.

20. Pirzer U, Schonhaar A, Fleischer B, et al. Reactivity of infiltrating T lymphocytes with microbial antigens in Crohn's disease. *Lancet.* 1991;338: 1238–1239.

21. Rosenberg E, Belew P. O Microbial factors in psoriasis. *Arch Dermatol.* 1982;118:143–144.

22. Juhlin L, Michaelsson G. Fibrin microclot in patients with acne. *Acta Derm Venereol.* 1984;63: 538–540.

23. Toskes PP. Bacterial overgrowth of the gastrointestinal tract. *Adv Intern Med.* 1993;38:387–407.

24. Parmely M, Gale A, Clabaugh M, Horvat R, Zhou WW. Proteolytic inactivation of cytokines by *Pseudomonas aeruginosa*. *Infect Immun.* 1990; 58(9):3009–3014.

25. Donaldson RM, Toskes PP. The relation of enteric bacterial populations to gastrointestinal function and disease. In: Sleisinger MH, Lordtran JS,

eds. *Gastrointestinal Disease.* 4th ed. Philadelphia: WB Saunders; 1989:107–131.

26. Moore WEC, Loore L. Intestinal floras of populations that have a high risk of colon cancer. *Appl Environ Microbiol.* 1995;61:3202–3207.

27. Kruis W, Forstmaier G, Sheurlein C, Stellard F. Effects of diets low and high in refined sugars on gut transit, bile acid metabolism, and bacterial fermentation. *Gut.* 1991;32:367–371.

28. Eaton KK. Sugars in food intolerance and gut fermentation. *J Nutr Med.* 1992;3:295–301.

29. Berghouse L, Hori S, Hill M, et al. Comparison between the bacterial and oligosaccharide content of ileostomy effluent in subjects taking diets rich in refined or unrefined carbohydrate. *Gut.* 1984;25:1071–1077.

30. Rowland IR, Mallett AK. Dietary fiber and the gut microflora-their effects on toxicity. In: Chambers PL, Gehring P, Sakai F, eds. *New Concepts and Developments in Toxicity.* Amsterdam: Elsevier; 1986:125–138.

31. Freudenheim J, Graham S, Horvath P. Risks associated with the source of fiber and fiber components in cancer of the colon and rectum. *Cancer Res.* 1990;50:3295–3300.

32. Newmark HL, Lupton JR. Determinants and consequences of colonic luminal pH: implications for colon cancer. *Nutr Cancer.* 1990;14:161–173.

33. Rowlkand IR. Factors affecting metabolic activity of the intestinal microflora. *Drug Metab Rev.* 1988;19:243–261.

34. Chung K-T, Fulk GE, Slein MW. Tryptophanase of fecal flora as a possible factor in the etiology of colon cancer. *J Natl Cancer Inst.* 1975;54: 1073–1078.

35. Malhotra SL. Faecal urobilinogen levels and pH of stools in population groups with different incidence of cancer of the colon, and their possible role in its aetiology. *J R Soc Med.* 1982;75: 709–714.

36. Steijns JM, van Hooijdonk AC. Occurrence, structure, biochemical properties and technological characteristics of lactoferrin. *Br J Nutr.* 2000; 84(suppl 1): S11–S17.

37. Gorard DA, Gomborone JE, Libby GW, Farthing MJG. Intestinal transit in anxiety and depression. *Gut.* 1996;39:551–555.

38. Gershon MD. Review article: roles played by 5-hydroxytryptamine in the physiology of the bowel. *Aliment Pharmacol Ther.* 1999;13(suppl 2): 15–30.

39. Yamahara J, Huang Q, Li Y et al. Gastrointestinal motility enhancing effect of ginger and its active constituents. *Chem Pharm Bull.* 1990;38:430–431.

40. Lizko NN. Stress and intestinal microflora. *Die Nahrung.* 1987;31:443–447.

41. Giannella RA, Broitman SA, Zamcheck N. Gastric acid barrier to ingested microorganisms: studies in vivo and in vitro. *Gut.* 1972;13:251–256.

42. Neal KR. Omeprazole as a risk factor for *Campylobacter* gastroenteritis: a case-control study. *BMJ.* 1996;312:414–415.

43. Chadwick RW, George SE, Claxton LD. Role of the gastrointestinal mucosa and microflora in the bioactivation of dietary and environmental mutagens or carcinogens. *Drug Metabol Rev.* 1992;24:425–492.

44. Bode JC, Rust S, Bode C. The effect of cimetidine treatment on ethanol formation in the human stomach. *Scand J Gastroenterol.* 1984;19:853–856.

45. Bhatnagar S, Bhan MJ, George C, et al. Is small bowel bacterial overgrowth of pathogenic significance in persistent diarrhea? *Acta Paediatr.* 1992;381(suppl):108–113.

46. Edman J, Sobel JD, Taylor ML. Zinc status in women with recurrent vulvovaginal candidiasis. *Am J Obstet Gynecol.* 1986;155(5):1082–1085.

47. Higgs JM. Chronic mucocutaneous candidiasis: iron deficiency and the effects of iron therapy. *Proc R Soc Med.* 1973;66(8):802–804.

48. Montes LF, Krumdieck C, Cornwell PE. Hypovitaminosis A in patients with mucocutaneous candidiasis. *J Infect Dis.* 1973;128(2):227–230.

49. Boyne R, Arthur JR. The response of selenium-deficient mice to *Candida albicans* infection. *J Nutr.* 1986;116(5):816–822.

50. Beeken WL. Remediable defects in Crohn's disease. *Arch Intern Med.* 1975;135:686–690.

51. Greenber GR. Nutritional support in inflammatory bowel disease: current status and future directions. *Scand J Gastroenterol.* 1992;27(suppl 192):117–122.

52. Hendricks KM, Walker WA. Zinc deficiency in inflammatory bowel disease. *Nutr Rev.* 1988;46:401–408.

53. Hinks LJ, Inwards KD, Lloyd B, Clayton B. Reduced concentrations of selenium in mild Crohn's disease. *J Clin Pathol.* 1988;41:198–201.

54. Mason JB. Folate, colitis, dysplasia, and cancer. *Nutr Rev.* 1989;47(10):314–317.

55. Smith BS, Summa MA. Does omeprazole cause fat malabsorption? *Nutr Clin Care.* 1999;2: 103–108.

56. Chen HC, Chang MD, Chang TJ. [Antibacterial properties of some spice plants before and after heat treatment.] *Chung Hua Min Kuo Wei Sheng Wu Chi Mien I Hsueh Tsa Chih.* 1985;18:190–195.

57. Schulick P. *Ginger: Common Spice & Wonder Drug.* Brattleboro, VT: Herbal Free Press; 1994.

58. Venugopal PV, Venugopal TV. Antidermatophytic activity of garlic (*Allium sativum*) in vitro. *Int J Dermatol.* 1995;34:278–279.

59. Farbman KS, Barnett ED, Bolduc GR, Klein JO. Antibacterial activity of garlic and onions: a historical perspective. *Pediatr Infect Dis J.* 1993;12:613–614.

60. Leung A. *Encyclopedia of Common Natural Ingredients Used in Foods, Drugs and Cosmetics.* New York. John Wiley & Sons; 1980:246–247.

61. Zohri AN, Abdel-Gawad K, Saber S. Antibacterial, antidermatophytic and antitoxigenic activities of onion (*Allium cepa* L.) oil. *Microbiol Res.* 1995;150:167–172.

62. Lutomski VJ, Kedzia B, Debska W. Effect of an alcohol extract and active ingredients from *Curcuma longa* on bacteria and fungi. *Planta Med.* 1974;26:17–19.

63. Leung A. *Encyclopedia of Common Natural Ingredients Used in Foods, Drugs and Cosmetics.* New York. John Wiley & Sons; 1980:313–314.

64. Bullerman LB. Inhibition of aflatoxin production by cinnamon. *J Food Sci.* 1974;13:1163–1165.

65. Beier RC. Natural pesticides and bioactive compounds in food. *Rev Environ Contam Toxicol.* 1990;113:113–137.

66. Beier RC. Natural pesticides and bioactive components in foods. *Rev Environ Contam Toxicol.* 1990;113:47–137.

67. El-Assal GS. Ancient Egyptian medicine. *Lancet.* 1972;2:272–274.

68. Hilton E, Isenberg HD, Alperstein P, et al. Ingested yogurt as prophylaxis for chronic candidal vaginitis. *Ann Intern Med.* 1992;116:353–357 (comment in: Drutz DJ. *Lactobacillus* prophylaxis for *Candida vaginitis. Ann Intern Med.* 1992;116:419–420).

69. Gorbach SL. The discovery or *Lactobacillus* GG. *Nutr Today.* 2001;31(suppl 1):2S–4S. The entire supplement is devoted to *Lactobacillus* GG.

70. Elmer GW, Surawicz CM, McFarland LV. Biotherapeutic agents. A neglected modality for the treat-

ment and prevention of selected intestinal and vaginal infections. *JAMA*. 1996;275:870–876.

71. Rayes N, Hansen S, Seehofew R, et al. Early enteral supply of fiber and lactobacilli versus conventional nutrition: a controlled trial in patients with major abdominal surgery. *Nutrition*. 2002;18:609–615.

72. Bjarnasson I, Macpherson A, Hollander D. Intestinal permeability: an overview. *Gastroenterology*. 1995;108:1566–1581.

73. Walker WA. Antigen absorption from the small intestine and gastrointestinal disease. *Pediatr Clin North Am*. 1975;22(4):731–746.

74. Gardener MLG. Gastrointestinal absorption of intact proteins. *Annu Rev Nutr*. 1988;8:329–350.

75. Deitch EA. The role of intestinal barrier failure and bacterial translocation in the development of systemic infection and multiple organ failure. *Arch Surg*. 1990;125:403–404.

76. Ohri SK, Bjarnason I, Pathi V, et al. Cardiopulmonary bypass impairs small intestinal transport and increases gut permeability. *Ann Thorac Surg*. 1993;55(5): 1080–1086.

77. Ohri SK, Somasundaram S, Koak Y, et al. The effect of intestinal hypoperfusion on intestinal absorption and permeability during cardiopulmonary bypass. *Gastroenterology*. 1994;106(2): 318–323.

78. Buchman AL, Moukarzel AA, Bhuta S, et al. Parenteral nutrition is associated with intestinal morphologic and functional changes in humans. *JPEN J Parenter Enteral Nutr*. 1995;19(6):453–460.

79. Halsted CH, Sheir S, Sourial N, Patwardhan VN. Small intestinal structure and absorption in Egypt. Influence of parasitism and pellagra. *Am J Clin Nutr*. 1969;22(6):744–754.

80. Mehta SK, Kaur S, Avasthi G, Wig NN, Chhuttani PN. Small intestinal deficit in pellagra. *Am J Clin Nutr*. 1972;25(6):545–549.

81. Cook GC. D-xylose absorption and jejunal morphology in African patients with pellagra (niacin tryptophan deficiency). *Trans R Soc Trop Med Hyg*. 1976;70(4):349–351.

82. Ballard ST, Hunter JH, Taylor AE. Regulation of tight-junction permeability during nutrient absorption across the intestinal epithelium. *Annu Rev Nutr*. 1995;15:35–55.

83. Saunders PR, Hanssen NP, Perdue MH. Cholinergic nerves mediate stress-induced intestinal transport abnormalities in Wistar-Kyoto rats. *Am J Physiol*. 1997;273(2 pt 1):G486–G490.

84. Katz KD, Hollander D, Vadheim CM, et al. Intestinal permeability in patients with Crohn's disease and their healthy relatives. *Gastroenterology*. 1989;97:927–931.

85. Hollander D, Vadheim CM, Brettholz E, et al. Increased intestinal permeability in patients with Crohn's disease and their relatives. A possible etiologic factor. *Ann Intern Med*. 1986;105(6): 883–885.

86. Fasano A. Regulation of intercellular tight junctions by zonula occludens toxin and its eukaryotic analogue zonulin. *Ann N Y Acad Sci*. 2000;915:214–222.

87. Bjarnason I, Smethurst P, Clark P, et al. Effect of prostaglandin on indomethacin-induced increased intestinal permeability in man. *Scand J Gastroenterol Suppl*. 1989;164:97–102.

88. Bjarnason I, Williams P, Smethurst P, et al. Effect of non-steroidal anti-inflammatory drugs on the human small intestine. *Drugs*. 1986;1:35–41.

89. Bjarnason I, Hayllar J, Smethurst P, et al. Metronidazole reduces intestinal inflammation and blood loss in non-steroidal anti-inflammatory drug-induced enteropathy. *Gut*. 1992;33:1204–1208.

90. Dearlove M, Barr K, Neumann V, et al. The effect of non-steroidal anti-inflammatory drugs on faecal flora and bacterial antibody levels in rheumatoid arthritis. *Br J Rheumatol*. 1992;31: 443–447.

91. Alarcon GS, Mikhail IS. Antimicrobials in the treatment of rheumatoid arthritis and other arthritides: a clinical perspective. *Am J Med Sci*. 1994; 309:201–209.

92. Kloppenburg M, Breedveld FC, Miltenburg AM, et al. Antibiotics as disease modifiers in arthritis. *Clin Exp Rheumatol*. 1993; 11(suppl 8):S113–S115.

93. Serrander R, Magnusson KE, Kihlstrom E, et al. Acute yersinia infections in man increase intestinal permeability for low-molecular weight polyethylene glycols (PEG 400). *Scand J Infect Dis*. 1986;18(5):409–413.

94. Serrander R, Magnusson KE, Sundqvist T. Acute infections with *Giardia lamblia* and rotavirus decrease intestinal permeability to low-molecular weight polyethylene glycols (PEG 400). *Scand J Infect Dis*. 1984;16(4):339–344.

95. Worthington BS, Meserole L, Syrotuck JA. Effect of daily ethanol ingestion on intestinal permeability to macromolecules. *Am J Dig Dis*. 1978; 23(1):23–32.

96. Lifschitz CH, Mahoney DH. Low-dose methotrexate-induced changes in intestinal permeability

determined by polyethylene glycol polymers. *J Pediatr Gastroenterol Nutr.* 1989;9(3):301–306.

97. André C, André F, Colin L. Effect of allergen ingestion challenge with and without cromoglycate cover on intestinal permeability in atopic dermatitis, urticaria and other symptoms of food allergy. *Allergy.* 1989;9:47–51.

98. André C, André F, Colin L. Effect of allergen ingestion challenge with and without cromoglycate cover on intestinal permeability in atopic dermatitis, urticaria and other symptoms of food allergy. *Allergy.* 1989;9:47–51.

99. André C, André F, Colin L, et al. Measurement of intestinal permeability to mannitol and lactulose as a means of diagnosing food allergy and evaluating therapeutic effectiveness of disodium cromoglycate. *Ann Allergy.* 1987;59(5 pt 2):127–130.

100. Barau E, Dupont C. Allergy to cow's milk proteins in mother's milk or in hydrolyzed cow's milk infant formulas as assessed by intestinal permeability measurements. *Allergy.* 1994;49(4):295–298.

101. Rooney PJ, Jenkins RT, Buchanan WW. A short review of the relationship between intestinal permeability and inflammatory joint disease. *Clin Exp Rheumatol.* 1990;8(1):75–83.

102. Walker WA. Antigen absorption from the small intestine and gastrointestinal disease. *Pediatr Clin North Am.* 1975;22(4):731–746.

103. Bloembergen P, Hofhuis FM, van Dijk H, et al. Endotoxin-induced autoimmunity in mice. I. Time and dose dependence of production and serum levels of antibodies against bromelain-treated mouse erythrocytes and circulating immune complexes. *Int Arch Allergy Appl Immunol.* 1987;84(3):291–297.

104. Hollander D, Vadheim CM, Brettholz E, et al. Increased intestinal permeability in patients with Crohn's disease and their relatives. A possible etiologic factor. *Ann Intern Med.* 1986;105(6):883–885.

105. Smith MD, Gibson RA, Brooks PM. Abnormal bowel permeability in ankylosing spondylitis and rheumatoid arthritis. *J Rheumatol.* 1985;12(2):299–305.

106. Juhlin L, Michaelsson G. Fibrin microclot formation in patients with acne. *Acta Derm Venereol.* 1983;63(6):538–540.

107. Juhlin L, Vahlquist C. The influence of treatment on fibrin microclot generation in psoriasis. *Br J Dermatol.* 1983;108(1):33–37.

108. Hamilton I, Fairris GM, Rothwell J, et al. Small intestinal permeability in dermatological disease. *Q J Med.* 1985;56(221): 559–567.

109. Jackson P.G, Lessof MH, Baker RW, et al. Intestinal permeability in patients with eczema and food allergy. *Lancet.* 1981;1(8233):1285–1286.

110. Paganelli R, Fagiolo U, Cancian M, et al. Intestinal permeability in irritable bowel syndrome. Effect of diet and sodium cromoglycate administration. *Ann Allergy.* 1990;64(4):377–380.

111. Tepper RE, Simon D, Brandt LJ, et al. Intestinal permeability in patients infected with human immunodeficiency virus. *Am J Gastroenterol.* 1994; 89:878–882.

112. Mack DR, Flick JA, Durie PR, et al. Correlation of intestinal lactulose permeability with exocrine pancreatic dysfunction. *J Pediatr.* 1992;120: 696–701.

113. Williamson RC. Intestinal adaptation (first of two parts). Structural, functional and cytokinetic changes. *N Engl J Med.* 1978;298(25):1393–1402.

114. Behrens RH, Lunn PG, Northrop CA, et al. Factors affecting the integrity of the intestinal mucosa of Gambian children. *Am J Clin Nutr.* 1987; 45(6):1433–1441.

115. Salminen E, Elomaa I, Minkkinen J, et al. Preservation of intestinal integrity during radiotherapy using live Lactobacillus acidophilus cultures. *Clin Radiol.* 1988;39:435–437.

116. van der Hulst RR, van Kreel BK, von Meyenfeldt MF, et al. Glutamine and the preservation of gut integrity. *Lancet.* 1993;341(8857):1363–1365.

117. Shive W, Snider RN, DuBilier B, et al. Glutamine in treatment of peptic ulcer. *Texas State J Med.* 1957;6:840–843.

118. Roediger W. The starved colon—diminished mucosal nutrition, diminished absorption, and colitis. *Dis Colon Rectum.* 1990;33:858–862.

119. Vanderhoof JA, Blackwood DJ, Mohammadpour H, et al. Effect of dietary menhaden oil on normal growth and development and on ameliorating mucosal injury in rats. *Am J Clin Nutr.* 1991; 54(2):346–350.

120. Ruthig DJ, Meckling-Gill KA. Both (n-3) and (n-6) fatty acids stimulate wound healing in the rat intestinal epithelial cell line, IEC-6. *J Nutr.* 1999; 129:1791–1798.

121. Stark JM, Jackson SK. Sensitivity to endotoxin is induced by increased membrane fatty-acid unsaturation and oxidant stress. *J Med Microbiol.* 1990;32(4):217–221.

122. Salminen E, Elomaa I, Minkkinen J, et al. Preservation of intestinal integrity during radiotherapy using live Lactobacillus acidophilus cultures. *Clin Radiol.* 1988;39:435–437.

123. Salminen E, Elomaa I, Minkkinen J, et al. Preservation of intestinal integrity during radiotherapy using live Lactobacillus acidophilus cultures. *Clin Radiol.* 1988;39:435–437.

124. Playford RJ, Woodman AC, Clark P, et al. Effect of luminal growth factor preservation on intestinal growth. *Lancet.* 1993;341(8849):843–848.

125. Yagi K, Ohishi N. Action of ferulic acid and its derivatives as anti-oxidants. *J Nutr Sci Vitaminol.* 1979;205:127–135.

126. McFarland V, Bernasconi P. A review of a novel biotherapeutic agent: *Saccharomyces boulardii. Microb Ecol Health Dis.* 1993;6:157–171.

127. Surawicz CM, McFarland LV, Elmer G, et al. Treatment of recurrent *Clostridium difficile* colitis with vancomycin and *Saccharomyces boulardii. Am J Gastroenterol.* 1989;84(10):1285–1287.

128. Surawicz CM, Elmer GW, Speelman P, et al. Prevention of antibiotic-associated diarrhea by *Saccharomyces boulardii:* a prospective study. *Gastroenterology.* 1989;96(4):981–988.

129. Buts J-P, Bernasconi P, Vaerman JP, et al. Stimulation of secretory IgA and secretory component of immunoglobulins in small intestine of rats treated with Saccharomyces boulardii. *Dig Dis Sci.* 1990; 35:251–256.

130. Machado Caetano JA, Parames MT, Babo MJ, et al. Immunopharmacological effects of *Saccharomyces boulardii* in healthy human volunteers. *Int J Immunopharmacol.* 1986;8:245–259.

131. Carlander D, Kollberg H, Wejaker PE, Larsson A. Perioral immunotherapy with yolk antibodies for the prevention and treatment of enteric infections. *Immunol Res.* 2000;21(1):1–6.

132. Eibl MM, Wolf HM, Furnkranz H, et al. Prophylaxis of necrotizing enterocolitis by oral IgA-IgG: review of a clinical study in low birth weight infants and discussion of the pathogenic role of infection. *J Clin Immunol.* 1990;10(6 suppl):77S–79S.

133. Playford RJ, MacDonald CE, Calnan DP, et al. Co-administration of the health food supplement, bovine colostrum, reduces the acute non-steroidal anti-inflammatory drug-induced increase in intestinal permeability. *Clin Sci (Lond).* 2001;100(6):627–633.

134. Spaeth G, Berg RD, Specian RD, et al. Food without fiber promotes bacterial translocation from the gut. *Surgery.* 1990;108(2):240–246.

135. Sundqvist T, Lindstrom F, Magnusson K-E, et al. Influence of fasting on intestinal permeability and disease activity in patients with rheumatoid arthritis. *Scand J Rheumatol.* 1982;11:33.

136. Shiau SY, Chang GW. Effects of certain dietary fibers on apparent permeability of the rat intestine. *J Nutr.* 1986;116(2):223–232.

137. Eisenhans B, Caspary WF. Differential changes in the urinary excretion of two orally administered polyethylene glycol markers (PEG 900 and PEG 4000) in rats after feeding various carbohydrate gelling agents. *J Nutr.* 1989;119:380–387.

138. Gyory CP, Chang GW. Effects of bran, lignin and deoxycholic acid on the permeability of the rat cecum and colon. *J Nutr.* 1983;113:2300–2307.

139. Langmead L, Rampton DS. Review article: herbal treatment in gastrointestinal and liver disease—benefits and dangers. *Aliment Pharmacol Ther.* 2001;15(9):1239–1252.

140. Fintelmann V. Modern phytotherapy and its uses in gastrointestinal conditions. *Planta Med.* 1991;57(7):S48–S52.

141. Di Stasi LC. Amoebicidal compounds from medicinal plants. *Parasitologia.* 1995;37(1):29–39.

142. Paulo A, Pimentel M, Viegas S, et al. Cryptolepis sanguinolenta activity against diarrhoeal bacteria. *J Ethnopharmacol.* 1994;44(2):73–77.

143. Elisabetsky E, Posey DA. Ethnopharmacological search for antiviral compounds: treatment of gastrointestinal disorders by Kayapo medical specialists. *Ciba Found Symp.* 1994;185:77–90; discussion 90–94.

144. Caceres A, Fletes L, Aguilar L, et al. Plants used in Guatemala for the treatment of gastrointestinal disorders. 3. Confirmation of activity against enterobacteria of 16 plants. *J Ethnopharmacol.* 1993;38(1):31–38.

145. Heinrich M, Rimpler H, Barrera NA. Indigenous phytotherapy of gastrointestinal disorders in a lowland Mixe community (Oaxaca, Mexico): ethnopharmacologic evaluation. *J Ethnopharmacol.* 1992;36(1):63–80.

146. Quinlan MB, Quinlan RJ, Nolan JM. Ethnophysiology and herbal treatments of intestinal worms in Dominica, West Indies. *J Ethnopharmacol.* 2002;80(1):75–83.

147. Iwalokun BA, Gbenle GO, Adewole TA, Akinsinde KA. Shigellocidal properties of three Nigerian medicinal plants: *Ocimum gratissimum,*

Terminalia avicennoides, and *Momordica balsamina. J Health Popul Nutr.* 2001;19(4):331–335.

148. Longanga Otshudi A, Vercruysse A, Foriers A. Contribution to the ethnobotanical, phytochemical and pharmacological studies of traditionally used medicinal plants in the treatment of dysentery and diarrhoea in Lomela area, Democratic Republic of Congo (DRC). *J Ethnopharmacol.* 2000;71(3):411–423.

149. Otshudi AL, Foriers A, Vercruysse A, Van Zeebroeck A, Lauwers S. In vitro antimicrobial activity of six medicinal plants traditionally used for the treatment of dysentery and diarrhoea in Democratic Republic of Congo (DRC). *Phytomedicine.* 2000;7(2):167–72.

150. Meckes M, Calzada F, Tapia-Contreras A, Cedillo-Rivera R. Antiprotozoal properties of Helianthemum glomeratum. *Phytother Res.* 1999;13(2): 102–105.

151. Vijaya K, Ananthan S. Microbiological screening of Indian medicinal plants with special reference to enteropathogens. *J Altern Complement Med.* 1997;3(1):13–20.

152. Haider R, Khan AK, Aziz KM, Chowdhury A, Kabir I. Evaluation of indigenous plants in the treatment of acute shigellosis. *Trop Geo Med.* 1991;43(3):266–270.

153. Hien TT, White NJ. Qinghaosu. *Lancet.* 1993;341: 603–608.

154. Kaneda Y, Tori N, Tanaka T, Aikawa M. In vitro effects of berberine sulfate on the growth and structure of *Entamoeba histolytica, Giardia lamblia* and *Trichomonas vaginalis. Ann Trop Med Parasitol.* 1991;85:417–425.

155. Subbaiah TV, Amin AH. Effect of berberine sulfate on *Entamoeba histolytica. Nature.* 1967;215: 527–528.

156. Yang LQ, Singh M, Yap EH, et al. In vitro response of *Blastocystic hominis* against traditional Chinese medicine. *J Ethnopharmacol.* 1996;55: 35–42.

157. Gupte S. Use of berberine in treatment of giardiasis. *Am J Dis Child.* 1975;129:866.

158. Mirelman D, Monheit D, Varon S. Inhibition of growth of *Entamoeba histolytica* by allicin, the active principle in garlic extract *(Allium sativum). J Infect Dis.* 1987;156:243–244.

159. Wright CW, Phillipson JD. Natural products and the development of selective antiprotozoan drugs. *Phytother Res.* 1987;4:1127–1139.

160. Soffar SA, Mokhtar GM. Evaluation of the anti-parasitic effect of aqueous garlic *(Allium sativum)* extract in hymenolepiasis nana and giardiasis. *J Egypt Soc Parasitol.* 1991;21(2):497–502.

161. Information on herbal medications for relief of gastrointestinal symptoms may be obtained by running a literature search on PubMed (www.pubmed.gov) using the name of the condition or the term "Gastrointestinal Diseases" AND "Plants, Medicinal" or "Medicine, Oriental Traditional" or "Drugs, Herbal." The *PDR for Herbal Medicines* (Montvale, NJ: Medical Economics Press.) provides a summary of data for herbs commonly used in the United States; those applied to gastrointestinal disorders can be found in the "Indications" index.

162. Whitehead WE. Behavioral medicine approaches to gastrointestinal disorders. *J Consult Clin Psychol.* 1992;60(4):605–12.

163. Li Y, Tougas G, Chiverton SG, Hunt RH. The effect of acupuncture on gastrointestinal function and disorders. *Am J Gastroenterol.* 1992;87(10): 1372–81.

164. Podolsky DK. Inflammatory bowel disease. *N Engl J Med.* 2002;347:417–429.

165. Evans JM, McMahon AD, Murray FE, et al. Non-steroidal anti-inflammatory drugs are associated with emergency admission to hospital for colitis due to inflammatory bowel disease. *Gut.* 1997;40: 619–622.

166. Sutherland L, Singlewton J, Sessions J, et al. Double-blind placebo-controlled trial of metronidazole in Crohn's disease. *Gut.* 1991;32:1071–1075.

167. Turunen UM, Farkkila MA, Hakala K, et al. Long-term treatment of ulcerative colitis with ciprofloxacin: a prospective, double-blind, placebo-controlled study. *Gastroenterology.* 1998;115(5): 1072–1078.

168. Darfeuille-Michaud A, Neut C, Barnich N, et al. Presence of adherent *Escherichia coli* strains in ileal mucosa of patients with Crohn's disease. *Gastroenterology.* 1998;115:1405–1413.

169. Swidinski A, Ladhoff A, Pernthaler A, et al. Mucosal flares in inflammatory bowel disease. *Gastroenterology.* 2002;122:44–54.

170. Fuss IJ, Neurath M, Boirivant M, et al. Disparate CD4+ lamina propria (LP) lymphokine secretion profiles in inflammatory bowel disease: Crohn's disease LP cells manifest increased secretion of IFN-gamma, whereas ulcerative colitis LP cells manifest increased secretion of IL-5. *J Immunol.* 1996;157:1261–1270.

171. Dionne S, D'Agata ID, Hiscott J, et al. Colonic explant production of IL-1 and its receptor antagonist in imbalanced in inflammatory bowel disease. *Clin Exp Immunol*. 1998;112:381–387.

172. Lih-Brody L, Powell SR, Collier KP, et al. Increased oxidative stress and decreased antioxidant defenses in mucosa of inflammatory bowel disease. *Dig Dis Sci*. 1996;41:2078–2086.

173. Buffinton GD, Doe WF. Altered ascorbic acid status in the mucosa from inflammatory bowel disease patients. *Free Radic Res*. 1995;22(2):131–143.

174. D'Odorico A, Bortolan S, Cardin R, et al. Reduced plasma antioxidant concentrations and increased oxidative DNA damage in inflammatory bowel disease. *Scand J Gastroenterol*. 2001;36(12):1289–1294.

175. Heaton KW. Dietary factors in the aetiology of inflammatory bowel disease. In: Allan RN, Keighley MRB, Alexander-Williams J, Hawkins CF, eds. *Inflammatory Bowel Diseases*. 2nd ed... Edinburgh, UK: Churchill Livingstone; 1990:165–169.

176. Ballegaard M, Bjergstrom A, Brondum S, et al. Self-reported food intolerance in chronic inflammatory bowel disease. *Scand J Gastroenterol*. 1997;32:569–571.

177. Robertson DA, Ray J, Diamond I, Edwards JG. Personality profile and affective state of patients with inflammatory bowel disease. *Gut*. 1989; 30(5):623–626.

178. von Wietersheim J, Kohler T, Feiereis H. Relapse-precipitating life events and feelings in patients with inflammatory bowel disease. *Psychother Psychosom*. 1992;58(2):103–112.

179. Levenstein S, Prantera C, Varvo V, et al. Psychological stress and disease activity in ulcerative colitis: a multidimensional cross-sectional study. *Am J Gastroenterol*. 1994;89(8):1219–1225.

180. Straub RH, Herfarth H, Falk W, Andus T, Scholmerich J. Uncoupling of the sympathetic nervous system and the hypothalamic-pituitary-adrenal axis in inflammatory bowel disease? *J Neuroimmunol*. 2002;126(1–2):116–125.

181. Turnbull GK, Vallis TM. Quality of life in inflammatory bowel disease: the interaction of disease activity with psychosocial function *Am J Gastroenterol*. 1995;90(9):1450–1454.

182. Maunder R, Esplen MJ. Facilitating adjustment to inflammatory bowel disease: a model of psychosocial intervention in non-psychiatric patients. *Psychother Psychosom*. 1999;68(5):230–240.

183. Dudley-Brown S. Prevention of psychological distress in persons with inflammatory bowel disease. *Issues Mental Health Nurs*. 2002;23(4): 403–422.

184. Maunder RG, Esplen MJ. Supportive-expressive group psychotherapy for persons with. inflammatory bowel disease. *Can J Psychiatry*. 2001; 46(7):622–6.

185. Jantschek G, Zeitz M, Pritsch M, et al. Effect of psychotherapy on the course of Crohn's disease. Results of the German prospective multicenter psychotherapy treatment study on Crohn's disease. German Study Group on Psychosocial Intervention in Crohn's Disease. *Scand J Gastroenterol*. 1998;33(12):1289–1296.

186. Schwarz SP, Blanchard EB. Evaluation of a psychological treatment for inflammatory bowel disease. *Behav Res Ther*. 1991;29(2):167–177.

187. Robinson A, Thompson DG, Wilin W, et al. Guided self-management and patient-directed follow-up of ulcerative colitis: a randomized trial. *Lancet*. 2001;358:976–981.

188. Peeters M, Ghoos Y, Maes B, et al. Increased permeability of macroscopically normal small bowel in Crohn's disease. *Dig Dis Sci*. 1994;39: 2170–2176.

189. Hollander D, Vadherim CM, Brettholz, et al. Increased intestinal permeability in patient's with Crohn's disease and their relatives, a possible etiologic factor. *Ann Intern Med*. 1986;105:883–885.

190. Hilsden RJ, Meddings J, Sutherland LR. Aspirin provokes an exaggerated increase in the lactulose-mannitol permeability index in first-degree relatives of Crohn's patients. *Gastroenterology*. 1995;108:A834.

191. Wyatt J, Vogelsgang H, Hubl W, et al. Intestinal permeability and the prediction of relapse in Crohn's disease. *Lancet*. 1993;341:1437–1439.

192. Simmonds NJ, Rampton SD. Inflammatory bowel disease—a radical view. *Gut*. 1993;34:865–868.

193. Matsui T, Mitsuo I, Fujishima M, et al. Increased sugar consumption in Japanese patients with Crohn's disease. *Gastroenterol Jpn*. 1990;25:271.

194. Martini GA, Brandes JW. Increased consumption of refined carbohydrates in patients with Crohn's disease. *Wien Klin Wochenschr*. 1976;54:367–371.

195. Thurnton JR, Emmett PM, Heaton KW. Diet and Crohn's disease: characteristics of the pre-illness diet. *Br Med J*. 1979;2:762–764.

196. Mayberry JF, Rhodfes J, Newcombe RC. Increased sugar consumption in Crohn's disease. *Digestion*. 1980;20:323–326.

197. Heaton KW, Thornton JR, Emmett PM. Treatment of Crohn's disease with an unrefined-carbohydrate, fiber-rich diet. *Br Med J.* 1979;2:764–766.

198. Elliott DE, Urban JF Jr, Argo CK, Weinstock JV. Does the failure to acquire helminthic parasites predispose to Crohn's disease? *FASEB J.* 2000; 14(12):1848–1855.

199. van den Bogaerde J, Kamm MA, Knight SC. Immune sensitization to food, yeast and bacteria in Crohn's disease. *Aliment Pharmacol Ther.* 2001;15(10):1647–1653.

200. North CS, Alpers DH, Helzer JE, Spitznagel EL, Clouse RE. Do life events or depression exacerbate inflammatory bowel disease? A prospective study. *Ann Intern Med.* 1991;114(5):381–386.

201. Barnes RMR, Allan S, Taylor-Robinson CH, et al. Serum antibodies reactive with Saccharomyces cerevisiae in inflammatory bowel disease: is IgA antibody a marker for Crohn's disease? *Int Arch Allergy Appl Immunol.* 1990;92:9–15.

202. Barclay GR, McKenzie H, Pennington J, Parratt D, Pennington CR. The effect of dietary yeast on the activity of stable chronic Crohn's disease. *Scand J Gastroenterol.* 1992;27(3):196–200.

203. Riordan AM, Hunter JO, Cowan RE, et al. Treatment of active Crohn's disease by exclusion diet: East Anglican multicentre controlled trial. *Lancet.* 1993;342:1131–1134.

204. Alun Jones V, Workman E, Freeman AH. Crohn's disease: maintenance of remission by diet. *Lancet.* 1985;ii:177–180.

205. Belluzzi A, Brignola C, Campieri M, et al. Effect of an enteric coated fish-oil preparation on relapses in Crohn's disease. *N Engl J Med.* 1996; 334:1557–1560.

206. Siguel EN, Lerman RH. Prevalence of essential fatty acid deficiency in patients with chronic gastrointestinal disorders. *Metabolism.* 1996;45:12–23.

207. Cunnane SC, Ainley CC, Keeling PWN, et al. Diminished phospholipids incorporation of essential fatty acids in peripheral blood leukocytes from patient's with Crohn's disease: correlation with zinc depletion. *J Am Coll Nutr.* 1986;5: 451–458.

208. Hendricks KM, Walker WA. Zinc deficiency in inflammatory bowel disease. *Nutr Rev.* 1988;46: 401–408.

209. Galland L. Nutritional therapy for Crohn's disease: disease modifying and medication sparing. *Altern Ther.* 1999;5:94–95.

210. Gottschall E. *Breaking the Vicious Cycle: Intesti-*
nal Health through Diet. Kirkton, Ontario: Kirkton Press; 1994.

211. Shanahan F. Probiotics and inflammatory bowel disease: from fads and fantasy to facts and future. *Br J Nutr.* 2002;88(suppl 1):S5–S9.

212. Giaffer MH, Hollingsworth CD. Effect of an elemental diet on the faecal flora of patients with Crohn's disease. *Scand J Gastroenterol.* 1989; 24(suppl):158.

213. Rembacken BJ, Snelling AM, Hawkey PM, et al. Non-pathogenic *E. coli* versus mesalazine for the treatment of ulcerative colitis: a randomized trial. *Lancet.* 1999;354:635–639.

214. Gionchetti P, Rizzello F, Venturi A, et al. Oral bacteriotherapy as maintenance treatment in patients with chronic pouchitis: a double-blind placebo-controlled trial. *Gastroenterology.* 2000; 119:305–309.

215. Venturi A, Gionchetti P, Rizzello F, et al. Impact on the composition of the faecal flora by a new probiotic preparation: preliminary data on maintenance treatment of patients with ulcerative colitis. *Aliment Pharmacol Ther.* 1999;13:1103–1108.

216. Stenson WF, Cort D, Rodgers J, et al. Dietary supplementation with fish oil in ulcerative colitis. *Ann Intern Med.* 1992;116:609–615.

217. Gupta I, Parihar A, Malhotra P, et al. Effects of gum resin of *Boswellia serrata* in patients with chronic colitis. *Planta Med.* 2001;67(5):391–395.

218. Robinson M. Medical therapy of inflammatory bowel disease for the 21st century. *Eur J Surg Suppl.* 1998;(582):90–98.

219. Ben-Ayre E, Goldin E, Wengrower E, et al. Wheat grass juice in the treatment of active distal alternative colitis. *Scand J Gastroenterol.* 2002;37: 444–449.

220. Bamba T, Kanauchi O, Andoh A, Fujiyama Y. A new prebiotic from germinated barley for nutraceutical treatment of ulcerative colitis. *J Gastroenterol Hepatol.* 2002;17(8):818–824.

221. Wright R, Truelove SC. A controlled trial of various diets in ulcerative colitis. *Br Med J.* 1965;2: 138–141.

222. Roediger WE, Duncan A, Kapaniris O, Millard S. Reducing sulfur compounds of the colon impair colonocyte nutrition: implications for ulcerative colitis. *Gastroenterology.* 1993;104(3):802–809.

223. Roediger WE. Decreased sulphur amino acid intake in ulcerative colitis. *Lancet.* 1998;351(9115): 1555.

224. Tucker PC, Webster PD, Kilpatrick ZM. Amebic

colitis mistaken for inflammatory bowel disease. *Arch Intern Med.* 1975;135(5):681–685.

225. Fung WP, Monteiro EH, Ang HB, Kho KM, Lee SK. Ulcerative postdysenteric colitis. *Am J Gastroenterol.* 1972;57(4):341–348.

226. Bolton RP. *Clostridium difficile* and its association with inflammatory bowel disease. *Int Med.* 1980;Oct:19–23.

227. Rosenberg SN. A comparison of the techniques used by specialized and general purpose laboratories for the detection of intestinal parasites. *Practical Gastroenterology.* 1996;Nov.

228. Pardo-Gilbert A, Perez-Alvarado N, Zavala B. Differential diagnosis of nonspecific and amebic ulcerative colitis: survey of 100 patients. *Dis Colon Rectum.* 1972;15(2):147–149.

229. Yang C, Yan H. Observation of the efficacy of acupuncture and moxibustion in 62 cases of chronic colitis. *J Tradit Chin Med.* 1999;19(2):111–114.

230. Zhang X. 23 cases of chronic nonspecific ulcerative colitis treated by acupuncture and moxibustion. *J Tradit Chin Med.* 1998;18(3):188–191.

231. Wu H, Chen H, Hua X, Shi Z, Zhang L, Chen J. Clinical therapeutic effect of drug-separated moxibustion on chronic diarrhea and its immunologic mechanisms. *J Tradit Chin Med.* 1997;17(4):1997;253–258.

232. Li Y, Tougas G, Chiverton SG, Hunt RH. The effect of acupuncture on gastrointestinal function and disorders. *Am J Gastroenterol.* 1998;87(10):1372–1381.

233. Maxwell PR, Mendall MA, Kumar D. Irritable bowel syndrome. *Lancet.* 1997;350:1691–1695.

234. Bueno L, Fioramonti J, Delvaux M, Frexinos J. Mediators and pharmacology of visceral sensitivity: from basic to clinical investigations. *Gastroenterology.* 1997;112(5):1714–1743.

235. Callahan MJ. Irritable bowel syndrome neuropharmacology. A review of approved and investigational compounds *J Clin Gastroenterol.* 2002;35(1 suppl):S58–S67.

236. Gershon MD. Review article: roles played by 5-hydroxytryptamine in the physiology of the bowel. *Aliment Pharmacol Ther.* 1999;13(suppl 2):15–30.

237. Spiller R. Pharmacotherapy: non-serotonergic mechanisms *Gut.* 2002;51(suppl 1):i87–i90.

238. Chey WY, Jin HO, Lee MH, Sun SW, Lee KY. Colonic motility abnormality in patients with irritable bowel syndrome exhibiting abdominal pain and diarrhea. *Am J Gastroenterol.* 2001;96(5):1499–1506.

239. Talley NJ, Spiller R. Irritable bowel syndrome: a little understood organic bowel disease? *Lancet.* 2002;360:555–564.

240. Wang Y, Reen DJ, Puri P. Is a histologically normal appendix following emergency appendicectomy always normal? *Lancet.* 1996;347(9008):1076–1079.

241. Alun Jones V, Shorthouse M, McLaughlin P, et al. Food intolerance: a major factor in the pathogenesis of irritable bowel syndrome. *Lancet.* 1982;2:1115–1117.

242. Hunter JO, Alun Jones V. Studies on the pathogenesis of irritable bowel syndrome produced by food intolerance. In: Read NW, ed. *The Irritable Bowel Syndrome.* New York: Grune & Stratton; 1985.

243. King TS, Elia M, Hunter JO. Abnormal colonic fermentation in irritable bowel syndrome. *Lancet.* 1998;352:1187–1189.

244. Zar S, Kumar D, Kumar D. Role of food hypersensitivity in irritable bowel syndrome. *Minerva Med.* 2002;93(5):403–412.

245. Sanders DS, Carter MJ, Hurlstone DP, et al. Association of adult celiac disease with irritable bowel syndrome: a case-control study in patients fulfilling Rome II criteria referred to secondary care. *Lancet.* 2001;358:1504–1508.

246. Holti G. Candida allergy. In: Winner HL, Hurley R, eds. *Symposium on Candida Infections.* London: Livingstone; 1966:73–81.

247. Pimentel M, Chow EJ, Lin HC. Eradication of small intestinal bacterial overgrowth reduces symptoms of irritable bowel syndrome. *Am J Gastroenterol.* 2000;95(12):3503–3506.

248. Hunnisett A, Howard J, Davies S. Gut fermentation (or the auto-brewery) syndrome: a new clinical test with initial observations and discussion of clinical and biochemical implications. *J Nutr Med.* 1990;1:33–38.

249. Chappell CL, Matson CC. Giardia antigen detection in patients with chronic gastrointestinal disturbances. *J Fam Pract.* 1992;35:49–53.

250. Giacometti A, Cirioni O, Fiorentini A, Fortuna M, Scalise G. Irritable bowel syndrome in patients with *Blastocystis hominis* infection. *Eur J Clin Microbiol Infect Dis.* 1999;18(6):436–9.

251. Collins SM, Barbara G, Vallance B. Stress, inflammation and the irritable bowel syndrome. *Can J Gastroenterol.* 1999;13(suppl A):47A–49A.

252. Uvnas-Moberg K, Arn I, Theorell T, Jonsson CO. Gastrin, somatostatin and oxytocin levels in patients with functional disorders of the gastrointestinal tract and their response to feeding and interaction. *J Psychosom Res.* 1991;35(4–5): 525–533.

253. Keefer L, Blanchard EB. The effects of relaxation response meditation on the symptoms of irritable bowel syndrome: results of a controlled treatment study. *Behav Res Ther.* 2001;39(7): 801–811.

254. Guthrie E, Creed F, Dawson D, Tomenson B. A controlled trial of psychological treatment for the irritable bowel syndrome. *Gastroenterology.* 1991; 100(2):450–457.

255. Guthrie E, Creed F, Dawson D, Tomenson B. A randomised controlled trial of psychotherapy in patients with refractory irritable bowel syndrome. *Br J Psychiatry.* 1993;163:315–321.

256. Blanchard EB, Schwarz SP, Suls JM, et al. Two controlled evaluations of multicomponent psychological treatment of irritable bowel syndrome. Behav Res Ther. 1992;30(2):175–189.

257. Blanchard EB, Scharff L, Payne A, Schwarz SP, Suls JM, Malamood H. Prediction of outcome from cognitive-behavioral treatment of irritable bowel syndrome. *Behav Res Ther.* 1992;30(6): 647–650.

258. Corney RH, Stanton R, Newell R, Clare A, Fairclough P. Behavioural psychotherapy in the treatment of irritable bowel syndrome. *J Psychosom Res.* 1991;35(4–5):461–469.

259. Boyce P, Gilchrist J, Talley NJ, Rose D. Cognitive-behaviour therapy as a treatment for irritable bowel syndrome: a pilot study. *Aust N Z J Psychiatry.* 2000;34(2):300–309.

260. Heymann-Monnikes I, Arnold R, Florin I, Herda C, Melfsen S, Monnikes H. The combination of medical treatment plus multicomponent behavioral therapy is superior to medical treatment alone in the therapy of irritable bowel syndrome. *Am J Gastroenterol.* 2000;95(4):981–994.

261. Greene B, Blanchard EB. Cognitive therapy for irritable bowel syndrome. *J Consult Clin Psychol.* 1994;62(3):576–582.

262. van Dulmen AM, Fennis JF, Bleijenberg G. Cognitive-behavioral group therapy for irritable bowel syndrome: effects and long-term follow-up. *Psychosom Med.* 1996;58(5):508–514.

263. Payne A, Blanchard EB. A controlled comparison of cognitive therapy and self-help support groups in the treatment of irritable bowel syndrome. *J Consult Clin Psychol.* 1995;63(5):779–86.

264. Sanders MR, Shepherd RW, Cleghorn G, Woolford H. The treatment of recurrent abdominal pain in children: a controlled comparison of cognitive-behavioral family intervention and standard pediatric care. *J Consult Clin Psychol.* 1994;62(2):306–314.

265. Whorwell PJ, Prior A, Faragher EB. Controlled trial of hypnotherapy in the treatment of severe refractory irritable-bowel syndrome. *Lancet.* 1984;2(8414);1232–1234.

266. Whorwell PJ, Prior A, Colgan SM. Hypnotherapy in severe irritable bowel syndrome: further experience. *Gut.* 1987;28(4):423–425.

267. Houghton LA, Heyman DJ, Whorwell PJ. Symptomatology, quality of life and economic features of irritable bowel syndrome—the effect of hypnotherapy. *Aliment Pharmacol Ther.* 1996;10(1): 91–95.

268. Vidakovic-Vukic M. Hypnotherapy in the treatment of irritable bowel syndrome: methods and results in Amsterdam. *Scand J Gastroenterol Suppl.* 1999;230:49–51.

269. Galovski TE, Blanchard EB. The treatment of irritable bowel syndrome with hypnotherapy. *Appl Psychother Biofeed.* 1998;23(4):219–232.

270. Anbar RD. Self-hypnosis for the treatment of functional abdominal pain in childhood. *Clin Pediatr.* 2001;40(8):447–451.

271. Disbrow EA, Bennett HL, Owings JT. Effect of preoperative suggestion on postoperative gastrointestinal motility. *West J Med.* 1993;158(5): 488–492.

272. Prior A, Colgan SM, Whorwell PJ. Changes in rectal sensitivity after hypnotherapy in patients with irritable bowel syndrome. *Gut.* 1990;31(8): 896–898.

273. Heymann-Monnikes I, Arnold R, Florin I, Herda C, Melfsen S, Monnikes H. The combination of medical treatment plus multicomponent behavioral therapy is superior to medical treatment alone in the therapy of irritable bowel syndrome. *Am J Gastroenterol.* 2000;95(4):981–994.

274. Chiarioni G, Scattolini C, Bonfante F, Vantini I. Liquid stool incontinence with severe urgency: anorectal function and effective biofeedback treatment. *Gut.* 1993;34(11):1576–1580.

275. Pager CK, Solomon MJ, Rex J, Roberts RA. Long-term outcomes of pelvic floor exercise and biofeedback treatment for patients with fecal

incontinence. *Dis Colon Rectum*. 2002;45(8): 997–1003.

276. Keck JO, Staniunas RJ, Coller JA, et al. Biofeedback training is useful in fecal incontinence but disappointing in constipation. *Dis Colon Rectum*. 1994;37(12):1271–1276.

277. Brazzelli M, Griffiths P. Behavioural and cognitive interventions with or without other treatments for defaecation disorders in children. *Cochrane Database Syst Rev*. 2001;(4):CD002240.

278. Heymen S, Jones KR, Ringel Y, Scarlett Y, Whitehead WE. Biofeedback treatment of fecal incontinence: a critical review. *Dis Colon Rectum*. 2001;44(5):728–736.

279. Keck JO, Staniunas RJ, Coller JA, et al. Biofeedback training is useful in fecal incontinence but disappointing in constipation. *Dis Colon Rectum*. 1994;37(12):1271–1276.

280. Brown SR, Donati D, Seow-Choen F, Ho YH. Biofeedback avoids surgery in patients with slow-transit constipation: report of four cases. *Dis Colon Rectum*. 2001;44(5):737–739.

281. Turnbull GK, Ritvo PG. Anal sphincter biofeedback relaxation treatment for women with intractable constipation symptoms. *Dis Colon Rectum*. 1992;35(6):530–536.

282. Loening-Baucke V. Persistence of chronic constipation in children after biofeedback treatment. *Dig Dis Sci*. 1991;36(2):153–160.

283. Humphreys PA, Gevirtz RN. Treatment of recurrent abdominal pain: components analysis of four treatment protocols. *J Pediatr Gastroenterol Nutr*. 2000;31(1):47–51.

284. Mayer DJ. Acupuncture: an evidence-based review of the clinical literature. *Annu Rev Med*. 2000;51:49–63.

285. Dundee JW, Ghaly G. Local anesthesia blocks the antiemetic action of P6 acupuncture. *Clin Pharmacol Ther*. 1991;50(1):78–80.

286. Zhao J. Acupuncture at huatuojiaji (extra 21) points for treatment of acute epigastric pain. *J Tradit Chin Med*. 1991;11(4):258.

287. Jiang R. Analgesic effect of acupuncture on acute intestinal colic in 190 cases. *J Tradit Chin Med*. 1990;10(1):20–21.

288. Diehl DL. Acupuncture for gastrointestinal and hepatobiliary disorders. *J Altern Complement Med*. 1999;5(1):27–45.

289. Dang W, Yang J. Clinical study on acupuncture treatment of stomach carcinoma pain. *J Tradit Chin Med*. 1998;18(1):31–38.

290. Xu S, Liu Z, Xu M. Treatment of cancerous abdominal pain by acupuncture on zusanli (ST 36)—a report of 92 cases. *J Tradit Chin Med*. 1995;15(3):189–191.

291. Chan J, Carr I, Mayberry JF. The role of acupuncture in the treatment of irritable bowel syndrome: a pilot study. *Hepatogastroenterology*. 1997;44(17): 1328–1330.

292. Klauser AG, Rubach A, Bertsche O, Muller-Lissner SA. Body acupuncture: effect on colonic function in chronic constipation. *Z Gastroenterol*. 1993;31(10):605–608.

293. Fireman Z, Segal A, Kopelman Y, Sternberg A, Carasso R. Acupuncture treatment for irritable bowel syndrome. A double-blind controlled study. *Digestion*. 2001;64(2):100–103.

294. Chester CA, Macmurray FG, Restifo MD, Mann O. Giardiasis as a chronic disease. *Dig Dis Sci*. 1985; 30:215–218.

295. Kane JG, Chretien JH, Garagusi VF. Diarrhoea caused by *Candida*. *Lancet*. 1976;1:335–336.

296. Brabinder JOW, Blank F. Intestinal moniliasis in adults. *Can Med Assoc J*. 1957;77:478–483.

297. Caselli M, Trevisani L, Bighi S, et al. Dead fecal yeasts and chronic diarrhea. *Digestion*. 1988;41: 142–148.

298. Durlach J, Bac P, Durlach V, Bara M, Guiet-Bara A. [Neurotic, neuromuscular and autonomic nervous form of magnesium imbalance.] *Magnes Res*. 1997;10(2):169–195.

299. Galland L. Magnesium, stress and neuropsychiatric disorders. *Magnes Trace Elements*. 1991;10: 287–301.

300. Lieberman AD, Craven MR. Reactive intestinal dysfunction syndrome (RIDS) caused by chemical exposures. *Arch Environ Health*. 1998;53(5): 354–358.

301. Kline R, Kline J, DiPalma J, et al. Enteric-coated, pH-dependent peppermint oil capsules for the treatment of irritable bowel syndrome in children. *J Pediatr*. 2001;138:125–128.

302. Sach JA, Chang L. Irritable bowel syndrome. *Curr Treat Options Gastroenterol*. 2002;5(4):267–278.

303. Odes HS, Madar Z. A double-blind trial of a celandine, aloe vera and psyllium laxative preparation in adult patients with constipation. *Digestion*. 1991;49(2):65–71.

304. Ishii Y, Tanizawa H, Takino Y. Studies of aloe. V. Mechanism of cathartic effect (4). *Biol Pharmaceut Bull*. 1994;17:651–653.

305. Bornet FRJ, Brounds F. Immune-stimulating and

gut health-promoting properties of short-chain fructooligosaccharides. *Nutr Rev.* 2002;60:326–334.

306. Mahdihassan S. Triphala and its Arabic and Chinese synonyms. *Indian J Hist Sci.* 1978;13(1): 50–55.

307. Yamahara J, Matsuda H, Huang Q, et al. Intestinal motility enhancing effect of *Atractyloides lancea* rhizome. *J Ethnopharmacol.* 1990;29: 341–344.

308. Bensoussan A, Talley NJ, Hing M, Menzies R, Guo A, Ngu M. Treatment of irritable bowel syndrome with Chinese herbal medicine: a randomized controlled trial. *JAMA.* 1998;280(18): 1585–1589.

309. Information about the classification of patients with IBS according to principles of traditional Chinese medicine is available over the Internet from the American Academy of Acupuncture and Oriental Medicine (AAAOM) at http://www.aaaom.org/HPIRRITABLE%20BOWEL.htm, and from the *Journal of Chinese Medicine* at http://www.jcm.co.uk/SampleArticles.phtml (see *Irritable Bowel Syndrome: Treatment by Traditional Oriental Medicine* by Andrew Pagon).

310. Moss FM, Legon S, Bishop AE, et al. Effect of *Helicobacter pylori* on gastric somatostatin in duodenal ulcer disease. *Lancet.* 1992;340:930–932.

311. Ainsworth MA, Hogan DL, Koss MA, Isenberg JI. Cigarette smoking inhibits acid-stimulated duodenal mucosal bicarbonate secretion. *Ann Intern Med.* 1993;119(9):882–886.

312. Shigemi J, Mino Y, Tsuda T. The role of perceived job stress in the relationship between smoking and the development of peptic ulcers. *J Epidemiol.* 1999,9(5):320–326.

313. Rodriguez-Hernandez H, Jacobo-Karam JS, Guerrero-Romero F. Risk factors for peptic ulcer recurrence. *Gac Med Mex.* 2001;137(4):303–310.

314. De Lazzari F, Mancin O, Plebani M, et al. High IgE serum levels and "peptic" ulcers: clinical and functional approach. *Ital J Gastroenterol.* 1994; 26(1):7–11.

315. Weisman SM, Graham DY. Evaluation of the benefits and risks of low-dose aspirin in the secondary prevention of cardiovascular and cerebrovascular events. *Arch Intern Med.* 2002;162(19): 2197–2202.

316. Suerbaum S, Michetti P. *Helicobacter pylori* infection. *N Engl J Med.* 2002;347:1175–1186.

317. Pounder RE. *Helicobacter pylori* and NSAIDs—the end of the debate? *Lancet.* 2002;358:3–4.

318. Kuipers EJ, Lundell L, Klinkenberg-Knol EC, et al. Atrophic gastritis and *Helicobacter pylori* infection in patients with reflux esophagitis treated with omeprazole or fundoplication. *N Eng J Med.* 1996;334(16):1018–1022.

319. Sivam GP. Protection against *Helicobacter pylori* and other bacterial infections by garlic. *J Nutr.* 2001;131(3s):1106S–1108S.

320. Chung JG, Chen GW, Wu LT, et al. Effects of garlic compounds diallyl sulfide and diallyl disulfide on arylamine N-acetyltransferase activity in strains of *Helicobacter pylori* from peptic ulcer patients. *Am J Chin Med.* 1998;26(3–4):353–364.

321. Cellini L, Di Campli E, Masulli M, Di Bartolomeo S, Allocati N. Inhibition of *Helicobacter pylori* by garlic extract *(Allium sativum).* *FEMS Immunol Med Microbiol.* 1996;13(4):273–7.

322. Sivam GP, Lampe JW, Ulness B, Swanzy SR, Potter JD. *Helicobacter pylori*—in vitro susceptibility to garlic *(Allium sativum)* extract. *Nutr Cancer.* 1997;27(2):118–121.

323. You WC, Zhang L, Gail MH, et al. *Helicobacter pylori* infection, garlic intake and precancerous lesions in a Chinese population at low risk of gastric cancer. *Int J Epidemiol.* 1998;27(6): 941–944.

324. Fleischauer AT, Poole C, Arab L. Garlic consumption and cancer prevention: meta-analyses of colorectal and stomach cancers. *Am J Clin Nutr.* 2000;72(4):1047–1052.

325. Takezaki T, Gao CM, Ding JH, Liu TK, Li MS, Tajima K. Comparative study of lifestyles of residents in high and low risk areas for gastric cancer in Jiangsu Province, China; with special reference to allium vegetables. *J Epidemiol.* 1999; 9(5):297–305.

326. Dorant E, van den Brandt PA, Goldbohm RA, Sturmans F. Consumption of onions and a reduced risk of stomach carcinoma. *Gastroenterology.* 1996;110(1):12–20.

327. Fahey JW, Haristoy X, Dolan PM, et al. Sulforaphane inhibits extracellular, intracellular, and antibiotic-resistant strains of *Helicobacter pylori* and prevents benzo[a]pyrene-induced stomach tumors. *Proc Natl Acad Sci U S A.* 2002 28;99(11): 7610–7615.

328. Zhang L, Yang L, Zheng X. A study of *Helicobacterium pylori* and prevention and treatment of chronic atrophic gastritis. *J Tradit Chin Med.* 1997;17(1):3–9.

329. Ma S, Liang F, Wang S, et al. Treatment of 910

cases of atrophic gastritis with wei you decoction. *J Tradit Chin Med*. 1990;10(3):168–171.

330. Zhang L, Yang L, Zheng X. A study of *Helicobacterium pylori* and prevention and treatment of chronic atrophic gastritis. *J Tradit Chin Med*. 1997;17(1):3–9.

331. Shimamoto C, Tokioka S, Hirata I, Tani H, Ohishi H, Katsu K. Inhibition of *Helicobacter pylori* infection by orally administered yolk-derived anti-*Helicobacter pylori* antibody. *Hepatogastroenterology*. 2002;49(45):709–714.

332. Borrelli F, Izzo AA. The plant kingdom as a source of anti-ulcer remedies. *Phytother Res*. 2000;14(8):581–591.

333. Davis EA, Morris DJ. Medicinal uses of licorice through the millennia: the good and plenty of it. *Mol Cell Endocrinol*. 1991;78(1–2):1–6.

334. Fintelmann V. Modern phytotherapy and its uses in gastrointestinal conditions. *Planta Med*. 1991; 57(7):S48–S52.

335. Zhgun AA, Aloiants GA. [Effect of dehydrated cabbage juice on the secretory, acid- and pepsin-forming function of the stomach.] *Voen Med Zh*. 1971;(4):36–38.

336. Walker AF, Middleton RW, Petrowicz O. Artichoke leaf extract reduces symptoms of irritable bowel syndrome in a post-marketing surveillance study. *Phytother Res*. 2001;15(1):58–61.

337. Kositchaiwat C, Kositchaiwat S, Havanondha J. *Curcuma longa Linn.* in the treatment of gastric ulcer comparison to liquid antacid: a controlled clinical trial. *J Med Assoc Thai*. 1993;76(11): 601–605.

338. Yeoh KG, Kang JY, Yap I, et al. Chili protects against aspirin-induced gastroduodenal mucosal injury in humans. *Dig Dis Sci*. 1995;40(3):580–583.

339. Kang JY, Yeoh KG, Chia HP, et al. Chili—protective factor against peptic ulcer? *Dig Dis Sci*. 1995;40(3):576–579.

340. Mathew A, Gangadharan P, Varghese C, Nair MK. Diet and stomach cancer: a case-control study in South India. *Eur J Cancer Prev*. 2000;9(2):89–97.

341. Takahashi S, Yoshikawa T, Naito Y, Minamiyama Y, Tanigawa T, Kondo M. Antioxidant properties of antiulcer Kampo medicines. *Free Radic Res Commun*. 1993;19(suppl 1):S101–S108.

342. Tatsuta M, Iishi H. Effect of treatment with liu-jun-zi-tang (TJ-43) on gastric emptying and gastrointestinal symptoms in dyspeptic patients. *Aliment Pharmacol Ther*. 1993;7(4):459–462.

343. Ichimaru Y, Moriyama M, Ichimaru M, Gomita Y. [Effects of gamma-oryzanol on gastric lesions and small intestinal propulsive activity in mice.] *Nippon Yakurigaku Zasshi*. 1984;84(6):537–542.

344. Han KS. The effect of an integrated stress management program on the psychologic and physiologic stress reactions of peptic ulcer in Korea. *J Holistic Nurs*. 2002;20(1):61–80.

345. Wilhelmsen I, Haug TT, Ursin H, Berstad A. Effect of short-term cognitive psychotherapy on recurrence of duodenal ulcer: a prospective randomized trial. *Psychosom Med*. 1994;56(5): 440–448.

346. Hu J. Acupuncture treatment of epigastric pain. *J Tradit Chin Med*. 1995;15(3):238–240.

347. Zhang J. Treatment with acupuncture at zusanli (St 36) for epigastric pain in the elderly. *J Tradit Chin Med*. 1992;12(3):178–179.

348. Chen Z. Treatment of chronic gastritis with acupuncture. *J Tradit Chin Med*. 1994;14(3): 233–235.

349. Chang CS, Ko CW, Wu CY, Chen GH. Effect of electrical stimulation on acupuncture points in diabetic patients with gastric dysrhythmia: a pilot study. *Digestion*. 2001;64(3):184–190.

350. Hesketh PJ, Clapp RW, Doos WG, Sprechler SJ. The increasing frequency of adenocarcinoma of the esophagus. *Cancer*. 1989;61:526–530.

351. Bollschweiler E, Wolfgarten E, Nowroth T, Rosendahl U, Monig SP, Holscher AH. Vitamin intake and risk of subtypes of esophageal cancer in Germany. *J Cancer Res Clin Oncol*. 2002; 128(10):575–580.

352. Lablenz J, Blum AL, Bayerdorffer E, et al. Curing *Helicobacter pylori* in patients with duodenal ulcer may provoke reflux esophagitis. *Gastroenterology*. 1997;112:1442–1447.

353. Boeckxstaens GE, Tytgat GN. More pathophysiologically oriented treatment of GORD? *Lancet*. 2002;359:1267–1268.

354. Fox JA, Daniel EE. Role of Ca^{2+} in genesis of lower esophageal sphincter tone and other active contractions. *Am J Physiol*. 1979;237(2): E163–E171.

355. Bortolotti M, Coccia G, Grossi G. Red pepper and functional dyspepsia. *N Engl J Med*. 2002;346: 947–948.

356. Washington N, Steele RJ, Jackson SJ, Washington C, Bush D. Patterns of food and acid reflux in patients with low-grade oesophagitis—the role of an anti-reflux agent. *Aliment Pharmacol Ther*. 1998;12(1):53–58.

CHAPTER 22

Integrative Approach to Neurology

JAY LOMBARD AND SAMUEL SHIFLETT

The current treatments of neurological disorders have increasingly become subspecialized. This subspecialization has occurred in parallel with the overall reductionistic movement of modern Western medicine and has emerged as a result of the growing complexity and depth of knowledge within each respective field of neurology. In the process, however, a whole field of integrative neuroscience has been neglected.

Integrative neuroscience is based upon the recognition that all brain processes are interrelated and that there may exist only a small number of key mechanisms that may underlie a diverse range of pathological brain processes. Thus, while the phenotypical features of a particular neurological disease may vary widely from one disorder to the next, the intrinsic mechanisms that bring forth the expression of these disorders may be remarkably similar. One example of this changing paradigm occurred after the recognition of the role of the immune system in neurological health and disease. Previous concepts that the brain was an immunologically privileged organ are no longer valid; we now know that inflammatory processes may underlie a host of neurodegenerative processes including Alzheimer's disease, Parkinson's disease, and amyotrophic lateral sclerosis.

In the model of an integrative approach to neurological disorders, an exogenous or endogenous trigger(s) may set off a pathological cascade that ultimately leads to the dysfunction or demise of a focal region of the central nervous system. Triggers that have been causally associated with neurological diseases include pesticides in Parkinson's disease, saturated fat consumption in Alzheimer's disease, psychic stress in multiple sclerosis, and possibly mercury in autism.

A critical component in this common pathological cascade is the role of excitatory processes involving glutamate neurotransmission. Glutamate is thought to mediate normal excitatory neurotransmission, but it is believed also to mediate the final common pathway of several neurological and psychiatric disorders, including Alzheimer's disease, amyotrophic lateral sclerosis, Parkinson's disease, epilepsy, and bipolar disease. A disruption in the stability of the glutamate system as a result of a heterogeneous class of initiating events leads to an array of detrimental molecular triggers, including excessive free radical production, mitochondrial calcium accumulation, activation of proinflammatory cytokines, and proteolytic enzymes that damage intracellular protein and DNA.

▶ **TABLE 22-1** INTEGRATIVE PERSPECTIVE ON NEUROSCIENCE

Stress (Physical or Psychological)

• Heavy metals (Parkinson's disease)
• Pesticides (Parkinson's disease)
• Dietary fats (Alzheimer's disease)
• Psychological stress (multiple sclerosis)

Stressor	Biochemical Changes	Pathology
Environmental	Increased glutamate	Site-specific degeneration
Psychic	Increased free radicals	
Physical	≠ Systolic calcium	
	≠ Proteolytic caspases	

The usefulness of this model is that it enables us to design interventional strategies effective across scale from single neurons to behavior. Patients presenting with neurological diseases should be assessed for both physical and psychological toxins, including dietary fat consumption, heavy metal exposure, betacarbolines, organochlorine pesticides, and psychosocial stressors. Table 22–1 outlines the elements of an integrative perspective on neuroscience.

▶ **ALZHEIMER'S DISEASE**

Pathophysiology

Alzheimer's disease is a progressive neuronal degenerative disorder that results in the loss of higher cognitive function. This condition is characterized by the formation of senile plaques and neurofibrillary tangles predominantly found in cortical association areas which mediate short-term memory. Plaques are composed of beta amyloid which is derived from proteolytic cleavage of amyloid precursor protein.[1] Beta-amyloid is toxic to neurons and may be the primary cause of neuronal degeneration in Alzheimer's disease. Proposed additional mechanisms of neuronal degeneration include immunological factors, oxidative insults, disturbances of mitochondrial metabolism, excitotoxicity, and vascular angiopathy.[2] These influ-

ences result in the degradation of cholinergic neurons in the basal forebrain (Figure 22–1).

Failure of recent memory is one of the earliest prominent symptoms of Alzheimer's disease and is frequently associated with distur-

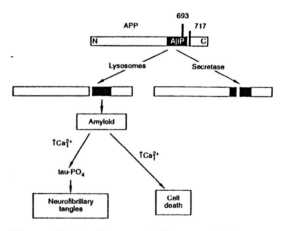

Figure 22-1. The amyloid cascade hypothesis. Processing of amyloid precursor protein (APP) can occur via two pathways: (1) Cleavage within AβP by the secretase, which generates peptide products that do not precipitate to form amyloid and (2) cleavage in the endosomal-lysosomal compartment, resulting in intact AβP that precipitates to form amyloid and, in turn, causes neurofibrillary tangles and cell death, the hallmarks of Alzheimer's disease. (Reproduced with permission from Hardy JA, Higgins GA. Alzheimer's disease: the amyloid cascade hypothesis. *Science.* 1992;256:184–185.)

bances in emotional behavior consisting most often of either a reduction in affect or an increase in anxiety. Focal neural psychological deficits may include difficulty in spatial relationships, anomia, and perseverations.

The diagnosis of Alzheimer's disease is made on clinical grounds that may be supported by neuroimaging studies including magnetic resonance spectroscopy, which demonstrates reduced N-acetyl aspartate levels in the hippocampus.[3]

The differential diagnosis of Alzheimer's disease includes multiinfarct dementia, drug intoxication, vitamin or hormonal deficiency, normal pressure hydrocephalus, and other neurodegenerative diseases such as Pick's disease and Lewy body disease.

Prevalence and Epidemiology

Alzheimer's disease afflicts an estimated 4 million Americans and is a leading cause of death. Approximately 10% of the population older than the age of 65 years and as much as 50% of the population older than age 85 years is believed to be affected by Alzheimer's disease.[1] Epidemiological studies have identified several factors involved in a higher incidence of Alzheimer's disease. These include advancing age, higher intake of total fat, saturated fat, and cholesterol, and an inverse relationship with both nonsteroidal antiinflammatory drug use, and hormone replacement therapy in women.[5]

▶ Case Example 1: Alzheimer's Disease

A 74-year-old woman presents with recent short-term memory loss and subtle personality changes. The history is provided mostly by family members as the patient lacks insight into her behavioral and cognitive disturbances. Initial symptoms began approximately 18 months prior to the consultation and were attributed to the recent death of her spouse. At that time, the patient exhibited some mild short-term memory loss characterized by perseverations and repeated questioning of recent events. Over the past several months she has become increasingly paranoid, believing strangers were entering her home and stealing her possessions. She is intermittently agitated and has a significant disruption of her sleep–wake cycle.

Previous medical history is remarkable for mild hypertension treated with an angiotensin converting enzyme (ACE) inhibitor. Neurological examination is grossly nonfocal with the exception of a mini-mental status examination score of 23 over 30. Routine laboratory data including a complete blood cell count, basic chemistry, lipid profile, thyroid profile, vitamin B_{12}, and folate are all within normal limits. Magnetic resonance imaging (MRI) of the brain reveals mild senile atrophy and age-related microvascular ischemic changes, but the primary diagnosis is Alzheimer's disease with the possibility of multiinfarct dementia being less likely. The family refuses apolipoprotein E testing and are requesting advice on therapeutic strategies to forestall dementia.

Conventional Treatment Approaches to Alzheimer's Disease

Conventional pharmacological approaches for treatment of Alzheimer's disease are based on the concept of a cholinergic deficiency syndrome, which has been proposed to be responsible for the memory impairments associated with Alzheimer's disease. Choline acetyltransferase, the enzyme responsible for the synthesis of acetylcholine, is decreased by 40–90% in the cortex and hippocampus of Alzheimer's disease patients.[6]

The nucleus basalis of Meynert also shows progressive neuronal loss in Alzheimer's disease.[7] The current pharmacological approach to augmenting cholinergic function in Alzheimer's disease is to inhibit the breakdown of acetylcholine by inhibiting the enzyme acetylcholinesterase. Current FDA-approved cholinesterase inhibitors include donepezil, rivastigmine, and galanthamine. Cholinesterase inhibitors are effective in the treatment of the cognitive, behavioral, and functional deficits of Alzheimer's disease. Caution should be used in prescribing cholinesterase inhibitors to patients with preexisting bradycardia, peptic ulcer disease, or chronic obstructive pulmonary disease. Nausea, vomiting, diarrhea, and anorexia are the most common side effects of cholinesterase inhibitors.[8]

Integrative Strategies in the Treatment of Alzheimer's Disease

The integrative approach to the treatment of Alzheimer's disease includes the use of antioxidants, antiinflammatory agents, neuroprotective agents, hormone replacement therapy, modulators of phospholipid and angiometabolism, and lipid-lowering strategies.

Nutritional and Hormonal Approaches

Antioxidants

The brain is rich in unsaturated fatty acids and is particularly susceptible to free radical injury. The importance of free radicals in the pathogenesis of Alzheimer's disease is supported by a number of biochemical abnormalities noted in this condition, which demonstrate oxidative stress in this disorder. These include reduced levels of the antioxidant enzymes superoxide dismutase, catalase, and glutathione peroxidase in Alzheimer's diseased brains.[9] Furthermore, in autopsy of Alzheimer's diseased brains, there is an increase in lipid peroxidation, a decline in polyunsaturated fatty acid, and an increase in 4-hydroxy-2-nonenal, a neurotoxic aldehyde of polyunsaturated fatty acid oxidation.[10] Furthermore, immunohistochemical studies show the presence of oxidative stress products in neurofibrillary tangles and senile plaques.[11] Isoprostanes, which are sensitive and specific markers of in vivo lipid peroxidation, are increased in the cerebrospinal fluid, blood, and urine of patients with a clinical diagnosis of Alz-heimer's disease.[12]

Vitamin E interferes with the effects of lipid peroxidation by trapping free radicals. Vitamin E prevents cell death caused by amyloid beta protein.[13] Because of this antioxidant potential, vitamin E has been investigated to slow the progression of Alzheimer's disease. A placebo-controlled clinical trial of vitamin E in patients with moderately advanced Alzheimer's disease was conducted by the Alzheimer's Disease Cooperative Study. The subjects in the vitamin E group were treated with vitamin E 2,000 IU daily, alone or in combination with selegiline 10 mg/d, and were compared against a placebo-controlled group. The primary outcome measures included institutionalization, loss of ability to perform activities of daily living, and severe dementia. There was significant delay in the time to primary outcome measures for patients treated with selegiline, alpha-tocopherol, or combination therapy, as compared to patients treated with placebo.[14]

There is evidence that increased blood concentrations of homocysteine may be a risk factor for Alzheimer's disease. There is a significant correlation between cerebrospinal fluid concentrations of homocysteine and 4-hyroxy-2-nonenal, a neurotoxic product of lipid peroxidation in Alzheimer's disease patients.[15] Furthermore, patients with Alzheimer's disease have significantly lower levels of folic acid in their cerebrospinal fluid as compared to age-matched controls.[16] Patients with mild to moderate dementia and elevated plasma homocysteine levels improve clinically after folic acid supplementation. Folic acid may exert its beneficial effects on cognition by improving endothelial function and reducing endothelial superoxide.[17]

Alzheimer's Disease and Estrogen Replacement Therapy

Recently, there has been a growing awareness of the importance of estrogen in brain function and cognition, as well as its possible protective effects against Alzheimer's disease. Estrogen acts as a nerve growth factor, facilitating the formation of synapses predominantly in the hippocampus.[18] Estrogen is also critical in the preservation of cholinergic neurons and acts as a cofactor in acetylcholine synthesis.[19]

Epidemiological studies support a role of estrogen as being a protective factor against dementia. Alzheimer's disease is more common in women than in men, and longitudinal studies demonstrate that women who take estrogen have a substantially lower risk of developing Alzheimer's disease than do those who have never used the hormone.[20]

To characterize the cognitive effects of high-dose estradiol for postmenopausal women with Alzheimer's disease, 20 postmenopausal women with Alzheimer's disease were randomized to receive 0.1 mg of estradiol or placebo for 8 weeks. Significant effects of estrogen treatment were observed on attention, verbal memory, and visual memory scores.[21]

Modulation of Phospholipid and Energy Metabolism

Membrane phospholipids determine neuronal membrane function by modulating receptor plasticity and signal transduction. In Alzheimer's disease there is a substantial increase in saturated fatty acids in neuronal cell membranes that is paralleled by a decrease in the polyunsaturated fatty acid components.[22] Human autopsy studies demonstrate that docosahexanoic acid (DHA), a polyunsaturated fatty acid, is significantly decreased in the hippocampus of Alzheimer's diseased brains.[23]

Phosphatidylserine, a major phospholipid in the brain, exerts a beneficial effect on acetylcholine neurotransmission and diminishes the atrophy of cholinergic neurons in the basal forebrain.[24] Thomas Crook reported that in a sample of 51 patients who met criteria for probable Alzheimer's disease, phosphatidylserine 300 mg exerted a mild therapeutic effect on cognitive scores over a 12-week period.[25]

Acetylcarnitine is structurally similar to acetylcholine and plays a fundamental role in brain lipid metabolism by acting as a carrier of medium-chain fatty acids across the inner mitochondrial membrane. Treatment with acetylcarnitine raises brain phosphocreatine levels measured by magnetic resonance spectroscopy.[26] Acetylcarnitine, in addition to modulating brain energy metabolism, enhances the production of essential neurotrophic factors and the stimulation of cholinergic synaptic pathways.[27]

In a double-blind, placebo-controlled study of 30 mild to moderately demented patients with probable Alzheimer's disease, acetylcarnitine 2.5 g over a 6-month period resulted in significantly less deterioration in some cognitive areas than in age-matched controls.[28]

Lipid-Lowering Strategies

Recent epidemiological studies report a relationship between dietary fat intake and dementia. In the Rotterdam study, different components of fat intake, including total fat, saturated fat, cholesterol, and polyunsaturated fatty acids were examined in a population-based study. High intake of total fat, saturated fat, and cholesterol were related to increased risk of dementia. Conversely, fish consumption was associated with a reduced risk of dementia.[29] The relationship of a high-fat diet to dementia may be explained by the correlation of elevated cholesterol and amyloid plaque deposition. Conversely, consumption of fish rich in omega-3 fatty acids increases plasma phospholipids including DHA. The elevation of

polyunsaturated fatty acids may help to reduce proinflammatory cytokines, which are
implicated in the pathogenesis of Alzheimer's
disease.[30]

Epidemiological studies demonstrate that
hypercholesterolemia is an independent risk
factor for the development of Alzheimer's disease. Recent evidence suggests that cholesterol
levels regulate amyloid plaque deposition.

Humans with elevated low-density lipoprotein (LDL) cholesterol were treated in a double blind randomized study with lovastatin
10–60 mg, a beta-hydroxy-beta-methylglutaryl-
coenzyme A (HMG-CoA) reductase inhibitor.
Serum concentrations of beta-amyloid peptide
were significantly reduced in the lovastatin
treatment group. Recent clinical reports also
described an association between statin therapy and a reduction in the occurrence of
Alzheimer's disease by as much as 70%.[31]

Botanical Medicine Approaches

Ginkgo biloba is a plant extract that has been
popularized as a memory-enhancing herb. Extracts from Ginkgo contain specific terpenoids
that possess antioxidant and free radical scavenging activity, reverse age-related loss of
neurotransmitter receptors, increase choline uptake, and downregulate the hippocampal glucocorticoid receptors.[32]

In a 1-year double-blind, placebo-controlled
study, ginkgo was found to produce symptomatic improvement in patients with dementia.[33] However, many methodological flaws
limit the interpretation of these findings, and
currently several multicenter double-blind,
placebo-controlled studies are underway to
confirm these preliminary findings.

Huperzine A is an alkaloid isolated from a
traditional Chinese herbal medicine used to treat
inflammation. It acts as a potent inhibitor of
acetylcholinesterase more selectively and possibly with less toxicity than the current FDA drugs
approved for Alzheimer's disease. Compared

with donepezil, huperzine A has a longer half-
life and appears to have additional pharmacological properties that make it an attractive candidate therapy for clinical trials. Huperzine A
also reduces neuronal cell death caused by its
toxic relative glutamate.[34]

In a double-blind study of 56 patients
with multiinfarct dementia and 104 patients with
Alzheimer's disease who were treated with huperzine A 50 μg twice daily or placebo, huperzine A treatment significantly improved memory in patients in both treatment groups.[35]

Mind–Body Approaches

There is increasing evidence that cortisol damages the hippocampus in primates. Hippocampal atrophy induced by cortical steroids may
play an important role in the pathogenesis of
a range of neuropsychiatric disorders including
Alzheimer's disease.[36] Plasma cortisol levels in
Alzheimer's disease subjects are significantly
elevated when compared to nondemented subjects. Furthermore, high plasma cortisol levels
are associated with a rapid decline in mini-
mental status examination scores over a 40-
month period.[37] Cortisol adversely affects cognition and is a risk factor for Alzheimer's
disease probably via its effects of impairing
hippocampal neurogenesis and glucose utilization. Mind–body approaches that are directed
at attenuating persistent elevated cortisol production are recommended for patients of all
ages to reduce cortisol and limit the loss of
hippocampal neurons.

Conclusions

When a diagnosis of Alzheimer's disease is clinically established and a reversible cause of dementia has been excluded, a combination of
symptomatic and neuroprotective strategies
should be initiated. Current FDA symptomatic
therapies include acetylcholin-esterase inhibitors

such donepezil, rivastigmine, and galanthamine. An alternative may be the use of huperzine A, which, in addition to inhibiting acetylcholinesterase, demonstrates neuroprotective effects in vitro and in vivo.

Neuroprotective strategies can also be recommended including the use of vitamin E 2,000 IU/d, and folic acid 800 μg/d. *Ginkgo biloba* should be used with caution, especially with patients on antiplatelet or anticoagulant therapies or with bleeding diatheses, because it can interfere with normal coagulation. Estrogen therapy should not be routinely recommended until further clinical studies establish a clear efficacy for hormone replacement therapy and then a benefit:risk ratio must be carefully assessed. Acetylcarnitine 2,000 mg/d and phosphatidylserine 300 mg/d are safe and potentially useful nutritional adjunctive therapies for Alzheimer's disease patients.

Lipid-lowering strategies are strongly recommended especially in patients with elevated low-density lipoprotein (LDL) levels. Dietary reduction of saturated fat and increased consumption of omega-3 fatty acids, such as those found in cold-water fish, should be part of a dietary strategy for Alzheimer's disease patients.

Statin therapy should also be considered in patients with Alzheimer's disease, especially in light of the recent findings that correlate high cholesterol with amyloid plaque deposition. Table 22–2 summarizes treatment strategies for Alzheimer's disease.

▶ PARKINSON'S DISEASE

Pathophysiology

Parkinson's disease is a movement disorder characterized by a progressive loss of dopaminergic neurons in the substantia nigra. Dopamine is involved in the control of movement, and depletion of this neurotransmitter results in a characteristic set of motor disturbances. In addition to the motor projections of dopaminergic neurons from the substantia nigra, dopamine is also found in cortical and subcortical regions. As a consequence, dopamine depletion as found in Parkinson's disease has a wide range of physical and emotional disturbances beyond simply motor disturbances.

The exact cause of Parkinson's disease is unknown. However, a variety of factors appears to

---

▶ TABLE 22–2 THERAPEUTIC REVIEW FOR ALZHEIMER'S DISEASE

- Diet
  Recommend to patients a dietary reduction of saturated fat and an increase in consumption of omega-3 fatty acids
- Supplements
  Vitamin E 2,000 IU/d
  Acetylcarnitine 2000 mg/d
  Phosphatidylserine 300 mg/d
- Botanicals
  Ginkgo biloba extract 240 mg/d
  Huperzine A 50–200 μg/d
- Mind–body exercises
  Stress reduction techniques including meditation
- Pharmaceuticals
  Acetylcholinesterase inhibitors including donepezil, galanthamine, and rivastigmine
- Lipid-lowering strategies (red yeast extract or other HMG-CoA reductase inhibitors)

contribute to a loss of dopamine containing neurons in the substantia nigra. These include environmental, genetic, and other biochemical factors. Epidemiological studies link Parkinson's disease to rural living, drinking well water, and exposure to pesticides. A large number of population studies suggest that people with jobs that expose them to pesticides have a greater risk of developing Parkinson's disease. Rotenone, a common environmental pesticide, produces selective degeneration of dopamine neurons in a Parkinson's-like syndrome in experimental animal models. Furthermore, rotenone-treated rats develop protein aggregates that are identical to alpha-synuclein, an abnormal protein associated with human forms of inherited Parkinson's disease.[38]

The mechanism by which dopaminergic neurons are selectively lost in Parkinson's disease is unknown but may also involve genetic factors. Genetic studies in families with a strong history of Parkinson's disease have identified mutations in genes that regulate how proteins are folded and broken down, resulting in alpha-synuclein aggregates.[39] The molecular mechanisms underlying these pathological effects appear to induce oxidative stress and impair mitochondrial function.

The concept of free radical-mediated injury in Parkinson's disease is currently a leading hypothesis for its pathogenesis. The free radical hypothesis of Parkinson's disease has received support from studies on postmortem brains. For example, reduced levels of glutathione are found in the substantia nigra of Parkinson's disease patients.[40] The markers of oxidative stress in Parkinson's disease patients include reduced levels of polyunsaturated fatty acids and an increase in levels of malondialdehyde in the central nervous system.[41] (Figure 22–2).

The substantia nigra is rich in iron and iron concentration increases in Parkinson's disease. Intracellular iron is normally sequestered as inorganic material complexed with ferritin. Recently, it was observed that there are decreased levels of ferritin in the substantia nigra of Parkinson's disease brains.[42] A consequence of

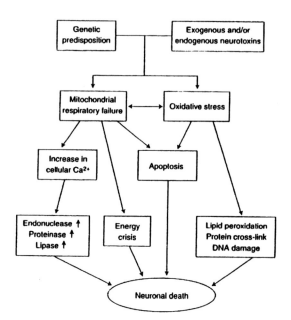

Figure 22–2. Representation of the mechanism of nigral neuronal death in Parkinson's disease. (Reproduced with permission from Mizuno Y, Yoshino H, Ikebe S, et al. Mitochondrial dysfunction in Parkinson's disease. *Ann Neurol.* 1998;44[3 suppl. 1]:S99–S109.)

decreased ferritin is liberation of iron from its carrier molecule into the cytoplasm with excessive free radical production. Free radical–mediated damage to proteins including 4-hydroxy-2-nonenal has been identified also by immunohistochemical studies in the substantia nigra of Parkinson's disease patients.[43]

Reduced glutathione is an important endogenous antioxidant. Recently, Jenner confirmed that the low levels of reduced glutathione in the substantia nigra in Parkinson's patients are disease specific.[44] This finding suggests that reduced levels of glutathione may be a fundamental and primary abnormality in Parkinson's disease.

Another postmortem finding in Parkinson's disease patients that is compatible with the free radical hypothesis is that of a deficiency in the enzyme mitochondrial complex-1. Schapira demonstrated the defect in complex-1 in

Parkinson's disease with a 70% decrease in this enzyme's activity.[45] This decrease appears to be regionally specific for the substantia nigra and for Parkinson's disease.

Prevalence and Diagnosis

Parkinson's disease is a common chronic disease of advancing age. It will become more prevalent in the coming years as the population continues to age. One million Americans are afflicted with Parkinson's disease and approximately 50,000 new cases are diagnosed each year. The average age of onset is 60 years, and between 5% and 10% of Parkinson's disease patients are younger than age 40 years.

Parkinson's disease is primarily a disease of the motor system. The four cardinal motor symptoms of Parkinson's disease include resting tremor, rigidity, akinesia or bradykinesia, and postural instability. The resting tremor in Parkinson's disease is an involuntary movement of a limb that is stationary. It may be unilateral or bilateral. For some patients, tremor is the major symptom; however, approximately 30% of patients with Parkinson's disease do not experience tremor. In addition to the motor abnormalities, patients with Parkinson's disease have common secondary symptoms that involve cognitive and affective disturbances. Depression and dementia are common in Parkinson's disease with a prevalence of approximately 50% of Parkinson's disease cases.[46] Other often underrecognized symptoms include sleep disturbances, oily skin, and increased sweating.

Parkinson's disease is a clinical diagnosis. There currently are no biological markers or laboratory blood tests to diagnose Parkinson's disease. Positron Emission Tomography (PET scan) uses a radioactive tracer technique that can measure dopamine markers in the basal ganglia. This test may prove useful for confirmation of the diagnosis of Parkinson's disease.

The differential diagnosis of Parkinson's disease includes other disorders of the extrapyramidal system, including progressive supranuclear palsy, olivopontocerebellar atrophy, and Shy-Drager syndrome. Vascular brain disease with subcortical involvement can also mimic some of the clinical symptoms of Parkinson's disease. Clinicians should also be alert to the possibility of iatrogenic causes of Parkinson's disease, including the use of neuroleptics in psychiatric practice.

▶ Case Example 2: Parkinson's Disease

A 67-year-old man has noticed an involuntary tremor involving his right hand for several years. Previously, it would wax and wane in severity, but more recently it became more noticeable and associated with a deterioration in his handwriting and diminished voice volume. He also notes some balance difficulties and has fallen on more than one occasion. His examination is remarkable for extrapyramidal stigmata including cogwheel rigidity, hypomimia, and retropulsion. A tentative diagnosis of Parkinson's disease is made.

Conventional Treatment Approaches to Parkinson's Disease

The two main pharmacological treatments for Parkinson's disease are either increasing dopamine levels or mimicking the effects of dopamine in the brain. The most common treatment for Parkinson's disease is dopamine replacement with levodopa. After ingestion levodopa enters the brain where it is converted to dopamine. Premature conversion of levodopa to dopamine prior to crossing the blood–brain barrier results in side effects including nausea and vomiting. Carbidopa prevents the peripheral decarboxylation of levodopa. Levodopa replacement therapy is extremely effective in controlling many of the symptoms of disability in Parkinson's disease, especially rigidity and hypokinesia. Because the progressive loss of dopamine neurons continues despite levodopa therapy, incremental dosing is often required. These increments result in dyskinesias and other complications, including unpredictable fluctuations in the ability to control movement and episodes of freezing. Of patients who take levodopa for 5–10 years, 50–90% experience on-off periods in which levodopa works (on) and does not work (off). In addition, recent data suggests that long-term exposure to levodopa may have a toxic effect on neurons. It has been speculated that levodopa damages dopamine-containing neurons via its contribution to the formation of free radicals.[47]

Dopamine agonists, such as amantadine, pergolide, bromocriptine, pramipexole, and ropinirole, are important in the treatment of Parkinson's disease. While the previous guidelines supported the use of levodopa as a first-line therapy, the most recent guidelines for treating Parkinson's disease advocate dopamine agonists as initial symptomatic therapy to treat Parkinson's disease. Although dopamine agonists result in less symptomatic improvement than levodopa therapy, they may also exhibit neuroprotective effects. Dopamine agonists stimulate autoreceptors, thereby decreasing dopamine synthesis. Dopamine agonists have also been demonstrated to inhibit hydroxyl, superoxide, and nitric oxide radicals and to increase superoxide dismutase levels in the substantia nigra.[48] A number of clinical studies are underway to determine if dopamine agonists exhibit neuroprotective effects clinically.

Surgical treatments for Parkinson's disease, including deep-brain stimulation, have gained wider acceptance. Deep-brain stimulation in the globus pallidus produces improvement in Parkinson's disease signs, including a reduction in tremor and dyskinesia.

Integrative Strategies in the Management of Parkinson's Disease

An ideal therapy for Parkinson's disease prevents or reduces the loss of dopamine-producing neurons. Dietary factors and certain supplements may be beneficial and considered as part of a neuroprotective strategy. Table 22–3 provides an overview of Parkinson's disease treatment.

Nutritional and Botanical Approaches

Isothiocyanates
The class of phytochemicals known as isothiocyanates has generated considerable attention. The beneficial effects of isothiocyanates appear to be mediated through the induction of cellular antioxidant defenses, including the induction of glutathione and the activation of glutathione transferase. The ability of phytochemicals such as isothiocyanates to augment antioxidant defenses raises the possibility that these agents may have a role in preventing neurological diseases associated with oxidative damage, including Parkinson's disease. The ability to augment central nervous system antioxidant enzyme activity by using small molecules such as isothiocyanates, which are known to cross the blood–brain barrier, has clear advantages over strategies that seek to deliver large antioxidants directly past the blood–brain barrier into the central nervous system.[49] Recommending three to five servings of cruciferous vegetables such as broccoli and cauliflower per day provides approximately 100 mg of isothiocyanates.

There is a strong theoretical benefit in recommending specific antioxidants as well as

▶ **TABLE 22-3** THERAPEUTIC OVERVIEW FOR PARKINSON'S DISEASE

- Diet
  Encourage food switch in isothiocyanates such as cruciferous vegetables like broccoli and cauliflower; current isothiocyanates are not found in supplemental form owing to their relative instability
- Supplements
  Lipoic acid 400–800 mg/d, preferably in sustained-release formulation
  Glutathione 600 mg/d (owing to its poor bioavailability, intravenous administration of glutathione is preferable)
  Coenzyme Q10 1,200 mg/d
  Tea polyphenols 100–200 mg/d
- Exercise modalities
  Occupational therapy
  Physical therapy
  Yoga and Tai Chi
- Pharmaceuticals
  Initiate carbidopa and levodopa when functional impairments are present
    Dopamine agonists may be used as first-line agents owing to their combined symptomatic and neuroprotective effects
    Selegiline may be used in combination with any of the above medications, but dose adjustments may be necessary

mitochondrial augmenting agents in the adjunctive treatment of Parkinson's disease patients. Antioxidants, including vitamin E, lipoic acid, polyphenols found in green and black tea, and glutathione, have been proposed as agents that potentially have the ability to prevent the progression of Parkinson's disease. Mitochondrial agents, including nicotinamide adenine dinucleotide (NADH) and coenzyme Q10, have also been studied in the management of Parkinson's disease.

Vitamin E

The deprenyl and tocopherol antioxidant therapy of Parkinsonism (Data Top trial) involving vitamin E was undertaken because of the data suggesting that oxidative stress plays a role in the pathogenesis of Parkinson's disease. Unfortunately, oral vitamin E given to early Parkinson's disease patients failed to result in symptomatic improvement or delay in clinical progression.[50] A recent study, however, showed that oral vitamin E failed to alter levels of alpha-tocopherol in ventricular spinal fluid of Parkinson's disease patients.[51] These studies suggested that vitamin E administered orally may have limited access across the blood–brain barrier, and thus may not increase brain vitamin E levels enough to observe clinically beneficial effects. These important observations raise questions about the validity of prior negative studies on the effects of antioxidant vitamins in the progression of Parkinson's disease.

Lipoic Acid

Lipoic acid is a thiol-based antioxidant that acts as a free radical scavenger as well as a potential metal chelator. It stimulates glutathione transferase activity which enhances glutathione production. Lipoic acid supplementation has been demonstrated to increase liver and plasma glutathione levels and protect against lipid peroxidation in a variety of animal studies.[52] In one human study, all administration of lipoic acid increased brain mitochondrial activity measured by magnetic resonance spectroscopy.[53] Dihydrolipoic acid was demonstrated to prevent some of the pathological changes in postmortem brains of Parkinson's disease patients.[54] Daily doses of lipoic acid 400–800 mg can be recommended, preferably in a sustained-release formulation.

Tea Polyphenols

Tea extracts have been reported to possess radical scavenger, iron chelating, and antiinflammatory properties in a variety of tissues. A recent study demonstrated a neuroprotective effect of tea extracts in a neuronal cell model of Parkinson's disease. Green tea and black tea extracts demonstrated highly potent antioxidant radical scavenging activity on brain mitochondrial membrane fraction against iron-induced lipid peroxidation. Neuroprotection was attributed to the potent antioxidant and iron-chelating actions of the polyphenolic constituents of tea extracts, which apparently prevent nuclear translocation and activation of cell-death-promoting nuclear factor-κB.[55]

Glutathione

Use of glutathione in Parkinson's disease is limited as a consequence of its poor absorption when given orally. Intravenous glutathione has been recommended by some physicians. An open-label study in a small sample of Parkinson's disease patients demonstrated a small but significant decline in disability scores in patients treated with glutathione 600 mg IV daily.[56]

Coenzyme Q10

Coenzyme Q10 is a fat-soluble quinone, which is responsible for assisting in the mitochondrial electron transport chain. In addition to its role in energy utilization, coenzyme Q10 may also function as a free radical scavenger, exerting beneficial effects on cell membrane stability. Oral coenzyme Q10 increases complex-1 activity and protects mitochondria from free radical damage.

Coenzyme Q10 has also been found to be protective to dopamine-producing neurons and is neuroprotective in animal models of Parkinson's disease.[57] In a recent multicenter study involving 80 patients with early Parkinson's disease, patients were randomly assigned to receive coenzyme Q10 at a dosage of 300, 600, or 1,200 mg/d or matching placebo. Coenzyme Q10 was well tolerated, and at the 1,200-mg dose was associated with significant slowing of the progression of Parkinson's disease.[58]

NADH

The use of NADH for Parkinson's disease was first suggested by Birkmayer, who demonstrated modest improvement in an open-label study involving 800 patients.[59]

NADH may increase complex-1 activity and stimulate tyrosine hydroxylase, the rate-limiting step in dopamine biosynthesis. Follow-up studies of NADH in Parkinson's disease patients have been equivocal, however, including a study by researchers in Sweden who found no significant benefit from treating patients with intravenous NADH.[60] This may be accounted for by the finding that NADH has been demonstrated to increase dopamine production in vitro but not in vivo.[61]

Physiotherapy in the Management of Parkinson's Disease

Despite existing therapies for Parkinson's disease, patients develop progressive disability. The role of physical therapy is to improve functional ability and minimize secondary complications through movement rehabilitation. Recently, the Cochrane Database analyzed 11 trials reported in the literature, assessing the benefits of physiotherapy in Parkinson's disease. Although 10 of the trials claimed a positive effect from physiotherapy, few outcomes measured were statistically significant. The studies illustrate that a wide range of approaches are being employed by physiotherapists to treat Parkinson's disease. Clearly, large well-designed, placebo-controlled, randomized controlled trials are needed to demonstrate the effectiveness and efficacy of best practice physiotherapy in Parkinson's disease.[62]

Mind–Body Approaches to Parkinson's Disease

Persistently elevated cortisol has an adverse effect on brain function. Serum cortisol levels are elevated in Parkinson's disease patients compared to controls, and there is an inverse relationship between cortisol levels and parkinsonian disability.[63] Clearly, any activity, such as meditation, that results in a reduction of serum cortisol levels will be of benefit as an adjunctive treatment in the management of Parkinson's disease.

▶ MULTIPLE SCLEROSIS

Pathophysiology

Multiple sclerosis is an autoimmune disorder of unknown etiology involving environmental factors, genetic factors, and immune dysfunction. Environmental factors include possible viruses that individuals may have been exposed to at some point in their lives. Viral candidates include herpes simplex 6 and Epstein-Barr virus, but there has never been a definitive established link between multiple sclerosis and a particular viral entity. *Chlamydia* infection has also been found to be associated with multiple sclerosis. Elevated titers of antichlamydia antibodies were detected in the cerebrospinal fluid in 13 of 66 (20%) patients with multiple sclerosis and only 1 of 25 (4%) of other neurological disease controls.[64] Human herpes virus type 6 and chlamydia are both known to induce experimental autoimmune encephalomyelitis in rats.

The presence of a genetic factor in multiple sclerosis is supported by the studies of monozygotic twins. When one twin gets multiple sclerosis, the other has approximately a 30% chance of also acquiring the disease. Results of genetic studies suggest a complex genetic etiology including multiple genes of small to moderate effect and probably genetic heterogeneity. Transcriptional analysis of brain plaques in multiple sclerosis has yielded proteins associated with an allergic response, including histamine receptors, prostaglandin D synthase, and osteopontin.[65]

Autoimmune factors are clearly implicated in multiple sclerosis. A variety of immune system abnormalities have been reported in multiple sclerosis patients including a predominant mixture of T lymphocytes and macrophages in the region of myelin affected by plaques in multiple sclerosis. Macrophages directly attack myelin and present fragments of myelin basic protein on their surface for T-cell recognition. T cells attack from a distance by secreting cytokines such as tumor necrosis factor and interleukin (IL)-12. They also induce beta cells to produce antibodies that destroy oligodendroglial cells, which, under normal circumstances, repair myelin (Figure 22–3).

Prevalence and Diagnosis

Multiple sclerosis is a common neurological disease that affects approximately 350,000 people in the United States. In about two-thirds of the cases, onset is between ages 20 and 40 years, and women are diagnosed about twice as frequently as men. There is a geographical predilection for people in higher latitudes, with 100 cases per 100,000 versus 10 per 100,000 in areas closer to the equator (Figure 22–4).

Multiple sclerosis can be a difficult diagnosis to make because many symptoms can be quite variable. This variability occurs because multiple sclerosis lesions can be randomly distributed in the subcortical white matter, resulting in diverse symptomatology. Common symptoms include paresthesias, sensory loss or pain, weakness, incoordination, or visual symptoms, such as optic neuritis or diplopia. Fatigue and memory loss

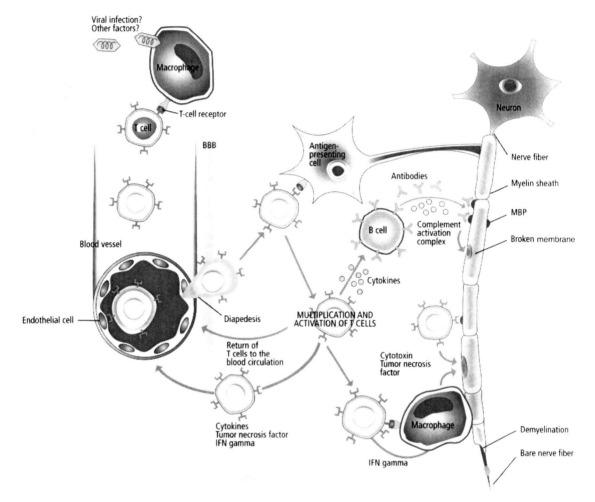

Figure 22-3. Autoimmunity and demyelination in multiple sclerosis. BBB = blood–brain barrier; IFN = interferon; MBP = myelin base protein. (Adapted from Steinman L. Multiple sclerosis: a coordinate immunological attack against myelis in the central nervous system. *Cell*. 1996;85[3]:299–302.)

are commonly overlooked symptoms that occur quite frequently in multiple sclerosis.

The paroxysmal and fluctuating nature of symptoms of multiple sclerosis also can make the diagnosis difficult. A diagnosis of multiple sclerosis can be confirmed by MRI of the neuraxis, and gadolinium enhancement will demonstrate active pathology. A lumbar puncture with cerebral spinal fluid elevation of gamma-globulin and the presence of oligoclonal bands may also be helpful to support a diagnosis.

The differential diagnosis for multiple sclerosis includes other demyelinating and dysmyelinating diseases of the central nervous system, including subcortical ischemic disease; other autoimmune diseases such as lupus and sarcoidosis; vitamin B_{12} deficiency; infectious etiologies, including HIV infection and Lyme disease; and congenital leukodystrophies. Complicated migraine with transient focal deficits may also be confused with a demyelinating disorder and may also be associated with white matter abnormalities.

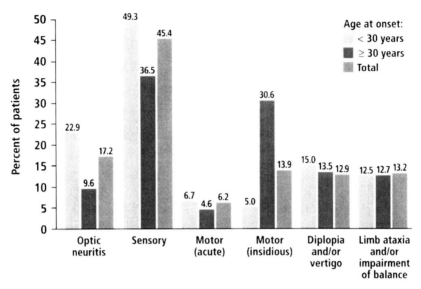

Figure 22-4. Initial presentation of multiple sclerosis symptoms in total clinic population. (Adapted from Weinshenker BG, Bass B, Rice GP, et al. The natural history of multiple sclerosis: a geographically based study. I. Clinical course and disability. *Brain.* 1989; 112:133–146.)

▶ Case Example 3: Multiple Sclerosis

A 31-year-old lawyer presents with a tentative diagnosis of multiple sclerosis. Two years earlier, she had noted visual loss in her right eye, which resolved spontaneously after 3 weeks. Ophthalmologic, neurologic, and MRI examinations at that time were unremarkable. She remained relatively asymptomatic except for severe fatigue until 1 month ago. At that time, she complained of severe stress related to work overload, and reported diffuse paresthesias in her limbs and recurrent loss of vision in her right eye. An MRI of the brain was obtained which revealed T2 hyperintensities in the subcortical white matter. Routine lab studies were normal, and lumbar puncture (LP) was acellular. Human herpes virus type 6 titers were markedly elevated, but the patient had negative Lyme titer, antinuclear antibody, and vitamin B_{12} levels.

Table 22–4 provides an overview of multiple sclerosis treatment.

Conventional Treatment Approaches to Multiple Sclerosis

Since 1993 the FDA has approved four medications for multiple sclerosis: Betaseron, Avonex, Copaxone, and Rebif. These drugs de-

crease the number and severity of relapses, slow the progression of the disease, and decrease the development of new lesions. Mitoxantrone (Novantrone) is the only drug approved for secondary progressive multiple sclerosis. It is available by intravenous infusion

▶ **TABLE 22-4** THERAPEUTIC OVERVIEW OF MULTIPLE SCLEROSIS

- Conventional therapies.
  Avonex, Betaseron, Copaxon, and Rebif.
    These therapies significantly reduce relapses and prevent subclinical signs of multiple sclerosis, including brain atrophy and silent white matter lesions. Side effects are often problematic, and neutralizing antibodies may inhibit the effectiveness of these agents.
- Nutritional approaches.
  Carefully monitor patient's lipid profile.
    If cholesterol and LDL levels are elevated, consideration should be given to statin therapy. Red yeast extract is used as an HMG-CoA reductase inhibitor. Statins reduce experimental forms of multiple sclerosis in animal studies, but have not been fully studied in human patients.
- Monitor vitamin D levels and supplement if deficient.
- Inosine 3 g/d (for investigational purposes only).
- Herbal approaches.
  Curcumin is a safe, available herbal supplement that can be recommended as an adjunctive therapy.
- Psychosocial issues should be addressed.
- Mind–body approaches.
  Biofeedback.
    There is a relationship between emotional stress and multiple sclerosis symptoms.
- Cooling garments.

---

only, and serious side effects have been reported, including myocardial toxicity with reduced left ventricular ejection function and neutropenia.

Interferons appear to modulate cytokines including tumor necrosis factor-alpha, intercellular adhesion molecule-1, and IL-12. Side effects include injection site reactions, elevated liver enzymes, leukopenia, and flu-like symptoms. Neutralizing antibodies interfere with receptor mediator function of interferon-beta and are associated with a loss of function in some of these agents. Avonex has a significantly lower incidence of production of neutralizing antibodies than other existing interferons.

In an animal model, Lovastatin, an HMG-CoA reductase inhibitor, reversed the paralysis and prevented the development of chronic relapsing multiple sclerosis.[66] The use of statins in MS may be a promising avenue of conventional treatment in the future.

Integrative Strategies for Treatment of Multiple Sclerosis

Approximately 60% of patients with multiple sclerosis use some form of alternative therapy.[67] Many of these therapies are untested despite the fact that exaggerated claims are frequently made about their efficacy in multiple sclerosis. It is this author's opinion that clinicians should avoid making recommendations regarding hyperbaric oxygen and the removal of dental amalgam. In regard to the suggestion that dental amalgam fillings that contain mercury may be a risk factor for multiple sclerosis, epidemiological studies have failed to find such an association.[68]

Nutritional Approaches

The association of multiple sclerosis with dietary fat has been suggested by epidemiological observations that consumption of saturated fat, especially animal fat, is higher in populations where multiple sclerosis is also higher. Furthermore, populations with a relatively high intake of polyunsaturated fatty acids appear to have a lower incidence of multiple sclerosis. However, a recent prospective study completed at Harvard Medical School examined two large cohorts of 92,000 women with 14 years of follow-up. The pooled multivariate relative risk comparing women in the highest consumption of total fat, animal fat, vegetable fat, saturated fat, and unsaturated fat were unrelated to the risk of development of multiple sclerosis. These findings do not support relationships between intakes of total fat or major specific types of fat and the risk of multiple sclerosis.[69]

Conversely, numerous studies demonstrate the relationship between plasma lipid profile and disease activity in multiple sclerosis. These studies have found a significant correlation between the mean number of enhancing lesions and the mean plasma level of total and low-density lipoprotein cholesterol.[70]

Significant attention has been paid to polyunsaturated fatty acids as a therapeutic strategy for multiple sclerosis. Polyunsaturated fatty acids include the omega-6 fatty acids and the omega-3 fatty acids. Linoleic acid is the precursor for the biochemical pathway of both omega-6 and omega-3 fatty acids. Regarding the effects of oral feeding of omega-6 fatty acid gamma-linoleic acid studies on acute and relapsing disease in experimental autoimmune encephalomyeli-tis (EAE), clinical incidents and histological manifestations of acute EAE in the clinical relapse phase of chronic relapsing EAE were markedly inhibited by omega-6 fatty acid feeding.[71]

Human data regarding the effects of omega-3 fatty acids in multiple sclerosis are conflicting and have not demonstrated clinically significant effects on disease activity. In one 2-year study involving 312 patients treated with 10 g of fish oil, 52% of patients in the untreated group worsened, while in the treated group, 43% worsened.[72]

Three studies have involved linoleic acid, an omega-6 polyunsaturated fatty acid, in people with multiple sclerosis. These studies yielded mixed results, and a combined analysis was published in 1984. The information on a total of 172 people from all three studies was pooled. With the combined analysis, linoleic acid treatment slowed the progression and reduced the length and severity of attacks.[73] Although a robust clinical effect has not been demonstrated with the use of linoleic acid in multiple sclerosis, the rationale for using this dietary fatty acid as an adjunctive therapy in multiple sclerosis is strong. This is based on observations that this dietary fat has anti-inflammatory properties including reductions in interferon-gamma, and reduced activity of cyclooxygenase, inducible nitrous oxide synthase, and tumor necrosis factor-alpha in macrophages.[74]

One of the most studied nutritional supplements as a treatment for multiple sclerosis has been vitamin D. The observation that vitamin D deficiency may be causally associated with multiple sclerosis was first made in 1997 by Hayes, Cantorna, and DeLuca. Based upon epidemiological studies that demonstrate a higher incidence of multiple sclerosis in northern hemispheres, it was speculated that low sunlight produced insufficient vitamin D,[75] and that this would have a permissive effect on autoimmune vulnerability.[76]

Vitamin D has physiological effects on cytokine production, and it may serve a protective role in multiple sclerosis. As mentioned earlier, multiple sclerosis is associated with increased IL-12, a proinflammatory cytokine, and diminished IL-10, an antiinflammatory cytokine. Vitamin D decreases IL-12 and increases IL-10, the two cytokines that are inversely related to multiple sclerosis exacerbations. In experimental animal models of multiple sclerosis, recent studies also support the notion that vitamin D may be protective. Vitamin D decreases macrophage accumulation in the central nervous system of mice with experimental autoimmune encephalomyelitis, an experimental animal model of multiple sclerosis. It also decreases the severity of EAE in this model.[77]

Human data is also suggestive. Vitamin D receptor gene polymorphisms have been reported in Japanese patients with multiple sclerosis,[78] and vitamin D deficiency commonly afflicts multiple sclerosis patients.[79] Although no controlled data are available that demonstrate a therapeutic effect of vitamin D administration in multiple sclerosis, routine measurements of vitamin D levels should be obtained in all multiple sclerosis patients and corrected when found to be deficient. Hypercalcemia with vitamin D supplementation is generally uncommon with doses less than 2,000 IU/d.

Peroxynitrite has been implicated in the pathogenesis of multiple sclerosis. Inosine, a purine nucleoside, that acts as a natural peroxynitrite scavenger, has been investigated in multiple sclerosis patients. The results of an open-label study of 11 patients treated with inosine demonstrated statistical improvement in three patients and disease stabilization in the remaining patients, as demonstrated by clinical examinations and MRI findings.[80]

Herbal Therapies

Many immune-enhancing herbs are prescribed to multiple sclerosis patients based on the faulty assumption that the immune system is weakened and needs to be enhanced. In fact, the opposite is true, and any potential herbal therapy should be based upon its ability to reduce harmful inflammatory mediators that are upregulated in multiple sclerosis.[81]

An especially promising herb in the treatment of multiple sclerosis is curcumin. Curcumin, the yellow-coloring ingredient of tumeric, is a naturally occurring polyphenolic phytochemical isolated from the rhizome of *Curcuma longa* (tumeric). It has antiinflammatory activity and has been used to treat inflammatory conditions. In one mouse study, treatment with curcumin significantly reduced the

duration and severity of experimental allergic encephalomyelitis, an experimental model of multiple sclerosis. Curcumin reduced IL-12 cytokine production from microglial cells and reduced other transcription factors involved in central nervous system inflammation.[82]

Mind–Body Approaches

There remains a strong consensus among both patients with and clinicians who treat multiple sclerosis that emotional trauma may precipitate the disorder. Furthermore, many multiple sclerosis patients hold a strong belief that emotional stress provokes attacks of their disease, and several studies show a strong correlation between multiple sclerosis symptoms and emotional factors and stress.[83] Stress may worsen multiple sclerosis by activating the hypothalamic pituitary adrenal axis. Corticotropin-releasing factor, a neuropeptide released by the hypothalamus, heightens the ability of immune cells at sites of inflammation. Therefore, clinicians should be aware of the relationship of stress to multiple sclerosis, and appropriate steps should be taken to reduce stress by various modalities.

A wide range of mind–body approaches have been applied in the treatment of multiple sclerosis. Mind–body approaches include biofeedback and meditation, which may attenuate the stress response. Biofeedback and meditation therapies are discussed in detail in Chapter 3. Although no clinical studies have examined the effects of these mind–body approaches in multiple sclerosis, it is this author's experience that relaxation training is especially helpful in reducing multiple sclerosis symptoms and in possibly preventing relapses.

Physical Modalities

Physical modalities used in the treatment of multiple sclerosis include cooling therapy and electromagnetic therapy. In regards to cooling therapy, it is well known that even a slight elevation of body temperature has an adverse effect on multiple sclerosis symptoms because of impaired myelin conduction. Cooling garments and various vest configurations are helpful in reducing multiple sclerosis symptomatology.[84]

► STROKE

Pathophysiology

A stroke is a cerebrovascular accident associated with an interruption of blood flow to a part of the brain as a result of arterial blockage or hemorrhage. Because cerebral metabolism depends on a fairly constant supply of blood and oxygen, deprivation of oxygen in the brain can result in extensive damage within 10–20 seconds and irreversible damage after 3–10 minutes.[85] The four major types of stroke are the following.

1. An *embolic stroke* is when a clot from a region outside the brain breaks loose and is carried in the bloodstream to an artery in the brain, plugging a blood vessel and cutting off the blood supply.
2. A *cerebral occlusion* is when a clot forms in an artery supplying blood to the brain, partially or totally obstructing blood flow.
3. A *lacunar stroke* is when multiple small cerebral infarcts affect subcortical regions.
4. A *hemorrhagic stroke* is when a break in the wall of a blood vessel results in blood spilling into brain tissue or into the area surrounding the brain.

Prevalence

Stroke is the third leading cause of death in the United States, and four of five families will be affected by stroke at some point. The more severe the stroke, the greater the likelihood of death, or of only limited recovery. In fact, stroke is a major cause of long-term disability, with 550,000 Americans annually experiencing a stroke and almost two-thirds of the survivors demonstrating some form of impairment.[86] Minimal to moderate strokes have excellent recovery curves, with patients often regaining a substantial amount of functional independence within 6 months, at which point recovery begins to plateau. Much of this recovery is attributed to the natural healing ability of the body, including the ability of the brain to develop new pathways to restore motor and other functions. When highly specialized areas of the brain are substantially damaged, full recovery may never occur, as is often the case with aphasia. Standard rehabilitation is designed to facilitate and augment this natural healing process.

Stroke Prevention and Prevention of Subsequent Stroke

Nearly all therapies that are recommended for reduction of cardiac risk are also appropriate for stroke prevention. Hence, exercise, stress reduction techniques, diet, appropriate supplements and herbs can all help in reducing the risk of stroke. In China, tai chi and Qi Gong exercises are routinely practiced by millions in the hope of maintaining good cardiovascular health.[87]

Diet and Nutrition
Epidemiologic evidence suggests that a daily diet high in fruits and vegetables has a protective effect against stroke. Ness and Powles conducted a review of studies published between 1966 and 1995 on the protective action of fruits and vegetables against cardiovascular disease. Of the 14 stroke studies, 9 showed that the consumption of fruits and vegetables had a significant protective association with stroke.[88] Similar results were found in a

17-year follow-up of 11,000 individuals who consumed a vegetarian diet in which daily consumption of fresh fruit was associated with significantly reduced mortality from cerebrovascular disease and ischemic heart disease.[89]

The protective action of fruits and vegetables is believed to be a result of their high content of dietary antioxidant vitamins (beta-carotene and vitamin C) and flavonoids. This hypothesis was examined in a 15-year study of 552 males.[90] The investigators found an inverse relation between the intake of dietary antioxidants and stroke incidence. Antioxidants prevent LDL oxidation, thereby reducing the subsequent formation of atherosclerotic plaques. Support for the protective antioxidant action of vitamin C was found in a review of the research literature between 1966 and 1996.[91] The review indicated a protective association between amount of vitamin C taken and cardiovascular disease. Although evidence was limited, there was support for the premise that vitamin C had a protective effect against stroke. Research suggests that garlic may also provide some protection against atherosclerosis, coronary thrombosis, and stroke, effects believed to be directly related to its ability to inhibit aggregation of blood platelets.[92] Furthermore, alcohol intake in moderation may decrease the incidence of cardiovascular disease[93] and stroke, although binge drinking or high intake of alcohol may increase the risk of stroke 10-fold.[94]

Nutritional supplementation has been suggested to reduce the risk of a subsequent occurrence of stroke. Although these recommendations are often based on a presumed protective mechanism of action within the body based on the biochemistry of the substance, little research exists directly relating these substances to effective treatment of neurologic conditions. When the limited studies are examined closely, there is often contradictory information. For example, although the belief that fish consumption reduces risk of stroke is supported by several retrospective studies,[95,96] a recent population-based retrospective study not only failed to support these earlier findings, but rather seemed to contradict them, finding a slightly higher level of stroke in men with the highest level of reported fish consumption.[97]

Ginkgo biloba Extract

A popular herb that has been recommended for a number of purposes, including reduction of risk of stroke, is *Ginkgo biloba* leaf. This herb, especially its standardized extract, has a number of qualities that have a positive effect on the cardiovascular system, including its ability to attenuate clotting via inhibition of platelet-activating factor and its association with increased vascular elasticity. The leaf of the Ginkgo tree (also known as maidenhair tree) has been part of the traditional Chinese pharmacopoeia for 500 years. A standardized extract of the Ginkgo leaf is widely used in Asia, Germany, France, and the United States. There are multiple active ingredients in the extract, including amino acids, flavonoids, flavonols, and steroids. *Ginkgo biloba* extract has been used in both animal and human models, showing promise in the treatment of some of the most important and debilitating symptoms associated with stroke, as well as traumatic brain injury, cerebral vascular insufficiency, and Alzheimer dementia.[98]

Evidence that *Ginkgo biloba* improves arterial and vascular elasticity, and also has antiplatelet aggregation effects supports its use in stroke patients.[99,100] These properties have been used to treat other vascular disorders as well; for example, a recent metaanalysis of ginkgo for intermittent claudication showed modest improvements in pain-free walking distance in patients taking ginkgo over placebo.[101] In animal subjects fed oral ginkgo extract, significant reductions in cerebral infarct volume, as well as improvements in neurological function, have been demonstrated.[102] Intravenous injection of ginkgo extract in human subjects increased cerebral blood flow.[103]

One placebo-controlled, double-blind study in patients with cerebrovascular disease demonstrated improvements in neurologic and psychometric variables in subjects who received

Ginkgo biloba extract.[104] There was a reduction in the proportion of theta waves in the electroencephalogram of the patients, suggesting a recovery in neurological function. A meta-analysis of eleven randomized placebo-controlled trials found clinical benefit in stroke patients taking ginkgo.[105] Thus although definitive conclusions are difficult to reach, there is in fact a large body of evidence to support the effects of ginkgo.[106] Nevertheless, controversy over both effectiveness and safety continues, and there is currently (2003) a major multisite clinical trial underway in the United States, funded by the National Institutes of Health (NIH), to study its anticoagulant ability.

Adverse effects from ginkgo extract are uncommon, but include headache, abdominal discomfort, rash, and palpitations.[107] Because of ginkgo's possible role as an anticoagulant due to its effects on antiplatelet-activating factor, it should not be routinely taken with other anticoagulants, including warfarin (Coumadin), heparin, or aspirin (when routinely taken for stroke prevention) except under a doctor's supervision. For the same reasons, it is also not recommended following a hemorrhagic stroke. A typical daily regimen for the treatment of cerebrovascular disease is 120–240 mg in divided doses.[108]

Coenzyme Q10

Another dietary supplement that may have some utility in the treatment of stroke patients is coenzyme Q10 (CoQ10 or ubiquinone). As a mitochondrial enzyme, CoQ10 is integral to many of the body's metabolic processes; it also has significant antioxidant properties. Studies show that it has beneficial effects in patients with congestive heart failure because of its positive effects on cardiac output and exercise tolerance.[109,110] Although there are no clinical trials to date investigating the effect of CoQ10 specifically on stroke patients, there are case reports of patients with MELAS (myopathy, encephalopathy, lactic acidosis, and stroke-like episodes) syndrome, a hereditary disease, who were treated with CoQ10 with improvement in their metabolic parameters.[111] It is possible that CoQ10 may be useful in limiting the ischemic injury sustained in stroke patients.

Meditation and Relaxation

Meditation and relaxation have been suggested for any number of medical conditions that are associated with stress reactions. In terms of stroke prevention, the most relevant finding is the success of meditation for reducing hypertension.[112–114] Evidence also indicates a reduction in the cholesterol level.[115–116] Although no studies were found that specifically address the issue of stroke prevention, it seems reasonable to conclude that meditation may be effective in reduction of risk for stroke through its success in reducing hypertension, a predisposing factor for stroke. For example, in a well-controlled, randomized study comparing several relaxation techniques,[117] regular practice of transcendental meditation by elderly nursing home residents was associated with significantly reduced systolic blood pressure and significantly increased 3-year survival rate when compared with the simple relaxation and no-treatment conditions. After 3 years, 100% of the transcendental meditation group were alive versus 68% of the no-treatment group.

Ethylenediaminetetraacetic Acid (EDTA) Chelation Therapy

Ethylenediaminetetraacetic acid (EDTA) chelation therapy is popularly believed to be helpful for the treatment and prevention of cardiovascular and cerebrovascular disorders. Despite many anecdotal reports of improvement in anginal symptoms and other parameters of cardiac disease following chelation, however, no controlled trials to date substantiate these claims, and its use is quite controversial. A multisite clinical trial is now underway (2003), sponsored by the NIH, to determine if chelation can be effective in reducing the risk of cardiovascular disorders.

A small amount of research evidence for chelation therapy does exist. In an uncontrolled trial, cerebral arterial occlusion was measured in 57 patients before and after treatment with from 10 to 46 sessions of EDTA chelation therapy; 88% improved (criteria for improvement not stated), and cerebral arterial stenosis reportedly was reduced from a mean 28% to 10%.[118] A retrospective analysis was conducted in Brazil of 2,870 patients who were treated with EDTA chelation therapy between 1983 and 1985.[119] These patients had a variety of vascular and degenerative diseases, with about 18% of the patients (504) being diagnosed with cerebrovascular disease or degenerative central nervous system disease. The investigators reported "marked recovery" in 24% of the patients and "good recovery" in 60%.

Recovery and Rehabilitation After Stroke

Once a stroke has occurred, treatment tends to focus on restoring a patient's ability to function independently. This approach is generally referred to as physical rehabilitation. Physical rehabilitation often embraces therapies that are outside of the conventional allopathic treatment options, and so sometimes there is a fine line between what is conventional rehabilitation and what is "alternative." Examples of "alternative" therapies that are routinely available in rehabilitation settings include heat therapy, hydrotherapy, various forms of physical manipulation, music therapy, pet therapy, and hippotherapy (use of horseback riding as a therapeutic tool). Some therapies focus on physical functioning, while others, such as pet therapy and music therapy, focus on social functioning. A small pilot study has shown that music therapy supplementing conventional rehabilitation protocols resulted in increases in social behaviors as rated by the therapists and patients' families.[120]

In the case of stroke, because brain cells controlling the body's function have died or been irreparably damaged, it is assumed that restoration of functioning involves creation of new pathways in the brain. A recently developed approach to facilitating this process is "constraint-induced movement therapy," a process in which the unaffected limb is constrained in order to force the patient to actively use the paretic limb. The results have been extremely encouraging, and in less than 5 years, this therapy has become available in most rehabilitation settings. The success of this therapy has been associated with cortical reorganization as detected by functional MRI.[121]

Research on the effectiveness of therapies in stroke recovery is often difficult because the effectiveness of the complementary therapy must be demonstrated in the context of the rapid natural healing that occurs along with the positive effects of conventional rehabilitation. Consequently, it may take larger sample sizes to detect effects if they are relatively small compared to the natural healing process that is also occurring.

Acupuncture

Acupuncture has been used for more than 3,000 years for the treatment of "windstroke" in traditional Chinese medicine. In general, acupuncture has been reported to work best when used as early as possible on stroke patients. Acupuncture appears to be more effective with stroke patients if their lesions are singular, shallow, and with a small focus instead of large, bilateral lesions with deep multiple foci.[122] Research support for most of these beliefs is, however, limited or nonexistent. Prior to the 1980s, a very limited amount of research evidence for the effectiveness of acupuncture had been published in the Chinese literature; until recently, this literature was virtually unavailable to Western biomedical scientists. These studies also were very limited in methodological rigor, so were of little use in determining acupuncture's true utility. As acupuncture has become better known in the West, more rigorous research has begun to appear in easily available biomedical journals.

The recent history of research on acupuncture and stroke is limited but encouraging. A research program directed by Margaret Naeser and colleagues at the Boston University Medical Center and Boston Veterans Administration (VA) hospital provided some evidence for the efficacy of acupuncture in the treatment of stroke under certain limiting conditions.[123] In a study comparing real versus sham acupuncture in the treatment of paralysis in acute stroke patients, 16 patients with right-side paralysis who had left hemisphere ischemic infarction were randomly assigned to receive either 20 real acupuncture treatments (11 points, some with electrical stimulation) or 20 sham acupuncture treatments (nonacupoints with no electrical stimulation) over 1 month beginning 1 to 3 months after stroke onset. The outcome measure was "good" versus "poor" response on the Boston Motor Inventory for upper and lower extremities. Results indicated that significantly more patients had a good response after real acupuncture than sham acupuncture when a computed tomography scan indicated that there was a lesion in half or less than half of the motor pathways involving the periventricular white matter ($P < .013$). A follow-up study demonstrated similar results with laser acupuncture; however, five of the seven patients in this study had been subjects in the 1992 acupuncture study.[124]

In another study of both chronic and acute stroke patients, eight chronic stroke patients were treated with acupuncture beginning 6 months to 8 years after stroke, and three acute stroke patients were treated with acupuncture beginning 2 months after stroke onset.[125] Patients received 20 or 40 acupuncture treatments over 2 to 3 months. All patients had good response, defined as improvement on at least four of six hand tests, which was sustained for at least 2 months after completion of the acupuncture treatments. The researchers concluded that acupuncture may be an additional beneficial treatment method for stroke patients with hand paresis, even when started

as late as 5 to 8 years after stroke. Although there was no control condition in this study, chronic patients were their own controls in the sense that their condition had been stable for 6 months or more before treatment. This same study also reported that patients exhibiting a beneficial response to treatment had damage to less than half of the motor pathway areas, as seen on computed tomography scans.

Two other randomized controlled trials of acupuncture treatment of stroke support the findings described above. In a study of ischemic stroke conducted in Taiwan, when compared with subjects receiving standard rehabilitation only, subjects receiving acupuncture in addition to standard care had significantly better functional outcomes as measured by the Barthel index at 1 month and 3 months after stroke. Subjects began receiving treatment within 36 hours after stroke and received 12 treatments over 4 weeks. Subjects with poor neurologic scores responded better to acupuncture than control subjects, whereas no difference was found in subjects with good neurologic scores. This finding suggests that acupuncture has an incrementally helpful effect only when the condition is serious enough that full recovery is not likely through spontaneous recovery or standard rehabilitation.[126] In a Norwegian study, 45 patients with cerebral infarction or cerebral hemorrhage were randomly entered into either a standard rehabilitation condition or the acupuncture plus standard rehabilitation condition. Six weeks after treatment, individuals receiving acupuncture had significantly better outcomes in activities of daily living and on the motor assessment scale and Nottingham Health Profile.[127]

In a well-controlled study conducted in Sweden,[128] 40 hemiparetic male and female patients who received 10 weeks of acupuncture, along with standard physical therapy and occupational therapy beginning 10 days after stroke, recovered faster and had significant improvements in activities of daily living (Barthel index), quality of life (Nottingham Health Profile), and balance/mobility (idiosyncratic motor function assessment scale) than did a control group of 38 patients who received only physical therapy and occupational therapy. A drawback to this study was the lack of a sham acupuncture condition; positive results could also be attributable to general sensory stimulation of the muscles surrounding the acupuncture point rather than acupuncture per se. In a follow-up of the 48 survivors in this study,[129] conducted approximately 3 years after the original treatment, subjects received perturbations (vibratory stimulation to the calf muscle or galvanic stimulation of the vestibular nerves) in three different tests, each with eyes open and closed. Significantly more of the treatment group (17 of 21) than the control group (9 of 25) could maintain stance on all six tests ($P <$ .0025). Based on these results, the researchers hypothesized that the sensory stimulation of traditional acupuncture points with needles and electrostimulation may promote the restructuring and consolidation of coordinated motor function of affected limbs in the stroke patient, thus serving to enhance the recovery of postural control.

More recently, Johansson et al.[130] evaluated acupuncture and transcutaneous nerve stimulation in a randomized controlled trial. While they concluded that there was no effect from acupuncture in aiding functional recovery, it has been suggested[131] that their statistical analysis did not treat the data adequately. Among various problems mentioned by Shiflett, the failure to correct for baseline deficit was most telling. Another recent study[132] seems to have a similar problem in dealing with baseline impairment and in terms of statistical treatment. In a prospective randomized controlled trial on 106 stroke patients, with treatments begun 3–15 days after stroke, the control group consisted of standard of care, including physical, occupational, and speech therapy, and the experimental group received acupuncture in addition to standard of care. Observations on functional measures (Barthel, Functional Independence Measure [FIM], and others) were

made just prior to commencing treatment, at 5 weeks into treatment, and when treatment was completed at week 10. This procedure differs in a very important way from other similar studies in that the measurements are made *during* and *immediately after* the treatment period, rather than after treatment is completed with one or more longer-term follow-ups, at 3, 6, and/or 12 months, as in most other studies of this type. In an early statistical analysis of their data, these researchers concluded that there was no difference in the groups. This conclusion that acupuncture had failed to improve recovery over standard of care resulted in the researchers' decision not to perform the follow-up evaluations, despite the fact that nearly all of the studies with longer term measurements found increasing differences over time between the control and acupuncture groups, and always in favor of acupuncture. Thus there was no opportunity to observe longer-term improvements, and a low-power statistical test (relative to analysis of variance) may have caused an erroneous conclusion to be drawn.

It should be obvious from the above discussion that research evidence for the use of acupuncture in the treatment of stroke is mixed. Park et al.[133] performed a systematic review of the pre-1990 literature and concluded that the majority of studies suffered from a variety of confounding factors, including etiology of the stroke, location of lesions, degree of neural damage, sample size, blinding, treatment scheduling, needle insertion protocol, and techniques. Sze[134] conducted a meta-analysis of 14 stroke studies and concluded that there was little evidence supporting acupuncture for motor recovery, but there was a small positive effect on disability. The problem with this type of analysis is that when underpowered statistics are used in the original studies, the meta-analysis will produce the same, potentially erroneous, conclusions. Thus, while the results of these reviews seem overly pessimistic and ignore the more positive evidence in several well-controlled studies, the fact remains that research on acupuncture and stroke will need to account more carefully for these factors. An overview of several of these studies suggests that strokes occurring in the moderate range of severity are most likely to respond best to acupuncture. If the stroke is relatively mild, natural recovery and standard rehabilitation appear to result in nearly full recovery. If it is too severe, or if there is too much damage in the brain, then acupuncture probably has little or no effect.

Massage and Other Manual Manipulations

Massage has been suggested to be a valuable adjunct in treatment regimens for hemiplegia.[135] Soothing massage before performing exercises can help reduce spasticity, and in patients with flaccid paralysis, more stimulating massage can help stimulate nerves and increase circulation.

Energy Healing

The term *subtle energy* encompasses any number of techniques that purport to use a form of nonphysical energy that is believed to exist within and around the body. Examples of this type of therapy are therapeutic touch, Qigong, and Reiki. The use of subtle energy healing for any medical condition is highly controversial because the putative underlying mechanism cannot at present be measured. Research supporting the effectiveness of this type of therapy is very limited and results are often attributed to placebo effects. Nevertheless, there is growing interest in this therapy, and it does seem to have a relaxing and calming effect on individuals. With respect to stroke, evidence is extremely limited. McGee and Chow relate a number of case studies on the success of Qigong for many different medical conditions, including stroke, paralysis, and cerebral palsy. A recently published randomized sham-controlled trial of Reiki on subacute stroke inpatients[136] showed no improvement in functional independence, measured by the FIM, over the sham treatment. There was, however, a tendency for Reiki to be associated with improved FIM scores in males, but not in females, perhaps because women seemed to improve on their own more than men did.[137]

Hyperbaric Oxygen Therapy

A problem for stroke patients is the deprivation of oxygen in key brain areas resulting from an interruption of blood flow. Hyperbaric oxygen therapy has been advocated in these patients because it may enhance neuronal viability by its ability to increase the amount of dissolved oxygen in the blood without changing blood viscosity.[138] This therapy is controversial, rarely, if ever, recommended by physicians, and supported by a very limited amount of research.

In one fairly large study by Neubauer and End,[139] 122 patients with thrombotic stroke were treated with hyperbaric oxygen in addition to standard treatment. In the bedridden group, 64% of the patients improved by showing an ability to use a wheelchair or to walk with or without aids. In the wheelchair group, 71% of the patients showed improved ambulation. In the group categorized as walking with aids, 56% of the patients improved enough to walk independently. However, in a study of hyperbaric oxygen therapy for acute ischemic stroke in patients with middle cerebral artery occlusion, the results were mixed.[140] In addition, although there have been a number of animal studies and isolated small clinical/case-based studies, no major study has shown the benefit of hyperbaric oxygen for wide-scale application. In general, existing research suggests that hyperbaric oxygen therapy in patients with stroke may be beneficial, but additional research is clearly needed.

Issues of safety and toxicity are a major concern surrounding hyperbaric oxygen therapy.[141] Adverse events, such as increased free-radical production and peroxidation, have been reported. However, serious side effects have been virtually eliminated by keeping pressures at 1.5–2.0 atmospheres, limiting exposure time, and following more rigorous procedures during compression and decompression.[112]

▶ CONCLUSION

Because it provides an opportunity to move beyond a reductionistic view of neurological disorders to a perspective that takes into account the complex nature of the influences on neurological function in the human organism, the integrative approach to neuroscience offers a great deal of promise. The connections now known to exist between neurological function, immune system, endocrinological function, digestive function, and psychological and spiritual state require an approach to prevention and treatment which is prepared to address the diverse natures of these systems. By identifying the triggers and mediators of neurological disease using data from conventional neuroscience literature, and then applying modalities from integrative medicine known potentially to influence these triggers and mediators— diet, botanicals, mind–body approaches, acupuncture—the integrative approach to neurology can greatly expand the options available to patients with a wide range of neurological disorders.

REFERENCES

1. Hardy J, Allsop D. Amyloid deposition as a central event in the etiology of Alzheimer's disease. *Trends Pharmacol Sci.* 1991;12:383–388.

2. Hardy J, Higgins G.. Alzheimer's disease: the amyloid cascade hypothesis. *Science.* 1992;256: 184–185.

3. Block, W, Jessen, F, Traber, F, et al. Regional N-acetyl aspartate reduction in the hippocampus detected with fast proton magnetic resonance spectroscopic imaging in patients with Alzheimer's disease. *Arch Neurol.* 2002;59(5): 828–834.

4. Kukull, W, Bowen, J. Dementia Epidemiology. *Med. Clin. North America.* 2002;86(3):573–590.

5. Calmijn S, Laurner L, Ott A, et al. Dietary fat intake and the risk of incident dementia in the Rotterdam study. *Ann Neurol.* 1997;42:776–782.

6. Boissiere F, Faucheux B, Agid Y. Choline acetyl transferase M R and A expression in the striatal neurons of patients with Alzheimer's disease. *Neurosci Lett.* 1997;225(3):169–172.

7. Mufson E, Ma S, Dills J, et al. Loss of basal forebrain immunoreactivity in subjects with mild cognitive impairment and Alzheimer's disease. *J Comp Neurol.* 2002;443(2):136–153.

8. Bonner L, Peskind E. Pharmacological treatments of dementia. *Med Clin North Am.* 2002;86(3): 657–674.

9. Repetto MG, Reides CG, Evelson P, et al. Peripheral markers of oxidative stress in probable Alzheimer's patients. *Eur J Clin Invest.* 1999;29(7): 643–649.

10. Selley M, Close D, Stern S. The effect of increased concentrations of homocysteine on the concentration of 4-hydroxy-2-nonenal in the plasma and cerebrospinal fluid of patients with Alzheimer's disease. *Neurobiol Aging.* 2002;23(3): 383–388.

11. Palmer A, Burns M. Selective increase in lipid peroxidation in the inferior temporal cortex in Alzheimer's disease. *Brain Res.* 1994;645:338–342.

12. Pratico D. F2 isoprostanes: sensitive and specific noninvasive indices of lipid peroxidation in vivo. *Atherosclerosis.* 1999;147:1–10.

13. Subramanian R, Koppal T, Green M, et al. The free radical antioxidant vitamin E protects cortical synaptosomal membranes from amyloid beta peptide toxicity but not from hydroxy nonenal toxicity: relevance to the free radical hypothesis of Alzheimer's disease. *Neurochem Res.* 1998; 23(11):1403–1420.

14. Sano M, Ernesto C, Thomas R, et al. A controlled trial of selegiline, alpha-tocopherol, or both as treatments for Alzheimer's disease. The Alzheimer's Disease Cooperative Study. *N Engl J Med.* 1997;336(17):1216–1222.

15. Selley M, Close D, Stern S. The effect of increased concentrations of homocysteine on the concentration of 4-HNE in the plasma and cerebrospinal fluid of patients with Alzheimer's disease. *Neurobiol Aging.* 2002;23(3):383–388.

16. Serot J, Christmann D, Dubost T, et al. CSF folate levels are decreased in late onset AD patients. *J Neural Transm.* 2001;108(1):93–99.

17. Doshi S, McDowell IF, Moat SJ, et al. Folate improves endothelial function in coronary artery disease—an effect mediated by reduction of in-

tracellular superoxide. *Arterioscler Thromb Vasc Biol*. 2001;21(7):1196–1202.

18. Solum D, Hand AR. Estrogen regulates the development of brain-derived neurotrophic factor MRNA and protein in the rat hippocampus. *J Neurosci*. 2002;22(7):2650–2659.

19. Horvath K, Hartig W, VanderVeen R, et al. Seventeen beta-estradiol enhances cortical cholinergic enervation and preserves synaptic density following excitotoxic lesions to the right nucleus basalis magnocellularis. *Neuroscience*. 2002; 110(3):489–504.

20. Paganini-Hill A, Henderson V. Estrogen deficiency and risk of Alzheimer's disease in women. *Am J Epidemiol*. 1994;140(3):256–261.

21. Asthana S, Baker L, Kraft L. High-dose estradiol improves cognition for women with Alzheimer's disease: results of a randomized study. *Neurology*. 2001;57(4):605–612.

22. Soderberg M, Edlund C, Kristensson K. The fatty acid composition of brain phospholipids in aging and in Alzheimer's disease. *Lipids*. 1991;26(6): 421–425.

23. Soderberg M, Edlund C, Kristensson K. The fatty acid composition of brain phospholipids in aging and in Alzheimer's disease. *Lipids*. 1991; 26(6):421.

24. Vannucchi M, Pepeu G. Effects of phosphatidylserine on acetyl-choline release and content in cortical slices from aging rats. *Neurobiol Aging*. 1987;8:403–407.

25. Crook T, Petrie W, Wells C. Effects of phosphatidylserine in Alzheimer's disease. *Psychopharmacol Bull*. 1992;28(1):61–65.

26. Aureli T, Dicocco ME, Kapuani G, et al. Effect of long-term feeding with acetyl-carnitine on the age related changes in rat brain lipid composition: a study of 31-P MNR spectroscopy. *Neurochem Res*. 2000;25(3):395–399.

27. Aureli T, Miccheli A, Ricciolini R. Aging brain: effect of acetyl-l-carnitine treatment on brain energy and phospholipid metabolism. A study by ^{31}P and HNMR spectroscopy. *Brain Res*. 1990; 526:108–112.

28. Sano M, Bell K, Cote L. Double-blind parallel-design pilot study of acetyl-carnitine in patients with Alzheimer's disease. *Arch Neurol*. 1992;49: 1137–1141.

29. Kalmiijn F, Launer A, Ott, A, et al. Dietary fat intake in the risk of incident dementia in the Rotterdam study. *Ann Neurol*. 1997;42:776–782.

30. Kalmiijn F, Launer A, Ott, A, et al. Dietary fat in-

take in the risk of incident dementia in the Rotterdam study. *Ann Neurol*. 1997;42:776–780.

31. Buxbaum JD, Cullen EI, Friedhoff LT. Pharmacological concentrations of the hmg coa reductase inhibitor lovastatin decreased the formation of the Alzheimer beta amyloid peptide in vitro and in patients. *Front Biosci*. 2002;7:50–59.

32. Loluo Y. Ginkgo biloba neuroprotection: therapeutic implications in Alzheimer's disease. *J Alzheimers Dis*. 2001;3(4):401–407.

33. Lebars P, Katz M, Berman N, et al. A placebo-controlled double-blind randomized trial of an extract of ginkgo biloba for dementia. North American EEG B Study Group. *JAMA*. 1997; 278(16):1327–1332.

34. Wang H, Tang X. Anticholinesterase effects of huperzine A, E2020 and tacrine in rats. *Zhongguo Yao Li Xue Bao*. 1998;19(1):27–30.

35. Xu F, Cai Z, Qu Z. Huperzine A in capsules and tablets for treating patients with Alzheimer's disease. *Zhongguo Yao Li Xue Bao*. 1999;20(6): 486–490.

36. Hoschl C, Hajek T. Hippocampal damage mediated by cortical steroids-a neuropsychiatric research challenge. *Eur Arch Psychiatric Clin Neurosci*. 2001;251(suppl 2):I181–I188.

37. Umegaki H, Ikari H, Nakahata H, et al. Plasma cortisol levels in elderly female subjects with Alzheimer's disease: a cross-sectional and longitudinal study. *Brain Res*. 2000;881(2):241–243.

38. Greenamyre JR, Betarbet R, Sherer T, et al. Chronic systemic complex 1 inhibition by pesticide causes selective nigra striatal degeneration with excytoplasmic inclusions. *Soc Neurosci*. 2000; 26:1026.

39. Xu J, Kao SY, Lee FJ, et al. Dopamine dependent neurotoxicity of alpha-synuclein: a mechanism for selective neurodegeneration in Parkinson's disease. *Nat Med*. 2002;8(6):600–606.

40. Perry TL, Godin DV, Hansen S. Parkinson's disease: a disorder due to nigra glutathione deficiency. *Neurosci Lett*. 1982;33:305.

41. Dexter DT, Carter CJ, Wells FR, et al. Basal lipid peroxidation in substantia nigra is increased in Parkinson's disease. *J Neurochem*. 1989;52:381.

42. Dexter DT, Carayon A, Vidailhet M, et al. Decreased ferritin levels in the brains of Parkinson's disease. *J Neurochem*. 1999;55:16.

43. Selley ML. 4-HNE may be involved in the pathogenesis of Parkinson's disease. *Free Radic Biol Med*. 1998;25(2):169–174.

44. Spencer JP, Jenner P, Daniel SE. Conjugates of

catecholamines with cysteine and GSH in Parkinson's disease: possible mechanisms of formation involving reactive oxygen species. *J Neurochem.* 1998;71(5):2112–2122.

45. Schapira AHV, Cooper JM, Dexter D, et al. Mitochondrial complex-1 deficiency in Parkinson's disease. *Lancet.* 1989;1:1269.

46. Burn DJ. Beyond the iron mask: towards better recognition and treatment of depression associated with Parkinson's disease. *Mov Disord.* 2002; 17(3):445–454.

47. Blin J, Bonnet AM, Agid Y. Does levodopa aggravate Parkinson's disease? *Neurology.* 1998; 38:1410.

48. Olanow CW, Jenner P, Brooks D. Dopamine agonists and neuroprotection in Parkinson's disease. *Ann Neurol.* 1998;44:S167.

49. Ratan R. Antioxidants in the treatment of neurological disease. In: Koliatsos V, Ratan R, eds. *Cell Death and Diseases of the Nervous System.* Totowa, NJ: Humana Press; 1999:649.

50. The Parkinson Study Group. Effects of tocopherol and deprenyl on the progression of disability in early Parkinson's disease. *N Engl J Med.* 1993;328:176–183.

51. Pappert EJ, Tangney CC, Goetz CG, et al. Alphatocopherol in the ventricular cerebrospinal fluid of Parkinson's disease patients: dose response study and correlates with plasma levels. *Neurology.* 1996;47(4);1037–1042.

52. Khanna S, Atalay M, Laaksonen DE, et al. Alphalipoic acid supplementation: tissue glutathione homeostatsis at rest and after exercise. *J Appl Physiol.* 1999;86:1191.

53. Barbiroli B, Mcdori R, Tritschler H.J, et al. Lipoic acid increases brain energy availability and skeletal muscle performance as shown by in vivo 31P MRS in a patient with mitochondrial cytopathy. *J Neurol.* 1995;242:471.

54. Spencer JP, Jenna P, Daniel SE, et al. Conjugates of catecholamines with cysteine and GSH in Parkinson's disease: possible mechanisms of formation involving reactive oxygen species. *J Neurochem.* 1998;5:2112.

55. Levites Y, Youdin MB, Maor G, et al. Attenuation of 6-hydroxy dopamine induced nuclear factor kappa beta activation and cell death by tea extracts in neuronal cultures. *Biochem Pharmacol.* 2002;63(1):21–29.

56. Sechi G, Deledda MG, Bua G, et al. Reduced intravenous glutathione in the treatment of early Parkinson's disease. *Prog Neuropsychopharmacol.* 1996;7:1159.

57. Schulz JB, Henshaw DR, Matthews RT, et al. Coenzyme Q10 and nicotinamide in a free radical spin trap protect against MPTP neurotoxicity. *Exp Neurol.* 1995;132:279–283.

58. Shults C, Oakes D, Kieburts K, et al. Effects of coenzyme Q10 in early Parkinson's disease. *Arch Neurol.* 2002;59:1541–1550.

59. Birkmayer JG, Vrecko C, Volc D, et al. Nicotinamide adenine dinucleotide (NADH)—a new therapeutic approach to Parkinson's disease: comparison of oral and parenteral application. *Acta Neurol Scand Suppl.* 1993;146:32.

60. Dizdar N, Kagedal B, Lindvall B. Treatment of Parkinson's disease with NADH. *Acta Neurol Scand.* 1994;90:345.

61. Pearl SM, Antinon MD, Stanwood GP, et al. The Effects of NADH on dopamine release in rats striatum. *Synapse.* 2000;36:95.

62. Deane KH, Jones D, Playford ED, et al. Physiotherapy for patients with Parkinson's disease: a comparison of techniques. *Cochrane Database Syst Rev.* 2001;(3):CD002817.

63. Charlett A, Dobbs RJ, Purkiss AG, et al. Cortisol is higher in parkinsonism and associated with gait deficit. *Acta Neurol Scand.* 1998;97(2): 77–85.

64. Hao Q, Miyashita N, Matsui M, et al. Chlamydia pneumonia infection associated with enhanced MRI spinal lesions in multiple sclerosis. *Mult Scler.* 2002;8(5):436–440.

65. Chabas D, Baranzini SE, Mitchell D, et al. The inflammation of the pro-inflammatory cytokine, osteopontin, on autoimmune demyelinating disease. *Science.* 2001;294(5547):1731–1735.

66. Stanislaus R, Singh A, Singh I. Lovastatin treatment decreases mononuclear cell infiltration into the CNS of Lewis rats with experimental allergic encephalomyelitis. *J Neurosci Res.* 2001;66(2): 155–162.

67. Berkman CS, Pignolti MG, Cavallo PF, et al. Use of alternative treatments by people with multiple sclerosis. *Neurorehab Neural Repair.* 1999;13: 243–254.

68. Casetta I, Invernizzi M, Granieri E. Multiple sclerosis and dental amalgam: case controlled study in Ferrara, Italy. *Neuroepidemiology.* 2001;20(2): 134–137.

69. Zhang SM, Willett WC, Hernan MA, et al. Dietary fat in relation to risk of multiple sclerosis among two large cohorts of women. *Am J Epidemiol.* 2000;152(11):1056–1064.

70. Giubilei F, Antonini G, Dilegge S, et al. Blood cholesterol and MRI activity in first clinical episodes suggestive of multiple sclerosis. *Acta Neurol Scand.* 2002;106(2):109–112.

71. Harbige L, Layward L, Dones M, et al. The protective effect of omega 6 fatty acids in experimental autoimmune encephalomyelitis in relation to transforming growth factor-beta 1, upregulation and increased prostaglandin E2 production. *Clin Exp Immunol.* 2000;122(3):445–452.

72. Bates D, Cartlidge N, French J, et al. A double-blind controlled trial of long-chain N-3 polyunsaturated fatty acids in the treatment of multiple sclerosis. *J Neurol Neurosurg Psychiatry.* 1989;52: 18–22.

73. Dworkin R, Bates D, Millar JHD, et al. Linoleic acid in multiple sclerosis: a re-analysis of three double-blind trials. *Neurology.* 1984;34:1441–1445.

74. Yu Y, Correl PH, Vanden Heuvel JP. Conjugated linoleic acid decreases production of pro-inflammatory products in macrophages: evidence for a PPAR gamma-dependent mechanism. *Biochem Biophys Acta.* 2002;1581(3):89–99.

75. Hayes CE, Cantorna MT, DeLuca HF. Vitamin D and multiple sclerosis. *Proc Soc Exp Biol Med.* 1997;216(1):21–27.

76. Nashold SE, Miller DJ, Hayes CE. 1,25-Dihydroxy vitamin D-3 treatment decreases macrophage accumulation in the CNS of mice with experimental autoimmune encephalomyelitis. *J Neuroimmunol.* 2000;103(2):171–179.

77. Bowling AC. *Alternative Medicine and Multiple Sclerosis.* New York: Demos Medical Publishing; 2001.

78. Fukazawa T, Yabe I, Kikuchi S, et al. Association of vitamin D receptor gene polymorphism with multiple sclerosis in Japanese. *J Neurol Sci.* 1999;166(1):47–52.

79. Kosman F, Nieves J, Komar L. Fracture history and bone loss in patients with multiple sclerosis. *Neurology.* 1998;51(4):1161–1165.

80. Spitsio S, Hooper PC, Leist T. Inactivation of peroxynitrite in multiple sclerosis patients with oral administration of inosine may signal approaches to therapy of the disease. *Mult Scler.* 2001;7(5): 313–319.

81. Huntley A, Ernst E. Complementary and alternative therapy for treating multiple sclerosis symptoms: a systematic review. *Complement Therap Medicine.* 2000;8(2):97–105.

82. Natarajn C, Bright JJ. Curcumin inhibits experimental allergic encephalomyelitis by blocking IL-12 signaling through Janus Kinase-Stat pathways in T lymphocytes. *J Immunol.* 2000;168(12): 6506–6513.

83. Warren S, Greenhill S, Warren K. Emotional stress and the development of multiple sclerosis: case control evidence of a relationship. *J Chronic Dis.* 1982;35:821–831.

84. Ku Y, Montgomery LD, Lee HC. Physiological responses of multiple sclerosis patients to body cooling. *Am J Phys Med Rehabil.* 2000;79(5): 427–434.

85. Sessler GJ. *Stroke: How to Prevent It/How to Survive It.* Englewood Cliffs, NJ: Prentice-Hall; 1981.

86. Matchar DB, Duncan PW, Samsa GP, et al. The Stroke Prevention Patient Outcome Research Team: goals and methods. *Stroke.* 1993;24: 2135–2142.

87. McGee CT, Chow EPY. *Miracle Healing from China . . . Qigong,* Coeur d'Alene, ID: MediPress; 1994.

88. Ness AR, Powles JW. Fruit and vegetables, and cardiovascular disease: a review. *Int J Epidemiol.* 1997;26(1):1–13.

89. Key TJ, et al. Dietary habits and mortality in 11,000 vegetarians and health-conscious people: results of a 17-year follow-up. *BMJ.* 1996;313(7060):775.

90. Keli SO, Hartog MG, Feskens EJ, Krombout D, et al: Dietary flavonoids, antioxidant vitamins, and incidence of stroke: the Zutphen study. *Arch Intern Med.* 1996;156:637.

91. Ness AR, Powles JW, Khaw KT. Vitamin C and cardiovascular disease: a systematic review. *J Cardiovasc Risk.* 1996;3(6):513.

92. Tyler VE. *The Honest Herbal.* 3rd ed. New York: Pharmaceutical Products Press; 1993.

93. Vogel RA. Alcohol, heart disease, and mortality: a review. *Rev Cardiovasc Med.* 2002;3:7–13.

94. Renaud SC. Diet and stroke. *J Nutr Health Aging.* 2001;5(3):167.

95. Jamrozik EK, Broadhurst RJ, Anderson CS, Stewart-Wynne EG, et al. The role of lifestyle factors in the etiology of stroke: a population-based case-control study in Perth, Western Australia. *Stroke.* 1994;25(1):51.

96. Keli SO, Feskens EJM, Kromhout D. Fish consumption and risk of stoke: the Zutphen study. *Stroke.* 1994;25(2):328.

97. Orencia AJ, Daviglus ML, Dyer AR, et al. Fish consumption and stroke in men: 30-year findings of the Chicago Western Electric Study. *Stroke.* 1996;27(2):204.

98. Diamond BJ, Shiflett SC, Feiwel N, et al. Ginkgo biloba extract: mechanisms and clinical indications. *Arch Phys Med Rehabil.* 2000;81:668.

99. Paubert-Braquet M, Koltai M, et al. Is there a case for PAF antagonists in the treatment of ischemic disease? *Trends Pharmacol Stud* 1989; 10:23.

100. Christen Y, Costentin J, Lacour M. Effects of ginkgo biloba extract (Egb 761) on the central nervous system. Paper presented at IPSEN Institute International Symposium; Montreaux, Switzerland; 20 April, 1991.

101. Pittler MH, Ernst E. Ginkgo biloba extract for the treatment of intermittent claudication: a meta-analysis of randomized trials. *Am J Med.* 2000; 108(4):276–281.

102. Clark WM, Rinker LG, Lessov NS, Lowery SL, Cipolla MJ. Efficacy of antioxidant therapies in transient focal ischemia in mice. *Stroke.* 2001; 32(4):1000–1004.

103. Agnoli A, Fiorani P, Pistoles GR. Preliminary results in the modifications of cerebral blood flow using Xenon-133 during administration of ginkgo-biloba. *Minerva Med* 1973;64(79 suppl): 4166–4173.

104. DeFeudis FV, Drieu K. Ginkgo biloba extract (EGb 761) and CNS functions: basic studies and clinical applications. *Curr Drug Target.* 2000; 1(1):25.

105. Hopfenmuller W. [Evidence for a therapeutic effect of ginkgo biloba special extract. Meta-analysis of 11 clinical studies in patients with cerebrovascular insufficiency in old age.] [German.] *Arzneimittelforschung.* 1994;44(9):1005–1013.

106. Diamond BJ, Shiflett SC, Feiwel N, et al. Ginkgo biloba extract: mechanisms and clinical indications. *Arch Phys Med Rehabil.* 2000;81:668.

107. Dermarderosian A, Beutler JA, eds. *Review of Natural Products: The Most Complete Source of Natural Product Information.* Philadelphia: Lippincott Williams & Wilkins; 2002.

108. Blumenthal M, Brinckmann J, Goldberg A, eds. *Herbal Medicine: Expanded Commission E Monographs.* Newton, MA: Integrative Medicine, 2000.

109. Tran TN, Christophersen BO. Studies on the transport of acetyl groups from peroxisomes to mitochondria in isolated liver cells oxidizing the polyunsaturated fatty acid 22:4n-6. *Biochim Biophys Acta.* 2001;1533(3):255–265.

110. Sacher HL, Sacher ML, Landau SW, et al. The clinical and hemodynamic effects of coenzyme Q10 in congestive cardiomyopathy. *Am J Ther.* 1997;4(2–3):66–72.

111. Abe K, Matsuo Y, Kadekawa J, Inoue S, Yanagihara T. Effect of coenzyme Q10 in patients with mitochondrial myopathy, encephalopathy, lactic acidosis, and stroke-like episodes (MELAS): evaluation by noninvasive tissue oximetry. *J Neurol Sci.* 1999;162(1):65–68.

112. Benson H. Systemic hypertension and the relaxation response. *N Engl J Med.* 1977;296:1152.

113. Hafner RJ. Psychological treatment of essential hypertension: a controlled comparison of meditation and meditation plus biofeedback. *Biofeedback Self Regul.* 1982;7:305.

114. Wallace RK, Silver J, Mills PJ, et al. Systolic blood pressure and long-term practice of the transcendental meditation and TM-Sidhi program: effects of TM on systolic blood pressure. *Psychosom Med.* 1983;45:41.

115. Cooper MJ, Aygen MM. A relaxation technique in the management of hypercholesterolemia. *J Human Stress.* 1979;5:24–27.

116. Cooper MJ, Aygen MM. Relaxation technique in the management of hypercholesterolemia. *J Human Stress* 1979;5:24–27.

117. Alexander CN, Langer EJ, Newman RI, et al. Transcendental meditation, mindfulness, and longevity: an experimental study with the elderly. *J Pers Soc Psychol.* 1989;57(6):950.

118. McDonagh EW, Rudolph CJ, Cheraskin E. An oculocerebrovasculometric analysis of the improvement in arterial stenosis following EDTA chelation therapy. In: Cranton EM, ed. *A Textbook on EDTA Chelation Therapy.* New York: Human Sciences Press; 1989:155.

119. Olszewer E, Carter JP. EDTA chelation therapy in chronic degenerative disease. *Med Hypotheses.* 1988;27(1):41.

120. Nayak S, Wheeler B, Shiflett SC, Agostinelli S. Music therapy in the rehabilitation of TBI and Stroke patients. *Rehabil Psychology.* 2000;45: 274–283.

121. Schaechter JD, Kraft E, Hilliard TS, et al. Motor recovery and cortical reorganization after con-

straint-induced movement therapy in stroke patients: a preliminary study. *Neurorehabil Neural Repair*. 2002;16(4):326–338.

122. Naeser MA, Alexander MP, Stiassny-Eder D, et al. Real versus sham acupuncture in the treatment of paralysis in acute stroke patients: a CT scan lesion site study. *J Neurol Rehabil*. 1992;6:163.

123. Naeser MA, Alexander MP, Stiassny-Eder D, et al. Acupuncture in the treatment of hand paresis in chronic and acute stroke patients: improvement observed in all cases. *Clin Rehabil*. 1994;8:127.

124. Naeser MA, Alexander MP, Stiassny-Eder D, et al. Laser acupuncture in the treatment of paralysis in stroke patients: a CT scan lesion site study. *Am J Acupunct*. 1995;23(1):13.

125. Naeser MA, Alexander MP, Stiassny-Eder D, et al. Acupuncture in the treatment of hand paresis in chronic and acute stroke patients: improvement observed in all cases. *Clin Rehabil*. 1994;8:127.

126. Wong AM, Su TY, Tang FT, Cheng PT, Liaw MY. Clinical trial of electrical acupuncture on hemiplegic stroke patients. *Am J Phys Med Rehabil*. 1999;78:117–122.

127. Sallstrom S. Acupuncture in the treatment of stroke patients in the subacute stage: a randomized, controlled study. *Complement Ther Med*. 1996;4:193.

128. Johansson K, Lindgren I, Widner H, et al. Can sensory stimulation improve the functional outcome in stroke patients? *Neurology*. 1993;43:2189.

129. Magnusson M, Johansson K, Johansson BB. Sensory stimulation promotes normalization of postural control after stroke. *Stroke*. 1994;25:1176–1180.

130. Johansson BB, Naker E, von Arbin M, et al. Acupuncture and transcutaneous nerve stimulation in stroke rehabilitation: a randomized, controlled trial. *Stroke*. 2001; 32(3):707.

131. Shiflett SC. Acupuncture and stroke rehabilitation. *Stroke*. 2001;32:1934.

132. Sze FK, Wong E, Or KK, Lau J, Woo J. Does acupuncture improve motor recovery after stroke? A meta-analysis of randomized controlled trials. *Stroke*. 2002;33:2604–2619.

133. Park J, Hopwood V, White AR, Ernst E. Effectiveness, of acupuncture for stroke: a systematic review. *J Neurol*. 2001;248: 558–563.

134. Sze FK, Wong E, Yi X, Woo J. Does acupuncture have additional value to standard poststroke motor rehabilitation? *Stroke*. 2002;33:186.

136. Shiflett SC, Nayak S, Bid C, Miles P, Agostinelli S. Effect of Reiki treatments on functional recovery in post-stroke rehabilitation patients: a pilot study. *J Altern Complement Med*. 2002;8:755–763.

137. Shiflett SC. Reiki and stroke. In: Leskowitz E, ed. *Complementary and Alternative Medicine in Rehabilitation*. St. Louis: Churchill-Livingstone; 2002:386–388.

138. Mink RB, Dutka AJ. Hyperbaric oxygen after global cerebral ischemia in rabbits does not promote brain lipid peroxidation. *Crit Care Med*. 1995;23(8):1398.

139. Neubauer RA, End E. Hyperbaric oxygenation as an adjunct therapy in strokes due to thrombosis: a review of 122 patients. *Stroke*. 1980;11(3):297.

140. Nighoghossian N, Trouillas P, Adeleine P, Salord F. Hyperbaric oxygen in the treatment of acute ischemic stroke. *Stroke*. 1995;26(8): 1369.

141. Rockswold GL, Ford SE, Anderson DC, et al. Results of a prospective randomized trial for treatment of severely brain-injured patients with hyperbaric oxygen. *J Neurosurg*. 1992;76:929.

142. Neubauer RA, Gottlieb SF, Pevsner H. Hyperbaric oxygen for treatment of closed head injury. *South Med J*. 1994;87(9):933.

CHAPTER 23

Integrative Approach to Oncology

Raymond Chang

Complementary and alternative medicine (CAM) is commonly sought by patients with cancer when conventional treatments are ineffective or inadequate. Patients are often moved to the use of CAM approaches in oncology because of the limited efficacy of conventional treatments, as well as their significant side effect potential. However there are also a great number of unsubstantiated claims regarding the applications of CAM to cancer therapy. Recent surveys cite a 31–83% prevalence of CAM use among cancer patients,[1,2] the majority of whom preferred an integrative approach.[3]

This chapter outlines some of the more common CAM modalities in oncology and illustrates the application of the basic principles behind their use. These basic principles for the integrative approach to cancer treatment are as follows:

1. *Biology Specific*—the CAM treatment should be appropriate for the specific type, site, and stage of cancer;
2. *Intent Specific*—the CAM treatment should be appropriate for the goal of treatment, that is, prevention, palliation, or survival;
3. *Cost:Benefit Specific*—the more efficacious and least costly (financially or physically in

terms of toxicity or side effects) therapy should be considered first; and
4. *Evidence Specific*—the above principles should be applied using an evidence-based approach whenever possible.

With attention to these basic principles, this chapter discusses the biology and intent-specific application of CAM in oncology by an overview of the range of therapeutic modalities followed by a clinical vignette to illustrate an evidence-based and cost:benefit specific implementation of a CAM program for a cancer patient.

► CAM MODALITIES IN ONCOLOGY

CAM modalities in oncology can be classified in different ways. The modalities are reviewed here based on therapeutic intent followed by a description of the various classes of modalities themselves. All CAM modalities in oncology should be firstly considered from an intent-specific perspective: that is, is it intended as a preventative, for palliation, or for enhanced survival? Then its application should be considered with evidence and cost:benefit considerations.

▶ CAM MODALITIES BASED ON INTENT OF TREATMENT

Cancer Prevention

This is the use of specific interventions to reduce the primary or secondary occurrence of cancer. This is an especially important role for CAM as there are few drug therapies indicated for prevention. Because prevention is by definition carried out in a healthy population over a period of time, it is important to use the least toxic and/or costly modalities. CAM approaches such as diet, in conjunction with judicious use of nutraceuticals and herbs that are relatively nontoxic, thus potentially can play a major role.

In the United States, unhealthy diet accounts for more cancer related deaths than any other environmental or genetic factor.[1] Dietary preventative programs include the ingestion of foods with known anticancer properties (Table 23–1), as well as the avoidance of foods that may be directly carcinogenic or encourage cancer growth (Table 23–2). Specific supplemental vitamins, nutraceuticals, and herbals that have preventa-

▶ **TABLE 23-1** SOME FOODS WITH KNOWN CANCER PREVENTATIVE COMPONENTS

Food	Bioactive Compound Class
Fish (deep sea, oily)	Omega fatty acids
Tea	Polyphenols, e.g., epigallocatechin gallate (EGCG)
Soy*	Isoflavones genistein and daidzein
Flax*	Omega-3 fatty acid, lignans
Mushrooms	Beta-1,3 glucans
Fruits and vegetables	Carotenoids, flavonoids, polyphenols
Whole grains	
Spice	Polyphenols
Red wine	Polyphenols

▶ **TABLE 23-2** SOME FOODS WITH POSSIBLE ASSOCIATED CANCER RISK

Alcohol[100]
Dairy[101]
Sugar and high glycemic foods[102]
Saturated fat[103]
Red meat, smoked and cured meats[104]

tive potential are usually those with known anticancer biological principles such as antioxidant, prodifferentiation, immunostimulatory, antiangiogenic, or specific hormonal properties. At the molecular level, modification of cancer risk may be mediated by an effect on cellular signaling molecules such as kinases, telomerase, cyclooxygenase-2, triggers of apoptosis, and transcription factors AP1, and nuclear factor-κB.

Despite a large body of research relating to individual micronutrients at the molecular and cellular levels and carcinogenesis, corroboration of an impact on cancer outcomes from clinical studies is relatively weak with a handful of supportive clinical trials, a few cohort studies and some case-control research. To date, randomized intervention trials involving more than 30,000 adults followed up to 12 years evaluating the effects of vitamin and mineral supplementation on cancer rates have been reported. Such trials included assessments of multiple vitamin and mineral combinations in an area of China with limited micronutrient intake and one of the world's highest cancer rates,[5] and of beta-carotene, vitamin E, or selenium in several more-well-nourished Western populations, some at very high risk of lung cancer. Unfortunately, few conclusive results have been obtained to date. Significantly lower cancer mortality has been found among those supplemented with a combination of beta-carotene, vitamin E, and selenium in the China trial, and among those with certain types of cancer who were supplemented with selenium in the United States,[6] but the risk of lung cancer was actually increased in a Finnish trial of adults provided with high-dose beta-carotene.[7] In light of available data, it seems that antioxidant supplementation may prevent certain cancers of the aerodigestive tract; selenium may specifically prevent lung, colorectal, and prostate cancer; and folate and calcium supplementation may prevent colorectal cancer.[8]

Such trials indicate that the relation between specific micronutrient intake and cancer risk is complex. Whereas specific micronutrients may not independently exert a marked chemopreventative effect, promising chemopreventative foods and beverages that contain a complex of micronutrients and macronutrients, such as cruciferous vegetables, tomato, fish, soy, tumeric, and tea, warrant further investigation.[9]

Palliation of Symptoms

This is the use of specific interventions to reduce side effects of conventional treatments or to palliate symptoms of the underlying malignancy and its complications. As mainstays of conventional cancer treatment, chemotherapy and radiation therapy carry significant morbidity. Such side effects frequently include fatigue; hair loss; mucositis; nausea and vomiting; marrow or immune suppression and consequent infection; and neuropathy. Although there are conventional treatments for such complications, those drugs themselves may have additional side effects and are not always effective. Some chemotherapy and radiation side effects have been demonstrated to be effectively treated by CAM. For example, acupuncture can reduce nausea and vomiting caused by chemotherapy[10] as well as xerostomia resulting from radiation.[11] Chinese herbs and herbal formulae are also useful in relieving a range of chemotherapy-associated side effects[12] and specific herbs, such as ginger, are useful for chemotherapy-induced nausea.[13] The amino acid L-glutamine is useful in the treatment or prevention of mucositis, immune suppression, myalgia, and neuropathy.[14] Other CAM modalities which may have application to reduce chemotherapy or radiation side effects include aromatherapy for nausea or fatigue, visualization, and meditation.

Enhancing Survival

The ultimate goal of cancer treatment is to enhance quality survival, and this is an area where there are many claims but relatively few clinical trials to document efficacy. Nonetheless, many patients pursue CAM because of a lack of conventional options, and it is important to be familiar with the mechanisms of action as well as the CAM modalities or agents that are commonly in use by cancer patients so as to properly advise them. CAM modalities that may enhance quality survival generally include those agents which have antiproliferative, antiangiogenic, apoptotic, immunostimulatory, or other yet unknown antineoplastic properties.

▶ RANGE OF CAM MODALITIES

There is a broad range of CAM modalities and agents commonly used by patients with cancer, including such nonconventional therapies as foreign drugs (e.g., Lentinan,[15] Clodronate[16]), off-label drugs (e.g., cyclooxygenase [COX]-2 inhibitors,[17] statins,[18] phenylbutyrate[19]), dietary approaches, nutraceuticals (vitamins and micronutrients), botanicals, mind–body approaches, spiritual approaches, and some less-well-documented approaches. It is important to recommend agents appropriate to the patient's diagnosis, stage, and prognosis, as well as agents that have the most documentation of efficacy while having the least side effects and cost. To facilitate this evidence-based approach, the University of Texas MD Anderson Cancer Center's Complementary/Integrative Medicine Education Resources (CIMER) web site (www.mdanderson.org/cimer) contains evidence-based reviews of complementary or alternative cancer therapies, as well as links to other authoritative resources. These reviews evaluate the designs and the results of published research on herbal, mind–body, energy, nutrition, and other biological/organic/pharmacological substance use in cancer.[20]

Dietary Approaches

Dietary strategies are perhaps the best noninvasive preventative for cancer. Dietary compounds can impede carcinogenesis in several ways:

1. They block the activation of enzymes involved in conjugative or oxidative reactions.
2. They increase metabolic detoxification reactions.
3. They provide alternative targets for electrophilic metabolites.

Additionally, phytonutrients increase the levels of glutathione and/or glucuronic transferases to facilitate quenching of reactive electrophiles and oxidants that may damage DNA. Table 23–1 lists some of the better-known dietary elements that are known to have preventative potential.

As for cancer therapy, there are many dietary approaches for cancer treatment. While many individual nutrients and dietary components show promise as preventatives for cancer via the above pathways, no particular dietary program has been proven definitively to improve survival. Well-known alternative dietary programs for cancer include macrobiotics,[21] Kelley's,[22] and Gerson's programs. As an example, Gerson's program[23] is based on the concepts that cancer patients have low immunoreactivity and generalized tissue damage, especially of the liver, and that when the cancer is destroyed, toxic degradation products appear in the bloodstream. The diet itself involves high potassium, low sodium, no fats or oils, and minimal animal proteins. Juices of raw fruits and vegetables and of raw liver are thought to provide enzymes that facilitate rehabilitation of the liver. Iodine and niacin supplementation is used. Coffee enemas cause dilation of bile ducts, which is believed to facilitate excretion of toxic cancer breakdown products and dialysis of toxic products from blood across the colonic wall. Although no randomized trial exists for these dietary approaches, the Gerson diet has been reported to improve 5-year melanoma survival when compared to historical controls.[24]

A similarly well-known alternative dietary, nutritional, and detoxification regimen[25] based on Kelley's, as well as Gerson's principles, was reported by Gonzalez to improve pancreatic cancer survival based on a small cohort study of 10 patients.[26] These regimens are usually elaborate to carry out and are exclusive of other alternative regimens. Such programs are not entirely based on modern scientific principles and have scant evidence of clinical efficacy to date; as such, they should not be generally recommended but may deserve further investigation.

Vitamins, Micronutrients, and Other Nutraceuticals

While vitamin treatments for cancer have been extensively studied and certain vitamins, such as ascorbic acid (vitamin C), are often used as a cancer therapeutic,[27,28] the use of specific vitamins and micronutrients as cancer preventatives and therapeutics has been somewhat limited by lack of conclusive clinical research.[29] Zinc,[30] selenium,[31] certain B[32,33] and E[34] vitamins, vitamin A[35] and carotenoids, vitamins K_2 and K_3,[36] and vitamin D_3 and analogues[37,38] have shown some promise as cancer preventatives or therapeutics (Table 23–3). Examples of specific nutraceuticals that may potentially be useful in preventing or treating cancer include inositol hexaphosphonate,[39] D-glucarate,[40] con-

▶ **TABLE 23–3** VITAMINS AND MICRONUTRIENTS WITH KNOWN ANTICANCER PROPERTIES

Vitamin B_9 (folic acid)
Vitamin B_{12}
Retinoids and vitamin A
Vitamin C
Vitamin D
Vitamin E
Vitamin K
Selenium
Zinc

jugated linolenic acid,[41] lactoferrin,[42] gamma-linolenic acid and certain omega-3 fatty acids,[43] resveratrol,[44] and melatonin.[45]

Botanical Medicines

Several important chemotherapeutic drugs, including paclitaxel, vincristine, and camptothecin, are plant derivatives, and research in this area is still very active. Moreover, many botanicals exhibit other therapeutic properties besides cytotoxicity, which may be useful for cancer prevention and treatment, such as antiangiogenesis, differentiation, and immunopotentiation. Some nonchemotherapy drugs of botanical origin, such as Lentinan,[46] have undergone rigorous clinical trials to demonstrate clinical efficacy. Some of the more well-known, although not necessarily proven, botanical approaches in alternative cancer care include Essiac tea and mistletoe[47] (Iscador). Essiac tea is one of the more popular herbal remedies and is not made of any single herb but a combination of herbs, some of which have individual antitumor activity. At its inception in 1922, when the Canadian nurse Rene Caisse began providing this herbal formula to cancer patients, it mainly consisted of Turkish rhubarb, sheep sorrel, slippery elm bark, and burdock root. Proof of its claim to anticancer efficacy has been limited to anecdotal reports; nevertheless, Essiac continues to be widely used by patients with cancer. Caisse reportedly altered the original formula some 40 years after its introduction and added watercress, blessed thistle, red clover, and kelp, although she never revealed the exact Essiac formulation.[48] The chemistry and biology of the herbs used in Essiac has been reviewed in the literature,[49] and although there is supporting laboratory evidence of anticancer activity of isolates of the individual herbs used in Essiac, there is no trial documenting Essiac's clinical efficacy in cancer.[50]

Medicinal mushrooms and fungal derivatives, including compounds derived from agaricus, coriolus, cordyceps, ganoderma, maitake, and shiitake, are used as drugs or nutraceuticals in the adjuvant treatment of cancer.[51] In addition, many traditional Chinese herbs have been studied for their antineoplastic potential.[52] A number of folk herbs such as noni *(Morinda citrifolia)*,[53] Pau D'Arco *(Tabebuia avellanedae)*,[54] and una de gato *(Uncaria tomentosa,* also known as "cat's claw")[55] are popular, although less proven, alternative remedies for cancer.

Mind–Body Approaches

This area as applied to cancer treatment includes such techniques as relaxation techniques, biofeedback, hypnosis, visualization, meditation, yoga, Qigong, and psychotherapies. These approaches have benefits in symptom management, stress relief, and perhaps survival. Beginning in the 1970s, researchers began to explore whether behavioral techniques could extend cancer survival, perhaps through affecting the immune system.[56] Spiegel's now classic randomized study demonstrating a survival advantage of group psychotherapy and hypnosis in breast cancer is widely quoted among those who are in favor of this approach,[57] although a recent trial cast doubts and resurrected controversy on the efficacy of psychotherapy for cancer patients.[58] Moreover, a recent systemic review of 627 relevant papers and 329 interventional trials of psychotherapy interventions for cancer yielded no conclusive results, in large part because of suboptimal study methodology.[59] Thus one could only suggest that such interventions should be further investigated, but recommendation of such nontoxic interventions should meanwhile be individualized.

Acupuncture

For the cancer patient, acupuncture is specifically useful for the relief of nausea secondary to chemotherapy,[4] treatment of cancer pain,[60] and in the treatment of postradiation xerostomia.[11] In a recent review of the integration of acupuncture in an oncology clinic for patients with various symptoms at a medical center, it was noted that a majority (60%) of patients reported at least 30% symptomatic improvement without untoward effects, while most of the patients (86%) considered it "very important" that the clinic continue to provide acupuncture services.[61]

Spirituality

This aspect of integrative care is often overlooked in the Western and conventional medical tradition, partly because of the philosophical schism between mind and body as well as between science and religion, yet "the ultimate cure" of death and disease may lie in this transcendent realm. Spirituality may confer on a patient a sense of well-being despite physical suffering, and the greater sense of meaning and purpose to life may allow a patient to better face and manage a cancer diagnosis. There are a paucity of clinical studies in this area, and although there are hints that use of a psycho-spiritual therapy program may be associated with survival,[62] ultimately, spirituality is a personal matter. Nevertheless, it is an area that deserves serious attention from the physician-healer.

Other Approaches

There are specific cancer therapeutics that cannot be easily categorized by modality or mechanism of action and may involve alternative theories of oncogenesis as well and are thus more controversial among various alternative therapies for cancer. Such treatments include antineoplastons,[63] Cancell,[64] immunoaugmentative therapy,[65] Hoxsey,[66] Livingston-Wheeler therapy,[67] and Naessens (714-X).[68] Although there are anecdotal reports supporting each approach, there is a relative lack of scientific or clinical support for them.

▶ Case Example: Breast Cancer

MJ is a 42-year-old premenopausal white female who is otherwise healthy except for mild hypercholesterolemia, which is under diet control, and mild depression, for which she takes St. John's wort. A right breast mass was discovered at screening mammography and a lumpectomy with node dissection yielded a $2 \times 2 \times 1.3$-cm ($0.8 \times 0.8 \times 0.5$-inch) infiltrating ductal carcinoma with 2 positive lymph nodes out of 16. Assay for estrogen receptor (ER) was positive. She was advised to undertake adjuvant doxorubicin and cyclophosphamide and chemotherapy for four cycles followed by paclitaxel for four cycles, then followed by local radiation and five subsequent years of tamoxifen. MJ never took medications in her life and is particularly fearful of radiation and chemotherapy, which she believes will "destroy" her immune system, but she is also afraid to stray from the conventional oncologist's recommendations. She seeks out CAM potentially to reduce the side effects of the chemo- and radiotherapy, as well to help her cope with the side effects of a premature menopause induced by chemotherapy and tamoxifen treatments. She is also interested in changing her diet and lifestyle in order to reduce the risk of recurrence.

Discussion: Overview

The incidence of newly diagnosed breast cancer is approximately 175,000 a year in the United States.[69] MJ is without major risk factors, and adjuvant chemotherapy followed by hormonal therapy is standard management in such a case as it confers a disease-free as well as an overall survival advantage.[70] Because MJ had breast-conserving surgery, locoregional radiation is routinely recommended to prevent local recurrence.

Estrogen blockade using a estrogen receptor modulator such as tamoxifen has also been convincingly demonstrated to enhance survival and reduce the risk of recurrence because her tumor was ER positive.[71]

INTEGRATIVE STRATEGIES

The use of CAM must take into consideration the whole patient (MJ is a healthy premenopausal female), the cancer type and stage (ER-positive and node-positive breast cancer), and the conventional treatments the patient will undertake (chemotherapy, radiation, and hormonal therapy), and should be programmed and synchronized to the various phases of the patient's conventional treatment. The consideration of the specific conventional agents used with the distinct goals of reducing side effects or otherwise enhancing those agents is especially important. There is also the importance of reducing the patient's risk of recurrence after the conventional treatments are completed. In MJ's case, consultations with the patient should take place parallel to the ongoing conventional treatments and CAM therapy and could be introduced in three phases:

Phase I   During chemotherapy
Phase II During radiation
Phase III Before and after initiating hormonal therapy

For each phase, the use of off-label drugs, supplements, herbs, acupuncture, diet, mind–body, and other approaches (in that order of priority) should be carefully considered and initiated with the cooperation of the treating oncologist and radiation oncologist and primary care physician.

PHASE I: DURING CHEMOTHERAPY

The patient is scheduled to receive Adriamycin (doxorubicin) and Cytoxan (cyclophosphamide) followed by paclitaxel.

These agents each have unique side effects in addition to the general chemotherapeutic side effects of fatigue, cytopenia, hair loss, nausea, and mucositis. As an example, doxorubicin is known to be cardiotoxic and can cause cardiomyopathy as well as heart failure. Paclitaxel, on the other hand, is known to be associated with arthralgias and myalgias following administration, as well as a potential for cumulative neuropathy. Specific nutritional supplements have been shown to reduce the side effects of such chemotherapies, and in the case of Adriamycin, the mitochondrial enzyme ubiquinone has been found to protect against anthracycline cardiac damage.[72,73] However, it is also important to note that there is a serious concern that certain nutritional supplements may interact adversely with chemotherapy. Because certain chemotherapeutic effects are thought to be mediated by free radicals, quenching free radicals by antioxidant supplementation may in theory reduce treatment efficacy.[74] However, not all antioxidants are the same and there are multiple determinants of antioxidant–chemotherapy interactions, thus there are exceptions to the rule (e.g., mesna, an antioxidant that is protective against methotrexate chemotoxicity without reducing chemoefficacy[75]). In general, however, it is probably safer to avoid supplemental antioxidant consumption by cancer patients during chemotherapy with alkylating agents, anthracyclines, bleomycin, etoposide, and mitomycin.

Aside from antioxidants, specific herbs or supplements, such as the St. John's wort that MJ takes for depression, may also adversely affect chemotherapy and should be avoided. In the case of St. John's wort, it induces the activity of the cytochrome P450 isozyme 3A4 (CYP3A4) pathway and can increase the metabolic clearance of chemotherapeutic drugs.[76] This herb should be discontinued in MJ's case with an appropriate replacement by an antidepressant drug therapy or other CAM treatments.

In the case of paclitaxel, the amino acid L-glutamine at a dose of 1500 mg/day has been studied and found to significantly reduce the associated arthralgia and myalgia, as well as neuropathy.[77,78] Apart from this, various Chinese herbal formulae and single herbs have been shown to reduce overall side effects of chemotherapy. Polysaccharide-containing Chinese herbs such as astragalus, Cordyceps, coriolus, ganoderma, glycyrrhiza (licorice), *Poria cocos,* and ginseng (Table 23–4) have all been studied and confirmed to be useful.[79] However, in MJ's case—with an ER-positive cancer—it is important to avoid including foods, herbs, or herbal formulae with phytoestrogenic activity (Table 23–5) as part of the supportive regimen.

Melatonin is a pineal hormone that has been studied extensively for its potential role as an adjuvant cancer therapeutic and has been found to be useful against ER-positive breast cancer.[80] Melatonin can also significantly reduce the side effects of chemotherapy.[81] Other less substantiated but mild and harmless remedies for specific conditions, such as mucositis, can be aloe vera or diluted tea-tree oil as a mouthrinse, and nausea can be treated with ginger tea.[82] Similarly, acupuncture may be used to reduce nausea and to support the immune system (see "Acupuncture" above). Lifestyle approaches that may be helpful include the use of aromatherapy to relax and/or reduce nausea and vomiting; a healthy diet (see "Dietary Approaches" above) to be adjusted to patient's appetite; visualizations; and support groups to provide psychosocial support.

PHASE II: RADIATION

Special care has to be taken in this phase to avoid antioxidants during radiotherapy as in chemotherapy because radiation efficacy against cancer is thought to be mediated by free radicals, and antioxidant supplementation may reduce treatment effects, although there are exceptions to the rule with antioxidant radioprotectants (e.g., amifostine) that maintain tumor radiosensitivity.[83] During this phase, it is possible to consider the concurrent off-label use of a COX-2 inhibitor such as celecoxib, as it has been shown to enhance tumor radiosenstivity[84] in addition to inhibiting breast cancer cell growth.[85] Otherwise, acupuncture and Chinese herbs started during chemotherapy phase can be

▶ **TABLE 23–4** COMMON POLYSACCHARIDE-CONTAINING BOTANICALS

Agaricus
Aloe
Astralgalus
Cordyceps
Coriolus
Echinacea
Ganoderma
Ginseng
Maitake
Shiitake

▶ **TABLE 23–5** COMMON ESTROGENIC BOTANICALS/FOODS/SUPPLEMENTS

Soy[105]
Flax[106]
Red Clover (*Trifolium pratense* L.)[107]
Chasteberry (*Vitex agnus-castus* L.)[108]
Hops (*Humulus lupulus* L.)[109]
Ginseng (*Panax ginseng*)[110]
American Ginseng (*Panax quinquefolius* L.)[111]
Licorice[112]
Dong Quai (*Angelica sinensis*)
DHEA[113] (dehydroepiandrosterone)
Boron[114]

continued in MJ, and certain supplements specifically helpful during radiation therapy, such as alkylglycerols,[86] can be added. Meanwhile supplements specific for chemotherapy such as ubiquinone and L-glutamine can be discontinued.

PHASE III: SECONDARY PREVENTION AND TAMOXIFEN-RELATED SIDE EFFECTS

This is actually the most complex part of MJ's treatment planning, as she completes the main conventional therapies and embarks on long-term use of tamoxifen for secondary prevention. One should work closely with the patient now to institute a preventative dietary and supplemental nutritional program as well as follow-up with the patient after hormonal therapy to discuss side effects of hormone deprivation in an otherwise premenopausal female.

In MJ's case, because she has been mildly depressed, the use of an selective serotonin reuptake inhibitor antidepressant may be helpful for her mood as well as for hot flashes related to estrogen deprivation.[87]

COX-2 inhibitors are currently in preventative trials in breast cancer[85] and one can consider their continuation in this phase for MJ. Other off-label drugs, such as statins, can be considered as well,[88] especially if MJ has borderline hyperlipidemia. In terms of supplements and herbs, the Chinese herbal formula that was used since chemotherapy can be continued as an immune adjuvant. Vitamins found to have preventative potential in breast cancer include vitamin E, including tocopherols and tocotrienols,[89] and vitamin D_3.[90] Supplements that are thought to be useful in an ER-positive case include such compounds as inositol hexaphosphate,[91] di-indolylmethane[92] and its precursor indole-3-carbinol,[93] and D-glucarate,[94] although the research is limited to laboratory or animal data. As above, all potentially

estrogenic supplements that contain phytoestrogens should be avoided, even though these agents may reduce the symptoms associated with estrogen deprivation such as hot flashes.

The discussion of an appropriate diet for breast cancer should probably be individualized and is otherwise beyond the scope of this chapter, but general dietary recommendations involve the principle of maintaining ideal body weight and following a low glycemic diet,[95] with an emphasis on fruits and vegetables and a healthy source of protein, as well as healthy fats. As usual, one should counsel the patient to avoid dietary substances which may interfere with the patient's drug therapy (e.g., grapefruit juice may reduce the efficacy of tamoxifen[96]). The same general principle of avoiding intake of estrogenic substances in an ER-positive patient would apply for diet, and MJ should avoid soy or flax-based foods (see Table 23–5).

Although controversial, some studies suggest that group psychotherapy enhances survival in breast cancer (see above). In the absence of conclusive trials, however, the author believes that mind–body aspects of MJ's care should be individualized and tailored to the patient's preference and lifestyle.

The treatment of estrogen deprivation-related symptoms secondary to hormonal drugs for ER-positive breast cancer is particularly difficult because of the need to avoid estrogenic substances. As alternatives, supplements such as vitamin E,[97] off-label drugs such as gabapentin,[98] selective serotonin receptor inhibitors, or other modalities such as acupuncture[99] could be tried for specific complaints such as hot flashes.

Conclusion

As the case of MJ illustrates, the integrative approach to the patient with cancer greatly expands the range of options available for palliation of symptoms related both to the disease and the treatment. In some cases, this approach may offer options with the potential to enhance survival as well. The distinction between curing and healing is uniquely important in cancer therapeutics, as even in the patient for whom the disease will be terminal, there is the potential in the integrative approach for improved quality of life and emotional and spiritual healing as part of the process.

REFERENCES

1. Ernst E, Cassileth BR. The prevalence of complementary/alternative medicine in cancer: a systematic review. *Cancer.* 1998;83(4):777–782.
2. Sparber A, Bauer L, Curt G, et al. Use of complementary medicine by adult patients participating in cancer clinical trials. *Oncol Nurs Forum.* 2000;27(4):623–630.
3. Coss RA, McGrath P, Caggiano V. Alternative care. Patient choices for adjunct therapies within a cancer center. *Cancer Pract.* 1998;6(3):176–181.
4. Doll R, Peto R. The causes of cancer: quantitative estimates of avoidable risks of cancer in the United States today. *J Natl Cancer Inst.* 1981;66(6):1191–1308.
5. Taylor PR, Li B, Dawsey SM, et al. Prevention of esophageal cancer: the nutrition intervention trials in Linxian, China. Linxian. Nutrition Intervention Trials Study Group. *Cancer Res.* 1994; 54(7 suppl):2029s–2031s.
6. Clark LC, Combs GF Jr, Turnbull BW, et al. Effects of selenium supplementation for cancer prevention in patients with carcinoma of the skin. A randomized controlled trial. Nutritional Prevention of Cancer Study Group. *JAMA.* 1996; 276(24):1957–1963.
7. Albanes D, Heinonen OP, Huttunen JK, et al. Effects of alpha-tocopherol and beta-carotene supplements on cancer incidence in the Alpha-Tocopherol Beta-Carotene Cancer Prevention Study. *Am J Clin Nutr.* 1995;62(6 suppl): 1427S–1430S.
8. Garay CA, Engstrom PF. Chemoprevention of colorectal cancer: dietary and pharmacologic approaches. *Oncology (Huntingt).* 1999;13(1): 89–97; discussion 97–100, 105.
9. Kelloff GJ, Crowell JA, Steele VE, et al. Progress in cancer chemoprevention: development of diet-derived chemopreventive agents. *J Nutr.* 2000; 130(suppl 2S):467S–471S.
10. Dundee JW, Ghaly RG, Fitzpatrick KT, Abram WP, Lynch GA. Acupuncture prophylaxis of cancer chemotherapy-induced sickness. *J R Soc Med.* 1989;82(5):268–271.
11. Johnstone PA, Niemtzow RC, Riffenburgh RH. Acupuncture for xerostomia: clinical update. *Cancer* 2002;94(4):1151–1156.
12. Wong R, Sagar CM, Sagar SM. Integration of Chinese medicine into supportive cancer care: a modern role for an ancient tradition. *Cancer Treat Rev.* 2001;27(4):235–246.
13. Ernst E, Pittler MH. Efficacy of ginger for nausea and vomiting: a systematic review of randomized clinical trials. *Br J Anaesth.* 2000;84(3):367–371.
14. Decker GM. Glutamine: indicated in cancer care? [review] *Clin J Oncol Nurs.* 2002;6(2):112–115.
15. Chihara G, Hamuro J, Maeda YY, et al. Antitumor and metastasis-inhibitory activities of lentinan as an immunomodulator: an overview. *Cancer Detect Prev Suppl.* 1987;1:423–443.
16. Hurst M, Noble S. Clodronate: a review of its use in breast cancer. *Drugs Aging.* 1999;15(2): 143–167.
17. Howe LR, Dannenberg AJ. A role for cyclooxygenase-2 inhibitors in the prevention and treatment of cancer. *Semin Oncol.* 2002;29(3 suppl 11): 111–119.
18. Wong WW, Dimitroulakos J, Minden MD, Penn LZ. HMG-CoA reductase inhibitors and the malignant cell: the statin family of drugs as triggers of tumor-specific apoptosis. *Leukemia.* 2002;16(4): 508–519.
19. Jung M. Inhibitors of histone deacetylase as new anticancer agents. *Curr Med Chem.* 2001;8(12): 1505–1511.
20. Richardson MA, White JD. Complementary/alternative medicine and cancer research. A national initiative. *Cancer Pract.* 2000;8(1):45–48.
21. Kushi LH, Cunningham JE, Hebert JR, et al. The macrobiotic diet in cancer. *J Nutr.* 2001;131(11 suppl):3056S–3064S.

22. Kelley WD. *One Answer to Cancer: An Ecological Approach to the Successful Management of Malignancy.* Winfield, KS: Wedgestone Press; 1969.

23. Gerson M. The cure of advanced cancer by diet therapy: a summary of 30 years of clinical experimentation. *Physiol Chem Phys.* 1978;10(5): 449–464.

24. Hildenbrand GL, Hildenbrand LC, Bradford K, Cavin SW. Five-year survival rates of melanoma patients treated by diet therapy after the manner of Gerson: a retrospective review. *Altern Ther Health Med.* 1995;1(4):29–37.

25. Green S. Nicholas Gonzalez treatment for cancer: gland extracts, coffee enemas. *Sci Rev Altern Med.* 1998;2(2):25–30.

26. Gonzalez NJ, Isaacs LL. Evaluation of pancreatic proteolytic enzyme treatment of adenocarcinoma of the pancreas, with nutrition and detoxification support. *Nutr Cancer.* 1999;33(2):117–124.

27. Cameron E, Pauling L. *Cancer and Vitamin C.* Philadelphia: Camino Books; 1993.

28. Head KA. Ascorbic acid in the prevention and treatment of cancer. *Altern Med Rev.* 1998;3(3): 174–186.

29. Moyad MA. Results and lessons from clinical trials using dietary supplements for cancer: direct and indirect investigations. *Semin Urol Oncol.* 2001;19(4):232–246.

30. Fong LY, Nguyen VT, Farber JL. Esophageal cancer prevention in zinc-deficient rats: rapid induction of apoptosis by replenishing zinc. *J Natl Cancer Inst.* 2001;93(20):1525–1533.

31. Kim YS, Milner J. Molecular targets for selenium in cancer prevention. *Nutr Cancer.* 2001;40(1): 50–54.

32. Prinz-Langenohl R, Fohr I, Pietrzik K. Beneficial role for folate in the prevention of colorectal and breast cancer. *Eur J Nutr.* 2001;40(3):98–105.

33. Choi SW. Vitamin B_{12} deficiency: a new risk factor for breast cancer? *Nutr Rev.* 1999;57(8): 250–253.

34. Theriault A, Chao JT, Wang Q, Gapor A, Adeli K. Tocotrienol: a review of its therapeutic potential. *Clin Biochem.* 1999;32(5):309–319.

35. Altucci L, Gronemeyer H. The promise of retinoids to fight against cancer. *Nat Rev Cancer.* 2001;1(3):181–193.

36. Okayasu H, Ishihara M, Satoh K, Sakagami H. Cytotoxic activity of vitamins K_1, K_2 and K_3 against human oral tumor cell lines. *Anticancer Res.* 2001;21(4A):2387–2392.

37. van den Bemd GJ, Chang GT. Vitamin D and vitamin D analogs in cancer treatment. *Curr Drug Targets.* 2002;3(1):85–94.

38. Hansen CM, Binderup L, Hamberg KJ, Carlberg C. Vitamin D and cancer: effects of $1,25(OH)_2D_3$ and its analogs on growth control and tumorigenesis. *Front Biosci.* 2001;6:D820–D848.

39. Jariwalla RJ. Inositol hexaphosphate (IP6) as an anti-neoplastic and lipid-lowering agent. *Anticancer Res.* 1999;19(5A):3699–3702.

40. Walaszek Z. Potential use of D-glucaric acid derivatives in cancer prevention. *Cancer Lett.* 1990; 54(1–2):1–8.

41. McCarty MF. Activation of PPAR gamma may mediate a portion of the anticancer activity of conjugated linoleic acid. *Med Hypotheses.* 2000;55(3): 187–188.

42. Tsuda H, Sekine K, Fujita K, Ligo M. Cancer prevention by bovine lactoferrin and underlying mechanisms—a review of experimental and clinical studies. *Biochem Cell Biol.* 2002;80(1): 131–136.

43. Das UN. Gamma-linolenic acid, arachidonic acid, and eicosapentaenoic acid as potential anticancer drugs. *Nutrition.* 1990;6(6):429–434.

44. Savouret JF, Quesne M. Resveratrol and cancer: a review. *Biomed Pharmacother.* 2002;56(2): 84–87.

45. Pawlikowski M, Winczyk K, Karasek M. Oncostatic action of melatonin: facts and question marks. *Neuroendocrinol Lett.* 2002;23(suppl 1): 24–29.

46. Taguchi T, Furue H, Kimura T, et al. Results of phase III study of Lentinan [in Japanese]. *Gan To Kagaku Ryoho.* 1985;12(2):366–378.

47. Kaegi E. Unconventional therapies for cancer: 3. Iscador. *Can Med Assoc J.* 1998;158(7): 1157–1159.

48. Thomas R. *The Essiac Report: The True Story of a Canadian Herbal Cancer Remedy and of the Thousands of Lives it Continues to Save.* 3rd ed. Los Angeles: Alternative Treatment Information Network; 1993.

49. Tamayo C, Richardson MA, Diamond S, Skoda I. The chemistry and biological activity of herbs used in Flor-Essence herbal tonic and Essiac. *Phytother Res.* 2000;14(1):1–14.

50. Kaegi E. Unconventional therapies for cancer: 1. Essiac. The Task Force on Alternative Therapies of the Canadian Breast Cancer Research Initiative. *Can Med Assoc J.* 1998;158(7):897–902.

51. Kidd, P. The use of mushroom glucans and proteoglycans in cancer treatment. *Altern Med Rev.* 2000;5(1):4–27.

52. Han R. Recent progress of traditional Chinese medicine and herbal medicine for the treatment and prevention of cancer. *Chin J Integ Tradit West Med.* 1995;194:242–248.

53. Wang MY, Su C. Cancer preventive effect of *Morinda citrifolia* (noni). *Ann N Y Acad Sci.* 2001;952:161–168.

54. Dinnen RD, Ebisuzaki K. The search for novel anticancer agents: a differentiation-based assay and analysis of a folklore product. *Anticancer Res.* 1997;17(2A):1027–1033.

55. Riva L, Coradini D, Di Fronzo G, et al. The antiproliferative effects of *Uncaria tomentosa* extracts and fractions on the growth of breast cancer cell line. *Anticancer Res.* 2001;21(4A): 2457–2461.

56. Achterberg J, Lawlis GF. *Imagery of Cancer.* Chicago: Institute of Personality and Ability Test; 1978.

57. Spiegel D, Bloom JR, Kraemer HC, Gottheil E. Effect of psychosocial treatment on survival of patients with metastatic breast cancer. *Lancet.* 1989;2(8668):888–891.

58. Goodwin PJ, Leszcz M, Ennis M, et al. The effect of group psychosocial support on survival in metastatic breast cancer. *N Engl J Med.* 2001;345(24):1719–1726.

59. Newell SA, Sanson-Fisher RW, Savolainen NJ. Systematic review of psychological therapies for cancer patients: overview and recommendations for future research. *J Natl Cancer Inst.* 2002; 94(8):558–584.

60. Xu S, Liu Z, Xu M. Treatment of cancerous abdominal pain by acupuncture on zusanli (ST 36)—a report of 92 cases. *J Tradit Chin Med.* 1995;15(3):189–191.

61. Johnstone PA, Polston GR, Niemtzow RC, Martin PJ. Integration of acupuncture into the oncology clinic. *Palliat Med.* 2002;16(3):235–239.

62. Cunningham AJ, Edmonds CVI, Philllips C, et al. A prospective longitudinal study of the relationship of psychological work and change to duration of survival in patients with metastatic cancer. *Psychooncology.* 2000;9:323–339.

63. Green S. Antineoplastons. An unproved cancer therapy. *JAMA* 1992;267(21):2924–2928.

64. The American Cancer Society. Questionable methods of cancer management: Cancell/Entelev. *CA Cancer J Clin.* 1993;43(1):57–62.

65. Office of Technology Assessment of the US Congress. *Unconventional Cancer Therapies.* Washington, DC: Project Cure; 1989.

66. Unproven methods of cancer management: Hoxsey method. *CA Cancer J Clin.* 1990;40(1): 51–55.

67. Livingston-Wheeler VC. The role of nutrition in the immunotherapy of cancer. *J Intl Acad Prev Med.* 1979;52(2):54–75.

68. Kaegi E. Unconventional therapies for cancer: 6. 714X. *Can Med Assoc J.* 1998;158:1621–1624.

69. Landis SH, Murray T, Bolden S, et al. Cancer statistics, 1999. *CA Cancer J Clin.* 1999;29:8–31.

70. Davidson N, O'Neill A, Vukov A, et al. Effect of chemohormonal therapy in premenopausal node (+), receptor (+) breast cancer: an Eastern Cooperative Oncology Group phase III Intergroup trial (E5188, INT00101) [abstract 249]. *Proc Am Soc Clin Oncol.* 1999;18:67a.

71. Early Breast Cancer Trialists' Collaborative Group. Tamoxifen for early breast cancer: an overview of the randomized trials. *Lancet.* 1998;351: 1451–1467.

72. Iarussi D, Auricchio U, Agretto A, et al. Protective effect of coenzyme Q10 on anthracyclines cardiotoxicity: control study in children with acute lymphoblastic leukemia and non-Hodgkin lymphoma. *Mol Aspects Med.* 1994;15(suppl): s207–s212.

73. Judy WV, Hall JH, Dugan W, et al. Coenzyme Q10 reduction of Adriamycin cardiotoxicity. In: Folkers K, Yamamura Y, eds. *Biomedical and Clinical Aspects of Coenzyme Q.* Vol. 4. Amsterdam: Elsevier/North Holland Biomedical Press; 1984:231–241.

74. Labriola D, Livingston R. Possible interactions between dietary antioxidants and chemotherapy. *Oncology.* 1999;13(7):1003–1008.

75. Gressier B, Lebegue S, Brunet C, et al. Pro-oxidant properties of methotrexate: evaluation and prevention by an anti-oxidant drug. *Pharmazie.* 1994;49(9):679–681.

76. Mathijssen RHJ. Modulation of irinotecan (CPT-11) metabolism by St. John's wort in cancer patients [abstract 2443]. American Association for Cancer Research; 93rd Annual Meeting; April 8, 2002; San Francisco, CA.

77. Savarese D, Boucher J, Corey B. Glutamine treatment of paclitaxel-induced myalgias and arthralgias. *J Clin Oncol.* 1998;16(12):3918–3919.

78. Vahdat L, Papadopoulos K, Lange D, et al. Reduction of paclitaxel-induced peripheral neuropathy with glutamine. *Clin Cancer Res.* 2001; 7(5):1192–1197.

79. Chang R. Bioactive Polysaccharides from traditional Chinese medicine herbs as anticancer adjuvants. *J Altern Complement Med.* 2002;8(5): 559–565.

80. Cos S, Mediavilla MD, Fernandez R, et al. Does melatonin induce apoptosis in MCF-7 human breast cancer cells in vitro? *J Pineal Res.* 2002; 32(2):90–96.

81. Lissoni P, Tancini G, Barni S, et al. Treatment of cancer chemotherapy-induced toxicity with the pineal hormone melatonin. *Support Care Cancer.* 1997;5:126–129.

82. Ernst E, Pittler MH. Efficacy of ginger for nausea and vomiting: a systematic review of randomized clinical trials. *Br J Anaesth.* 2000;84(3):367–371.

83. Curran WJ. Radiation-induced toxicities: the role of radioprotectants. *Semin Radiat Oncol.* 1998;8(4 suppl 1):2–4.

84. Kishi K, Petersen S, Petersen C, et al. Preferential enhancement of tumor radioresponse by a cyclooxygenase-2 inhibitor. *Cancer Res.* 2000; 60(5):1326–1331.

85. Howe LR, Subbaramaiah K, Brown AM, Dannenberg AJ. Cyclooxygenase-2: a target for the prevention and treatment of breast cancer. *Endocr Relat Cancer.* 2001;8(2):97–114.

86. Pugliese PT, Jordan K, Cederberg H, Brohult J. Some biological actions of alkylglycerols from shark liver oil. *J Altern Complement Med.* 1998; 4(1):87–99.

87. Weitzner MA, Moncello J, Jacobsen PB, Minton S. A pilot trial of paroxetine for the treatment of hot flashes and associated symptoms in women with breast cancer. *J Pain Symptom Manage.* 2002;23(4):337–345.

88. Chlebowski RT. Breast cancer risk reduction: strategies for women at increased risk. *Annu Rev Med.* 2002;53:519–540.

89. McIntyre BS, Briski KP, Gapor A, Sylvester PW. Antiproliferative and apoptotic effects of tocopherols and tocotrienols on preneoplastic and neoplastic mouse mammary epithelial cells. *Proc Soc Exp Biol Med.* 2000;224(4):292–301.

90. Bortman P, Folgueira MA, Katayama ML, Snitcovsky IM, Brentani MM. Antiproliferative effects of 1,25-dihydroxyvitamin D_3 on breast cells: a mini review. *Braz J Med Biol Res.* 2002;35(1):1–9.

91. Shamsuddin AM, Vucenik I. Mammary tumor inhibition by IP6: a review. *Anticancer Res.* 1999; 19(5A):3671–3674.

92. McDougal A, Gupta MS, Morrow D, et al. Methyl-substituted diindolylmethanes as inhibitors of estrogen-induced growth of T47D cells and mammary tumors in rats. *Breast Cancer Res Treat.* 2001;66(2):147–157.

93. Meng Q, Goldberg ID, Rosen EM, Fan S. Inhibitory effects of indole-3-carbinol on invasion and migration in human breast cancer cells. *Breast Cancer Res Treat.* 2000;3(2):147–152.

94. Curley RW Jr, Humphries KA, Koolemans-Beynan A, Abou-Issa H, Webb TE. Activity of D-glucarate analogues: synergistic antiproliferative effects with retinoid in cultured human mammary tumor cells appear to specifically require the D-glucarate structure. *Life Sci.* 1994;54(18): 1299–1303.

95. Augustin LS, Dal Maso L, La Vecchia C, et al. Dietary glycemic index and glycemic load, and breast cancer risk: a case-control study. *Ann Oncol.* 2001;12(11):1533–1538.

96. Depypere HT, Bracke ME, Boterberg T, et al. Inhibition of tamoxifen's therapeutic benefit by tangeretin in mammary cancer. *Eur J Cancer.* 2000;36(suppl 4):S73.

97. Barton DL, Loprinzi CL, Quella SK, et al. Prospective evaluation of vitamin E for hot flashes in breast cancer survivors. *J Clin Oncol.* 1998;16(2): 495–500.

98. Guttuso TJ Jr. Gabapentin's effects on hot flashes and hypothermia. *Neurology.* 2000;54(11): 2161–2163.

99. Towlerton G, Filshie J, O'Brien M, Duncan A. Acupuncture in the control of vasomotor symptoms caused by tamoxifen. *Palliat Med.* 1999; 13(5):445.

100. Singletary KW, Gapstur SM. Alcohol and breast cancer: review of epidemiologic and experimental evidence and potential mechanisms. *JAMA.* 2001;286(17):2143–2151.

101. Outwater JL, Nicholson A, Barnard N. Dairy products and breast cancer: the IGF-I, estrogen, and bGH hypothesis. *Med Hypotheses.* 1997;48(6): 453–461.

102. Augustin LS, Dal Maso L, La Vecchia C, et al. Dietary glycemic index and glycemic load, and breast cancer risk: a case-control study. *Ann Oncol.* 2001;12(11):1533–1538.

103. Meyer F, Bairati I, Shadmani R, Fradet Y, Moore L. Dietary fat and prostate cancer survival. *Cancer Causes Control.* 1999;10(4):245–251.

104. Bingham SA. High-meat diets and cancer risk. *Proc Nutr Soc.* 1999;58(2):243–248.

105. Doerge DR, Sheehan DM. Goitrogenic and estrogenic activity of soy isoflavones. *Environ Health Perspect.* 2002;110(suppl 3):349–353.

106. Stark A, Madar Z. Phytoestrogens: a review of recent findings. *J Pediatr Endocrinol Metab.* 2002;15(5):561–572.

107. Burdette JE, Liu J, Lantvit D, et al. *Trifolium pratense* (red clover) exhibits estrogenic effects in vivo in ovariectomized Sprague-Dawley rats. *J Nutr.* 2002;132(1):27–30.

108. Liu J, Burdette JE, Xu H, et al. Evaluation of estrogenic activity of plant extracts for the potential treatment of menopausal symptoms. *J Agric Food Chem.* 2001;49(5):2472–2479.

109. Milligan S, Kalita J, Pocock V, et al. Oestrogenic activity of the hop phyto-oestrogen, 8-prenylnaringenin. *Reproduction.* 2002;123(2):235–242.

110. Punnonen R, Lukola A. Oestrogen-like effect of ginseng. *Br Med J.* 1980;281(6248):1110.

111. Duda RB, Taback B, Kessel B, et al. pS2 expression induced by American ginseng in MCF-7 breast cancer cells. *Ann Surg Oncol.* 1996;3(6):515–520.

112. Tamir S, Eizenberg M, Somjen D, Izrael S, Vaya J. Estrogen-like activity of glabrene and other constituents isolated from licorice root. *J Steroid Biochem Mol Biol.* 2001;78(3):291–298.

113. Labrie F, Luu-The V, Labrie C, Simard J. DHEA and its transformation into androgens and estrogens in peripheral target tissues: intracrinology. *Front Neuroendocrinol.* 2001;22(3):185–212.

114. Sheng MH, Taper LJ, Veit H, Qian H, Ritchey SJ, Lau KH. Dietary boron supplementation enhanced the action of estrogen, but not that of parathyroid hormone, to improve trabecular bone quality in ovariectomized rats. *Biol Trace Elem Res.* 2001;82(1–3):109–123.

CHAPTER 24

Integrative Approach to Osteoporosis

GEORGE KESSLER

---

*"Anyone can find disease; it is the job of the physician
to find health."*

—ANDREW STILL, FOUNDER OF OSTEOPATHIC MEDICINE

Osteoporosis is a condition characterized by compromised strength of the bone, which predisposes the bone to an increased risk of fracture. Because the major morbidities and mortality of this disease are related to bone phenomena, it is typically thought of as a disease of the bone. In part, this notion has been fostered by numerous reports on increased morbidity with respect to hip fractures. A more integrative view of osteoporosis, however, frames osteoporosis as a manifestation of an integrated disorder of metabolism in conjunction with influence from one's lifestyle rather than solely a disease of the bones. Even when osteoporosis is present, the bones are correctly performing the tasks they are directed to do by the messages and instructions they receive from the rest of the body.

The bones provide structural support, facilitate self-propelled locomotion, and stimulate and direct the growth and formation of mus-

cle, nerve, and blood vessels during embryonic development. However, perhaps the most important function of the bones is to act as a reservoir for essential nutrients of the body (absorbing, storing, and releasing these nutrients as directed by the whole body). It follows then that osteoporosis is a consequence of the bones having responded properly to systemic demands for nutrients at the expense of their own long-term health and integrity. The implication of this perspective brings new imperatives in assessing the nutritional status of those with osteoporosis or those at risk for it. Thus, the integrative approach to osteoporosis seeks to restore the adequate nutritional reserves and the proper homeodynamic balance between bone and other body systems to promote general health. This larger perspective involves the health of the digestive tract, the endocrine system, and the mind and spirit in the overall treatment strategy.

▶ PATHOPHYSIOLOGY

The average life cycle of normal bone is approximately 200 days. During this cycle, both formation and resorption occur. This process of continuous bone remodeling occurs at all stages in life.[1] The remodeling cycle begins with differentiation and activation of osteoclasts.[2] The osteoclast is a multinucleated giant cell derived from hematopoietic monocytes. These cells lay down an acidic environment on the bone surface allowing proteolytic enzyme activities to degrade the bone matrix. Osteoclasts are activated by any number of local and systemic factors, including macrophage colony-stimulating factors, cytokines, calcitrophic hormones, prostaglandin E_2, 1,25-dihydroxyvitamin D, mechanical forces or microfractures, and many others.[3] Osteoclasts do not appear to have receptors for parathyroid hormone (PTH) and vitamin D.

The osteoblast arises from mesenchymal stem cells in the bone marrow. These cells differentiate to carry PTH, estrogen, and vitamin D receptors, and express bone matrix genes, including type I collagen, osteocalcin, and bone-specific alkaline phosphatase.[4] These cells line the surface of bone for the purpose of laying down new uncalcified bone using the nutrient available to them. Osteoblasts are affected by local and systematic factors, including the following:

- Skeletal growth factor
- Insulin-like growth factors I and II
- Fibroblast growth factor
- Platelet-derived growth factor
- Bone morphogenetic proteins
- Hematopoietic factors
- Transforming growth factor
- Acidic and basic fibroblast growth factors
- Interleukins-1, -3, and -6
- Granulocyte colony-stimulating factors
- Granulocyte-macrophage colony-stimulating factors

The osteocyte is an osteoblast that was trapped and embedded within the bone during the re-modeling process. These cells play a role in mobilizing minerals to move in and out of the bone.

Cortical bone makes up approximately 80% of the skeletal mass and trabecular bone makes up approximately 20%.[5] Cortical bone is remodeled from within and trabecular bone remodeling occurs on the surface. Cortical bone's turnover state is as high as 5% per year at age 2 years and declines to 2% per year in the elderly (over age 60). Trabecular bone, because of its large surface-to-volume ratio, has a yearly turnover rate 5–10 times higher than that of cortical bone.[6,7] This is why trabecular bone is lost more rapidly during osteoporosis.[6]

Osteoporosis develops either because the individual failed to reach peak bone density by age 30 years or because resorption exceeded formation from any cause at any age. Hormone imbalance and menopause can exaggerate this process of increased resorption and decreased formation.[8-16]

At every stage of life, the balance of formation to resorption is affected by local and systemic signals. When minerals are needed in areas of the body other than bone, remodeling will be stimulated, which should stimulate formation of new bone. In a perfect situation, the ratio of formation would equal resorption. In childhood, we accept that formation outpaces resorption.

Presently, we see four phases of bone formation. Table 24–1 outlines these stages. We have always accepted this as normal, just as

▶ **TABLE 24–1** PHASES OF BONE FORMATION

	Age (yr)	Formation	Resorption
Phase I	0–20	≠ ≠ ≠	≠
Phase II	20–30	≠ ≠	≠
Phase III	35–50	≠	≠ ≠
Phase IV	60+	≠	≠ ≠ ≠

we accept other chronic diseases as a normal part of aging. However, although menopause and increased bone turnover may be a normal part of the life cycle, the hormone imbalance that contributes to bone loss in many patients is not.[17–20]

Bone loss is increased by estrogen or testosterone deficiency from any cause at any time.[21–29] Trabecular bone is affected 2.5 times more than cortical bone in the postmenopausal years.[30,31] Table 24–2 lists other signals typically contributing to bone loss or bone formation.

Osteoporosis can be defined either by pathological fracture or by score on a dual-energy x-ray absorptiometry (DEXA) scan of bone mineral density (BMD). The most usual fractures occur in the spinal vertebrae, the hip, and the radial bones. Osteoporotic fractures, however, can occur in any bone. When a patient presents with multiple fractures of any bones, over time, osteoporosis should be considered.

BMD is expressed as T score and Z score, representing the patient's bone density when compared to young controls and to age- and sex-matched controls. When resorption overtakes formation, net bone loss occurs. When this situation presents with a T score of less than −0.1, this is defined as osteopenia. When the T score is below −2.5, this is defined as osteoporosis.

▶ PREVALENCE

Gradual bone loss begins in both sexes between the ages of 30 and 40 years.[32] Based on the 2000 US Census, the National Osteoporosis Foundation estimates that more than 55% of Americans age 50 years or older either have osteoporosis or low bone mass. This figure is expected to rise approximately 15% by 2010. The number of people with osteoporosis is expected to rise 20% by 2010. Over an average lifetime, a woman loses 30–40% of her total bone mass. By age 80 years, many women have lost two-thirds of their skeletal bone mass.[33]

It is estimated that 30% of 50-year-old women already have osteoporosis. At age 65 years, 50% of women and 20% of men already have osteoporosis, and by age 75 years, 70% of men and women will have osteoporosis.[34]

The cost of osteoporosis to society is staggering. The costs represent dollars spent and human or quality of life costs. In the United States, approximately 15 billion dollars is spent annually for treatment of osteoporosis factors. Approximately 1 million Americans will suffer fractures each year. There will be an estimated 250,000 hip fractures in women, 500,000 vertebral fractures in women, and 250,000 fractures in men.[35]

Approximately 25% of patients who fracture a hip will die within 1 year of that fracture. Up to a third of patients who fracture a hip will require nursing home care in which the average length of stay is 7 years. Up to 67% of patients who experience a fracture will not regain their prefracture level of function.[36]

In people younger than age 55 years, men are more likely to have a hip fracture than women. However, the average American woman loses approximately 1–2% of her cortical bone per year after the age of 40–50 years. Three to

▶ **TABLE 24–2** SIGNALS FOR BONE FORMATION/ABSORPTION

Local Signals	Systematic Signals
Insulin-like growth factor	Calcitonin
β_2-Microglobulin	Parathyroid hormone
Transferring growth factor	Insulin
Fibroblast growth factor	Growth hormone
Platelet-derived growth factor	Steroid hormones
Tumor necrosis factor	Calcitrol
Prostaglandin	Glucocorticoids
Inteferons	Sex hormones
Interleukins-1 and -6	Thyroid hormones
	Prostaglandin

seven times more bone is lost the first 7 to 10 years after the onset of menopause.[37] Thus in those over 55, women are at much greater risk of significant fractures than are men.

The burden of osteoporosis in men is not widely discussed, but is nevertheless significant. Osteoporosis begins 5 to 10 years later in men than in women. It is estimated that 20% of 65-year-old men already have osteoporosis.[38] The probability that a 50-year-old man will have a hip fracture is approximately 5–6%. However, approximately 25% of men older than age 60 years will have an osteoporotic hip fracture.[39] Approximately 33% of all hip fractures and 20% of vertebral fractures occur in men[40]; the lower frequency of these fractures in men is thought to be because men in general have more muscles and bigger bones than women. Mortality from fracture is higher in men.[41,42] If fracture is the benchmark for the risk of os-

teoporosis, then the lifetime risk for men is 13–25% as compared to 50% in women.[43]

There are many risk factors associated with the development of osteoporosis. Risk results from issues in our past and in our present lives including genetics, lifestyle choices, medications, diseases, and others. Tables 24–3 and 24–4 outline some of these risk factors.

Inadequate nutrition is obviously an important risk factor for poor bone health as well. The General American Diet (especially in childhood) consists of highly processed food rich in saturated fats, salt, carbohydrates, and refined sugars, and low in whole grains, fruits, vegetables, and fibers. Only approximately 25% of boys and 10% of girls ages 9–17 years are getting adequate calcium in their diet. The foods we eat contain environmental pollutants, antibodies, hormones, and other things, which have an adverse affect on our bones.

▶ **TABLE 24–3** SELECTED RISK FACTORS FOR OSTEOPOROSIS[44–64]

Risk Factor	Comments
Ethnicity	↑ in whites and Hispanics
Size of frame	Petiteness is a risk factor
Age	
Gender	Females greater than males
Early menopause	Primary or secondary
Multiple pregnancies	Nutrients prioritized to the baby
Breast-feeding	Nutrients prioritized to the baby
Hypogonadism	Hormone imbalances
Hypercortisolism	↓ collagen synthesis, ↓ intestinal absorption of calcium, corticosteroid induced, osteoporosis is greater during the first 6–12 months of exogenous use (especially in children).
Hyperthyroid	Thyroid hormone directly ↑ bone resorption and affects calcium metabolism in the bone
Hyperparathyroid	Interferes with bone function and resorption
Diabetes mellitus	Results in ↓ formation
Connective tissue disorder	Abnormal collagen metabolism
Tobacco use	Causes ↑ estrogen metabolism, ↓ O_2; creates free radicals Smokers bone density averages 20–30% lower than that of nonsmokers; up to 20% of all hip fractures are attributed to smoking
Exercise/immobility	Lack of childhood exercise or sedentary adult life style
Associated diseases	Scoliosis, cirrhosis, chronic obstructive pulmonary disease, kidney stones (especially calcium), surgical excision of part of stomach or small bowel, irritable bowel syndrome

▶ **TABLE 24-4** NUTRITIONAL RISK FACTORS FOR BONE LOSS

Caffeine	1 cup of brewed coffee takes 40 mg of calcium out of the bones
Protein (excess)	1 oz animal protein requires 25 mg of calcium to buffer the acid it is metabolized into
Soda	Interferes with calcium/phosphorous balance
	Phosphorus binds with calcium, leaving the calcium unavailable to the body. This results in calcium being drawn from the bones to meet the body's demands
Sugar	↓ absorption of calcium and magnesium and ≠ renal excretion of calcium and magnesium
Salt	Increased calcium excretion; 500 oz of salt results in 10 oz of calcium being lost
Malnutrition	Lack of raw materials to make and support bone; poor diet, any disease of malabsorption, eating disorder, poor quality of nutrients
Alcohol consumption	Interferes with calcium absorption and is toxic to osteoblasts

▶ Case Example: Osteoporosis

Emily, a 39-year-old white female is 157.5 cm (5′2″) tall and weighs 49.9 kg (110 lb). She is a high-powered executive who is driven to be #1. Her work week is about 60 hours long. She works out very hard 5 mornings a week and she eats a good breakfast on the 2 days that she doesn't work out. Lunch is a sandwich on the run at her desk 5 days a week. Emily orders out for dinner (unless she has a business dinner) and eats before she "crashes." Emily takes a multivitamin and calcium 1,000 mg/d. Her menstrual cycle has been irregular for 3 years. Emily recently took her first DEXA scan because her mother, who has osteoporosis, kept insisting that she should know her bone density. The DEXA scan revealed significant osteopenia of the spine and hip.

Conventional Treatment Approach

Conventional therapy begins with patients being told to take calcium and vitamin D. Exercise is generally recommended to stimulate bone growth. The mainstay of therapy in most cases is antiresorptive medications. Didronel (etidronate) is an older and less-used medication. The newer bisphosphonates are Fosamax (alendronate) and Actonel (risedronate). Miacalcin (calcitonin) nasal spray can be effective. Aredia, an intravenous medication (pamidronate disodium), also has antiresorptive properties. Because it is given intravenously, it can be used when oral medications cannot be used. It can also be used when rapid onset of action and aggressive therapy is needed. PTH, given by injection, is a newly available agent that can stimulate bone growth. Rocaltrol (calcitriol), a vitamin D analogue, can be used to increase absorption of calcium through the gut. This is especially useful in patients who cannot tolerate higher doses of oral calcium, or who have hypocalcemia from other causes.

Estrogen is frequently prescribed at or around menopause. Serum estrogen receptor modulators (SERMS) are also prescribed. SERMS are estrogen agonists and antagonists that can stimulate bone growth while decreasing the risk of breast cancer. Recent concerns regarding the potential for increased breast cancer risk with the use of certain estrogens have called into question the safety of this approach, at least when the combination of Premarin and Provera is used.

Thiazide diuretics are useful in high-turnover osteoporosis with hypercalciuria and secondary hyperparathyroidism.

Less-studied and less-recommended substances include anabolic steroids, and the statin drugs, which seem to stimulate bone growth. Human growth hormone is being studied as well, with mixed results to date. Treatment of osteoporosis specifically in men has been much less studied than in women. The therapies in men should be geared at recreating homeostatic balance as we do in women.

Integrative Medicine Approach

One reason that the epidemic of osteoporosis is growing is that many women now are never achieving an optimal peak bone mass. The causes of this are multifactorial and, among others, include the poor American diet, a sedentary lifestyle, an inability to manage stress, and environmental factors such as the use of pesticide, antibiotics, hormones in our food chain, and other toxic substances in our water, air, soil, and food supply. In viewing osteoporosis as the result of disease in the homeodynamic mechanism, our treatment goal should be to recreate balance and health in the person. We need to do more than just stimulate bone formation or to slow resorption. We can and should be very specific to the patient's individual needs.

The first step in developing an individualized treatment approach is to go beyond simple recommendations based only on the T and Z score of an individual. We must also know the patient's ability to form bone and the rate at which bone resorption takes place. By knowing whether formation needs to be increased, resorption slowed, or both, we can develop a plan to address the specific needs of a patient.

By measuring the products of formation and resorption and knowing the T score, we now have a general idea of the scope of the patient's problem. To get more specific as to the source of the patient's problem, we should assess hormone levels (individual and in relation to each other), nutrients available and our ability to absorb and use them, and other factors that affect the patient's ability to form and keep bone. By knowing the specifics of the individual patient, we can then tailor a diet and nutrients, exercise, hormone, and stress control plan to address the needs and imbalances found.

Laboratory Testing

There are a number of laboratory tests that can be helpful in developing a more individualized treatment approach to osteoporosis. Laboratory tests, like imaging studies, are objective measures of bone metabolism and risk factors contributing to osteoporosis.

There are tests specific to bone metabolism, such as the markers that measure for products of bone resorption and bone formation. These are listed in Table 24–5. Table 24–6 lists other laboratory measurements and nutrients of substances that do not directly measure bone formation or resorption, but that can have a direct or indirect effect on these processes.

Nutritional Approaches

The raw materials needed to carry out our cellular functions come from outside our body. If the raw materials are not at hand when the demand for them is made, we can only turn to our stored nutrients. If they are not available, then we will sacrifice other, less-essential, sources of the material so that the more essential functions can be maintained. The generalized adaptation syndrome, or the stress response, is an example of this type of process. When stress is chronic, we need a constant supply of nutrients to feed the demand placed on our bodies. If the exogenous supply is inadequate, we will turn to the internal stores for our needs. If our ready stores are being de-

▶ **TABLE 24-5** LABORATORY TESTING FOR OSTEOPOROSIS[65-84]

Bone Resorption Urine	Serum
24-Hour calcium	Plasma tartrate-resistant acid phosphatase
Hydroxyproline	
Hydroxylysine	
Pyridinoline	
Deoxypyridinoline	
N-telopeptide of cross-linked type I collagen	

Bone Formation Serum
Serum alkaline phosphatase
Serum bone-specific alkaline phosphatase
Procollagen I extension peptides
Osteocalcin

pleted, we will then sacrifice less-essential functions to fuel more essential ones.

Calcium is the most abundant mineral in the body and 98% of it is found in the bones. Of the total bone mass, 20% is calcium. Seventy-five percent of Americans are deficient in calcium, and an average 50-year-old American gets less than 50% of what he or she needs.[85] If calcium intake is inadequate, the body will turn to the reservoir of calcium in the bones to find what it needs. Table 24–7 lists the FDA's daily calcium recommendations,[86,87] and Table 24–8 lists food sources of calcium.

▶ **TABLE 24-6** LABORATORY MARKERS INFLUENCING BONE FORMATION AND RESORPTION

Hormonal Markers	Other
Estrogen	Serum calcium
Progesterone	Serum PO_4
Testosterone	Urinary magnesium (24-hour)
Cortisol	Red blood cell magnesium
Estradiol	Liver function tests
Estriol	Complete blood cell count
Estrone	Urinalysis
2-Hydroxyestrone	Cholesterol
16-α Hydroxyestrone	Triglycerides/high-density lipoprotein/low-density
Parathyroid hormone	lipoprotein
Insulin	Thyroid antibodies
Thyroid-stimulating hormone	
Follicle-stimulating hormone	
Luteinizing hormone	
Dehydroepiandrosterone	

▶ **TABLE 24-7** RECOMMENDED DAILY
CALCIUM INTAKE

Age (yr)	Calcium Needed (mg)
1–3	500
4–8	800
9–18	1,300
19–50	1,000
51+	1,200

There are an endless number of calcium supplements and fortified foods available in the marketplace. However, calcium intake per se is only one aspect of preventing and/or treating osteoporosis. Calcium can only be absorbed in an acidic environment. Many patients have low stomach acid, and by age 60 years approximately 40% are deficient enough to alter calcium absorption. This is complicated by the intake of a large number of substances that either increase calcium excretion or decrease calcium absorption or both.

Another important factor is that calcium cannot be absorbed into the bone or bind to the collagen matrix without a host of other nutrients already present and in proper proportions,[85] including vitamin D, magnesium, copper, and boron. Supplementing these other nutrients can be a critical part of the integrative treatment program.

Medications can also exert a significant influence on bone metabolism, as outlined in Table 24–9. Identifying the use of medications that have a negative impact on bone density and finding other effective approaches to replace these can have a significant impact on treatment.

Probably the most important nutritional factors after calcium are vitamin D and magnesium. Half of all magnesium in the body is found in the bones. Fifty percent or more of women older than age 40 years are lacking adequate magnesium in their diet[88]; furthermore, by age 70 years, absorption of magnesium in the gastrointestinal tract has decreased to less than a third of what is absorbed in young adults (up to age 30).[89] Boron also plays an important role, and can increase calcium and magnesium absorption in the bowel and lower excretion through the kidney. Boron activates estrogen and other hormones and helps to activate vitamin D.[90] Copper slows bone resorption and is needed in order for two collagen molecules to bind together.[91-94]

Folic acid, manganese, selenium, silicon, strontium, pyridoxine (B$_6$), vitamin B$_{12}$, vita-

▶ **TABLE 24-8** SOME FOODS RICH IN CALCIUM

Food	Available Calcium (mg)	Food	Available Calcium (mg)
Yogurt (8 oz.)	345	Collards, frozen (0.5 cup)	179
Lowfat milk (1 cup)	300	Spinach (0.5 cup)	138
Lowfat chocolate milk (1 cup)	285	Tofu (120 g)	133
Swiss cheese (1 oz.)	272	White beans (0.5 cup)	96
Provolone cheese (1 oz.)	214	Kale, frozen (0.5 cup)	90
Cheddar cheese (1 oz.)	204	Large orange	72
Cheese pizza slice	117	Broccoli, frozen (0.5 cup)	47
Oatmeal with milk	313	Sardines (3 oz.)	325
Cereal* with milk	250	Canned salmon (3 oz.)	181
Cornbread (1 pc.)	162	Atlantic perch (3 oz.)	116
Pancakes, butter	128	Halibut (half fillet)	95

*These may vary widely; check the label.

▶ **TABLE 24-9** INFLUENCE OF SELECTED MEDICATIONS ON CALCIUM METABOLISM

Steroids	≠ resorption, ↓ formation, ↓ intestinal absorption of calcium, ≠ renal excretion of calcium, ↓ gonadal function
Thyroid	Stimulates resorption
Heparin	Inhibits vitamin K, prevents osteocalcin metabolism
Anticoagulants	Reduced vitamin D levels, secondary hyperparathyroidism, ↓ intestinal calcium transport, ↓ osteoblast function
Antacids (especially with aluminum)	↓ stomach acid, interfere with absorption of calcium
Long-term antibiotic	↓ intestinal absorption of nutrients

min E with tocotrienols, vitamin C, zinc, and vitamin K, among others, are also needed for bones to be healthy. All of these nutrients are found in healthy bone in varying amounts and all play a role in bone metabolism. Vitamin C is needed to form and repair cartilage, collagen, and other organic components of bone; it also increases calcium absorption. Vitamin K activates osteocalcin, which is needed to form new bone. Studies show that women who take vitamin K 100 mg/d have one third fewer fractures than those who do not use it.[95-98]

If we are healthy at a very young age, then we should be able to get the nutrients we need just from food. If, however, we are less than healthy, we may not be able to eat enough to catch up and supplements may be needed until our intake meets our demands. It is unlikely that we will get children to eat sardines, kale, turnip greens, and okra for dinner. Children, however, can be helped with other easy meth-

ods. One study of identical twins ages 6–14 years showed that twins given calcium 1,800 mg/d at puberty had 5% denser bones than did twins given 900 mg/d. That 5% increase translates into a 40% drop in fracture risk later in life.[99]

Table 24–10 provides a complete set of recommendations for nutritional supplementation to promote healthy bone formation.

Hormone Replacement

Progesterone and testosterone are potent stimulators of bone formation and, to a lesser extent, slow bone resorption. DHEA also significantly stimulates bone formation where estrogen has a more potent effect on bone resorption than on formation.[100-110] Endogenous cortisol has similar effects on our bones as exogenous cortisol. Cortisol interferes with calcium absorption and promotes calcium excretion, which results in bone loss. Excess cortisol also causes a decrease

▶ **TABLE 24-10** DAILY DOSE OF NUTRITIONAL SUPPLEMENTS TO PREVENT AND REVERSE OSTEOPOROSIS

Calcium	1,200–1,500 mg	Boron	3–12 mg
Folic acid	400 μg	Copper	25–50 mg
Pyridoxine	25 mg	Magnesium	600–1,000 mg
Vitamin B$_{12}$	1,000 μg	Manganese	5–10 mg
Vitamin C	1,000 mg	Selenium	200 μg
Vitamin D	400–800 IU	Zinc	50–100 mg
Vitamin K	100–300 μg	Strontium	0.5–3 mg
Silicon	1–2 mg		

in gonadal functions and a decrease in bone formation.

Hormones are important individually but their proper balance with each other is crucial. This is why the widespread use of hormones in meat and dairy food production is of such significant concern. Estrogen dominance—perhaps related in part to the estrogens being artificially added to our food supply—is a major health problem in the United States, and it is one reason why so many of our young women have low bone density and other problems. Tables 24–11 through 24–14 outline some of the signs and symptoms that can alert the clinician to a subtle hormonal imbalance, which may need treatment as part of preventing or reversing bone loss.

The relative risks and benefits of using synthetic hormones, which are chemically and structurally unrelated to our natural hormones, versus natural hormones, which are closely related to our circulating hormones, need further study. Recent data from the Women's Health Initiative study has raised concerns about the role of the combination of Premarin and Provera (Prempro) in increasing women's risk of breast cancer. Whether or not the "bioidentical" hormones currently being recommended by some integrative practitioners for osteoporosis prevention and treatment convey a similarly increased risk of breast cancer is unknown at this point. A number of supplements other than estrogens are used as "hormone replacement therapy" in the integrative model, with the goal being to restore the age-appropriate physiological level of all systematic hormones from cholesterol to cortisol.

In addition to hormones, natural or synthetic, there are many plants that have hormone-like properties, including foods such as yams with its progesterone-like properties and soy with its estrogen-like properties.[107-110] Soy and its derivative isoflavones, including genistein, daidzein, and ipriflavone, have direct effects on bone density.[111-119] The soy isoflavones also have adaptogenic effects on

▶ **TABLE 24–11** SYMPTOMS OF ESTROGEN IMBALANCE

Estrogen Deficiency	Estrogen Excess
Vaginal dryness	Foggy thinking
Night sweats	Gallbladder problems
Bladder infections	Weepiness
Incontinence	Fibrocystic breast
Sleep disturbance	Water retention (hips)
Painful intercourse	Puffiness and bloating
Memory problems	Breast tenderness
Hot flashes	Rapid weight gain (hips)
Lethargic depression/tearful	Mood swings (PMS)
Foggy thinking	Heavy menstrual bleeding
Bone loss	Anxiety/depression/irritable
Palpitations	Migraine headaches
	Cervical dysplasia (abnormal PAP smear)
	Fibroids
	Red flush on face
	Insomnia

Estrogen Dominance
Combination of symptoms in estrogen excess and progesterone deficiency

▶ **TABLE 24–12** SYMPTOMS OF ANDROGEN IMBALANCE

Androgen Deficiency	Androgen Excess
Decreased libido	Acne
Fatigue	Polycystic ovary
Depression	syndrome
Sleep disturbances	Excessive hair on
Bone loss	face and arms
Decreased muscle	Ovarian cysts
mass	Hypoglycemia or
Vaginal dryness	unstable sugar
Foggy thinking/	Midcycle pain
memory lapses	Infertility
Aches and pain	
Incontinence	
Thinning skin	

estrogen receptors and can act as estrogen agonists or antagonists.[120–125] The isoflavones show promise for treatment and prevention of osteoporosis, although there remains some the-

▶ **TABLE 24–13** SYMPTOMS OF PROGESTERONE IMBALANCE

Progesterone Deficiency	Excess Progesterone
PMS	Breast swelling/
Insomnia	tenderness
Early miscarriage	Mild depression
Vaginal dryness	Decreased libido
Unexplained weight	Yeast infection
gain	
Foggy thinking	
Water retention	
Early bone loss	
Memory lapses	
Hot flashes	
Incontinence	
Anxiety	
Heart palpitations	
Painful and/or	
lumpy breasts	
Tearful	
Cyclical headaches	
Infertility	

▶ **TABLE 24–14** SYMPTOMS OF CORTISOL IMBALANCE

Cortisol Deficiency	Cortisol Excess
Debilitating fatigue	Sleep disturbance
Sugar craving	Fatigue
Unstable blood	Depression
sugar	Thinning skin
Allergies	Bone loss
Chemical sensitivity	Decreased
muscle	
Stress	mass
Foggy thinking	
Low blood pressure	
Thin and/or dry	
skin	
Intolerance to	
exercise	
Brown spots on	
face	
Cold body	
temperature	
Palpitations	
Aches and pains	

oretical concern about their impact on breast tissue.

Mind–Body Approaches

Although no studies have specifically examined the role of mind–body approaches in osteoporosis, it is reasonable to assume, based on what we know of psychoneuroimmunology and the intracellular signaling systems associated with chronic stress, that these therapies can most likely affect the balance between bone formation and bone resorption. Balancing of stress hormones such as cortisol and dehydroepiandrosterone can directly affect bone health. As discussed earlier, levels of our sex hormones, which can be affected by cortisol levels and other mediators of stress, also directly affect bone health.

Exercise

Weight-bearing exercises such as weight lifting, jogging, swimming, jumping rope, exercise with Thera-Band, and Cybex-type machines can directly stimulate bone growth.[126–135] Activities such as yoga and Qigong combine both meditation and resistance exercise. Exercise recommendations must be tailored to an individual's needs and abilities, keeping in mind other coexisting medical conditions. If indicated by a BMD scan showing differential bone loss in the spine, hip, or elsewhere, an exercise program can be designed specifically to emphasize one or another area of the body. In general, the more large muscle groups regularly involved in the exercise program, the more effective the program will be in building bone. Specific exercise approaches to osteoporosis are discussed in detail in Chapter 13.

Manipulative Approaches

Although there are no specific studies demonstrating its efficacy, osteopathic manipulative therapy and other manipulative disciplines may have a role in treatment and prevention of osteoporosis.[137,138] By promoting proper alignment and structural integration, these therapies can lead to improved balance and proprioception. Via its effects on circulation and nervous system function, manipulative therapy, like Eastern medicine, ayurvedic medicine, and yoga, can be a powerful means of eliminating obstructions to the flow of nutrients and oxygen through blood, lymph, and interstitial fluids.

Environmental Strategies

Environmental strategies include efforts to clean our air, soil, water, and food chain. Removing random exogenous sources of pollutants, toxins, xenobiotics, antibiotics, nonhuman hormones, and other substances foreign to our natural bodily functions will reduce the risk of real or potential toxicity to our health.

Herbal Medicines

Herbs, per se, are not treatments for osteoporosis. There are herbs that can have a great effect on our bodies and help to eliminate conditions that promote osteoporosis. In particular, herbals can play an important role in maintaining normal digestive function, promoting healthy sleep, and managing excessive stress.

▶ Case Example: Osteoporosis Conclusion

Stress reduction is paramount for Emily; not only the emotional stress of having to be perfect in every area of her life, but also the physical stress of excessive exercise and severe work demands. Fueling her stress response requires nutrients she does not get in adequate amounts from her diet or from her supplements. Finding out if her menses are irregular because of ovarian failure or secondary to fueling the stress response is very important. Taking calcium 1,000 mg only helps her bones if it gets into and stays in the bones. Chronic stress is associated with bone loss for many reasons. By doing an adequate work-up, we can identify Emily's specific biochemical derangements and help to correct them. Her new stress-reduction program, exercise regimen, and diet will eventually be adequate to maintain health. Until then, supplementation with appropriate nutrients, herbs, and hormones—based on her unique history and biochemical/hormonal profile—may be helpful in beginning to restore both the health of her bones and her health overall. Specific therapy for specific needs is the key to success.

REFERENCES

1. Mirsky EC, Einhorn TA. Bone densitometry in orthopedic practice. *J Bone Joint Surg.* 1998;80A: 1687–1698.

2. Yoshida H, Hayashi S, Kunisada T, et al. The murine mutation osteoporosis is in the coding region of the macrophage colony stimulating factor gene. *Nature.* 1990;345:442–444.

3. Manolagas SC, Jilka RL. Bone marrow, cytokines, and bone remodeling: emerging insights into the pathophysiology of osteoporosis. *N Engl J Med.* 1995;332:305–311.

4. Recker RR, Davies MM, Hinders SM, et al. Bone gain in young adult women. *JAMA.* 1992;268: 2403–2408.

5. Gilsanz V, Boechat MI, Roe TF, Loro ML, Sayre JW, Goodman WG. Gender differences in vertebral body sizes in children and adolescents. *Radiology.* 1994;190:673–677.

6. Prior JC, Vigna YM, Schechter MT, et al. Spinal bone loss and ovulatory disturbances. *N Engl J Med.* 1990;323:1221–1227.

7. Riggs BL, Wahner W, Seeman E, et al. Changes in bone mineral density of the proximal femur and spine with aging: differences between the postmenopausal and senile osteoporosis syndromes. *J Clin Invest.* 1982;70:716–723.

8. Marshall D, Johnell O, Wdel H. Meta-analysis of how well measures of bone mineral density predict occurrence of osteoporotic fractures. *BMJ.* 1996;312:1254–1259.

9. Miller PD, Bonnick SL. Clinical application of bone density. In: Favus MJ, ed. *Primer on the Metabolic Bone Diseases and Disorders of Mineral Metabolism.* 4th ed. Philadelphia: Lippincott, Williams & Wilkins; 1999:152–159.

10. Nieves JW, Komar L, Cosman F, et al. Calcium potentiates the effect of estrogen and calcitonin on bone mass: Review and analysis. *Am J Clin Nutr.* 1998;67:18–24.

11. Pacifici R, Avioli L. Effects of aging on bone structure and metabolism. In: Avioli LV, ed. *The Osteoporotic Syndrome.* 4th ed. San Diego, CA: Academic Press; 2000:25–34.

12. US Congress Office of Technology Assessment. *Effectiveness and Costs of Osteoporosis Screening and Hormone Replacement Therapy,* Vol. II: *Evidence on Benefits, Risks, and Costs.* OTA-BP-H-144. Washington DC: US Government Printing Office; 1995.

13. Mirsky EC, Einhorn TA. Bone densitometry in orthopedic practice. *J Bone Joint Surg.* 1998;80A: 1687–1698.

14. Parfitt AM, Matthewa CHE, Villaneuva AR, et al. Relationships between surface, volume, and thickness of iliac trabecular bone in aging and in osteoporosis: implications for the micro anatomic and cellular mechanisms of bone. *J Clin Invest.* 1983;72:1396–1409.

15. Gilsanz V, Gibbens DT, Roe TF, et al. Vertebral bone density in children: effect of puberty. *Radiology.* 1988;166:847–850.

16. Bonjour JP, Theintz G, Buchs B, Slosman B, Rizzoli R. Critical years and stages of puberty for spinal and femoral bone mass accumulation during adolescence. *J Clin Endicrinol Metab.* 1991; 73:555–563.

17. Matkovic V, Jelic T, Wardla GM, et al. Timing of peak bone mass in Caucasian females and its implication for the prevention of osteoporosis. *J Clin Invest.* 1994;93:799–808.

18. Steiniche T, Eriksen EF. Age-related changes in bone remodeling. In: Orwell E, ed. *Osteoporosis in Men.* San Diego, CA: Academic Press; 1999: 299–312.

19. Cummings SR, Nevitt MC, Browner WS, et al. Risk factors for hip fracture in white women: study of Osteoporotic Fractures Research Group. *N Engl J Med.* 1995;332:767–773.

20. Hannan MT, Felson DT, Anderson JJ. Bone mineral density in elderly men and women: results from the Framingham osteoporosis study. *J Bone Miner Res.* 1992;7:547–553.

21. Katznelson L, Finkelstein JS, Schoenfeld DA, et al. Increase in bone density and lean body mass during testosterone administration in men with acquired hypogonadism. *J Clin Endocrinol Metab.* 1996;81:4385–4365.

22. Chapuy MC, Arlot ME, Duboef F, et al. Vitamin D3 and calcium to prevent hip fractures in elderly women. *N Engl J Med.* 1992;327: 1637–1642.

23. Finkelstein JS, Klibanski A, Neer RM, et al. Increases in bone density during the treatment of men with idiopathic hypogonadotropic hypogonadism. *J Clin Endocrinol Metab.* 1989;69: 776–783.

24. Finkelstein JS, Klibanski A, Neer RM, et al. Osteoporosis in men with idiopathic hypogonadotrophic hypogonadism. *Ann Intern Med.* 1987; 106:354–361.

25. Finkelstein JS, Klibanski A, Biller BMK, et al. Osteopenia in men with a history of delayed puberty. *N Engl J Med.* 1992;326:600–604.

26. Jackson JA, Riggs MW, Spiekerman AM. Testosterone deficiency as a risk factor for hip fracture in men: a case control study. *Am J Med Sci.* 1992; 304:4–8.

27. Gasperino J. Androgenic regulation of bone mass in women. *Clin Orthop.* 1995;311:278–286.

28. Murphy S, Khaw K, Cassidy A, et al. Sex hormones and bone mineral density in elderly men. *Bone and Mineral.* 1993;20:133–140.

29. Buchanan JR, Myers C, Lloyd T, et al. Determinants of peak trabecular bone density in women: the role of androgens, estrogen, and exercise. *J Bone Miner Res.* 1988;3:673–680.

30. Rockoff SD, Sweet E, Bleustein J. The relative contribution of trabecular and cortical bone to the strength of human lumbar vertebrae. *Calcif Tissue Res.* 1969;3:163–175.

31. Parfitt AM, Matthewa CHE, Villanueva AR, et al. Relationships between surface, volume, and thickness of iliac trabecular bone in aging and in osteoporosis: implications for the micro anatomic and cellular mechanisms of bone. *J Clin Invest.* 1983;72:1396–1409.

32. NIH Consensus Development Panel. Osteoporosis prevention, diagnosis, and therapy. *JAMA.* 2001;285:785–795.

33. NIH Consensus Development Panel. Osteoporosis prevention, diagnosis, and therapy. *JAMA.* 2001;285:785–786.

34. NIH Consensus Development Panel. Osteoporosis prevention, diagnosis, and therapy. *JAMA.* 2001;285:785–795.

35. NIH Consensus Development Panel. Osteoporosis prevention, diagnosis, and therapy. *JAMA.* 2001;285:785–795.

36. NIH Consensus Development Panel. Osteoporosis prevention, diagnosis, and therapy. *JAMA.* 2001;285:785–795.

37. Garnero P, Hausherr E, Chapuy M-C, et al. Markers of bone resorption predict hip fracture in elderly women: The EPIDOS prospective study. *J Bone Miner Res.* 1996;11:1531–1538.

38. Orwoll ES. Osteoporosis in men. *Endocrinol Metab Clin North Am.* 1998;27:349–367.

39. American Medical Association. *Managing Osteoporosis: Update in Pain Management.* Chicago: American Medical Association; 2001.

40. Eastell R, Boyle IT, Compston J. Management of male osteoporosis: report of the UK Consensus Group. *QJM.* 1988;91:71–92.

41. Davidson CW, Merrilees MJ, Wilkinson TJ, et al.

Hip fracture mortality and morbidity: can we do better? *N Z Med J.* 2001;114:329–332.

42. Center JR, Nguyen TV, Schneider D, et al. Mortality after all major types of osteoporotic fracture in men and women: an observational study. *Lancet.* 1999;353:878–882.

43. Looker AC, Orwoll ES, Johnston CC Jr, et al. Prevalence of low femoral bone density in older US adults from NHANES III. *J Bone Miner Res.* 1997;12:1761–1768.

44. Burger H, de Laet CE, van Daele PL, et al. Risk factors for increased bone loss in an elderly population: the Rotterdam Study. *Am J Epidemiol.* 1998;147:871–879.

45. Villa ML, Nelson L. Race ethnicity and osteoporosis. In: Feldman MR, Kesley J, eds. *Osteoporosis.* San Diego, CA: Academic Press; 1996: 435–444.

46. Aloia JF, Mikhail M, Pagan CD, Arunachalam A, Yeh JK, Flaster E. Biochemical and hormonal variables in black and white women matched for age. *J Lab Clin Med.* 1998;132:383–389.

47. Ross PD, Fujiwara S, Huang C, et al. Vertebral fracture prevalence in women in Hiroshima compared to Caucasians or Japanese in the US. *Int J Epidemiol.* 1995;24:1171–1177.

48. Guzman B. The Hispanic population 2000. Census 2000 brief. US Dept. of Commerce, Economics, and Statistics Administration, US Census Bureau; 2001. Available at: http://www.census.gov/prod/2001pubs/c2kbr01-3.pdf-. Accessed October 15, 2002.

49. Barnes JS, Bennett CE. The Asian population: 2000. Census 2000 brief. US Dept. of Commerce, Economics, and Statistics Administration, US Census Bureau; 2002. Available at: http://www.census.gov/prod/2002pubs/c2kbr01-16.pdf-. Accessed October 15, 2002.

50. Ward KD, Klesges RC. A meta-analysis of the effects of cigarette smoking on bone mineral density. *Calcif Tissue Int.* 2001;68:259–270.

51. Booth F, Gordon SE, Carlson CJ, Hamilton MT. Waging war on modern chronic diseases: primary prevention through exercise biology. *J Appl Physiol.* 2000;88:774–787.

52. Khan KM, McKay HA, Happasalo H, et al. Does childhood and adolescence provide a unique opportunity for exercise to strengthen the skeleton? *J Sci Med Sport.* 2000;3:160–164.

53. Bass S, Pearce G, Bradney M, et al. Exercise before puberty may confer residual benefits in bone

density in adulthood: studies in active prepubertal and retired female gymnasts. *J Bone Miner Res.* 1998;13:500–507.

54. Bradney M, Pearce G, Naughton G, et al. Moderate exercise during growth in pubertal boys: changes in bone mass, size, volumetric density, and bone strength: a controlled prospective study. *J Bone Miner Res.* 1998;13:1814–1821.

55. Heininen A, Sievanen H, Kannus P, Pasanen M, Vuori I. High impact exercise and bones of growing girls: a nine month controlled trial. *Osteoporosis Int.* 2000;11:1010–1017.

56. Blimkie C, Rice S, Webber C, Marting J, Levy D, Gordon C. Effects of resistance training on bone mineral content and density in adolescent females. *Can J Physiol Pharmacol.* 1996;74(9):1025–1033.

57. Ferrari S, Rizzoli R, Slosman D, Bonjour JP. Familial resemblance for mineral mass is expressed before puberty. *J Clin Endocrinol Metab.* 1998;83: 358–361.

58. Sainz J, van Tornout JM, Sayre J, Kaufman F, Gilsanz V. Association of collagen type 1 a1 gene polymorphism with bone density in early childhood. *J Clin Endocrinol Metab.* 1999;84:853–855.

59. Mosekilde L. Sex differences in age-related loss of vertebral trabecular bone mass and structure—biomechanical consequences. *Bone.* 1989;10: 425–432.

60. Buchanan JR, Myers C, Lloyd T, et al. Early vertebral trabecular bone loss in normal premenopausal women. *J Bone Miner Res.* 1988;3: 583–587.

61. Ettinger B, Genant HK, Cann CE. Postmenopausal bone loss is prevented by treatment with low-dosage estrogen with calcium. *Ann Intern Med.* 1987;106:40–45.

62. Forsen L, Bjorndal A, Bjartveit K, et al. Interaction between current smoking, leanness, and physical inactivity in the prediction of hip fracture. *J Bone Miner Res.* 1994;9:1671–1678.

63. Krolner B, Toft B. Vertebral bone loss: an unheeded side effect of therapeutic bed rest. *Clin Sci.* 1983;64:537–540.

64. Prior JC, Vigna YM, Schechter MT, et al. Spinal bone loss and ovulatory disturbances. *N Engl J Med.* 1990;323:1221–1227.

65. Chestnut CH 3d, Bell NH, Clark GS. Hormone replacement therapy in postmenopausal women: urinary N-telopeptide of type I collagen monitors therapeutic effect and predicts response of bone mineral density. *Am J Med.* 1997;102:29–37.

66. Garnero P, Hausherr E, Chapuy M-C, et al. Markers of bone resorption predict hip fracture in elderly women: the EPIDOS prospective study. *J Bone Miner Res.* 1996;11:1531–1538.

67. Garnero P, Sornay-Rendu E, Chapuy MC, et al. Increased bone turnover in late postmenopausal women is a major determinant of osteoporosis. *J Bone Miner Res.* 1996;11:337–349.

68. Rockoff SD, Sweet E, Bleustein J. The relative contribution of trabecular and cortical bone to the strength of human lumbar vertebrae. *Calcif Tissue Res.* 1969;3:163–175.

69. Rosen CJ, Chestnut CH 3d, Mallinak NJ. The predictive value of biochemical markers of bone turnover for bone mineral density in early postmenopausal women treated with hormone replacement or calcium supplementation. *J Clin Endocrinol Metab.* 1997;82:1904–1910.

70. Ross PD, Knowlton W. Rapid bone loss is associated with increased levels of biochemical markers. *J Bone Miner Res.* 1998;13(2):297–302.

71. Cole H, ed. *Managing Osteoporosis: Part 1. Detection and Clinical Issues in Testing.* Chicago: American Medical Association; 1999:3.

72. Marshall D, Johnell O, Wedel H. Meta-analysis of how well measures of bone mineral density predict occurrence of osteoporotic fractures. *BMJ.* 1996;312:1254–1259.

73. Miller PD, Bonnick SL. Clinical application of bone density. In: Favus MJ, ed. *Primer on the Metabolic Bone Diseases and Disorders of Mineral Metabolism.* 4th ed. Philadelphia: Lippincott, Williams & Wilkins; 1999:152–159.

74. Miller PD, Bonnick SL, Rosen CJ. Consensus of an international panel on the clinical utility of bone mass measurements in the detection of low bone mass in the adult population. *Calcif Tissue Int.* 1996;58:207–214.

75. Miller PD, Zapalowski C, Kulak CA, et al. Bone densitometry: the best way to detect osteoporosis and to monitor therapy. *J Clin Endocrinol Metab.* 1999;84:1867–1871.

76. Nieves JW, Komar L, Cosman F, et al. Calcium potentiates the effect of estrogen and calcitonin on bone mass: review and analysis. *Am J Clin Nutr.* 1998;67:18–24.

77. Pacifici R, Avioli L. Effects of aging on bone structure and metabolism. In: Avioli LV, ed. *The Osteoporotic Syndrome.* 4th ed. San Diego, CA: Academic Press; 2000:25–34.

78. Boonen S, Broos P, Verbeke G, et al. Calciotrophic

hormones and markers of bone remodeling in age-related (type II) femoral neck osteoporosis: alterations consistent with secondary hyperparathyroidism-induced bone resorption. *J Gerontol Med Sci.* 1997;52:M286–M293.

79. Prestwood KM, Pilbeam CC, Burleson JA, et al. The short-term effects of conjugated estrogen on bone turnover in older women. *J Clin Endocrinol Metab.* 1994;79:366–371.

80. Dresner-Pollak R, Parker RA, Poku M, et al. Biochemical markers of bone turnover reflect femoral bone loss in elderly women. *Calcif Tissue Int.* 1996;59:328–333.

81. Calvo MS, Eyre DR, Gundberg CM. Molecular basis and clinical application of biological markers of bone turnover. *Endocr Rev.* 1996;17:333–368.

82. Kleerekoper M, Nelson DA, Peterson EL, et al. Reference data for bone mass, calciotrophic hormones, and biochemical markers of bone remodeling in older (55–75) postmenopausal white and black women. *J Bone Miner Res.* 1994;9: 1267–1276.

83. Looker AC, Bauer DC, Chestnut III C, et al. Clinical use of biochemical markers of bone remodeling: current status and future directions. *Osteoporosis Int.* 2000;11:467–480.

84. Kleerekoper M. Biochemical markers of bone turnover: why theory, research, and clinical practice are still in conflict. *Clin Chem.* 2001;47: 1347–1349.

85. NIH Consensus Development Panel. Osteoporosis prevention, diagnosis, and therapy. *JAMA.* 2001;285:785–795.

86. Food and Nutrition Board, Institute of Medicine. *Dietary Reference Intakes for Calcium, Magnesium, Phosphorus, Vitamin D, and Fluoride.* Washington, DC: National Academy Press; 1997.

87. NIH Consensus Conference. Optimal calcium intake. *JAMA.* 1994;272:1942–1948.

88. Morgan KJ, Stampley GL, Zabik ME, Fischer DR. Magnesium and calcium dietary intakes of the U.S. population. *J Am Coll Nutr.* 1985;4:195–206.

89. Morgan KJ, Stampley GL, Zabik ME, Fischer DR. Magnesium and calcium dietary intakes of the U.S. population. *J Am Coll Nutr.* 1985;4:195–206.

90. Nielsen FH, Hunt CD, Mullen LM, Hunt JR. Effect of dietary boron on mineral, estrogen, and testosterone metabolism in postmenopausal women. *FASEB J.* 1987;1(5):394–397.

91. Davis GK, Mertz W. Copper. In: Mertz W, ed. *Trace Elements in Human and Animal Nutri-*

tion. 5th ed. Vol. I. Orlando, FL: Academic Press; 1986:301–364.

92. Schmidt H, Herwig J, Greinacher I. The skeletal changes in premature infants with copper deficiency. *Rofo Fortschr Geb Rontgenstr Neuen Bildgeb Verfahr.* 1991;155:38–42.

93. Buchman L, Keen CL, Vinters HJV, et al. Copper deficiency secondary to a copper transport defect: a new copper metabolic disturbance. *Metabolism.* 1994;43:1462–1469.

94. Strain JJ. A reassessment of diet and osteoporosis: possible role for copper. *Med Hypotheses.* 1988;27:333–338.

95. Hodges SJ, Pilkington MJ, Stamp TCB, et al. Depressed levels of circulating menaquinones in patients with osteoporotic fractures of the spine and femoral neck. *Bone.* 1991;12:387–389.

96. Knapen MHJ, Hamulyak K, Vermeer C. The effect of vitamin K supplementation on circulating osteocalcin (bone gla protein) and urinary calcium excretion. *Ann Intern Med.* 1989;111: 1001–1005.

97. Vermeer C, Hamulyak K. Pathophysiology of vitamin K-deficiency and oral anticoagulants. *Thromb Haemost.* 1991;66:153–159.

98. Feskanich D, Weber P, Willett WC, et al. Vitamin K intake and hip fractures in women: a prospective study. *Am J Clin Nutr.* 1999;69:74–79.

99. Anonymous. Maximizing peak bone mass: calcium supplementation increases bone mineral density in children. *Nutrition Rev.* 1992;50(11): 335–337.

100. Burnett CC, Reddi AH. Influence of estrogen and progesterone on matrix-induced endochondral bone formation. *Calcif Tissue Int.* 1938;35: 609–614.

101. Albright F. The effect of hormones on osteogenesis in man. *Recent Prog Horm Res.* 1947;1: 293–353.

102. Longcope C. The endocrinology of the menopause. In: Lobo RA, ed. *Treatment of the Postmenopausal Women: Basic and Clinical Aspects.* Vol. 4. Baltimore, MD: Lippincott, Williams & Wilkins; 1999:35–42.

103. Jilka RL. Cytokines, bone remodeling, and estrogen deficiency: a 1998 update. *Bone.* 1998;23: 75–18.

104. Ernst M, Schmid C, Froesch ER. Enhanced osteoblast proliferation and collagen gene expression by estradiol. *Proc Natl Acad Sci U S A.* 1988;85:2307–2310.

105. Hoffman A, Grobbee DE, de Jong PT, van den Ouweland FA. Determinants of disease and disability in the elderly: the Rotterdam Elderly Study. *Eur J Epidemiol.* 1991;7:403–422.

106. Klibanski A, Neer RM, Beitins IZ, Ridgeay C, Zervas NT, Mac Arthur J. Decreased bone density in hyperprolactinemic women. *N Engl J Med.* 1980; 305:1511–1514.

107. Anderson JJ, Anthony MS, Cline JM, et al. Health potential of soy isoflavones for menopausal women. *Public Health Nutr.* 1999;2:489–504.

108. Tham DM, Gardner CD, Haskell WL. Clinical review 97: potential health benefits of dietary phytoestrogens: a review of the clinical, epidemiological, and mechanistic evidence. *J Clin Endocrinol Metab.* 1998;83:2223–2235.

109. Messina MJ. Legumes and soybeans: overview of their nutritional profiles and health effects. *Am J Clin Nutr.* 1998;68:1375S–1379S.

110. Miksicek RJ. Commonly occurring plant flavonoids have estrogenic activity. *Mol Pharmacol.* 1993;44:37–43.

111. Scheiber MD, Rebar RW. Isoflavones and postmenopausal bone health: a viable alternative to estrogen therapy? *Menopause.* 1999;6:133–241.

112. National Osteoporosis Foundation. Available at: http://www.nof.oeg/osteoporosis/stats.htm. Accessed October 15, 2002.

113. Messina M, Messina V. Soy foods, soybean isoflavones, and bone health: a brief overview. *J Ren Nutr.* 2000;10:63–68.

114. Arjmandi BH, Alekel L, Hollis BW, et al. Dietary soybean protein prevents bone loss in an ovariectomized rat model of osteoporosis. *J Nutr.* 1996;126:161–167.

115. Alekel DL, Germain AS, Peterson CT, et al. Isoflavone-rich soy protein isolate attenuates bone loss in the lumbar spine of perimenopausal women. *Am J Clin Nutr.* 2000;72:844–852.

116. Anderson JJ, Garner SC. Phytoestrogens and bone. *Baillieres Clin Endocrinol Metab.* 1998;12: 543–557.

117. Sugimoto E, Yamaguchi M. Stimulatory effect of daidzein in osteoblastic MC3T3-E1 cells. *Biochem Pharmacol.* 2000;59;5:471–475.

118. Arjmandi BH, Getlinger MJ, Goyal NV, et al. Role of soy protein with normal or reduced isoflavone content in reversing bone loss induced by ovarian hormone deficiency in rats. *Am J Clin Nutr.* 1998;68:1358S–1363S.

119. Fanti P, Monier-Faugere MC, Geng Z, et al. The phytoestrogen genistein reduces bone loss in short-term ovariectomized rats. *Osteoporosis Int.* 1998;8:274–281.

120. Ettinger B, Grady D. The waning effect of postmenopausal estrogen therapy on osteoporosis. *N Engl J Med.* 1993;329:1192–1193.

121. Knight DC, Eden JA. A review of the clinical effects of phytoestrogens. *Obstet Gynecol.* 1996;87: 897–904.

122. Kuiper GG, Carlsson B, Grandien K, et al. Comparison of the ligand binding specificity and transcript tissue distribution of estrogen receptors alpha and beta. *Endocrinology.* 1997;138: 863–870.

123. Vincent A, Fitzpatrick LA. Soy isoflavones: are they useful in menopause? *Mayo Clinic Proc.* 2000;75:1174–1184.

124. Arjmandi BH, Birnbaum R, Goyal NV, et al. Bone-sparing effect of soy protein in ovarian hormone-deficient rats is related to its isoflavone content. *Am J Clin Nutr.* 1998;68:1364S–1368S.

125. Ishimi Y, Miyaura C, Ohurma M, et al. Selective effects of genistein, a soybean isoflavone on B-lymphopoiesis and bone loss caused by estrogen deficiency. *Endocrinology.* 1999;140:1893–1900.

126. Bailey DA, McKay HA, Mirwald RL, Crocker PRE, Faulkner RA. The University of Saskatchewan Bone Mineral Accrual Study: a six-year longitudinal study of the relationship of physical activity to bone mineral accrual in growing children. *J Bone Miner Res.* 1994;14:1672–1679.

127. Prince R, Devine A, Dick I, et al. The effects of calcium supplementation (milk powder or tablets) and exercise on bone density in postmenopausal women. *J Bone Miner Res.* 1995;10: 1068–1075.

128. Anonymous. ACSM position stand on osteoporosis and exercise. American College of Sports Medicine. *Med Sci Sports Exerc.* 1995;27:i–vii.

129. Greendale GA, Barrett-Connor E, Edelstein S, et al. Lifetime leisure exercise and osteoporosis: The Rancho Bernardo study. *Am J Epidemiol.* 1995;141:951–959.

130. Booth F, Gordon SE, Carlson CJ, Hamilton MT. Waging war on modern chronic diseases: primary prevention through exercise biology. *J Appl Physiol.* 2000;88:774–787.

131. Khan KM, McKay HA, Happasalo H, et al. Does childhood and adolescence provide a unique opportunity for exercise to strengthen the skeleton? *J Sci Med Sport.* 2000;3:160–164.

132. Bass S, Pearce G, Bradney M, et al. Exercise before puberty may confer residual benefits in bone density in adulthood: studies in active prepubertal and retired female gymnasts. *J Bone Miner Res.* 1998;13:500–507.

133. Bradney M, Pearce G, Naughton G, et al. Moderate exercise during growth in pubertal boys: changes in bone mass, size, volumetric density, and bone strength: a controlled prospective study. *J Bone Miner Res.* 1998;13:1814–1821.

134. Heininen A, Sievanen H, Kannus P, Pasanen M, Vuori I. High impact exercise and bones of growing girls: a nine month controlled trial. *Osteoporosis Int.* 2000;11:1010–1017.

135. Blimkie C, Rice S, Webber C, Marting J, Levy D, Gordon C. Effects of resistance training on bone mineral content and density in adolescent females. *Can J Physiol Pharmacol.* 1996;74(9):1026.

136. O'Connell JA. Application of osteopathic manipulative medicine in the diagnosis and treatment of osteoporosis. *J Am Osteopath Assoc.* 1997;97:2–15.

137. Cavalier TA. Management of osteoporosis in the new millennium. *J Am Osteopath Assoc.* 2000;100:516–520.

CHAPTER 25

Integrative Approach to Otolaryngology

SEZELLE GEREAU HADDON

Any general medical practitioner will encounter numerous complaints referable to the ear, nose, and throat (ENT) during the course of routine practice. Krouse and Krouse have noted that 78% of patients sought the care of a primary care physician, prior to seeking an otolaryngologist's opinion, regarding the treatment of their sinusitis. Most of these patients had had symptoms for an average of 3.5 years before consulting a specialist.[1] A practitioner's ability to handle these common diseases, prior to seeking the advice of a specialist, is an asset. First-line practitioners must consider a variety of ways to treat these illnesses effectively, without prematurely exposing patients to undue morbidity from the side effects of medications or surgical interventions.

As in other medical specialties, otolaryngologic patients themselves have begun to seek out alternative treatments instead of, or in addition to, allopathic medicine. In a review of 300 patients with asthma and/or sinusitis, some 42% reported using complementary modalities. Herbal treatments were sought most frequently.[2] Krouse noted that prior to presenting to an otolaryngologist, medication, such as antibiotics, antihistamines and decongestants, were the most frequently used treatment for chronic sinusitis.[1] In a subsequent study,

Krouse surveyed 84 patients derived from a community ENT practice who had been diagnosed with chronic sinusitis by computed tomography or nasal endoscopy.[3] Some 5 years after treatment by an otolaryngologist, 81% of these patients reported that exercise was more helpful in controlling their symptoms than were antibiotics or decongestants. They also noted equivalent frequency of use of antihistamines, dietary supplements, and decongestants for symptom control.

Despite these findings, there is scant research available regarding the efficacy of complementary therapies for diseases of the ear, nose, and throat.[3,4] As Asher states, "The difficulty in assessing these therapies often lies in their multimodal complexity (diet, lifestyle changes, and herbs) or the fact that the concept of disease origin is radically different from conventional medicine (traditional Chinese medicine, homeopathy, Ayurveda)."[4]

This chapter discusses what is currently known of complementary treatments in otolaryngology. In certain cases, these treatments are discussed in a theoretical context, as they could hold promise for otolaryngology, because they have the potential to affect the pathophysiology that results in the diseases discussed. Unfortunately, many of these treatments have not been subjected to appropriate clinical trials to allow them to be accepted in the allopathic medical community. The specific illnesses focused on are otitis media, sinusitis, adenotonsillar disease, obstructive sleep apnea, tinnitus, vertigo, and balance disorders.

Allergies underlie many ENT illnesses, and appropriate treatment for allergic symptoms should always be considered. The integrative approach to allergy is covered in Chapter 17 and is not discussed here. Also, remembering that general principles apply, disorders such as head and neck malignancies may be handled according to the principles of integrative oncology described in Chapter 23.

▶ ILLNESSES THAT REQUIRE PROMPT REFERRAL

It is important first to screen for those illnesses that are potentially life threatening, and then determine a course of treatment. Many illnesses that affect the head and neck will not result in death or significant disability. But these same disorders can become major quality-of-life issues for patients, as they interfere with one's interaction with the world in general, as in hearing loss from otitis media, hoarseness resulting from postnasal drip, or headaches associated with chronic sinusitis.

While many head and neck illnesses do not result in mortality or significant morbidity, the practitioner must remain alert for signs and symptoms that could signal more sinister disease. The following clinical presentations warrant consideration of quick referral for otolaryngologic consultation. This list is not meant to be inclusive of all illness that should be referred, but provides guidelines for the general practitioner who would like to consider conservative treatment in appropriate situations without precipitating untoward results.

- *Complications of otitis media*—Consultation by a specialist should be sought for any suspected complication of otitis media, in-cluding mastoiditis, facial nerve paralysis, meningitis, brain or epidural abscess, and otitic hydrocephalus.

- *Complications of sinusitis*—Periorbital abscess, meningitis, and brain abscess can all result from untreated sinusitis. Prior to initiating integrative treatment, care should be taken to screen patients presenting with sinusitis for signs and symptoms of orbital or intracranial extension.

- *Cranial neuropathies*—Any new onset of cranial nerve paresis or paralysis warrants evaluation by an otolaryngologist or neurologist.

- *Unilateral serous otitis media in an adult*—Adults can present with otitis media, but it remains primarily a disease of childhood, as most children will outgrow this illness by early adolescence. Unilateral presentation of otitis in an adult may be benign, but could also result from nasopharyngeal carcinoma. The best screening tool for this disease is flexible endoscopy of the nasopharynx by a skilled observer. Most otolaryngologists have flexible nasopharyngoscopes in the office, and within minutes can perform this noninvasive examination (Figure 25–1).

- *Sudden-onset sensorineural hearing loss*—Sudden-onset deafness can be unilateral or bilateral, and warrants immediate ENT evaluation. Potential etiologies include infectious, neoplastic, traumatic, ototoxic, immunologic, vascular, developmental, and psychogenic causes.[5] Although the vast majority of cases of sudden-onset deafness are idiopathic in origin, in some cases, prompt diagnosis and treatment can stabilize or reverse hearing loss.

- *Vertigo*—Any vertigo of suspected central etiology should be referred for prompt evaluation.

- *Stridor or persistent hoarseness*—Stridor in a child or adult could signal airway compromise and necessitates immediate evaluation of the upper aerodigestive tract. The differential diagnosis of hoarseness is extensive,

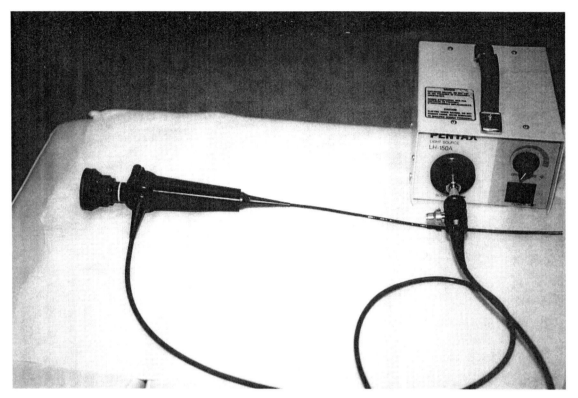

Figure 25-1.   Flexible nasopharyngoscope, which is used to examine the nasopharynx and the larynx.

including gastroesophageal reflux, vocal abuse, and postnasal drip. Treatment varies according to the underlying cause. In the adult, or smoker who does not respond promptly to treatment, the larynx should be examined thoroughly to rule out malignancy. Children who present with hoarseness in infancy should be screened with flexible endoscopy for laryngeal papillomatosis or congenital laryngeal anomalies.

- *Suspected malignancy*—Patients with neck masses, suspicious lymphadenopathy, or lesions of the face, head, or necks should be considered for further evaluation. Patients who have a history of tobacco usage or alcohol abuse are at even greater risk for malignancies of the pharynx and larynx. These individuals obviously need the urgent attention of a head and neck specialist.

▶ OTITIS MEDIA AND SINUSITIS

The pathophysiologies of otitis and sinusitis have marked similarities. The pathophysiology and ensuing treatment shared by the two conditions is discussed first, followed by a separate discussion of each disorder.

Obstruction of the natural outflow tract causes stasis of normal mucociliary transport or lack of aeration within the sinus or middle ear. This blockage results in edema of the mucosal lining of the cavities and buildup of secretions. Obstruction occurs at the level of the Eustachian tube orifice, that is, the nasopharynx, to result in otitis media, or in the nasal cavity, particularly under the middle turbinate, in the case of sinusitis (Figure 25–2). This fluid then becomes infected and causes acute otitis media (AOM) or acute sinusitis. The most common

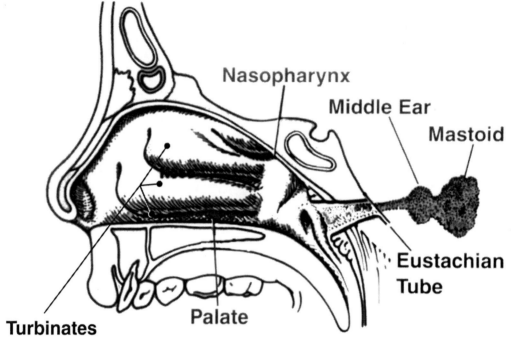

Figure 25-2. Nasopharynx, eustachian tube, and middle ear.

causative organisms in both cases are *Streptococcus pneumoniae,* nontypable *Haemophilus influenzae, Moraxella (Branhamella) catarrhalis,* and various viruses.[5] When this process becomes chronic, secondary changes persist in the mucosa lining the middle ear or sinus cavity. Chronic inflammatory changes occur, and result in the signs and symptoms of chronic serous otitis and chronic sinusitis. Allopathic treatment includes antibiotics, steroids, antihistamines, decongestants, and surgery.

Integrative Medicine Approaches

Environmental Factors
Passive smoke and environmental air pollutants cause structural and physiological changes in the mucosa of the upper and lower respiratory tract. Goblet cell hyperplasia, excess mucus secretion, ciliostasis, and a reduction in mucociliary transport have all been reported. These changes may affect the protective capabilities of the respiratory tract.[6] Proposed avoidance of cigarette smoke and air pollutants or treatment with air purifiers and negative ion generators seem to make sense in this context. Symptoms of sinusitis were reduced in 90 children treated for 3 years with an air purifier.[7] Studies in children with otitis and higher levels of urinary cotinine, a nicotine by-product, have been mixed, but suggest a role for passive smoke in the etiology of otitis media.[6]

Immune Modulation
Upper respiratory tract infections (URIs) can precipitate both otitis and sinusitis. As such, integrative treatment has focused on boosting the

immune system. Epidemiological evidence exists that regular exercise at moderate intensity can prevent upper respiratory tract infections.[8] Sedentary individuals were found to be at moderate risk, and elite athletes at high risk for URIs.

Numerous studies have examined the role of echinacea in the treatment of infections of the upper respiratory tract.[9-16] Extracts have been prepared from the roots, flowers, and leaves of *Echinacea purpurea* and related species *E. pallida* and *E. angustifolia*. This herbal remedy has been found both in vitro and in vivo to be an effective immune modulator, enhancing both primary and secondary immunoglobulin (Ig) G responses, T cells, cytokines, and phagocytosis. Some antiinflammatory and weak antiviral properties have also been demonstrated.[14,15] A number of its ingredients have been studied, including alkyl-amides, echinacosides, chicoric acid derivatives, and polysaccharides.[15,17]

Two comprehensive, systematic reviews of existing studies on echinacea for treatment of acute URIs have been performed.[9,10,13] Most studies reviewed found a modest, but statistically significant benefit when used within days of the onset of symptoms and continued for 8-10 days.[15] Four trials looked at *Echinacea* preparations for prevention of upper respiratory infections, and failed to find a statistically significant effect.[10]

A newly published randomized, placebo-controlled, double-blind study did not find any benefit with dried, encapsulated *E. angustifolia* root and whole-plant *E. purpurea* when used in a population of college students self-reporting symptoms of URI.[18] The authors suggest that both the type of preparation and the relatively healthy population may have skewed results. Further study was recommended.

Echinacin (Madaus AG) is the brand studied most in Germany. It is imported into the United States as Echinaguard by Nature's Way and has been used in clinical trials here. It is formulated from the pressed juice of *E. purpurea*. The recommended dose for children is 3.5 mL BID for 2-6-year-olds and 5 mL BID for 6-12-year-olds. Both the *E. purpurea* herb and *E. pallida* root may be superior preparations to *E. angustifolia* and *E. purpurea* root.[19]

Side effects are rare among users in Germany and the United States, but cases of anaphylaxis, including asthma, angioedema, and erythema nodosum, have been reported.[19,20] There is no good scientific evidence to suggest harm in nonallergic individuals or tolerance with 8 weeks of continuous usage.[21]

When echinacea is combined with goldenseal *(Hydrastis canadensis)*, an IgM response is also noted within the first 2 weeks of treatment.[14] Goldenseal's effectiveness has been attributed to its isoquinoline alkaloids berberine, hydrastine, and canadine. There are no clinical trials using goldenseal or its crude herbal extracts.[15] Clinical research has used the berberine alone, which was frequently isolated from other plants containing this compound. In vitro activity has been demonstrated against gram-positive and gram-negative bacteria, fungi, protozoa and other parasites.[22-24] It is not highly regarded, however, as an antiviral, and it is not well-absorbed systemically.[15,25] In vitro, it inhibits the cytochrome P450–3A4 system for drug metabolism.[26] These factors, coupled with the fact that goldenseal remains an endangered species, make it inappropriate for use in the treatment of otitis or sinusitis.

Other immune-enhancing herbs to consider are *Astragalus membranaceous* and elderberry *(Sambucus nigra)*. Either of these herbs can be used early in the onset of an upper respiratory infection to prevent development of an acute otitis or sinusitis. Astragalus may stimulate production of interferon, B lymphocytes, and macrophages. Its active constituents are thought to be astragalosides and other related triterpene saponins. A number of polysaccharides and flavonoids have also been isolated. It is not clear which of these lends to its therapeutic value.[15] In a study using an herbal mixture containing astragalus and interferon, a statistically significant reduction in the incidence and duration of upper respiratory symptoms was noted when compared with interferon alone or placebo.[27] It is also thought to increase IgA and IgM production in human nasal secretions.[15]

Elderberry has been used in Europe for the treatment of URIs and fever. Leaves, flowers, and seeds have been studied; they contain more than 60 compounds (glycosides, anthocyanins, flavonoids, sterols, and lectins).[15] In vivo elderberry increases cytokine production and functions as an anticatarrhal, diaphoretic, and antiinflammatory.[19,28,29] It has an effect on acute symptoms of influenza when compared to placebo.[29] In Germany, elderberry is used in a combination product, Sinupret, which contains elder flowers combined with gentian root, primrose flowers (*Primula vulgaris*), sourdock (*Rumex areticus*) and vervain (*Verbena officinalis*).[30] Two separate trials showed efficacy for sinusitis, demonstrating improvement in both headache symptoms and radiological findings.[30]

Vitamin C intake has also been cited as treatment for URIs. A meta-analysis of some 30 trials of vitamin C for both treatment and prevention of the common cold failed to show its usefulness in preventing attacks. Research does suggest that there is some benefit from high-dose supplementation with the onset of symptoms.[31]

Natural Antiinflammatories

Because inflammation of the nasal cavity, nasopharynx, and middle ear plays such a critical role in the development of sinusitis and otitis, it stands to reason that antiinflammatory agents can be used to treat both. Takoudes and Haddad have demonstrated formation of hydrogen peroxide, a free radical intermediate, in the ears of guinea pigs injected with *S. pneumoniae*.[32] Lipoperoxidation persists in experimental models of otitis media for at least 30 days after infection.[33] As treatment options, Western medicine uses nasal and systemic steroids, and in nonintact ears, steroid-containing drops.

Studies have examined complementary agents with antiinflammatory properties, mostly from the perspective of sinusitis. Bromelains

are enzymes that have antiinflammatory, proteolytic, and antiedematous properties.[34] They are derived from the pineapple plant (*Ananas comosus*). Studies performed in the 1960s examined the role of bromelains in the treatment of sinusitis. While these clinical trials were well constructed and showed statistical efficacy, state-of-the-art radiographic documentation of sinusitis was not included.[4] These studies have not since been reproduced.

Natural Antihistamines

Herbal antihistamines and decongestants have also been proposed as treatments for the allergic etiology of both otitis and sinusitis. Stinging nettles (*Urtica dioica*), ephedra (*Ephedra sinica*), and homeopathic preparations have all been used for this reason. Integrative treatment for allergy is covered more thoroughly in Chap. 17.

Otitis Media

Pathophysiology and Conventional Treatment

It is important to differentiate acute from chronic disease when selecting therapeutic options for otitis. Acute disease presents with pain, fever, and hearing loss. The tympanic membrane has a bulging, erythematous appearance. It is generally thought to be associated with an infectious etiology, and is treated with antibiotics. Research suggests that even placebo will benefit at least 60% of children and that spontaneous resolution will occur in 81% of children within 7 days.[35,36] While acute otitis media is thought to be associated with an infectious agent, up to 40 % of aspirates fail to grow a causative agent.[5]

Because of the high degree of antibiotic resistance that has developed over the past several years, many European countries have adopted watchful waiting as an option for an uncomplicated course of otitis in an otherwise healthy child (Table 25–1). In Holland, only 30% of children receive antibiotics for acute otitis media, and the rate of drug resistance is

▶ **TABLE 25–1** GUIDELINES FOR MANAGEMENT OF ACUTE OTITIS MEDIA—DUTCH COLLEGE OF GENERAL PRACTITIONERS

Patients age 2 years and older
  Analgesia; perhaps decongestive nose drops
    Parent instructions:
      Recovery within 3 days, no follow-up
      Return if symptoms persist or worsen (pain ± fever ± sickness)
      If ear drum perforates, follow-up 2 weeks after onset of running ear
  If earache + fever persist, amoxicillin (if contraindicated, erythromycin) for 7 days
    Parent instructions:
      Reevaluate if no improvement after 48 hours of drug
      If no improvement in ear signs, referral
Patients age 6 months to 2 years
  Act as for older children, but more active attitude related to higher probability of deterioration
  Visit or phone contact 24 hours after initial examination
  If no improvement, another 24 hours of observation or amoxicillin (if contraindicated,
    erythromycin) for 7 days
  Contact 24 hours later; exam if necessary
    If no improvement, referral
Special patients
  Younger than age 6 months, recurrent episodes (3 or more within 1 year), immunocompromised hosts
  Start amoxicillin (or erythromycin) for 7 days
  Reevaluate at 24 hours
    Refer if patient deteriorates
  Follow-up 2 weeks after evaluation

Reprinted with permission from Bluestone CD, Klein JO. Otitis Media in Infants and Children. Philadelphia: WB Saunders; 2001:223, Table 8-17.

1%. There, the observation option advocates deferring antibiotic treatment of certain children for up to 72 hours. During this period of observation, management is solely supportive. The New York Regional Otitis Project offers a tool kit for those wishing to utilize the observation option, which can be found at: www.health. state.ny.us/nysdoh/antibiotic/.[37] Other allopathic treatments include decongestants, antihistamines, corticosteroids, immunizations, and allergy desensitization injections.[6,39] More recently, immunization against *S. pneumoniae* has held promise in preventing recurrent disease.[6]

Recurrent acute otitis media is defined as three or more attacks of otitis within 6 months, or four attacks within 1 year.[5] This disease remains difficult to treat. Previous treatment modalities have included prophylactic antibi-

otics (half the daily dose taken once daily for up to 6 months) with or without adenoidectomy and/or tympanostomy tubes. As prophylaxis has contributed significantly to antibiotic resistance, it is no longer recommended for widespread use.[5,6]

Chronic serous otitis media with middle ear effusion is most commonly preceded by acute disease, but can also be found asymptomatically on routine physical examination. The tympanic membrane is dull in appearance, hypomobile on pneumatoscopy, and the child may have some discomfort. There is no fever. While an infectious etiology may trigger the initial formation of fluid, culture of serous fluid yields a bacterial agent in only 40–60% of middle ear effusion cases.[5] Chronic antigenic stimulation of the middle ear and viral etiology have both been proposed as contributing to persistence of fluid.

Suggested treatment is similar to that for acute otitis. Observation remains an option, especially in the child already treated with antibiotics for an acute episode. Ninety percent of cases will clear within 3 months with no intervention. Typically, any child with serous otitis that persists for more than this amount of time, and is associated with significant hearing loss, is considered for placement of tympanostomy tubes. The New York State Department of Health has published guidelines for management of serous otitis that can be accessed at: www.health.state.ny.us/nysdoh/antibiotic. html.

Integrative Medicine Approaches

Homeopathy

Homeopathy has been suggested as treatment for acute otitis. In a nonrandomized, observational study, homeopathy was compared to conventional treatment in the treatment of acute otitis media (AOM). Table 25–2 lists the agents used.[40] Patients treated with homeopathic preparations had a tendency toward earlier pain relief, shorter duration of therapy, and fewer recurrences than did those treated with antibiotics or placebo. In most studies, homeopathic preparations will have an effect within the first 24 to 72 hours. Fewer than 10% of patients were referred for antibiotics in this and other studies.[40–43] This trend toward fewer treatment failures and less pain was supported in a more recent study by Jacobs et al.[44] Homeopathic remedies employed in this study included pulsatilla (62.7%), chamomilla (10.7%), sulfur (9.3%), and calcarea carbonica (5.3%).

Randomized clinical trials exist that examine the use of homeopathy for otitis media.[45] These look mostly at single agents, and suggest that homeopathic preparations can be useful in the treatment of acute otitis. A large study

▶ **TABLE 25–2** HOMEOPATHIC REMEDIES COMMONLY USED TO TREAT OTITIS MEDIA

Remedy/Potency/Form	Indications
Aconitum 30x, globules	Sudden onset of condition; fever, sequel of exposure to wind
Apis mellifica 6x, globules	If the child likes ice on the ear
Belladonna 30x, globules	Inflamed red ear drum, often combined with reddened throat, cold extremities, high fever, throbbing pains in the ear(s)
Capsicum 6x, tablets	High fever, very pronounced pains in the ear(s)
Chamomilla 3x, globules	Otitis media as a sequel to teething problems
Kalium bichronicum 4x, tablets	Increased temperature, yellow nasal secretion, moderate pains in the ear(s), diffuse headache
Lachesis 12x, globules	High, continuous fever, otitis media starts on the left side, then on the right
Lycopodium 6x, tablets	Otitis media starts on the right side, then on the left
Mercurius solubilis 12x, tablets	Pronounced sensitivity to cold (freezing sensation), otitis media combined with purulent tonsillitis, pronounced soreness in the throat, and fever
Okoubaka 3x, globules	Following an unsuccessful therapy with antibiotics, intermediate administration for approximately 2 days
Pulsatilla 2x, globules	Fever, pronounced pains in the ear(s), generally administered after aconitum (see above)
Silicea 6x, tablets	If progress is protracted, if purulent otorrhea occurs, mild pains in the ear(s), generally no fever

Reprinted with permission from Friese, et al. The homeopathic treatment of otitis media in children. Int J Clin Pharm Therapeutics. 1997;35(7):297.

is currently being performed at the University of Seattle.

Homeopathy may be an option for families who choose a conservative route of treatment for acute otitis. It may be considered early in an uncomplicated bout of the disease, when watchful waiting is an option. Homeopathy has also been suggested for use in chronic serous otitis, but the evidence here has been less-well established, and larger clinical trials are needed.[42]

Nutritional Approaches

Breast-feeding is well accepted as reducing the incidence of middle ear disease in children.[5] While studies do not provide reasons for the decreased number of ear infections in breast-fed infants, a number of theories have been proposed, including immunologic factors, allergy to cow's milk, antiviral and antibacterial properties in breast milk, positioning of the child, development of the facial musculature, and aspiration of fluids into the middle ear space. Modification of the diet to consider food allergies, antiinflammatory types of foods, and probiotics should also be considered. These interventions are covered in greater depth in other chapters.

Xylitol has been studied both in vitro and in vivo. It is a polyol sugar alcohol naturally available in birch trees, plums, and certain berries. In the laboratory, xylitol inhibits growth of both *S. pneumoniae* and *S. mutans*.[46] In a randomized, controlled clinical trial of 306 Finnish children in day care, xylitol-containing chewing gum was compared to sucrose-containing gum in prevention of otitis media.[47] This study controlled for many variables associated with increased frequency of otitis media, including passive smoke exposure, breast-feeding, pacifier use, family history of otitis, and previous history of ear infections. A clear decrease in the occurrence of infections was demonstrated with the xylitol gum. The only side effect noted was diarrhea in a small percentage of patients. Of note is that frequent usage of xylitol gum (two pieces five times a day

after meals) was recommended in this clinical trial.

A small but promising study looked at use of lemon-flavored cod liver oil and multivitamin supplementation in prevention of recurrent acute otitis media.[48] This study proposes that vitamin A, trace minerals (especially selenium) and omega-3 fatty acids have important effects on immune functions. In a small sample of otitis-prone children, prescreened for deficiencies in vitamin A and selenium, administration resulted in fewer days of otitis during supplementation, as compared to the period prior to supplementation. This study only included eight participants, and was not double-blinded, placebo-controlled, or randomized, but a larger study is planned for the near future.[48]

Manipulative Medicine

Osteopathic manipulations have long been described as treatment for otitis media. They are thought to work on multiple levels. Anatomical treatment involves lysis of theoretical adhesions around the eustachian tube. Normalization of function of the musculature surrounding the hyoid muscle has also been described.[49] Neurological realignment of cranial nerves V (trigeminal) and IX (glossopharyngeal) has also been offered as an effect of treatment. Lymphatic drainage techniques are thought to be an effective augmentation of the immune response.[50,51] Early treatment is recommended prior to fusion of the cranial bones. Primary prevention of otitis in children prone to middle ear disease is recommended by 2 months of age.[25]

A retrospective study of 100 cases of head and neck abnormalities treated with osteopathy describes both techniques and case reports.[52] Review of the literature failed to reveal properly conducted clinical studies to support these claims. A National Institutes of Health (NIH)-sponsored clinical trial examining the efficacy of osteopathic manipulations, with and without echinacea, in children with recurrent acute otitis media is ongoing at the University of Arizona.[53] This study may soon yield more information regarding both of these therapies for treatment of otitis.

Sinusitis

Pathophysiology and Conventional Treatment

There are four pairs of sinuses, each named after the skull bones in which it is located: maxillary, ethmoid, frontal, and sphenoid. The sinuses are similar in that they all contain air and are lined by the typical ciliated respiratory mucosa. The sinuses drain into the nose, under the turbinates, which are structures that exist within the nose to humidify, warm, and filter air prior to presentation to the upper respiratory tract. Maxillary, ethmoid, and frontal sinuses drain under the middle turbinate. The sphenoid sinus drains into the sphenoethmoid recess above the superior concha. Figure 25–3 demonstrates a normal computed tomography (CT) scan of the sinuses, compared to Figure 25–4 which demonstrates the sinuses of a patient with sinusitis.

Any obstruction of the usual sinus outflow tract can result in sinusitis. In some cases this obstruction is physiological, and as with otitis media, an antecedent upper respiratory tract infection is the most common predisposing factor. Other factors to consider are environmental pollutants such as ozone, sulfur dioxide, nitrogen dioxide, carbon monoxide, and lead; seasonal and perennial allergies; gastroesophageal reflux; and immune deficiency. Anatomic abnormalities also result in sinusitis. Polyps or bony deformities of the nose and sinuses can all result in obstruction of the outflow tract, and thus result in acute or chronic sinusitis.[5]

Symptoms include facial, head, and tooth pain, nasal drainage and congestion. Sinus

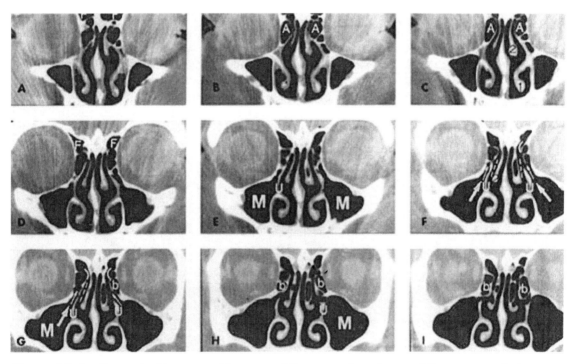

Figure 25–3. Computed tomographic scan of the normal anatomy of the paranasal sinuses.

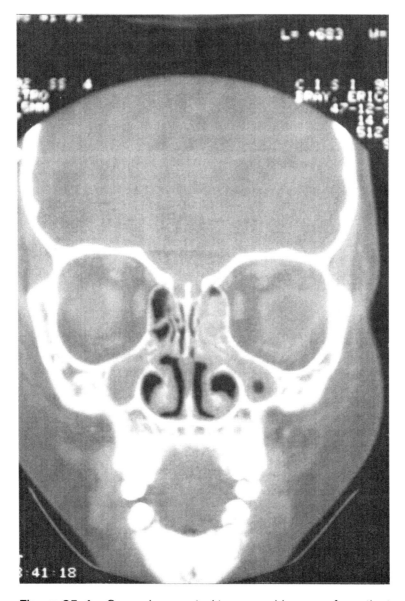

Figure 25–4. Coronal computed tomographic scan of a patient with sinusitis. Note changes in the maxillary and ethmoid sinuses.

symptoms lasting more than 6–12 weeks can be considered chronic. When infections do occur, the organisms are the same as those that cause otitis media. Traditional treatment involves administration of antibiotics, decongestants, mucolytics, and systemic or topical steroids. Surgery should be considered in patients who fail to respond to conservative therapy, develop recurrent or chronic disease, or who have complications of sinusitis.[5]

Integrative Medicine Approaches

Nasal Irrigation

Hypertonic nasal saline irrigations can be prepared at home cheaply and are easily administered to both children and adults.[54] Table 25–3 contains instructions for preparation of this solution. A neti pot, bulb syringe, and Water Pik can all be used to deliver the irrigant to the nasal cavity.[7] The saline solution serves as

▶ **TABLE 25–3** INSTRUCTIONS FOR PREPARATION AND USE OF HYPERTONIC SALINE SOLUTION

New York Weil Cornell Medical Center 525 East 68th Street New York, N.Y. 10021	Columbia Presbyterian Medical Center 622 West 168th Street New York, N.Y. 10032

Health Matters

Hypertonic Saline Nasal Irrigation

What is hypertonic saline nasal irrigation?
Hypertonic saline is very salty water. Irrigation means to wash out. Irrigating the nose with hypertonic saline dissolves mucous crusts. It pulls fluid out of swollen nasal membranes and shrinks them. This makes it easier to breathe. Very salty water also speeds up the movement of hairs in your nose to clear it.

How do I prepare the solution?
1. Clean a 1-quart glass jar and fill it with tap water.
2. Add 2 teaspoons kosher, pickling, sea, or canning salt. Do not use table salt or salt with iodine. Add 1 teaspoon baking soda.
3. Put on the jar lid and shake it well.
4. Write "Hypertonic Saline" and the date on the jar.
5. Throw the solution away after 1 week.
6. Store it at room temperature. Do not refrigerate it.
   If the solution is too strong for you, use 1½ teaspoons of salt the first time, then use 2 teaspoons the next time you make it.

For children, start with 1½ teaspoons of salt, and use 2 teaspoons the next time. You may go back to the weaker solution if it is too strong for your child.

How is the irrigation done?
Use a bulb-style ear syringe. This can be bought in any drug store. Irrigate 2 or 3 times a day before using any nose drops or sprays.
1. Pour about 1 cup of solution into a clean bowl.
2. Fill the bulb syringe with the solution.
3. Standing over the sink or in the shower, squirt the solution into one nostril then spit it out.
4. Repeat this for the other nostril.
5. Do this for each nostril 2 or 3 times, or until your nose clears.
6. Blow your nose.
   For young children, you can spray the solution into the nostrils. Fill a clean pump spray container with the solution. Write "Hypertonic Saline" on it along with the date you made it. Have your child sit or stand. Squirt 4 or 5 times into each nostril.

If you have any questions, call your doctor or clinic at _____.

This material gives you brief, general information about this health care topic. It does not take the place of instructions you receive from your health care providers. For answers to other questions, talk to your doctor or other health care provider.

a mucolytic agent. In a prospective, controlled study of 211 patients with sinonasal disease (allergic rhinitis, aging rhinitis, atrophic rhinitis, and postnasal drip), improvement in most parameters was noted, when compared to controls, with 3–6 weeks of twice-daily irrigations.[55]

Other mucolytic agents include horseradish and increased fluid intake.[39] Herbal mucolytic agents that can be considered are marshmallow *(Althaea officinalis)* and slippery elm *(Ulmus rubra),* both of which have a high mucilage content and can be found in various preparations for upper respiratory tract irritation, and neither of which has been subjected to clinical trials. Ivker's *Sinus Survival* has many suggested alternatives to traditional therapy for acute and chronic sinusitis.[7] Among other treatments, he recommends inhaled steam with or without the addition of eucalyptus *(Eucalyptus globules)* and menthol *(Mentha arvensis).* These essential oils improve flow of nasal secretions and prevent drying of the nasal mucosa. They also stimulate cold receptors in the nose, which leads to a perceived improvement in symptoms.[19]

Homeopathy

Weiser and Clasen examined the use of a homeopathic nasal spray *(Euphorbium compositum S)* in a prospective, randomized, placebo-controlled, double-blind study of 155 patients. While only subjective parameters were examined, a statistically significant improvement was noted in nasal obstruction, headache, and sinus pressure.[55]

Acupuncture

Acupuncture has also been offered as treatment for sinusitis. Pothman describes a small group of patients with chronic maxillary sinusitis. They received symptomatic relief for 3 months or greater from acupuncture when compared to antibiotics and laser acupuncture. This study was randomized, but not placebo-controlled, and radiographic evidence of sinusitis was not applied.[56] In a small case series of six patients, Asher found no improvement.[4]

Manipulative Medicine

Osteopathic and intranasal chiropractic techniques have been employed to treat sinusitis.[57,58] No appropriate clinical trials were found that evaluated either of these techniques.

▶ ADENOTONSILLAR DISEASE

Pathophysiology

The tonsils and adenoids comprise the Waldeyer ring, which is part of the secondary immunologic system. They produce predominantly B cells (50–65%) and a smaller portion of T cells (40%), and as such play a role in both the local and systemic immune responses. Their role is most prominent between 4 and 10 years of age, with involution occurring after puberty. While immunologic changes do occur after adenotonsillectomy, they do not appear to be clinically significant.[5]

Group A β-hemolytic *S. pneumoniae* is the most common bacterial pathogen to cause acute pharyngitis. Patients typically present with exudative tonsillar changes, fever, malaise, and cervical adenopathy. Other infectious agents that can cause pharyngitis are *Neisseria gonorrheae* and *Candida albicans,* especially in immune-compromised patients. Other causes of sore throat include viruses, allergies, and reflux esophagitis.[5]

Conventional Treatment Approach

After diagnosis of streptococcal pharyngitis, patients should be treated with antibiotics because of the potential for rheumatic heart disease or glomerulonephritis. Should testing for this pathogen prove to be negative, pharyngitis may be managed conservatively. Recurrent bacterial or viral pharyngitis might cause one to consider adenotonsillectomy. While this operation remains one of the most common surgical procedures of childhood, indications for surgery have changed, and it is not performed as commonly as it was in the past. Certainly any patient who fails conservative treatment for recurrent pharyngitis, and has significant associated morbidity, should be considered for this operation.

Integrative Medicine Approaches

Any of the immune-enhancing or antiinflammatory preparations discussed above under otitis media and sinusitis can theoretically be used in the treatment of pharyngitis.

Nutritional Approaches
Zinc gluconate lozenges have long been held to be effective in the treatment of sore throats and in alleviating other symptoms of the common cold. A randomized, double-blind, placebo-controlled study was performed on 100 employees of the Cleveland Clinic, who developed symptoms of the common cold. Half received zinc lozenges, the other half received a lozenge containing 5% calcium lactate pentahydrate as placebo. Daily subjective scores for cough, headache, hoarseness, muscle ache, nasal drain-age, nasal congestion, scratchy throat, sore throat, sneezing, and fever were obtained. The zinc group had shorter time to complete resolution and fewer days with coughing, headache, hoarseness, nasal congestion, nasal drainage, and sore throat than did the placebo group. The zinc group also had a higher rate of side effects, including nausea and bad taste in the mouth.[59]

Botanical Approaches
A number of herbal preparations have been used for properties that ease the symptoms of sore throat and cough. Many of these are approved by the German Commission E, and have many years of clinical usage for this indication. While most of these do not have well-constructed human studies to support their claims, their mechanism of action and safety profile make them a consideration for patients with sore throat and upper respiratory symptoms.

DEMULCENTS
Most demulcents are high in mucilage content. Ex vivo evidence using buccal mucosa has shown the bioadhesive effect of polysaccharide-containing herbs.[60] They serve as antitussives and reduce irritation of the throat. They may be used as teas, tinctures, and lozenges.

- Marshmallow *(Althaea officinalis)* leaf and root—Animal studies show that the herb and isolated polysaccharides can reduce both the intensity and duration of cough, comparable to that of nonnarcotic cough suppressants.[61]
- Licorice *(Glycyrrhiza glabra)*—Glycyrrhizin stimulates mucus production in the trachea, contributing to its demulcent and expectorant effects. Licorice also has antiinflammatory and antiviral properties that have been demonstrated in vitro.[62]
- Mullein *(Verbascum densiflorum)*—While no controlled clinical studies have been performed on mullein and its individual constituents, it is a harmless herb that appears to soothe the oropharyngeal cough receptors.[15]
- Slippery elm *(Ulmus rubra)*—This is extracted from the bark of the red elm tree, and has been used for years in American herbal remedies. Today, slippery elm is used mostly in preparations for pharyngitis.[15]
- Plantain *(Plantago lanceolata)*—Approved by the German Commission E for treatment of cough associated with bronchitis and upper respiratory infections, human trials have suggested its efficacy as a treatment for chronic bronchitis.[63]

CHINESE HERBALS
Certain herbs are common in Chinese medical formulations. There is little clinical evidence in the Western literature for their efficacy. Hon-

eysuckle *(Lonicera japonica)* is one of these herbs. This herb used in China to treat sore throats, colds, flu, and other upper respiratory illnesses. One study of 425 Chinese students with URI used dried honeysuckle flowers and other antiseptic components of the honeysuckle plant, along with blackberry lily roots, with reduction of symptoms.[61]

ESSENTIAL OILS

Essential oils can be used as a tincture or added to mouthwash.

- Wintergreen—When freshly harvested, wintergreen contains gaultherin, which converts to methyl salicylate with drying.[65] This component, along with its soothing properties, promotes its use in sore throat. As with other salicylate-containing compounds, fresh preparations of wintergreen should not be used in children with suspected viral sore throat, as they could potentially develop Reye syndrome.
- Mints *(Mentha arvensis)*—In vitro studies suggest that mint oils have mild antiviral and antibacterial properties. While menthol vapors subjectively seem to open congested nasal passages, this has been shown experimentally not to be caused by a physical effect. In fact, menthol in high concentrations may impair ciliary motility and increase nasal congestion. Menthol does, however, seem to lessen cough when administered in eucalyptus oil.[15]
- Eucalyptus *(Eucalyptus globulus)*—Used as a volatile oil, eucalyptus has been reported to have antiseptic and expectorant activities. Strong antibacterial action has been demonstrated against several strains of *Streptococcus.*[19]
- Myrrh *(Commiphora molmol)*—Myrrh contains essential oil and mucilage that has antimicrobial and antiinflammatory properties. These components make it useful for sore throat.[19]

Homeopathy

Numerous homeopathic remedies have been proposed for use in sore throat. Some of the agents used are:

Ferrum phosphoricum 6×
Apis mellifica 30× or 9c
Belladonna 30× or 9c
Hepar sulphuris 30× or 9c
Lachesis 30× or 9c[66]

Please see Chapter 12 for a more comprehensive discussion of homeopathic treatment of upper respiratory tract disease.

► OBSTRUCTIVE SLEEP APNEA

Pathophysiology

The science of sleep-disordered breathing is now recognized as an area of medical specialty.[67] Apnea is defined as a cessation of breathing for 10 seconds or longer and can be as long as 2 minutes in duration. At the end of the obstructive component, hypoxemia and hypercapnia cause an arousal.[5] Patients with greater than one apnea episode per hour, or who have significant hypoventilation with apneas, are defined as having obstructive sleep apnea syndrome (OSAS).

Children have a higher baseline oxygen consumption, and a tendency toward lower functional residual capacity during sleep. This scenario can cause them to desaturate with even shorter apneas. Any apnea that lasts for at least two breaths is considered significant in children.[5]

Diagnosis of obstructive apnea is made on history and physical examination. Loud snoring is ubiquitous in patients with OSAS and is reported by parents or bed partners. Other symptoms include excessive daytime sleepiness, unusual sleeping positions, and, in children, failure to thrive, enuresis, and poor school performance. Adults may present with signs of right-heart failure. They may also have morning headaches, inattentiveness, difficulty concentrating, or intellectual deterioration. In adults, thyroid and sex hormones are thought to play a role in supporting ventilation, which may explain the male preponderance of this disease.[68] Obstructive apnea is confirmed by polysomnography. Table 25-4 describes the parameters examined on polysomnography.

Conventional Treatment Approach

Once the diagnosis of OSAS is made, children are treated differently than adults. Adults with OSAS are usually obese. Treatment focuses on weight loss, and on the sites of upper airway obstruction, such as the nose, palate, base of the tongue, or mandible. Continuous positive airway pressure (CPAP) is found to be useful to many adults with OSAS who are not surgical candidates. Unlike adults, the vast majority of children with OSAS will respond to adeno-tonsillectomy.

Integrative Medicine Approach

Hypnotherapy

Any treatment for obesity in adults might apply for OSAS. Stradling describes hypnotherapy for weight loss in patients with known OSAS. Fifteen patients were randomized to three limbs of the study. The first limb included patients who only obtained dietary advice. The second limb also included hypnotherapy and specific stress-reduction techniques. The third limb looked at subjects who had both dietary advice and hypnotherapy, as well as specific dietary suggestions. The only group to maintain their weight loss for 18 months was the stress-reduction group. None of the patients in this study lost enough weight to discontinue their use of nasal CPAP.[69]

Miscellaneous Other Treatments

Other alternative medical treatments proposed for OSAS include nasal strips, nose drops, pillows, and magnetic therapy. There is no evidence in the literature for their efficacy.[67] Homeopathy has been studied in children scheduled for adenoidectomy. Eighty-two children participated in a randomized, double-blind clinical trial. Homeopathic preparations used included *Nux vomica,* Okaubaka, tuberculinum, and *Barium jodatum* D4 and D6 versus placebo. At the end of the study period, no surgery was necessary in 70.7% of the placebo-treated children and in 78% of the homeopathic treated children. This difference was not statistically significant.[70] A single case of sleep apnea treated by "vital energy" transfusion was described in the *Chinese Medical Journal* in 1980.[71]

▶ **TABLE 25-4** POLYSOMNOGRAPHY FOR OBSTRUCTIVE SLEEP APNEA SYNDROME IN CHILDREN

Sleep state
  Electroencephalogram
  Electro-oculogram (right and left)
  Electromyogram (submental)
Respiratory variables
  Abdominal and chest wall movement
    (strain gauges, inductive
    plethysmography)
  Oronasal airflow (thermistor)
  End-tidal CO_2
  Arterial oxygen saturation with pulse
    oximetry
Nonrespiratory variables
  Electrocardiogram
  Electromyogram (tibial) to document
    movements and arousals
  Recommended but not required
  Audiovideo recording

Reprinted with permission from Bluestone CD. Pediatric Otolaryngology, Head and Neck Surgery, *3rd ed. St. Louis, MO: Elsevier Science; 1998:220, Table 13-2.*

▶ TINNITUS

Pathophysiology

Tinnitus is a perception of ringing in the head. One-third of persons aged 65 and older have tinnitus. Cochlear hearing loss–related tinnitus is the type most frequently seen in clinical practice, but tinnitus can occur in patients with normal hearing.[5] The quality of the tinnitus can lead one to an underlying pathology; a venous hum, for example, may be caused by cervical compression of the jugular vein or by high cardiac output, such as is seen with anemia or thyrotoxicosis.

Many common medications, such as salicylates, certain antibiotics, and antihypertensive medications, can cause tinnitus (Table 25–5). Any patient with tinnitus should have a full workup, including audiogram and otoneurologic examination.[39] In the absence of a specific medical condition, the etiology of tinnitus is unknown.

Conventional Treatment Approach

There are few effective allopathic medical treatments for tinnitus. These treatments range from intravenous lidocaine to ultrasonography (Table 25–6). As such, patients with significant disability from tinnitus often seek alternative medicine as a last resort.

▶ TABLE 25-5 SOME COMMON MEDICATIONS THAT CAN CAUSE TINNITUS

ACE inhibitors: enalapil, fosinopril (Monopril)
Anesthetics: dyclonine, bupivacaine (Marcaine, Sensorcaine), lidocaine
Antibiotics: aztreonam, ciprofloxacin, erythromycin, estolate, erythromycin-ethylsuccinate/sulfasoxazole (Pediazole), gentamicin (Garamycin), imipenem-cilastatin (Primaxin), sulfasoxazole (Gantrisin), trimethoprim-sulfamethoxazole, vancomycin
Antidepressants: alprazolam (Xanax), amitriptyline (Elavil), desipramine, doxepin, fluoxetine (Prozac), imipramine (Tofranil), maprotiline (Ludiomil), nortriptyline (Pamelor)
Antihistamines: aspirin-promethazine-pseudophedrine (Phenergan), chlorpheniramine-phenylpropanolamine (Triaminic), clemastine (Tavist), pseudophedrine-chlorpheniramine (Deconamine), pseudophedrine-triprolidine (Actifed)
Antimalarials: chloroquine, pyrimethamine-sulfadoxine (Fansidar)
Beta-blockers: betaxolol (Kerlone), cateolol (Catrol), metoprolol (Lopressor), nadolol (Corgard), timolol (Timoptic)
Calcium channel blockers: diltiazem (Cardizem), nicardipine (Cardene), nifedipine (Procardia)
Diuretics: acetazolamide (Diamox), amiloride, ethacrynic acid
Narcotics: dezocine (Dalgan), pentazocine (Talwin)
NSAIDs: diclofenac (Voltaren), diflunisal (Dolobid), flurbiprofen (Ansaid), ibuprofen, indomethacin, meclofenamate (Meclomen), naproxen (Naprosyn), sulindac (Clinoril), tolemtin (Tolectin)
Sedatives/hypnotics/anxiolytics: azatadine (Optimine), buspirone (Buspar), chlorpheniramine-phenylpropanolamine (Ornade)
Miscellaneous: albuterol (Proventil), allopurinol, bismuth subsaliclate (Pepto Bismol), carbamazepine (Tegretol), cyclobenzaprine (Flexeril), cyclosporine, diphenhydramine (Benadryl), flecainide, hydroxychloroquine (Plaquenil), iohexol (Omnipaque), isotretinoin (Accutane), lithium, methylergonovine (Methergine), nicotine polacrilex (Nicorette), prazosin, omeprazole (Prilosec), quinidine, recombinant hepatitis B vaccine (Recombivax), salicylates, sodium nitroprusside (Nipride), sulfasalazine (Azulfidine), tocanide

Abbreviations: ACE = angiotensin-converting enzyme; NSAIDs = nonsteroidal antiinflammatory drugs.
Reprinted with permission from Jafek BW, Stark AK. ENT Secrets. 1st ed. Philadelphia: Hanley & Belfus; 1996:59.

▶ **TABLE 25–6** TREATMENTS FOR TINNITUS

Tocanide, related drugs
Carbamazepine
Benzodiazepines
Tricyclics
Iontophoresis (lidocaine)
Amino-oxy-acetic acid
Ginkgo
Miscellaneous drugs
Psychotherapy
Electrical/magnetic
Acupuncture
Masking
Biofeedback
Hypnosis
Ultrasonography
Miscellaneous nondrug: massage,
  temporomandibular joint, laser, yoga

Adapted from Dobie RA. A review of randomized clinical trials of tinnitus. Laryngoscope. 1999;109:1203, Table 1, with permission from Lippincott, Williams & Wilkins.

Integrative Medicine Approach

Botanical Approaches

Ginkgo biloba is an herbal extract that is widely used in Europe and United States for its neuroprotective ability, and as an aid in vascular insufficiency of various sorts. This herb has been examined as a possible treatment for tinnitus in a number of prospective studies. In patients without symptoms of cerebral insufficiency, results have been mixed. Many of these studies were small in size, and lacked adequate controls.[72] A recent matched-pair study, performed in a prospective randomized fashion, failed to show any benefit in some 489 pairs of patients. This study used a dose of 50 mg QD.[73] It is possible that the dose of ginkgo used was not high enough, as 80–120 mg/d is the recommended dose, with some studies for vascular insufficiency using up to 240 mg/d.[19,74] One study of 99 patients using 120 mg/d showed a reduction in the sound volume of the tinnitus at 8 and 10 weeks.[75] Standardiza-

tion of the preparation is critical in the use of ginkgo, and brand name is important. Researched brands include Ginkgold by Nature's Way and Ginkoba by Pharmaton.

Hypnotherapy and Biofeedback

Another proposed tinnitus treatment is hypnotherapy. It as effective as counseling, and works best in those without an accompanying severe hearing loss.[76,77] Biofeedback has also been proposed as a treatment. Both of these techniques appear at a minimum to modify the patient's reaction to the tinnitus, even if the physical symptom itself is not affected.[5] As there is no diagnostic test to quantify tinnitus, clinical response is difficult to monitor.

Acupuncture

Acupuncture has been examined as a possible treatment for tinnitus. Results again are mixed, with two well-performed studies failing to show effectiveness.[5,78,79] Noise-induced tinnitus does not appear to respond to acupuncture.[80]

▶ VERTIGO

Pathophysiology

Vertigo is the sensation of rotatory movement. Vertigo may or may not be accompanied by tinnitus and hearing loss. There are multiple peripheral and central nervous system reasons for vertigo. It is critical to differentiate between these. The most common peripheral causes of vertigo are benign positional vertigo, the Ménière triad, and vestibular neurolabyrinthitis. Central causes of vertigo include migraine headaches, stroke, multiple sclerosis, and brain tumor. Any patient suspected as having vertigo of central etiology needs referral to a specialist.

Benign positional vertigo is thought to be secondary to heavy particles (otoconia) near the ampulla of the posterior semicircular canal. Attacks occur with head movement involving neck rotation or extension. Vertigo traditionally lasts for seconds. It is diagnosed by a Hallpike-Dix maneuver, which precipitates vertigo when the patient is positioned appropriately.

Ménière's disease involves a triad of symptoms: episodic vertigo, sensorineural hearing loss, and fluctuating tinnitus. Aural fullness is also commonly associated. Vertigo lasts minutes to hours. Experimentally, a distortion of the membranous labyrinth, endolymphatic hydrops, caused by blockage of the endolymphatic duct, results in this constellation of symptoms. Ménière's disease is generally thought to be an autoimmune phenomenon.[5] Diagnosis is made by presentation and complete history. Overall guidelines of treatment focus on reducing the amount of endolymph present in order to directly alleviate vertigo.

Viral labyrinthitis can occur with or without an antecedent viral illness. Vertigo lasts for hours to days. Hearing loss can accompany symptoms. If there is no hearing loss, the disease is termed vestibular neuritis.

Conventional Treatment Approaches

For benign positional vertigo, the most commonly employed traditional treatments are the Epley maneuver and physical therapy. The Epley maneuver, or canalith repositioning technique, is thought to alter the position of these otoconia, resolving the attacks[81-83] (Figure 25–5). Physical therapy includes repeated intentional precipitation of attacks of vertigo, which allows the peripheral nervous system to habituate. Both of these treatments are safe and effective, with reported rates of resolution as high as 91.3% with the Epley maneuver.[82,83] There is some potential for recurrence, which has been reported at 15% per year.[82]

Overall guidelines of treatment focus on reducing the amount of endolymph present in order to directly alleviate vertigo. Thus, most treatment protocols for Ménière's triad involve some form of dietary intervention, salt restric-

tion, and diuretics. Lipoflavonoids and bioflavonoids have been proposed, but have not been subjected to appropriate clinical studies, and the mechanism of action is unclear (Table 25–7). Other treatments focus on improving the microcirculation of the inner ear. Betahistine is a structural analogue of histamine with potent H_3-receptor antagonist properties. It is thought to peripherally balance the sensory vestibular organs and increase blood flow to the stria vascularis.[81] One review of the medical treatments for Ménière's disease found that only betahistine and diuretics have been proven in double-blind studies to control vertigo long term.[85] The Cochrane Review looked specifically at studies of betahistine for Ménière's syndrome, and concluded that the evidence is insufficient to state that it is an effective treatment.[86] Surgical treatment can be considered if Ménière's disease is disabling. The approach is determined by whether or not the patient has serviceable hearing.

For viral labyrinthitis, treatment is symptomatic or directly aimed at suppressing the vestibular hyperresponsiveness. Sedatives such as meclizine, diazepam, and promethazine have been used.[39]

Integrative Medicine Approaches

Botanical Therapies

Many of the same treatments that have been proposed for tinnitus also have been used for vertigo, with similar results. Powdered ginger root was employed in eight healthy volunteers with artificially produced vertigo. It was thought to be better than placebo, but no statistically significant change in nystagmus was demonstrated.[87] In alcoholics with low blood levels of magnesium, improvement in their vertiginous symptoms was noted with magnesium supplementation.[88] Hawthorn berry *(Crataegus mono-gyna)*, beneficial for atherosclerosis and heart disease, has a mildly sedating effect. Its vasodilatory properties combined with its

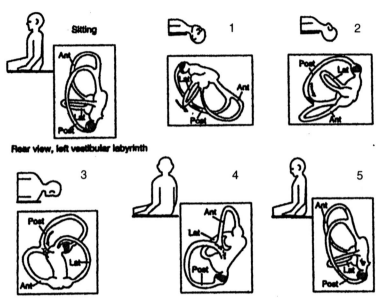

Beginning with patient in seated position, head and body are moved into Dix-Hallpike position with affected ear downward; head is rotated to opposite Dix-Hallpike position; keeping head downward, head and body are turned onto the side opposite affected ear; keeping head in same orientation in relation to the body, patient is raised to a sitting position; head is tilted forward 20 degrees. Positions 1 through 5 are held for the time of the latency plus the duration of the response. Cycles are repeated until there is no nystagmus in any position.

Figure 25-5. The canalith repositioning technique (Epley maneuver). *(From Lynn S, Pool A, Rose D, Brey R, Suman V. Randomized trial of the canalith repositioning procedure.* Otolaryngol Head Neck Surg. *1995; 113(6):712–720.)*

sedative qualities could be useful for treating vertigo, although clinical trials have not been performed.[4]

Homeopathy

Various homeopathic preparations have been used as treatment for the patient with dizzyness. Vertigoheel (ambra grisea D6, anamirta cocculus D4, conium maculatum D3, and petroleum rectificatum D8) has been studied and compared to betahistine in control of vertigo. During a 6-week treatment period, 119 patients were observed in 15 centers. The study was randomized, double-blinded, and placebo-controlled. Patients were not stratified or control matched by underlying diagnosis. A clinically relevant reduction in mean frequency, duration, and intensity of the attacks was noted.[89]

Tai Chi

Tai chi was offered to 22 persons with balance disorders. Objective measurements of imbalance were taken before and after an 8-week training period. A clinically significant improvement in symptoms was noted.[90]

► **TABLE 25-7** CONTENTS
OF LIPOFLAVONOID CAPSULE

Lemon bioflavonoid complex (bioflavonoids)	300 mg
Ascorbic Acid	300 mg
Choline	344 mg
Inositol	344 mg
DL-Methionine	84 mg
Thiamine	1 mg
Niacin	10 mg
Pyridoxine hydrochloride (B_6)	1 mg
Cyanocobalamin (B_{12}) concentrate	5 mg
Pantothenic acid	5 mg
Riboflavin	1 mg

*Reprinted from Slattery WH, Fayad JN. Medical
treatment of Ménière's disease. Otolaryngol Clin
North Am. 1997;30:1027–1037, with permission from
Elsevier Science.*

► **CONCLUSIONS**

Integrative treatment of various disorders of
the ear, nose, and throat includes a variety of
types of modalities. While some of these have
been subjected to rigorous clinical trials, others
have not. Whether or not one opts to offer
these to patients as treatment options depends
on the preponderance of the evidence, the individual patient, and whether or not a therapy
makes intrinsic sense in the mind of the practitioner with guidance and input from the client.
Even if the clinical studies have not yet been
performed, therapies that seem promising and
have minimal untoward effects can certainly be
attempted. Indeed, in many of these disorders,
allopathic treatments have little to offer, and
here integrative treatments may hold even more
promise.

As in all fields of integrative medicine, treatment becomes a dialogue between the practitioner and patient. Open communication with
patients regarding available treatments, alternatives, and consequences is part of the
therapeutic relationship. Knowledge of both
allopathic and integrative protocols allows us
to truly assist our patients as they maneuver
through the medical options for their illnesses.

Acknowledgment

*Many thanks to Dr. Joseph Haddad, Jr., for his
assistance in the preparation of this manuscript.*

REFERENCES

1. Krouse JH, Krouse J. Patient use of traditional
   and complementary therapies in treating rhinosinusitis before consulting an otolaryngologist.
   Laryngoscope. 1999;109:1223–1227.
2. Blanc PD, Trupin L, Earnest G, et al. Alternative
   therapies among adults with a reported diagnosis of asthma or rhinosinusitis. *Chest.* 2001;120:
   1461–1467.
3. Krouse J, Krouse JH. Complementary therapeutic practices in patients with chronic sinusitis.
   Clin Excel Nurse Pract. 1999;3:346–352.
4. Asher BF, Seidman M, Snyderman C. Complementary and alternative medicine in otolaryngology. *Laryngoscope.* 2001;111:1383–1389.
5. Cummings CW, Fredrickson JM, Harker LA, et al.
   Otolaryngology—Head and Neck Surgery. St.
   Louis, MO: Mosby; 1998.
6. Bluestone CD, Klein JO. *Otitis Media in Infants
   and Children.* Philadelphia: WB Saunders; 2001.
7. Ivker RS. *Sinus Survival: The Holistic Medical
   Treatment for Allergies, Asthma, Bronchitis, Colds
   and Sinusitis.* New York: Putnam Books; 1995.
8. Peters EM. Exercise, immunology and upper
   respiratory tract infections. *Int J Sports Med.* 1997;
   18:S69–S77.
9. Barrett BP, Vohmann M, Calabrese. Echinacea for
   upper respiratory infection. *J Fam Pract.* 1999;48:
   628–635.
10. Barrett BP. Echinacea for upper respiratory in-
    fection: an assessment of randomized trials.
    Healthnotes Rev Complem Integr Med. 2000;7:
    211–218.
11. Melchart D, Linde K, Worku F, et al. Results of
    five randomized studies on the immunomodula-
    tory activity of preparations of *Echinacea. J Al-
    tern Complement Med.* 1995;1:145–160.
12. Percival SS. Use of echinacea in medicine.
    Biochem Pharmacol. 2000;60:155–158.
13. Melchart D, Linde K, Fischer P, et al. Echinacea
    for preventing and treating the common cold.
    Cochrane Database Syst Rev. 2001;3.
14. Rehman J, Dillow JM, Carter SM, et al. Increased
    production of antigen-specific immunoglobulins

G and M following in vivo treatment with the medicinal plants *Echinacea angustifolia* and *Hydrastis canadensis*. *Immunol Lett*. 1999;68: 391–395.

15. Rotblatt M, Ziment I. *Evidence-Based Herbal Medicine*. Philadelphia: Hanley & Belfus; 2002.

16. Melchart D, Walther E, Linde K, et al. Echinacea root extracts for the prevention of upper respiratory tract infections: a double-blind, placebo-controlled randomized trial. *Arch Fam Med*. 1998; 7:541–545.

17. Chavez M, Chavez P. Echinacea. *Hosp Pharm*. 1998;33:180–188.

18. Barrett, BP, Brown RL, Locken K. Treatment of the common cold with unrefined *Echinacea*. *Ann Inernt Med*. 2002;137:12:939–946.

19. Blumenthal M, Goldberg A, Brinckmann J, et al. *Herbal Medicine Expanded Commission E Monographs*. Newton, MA: American Botanical Council; 2000.

20. Mullins RJ. Echinacea-associated anaphylaxis. *Med J Aust*. 1998;168:170–171.

21. McGruffin M, Upton R, Goldberg A, et al. *American Herbal Products Association's Botanical Safety Handbook*. Boca Raton, FL: CRC Press; 1997:146.

22. Gentry E, Jampani H, Keshavarz-Shokri A, et al. Antitubercular natural products: berberine from the roots of commercial *Hydrastis canadensis* powder. Isolation of inactive 8-oxotetrahydrothalifendine, canadine, β-hydrastine, and two new quinic acid esters, hycandinic acid esters-1 and-2. *Nat Prod*. 1998;61:1187–1193.

23. Scazzocchio, F, Cometa, M, Pallmery M. Antimicrobial activity of *Hydrastis canadensis* extract and its major isolated alkaloids. *Fitoterapia*. 1998;69(suppl 5):58–59.

24. Birdsall T, Kelly G. Berberine: therapeutic potential of an alkaloid found in several medicinal plants. *Altern Med Rev*. 1997;2:94–103.

25. Kohatsu W. *Complementary and Alternative Medicine Secrets*. Philadelphia: Hanley & Belfus; 2002.

26. Budzinski J, Foster B, Vandenhoek S, et al. An in vitro evaluation of human cytochrome P450–3A4 inhibition by selected commercial herbal extracts and tinctures. *Phytomedicine*. 2000;7:273–282.

27. Hou YD, Ma GL, Wu SH, et al. Effect of *Radix Astragali seu Hedysari* on the interferon system. *Chin Med J (Engl)*. 1981;94:35–40.

28. Barak V, Birkenfeld S, Halperin T, et al. The effect of herbal remedies on the production of

human inflammatory and anti-inflammatory cytokines. *Isr Med Assoc J*. 2002;4(suppl 11): 919–922.

29. Azkay-Rones Z, Varsano N, Zlotnik M, et al. Inhibition of several strains of influenza virus in vitro and reduction of symptoms by an elderberry extract (*Sambucus nigra* L.) during an outbreak of influenza B Panama. *J Altern Complement Med*. 1995;4:361–369.

30. Schulz V, Hansel R, Tyler V. *Rational Phytotherapy: A Physician's Guide to Herbal Medicine*. New York: Springer; 2001.

31. Douglas R, Chalker E, Treacy B. Vitamin C for preventing and treating the common cold. *Cochrane Database Syst Rev*. 2002;2.

32. Takoudes T, Haddad J. Hydrogen peroxide in acute otitis media in guinea pigs. *Laryngoscope*. 1997;107:207–210.

33. Haddad J. Lipoperioxidation as a measure of free radical injury in otitis media. *Laryngoscope*. 1998;108:525–530.

34. Maurer HR. Bromelain: biochemistry, pharmacology and medical use. *Cell Mol Life Sci*. 2001;58: 1234–1245.

35. Del Mar C, Glasziou P. Are antibiotics indicated as initial treatment for children with acute otitis media? A meta-analysis. *BMJ*. 1997;314: 1526–1529.

36. Rosenfeld RM, Vertrees JE, Carr J, et al. Clinical efficacy of antimicrobial drugs for acute otitis media: metaanalysis of 5400 children from thirty-three randomized trials. *J Pediatr*. 1994;124: 355–367.

37. New York Regional Otitis Project. *Observation Option Toolkit for Acute Otitis Media*. State of New York, Department of Health, Publication #4894, March 2002. Available at: http://www.health.state.ny.us/nysdoh/antibiotic/toolkit.pdf. Accessed 9/11/03.

38. Stool SE, Berg AO, Berman S, et al. *Otitis Media with Effusion in Young Children. Clinical Practice Guideline, Number 12*. AHCPR Publication No. 94-0622. Rockville, MD: Agency for Health Care Policy and Research, Public Health Service, US Department of Health and Human Services; July 1994. Available at: http://www.http://hstat.nlm. nih.gov. Accessed 9/11/03.

39. Jafek BW, Stark AK. *ENT Secrets*. 1st ed. Philadelphia: Hanley & Belfus; 1996.

40. Friese KH, Kruse S, Ludtke R, et al. The homeopathic treatment of otitis media in children—

comparisons with conventional therapy. *Int J Clin Pharmacol Ther.* 1997;35:296–301.

41. Barnett ED, Levitin JL, Chapman EH, et al. Challenges of evaluating homeopathic treatment of acute otitis media. *Pediatr Infect Dis J.* 2000;19: 273–275.

42. Harrison H, Fixen A, Vickers A. A randomized comparison of homeopathic and standard care for the treatment of glue ear in children. *Complement Ther Med.* 1999;7:132–135.

43. Frei H, Thurneysen A. homeopathy in acute otitis media in children: treatment effect or spontaneous resolution? *Br Homeopath J.* 2001;90: 180–182.

44. Jacobs J, Springer DA, Crothers D. Homeopathic treatment of acute otitis media in children: a preliminary randomized placebo-controlled trial. *Pediatr Infect Dis J.* 2001;20:177–183.

45. Kleijnen J, Knopschild P, ter Riet G. Clinical trials of homeopathy. *BMJ.* 1991;302:316–323.

46. Kontiokari T, Uhari M. Koskela M. Effect of xylitol on growth of nasopharyngeal bacteria in vitro. *Antimicrob Agents Chemother.* 1995;39: 1820–1823.

47. Uhari M, Kontiokari T, Koskela M, et al. Xylitol chewing gum in prevention of acute otitis media: double-blind randomized trial. *BMJ.* 1996; 313:1180–1183.

48. Linday L, Dolitsky J, Shindledecker R, et al. Lemon-flavored cod liver oil and a multivitamin-mineral supplement for the secondary prevention of otitis media in young children: pilot research. *Ann Otol Rhinol Laryngol.* 2002;111(7): 642–652.

49. Kuchera M, Kuchera WA. *Osteopathic Considerations in Systemic Dysfunction.* 2nd ed. Kirksville, MO: Greyden Press; 1994.

50. Measel JW Jr. The effect of the lymphatic pump on the immune response: I. Preliminary studies on the antibody response to pneumococcal polysaccharide assayed by bacterial agglutination and passive hemagglutination. *J Am Osteopath Assoc.* 1982;82(1):28–31.

51. Pratt-Harrington D. Galbreath technique: a manipulative treatment for otitis media revisited. *J Am Osteopath Assoc.* 2000;100:635–639.

52. Schmidt IC. Osteopathic manipulative therapy as a primary factor in the management of upper, middle and pararespiratory infections. *J Am Osteopath Assoc.* 1982;81:82–89.

53. Aldous M. A randomized controlled trial of the use of craniosacral osteopathic manipulative treatment and of botanical treatment in recurrent otitis media in children. Description available at: http://nccam.nih.gov/clinicaltrials/diseasecondition.htm. Accessed 9/16/03.

54. Tomooka LT, Murphy C, Davidson TM. Clinical study and literature review of nasal irrigation. *Laryngoscope.* 2000;110(7):1189–1193.

55. Weiser M, Clasen BPE. Controlled double-blind study of a homeopathic sinusitis medication. *Biol Ther.* 1995;13(1):4–11.

56. Pothman R, Yeh, HL. The effects of treatment with antibiotics, laser and acupuncture upon chronic maxillary sinusitis in children. *Am J Chin Med.* 1982;10:55–58.

57. Shrum KM, Grogg SE, Barton P, et al. Sinusitis in children: the importance of diagnosis and treatment. *J Am Osteopath Assoc.* 2001;101:S8–S13.

58. Folweiler DC, Lynch OT. Nasal specific technique as part of chiropractic approach to chronic sinusitis and sinus headaches. *J Manipulative Physiol Ther.* 1995;18:38–41.

59. Mossad SB, Macknin ML, Medendorp SV, et al. Zinc gluconate lozenges for treating the common cold. A randomized, double-blind, placebo-controlled study. *Ann Intern Med.* 1996;15;125(2): 81–88.

60. Schmidgall J, Schnetz E, Hensel A. Evidence for bioadhesive effects of polysaccharides and polysaccharide-containing herbs in an ex vivo bioadhesion assay on buccal mucosa. *Planta Med.* 2000;66(1):48–53.

61. Nosal'ova G, Strapkova A, Kardosova A, et al. [Antitussive action of extracts of polysaccharides of marsh mallow (*Althea officinalis* L., var. robusta*)]. *Pharmazie.* 1992;47(3):224–226.

62. Snow JM. *Glycyrrhiza glabra* L. (Leguminoseae). *Protocol J Botan Med* found at http://www.herbalgram.org/herbclip. 1998;HC#011982–129. Accessed 9/19/03.

63. Matev M, Angelova I, Koichev A, et al. Clinical trial of *Plantago major* preparation in the treatment of chronic bronchitis. [In Bulgarian] *Vutr Boles* 1982;21(2):133–137.

64. Duke JA. *The Green Pharmacy.* New York: St. Martin's Press; 1997.

65. Jellin JM, Gregory P, Batz F, et al. *Pharmacist's Letter/Prescriber's Letter Natural Medicines Comprehensive Database.* 3rd ed. Stockton, CA: Therapeutic Research Faculty; 2000.

66. Zand J, Walton R, Rountree B. *Smart Medicine*

for a Healthier Child. Garden City Park, NY: Avery Publishing Group; 1994.

67. Dexter D. Magnetic therapy is ineffective for the treatment of snoring and obstructive sleep apnea syndrome, *Wisc Med J.* 1997;March:35–37.

68. Block AJ, Boysen PG, Wynne JW, et al. Sleep apnea hypopnea and oxygen desaturation in normal subjects: a strong male predominance. *N Engl J Med.* 1979;300:513–517.

69. Stradling J, Roberts D, Wilson A, et al. Controlled trial of hypnotherapy for weight loss in patients with obstructive sleep apnea. *Int J Obes.* 1998; 22(3):278–281.

70. Friese KH, Feuchter U, Moeller H. Homeopathic treatment of adenoid vegetations. Results of prospective, randomized double-blind study [in German]. *HNO.* 1997;45(8):618–624.

71. Songshan Zhu. Successful treatment of sleep apnea syndrome by transfusion of "vital energy." *Chin Med J.* 1980;93(4):279–280.

72. Ernst E, Stevinson C. Ginkgo biloba for tinnitus: a review. *Clin Otolaryngol.* 1999;24:164–167.

73. Drew S, Ewart D. Effectiveness of Ginkgo biloba: double blind, placebo controlled trial. *BMJ* 2001; 322:1–6.

74. Cordey JP. Re: Dose. Found as a rapid response to Ref. 73. *BMJ* 2001;322:7.

75. Morgenstern C, Biermann E. Ginkgo biloba special extract Egb761 in the treatment of tinnitus aurium: results of a randomized, double-blind, placebo-controlled study. *Fortschr Med.* 1997; 115(4):7–11.

76. Mason J, Rogerson DR, Butler JD. Client-centered hypnotherapy in the management of tinnitus—is it better than counseling? *J Laryngol Otol.* 1996;110(2):117–120.

77. Mason J, Rogerson DR. Client-centered hypnotherapy for tinnitus: who is likely to benefit? *Am J Clin Hypn.* 1995;37(4):294–299.

78. Park J, White AR, Ernst E. Efficacy of acupuncture as a treatment for tinnitus: a systematic review. *Arch Otolaryngol Head Neck Surg.* 2000; 126:489–492.

79. Dobie RA. A review of randomized clinical trials in tinnitus. *Laryngoscope.* 1999;109:1202–1211.

80. Axelsson A, Andersson S, Li-De G. Acupuncture in the management of tinnitus: a placebo-controlled study. *Audiology.* 1994;33:351–360.

81. Cohen HS, Jerabek J. Efficacy of treatments for posterior canal benign paroxysmal positional vertigo. *Laryngoscope.* 1999;109:584–590.

82. Nunez RA, Cass SP, Furman JM. Short- and long-term outcomes of canalith repositioning for benign paroxysmal positional vertigo. *Otolaryngol Head Neck Surg.* 2000;122(5):647–652.

83. Lynn S, Pool A, Rose D, et al. Randomized trial of the canalith repositioning procedure. *Otolaryngol Head Neck Surg.* 1995;113(6):712–720.

84. Lacour M, Sterkers O. Histamine and betahistine in the treatment of vertigo: elucidation of mechanisms of action. *CNS Drugs.* 2001;15(11): 853–870.

85. Claes J, Van de Heyning PH. A review of medical treatment for Ménière's disease. *Acta Otolaryngol Suppl.* 2000;544:34–39.

86. James AL, Burton JM. Betahistine for Ménière's disease or syndrome. *Cochrane Database Syst Rev.* 2002;2.

87. Grontved A, Hentzer E. Vertigo-reducing effect of ginger root. A controlled clinical study. *ORL J Otorhinolaryngol Relat Spec.* 1986;48(5):282–286.

88. Altura BM, Altura BT. Association of alcohol in brain injury, headaches and stroke with brain-tissue and serum levels of ionized magnesium: a review of recent findings and mechanisms of action. *Alcohol.* 1999;19:119–130.

89. Weiser M, Strosser W, Klein P. Homeopathic vs conventional treatment of vertigo: a randomized double-blind controlled clinical study. *Arch Otolaryngol Head Neck Surg.* 1998;124(8):879–885.

90. Hain TC, Fuller L, Weil L, et al. Effects of T'ai Chi on balance. *Arch Otolaryngol Head Neck Surg.* 1999;125:1191–1195.

CHAPTER 26

Integrative Approach to Pain

James N. Dillard

Acute and chronic pain syndromes, and their concomitant disability and life disruption, have an enormous negative impact on individuals and society in general. It is conservatively estimated that as many as 75 million Americans live with chronic pain.[1] Twenty-two percent of patients in primary care practice report poorly controlled pain.[2] Unofficially, it is estimated to be the third greatest health problem in the United States behind heart disease and cancer, but pain disables more individuals than heart disease and cancer put together.

Chronic pain is among the most costly national and global health problems. Chronic pain is reported by 70 million Americans, and approximately 10 percent of the US population has pain more than 100 days per year. Seven million people experience low back pain in any given year.[3] Medical costs, lost workdays, and compensation payments are conservatively estimated at 70 billion dollars per year according to 1989 statistics.[4]

Pain has traditionally been poorly treated in hospitals and by physicians, which has prompted the Joint Commission on Accreditation of Hospitals Organization (JCAHO) to mandate guidelines for the appropriate assessment and treatment of pain in accredited hospitals.[5] As of 2001, pain is considered the fifth vital sign, and must be given due consideration by all those who work in the clinical setting. De-

spite these mandates, many pain specialists continue to observe poor pain management practices (such as consistent underdosing, failure to reassess for pain, and inappropriate choices of medications, such as repeated use of meperidine injections for pain control), and those of us who integrate complementary therapies into our approach to pain medicine might wish to see improvement in conventional pain practice even before we would wish for extensive complementary and alternative care medicine (CAM) integration into conventional pain care.

Until recently, physicians were reluctant to prescribe the narcotic opioid class of medications for fear of prosecution by state and federal authorities, and in a misguided desire to avoid causing addiction. More recent evidence indicates that new "addiction" rates from the appropriate prescribing of opioid medications in acute and postoperative setting are almost immeasurably small.[6] The development of opioid "addiction" behavior in the general chronic pain population (illicit diversion, recreational drug seeking, manipulation of the prescriber) is no higher than background rates of substance abuse, and state and federal authorities have given wider latitude to the prescription of schedule II medications in appropriate clinical settings.

While this increased availability of the most powerful of pain medications has eased the suffering of many, studies still indicate that only 57% of a patient's pain is relieved on average with even the best prescribing practices.[7] This remaining 43%, in the absence of a clear surgical or other invasive option, presents an opportunity for the application of nonpharmacological and complementary therapies to provide additional relief.

The use of pharmacotherapy as the sole intervention for pain often presents challenges in and of itself. The common myriad adverse reactions and side effects with both opioid and nonopioid adjuvants can confound the practitioner's ability to provide adequate relief. Opioid medications carry with them societal stigma and patient resistance; the persistent problems of constipation, nausea, euphoria, and sedation; the ever-present threat of withdrawal syndrome should the medication dosing be delayed; the potential risk of illicit drug diversion; the potential to worsen depression; opioid-induced hyperalgesia that can produce intense pain flares if medication is inadequate or reduced; need for opioid rotation because of genetic expression of opioid receptor splice variants; and challenges in access to appropriate opioid medications because of pharmacy unavailability.

Other classes of common pain medications and adjuvants carry their own adverse reactions and risks, not the least of which is the estimated 16,000 Americans who die each year as a result of adverse reactions from the nonsteroidal antiinflammatory medications. Pharmaceutical companies continue to search for pain-relieving drugs that can address issues of both effectiveness and tolerance. However, new drug development is expensive, slow, and often costly to the patient. Because of this, a current trend is to investigate new uses of known drugs. For example, antidepressant drugs are being used in the treatment of some specific chronic pain conditions, and anticonvulsant drugs are presently the most beneficial nonsurgical therapy for trigeminal neuralgia and other neuropathic conditions. Most such uses for these drugs are still in the developmental stage, however, and it remains to be seen how effective they will be in relieving many other chronic pain conditions. The incorporation of nonpharmacological therapies where applicable would thus appear appropriately conservative, humanistic, and safety conscious.

Appropriate nondrug therapies include physical and occupational therapy, exercise prescription, transcutaneous electrical nerve stimulation (TENS), conventional psychotherapy and psychoanalysis, cognitive and behavioral therapy, biofeedback, hypnosis, and others. These and other medical interventions, including surgical procedures such as trigger-point injections; epidural steroid injections; sympathetic ganglion blockade; lidocaine infusions; spinal disk procedures such as discography; intradiscal electrothermal annuloplasty and laser disk ablation; epidural catheter and indwelling intrathecal pump placement; and spinal cord stimulator placement, can all be very helpful in carefully selected patients. These are well covered in other texts solely devoted to this subject and are beyond the scope of this chapter.

There are several important clinical scenarios in which conventional pharmacological management of pain may be problematic or virtually impossible. Children and infants may not respond consistently to pain medications, and adverse reactions may be difficult to manage. Dosages and dosing schedules may be difficult to establish and maintain. The use of simple nonpharmacological therapies, such as distraction,[8] massage, guided imagery, humor therapy, and relaxation routines, may serve to augment the conventional pediatric pain treatment program. Pregnancy presents another consistent challenge to the prescription of pharmaceuticals. The use of conventional nonpharmaceutical therapies along with hands-on therapies, massage, acupuncture, mind–body routines, and relaxation may present the only treatments possible during pregnancy.[9] In addition, adding one or more pain medications to the often-lengthy drug list of an elderly person can present additional complications and unacceptable side effects. These clinical settings lend additional justification for an integrative model for the treatment of pain.

Alternative forms of therapy offer hope to many patients with chronic pain. Types of pain that frequently drive patients to seek nonconventional treatments include back pain, myofascitis, recurrent headaches, arthritis, and dental and postoperative pain, as well as pain associated with chronic fatigue syndrome and fibromyalgia. Alternative and complementary therapies range from simple massage treatments to complex systems of medicine, such as traditional Chinese medicine, which typically incorporates Chinese herbal formulas, dietary modifications, exercise, and acupuncture. Other systems of healing include Ayurvedic medicine, traditional Tibetan medicine, and other comprehensive healing traditions.

National surveys indicate that pain conditions comprise the leading reason for the use of CAM.[10] This fact, coupled with the unacceptably high prevalence rates of poorly treated pain, begs the exploration of opportunities to improve pain symptom and function outcomes by the sensible combination of conventional with unconventional pain therapies. Unfortunately, little substantive research exists to support this potential opportunity beyond cited studies on individual therapeutic modalities.

▶ PAIN FUNDAMENTALS

Pain has traditionally been defined by several different classification systems, the simplest of which is by time. We speak of acute pain, subacute pain, and chronic pain, with acute pain being that which lasts shorter than 6 weeks, and chronic pain being that which lasts longer than 6 months. Pain is also classified by the source of the pain, such as cancer or malignant pain versus nonmalignant pain syndromes. The type of pain, such as nociceptive pain, neuropathic pain, sympathetically maintained pain, and central pain, can also be used to classify pain. These classifications may aid in diagnosis and treatment.

Perhaps no other problem poses such a challenge to current medical practitioners, who are often at a loss as to how to treat chronic pain. Traditionally, physicians are trained to search for the organic disorder or pathophysiology, so that it may be surgically or medically cured. Unfortunately, for many disabling nonmalignant pain conditions, the pain-generating tissue of origin remains obscure or untreatable. This leaves the conventional practitioner at a loss for a treatment plan.

Occasionally, a treatable diagnosis can be missed in the chronic pain sufferer, obscured by the complexity of the symptomatology and clinical scenario. When pain stems from a disorder that is not well understood, such as fibromyalgia, treatment to relieve pain may mask symptoms of an undiscovered life-threatening disorder. To complicate matters, the relationship between organic causes and pain is often murky at best; for example, spinal abnormalities commonly show up in radiographs and scans of patients who suffer from severe back pain as well as of individuals who are pain-free. Conversely, there are those who live with constant back pain but who show no abnormalities whatsoever. Understanding these challenges, the modern pain practitioner can make judicious use of diagnostic tools and algorithms, even while being called upon to treat pain and symptoms of obscure origin. Often one must give up the search for a treatment to "cure" the pain, and accept that the pain has "taken on a life of its own," without treatable pathology or altered anatomy present.

A new understanding of pain mechanisms can explain how pain takes on a life of its own, and can inform the pain practitioner of the substrates for new strategies in pain control. The classic description of how pain travels from a burned foot directly to the brain, as illustrated by Descartes, implies that pain signals ascend from the peripheral nociceptor to the brain as if conducted by copper wire. This has been replaced by an ever-expanding understanding of the complex conversations that exist in major pain pathways and interneurons at the various signal processing "way stations" between the periphery and the brain. Moving past the gate control theory of Melzak and Wall,[11,12] we now see a potential barrage of inhibitory signals descending from the rostral medulla and para-aqueductal gray regions of the brain down into the spinal cord to moderate painful sensation. The new understanding of central nervous system pain sensitization clarifies persistent and apparently amplified pain.[13] In addition, the simple neurotransmitter systems of even a decade ago have been replaced by ever-more complex models of neurochemistry and neural receptor regulatory mechanisms.[14]

Pain also lives in the internal structure of the person's life, and can greatly modify and be modified by the individual's emotional, spiritual, and psychic identity. Chronic pain cannot be treated in a vacuum, as if it were a broken bone or a clogged artery. The conventional discipline of pain medicine has already embraced a multidisciplinary and "holistic" approach, that is, taking stock of the whole person rather than simply treating the manifest condition.[15,16] The National Institutes of Health (NIH) has published a Consensus Statement endorsing a multidisciplinary approach to pain,[17] but this guide for practice is often not followed by practitioners. The challenge remains for primary care, specialist, and pain physicians to adequately assess and treat the immensely important psychological and psychosocial factors typically present in the chronic pain patient.

► MIND–BODY TREATMENT APPROACHES

Many types of mind–body treatment approaches are used to reduce pain. Precise mechanisms for pain reduction using these practices are not completely understood, but they may involve the activities of neurotransmitters, serotonin, and catecholamines that influence the mind's perception of pain. Hypnosis, biofeedback, and relaxation techniques, such as meditation and autogenic training, are

the primary forms. In some cases, these methods have been found not only to be beneficial but economical as well. Of all the alternative therapies used for pain relief, these three techniques are the most widely accepted and are taught in medical schools and are available at many hospitals and outpatient clinics.

Numerous research studies support the benefits of mind–body treatment approaches. In 1995, a 35-member NIH panel was convened to determine the value of specific mind–body techniques for treating pain.[18] In particular, the panel found biofeedback to be effective in the treatment of tension headaches and other types of chronic pain, and hypnosis to be useful in adjunctive treatments for cancer pain, irritable bowel syndrome, temporomandibular joint syndrome, tension headaches, and chronic inflammatory disorders.

Systematic reviews of the literature indicate that mind–body interventions can be effective for health conditions that are caused or made worse by stress.[19] Furthermore, relaxation techniques can be helpful for pain control,[20] and visualization techniques may also be of benefit.[21] These simple techniques can be easily taught in the office or at the bedside, and may provide the pain sufferer with additional pain and symptom relief, as well as an enhanced sense of self-efficacy in the setting of chronic pain.

In a 1998 systematic review of chronic pain studies, nine randomized, placebo-controlled trials obtained through on-line databases singled out three studies in favor of using relaxation therapy to reduce chronic pain associated with cancer, rheumatoid arthritis, or ulcerative colitis.[22] The same reviewers, in a systematic review of acute pain management, found that in three of seven trials, relaxation methods reduced acute pain.[23] A recent NIH statement on management of cancer-related pain, depression, and fatigue[24] documents the high prevalence of these symptoms, and concludes that they are inadequately detected and treated. The statement suggests that integrative approaches may be helpful, but more research is needed. Relaxation techniques may be a valuable contribution to the control of cancer pain.[25,26] Guided imagery may also be useful.[27,28] Pediatric patients and older patients, particularly with some cognitive impairment, may respond better to passive distractions for pain relief such as an engaging movie or familiar music than to active mind–body therapies.

▶ MASSAGE, BODYWORK AND POSTURAL THERAPIES

Massage is a common and ancient bodywork technique for relieving pain. Massage has been used since the time of Hippocrates, and has variously been part of mainstream medical practice or considered unconventional. The techniques in massage very widely, but most involve stroking, kneading, and pressing on muscles and connective tissue. It is generally considered extremely safe, although rare adverse events, such as skin reactions, bruising, or fracture, have been reported.

In earlier randomized, controlled trials, the effects of massage for pain were found to be no different than the effects of a placebo. However, more recent studies and systematic reviews show clear benefit from massage over control interventions.[29–31] In 2002, Bascom reviewed more than 60 papers in CAM therapies for occupational health problems and concluded that massage therapy was a reasonable option for pain of occupational origin.[32] Cherkin et al. showed that massage therapy was superior to acupuncture for back pain, with a longer therapeutic effect,[33] although Carlsson and Sjolund also showed long-term benefits from acupuncture.[34]

A number of other recent studies find massage effective for pain in a variety of settings. Richards et al. reviewed 22 massage papers and concluded that it was effective for relaxation, pain, and insomnia in the acute care setting.[35] Field et al. conducted a prospective study of 26 pregnant women, comparing massage to relaxation therapy, showing the massage group to have less pain and fewer postnatal complications,[36] and in another study, showed reduced labor pain in the massage group.[37] Kober et al. showed acupressure massage to be effective in relieving pain in trauma patients.[38] Brattberg randomized 48 fibromyalgia sufferers into massage and control groups, and showed positive effects that lasted several months.[39] Hernandez-Reif has shown massage therapy was superior to a wait list in 26 migraine sufferers.[40]

Some theorists postulate that massage helps control pain by increasing pain-reducing neurochemicals, such as endorphins and serotonin in the brain and spinal cord. Variations of Swedish, deep-tissue, sports, and neuromuscular methods are frequently used. Newer methods incorporate theories from reflexology, zone therapy, and acupressure. Combinations of techniques are also effective in pain treatment. In one study, pain patients who were given Swedish massage, shiatsu, and trigger-point suppression experienced acute and chronic pain relief and increased flexibility.

Other types of bodywork used in pain treatment are the Alexander technique, the Trager method, and the Feldenkrais method. These are postural bodywork therapies that teach patients how to realign their bodies, improve posture and movement, and reduce structural stress. Although few controlled studies have been done on these techniques, and most of the reported benefits are subjective, each method is nevertheless used to treat chronic back pain, sports injury-related pain, headaches, and joint pain. These practitioners are generally unlicensed and relatively unregulated.

As discussed in Chapter 11, yoga is another body-oriented therapy commonly practiced for back, neck, and joint pain, although the research base remains sparse.[41] Practitioners believe that a combination of stretching postures with controlled rhythmic breathing create a combined effect of physical toning and a mind–body therapy that may be effective for musculoskeletal and stress-related symptoms.

▶ ALTERNATIVE SYSTEMS OF MEDICINE

Chinese Medicine

Traditional Chinese medicine is based upon descriptive metaphors for human bioenergetic properties that do not translate well or directly into the English terms used for them. These concepts are reviewed in depth in Chapter 9. Many of the internal bioenergetic properties assessed have a relationship with external and environmental factors. According to traditional Chinese medicine, pain is caused by a conflict between blood and Qi (or Chi, the life force that permeates the body), which, in turn, results in stagnation. Relieving this stagnancy, balancing the energy, nourishing the blood, and building up deficient blood are all ways that Chinese medicine uses to treat pain. Traditional Chinese doctors use acupuncture techniques to correct the flow of Qi; in addition they use herbal medicines to reestablish balanced Qi, blood, and moisture in organ networks in order to avert excess wind, heat, cold, dryness, and dampness. These sorts of metaphors form the basis of the descriptive and diagnostic systems in traditional Chinese medicine.

Studies support the use of acupuncture for the treatment of acute and chronic types of pain, including osteoarthritis, back pain, dysmenorrhea, and migraines.[42] In an effort to determine precisely how acupuncture works, researchers have isolated changes in the immune, neurochemical, and hormone functions as well as in pain pathways following acupuncture treatment, but the exact mechanisms of action from a Western perspective remain elusive. Acupuncture may act as a pain preventative, theoretically, by acting on the sympathetic nervous system. Chinese bodywork therapies, such as shiatsu and acupressure, may help to reduce pain through processes that combine massage with acupuncture principles.

Acupuncture research has progressed substantially in the last 10 years, although evidence regarding its mechanisms and efficacy for painful conditions is far from ironclad. Some of the best data to date has more strongly supported acupuncture for indications other than pain, such as nausea.[43] Research methodologies for studying acupuncture remain challenging,[44] as discussed in detail in Chapter 9. The equivocal benefit demonstrated for pain in most of the clinical trials literature, as discussed below, remains difficult to reconcile with the clinical experience of many practitioners who frequently refer to acupuncture for pain problems.

There is good evidence that acupuncture can be useful for facial and dental pain; Ernst and Pittler showed that in 14 of 16 high-quality, randomized, controlled trials, acupuncture was superior to sham acupuncture.[45] The evidence regarding low back pain is less definitive. Some studies have been fairly positive,[46,47] and others less so. In their meta-analysis of acupuncture trials for low back pain, Ernst et al. concluded that acupuncture was more effective than control interventions, although not clearly superior to placebo.[48] Other studies have been more negative,[49,50] and still others have found that sham acupuncture seems to work as well as real acupuncture for low back pain.[51] Certainly there is a need for more research on this question, although the current evidence tends to indicate that acupuncture is not clearly more effective for low back pain than other conservative treatments.

Similarly equivocal results have been found for acupuncture and neck pain,[52] although some have disagreed with these conclusions on methodological grounds.[53] Others have obtained more positive results.[54] Smith et al. have concluded that there is inadequate evidence to support the use of acupuncture for back or neck pain,[55] although this conclusion remains controversial. Again, the research literature seems at odds with the common clinical experience of acupuncture's utility.

The use of acupuncture for a number of other pain syndromes has been studied as well, although methodological challenges again have made conclusions difficult. Melchart et al. studied 22 trials of acupuncture for headache in a systematic review and concluded that acupuncture could be helpful, but that the evidence was not fully convincing.[56] White et al. randomized 50 headache patients to real and sham acupuncture and found it to be ineffective,[57] although other studies have been more positive. Knee osteoarthritis may be helped by acupuncture.[58] There is some reasonable evidence that acupuncture may be helpful with patients suffering from fibromyalgia.[59] Lastly, Lin et al. have shown that electroacupuncture can reduce postoperative analgesic requirements and associated side effects in patients undergoing lower abdominal surgery.[60]

Acupuncture is not often used in the pediatric population, but Kemper et al. studied 47 families in which acupuncture was used on children. A clear majority of children and parents reported that the treatments were helpful and well tolerated.[61] Other studies show that acupuncture can be helpful for the pain of labor, and may improve outcomes.[62]

In multiple papers, Paul White and colleagues have shown that a nontraditional dermatomally based electroacupuncture techniques called peripheral electroacupuncture nerve stimulation is effective for low back pain,[63] painful diabetic neuropathy,[64] headache,[65] and other conditions. This technique may not be acupuncture in the strictest sense, but the body of research is intriguing.

Chinese herbs for pain treatment often have analgesic properties, some of which are extremely potent. In China, as here, herbal medicines are typically taken as teas, capsules, tablets, or extracts. But depending upon the type and severity of the pain, some preparations in China are given in hospitals intravenously or subcutaneously. *Corydalis yanhusuo*, or corydalis tuber, is an example of a potent Chinese herb used for neuralgia, painful menstruation, and gastrointestinal spasm. Corydalis contains numerous potent alkaloids that inhibit activity in the brain stem associated with pain perception, and it has sedating properties—the powdered drug has a potency 1% that of opium. One of the predominant alkaloids responsible for these effects is tetrahydropalmatine, which has been isolated and tested on mice to determine its tranquilizing effects. It appears to inhibit postsynaptic dopaminergic receptors and simultaneously to increase the availability of gamma-aminobutyricacid receptors. These actions both reduce pain and relieve anxiety.

Arnold and Thornbrough recently reviewed from the Western perspective the applications of Chinese botanicals for musculoskeletal pain.[66] For those interested, reading this review added insight into pharmacologic use.

Ayurveda

Ayurveda attributes pain syndromes to imbalances and stagnation in constitutional types, known as doshas. The three doshas are vata, kapha, and pitta. The location and type of pain are believed to be dependent on which of three constitutional types is aggravated or stagnant, which, in turn, determines the treatment. Often, such treatment is herbal as well as dietary and involves giving patients botanical substances or foods that either stimulate or soothe the constitutional imbalance. These preparations are characterized as sweet, sour, salty, bitter, astringent, or pungent and are often combinations of these types.

For example, vata, which is normally dry, cold, and light in quality, is balanced with substances that are wet, warm, and dark. In Ayurvedic practice, such substances are usually sweet. But in the case of obstructive vata, sweet substances are thought likely to exacerbate blockage, so these patients are given pungent herbs and foods to stimulate the movement of vata. The Ayurvedic approach to treatments is discussed in detail in Chapter 10.

Triphala and Trikatu are two Ayurvedic herbal standards that may be recommended by a practitioner to relieve blockages that cause pain. Trikatu is a blend of black pepper, ginger, and Indian pepper. The Indian pepper used in Trikatu (long pepper; pippali) contains elements similar to capsaicin in cayenne pepper. It is used as a topical painkiller for arthritic conditions and is thought to stimulate and then inhibit pain by destroying substance P. Furthermore, constituents in the ginger can block the cyclooxygenase pathway, preventing the formation of inflammatory prostaglandins.[67] More recently, researchers found that ginger extracts can have a beneficial effect on osteoarthritis of the knee.[68]

Few randomized or double-blind trials have been conducted in the United States to determine the effects of Ayurvedic or Indian herbal treatments on pain. However, one recent study recognized the potential of a species of frankincense *(Boswellia serrata)*, which contains constituents known to interrupt leukotriene formation and to inhibit pain associated with polyarthritis. Because of the small number of participants, the researchers were unable to recommend *Boswellia serrata* for the treatment of polyarthritis based on the outcome of one study; however, they felt future research with more participants might be more conclusive.[69]

Homeopathy

Because classic homeopathy depends on the assessment of a patient's specific clinical pattern and relies on individualized treatment strategies, generalizations about this approach can be misleading. Nevertheless, evidence for reasonable applications of homeopathic remedies does exist for dental pain, sports injury, and some types of arthritis. Homeopathic remedies for pain may be taken either internally or externally. Homeopathic arnica ointment, for example, has long been recommended for sports-related injuries, such as sprains.

A double-blind, placebo-controlled crossover trial demonstrated that homeopathic *Rhus toxicodendron* (poison oak) reduced tender points by 25% in patients with fibromyalgia following 4 weeks of treatment.[70] However another recent study of homeopathy and rheumatoid arthritis was negative for effect.[71] Swiss

researchers recently published a positive trial of homeopathy in back pain,[72] and another study was positive for a homeopathic gel.[73]

Several studies have been positive for homeopathic treatment of headache and migraine frequency,[74] as well as chronic headache.[75] A study of 100 women with metastatic cancer showed no effect on pain, but positive effects on hot flashes and fatigue.[76]

Osteopathy and Chiropractic

Spinal manipulation as now performed has extraordinary heterogeneity, thus making it impossible to form sweeping conclusions about its efficacy.[77] A wide range of techniques are used, varying from extremely gentle contacts or mobilizations to very forceful manipulations. The most common and most studied form is referred to as high-velocity low-amplitude mobilization, where the slack is taken out of a spinal joint and a very rapid short thrust is applied to gap the joint. An audible click is often heard. This is the form studied in the cited research for this chapter. These manipulations, using either osteopathic or chiropractic techniques, show considerable effectiveness for the treatment of various types of back pain. In 1992, a literature review of spinal manipulations for low back pain determined that the techniques are helpful when acute and subacute low back pain occurs with or without mild neurological involvement or sciatic nerve irritation.[78]

In 1994, the Agency for Health Care Policy and Research (AHCPR), a federal research and information agency organized in 1989, released its guidelines for the treatment of acute low back pain. The guidelines recommend spinal manipulation, either osteopathic or chiropractic, above more typical forms of physical therapy (including traction, diathermy, TENS, and ultrasonography). Osteopathic and chiropractic treatments were found to have benefits that were equal to or superior to placebo. While the specific physiologic effects of spinal manipulation are largely unknown, the AHCPR guidelines acknowledge that the methods used often meet with positive results. National treatment guidelines in Canada and England also recommend chiropractic manipulation as first-line therapy for neck and back pain. Several positive meta-analyses and systematic reviews have been done on chiropractic manipulative therapy, but the final evidence of its efficacy remains dependent to some degree on the relative quality of the studies done.[79–81] Spinal manipulation remains immensely popular for back pain, and the safety of the procedure is quite good.[82]

There is some evidence for the efficacy of spinal manipulation in neck pain[83–86] and headache,[87,88] although some would argue that the risks of catastrophic neurological injury are too great.[89–91] The safety issues in cervical manipulation are reviewed in detail in Chapter 8. Some authors suggest that manipulation may be helpful in rheumatologic illness,[92] although the loosening of spinal ligaments in the cervical spine caused by inflammatory arthritis would be a contraindication to the use of any sort of aggressive techniques.

Osteopathic treatment of acute low back pain has been supported by some positive findings in randomized controlled trials, although most recent studies tend to show little effect.[93] Because of its universal popularity, chiropractic care is sometimes considered the first line of alternative therapy for various types of pain, including fibromyalgia and neck and back pain. Many medical practitioners are now willing to send spinal pain patients for a trial of spinal manipulative therapy, although most would limit the trial to no more than six to eight treatments before wanting to reassess the patient.

▶ NUTRITIONAL AND BOTANICAL SUPPLEMENTS

Dietary Supplements

Calcium and magnesium are the two minerals most often recommended for supplementation in the treatment of pain syndromes. Calcium is recommended for conditions such as osteoarthritis, more as a preventative or corrective supplement than as a painkiller. Recently, it was reported in the *American Journal of Obstetrics and Gynecology* that pain from premenstrual syndrome was reduced by half in women given supplemental calcium.[94] Usual daily dosage is 1,000–1,200 mg.

Magnesium, a mineral required for musculoskeletal maintenance and health, is recommended for osteoporosis and has long been valued in treating migraines. Because it relaxes skeletal and smooth muscles after they contract, magnesium is considered a relaxation-promoting mineral. The recommended daily allowance (RDA) for magnesium is 350 mg of elemental magnesium, but dosages up to 1,000 mg/d appear to be safe in those with no significant medical problems.

Current trends in supplement treatment of pain conditions also include use of essential fatty acids (EFAs)—particularly gamma-linolenic acid (omega-6) and fish-derived eicosapentaenoic acid (omega-3)—and glucosamine sulfate. Essential fatty acids are the starting point from which the body makes both prostaglandins and leukotrienes. Omega-6 fatty acids convert to series 1 or 2 prostaglandins and to the substances similar to prostaglandin called leukotrienes. The series 1 prostaglandins are considered beneficial. They appear to inhibit inflammation, lower cholesterol, and reduce blood pressure. However, the series 2 prostaglandins, along with certain of the leukotrienes, are associated with pain and inflammation. The reduction or alteration in synthesis of these pro-inflammatory compounds promoted by adjusting EFA intake may help with the inflammation and pain resulting from the series 2 prostaglandin end points.[95] Omega-3 fatty acids, found in marine animal fats and some vegetable oils, are converted to series 3 prostaglandins (generally antiinflammatory in effect) and to a less noxious form of leukotriene. The combination of omega-3 and omega-6 oils may be especially beneficial, as the presence of omega-3 fatty acids tends to prevent the omega-6 oils from being converted to less favorable end points (Figure 26–1).

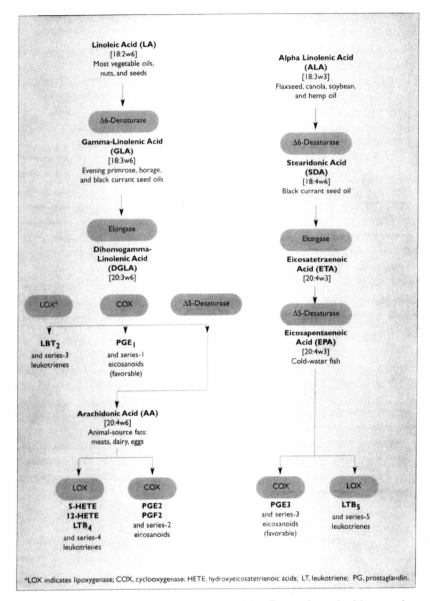

Figure 26–1. Biosynthesis of eicosanoids. Reproduced with permission from Modulation of the inflammatory cascade. *Int J Integrative Med.* 2002;4(5):6–29.

Fish oil and flax seed oil both provide omega-3 fatty acids. Fish oil is beneficial in the treatment of arthritis[96–98]; the benefits of flax seed oil are less clear because there is more interaction with other vegetable oils. Evening primrose oil, black currant oil, and borage oil are sources of omega-6 and are also effective in reducing pain, although results are equivocal and more study is warranted. EFA supplements can become rancid, and patients are urged to make sure the products they choose are fresh and well protected from the elements.

It is best to use expeller-pressed oils, check expiration dates, and keep oils refrigerated in opaque containers.

Finally, glucosamine sulfate is more effective in reducing osteoarthritic pain than nonsteroidal antiinflammatory drugs, shark cartilage, chondroitin sulfate, or placebo; some investigators feel glucosamine may have disease-modifying properties in osteoarthritis and actually slow the deterioration of joints characteristic of this condition.[99,100] Glucosamine typically takes 4–6 weeks to take effect. At doses of 500 mg three times a day, glucosamine sulfate is considered safe, although mild stomach discomfort and elevation of blood pressure as a consequence of salt content is sometimes reported.

Botanical Medicine

Pain-reducing botanicals are typically spoken of in terms of their mechanisms of action or in terms of the actions of their constituents, in the same manner as pharmaceutical drugs. In the context of pain treatment, these actions might inhibit platelet-activating factor, prostaglandin formation, cyclooxygenase, or arachidonase. For example, a constituent in garlic demonstrates the ability to block each of these pathways, and feverfew *(Tanacetum parthenium)*—which is thought to be helpful in relieving migraine headaches—appears to either prevent vasospasm or block cyclooxygenase, a metabolite of arachidonic acid that triggers the formation of prostaglandins. Like feverfew, black willow bark *(Salix nigra)*, ginger root, and Jamaican dogwood bark *(Piscidia piscipula)* extracts block cyclooxygenase, as does aspirin, which was originally derived from willow bark. However, phytochemists (plant chemists) are just beginning to develop our understanding of these mechanisms of action, and it may be quite some time before the full therapeutic potential of many botanicals is determined.

Long et al. have reviewed herbal medicines for treatment of osteoarthritis,[101] Ernst and Chrubasik have reviewed antiinflammatory herbs,[102] and Almeid and colleagues have summarized botanical products that have centrally acting analgesic properties.[103] Literally hundreds of plants have been found to have antinociceptive and antiinflammatory properties, including those traditionally thought of for other medicinal purposes.[104,105] It remains to be seen which plant products will be borne out for safety, efficacy, and tolerability in human clinical trials.

In a study of 174 low back pain patients, Laudahn and Walper showed positive effects for devil's claw *(Harpagophytum prothrombens)* for back pain with few adverse reactions.[106] White willow bark has been studied for pain with some success.[107] Other painkilling herbs include cayenne, which can be taken either internally or rubbed onto painful arthritic joints, and ginkgo, an extract formula that is also gaining popularity as a possible deterrent to Alzheimer disease and other types of dementia. One recent trial showed that Reumalex, a proprietary herbal formula, helped reduce chronic arthritis pain.[108] *Ginkgo biloba* extracts have been proven to reduce leg pain associated with intermittent claudication.[109]

In general, herbal treatments for pain are used topically or internally. One useful topical agent, cajeput oil, is usually administered in combination with other oils, such as peppermint, clove, menthol, eucalyptus, St. John's wort, cayenne, or arnica oil. It relieves musculoskeletal pain, headache, hemorrhoid pain, neuralgia, rheumatic pain, and pain resulting from sports injuries.

▶ BIOELECTROMAGNETICS

The theory behind bioelectromagnetics is that nonionizing electromagnetic fields, in the extremely low-frequency range, may benefit certain conditions as a consequence of electromagnetic changes to ligand-receptor interactions at the cell membrane.[110,111] The effects of bioelectromagnetics are thought to result from a change in membrane transport and gene expression. Bioelectromagnetics may one day prove to be the effectual factor in therapies that use energetic healing techniques, such as therapeutic touch.

Techniques of nonionizing bioelectromagnetics are either thermal (heat producing in biologic tissue) or nonthermal. Thermal methods are used with laser and radio frequency surgery, radio frequency diathermy, and radio frequency hyperthermia. However, the nonthermal applications are more prevalent in alternative medicine. Microwave resonance therapy is a method of nonthermal nonionizing bioelectromagnetics used extensively in Russia. Microwave resonance therapy incorporates low-intensity sinusoidal microwave radiation and has had favorable results in treating many conditions, including arthritis, pain, and hypertension. Often, microwave resonance therapy is applied to acupuncture points.

Transcranial electromagnetic stimulation of the prefrontal cortex has been shown in multiple studies to have an effect on pain, but this is probably not an alternative or complementary technique.[112] Stationary magnets have been studied for pain with some success for knee pain,[113,114] chronic pelvic pain,[115] and postpoliomyelitis pain.[116] Other studies of stationary magnets have found a positive effect for carpal tunnel pain,[117] no effect on wrist pain,[118] weak results in fibromyalgia,[119] and no effects in a small study for low back pain.[120] Electromagnetic stimulation has been shown to help with knee pain.[121,122] Trock and Vallbona have reviewed this literature.[123,124] The efficacy of magnetic fields for pain remains an area of controversy, although generally pulsed electromagnetic fields seem to be more supported by the literature than are static magnetic fields.

▶ COMPLEMENTARY THERAPIES IN PALLIATIVE CARE

Attention to palliation in the setting of terminal illness has only recently come to the conventional medical community from its origins in mid-twentieth century England. Although hospice services are widely available, most US hospitals still do not have a palliative care service, including many of the oldest and most prestigious medical institutions. Efforts to remedy this are currently underway in many medical centers.

Palliative care is by definition multidisciplinary. The emphasis in palliative care on the social, spiritual, and psychological needs of the patient is inherently a "holistic" approach. Integration of complementary therapies for pain and other symptoms is a natural extension of this multidisciplinary foundation, both in the hospice setting and in the hospital units. Although it is clearly not possible to do everything for every patient, selective complementary therapies may be helpful to patients approaching the end of life. Conventional nursing, pastoral care, and psychological services may be appropriately augmented by mind–body therapies, massage, aromatherapy, acupuncture, yoga, or other techniques.

Shumay and colleagues studied the existing use of CAM techniques in the cancer population, finding more use among women who were better educated, white, and had greater severity of symptoms, particularly nausea and vomiting.[125] Pan and colleagues reviewed 21 studies of CAM therapies and concluded that although there is still a paucity of data, some CAM therapies are probably useful for the terminally ill.[126] DiGianni and colleagues studied women with breast cancer and concluded that little evidence exists to support CAM use beyond somewhat helpful psychosocial interventions.[127] Finally, Power et al. studied the use of CAM therapies in the HIV-infected population.[128]

Although the evidence base may not currently be strong enough to justify the use of complementary therapies with the terminally ill, many patients do request these approaches, and some seem to find benefit from them. This is a relatively unstudied field, and from a research viewpoint, that which is unproven is not disproved. One or more of the CAM therapies may be of benefit in the palliative care setting, despite the lack of solid evidence at this time.

▶ CONCLUSION

Complementary and alternative therapies are widely used for painful conditions despite the lack of strong research supporting this use for many clinical problems and therapies. Despite this lack, one could conclude that questioning the absolute validity of a therapy and dismissing responses as placebo effects may be irrelevant in the subject of pain, for if the patient feels better, feels comforted, feels less stressed, and is more functional in life, then the desired outcome has been achieved. The only caveat would be that an as-yet-unproven therapy should be relatively or very inexpensive and extremely safe, as is the case with many of the complementary therapies reviewed. There is no measurable result, such as the glycosylated hemoglobin in diabetes, to objectively measure salutary effects from the use of regulated breathing, meditation, guided imagery, or a massage for a pain sufferer. A personal outcome for the individual in an improved sense of well-being and empowerment in the face of suffering and despair may be proof enough.

The foundations of good nutrition, exercise, stress reduction, and reengagement in life can contribute much to restoring the quality of life to a pain patient. Adding conventional nondrug therapies such as physical therapy, cognitive behavior therapy, TENS, hypnosis, biofeedback, and psychotherapy can complete the conventional picture. Adding touch therapies, acupuncture, and herbal and nutritional approaches may be appropriate in select cases, and depending on the circumstances, may significantly enhance the conventional pain management program.

REFERENCES

1. Schnitzer TJ. Non-NSAID pharmacologic treatment options for the management of chronic pain. *Am J Med.* 1998;105:45S–52S.
2. Guueje O, et al. Persistent pain and well-being: a World Health Organization study in primary care. *JAMA.* 1998;280:147–151.
3. Osterweis M, Kleinman A, Mechanic D. Pain and Disability: Clinical, Behavioral, and Public Policy Perspectives. Washington, DC: National Academy Press; 1987.
4. Schwartz GE, Watson SD, Galvin DE, Lipoff E. *The Disability Management Sourcebook,* Vol. 6, Washington, DC: Washington Business Group on Health and Institute for Rehabilitation and Disability Management; Fall 1989.
5. http://www.jcaho.org/. Accessed January 25, 2003.
6. Porter J, Jick H. Addiction rare in patients treated with narcotics. NEJM. 302;123, 1980.
7. Passik S. Chronic opioid therapy. Presentation at American Pain Society meeting; March 23, 2002; Baltimore, MD.
8. Kleiber C, Harper DC. Effects of distraction on children's pain and distress during medical procedures: a meta-analysis. *Nurs Res.* 1999;48(1):44–49.
9. Gentz BA. Alternative therapies for the management of pain in labor and delivery. *Clin Obstet Gynecol.* 2001;44(4):704–732.
10. Eisenberg DM, Davis RB, Ettner SL, et al. Trends in CAM use in the United States 1990–1997. Results of a follow-up national survey. *JAMA.* 1998;280:1569–1575.
11. Melzack R, Wall PD. Pain mechanisms: a new theory. *Science.* 1965;150(3699):971–979.
12. Wall PD. The gate control theory of pain mechanisms. A re-examination and re-statement. *Brain.* 1978;101(1):1–18.
13. Woolf CJ, Walters ET. Common patterns of plasticity contributing to nociceptive sensitization in mammals and Aplysia. *Trends Neurosci.* 1991;14(2):74–78.
14. Woolf CJ, Max MB. Mechanism-based pain diagnosis: issues for analgesic drug development. *Anesthesiology.* 2001;95(1):241–249.
15. Fordyce WE. *Behavioral Methods for Pain and Chronic Illness.* St. Louis, MO: Mosby; 1976.
16. Turk DC, Okifuji A. Evaluating the role of physical, operant, cognitive, and affective factors in the pain behaviors of chronic pain patients. *Behav Mod.* 1997;21(3):259–280.
17. Integrated Approach to the Management of Pain. NIH Consensus Statement; Vol. 6, No. 3; May

19–21, 1986. Available at: http://consensus.nih.gov/cons/055/055_intro.htm. Accessed 2000.

18. *Integration of Behavioral and Relaxation Approaches into the Treatment of Chronic Pain and Insomnia.* Bethesda, MD: NIH Tecnology Assessment Statement. 1995;October 16–18: 1–34.

19. Jacobs GD. Clinical applications of the relaxation response and mind–body interventions. *J Altern Comp Med.* 2001;7(suppl):S93–S101.

20. Cole BH, Brunk Q. Holistic interventions for acute pain episodes: an integrative review. *J Holistic Nurs.* 1999;17(4):384–396.

21. Hoffart MB, Keene EP. The benefits of visualization. *Am J Nurs.* 1998;98(12):44–47.

22. Carroll D, Seers K. Relaxation for the relief of chronic pain: a systematic review. *J Adv Nurs.* 1998;27(3):476–487.

23. Carroll D, Seers K. Relaxation techniques for acute pain management: a systematic review. *J Adv Nurs.* 1998;27(3):466–475.

24. *NIH State-of-the-Science Conference Statement on Symptom Management in Cancer: Pain, Depression and Fatigue;* July 15–17, 2002. Available at: http://odp.od.nih.gov/consensus/ta/022/022_intro.htm. Accessed 2003.

25. Bauer-Wu SM. Psychoneuroimmunology. Part II: Mind–body interventions. *Clin J Oncol Nurs.* 2002;6(4):243–246.

26. Luebbert K, Dahme B, Hasenbring M. The effectiveness of relaxation training in reducing treatment-related symptoms and improving emotional adjustment in acute non-surgical cancer treatment: a meta-analytical review. *Psycho-oncology.* 2001; 10(6):490–502.

27. Wallace KG. Analysis of recent literature concerning relaxation and imagery interventions for cancer pain. *Cancer Nurs.* 1997;20(2):79–87.

28. Syrjala KL, Donaldson GW, Davis MW, Kippes ME, Carr JE. Relaxation and imagery and cognitive-behavioral training reduce pain during cancer treatment: a controlled clinical trial. *Pain.* 1995;63(2):189–198.

29. Furlan AD, Brosseau L, Imamura M, Irvin E. Massage for low-back pain: a systematic review within the framework of the Cochrane Collaboration Back Review Group. *Spine.* 2002;27(17): 1896–1910.

30. Field T. Massage therapy. *Med Clin North Am.* 2002;86(1):163–171.

31. Ernst E. Massage therapy for low back pain: a

systematic review. *J Pain Symptom Manage.* 1999;17(1):65–69.

32. Bascom A. Complementary and alternative therapies in occupational health. Part II—specific therapies. *AAOHN J.* 2002;50(10):468–477.

33. Cherkin DC, Eisenberg D, Sherman KJ, et al. Randomized trial comparing traditional chinese medical acupuncture, therapeutic massage, and self-care for chronic low back pain. *Arch Intern Med.* 2001;161:1081–1088.

34. Carlsson CPO, Sjolund BH. Acupuncture for chronic low back pain: a randomized placebo-controlled study with long-term follow-up. *Clin J Pain.* 2001;17(4):296–305.

35. Richards KC, Gibson R, Overton-McCoy AL. Effects of massage in acute and critical care. *AACN Clin Issues.* 2000;11(1):77–96.

36. Field T, Hernandez-Reif M, Hart S, Theakston H, Schanberg S, Kuhn C. Pregnant women benefit from massage therapy. *J Psychosom Obstet Gynaecol.* 1999;20(1):31–38.

37. Field T, Hernandez-Reif M, Taylor S, Quintino O, Burman I. Labor pain is reduced by massage therapy. *J Psychosom Obstet Gynaecol.* 1997;18(4): 286–291.

38. Kober A, Scheck T, Greher M, et al. Prehospital analgesia with acupressure in victims of minor trauma: a prospective, randomized, double-blinded trial. *Anesth Analg.* 2002;95(3):723–727.

39. Brattberg G. Connective tissue massage in the treatment of fibromyalgia. *Eur J Pain.* 1999;3: 235–245.

40. Hernandez-Reif M, Dieter J, Field T, Swerdlow B, Diego M. Migraine headaches are reduced by massage therapy. *Int J Neurosci.* 1998;96(1–2): 1–11.

41. Ott MJ. Yoga as a clinical intervention. *Adv Nurse Pract.* 2002;10(1):81–83, 90.

42. Kaptchuk TJ. Acupuncture: theory, efficacy, and practice. *Ann Intern Med.* 2002;136(5):374–383.

43. Vickers A. Can acupuncture have specific effects on health? A systematic review of acupuncture antiemesis trials. *J R Soc Med.* 1996;89:303–311.

44. White AR, Filshie J, Cummings TM. Clinical trials of acupuncture: consensus recommendations for optimal treatment, sham controls and blinding. *Complement Ther Med.* 2001;9(4):237–245.

45. Ernst E, Pittler MH. The effectiveness of acupuncture in treating acute dental pain: a systematic review. *Br Dent J.* 1998;184(9):443–447.

46. Carlsson CP, Sjolund BH. Acupuncture for chronic low back pain: a randomized placebo-controlled

study with long-term follow-up. *Clin J Pain.* 2001;17(4):296–305.

47. Molsberger AF, Mau J, Pawelec DB, Winkler J. Does acupuncture improve the orthopedic management of chronic low back pain—a randomized, blinded, controlled trial with 3 months follow up. *Pain.* 2002;99(3):579–587.

48. Ernst E, White AR, Wider B. Acupuncture for back pain: meta-analysis of randomised controlled trials and an update with data from the most recent studies (in German). *Schmerz.* 2002; 16(2):129–139.

49. van Tulder MW, Cherkin DC, Berman B, Lao L, Koes BW. The effectiveness of acupuncture in the management of acute and chronic low back pain. A systematic review within the framework of the Cochrane Collaboration Back Review Group. *Spine.* 1999 1;24(11):1113–1123.

50. Tulder MW, Cherkin DC, Berman B, Lao L, Koes BW. Acupuncture for low back pain. *Cochrane Database Syst Rev.* 2000;(2):CD001351.

51. Leibing E, Leonhardt U, Koster G, et al. Acupuncture treatment of chronic low-back pain-a randomized, blinded, placebo-controlled trial with 9-month follow-up. *Pain.* 2002;96(1–2):189–196.

52. White AR, Ernst E. A systematic review of randomized controlled trials of acupuncture for neck pain. *Rheumatology (Oxford).* 1999;38(2): 143–147.

53. White P, Lewith G, Berman B, Birch S. Reviews of acupuncture for chronic neck pain: pitfalls in conducting systematic reviews. *Rheum.* 2002; 41(11):1224–1231.

54. Irnich D, Behrens N, Molzen H, et al. Randomised trial of acupuncture compared with conventional massage and "sham" laser acupuncture for treatment of chronic neck pain. *BMJ.* 2001;322(7302): 1574–1577.

55. Smith LA, Oldman AD, McQuay HJ, Moore RA. Teasing apart quality and validity in systematic reviews: an example from acupuncture trials in chronic neck and back pain. *Pain.* 2000;86(1–2): 119–132.

56. Melchart D, Linde K, Fischer P, et al. Acupuncture for recurrent headaches: a systematic review of randomized controlled trials. *Cephalalgia.* 1999;19(9):779–786; discussion 765.

57. White AR, Resch KL, Chan JCK, et al. Acupuncture for episodic tension-type headache: a multicentre randomized controlled trial. *Cephalalgia.* 2000;20(7):632–637.

58. Ezzo J, Hadhazy V, Birch S, et al. Acupuncture for osteoarthritis of the knee: a systematic review. *Arthritis Rheum.* 2001;44(4):819–825.

59. Berman BM, Ezzo J, Hadhazy V, Swyers JP. Is acupuncture effective in the treatment of fibromyalgia? *J Fam Pract.* 1999;48(3):213–218.

60. Lin JG, Lob MW, Wen YR, Hsieh CL, Tsai SK, Sun WZ. The effect of high and low frequency electroacupuncture in pain after lower abdominal surgery. *Pain.* 2002;99(3):509–514.

61. Kemper KJ, Sarah R, Silver-Highfield E, Xiarhos E, Barnes L, Berde C. On pins and needles? Pediatric pain patients' experience with acupuncture. *Pediatrics.* 2000;105(4 suppl S):941–947.

62. Skilnand E, Fossen D, Heiberg E. Acupuncture in the management of pain in labor. *Acta Obstet Gynecol Scand.* 2002;81(10):943–948.

63. Ghoname ESA, Craig WF, White PF, et al. Percutaneous electrical nerve stimulation for low back pain—a randomized crossover study. *JAMA.* 1999;281(9):818–823.

64. Hamza MA, White PF, Craig WF, et al. Percutaneous electrical nerve stimulation—a novel analgesic therapy for diabetic neuropathic pain. *Diabetes Care.* 2000;23(3):365–370.

65. Ahmed HE, White PF, Craig WF, Hamza MA, Ghoname ESA, Gajraj NM. Use of percutaneous electrical nerve stimulation (PENS) in the short-term management of headache. *Headache.* 2000;40(4):311–315.

66. Arnold MD, Thornbrough LM. Treatment of musculoskeletal pain with traditional Chinese herbal medicine. *Phys Med Rehabil Clin N Am.* 1999;10(3):663–71, ix–x.

67. Suekawa M, Ishige A, Yuasa K, Sido K, Aburada M, Hosoya E. Pharmacological studies on ginger 1. Pharmacological actions of pungent constituents, [6]-gingerol and [6]-shogaol. *Pharmacobiodyn.* 1984;7:836–848.

68. Altman RD, Marcussen KC. Effects of a ginger extract on knee pain in patients with osteoarthritis. *Arthritis Rheum.* 2001;44(11):2 531–2538.

69. Sander O, Herborn C, Rau R. Is H15 (resin extract of *Boswellia serrata*, "incense") a useful supplement to established drug therapy of chronic polyarthritis? results of a double-blind pilot study. *Z Rheumatol.* 1998;57(1):11–16.

70. Fisher PA, Greenwood A, Huskisson EC, Turner P, Belon P. Effect of homeopathic treatment on fibrosis (primary fibromyalgia). *BMJ.* 1989; 299(6695):365–366.

71. Fisher P, Scott DL. A randomized controlled trial of homeopathy in rheumatoid arthritis. *Rheumatology (Oxford).* 2001;40(9):1052–1055.

72. Gmunder R, Kissling R. The efficacy of homeopathy in the treatment of chronic low back pain compared to standardized physiotherapy. *Z Orthop Ihre Grenzgeb.* 2002;140(5):503–508.

73. Stam C, Bonnet MS, van Haselen RA. The efficacy and safety of a homeopathic gel in the treatment of acute low back pain: a multi-centre, randomised, double-blind comparative clinical trial. *Br Homeopath J.* 2001;90(1):21–28.

74. Straumsheim P, Borchgrevink C, Mowinckel P, Kierulf H, Hafslund O. Homeopathic treatment of migraine: a double-blind, placebo-controlled trial of 68 patients. *Br Homeopath J.* 2000; 89(1):4–7b

75. Walach H, Lowes T, Mussbach D, et al. The long-term effects of homeopathic treatment of chronic headaches: 1-year follow-up. *Cephalalgia.* 2000; 20(9):835–837.

76. Thompson EA, Reilly D. The homeopathic approach to symptom control in the cancer patient: a prospective observational study. *Palliat Med.* 2002;16(3):227–233.

77. Gatterman MI, Cooperstein R, Lantz C, Perle SM, Schneider MJ. Rating specific chiropractic technique procedures for common low back conditions. *J Manipulative Physiol Ther.* 2001;24(7): 449–456.

78. Shekelle PC, Adams AH, Chassin MR, Hurwitz EL, Brook RH. Spinal manipulation for low-back pain. *Ann Intern Med.* 1992;117(7):590–598.

79. Bronfort G. Spinal manipulation: current state of research and its indications. *Neurol Clin.* 1999;17(1):91–111.

80. Koes BW, Assendelft WJ, van der Heijden GJ, Bouter LM. Spinal manipulation for low back pain. An updated systematic review of randomized clinical trials. *Spine.* 1996;21(24):2860–2871; discussion 2872–2873.

81. van Tulder MW, Koes BW, Bouter LM. Conservative treatment of acute and chronic nonspecific low back pain. A systematic review of randomized controlled trials of the most common interventions. *Spine.* 1997;22(18):2128–2156.

82. Haldeman S. Neurological effects of the adjustment. *J Manipulative Physiol Ther.* 2000;23(2): 112–114.

83. Hoving JL, Gross AR, Gasner D, et al. A critical appraisal of review articles on the effectiveness of conservative treatment for neck pain. *Spine.* 2001;26(2):196–205.

84. Hurwitz EL, Aker PD, Adams AH, Meeker WC, Shekelle PG. Manipulation and mobilization of the cervical spine. A systematic review of the literature. *Spine.* 1996;21(15):1746–1759; discussion 1759–1760.

85. Aker PD, Gross AR, Goldsmith CH, Peloso P. Conservative management of mechanical neck pain: systematic overview and meta-analysis. *BMJ.* 1996;313(7068):1291–1296.

86. Bronfort G, Evans R, Nelson B, Aker PD, Goldsmith CH, Vernon H. A randomized clinical trial of exercise and spinal manipulation for patients with chronic neck pain. *Spine.* 2001;26(7): 788–797; discussion 798–799.

87. Vernon H, McDermaid CS, Hagino C. Systematic review of randomized clinical trials of complementary/alternative therapies in the treatment of tension-type and cervicogenic headache. *Complement Ther Med.* 1999;7(3):142–155.

88. Bronfort G, Assendelft WJ, Evans R, Haas M, Bouter L. Efficacy of spinal manipulation for chronic headache: a systematic review. *J Manipulative Physiol Ther.* 2001;24(7):457–466.

89. Haldeman S, Kohlbeck FJ, McGregor M. Risk factors and precipitating neck movements causing vertebrobasilar artery dissection after cervical trauma and spinal manipulation. *Spine.* 1999; 24(8):785–794.

90. Ernst E. Spinal manipulation: its safety is uncertain. *CMAJ.* 2002;166(1):40–41.

91. Ernst E. Prospective investigations into the safety of spinal manipulation. *J Pain Symptom Manage.* 2001;21(3):238–242.

92. Fiechtner JJ, Brodeur RR. Manual and manipulation techniques for rheumatic disease. *Med Clin North Am.* 2002;86(1):91–103.

93. Andersson GB, Lucente T, Davis AM, et al. A comparison of osteopathic spinal manipulation with standard care for patients with low back pain. *N Engl J Med.* 1999;314:1426–1431.

94. Thys-Jacobs S, Starkey P, Bernstein D, et al. Calcium carbonate and the premenstrual syndrome: effects on premenstrual and menstrual symptoms. *Am J Ob Gyn.* 1998;179(2):444–452.

95. McCarthy GM, Kenny D. Dietary fish oil and rheumatic diseases. *Semin Arthritis Rheum.* 1992; 21(6):368–375.

96. Gibson RA. The effect of diets containing fish

and fish oils on disease risk factors in humans. *Aust N Z J Med.* 1988;18(5):713–722.

97. Cathcart ES, Gonnerman WA. Fish oil fatty acids and experimental arthritis. *Rheum Dis Clin North Am.* 1991;17(2):235–242.

98. Henderson CJ, Panush RS. Diets, dietary supplements, and nutritional therapies in rheumatic diseases. *Rheum Dis Clin North Am.* 1999;25(4): 937–968.

99. Pavelka K, Gatterova J, Olejarova M, Machacek S, Giacovelli G, Rovati LC. Glucosamine sulfate use and delay of progression of knee osteoarthritis—a 3-year, randomized, placebo-controlled, double-blind study. *Arch Intern Med.* 2002;162(18):2113–2123.

100. McAlindon TE, LaValley MP, Gulin JP, Felson DT. Glucosamine and chondroitin for treatment of osteoarthritis—a systematic quality assessment and meta-analysis. *JAMA.* 2000;283(11):1469–1475.

101. Long L, Soeken K, Ernst E. Herbal medicines for the treatment of osteoarthritis: a systematic review. *Rheumatology.* 2001;40(7):779–793.

102. Ernst E, Chrubasik S. Phyto-anti-inflammatories— a systematic review of randomized, placebo-controlled, double-blind trials. *Rheum Dis Clin North Am.* 2000;26(1):13–27.

103. Almeid RN, Navarro DS, Barbosa-Filho JM. Plants with central analgesic activity. *Phytomedicine.* 2001;8(4):310–322.

104. Kim SJ, Kim MS. Inhibitory effects of cimicifugae rhizoma extracts on histamine, bradykinin and COX-2 mediated inflammatory actions. *Phytother Res.* 2000;14(8):596–600.

105. Nah JJ, Hahn JH, Chung S, Choi S, Kim YI, Nah SY. Effect of ginsenosides, active components of ginseng, on capsaicin-induced pain-related behavior. *Neuropharmacology.* 2000;39(11): 2180–2184.

106. Laudahn D, Walper A. Efficacy and tolerance of Harpagophytum extract LI 174 in patients with chronic non-radicular back pain. *Phytother Res.* 2001;15(7):621–624.

107. Schmid B, Ludtke R, Selbmann HK, et al. Efficacy and tolerability of a standardized willow bark extract in patients with osteoarthritis: randomized placebo-controlled, double blind clinical trial. *Phytother Res.* 2001;15(4):344–350.

108. Mills SY, Jacoby RK, Chacksfield M, Willoughby M. Effect of a proprietary herbal medicine on the relief of chronic arthritic pain: a double-blind study. *Br J Rheum.* 1996;35(9):874–878.

109. Pittler MH, Ernst E. Ginkgo biloba extract for the treatment of intermittent claudication: a meta-analysis of randomized trials. *Am J Med.* 2000;108(4):276–281.

110. Rubik B, Becker R, Fowler R, Hazlewood C, Liboff A, Walleezek J. Bioelectromagnetics: applications in medicine. In: *Alternative Medicine: Expanding Medical Horizons. A Report to the National Institutes of Health on Alternative Medical Systems and Practices in the United States.* Workshop on Alternative Medicine; Chantilly, VA; 1994.

111. Rubik B. Bioelectromagnetics and the future of medicine. *Admin Radiol J.* 1997;16(8):38–46.

112. Lefaucheur JP, Drouot X, Keravel Y, Nguyen JP. Pain relief induced by repetitive transcranial magnetic stimulation of precentral cortex. *Neuroreport.* 2001;12(13):2963–2965.

113. Hinman MR, Ford J, Heyl H. Effects of static magnets on chronic knee pain and physical function: a double-blind study. *Altern Ther Health Med.* 2002;8(4):50–55.

114. Segal NA, Toda Y, Huston J, et al. Two configurations of static magnetic fields for treating rheumatoid arthritis of the knee: a double-blind clinical trial. *Arch Phys Med Rehabil.* 2001;82(10): 1453–1460.

115. Brown CS, Ling FW, Wan JY, Pilla AA. Efficacy of static magnetic field therapy in chronic pelvic pain: a double-blind pilot study. *Am J Obstet Gyncol.* 2002;187(6):1581–1587.

116. Vallbona C, Hazlewood CF, Jurida G. Response of pain to static magnetic fields in postpolio patients: a double-blind pilot study. *Arch Phys Med Rehab.* 1997;78(11):1200–1203.

117. Weintraub MI, Cole SP. Neuromagnetic treatment of pain in refractory carpal tunnel syndrome: an electrophysiological and placebo analysis. *J Back Musculoskel.* 2000;15(2–3):77–81.

118. Carter R, Aspy CB. Mold J. The effectiveness of magnet therapy for treatment of wrist pain attributed to carpal tunnel syndrome. *J Fam Pract.* 2002;51(1):38–40.

119. Alfano AP, Taylor AG, Foresman PA, et al. Static magnetic fields for treatment of fibromyalgia: a randomized controlled trial. *J Altern Complement Med.* 2001;7(1):53–64.

120. Collacott EA, Zimmerman JT, White DW, Rindone JP. Bipolar permanent magnets for the treatment of chronic low back pain: a pilot study. *JAMA.* 2000;283(10):1322–1325.

121. Jacobson JI, Gorman R, Yamanashi WS, Saxena BB, Clayton L. Low-amplitude, extremely low-frequency magnetic fields for the treatment of osteoarthritic knees: a double-blind clinical study. *Altern Ther Health Med.* 2001;7(5):54–64, 66–69.

122. Pipitone N, Scott DL. Magnetic pulse treatment for knee osteoarthritis: a randomised, double-blind, placebo-controlled study. *Curr Med Res Opin.* 2001;17(3):190–196.

123. Trock DH. Electromagnetic fields and magnets. Investigational treatment for musculoskeletal disorders. *Rheum Dis Clin North Am.* 2000;26(1): 51–62, viii.

124. Vallbona C, Richards T. Evolution of magnetic therapy from alternative to traditional medicine. *Phys Med Rehabil Clin North Am.* 1999;10(3): 729–754.

125. Shumay DM, Maskarinec G, Gotay CC, Heiby EM, Kakai H. Determinants of the degree of complementary and alternative medicine use among patients with cancer. *J Altern Complement Med.* 2002;8(5):661–671.

126. Pan CX, Morrison RS, Ness J, Fugh-Berman A, Liepzig RM. Complementary and alternative medicine in the management of pain, dyspnea, and nausea and vomiting near the end of life: a systematic review. *J Pain Sympt Manage.* 2000; 20(5):374–387.

127. DiGianni LM, Garber JE, Winer EP. Complementary and alternative medicine use among women with breast cancer. *J Clin Oncol.* 2002;20(18 suppl S):34S–38S.

128. Power R, Gore-Felton C, Vosvick M, Israelski DM, Spiegel D. HIV: effectiveness of complementary and alternative medicine. *Prim Care.* 2002;29(2):361–378.

CHAPTER 27

Integrative Approach to Pulmonary Disorders

Benjamin Kligler

From both the conventional and the integrative perspective, proper function of the respiratory system is critical to good health. This chapter discusses in depth the integrative approach to asthma and to chronic obstructive pulmonary disease (COPD). Although there are many other important pulmonary conditions, including pneumonia, sarcoidosis, and environmental lung diseases, there is insufficient published evidence on any of the nonconventional approaches to these conditions allow for any in-depth discussion of an integrative approach. Diseases of the sinuses and upper respiratory tract are covered in Chapter 25.

Integrative medicine is an approach that addresses many dimensions of disease and health that may be ignored in Western medicine. With respect to pulmonary conditions, one concept of this approach to problems of respiration, regardless of the specific disease, is the notion from East Asian medicine that the lungs are the seat of the emotion of grief. Thus, the integrative approach to many pulmonary diseases incorporates an examination of unresolved grief in the patient's life and its impact on the patient's health. One of the many studies from the Western literature that may reflect

this convergence of thinking is the work by Smyth et al. on using journaling as a therapy for asthma.[1] In this study patients were asked to write for an hour on three successive days about their most painful past experience. Controls wrote about a nontraumatic memory or a life event. Treatment and control groups were similar in all important respects. The authors found that the treatment group participants had a reduction in medication use and symptom scores that lasted through the 6-month follow-up period. Further research is needed both to replicate this finding and to determine through what intracellular mediators such an effect might be created; the potential relevance for the integrative approach to pulmonary disease, and possibly to inflammatory disease in general, however, is clear.

▶ ASTHMA

Pathophysiology

Asthma is a recurrent condition caused by inflammation and obstruction of the small- and medium-sized airways as a consequence of

609

airway hyperresponsiveness to a variety of stimuli. Triggers of asthma exacerbation can include environmental, infectious, dietary, and psychoemotional stimuli; exercise is often also a stimulus. Clinical manifestations include recurrent shortness-of-breath, cough, and wheezing. In severe cases, the recurrent inflammation and obstructive characteristic of asthma can come to resemble the pattern of diminished pulmonary function seen in certain types of chronic obstructive pulmonary disease. The edema and inflammation of asthma are thought to be mediated largely by the leukotriene-4 series, which are produced in response to certain inflammatory mediator molecules released in the degranulation of mast cells in response to the asthma trigger.

Prevalence

The incidence and prevalence of asthma have risen dramatically over the past 30 years in the United States. For example, between 1971 and 1980, the prevalence of asthma in children age 6–11 years nearly doubled.[2] Hospital admissions and deaths from asthma also rose over this time period.[3] The reason for this increase in prevalence and severity is not known, although there is a dramatic concentration of disease in urban populations of lower socio-economic status. A number of factors have been proposed to explain this phenomenon, including the possible roles of poor air quality, exposure to cigarette smoke, crowded living conditions, and poor diet in this population.

▶ Case Example: Asthma

M.P. is a 34-year-old woman with a history of mild asthma since childhood. In her teenage years, she had symptoms primarily on exertion and was managed with PRN bronchodilators. Since age 28 years she has been experiencing more continuous symptoms, and under the care of her current doctor, is now maintained on twice-daily steroid inhaler, leukotriene antagonist, and PRN beta-agonist inhalers. She has only been hospitalized for the asthma once, 5 years ago, but has required courses of oral steroids two to four times yearly in the past 3 years, and has had several emergency room visits. She is uncomfortable with the level of medication she currently requires and is concerned that her asthma seems to be increasing in severity as time goes by rather than improving. She is also concerned about the recurrent need for oral steroids, given a strong family history of osteoporosis in her mother and two aunts.

Conventional Treatment Approach

The conventional medicine approach to asthma emphasizes the use of inhaled bronchodilators and steroid medication. The steroids are thought to address the inflammatory component of the condition. Recently, the use of oral leukotriene antagonists has added to the ability to control symptoms. Exacerbations are typically handled with systemic steroids and bronchodilators delivered via nebulizer.

Environmental assessment is also an important part of conventional asthma management, with particular emphasis on the role of triggers such as molds, insects, and pets. Cigarette smoking in the household has been clearly linked with increased risk of asthma in childhood.

Integrative Strategies

The integrative approach to asthma typically combines a number of different treatment strategies. A unifying principle in this approach is the view of asthma as an inflammatory condition—a view that has come to be shared by conventional medicine as first-line treatment options have shifted toward use of antiinflammatory agents such as steroids and leukotriene antagonists. The integrative approach uses "antiinflammatory" strategies from the realms of nutrition, herbal medicine, and mind–body medicine as the cornerstones of asthma treatment.[4,5] This approach is complemented by a more in-depth environmental assessment, including the role of the family and the psychospiritual state of the patient in this overview.

NUTRITIONAL APPROACHES

Nutritional treatment of asthma runs along two parallel tracks. First is the notion that certain foods may be triggers of airway inflammation through a process of food allergy or sensitivity. Second is the notion that deficiencies of certain nutrients, such as omega-3 essential fatty acids, certain antioxidants, and magnesium, may also exert significant influence on exacerbating this condition.

Conventionally, food allergy has been defined as response to certain food antigens on skin testing or on radioallergosorbent test blood testing. Some cases of asthma certainly manifest as a result of this type of allergy, and once the offending food is identified, symptoms are usually greatly improved by avoidance of this food. More controversial is the role of food "sensitivity" in asthma, a response which is believed to be triggered by exposure of the gut-associated lymphoid tissue to certain food antigens and then mediated by inflammatory cytokines, interleukin, and tumor necrosis factor. This type of sensitivity (described in detail in Chapters 4 and 17) does not manifest on conventional allergy testing and can be difficult to diagnose other than through a process of food elimination with concomitant symptom monitoring. A number of studies have examined the use of elimination diet in both children and adults with asthma with mixed results.[6–10] Some authors believe that the role of food sensitivities

has been overstated, and that most reported sensitivities do not stand up to the "gold-standard" test of randomized double-blind food challenge.[11] However, in clinical practice, elimination diet remains a useful tool in the treatment of asthma. Common causes of food sensitivity in children include dairy foods, eggs, citrus, peanuts, soy, wheat, and chocolate.[12]

A subgroup of patients can have their asthma triggered by exposure to some of the common food additives, including tartrazine, sulfites, and certain food dyes.[13–16] This possibility can be addressed with an intervention that is simpler than an elimination trial, especially in children: a trial of a "whole-food," additive-free diet with symptom monitoring. A low-salt diet also reduces symptoms in certain patients.[11,12]

Two other potential nutritional interventions bear mention here. The first is that weight loss programs have an important role in asthma treatment for those with accompanying obesity: a Finnish group found that a 14.5% weight loss in obese subjects led to significant improvements in forced expiratory volume at 1 second (FEV_1) and forced vital capacity (FVC), and to reductions in medication use, frequency of exacerbation, and subjective experience of dyspnea.[17] This benefit persisted over a year of follow-up. The second is evidence from a meta-analysis involving more than 8,000 subjects clearly showing that breast-feeding during the first 3 months of life significantly reduced the likelihood of developing asthma by 30–50%.[18] This effect was most pronounced in children with a family history of atopy. The mechanism for this protective effect was not known.

The nutritional supplements that have been looked at most rigorously for a role in the treatment of asthma are magnesium, antioxidants such as vitamin C, lycopene, selenium, and fish oils. Magnesium supplementation, particularly intravenously, is helpful in the treatment of acute asthma exacerbation, reducing in several studies the likelihood of admission when used in the emergency room.[19–22] It does not appear to have a role as an oral supplement in acute exacerbation or in either form for the management of chronic asthma. The proposed mechanism for its effect in acute asthma is a short-term but potent relaxation of the bronchial smooth muscle; animal models do support this as a potential mechanism.[11]

Antioxidants, including vitamin C, selenium, and lycopene, have been examined for a role in asthma treatment based on the notion that the recurrent and/or chronic state of inflammation in the airways creates a higher level of oxidative stress for the bronchial cells, thus leading, in turn, to a vicious cycle of ongoing release of inflammatory mediators, increased edema in the bronchial wall, and increased asthma symptoms. The conclusion regarding vitamin C is that it does have a modest effect in protecting the airways from hyperresponsiveness to provocative stimuli.[23–27] Vitamin C may also have a role in antagonizing prostaglandin-induced bronchoconstriction.[28] Population studies also confirm that adults with the lowest serum levels of vitamin C have the highest risk of bronchial reactivity.[29] Long-term benefit of vitamin C therapy in reducing asthma symptoms has not been demonstrated. Also, the question remains as to whether supplementation with vitamin C will confer the same benefit in terms of decreased airway sensitivity that has been suggested by epidemiological studies of a high-dose vitamin C diet. Of the other antioxidants, lycopene appears to be the most promising, with one study demonstrating a significant protection from exercise-induced asthma symptoms with a daily dose of lycopene 30 mg.[30] Similarly, selenium supplements may also have a role in reducing bronchial hypersensitivity.[31]

The final category of supplements that have been looked at extensively for treatment of asthma are the omega-3 polyunsaturated essential fatty acids, such as fish oils. As discussed in Chapter 26, these compounds have an important role in the treatment of certain inflammatory disorders, as they modulate the arachidonic acid cascade in the direction of the antiinflammatory series 5 leukotrienes. As such, it was anticipated that fish oils would have an important role to play in the treatment of asthma. For unclear reasons, however, the literature, including a recent Cochrane Collaborative analysis on this question, does not demonstrate any significant improvement in asthma patients using the omega-3 essential fatty acids.[32–38] The one scenario in which essential fatty acid supplementation may hold promise is in children if used in combination with dietary manipulation.[38] In addition, the possibility remains that essential fatty acid supplementation could be effective as one component of an integrative approach but not alone.

MIND–BODY APPROACHES

A number of mind–body approaches have been studied for their application in asthma, including biofeedback, cognitive behavior therapy, relaxation training, yoga, and numerous others. Conventional psychotherapy, particularly family therapy, addressing such issues as the sick role and the effect of family stress on health, has shown some benefit, particularly in children with asthma.[39] As mentioned above, Smyth et al. examined the potential role of using journaling to release unresolved trauma or grief with substantial benefit to their subjects.[1]

At least two studies show that yoga training, in which patients are typically taught a breath-slowing exercise, has a positive impact on medication use, frequency of attacks, and peak flow rates.[10,11] Aside from yoga, a number of other breathing techniques have been used to slow breathing on the theory that the hyperventilation and hypocapnia that normally accompany airway narrowing contribute to the vicious cycle of asthma exacerbation. These techniques, such as the Buteyko and Hale methods, teach a slower breathing strategy, which is believed by their proponents to eliminate this trigger for bronchoconstriction by producing hypercapnia, potentially reversing the asthma attack. The Buteyko breathing approach, as taught via video, has shown promise in at least one study, which found decreased medication use and improved quality of life in those practicing the technique, although without objective change in pulmonary function.[12] The use of breathing techniques in the treatment of asthma requires further study before any definitive conclusions can be drawn regarding their utility.

Biofeedback has been proposed as a strategy for reducing asthma symptoms, particularly in patients in whom stress has been identified as a trigger. One study which used electromyelographic biofeedback to teach relaxation of the facial muscles demonstrated both short and long-term (8 months) improvement in FEV_1/FVC in a group of asthmatic children, as well as a reduction in anxiety and an improvement in their attitudes toward their asthma.[13] The authors propose that this benefit is mediated by a reflex link connecting trigeminal function with vagal function, thus leading to bronchodilatation.

Hypnotic suggestion has been shown to be effective in at least one study in reducing airway hyperresponsiveness and in attenuating the exercise-induced bronchoconstriction experienced by patients with exercise-induced asthma. Ewer and Stewart showed in a prospective randomized trial that a 6-week course of hypnotherapy produced a 75% reduction in response to methacholine challenge, as well as improvements in symptom score and reduced medication use.[14] This benefit, however, was confined to those subjects who scored high on susceptibility to hypnosis; subjects who scored low in this regard did not experience a significant benefit from the intervention. Hypnotherapy is felt by some to be most effective in childhood asthma, perhaps because of children's tendency toward susceptibility to suggestion.[39]

MANIPULATIVE APPROACHES

Many clinicians believe that there may be a structural problem in asthmatic patients that can be addressed, at least in part, by chiropractic or osteopathic manipulation. There are very few studies of manipulative approaches for asthma in the medical literature; the 1998 trial published in the *New England Journal of Medicine*, which looked at chiropractic as an adjunctive treatment for children with asthma, failed to find a significant benefit.[15] A second trial that compared active with sham chiropractic in adults in a crossover design also found no significant effect of manipulation on pulmonary function measures, medication use, or symptom scores.[16] Osteopathic techniques, such as lymphatic pump, which is commonly used in treatment of asthma, have also not been examined in well-controlled trials.

The evidence in the literature to date does not support a role for manipulation in the treatment of asthma. Given the clinical experience of benefit in some cases, however, it may be that this approach is useful in certain subgroups where there is a musculoskeletal component, and that research needs to focus on how to identify this subgroup for referral for manipulation.

The single published study of massage therapy in children with asthma, in which parents were taught massage therapy and then practiced this with their children for 20 minutes before bedtime, did find a significant reduction in anxiety levels and cortisol levels with an improvement in peak flow. This effect was more pronounced in the 4–8-year-old group than in the 9–14-year-old group.[17]

ENVIRONMENTAL STRATEGIES

The conventional assessment of asthma has typically included environmental evaluation for triggers: pets, smokers at home, wall-to-wall carpets, cockroaches, and the like. The integrative assessment takes this one step further to include the potential role of solvents, molds, and chemical sensitivities in asthma.[18] A common approach—although one not conclusively substantiated by data to date—is the use of high-efficiency particulate air (HEPA) filtration and ion generators in treating the home environment. The single published trial on this approach did show a decrease in rhinitis and asthma symptoms with the use of HEPA filtration in the home.[19]

Homeopathic treatment has been explored as a strategy for the patient with environmental asthma triggers using a technique called isopathy, or homeopathic immunotherapy. Reilly et al. demonstrated the efficacy of this technique, in a large trial of treatment for allergic rhinitis[50] in which patients were treated with homeopathic dilutions of the environmental trigger. These results have been reproduced, and a recent review comprising a total of 350 treated patients confirmed this efficacy.[51] Proponents have suggested that a similar approach should be effective in asthma that is environmental in origin.

BOTANICAL MEDICINES

The botanicals most extensively studied for asthma to date are *Tylophora indica* and *Coleus forskohlii*, both Ayurvedic medicines used in asthma. *Tylophora*, in particular, has shown promise, with at least three randomized double-blind trials demonstrating a decrease in symptoms in the treatment group.[52-54] However, this herb frequently causes vomiting, limiting its use; neither *Tylophora* nor *Coleus* is currently widely available in the United States. A third Ayurvedic herb—*Boswellia serrata*—has been shown in one randomized trial to reduce asthma symptoms and frequency of attacks in 70% of treatment subjects, compared to similar improvement in 27% of controls.[55] The treatment group also demonstrated significant improvement in pulmonary function testing when compared to placebo. This herb contains boswellic acids, which inhibit leukotriene synthesis, and is purported to work via this mechanism. This study was only 6 weeks in duration, and longer-term studies are needed of this potentially promising herbal treatment.

A number of herbs from the Chinese pharmacopeia may also have a role in asthma, including ma huang (the source of ephedrine), ginkgo, and licorice. Ma huang is a fairly potent bronchodilator; however, its adrenergic agonist effects are not specific and in large doses it can cause significant blood pressure elevation and potentially dangerous arrhyth-

mias. A number of deaths have been reported from ma huang, although it should be noted that in most of these deaths, the herb was being used at far above the therapeutic level typically used in Chinese herbal formulae, and also without any appropriate medical supervision.[56] Licorice, which should be used with caution in anyone with elevated blood pressure because of an aldosterone-like effect may potentiate the effect of endogenous cortisol, thus acting as an antiinflammatory agent in some cases.[57] Ginkgo extract, which in animal studies inhibits platelet-activating factor-induced bronchoconstriction, has been studied in one small trial (8 subjects); the study showed a decrease in bronchoconstriction and hyperreactivity in response to allergen challenge. Saiboku-Tu, a Japanese herbal formula containing licorice and nine other herbs, has also shown promise in preliminary studies, particularly as a strategy to reduce steroid dosage in steroid-dependent asthmatics.[58]

Many other herbs have been used in the treatment of asthma, including belladonna (*Atropa belladonna LINN*), lobelia (*Lobelia inflatal*), marijuana (*Cannabis sativa*), sorrel (*Rumex acetosa*), and others; however, to date, none of these has been examined systematically for efficacy.[59,60]

TRADITIONAL SYSTEMS: ACUPUNCTURE

In a meta-analysis from 1991, Kleijne et al. found that trials of acupuncture for asthma up to that time had failed to demonstrate conclusively any benefit. Most of the trials at that point were poorly controlled, and thus did not have the power to demonstrate any effect.[61] There have been at least two well-done trials that have shown a significant improvement in pulmonary function with acupuncture in the treatment of acute exacerbation[62,63]; at least two others, however, failed to show such an effect.[64] The data in the treatment of chronic asthma is even less compelling; when Tashkin et al. expanded the treatment protocol they had found to be effective in acute exacerbation to an eight-session treatment and compared it to sham acupuncture in a blinded crossover design, they found no significant impact on lung function, medication use, or symptom scores.[65] Biernacki and Peake used a crossover double-blind design and similarly found no difference between real and sham acupuncture, although both showed a significant benefit over no treatment.[66] There does appear to be a significant but nonspecific benefit to needling in terms of reported symptoms, although not in terms of pulmonary function. This benefit may stem from the nonspecific release of endorphins, which has been documented to accompany acupuncture treatment whether needles are placed in real or sham locations.

The methodological challenges of studying acupuncture using conventional research designs are addressed elsewhere in Chapter 9. The Chinese literature on asthma treatment, which in general consists of uncontrolled studies, many of which use herbal treatments in combination with acupuncture, tends to show much more positive results.[67] Although this may be a consequence of examiner expectations and unblinded design, it could also be that acupuncture alone—particularly the standardized point protocols used in the blinded studies—is not as effective as the traditional combination of herbal and acupuncture approaches. In clinical practice, acupuncture in fact does often prove useful in acute asthma treatment.

► Case Study: Asthma Conclusions

Given the dramatic worsening of symptoms reported by M.P. around age 28 years, you decide to inquire regarding triggers from that time. There is no specific unresolved trauma or grief from that time period. She does, however, report a move from an urban apartment to an old Victorian suburban house at that time, which she and her husband have been renovating. She also reports a significant increase in work stress over the past 3 years, with increasing responsibility

at her law firm and a longer commute. Her diet is not significantly changed.

Your recommendations for M.P. at this point could include the use of a HEPA filter at home to address possible environmental triggers; the incorporation of a daily yoga practice as a strategy for both improved breathing control and overall reduction of stress and sympathetic tone; and a trial of *Boswellia serrata* at 300 mg TID as a substitute for her leukotriene antagonist.

► CHRONIC OBSTRUCTIVE PULMONARY DISEASE (COPD)

Pathophysiology

The term COPD describes a group of conditions that all share the quality of airflow obstruction. Although asthma and bronchiectasis are often included in this constellation of conditions, the focus here is on emphysema and chronic bronchitis, the two diseases most commonly considered to comprise the entity known as COPD. Chronic bronchitis represents the majority of COPD cases and is characterized by recurrent airway inflammation and severe, long-lasting episodes of productive cough. Emphysema, thought to comprise approximately 15% of cases,[68] is caused by a loss of elastic recoil in the lungs as a result of destruction of alveoli and the small airways. Both conditions can lead to severe, chronic compromise in respiratory function.

Smoking is the major risk factor for COPD. Environmental or occupational exposures, genetic factors (including α_1-antitrypsin deficiency), passive smoke exposure, and air pollution may all play a role in a minority of cases.

Prevalence

More than 16 million adults in the United States are believed to be affected by COPD. Onset of symptoms from COPD is typically in the fifties and sixties, and the disease is generally progressive. Each year approximately 110,000 people in the United States will die from COPD, making it the fourth leading cause of death in this country, exceeded only by heart disease, cancer, and stroke.[69]

Conventional Treatment Approach

Acute exacerbations of COPD are generally treated with systemic steroids; antibiotics, either oral or parenteral, are often used as well. The mainstays of maintenance therapy for COPD are inhaled corticosteroids and inhaled ipratropium, which are generally given on a daily basis. Many patients with severe COPD require long-term oral steroid treatment; although this approach is often effective in controlling the dyspnea and other symptoms of the disease, patients frequently suffer other long-term sequelae of the treatment, including osteoporosis and steroid-induced diabetes. Pulmonary rehabilitation and exercise programs to improve functional capacity have also become an important part of conventional treatment for COPD in recent years.

Integrative Strategies

Although the published literature on unconventional approaches to COPD is not nearly as extensive as that on asthma, there are a number of small but suggestive studies in the areas of mind–body medicine, as well as an emerging literature on nutritional approaches. The use of breathing retraining is also discussed, although this is often done in the mainstream setting as part of pulmonary rehabilitation programs.

Mind–Body Approaches
A number of studies, mostly from the nursing literature, have looked at the role of relaxation therapies in reducing symptoms of COPD. In one of these, the effectiveness of a taped relaxation message was studied in reducing dyspnea and anxiety in 26 adult patients with COPD. The intervention group was instructed in relaxation therapy using a prerecorded tape; the control group was instructed to sit quietly. Skin temperature, heart rate, and respiratory rate, as well as anxiety and dyspnea, were recorded for all subjects during a total of four weekly sessions. Dyspnea and anxiety were both significantly reduced in the relaxation group, while the controls either showed no improvement or became worse.[70]

A second study examined the effects of guided imagery in 19 patients with COPD, using as outcome measures functional status, fatigue, dyspnea, depression, mastery, quality of life, perceived health status, and inspiratory muscle strength. In this study, guided imagery significantly improved subjects' perceived quality of life.[71] Although this study was small and uncontrolled, the results suggest further study in this area is needed given the low cost and complete safety of the intervention.

A third study examined the feasibility of using music to reduce dyspnea and anxiety in patients with COPD. Twenty-four participants who experienced dyspnea at least once a week were studied over a 5-week period. Although this study found significant decreases in dyspnea and anxiety at specific points during the treatment period, this effect did not appear to be long-lasting, and no significant change in either dyspnea or anxiety was reported at the end of the 5-week period.[72]

Nutritional Approaches

Based on epidemiologic studies showing that diets high in consumption of fruits, vegetables, and fish seem to be protective against COPD, the role of antioxidants and fish oils in treatment or prevention of this condition has attracted attention in recent years. The MORGEN study from the Netherlands, which collected data on 13,651 men and women between the ages of 20 and 60 years, found that higher intake of both fruit and whole grains was protective against COPD as measured in this study by FEV_1. The amount of fruits required to show this benefit was more than 180 g/d, and the amount of whole grains more than 45 g/d. In this particular study, fish and vegetable intake did not show independent beneficial associations with COPD.[73]

As discussed above in the asthma section, evidence for a role of diet in asthma and chronic obstructive pulmonary disease (COPD) has been accumulating rapidly over the past decade. Various studies have reported possible associations between the intake of fruit, fish, antioxidant vitamins, fatty acids, sodium or magnesium, and indicators of asthma and COPD.[74]

Although intervention trials have not been done to date on nutritional approaches to COPD, the epidemiologic literature suggests that increased consumption of fruits and vegetables, as well as supplementation with antioxidant vitamins, particularly vitamin C and, to a lesser extent, vitamin E, may be the most promising interventions for future study. By decreasing oxidant insults to the lung, antioxidants could decrease the long-term impact of chronic inflammatory processes and potentially slow the progression of COPD or perhaps even prevent its inception.[75]

Chinese Medicine/Acupuncture

Although acupuncture has not been studied in detail for treatment of COPD per se, a number of studies have been published on the use of acupuncture to treat "disabling breathlessness."

Jobst et al. studied the impact of acupuncture treatment on 12 matched pairs of patients with COPD, with controls receiving placebo acupuncture. At week 3 of treatment, the active treatment group showed significant improvement in both subjective report of dyspnea and in 6-minute walking distance, despite the lack of any measurable change in measures of lung function. The authors here speculate that this effect may be mediated by endogenous endorphin release, because in clinical practice, use of morphine improves the subjective experience of dyspnea without a change in objectively measured lung function.[76]

A review of this approach, in 1995, examined 16 studies, including a total of 320 patients. Although the quality of the studies was highly variable, the authors of this review concluded that in 13 of 16 studies, acupuncture led to significant improvement in the subjective experience of dyspnea. In 10 of 11 studies that examined medication use, acupuncture subjects had significantly reduced rates of medication use when compared to controls.[77] Although the mechanism remains unclear and the effect perhaps not demonstrable on objective tests of pulmonary function, it appears that acupuncture may have an important role as an adjunctive treatment for patients with COPD.

Breathing Techniques

The impact of breathing retraining for patients with COPD has been debated for some time. The two techniques most widely studied and still offered as part of some pulmonary rehabilitation programs are "diaphragmatic breathing" and "pursed-lip" breathing. In diaphragmatic breathing, patients are taught to relax the accessory muscles of breathing and to use more abdominal and diaphragmatic breathing to theoretically decrease the work of respiration and improve dyspnea and ventilation. Although early studies suggested some subjective benefit from this technique, more recent studies show that diaphragmatic breathing may, in fact, increase inspiratory muscle work and dyspnea and actually be detrimental.[78]

In "pursed-lip" breathing, which is used for the relief of dyspnea at rest as well as during or after exercise, the patient is taught to exhale more slowly than usual over a 4–6-second period through the mouth while holding the lips in a "whistling" position. This strategy changes the ratio of inspiratory to expiratory time, and, although the mechanism remains unclear, appears, in some studies, to provide some measure of relief from dyspnea.[79] A variety of approaches to training patients in this technique have been studied including the use of visual and electromyographic biofeedback techniques; although further study is needed, Collins et al. conclude that although "activities learned during a resting state (including biofeedback training) are unlikely to transfer to periods of activity . . . a properly designed breathing retraining program in which patients with COPD learn to control their pattern of breathing under the stress of performing different modes of exercise at increasing intensity and duration may markedly decrease dyspnea and improve gas exchange."[79]

Conclusion

Although the research literature on integrative approaches to COPD is not as extensive as that on asthma, there is preliminary evidence to suggest that a number of modalities, including Chinese medicine, nutritional intervention, and mind–body approaches, may significantly improve the quality of life for patients with COPD.

REFERENCES

1. Smyth JM, Stone AA, Hurewitz A, et al. Effects of writing about stressful experiences on symptom reduction in patients with asthma or rheumatoid arthritis. *JAMA*. 1999;281:1304–9.
2. Gergen PJ, Mullally DI, Evans R III. National survey of prevalence of asthma among children in the United States, 1976 to 1980. *Pediatrics*. 1988; 81:1–7.
3. McWhorter WP, Polis MA, Kaslow RA. Occurrence, predictors and consequences of adult asthma in NHANES 1 and follow-up survey. *Am Rev Respir Dis*. 1989;139:721–724.
4. Ernst E. Complementary therapies in asthma: what patients use. *J Asthma*. 1998;35:667–671.
5. Lewith GT, Watkins AD. Unconventional therapies in asthma: an overview. *Allergy*. 1996;51:761–769.
6. Bock SA. Prospective appraisal of complaints of adverse reactions to foods in children during the first 3 years of life. *Pediatrics*. 1987;79:683–688.
7. Oehling A, Garcia B, Santos F, et al. Food allergy as a cause of rhinitis and/or asthma. *J Investig Allergol Clin Immunol*. 2:78–83, 1992.
8. Onorato J, Merland N, Terral C, Michel FB, Bousquet J. Placebo-controlled double-blind food challenge in asthma. *J Allergy Clin Immunol*. 1986; 78:1139–1146.
9. James JM, Bernhisel-Broadbent J, Sampson HA. Respiratory reactions provoked by double-blind food challenges in children. *Am J Respir Crit Care Med*. 1994;149:59–64.
10. Pelikan Z, Pelikan-Filipek M. Bronchial response to the food ingestion challenge. *Ann Allergy*. 1987;58:164–172.
11. Manteleone CA, Sherman AR. Nutrition and asthma. *Arch Intern Med*. 1997;157(1):23–34.
12. Baker JC, Ayres JG. Diet and asthma. *Respir Med*. 2000; 94:925–934.
13. Lockley SD. Hypersensitivity to tartrazine and other dyes and additives present in foods and pharmaceutical products. *Ann Allergy*. 1977;38: 206–10.
14. Stenius BSM, Lemola M. Hypersensitivity to acetylsalicylic acid and tartrazine in patients with asthma. *Clin Allergy*. 1976;6:119–29.
15. Baker GJ, Collett P, Allern DH. Bronchospasm induced by metabisulphite-containing food and drugs. *Med J Aust*. 1981;ii:614–616.
16. Stevenson DD, Simon RA. Sensitivity to ingested metabisulphites in asthmatic subjects. *J Allergy Clin Immunol*. 1981;68:26–32.
17. Stenius-Aarniala B, Poussa T, Kvarnstrom J, et al. Immediate and long-term effects of weight reduction in obese people with asthma: randomized controlled study. *BMJ*. 2000;320:827–832.
18. Gdalevich M, Mimouni D, Mimouni M. Breast-feeding and the risk of bronchial asthma in childhood: a systematic review with meta-analysis of prospective studies. *Pediatrics*. 2001;139:261–266.
19. Skobeloff EM, Spivey WH, McNamara RM, Greenspon L. Intravenous magnesium sulfate for the

treatment of acute asthma in the emergency department. *JAMA*. 1989;262:1210–1213.

20. Noppen M, Vanmaele L, Impens N, Schandevyl W. Bronchodilating effect of intravenous magnesium sulfate in acute severe bronchial asthma. *Chest*. 1990;97:373–376.

21. Tiffany BR, Berk WA, Todd IK, White SR. Magnesium bolus or infusion fails to improve expiratory flow in acute asthma exacerbations. *Chest*. 1993;104:831–834.

22. Britton J, Pavord I, Richards K, et al. Dietary magnesium, lung function, wheezing and airway hyperreactivity in a random adult population sample. *Lancet*. 1994;344:357–362.

23. Bielory L. Gandhi R. Asthma and vitamin C. *Ann Allergy*. 1994;73 (2):89–96.

24. Ting S, Mansfield LE, Yarbrough J. Effects of vitamin C on pulmonary functions in mild asthma. *J Asthma*. 1983;20:39–42.

25. Schachter EN, Schlesinger A. The attenuation of exercise: induced bronchospasm by vitamin C. *Ann Allergy*. 1982;49:146–151.

26. Kordansky DW, Rosenthal RR, Norman PS. The effect of vitamin C on antigen-induced bronchospasm. *J Allergy Clin Immunol*. 1979;63:61–64.

27. Malo JL, Cartier A, Pineau L, L'Archeveque J, Ghezzo H, Martin RR. Lack of acute effects of vitamin C on spirometry and airway responsiveness to histamine in subjects with asthma. *J Allergy Clin Immunol*. 1986;78:1153–1158.

28. Ogilvy CS, DuBois AB, Douglas JS. Effects of vitamin C and indomethacin on the airways of healthy male subjects with and without induced bronchoconstriction. *J Allergy Clin Immunol*. 1981;67:363–369.

29. Schwartz J, Weiss ST. Relationship between dietary vitamin C intake and pulmonary function in the First National Health and Nutrition Examination Survey (NHANES 1). *Am J Clin Nutr*. 1994;59: 110–114.

30. Neuman I, Nahum H, Ben-Amotz A. Reduction of exercise-induced asthma oxidative stress by lycopene, a natural antioxidant. *Allergy*. 2000;55: 1184–1189.

31. Hasselmark L, Malmgren R, Zetterstrom O, Unge G. Selenium supplementation in intrinsic asthma. *Allergy*. 1993;48:3026.

32. Kirsch CM, Payan DG, Wong MYS, et al. Effect of eicosapentaenoic acid in asthma. *Clin Allergy*. 1988;18:177–187.

33. Arm JP, Horton CE, Mencia-Huerta JM, et al. Ef-

fect of dietary supplementation with fish oil lipids on mild asthma. *Thorax*. 1988;43:84–92.

34. Dry J, Vincent D. Effect of a fish oil diet on asthma: results of a 1-year double blind study. *Int Arch Allergy Immunol*. 1991;95:156–157.

35. Arm JP, Horton CE, Spur BW, Mencia-Huerta JM, Lee TH. The effects of dietary supplementation with fish oil lipids on the airways response to inhaled allergen in bronchial asthma. *Am Rev Respir Dis*. 1989;139:1395–1400.

36. Picado C, Castillo JA, Schinca N, et al. Effects of a fish oil-enriched diet on aspirin-intolerant asthmatic patients: a pilot study. *Thorax*. 1988;43: 93–97.

37. Broughton KS, Johnson CS, Pace BK, et al. Reduced asthma symptoms with n-3 fatty acid ingestion are related to 5-series leukotriene production. *Am J Clin Nutr*. 1997;65(4):1011–1107.

38. Woods RK, Thien FCK Abramson MJ. Dietary marine fatty acids (fish oil) for asthma (Cochrane review). In: *The Cochrane Library*, Issue 4. Oxford: Update Software, 2001.

39. Lehrer PJ. Emotionally triggered asthma: a review of research literature and some hypotheses for self-regulation therapies. *Appl Psychophysiol Biofeedback*. 1998;23(1):13–41.

40. Nagarathna R, Nagendra HR. Yoga for bronchial asthma: a controlled study. *BMJ*. 1985;291:172–174.

41. Singh V, Wisniewski A, Britton J, et al. Effect of yoga breathing exercises (pranayama) on airway reactivity in subjects with asthma. *Lancet*. 1990; 335:1381–1383.

42. Opat AJ, Cohen MM, Bailey MJ, et al. A clinical trial of the Buteyko breathing technique in asthma as taught by a video. *J Asthma*. 2000; 37(7):557–564.

43. Kotses H, Harver A, Segreto J, et al. Long-term effects of biofeedback-induced facial relaxation on measures of asthma severity in children. *Biofeedback Self-Regul*. 1991;16(1):1–21.

44. Ewer TC, Stewart DE. Improvement in bronchial hyper-responsiveness in patients with moderate asthma after treatment with a hypnotic technique: a randomised controlled trial. *BMJ*. 1986;293: 1129–1132.

45. Nielsen NH, Bronfort G, Bendix T, et al. Chronic asthma and chiropractic spinal manipulation: a randomized clinical trial. *Clin Exp Allergy*. 1995; 25(1):80–88.

46. Balon J, Aker P, Crowther E, et al. A comparison of active and simulated chiropractic manipulation

as adjunctive treatment for childhood asthma. *N Engl J Med.* 1998;339:1013–1020.

47. Field T, Henteleff T, Hernandez-Reif M, et al. Children with asthma have improved pulmonary functions after massage therapy. *Pediatrics.* 1998; 132(5):854–858.

48. Peat JK. Prevention of asthma. *Eur Respir J.* 1996; 9:1545–1555.

49. Reisman RE, Mauriello PM, Davis GB, et al. A double-blind study of the effectiveness of a high-efficiency particulate air (HEPA) filter in the treatment of patients with perennial allergic rhinitis and asthma. *J Allergy Clin Immunol.* 1990;85: 1050–1057.

50. Reilly DT, Taylor MA, McSharry C, et al. Is homeopathy a placebo response? Controlled trial of homeopathic potency, with pollen in hayfever as a model. *Lancet.* 1986;2:881–886.

51. Linde K, Clausius N, Ramirez G, et al. Are the clinical effects of homeopathy placebo effects? A meta-analysis of placebo-controlled trials. *Lancet.* 1997; 350:834–843.

52. Shivpuri DN, Singal SC, Parkash D. Treatment of asthma with an alcoholic extract of Tylophora indica: a crossover, double-blind study. *Ann Allergy.* 1972;30:407–412.

53. Mathew KK, Shivpuri DN. Treatment of asthma with alkaloids of *Tylophora indica:* a double-blind study. *Aspects Allergy Appl Immunol.* 1974;7: 166–179.

54. Gupta S, George P, Gupta V, et al. Tylophora indica in bronchial asthma: a double-blind study. *Indian J Med Res.* 1979;69:981–989.

55. Gupta I, Gupta V, Parihar A, et al. Effects of *Boswellia serrata* gum resin in patients with bronchial asthma: results of a double-blind, placebo-controlled, 6-week clinical study. *Eur J Med Res.* 1998;3:511–514.

56. Haller CA, Benowitz NL. Adverse cardiovascular and central nervous system events associated with dietary supplements containing ephedra alkaloids. *N Engl J Med.* 2000;343(25):1833–1838.

57. Graham DM, Blaiss MS. Complementary/alternative medicine in the treatment of asthma. *Ann Allergy Asthma Immunol.* 2000;85:438–449.

58. Egashira Y, Nagano H. A multicenter clinical trial of TJ-96 in patients with steroid-dependent bronchial asthma. A comparison of groups allocated by the envelope method. *Ann N Y Acad Sci.* 1993;685:580–583.

59. Bielory L, Lupoli K. Review article: herbal interventions in asthma and allergy. *J Asthma.* 1999; 36:1–65.

60. Huntley A, Ernst E. Herbal medicines for asthma: a systematic review. *Thorax.* 2000;55(11):925–929.

61. Kleijnen J, ter-Reit G, Knipschild P. Acupuncture and asthma: a review of controlled trials. *Thorax.* 1991;46:799–802.

62. Tashkin DP, Bresler DE, Kroening RJ. Comparison of real and simulated acupuncture and isoproterenol in methacholine-induced asthma. *Ann Allergy.* 1977;39:379–387.

63. Takishima T, Mue S, Tamura G. The bronchodilating effect of acupuncture in patients with acute asthmas. *Ann Allergy.* 1982;48:44–49.

64. Christensen PA, Laursen LC, Taudorf E. Acupuncture and bronchial asthma. *Allergy.* 1984;39: 379–385.

65. Tashkin DP, Kroening RJ, Bresler DE. A controlled trial of real and stimulated acupuncture in the management of chronic asthma. *J Allergy Clin Immunol.* 1985;76:855–864.

66. Biernacki W, Peake MD. Acupuncture in treatment of stable asthma. *Respir Med.* 1998;92: 1143–1145.

67. Shao JM, Ding YD. Clinical observation of 111 cases of asthma treated by acupuncture and moxibustion. *J Tradit Chin Med.* 1985;5:23–5.

68. McCrory DC, Brown C, Gelfand SE, Bach PB. Management of acute exacerbations of COPD: a summary and appraisal of published evidence. *Chest.* 2001;119(4):1190–1209.

69. Department of Commerce. Statistical abstract of the United States 1997; US Department of Commerce, Bureau of the Census. Washington, DC: Department of Commerce; 1997.

70. Gift AG, Moore T, Soeken K. Relaxation to reduce dyspnea and anxiety in COPD patients. *Nurs Res.* 1992;41(4):242–246.

71. Moody LE, Fraser M, Yarandi H. Effects of guided imagery in patients with chronic bronchitis and emphysema. *Clin Nurs Res.* 1993;2(4):478–486.

72. McBride S, Graydon J, Sidani S, Hall L. The therapeutic use of music for dyspnea and anxiety in patients with COPD who live at home. *J Holistic Nurs.* 1999;17(3):229–250.

73. Tabak C, Smit HA, Heederik D, et al. Diet and chronic obstructive pulmonary disease: independent beneficial effects of fruits, whole grains, and alcohol (the MORGEN study). *Clin Exper Allergy.* 2001;31(5):747–755.

74. Smit HA. Chronic obstructive pulmonary disease, asthma and protective effects of food intake: from hypothesis to evidence. *Respir Res.* 2001;2(5): 261–264.

75. Romieu I, Trenga C. Diet and obstructive lung diseases. *Epidemiol Rev.* 2001;23(2):268–287.

76. Jobst K, Chen JH, McPherson K, et al. Controlled trial of acupuncture for disabling breathlessness. *Lancet.* 1986;2(8521–22):1416–1419.

77. Jobst KA. A critical analysis of acupuncture in pulmonary disease: efficacy and safety of the acupuncture needle. *J Altern Complement Med.* 1995;1(1):57–85.

78. Cahalin LP, Braga M, Matsuo Y, Hernandez E. Efficacy of diaphragmatic breathing in persons with chronic obstructive pulmonary disease: a review of the literature. *J Cardiopulm Rehabil.* 2002;22(1): 7–21.

79. Collins EG, Langbein WE, Fehr L, Maloney C. Breathing pattern retraining and exercise in persons with chronic obstructive pulmonary disease. *AACN Clin Issues.* 2001;12(2):202–209.

CHAPTER 28

Integrative Approach to Psychiatry

LEWIS MEHL-MADRONA

The current state of mainstream medicine and psychiatry is one in which pharmacology has become the standard treatment for most nonsurgical conditions. Throughout history, the healing arts have included many other types of treatment. This is particularly important in psychiatry, whose disorders are among the most important contributors to the worldwide health burden.[1]

Integrative psychiatry is the treatment of systems—humans, families, and communities. The molecular level is important, but so are all the others. Of equal importance, even on the molecular level, is the need to discover what works and causes the fewest side effects. If nutritional therapies reduce the dosage of neuroleptic medications, perhaps we can prevent some of the tardive dyskinesias, the neuroleptic malignant syndromes, the blood dyscrasias, and the other serious side effects of these medications.

Integrative psychiatry also calls for the study of the process of care. These factors are often called the nonspecific factors of the treatment situation, because they are not specific to any illness. As such, integrative psychiatry has much to say to the other specialties of medicine. Our concern is how these nonspecific factors affect physical disease and its healing. Does the intent of the doctor affect the action of drugs? What are the effects of the quality of the doctor–patient relationship, the patient's expectations for results, the culture within which the treatment takes place—all the more important when different cultures meet in the treatment room—and the role the illness plays in the family dynamic?

Future research efforts may need to be redirected toward discovering what it is that patients and clinicians do when they experience large improvements, comparing these findings to what can be observed about relationships and interventions when small or no improvements occur. Current research methods are generally not adequate to study what actually happens in clinical practice. Research aims at short studies of single therapies, while practice invokes multiple therapies over periods of years. More prospective, observational studies are needed for us to discover the wisdom of clinicians who help patients and to understand the mysteries of clinical improvement.

We can draw parallels from indigenous cultures for our further understanding of integrative psychiatry. Cherokee medicine, for example, included seven major categories of healing, each reflecting a separate level of intervention. These levels included

- Dietary therapies and herbs;
- Water cures (hydrotherapy), movement, and lifestyle;
- Energy medicine (acupuncture with porcupine quills and thorns, crystal healing, hands-above-the-body healing);
- Psychological therapies;
- Body therapies (manipulative medicine);
- Family and community therapies; and
- Spiritual therapies, including ritual and ceremony.

The psychiatry of indigenous cultures uses interventions from all of these categories, which is distinctly different from current academic psychiatry, which strives to treat only on the molecular level with single, pure substances. Unfortunately, in the practice of psychiatry, some patients receive eight or more medications, suggesting that the realities of psychiatry and the science of psychopharmacology do not mesh as closely as desired.

Psychological therapies have always had a role in psychiatry, although their emphasis has diminished in recent years to the extent that sometimes they are almost considered alternative or complementary therapies.

The Cherokee believed that mild illnesses could be treated with an intervention from any one of the seven levels, that moderate illness required addressing three or four different levels, and that a serious illness required all seven levels delivered simultaneously. Their practice reflected a basic understanding of the concept of synergy: that addressing separate levels simultaneously may produce results beyond the simple sum of the effects of each level taken independently. Synergy is implicit in the understanding that humans are systems and are embedded in larger systems called families and communities. The behavior of systems cannot be predicted from an understanding of the parts. The very definition of a system is a "whole that is greater than the sum of its parts."

Table 28–1 outlines most of the therapies to be discussed in this chapter and the conditions in which they have been effective.

▶ INTEGRATIVE PSYCHIATRY IN CONVENTIONAL CONTEXTS

Psychiatry has long attempted a kind of integration beyond the mere use of medication. For example, home-based intervention by a psychogeriatric team provided more benefit than what was found for medication alone.[2] The team provided an individualized package of care optimized for each client, focused upon problem-solving psychotherapy, development of social support, and community intervention. Data were analyzed on an intention to treat basis. Nineteen (58%) of the patients in the intervention group recovered, as compared with only nine (25%) of the control group, a difference of 33%. Even after controlling for possible confounders in logistic regression analysis, patients of the geriatric team were nine times more likely to recover than were patients receiving medication alone. The odds of recovering with medication alone was only 0.3%. Critical elements of what the geriatric team did, above and beyond its use of medications, contributed to patient improvement, emphasizing the importance of the human aspect of care.

Other studies in the conventional psychiatric literature have criticized models that fragment care and dilute the doctor–patient relationship. In one representative study, depressed patients receiving split care, in which pharmacotherapy was provided by a psychiatrist and psychotherapy by a nonphysician psychotherapist, did not do as well as patients receiving integrated care, in which both psychotherapy and pharmacotherapy were provided by the same psychiatrist.[3] Patients receiving integrated treatment were seen more often when necessary, had longer periods of no sessions, and used significantly fewer outpatient sessions overall as compared to patients receiving split care. Their treatment costs were, on average,

▶ **TABLE 28-1** SUMMARY OF INTEGRATIVE APPROACHES TO PSYCHIATRIC DISORDERS

Treatment	Depression	Anxiety	Schizophrenia	Bipolar
Acupuncture	±	+	±	
Antioxidants	+			
Behavior therapies	+	+		
Biofeedback/neurofeedback	±	+		
Body therapies (touch)				
Chinese herbs	+		±	
Cognitive behavior therapy	+	+		
Comprehensive vitamin program			−	+
Cranial electrical stimulation	±			
Dehydroepiandrosterone	±			
Elimination diet		±		
Evening primrose oil		−		
Exercise	+	+		
Fish consumption	+		+	
Folic acid	+		+	
Gluten/casein			±	
Hypnosis	±	+		
Inositol	+	+		
Kava kava		+		
Light therapy	+			±
Magnesium	±			
Medication	+	+	+	+
Melatonin	+			
Negative ions	+			
Niacinamide		+		
Omega-3 fatty acids	±		+	
Phenylalanine + pyridoxine			±	
Problem-solving psychotherapy	+			
Process psychotherapy	±			
Relaxation/meditation		+		
S-adenosylmethionine	+			
St. John's wort	+			
Supportive psychotherapy	+			
Therapeutic touch		+		
Thiamin		+	±	
Tryptophan and 5-OH tryptophan	+			
Valerian		+		
Vegetarian diet	+	+		
Vitamin A				
Vitamin B$_6$	+		±	
Vitamin B$_{12}$	+			
Vitamin C			±	
Zinc				

+ = effective; ± = both effective and ineffective.

lower than those of split treatment. The authors concluded that the results did not support the prevailing assumption that integrated treatment is more costly than split treatment in a managed care network. This study also suggested a value in a more concentrated relationship rather than in a fragmented relationship.

The prevailing assumptions of managed care and of modern psychiatry are that medication is more cost effective than relationship-based therapies. While collaborative care in which patients received both psychotherapy and medication costs more for treating depression, it was also more cost effective.[4] Collaborative care included brief cognitive behavior therapy and enhanced patient education. Other studies underscore this, often with savings seen in medical visits (although not in all studies).

Conventional psychiatry presents the rest of medicine with an important example of synergistic therapies when it shows that the addition of psychotherapy helps patients who are not responding to antidepressant medications.[5] Conventional psychiatry typically studies time-limited interpersonal, behavioral, and cognitive behavior therapies. Effective strategies emphasize individualized assessment, psychoeducation, a high level of structure and therapist activity, operationalized short-term goals, self-help and homework activities, and an empirical–collaborative approach to treatment.

Most interestingly, an early direction of research in psychiatry, which was, unfortunately, not pursued, concerned the role of the doctor's attitude and expectations upon patients' responses to medication.[6] Kast and Loesch[7] had suggested that drug effect was not a simple sum of biological activity and placebo activity (as is currently still assumed), but rather was affected by the physicians' attitudes toward the drugs. They hypothesized that drug effects were greater when physicians' attitudes were more favorable toward drugs. Further supporting this idea were the observations of Uhlenhuth et al.[8] that drug effects greater than placebo were observed among patients whose doctors expected a drug–placebo difference, but not among patients whose doctors were noncommittal. Uhlenhuth, et al.[6] designed an experiment of 15 patients in each of 12 different cells. Three clinics were represented—one at Johns Hopkins University in Baltimore, and two affiliated with the University of Pennsylvania in Philadelphia. For each clinic, patients were treated by a physician who was positive and enthusiastic about the medication being used (meprobamate) or by one who held an experimental and noncommittal attitude. Within each of these six groups, subjects either received placebo or active drug. The study lasted 6 weeks. Psychometric tests were used along with patient and physician ratings of anxiety. Patients receiving active drug from enthusiastic physicians experienced more relief than patients taking placebo. On the contrary, patients taking active drug with noncommittal physicians felt less relief than those taking placebo.

▶ DEPRESSION

Depression is the most common psychiatric disorder.[9] Although everyone seems to know what they mean by depression, DSM-IV (*Diagnostic and Statistical Manual of Mental Disorders,* 4th ed. [1994]) provides strict diagnostic criteria that will not be reviewed here, but defines the depression that is discussed in this section. In brief, the symptoms of depression, according to the National Mental Health Association, include

- A persistent sad, anxious or "empty" mood
- Sleeping too little or sleeping too much
- Reduced appetite and weight loss, or increased appetite and weight gain
- Loss of interest or pleasure in activities once enjoyed
- Restlessness or irritability
- Persistent physical symptoms that do not respond to treatment (such as headaches, chronic pain, or constipation and other digestive disorders)

- Difficulty concentrating, remembering, or making decisions
- Fatigue or loss of energy
- Feeling guilty, hopeless, or worthless
- Thoughts of death or suicide[10]

When untreated, this disorder may result in increased morbidity and mortality or suicide.

Pathophysiology

Biochemistry
One line of theoretical research delineates two subgroups of depressed patients.[11] One group has low levels of the norepinephrine metabolite MHPG (3-methoxy-4-hydroxyphenylglycol). This group does not respond to amitriptyline, but does respond to desipramine and imipramine, which raise norepinephrine, but not serotonin, levels. This group exhibits mood elevation with dextroamphetamine. The second group has normal or high urinary MHPG and does not respond to desipramine and imipramine but does respond to amitriptyline (which tends to raise serotonin levels). These patients do not experience mood elevation with dextroamphetamine. The first group would theoretically respond better to drugs such as venlafaxine that affect norepinephrine, while the second group would do better with the selective serotonin reuptake inhibitors.

Another intriguing line of investigation is that of Dr. Owen Wolkowitz, professor of psychiatry at the University of California, San Francisco, who suggests that some cases of depression may result from the endocrine system. Under conditions of stress, plus genetic susceptibility, excess adrenal cortisol feeds back to the brain to cause depression. High levels of cortisol actually deplete neurotransmitters such as serotonin. The two abnormalities may feed on each other. If so, lowering stress could improve depression.[12] Endocrine system hormones also affect cognitive processes. In state-dependent retrieval, we remember memory stored within the same affective state best when we are accessing those feelings. This means that sad feelings cause us to recall more sad feelings, in a kind of vicious cycle.

Psychological Theories
Depression has been associated with suppressed emotions, self-directed anger and/or loss, and aggression that is psychologically repressed and turned inward. In this theory, repressed aggression is associated with guilt-feelings and somatic symptoms with pain. The theory states that those who anxiously repress their aggressive impulses simultaneously repress all their energy and activity, become depressed, and thus avoid taking responsibility. A number of studies have found that episodes of depression are almost always preceded by a major life event.[13]

Incidence and Prevalence

While incidence and prevalence data for depression exist for the United States, the most reliable estimates come from the United Kingdom because of long-term data collection efforts and universal health coverage. Estimates from the United States are based upon population samples from specific studies and then extrapolated to the entire population, whereas UK figures are based upon total population figures from National Health Service data. Nevertheless, the mean weekly incidence rate, per 100,000 population, for England and Wales, for the year 1998 (Table 28–2), is remarkably similar to that found in the United States,[14] as is the prevalence rate (Table 28–3).[15] The importance of depression in childhood is underscored in these tables, which show a decreasing incidence and increasing prevalence with age, suggesting that depression can be a long-term problem for many people, even life-long.

The incidence of depression in the United States has risen every year since the early twentieth century;[16] at this point 1 in 6 people experience a depressive episode during their lifetime. Only 50% of the people who meet the criteria for diagnosis seek treatment, which affects estimates of incidence and prevalence.

► **TABLE 28-2** INCIDENCE OF DEPRESSION (INCLUDING CHILDHOOD AND ANACLITIC DEPRESSION) BY AGE GROUP FOR ENGLAND AND WALES, 1998, PER 100,000 PEOPLE

Age (Years)	0–4	5–14	15–44	45–64	65+	Male, All Ages	Female, All Ages	Male and Female
Rate	90.46	61.79	30.99	24.78	23.86	33.84	37.99	35.95

The reported prevalence of depressive disorders varies throughout the world. The lowest rates are reported in Asian and Southeast Asian countries. Taiwan reports less than a 2% lifetime probability that a person will experience a depressive episode lasting over 1 year, and Korea reports 3%. Western countries report higher rates, such as Canada, 7%; New Zealand, 11%; and France, 16%. Countries plagued by protracted war, like Bosnia and Northern Ireland, report higher rates of depression. Culturally based differences in the perception of symptoms of depression also influence statistics. Asian people may describe depression as a series of pains, loss of focus, or an imbalance in their energy, rather than as a mental health disorder.

Women have a prevalence rate for depression up to twice that of men.[17,18] Women in the United States are two-thirds more likely than men to be depressed,[19] with similar statistics in Britain.[20] Gender differences in depression are at their greatest during reproductive years,[17] suggesting hormonal influences.

Conventional Treatment Approaches

Effective conventional therapeutic options for depression include psychotherapy and pharmacotherapy.[21] Short-term, highly focused forms of psychotherapy are thought helpful for elderly patients who are reluctant to take, or unable to tolerate, antidepressant medication. Because of their favorable adverse effect profiles and safety in cases of overdose, the selective serotonin reuptake inhibitors have, in most cases, replaced tricyclic antidepressants as first-line therapy when antidepressants are indicated. Psycho-stimulants may be helpful for medically ill elderly patients with depressive symptoms. Electroconvulsive therapy is thought to offer a safe and effective alternative for patients refractory to or unable to tolerate antidepressant medication.

Factors compromising the effectiveness of pharmacological treatments include noncompliance, nonresponse, and relapse of depression. Psychological therapies, such as cognitive ther-

► **TABLE 28-3** PREVALENCE OF DEPRESSION (INCLUDING CHILDHOOD AND ANACLITIC DEPRESSION) BY AGE GROUP FOR ENGLAND AND WALES, 1996, PER 100,000 PEOPLE

Age (Years)	0–4	5–15	16–24	25–34	35–44	45–54	55–64	65–74	75–84	85+	Crude Rate (All Ages)	APR (All Ages)[15]
Male Rate	0.1	0.9	17.4	34.8	47.1	57.7	62.8	60.9	77.1	86.6	38.3	36.2
Females Rate	0.1	1.3	45.3	85.2	109.9	127.6	132.2	140.9	160.5	160.1	91.0	81.9

APR = adjusted prevalence rate.

apy, are effective and may prevent relapse, but are not available to the majority of depressed patients seen in primary care. Existing evidence demonstrates that primary care staff can be trained in effective psychological interventions for depression, but interventions need to be developed that are sufficiently brief to be incorporated into routine treatment. Consistent provision of information about depression, coping strategies, and sources of support may improve compliance with treatment and subsequent outcome.

Conventional Psychotherapy
SUPPORTIVE PSYCHOTHERAPY

In southeast London, Bannerjee et al.[22] examined the effect of an intervention by a psychogeriatric team in the treatment of depression in 69 elderly disabled, depressed (according to the standardized automatic geriatric examination for computer-assisted taxonomy or AGECAT) people receiving home care from their local authority. Subjects were randomized to an intervention group and to a control group. Members of the intervention group received an individual package of care that was formulated by the community psychogeriatric team in their catchment area and implemented by a researcher working as a member of that team. The control group received normal general practitioner care. Data were analyzed on an intention to treat basis. Nineteen (58%) of the intervention group recovered, as compared with only nine (25%) of the control group, a difference of 33% (95% confidence interval, 10–55%). This powerful treatment effect persisted after controlling for possible confounders in logistic regression analysis, with members of the intervention group more likely than members of the control group to have recovered at follow-up (odds ratio 9.0 [2.0–41.5]). This did not seem to be a simple effect of antidepressant prescription: use of antidepressants at follow-up did not have a significant effect.

PROBLEM-SOLVING PSYCHOTHERAPY

Brief, telephone-based treatment for minor depression in a family practice setting has been shown to be an efficient and effective method to decrease symptoms of depression and improve functioning.[23] Nurses in these settings with appropriate training and supervision can provide this treatment. Patients in a family practice residency practice were evaluated through the Medical Outcomes Study Depression Screening Scale and the Diagnostic Interview Schedule to identify those with subthreshold or minor depression. Twenty-nine subjects were randomly assigned to either a treatment or comparison group. Initial scores on the Hamilton Depression Rating Scale were equivalent for the groups and were in the mildly depressed range. Six problem-solving therapy sessions were conducted over the telephone by graduate student therapists supervised by a psychiatrist. The treatment group subjects had significantly lower postintervention scores on the Hamilton Depression Rating Scale, as compared with their preintervention scores ($p < .05$). Scores did not differ significantly over time in the comparison group. Postintervention, the treatment group subjects also had lower Beck Depression Inventory scores than did the comparison group $p < .02$), as well as more positive scores for social health ($p < .002$), mental health ($p < .05$), and self-esteem ($p < .05$) on the Duke Health Profile.

COGNITIVE BEHAVIOR THERAPY AND DEPRESSION

Meta-analyses of 78 controlled, clinical trials from 1977 to 1996 have shown that cognitive behavior therapy (CBT) is effective in patients with mild or moderate depression.[21] The meta-analysis included 48 high-quality controlled trials of 2,765 patients presenting with nonpsychotic and nonbipolar major depression, or dysthymia of mild to moderate severity. CBT appeared significantly better than waiting-list, antidepressants ($p < .0001$), and a group of miscellaneous therapies ($p < .01$), but was equal to behavior therapy. A review of eight follow-up studies comparing CBT with antidepressants suggested that CBT may prevent relapses in the long-term, with higher relapse rates found for antidepressants in naturalistic studies.

The Use of Alternative Medicine by People Who Are Depressed

The use of alternative medicine among patients with major depression is increasing.[25] Using data from the 1994–1995 and 1996–1997 Canadian National Population Health Surveys, subjects were selected with major depression according to the Composite International Diagnostic Interview Short Form for Major Depression (CIDI-SFMD). The prevalence of alternative medicine and conventional health service use by the subjects was calculated for each survey and was stratified by province. The prevalence of alternative medicine use among subjects with major depression was 7.8% in 1994–1995 and 12.9% in 1996–1997. Female sex, having more than 12 years' education, and having one or more long-term medical conditions were associated with an increased likelihood of using alternatives. The sex difference in the use of alternative medicine had disappeared among the younger age groups by 1996–1997.

Complementary and alternative therapies were used more than conventional therapies by people with self-defined anxiety attacks and severe depression.[26] Most patients visiting conventional mental health providers for these problems also used complementary and alternative therapies. The data came from a nationally representative survey of 2,055 respondents (1997–1998) that obtained information on the use of 24 complementary and alternative therapies for the treatment of specific chronic conditions. A total of 9.4% of the respondents reported suffering from "anxiety attacks" in the past 12 months and 7.2% reported "severe depression." A total of 56.7% of those with anxiety attacks and 53.6% of those with severe depression reported using complementary and alternative therapies to treat these conditions during the past 12 months. Only 20.0% of those with anxiety attacks and 19.3% of those with severe depression visited a complementary or alternative therapist. A total of 65.9% of the respondents seen by a conventional provider for anxiety attacks and 66.7% of those seen by a conventional provider for severe depression also used complementary and alternative therapies to treat these conditions. The perceived helpfulness of these therapies in treating anxiety and depression was similar to that of conventional therapies.

High rates of use of complementary and alternative medicine were found among respondents who met criteria for common mental disorders in data from a national household telephone survey conducted in 1997–1998 ($N = 9,585$).[27] Structured diagnostic screening interviews were used to establish diagnoses of probable mental disorders. Use of complementary and alternative medicine during the past 12 months was reported by 16.5% of the respondents. Of those respondents, 21.3% met diagnostic criteria for one or more mental disorders as compared to 12.8% of respondents who did not report use of alternative medicine. Individuals with panic disorder and major depression were significantly more likely to use alternative medicine than were individuals without those disorders. Respondents with mental disorders who reported use of alternative medicine were as likely to use conventional mental health services as respondents with mental disorders who did not use alternative medicine.

Integrative Treatment Approaches

Dietary Therapies

Less anxiety and depression has been reported among vegetarians when compared to nonvegetarians. Diet analysis found higher nutritional antioxidant agents levels in the vegetarian group in comparison with the nonvegetarian group, suggesting a role for antioxidants in the prevention and treatment of depression.[28] Slow weight reduction in overweight women can help to elevate mood. Eating breakfast regularly leads to improved mood, better memory, more energy, and feelings of calmness. Eating regular meals and nutritious afternoon snacks improves cognitive performance.[29]

Higher levels of fish consumption are associated with less depression and suicide among large populations.[30] Geographic areas where consumption of docosahexaenoic acid is high are associated with decreased rates of depression. Docosahexaenoic acid deficiency states, such as alcoholism and the postpartum period, also are linked with depression.[31]

Nutritional Supplements

A number of nutritional supplements have been examined for efficacy in the treatment of depression. Those with supportive data are reviewed below.

DEHYDROEPIANDROSTERONE

Dehydroepiandrosterone (DHEA) supplementation can be beneficial for major depression, although the exact physiological mechanism is unknown.[32] One study of women over age 70 years reported positive effects of DHEA administration on several neuropsychological symptoms. Positive effects on sexual interest and satisfaction and sense of well-being are more consistent in elderly women than in men. The recommended administered dose is 25–50 mg once a day in women and 100 mg in men. Androgenic effects (greasy skin, acne, increased growth of body hair) are frequent but reversible side effects. The treatment should be taken under close medical supervision in order to detect a possible hormone-dependent cancer such as breast cancer in women and prostate cancer in men. Many authorities recommend active screening for breast and prostate cancers before starting DHEA, as well as ongoing monitoring. Levels should be monitored as well during the course of treatment.

S-ADENOSYLMETHIONINE

S-adenosylmethionine (SAMe) is a substance found naturally in the human body which serves as a methyl donor in many synthetic reactions, and may contribute to an increase in the levels of certain neurotransmitters when given in supplemental form. Although definitive data is still lacking on efficacy, SAM-e appears to have enough of an antidepressant effect to warrant further research.[33] Fetrow and Avila[34] reviewed studies on SAMe and depression in 2001. These authors found that the sample sizes and dosages used in these trials varied considerably. Several reviews and at least two meta-analyses examined the available evidence surrounding SAMe in the therapy of depression for trials completed prior to 1994 and concluded that SAMe was superior to placebo in treating depressive disorders and approximately as effective as standard tricyclic antidepressants. However, much of this information existed in the form of isolated case reports or solitary clinical trials. SAMe appears to be well tolerated, with the majority of adverse effects presenting as mild to moderate gastrointestinal complaints. Di Rocco et al.[35] reported a pilot study of SAMe in 13 depressed patients with Parkinson's disease. All patients had been previously treated with other antidepressant agents without significant benefit or with intolerable side effects. SAMe was administered in doses of 800–3,600 mg/d for a period of 10 weeks. Eleven patients completed the study, and 10 had at least a 50% improvement on the Hamilton Depression Scale. Although uncontrolled and preliminary, this study suggested that SAMe is well tolerated and may be a safe and effective alternative to the antidepressant agents currently used in patients with Parkinson's disease.

B VITAMINS

B vitamins have been examined for a role in depression as well, in particular vitamin B_6 and folic acid. Depression has been related to oral contraceptive use, presumably through B_6 depletion.[36] In a double-blind crossover study, depressed patients were given 250 mg BID of vitamin B_6 and a placebo, each separately for 2 months. Subjects who were B_6 deficient were significantly less depressed during the B_6 phase ($P < .01$). Those who were non-B_6 deficient showed no benefit.

One-third of depressed patients have low folic acid levels, with treatment improving their depression.[37] Low serum folate and B_{12} levels predict refractory responses to antidepressant medication.[38,39] Neither macrocytosis nor anemia were predictive. Among unmedicated outpatients with major depression, medication responders had a significantly higher mean serum folate at baseline (nonresponders = 13.8 nmol/L; responders = 17.7 nmol/L). Red blood cell folate levels showed a significant inverse correlation with severity of depression and a significant positive correlation with age of onset of illness. After 5 weeks of treatment with desmethylimipramine, the change in the severity of depression was significantly correlated with the change in red blood cell folate levels. Significantly more responders than nonresponders had an increase in red blood cell folate levels.

Among inpatients with severe depression, 52% had elevated total plasma homocysteine accompanied by significant reductions of serum, red cell, and cerebrospinal fluid folate, cerebrospinal fluid S-adenosylmethionine, and all three cerebrospinal fluid monoamine metabolites. Total plasma homocysteine was significantly negatively correlated with red cell folate in depressed patients, but not controls.[40] In one representative study, fluoxetine 20 mg/d was given for 8 weeks to 213 outpatients with major depressive disorder. Subjects with low serum folate levels were more likely to have melancholic depression and were significantly less likely to respond to fluoxetine.[41]

The psychiatric symptoms of folate deficiency are found among 25% of hospitalized patients, and include anorexia, insomnia, fatigue, hyperirritability, apathy, withdrawal, confusion, lack of motivation, anxiety, depression, delusions, dementia, slowed cerebration, forgetfulness, and disorientation. Prevention requires 50–1,000 μg/d and oral treatment consists of 2–5 mg/d.

Inositol is a vitamin found in cell membranes (phosphatidylinositol) where it functions closely with choline.[42] Inositol is required for the proper function of several brain neurotransmitters and works together with other methyl donors including SAMe. The usual dose is 3 g given four times daily for a total of 12 g/d. Nine of 11 depressed patients, resistant to previous antidepressant medications, improved with inositol 6 g/d in an open trial. Mean Hamilton Depression Rating Scale scores decreased from 31.7 to 16.2.[13] In another study, inositol was equivalent to single-drug therapy for depression and panic disorder ($p = .043$).[11]

OTHER SUPPLEMENTS

In 1991, Shealy[15] reported that 75% of depressed patients are magnesium deficient with another 9% at borderline levels. He reported efficacy from magnesium supplementation. Melatonin has also been reported effective in some cases with up to 84% of depressed patients showing abnormal levels.[27,15] Melatonin may work in a similar fashion as light therapy in depressed patients.[17]

Amino acid supplementation has been reported to be helpful in some patients with depression. In one open trial of 351 depressed patients who had failed antidepressant drug treatment, 85% experienced significant improvement in 2 weeks from a combination of amino acids—tryptophan, taurine, and others.[18] Seventy percent remained consistently improved, based on scores on the Zung Depression Test. The authors also included vitamin B_6 and magnesium. Tryptophan has long been reported to be effective for depression, often in combination with vitamins B_3 and B_6.[19] Tryptophan has been compared to amitriptyline in a randomized, controlled trial.[50] One hundred fifteen general practice patients were enrolled in a 12-week double-blind study using the Hamilton Depression Scale before and after treatment to assess the level of depression. The four treatment groups were (1) tryptophan 1 g TID; (2) tryptophan 1 g TID and amitriptyline 25 mg TID raised later to 50 mg TID; (3) amitriptyline 25 mg TID, later raised to 50 mg TID; and (4) placebo TID. All treatments were significantly better than placebo ($p < .05$). Far more of the placebo group withdrew during the study than withdrew from the other three groups ($p < .0004$). Amitriptyline significantly relieved depression ($p < .001$) as did tryptophan ($p < .01$). The combination was better than either alone ($p < .05$), demonstrating synergy. Side effects of tryptophan were significantly less than amitriptyline.

Amino acid supplementation has also been examined as a strategy for preventing depression in genetically susceptible individuals. One double-blind crossover study enrolled 20 men, ages 18 to 30 years with no prior episodes of depression but with a multigenerational family history of major affective disorders, and compared them to a group of 19 men without a personal or family history of psychiatric illness. All were placed on a tryptophan-deficient amino acid mixture and alternatively a nutritionally balanced amino acid formula including tryptophan.[51] Plasma levels of tryptophan were reduced 89% at 5 hours after administration of the tryptophan-deficient amino acid mixture. At that point, 6 of 20 subjects with a family history showed a 10-point or greater increase in depressed mood, as assessed by the Profile of Mood States Depression Scale, as compared to no change in the controls with a negative family history ($p = .012$). Further research is needed about the possible preventive role of nutritional supplements in those at high risk for depression.

OMEGA-3 FATTY ACIDS

Essential fatty acid (EFA) supplementation may have an important role in the nutritional approach to depression. Phospholipids make up 60% of the dry weight of the brain. They are essential for neuronal, and especially for synaptic, structure and play key roles in the signal transduction responses to dopamine, serotonin, glutamate, and acetyl choline. The unsaturated fatty acid components of phospholipids are abnormal in depression, with deficits of eicosapentaenoic acid and other omega-3 fatty acids, and excesses of the omega-6 fatty acid arachidonic acid.[52] Correction of this abnormality by treatment with eicosapentaenoic acid improves depression.[53] The fatty acid abnormalities also provide a rational

explanation for the associations of depression with cardiovascular disease, immunological activation, cancer, diabetic complications, and osteoporosis. The abnormalities in EFA balance in depressed patients cannot be explained only by diet, although diet may attenuate or exacerbate their consequences. A number of enzyme abnormalities may explain the phenomena with phospholipase A_2, and coenzyme A-independent transacylase being strong candidates. Nevertheless, the field is still unfolding, and despite a clear correlation between low omega-3 levels and depression, the efficacy of EFA supplementation has not been clearly demonstrated.[51]

Botanical Therapies
ST. JOHN'S WORT

The first report on St. John's wort, *Hypericum perforatum*, to appear in the scientific literature described six women with depression, age 55–65 years, treated in an open trial with an active hypericin complex, a derivative of St. John's wort. A significant increase in the urinary output of 3-methoxy-4-hydroxyphenylglycol, a metabolite of norepinephrine and dopamine (both considered indicative of an antidepressant action) followed. After 4 weeks of treatment, the Clinical Assessment Geriatric Scale and Depression Status Inventory scores for these patients showed significant improvement in anxiety, dysphoric mood, loss of interest index, anorexia, hypersomnia, insomnia, obstipation, and feelings of worthlessness ($p < .01$ to $p < .05$).[56]

As of 1996, 25 controlled studies of the antidepressant action of hypericum (St. John's wort) had accumulated.[57] A meta-analysis of these 25 studies covered 1,600 patients. Doses ranged from 300 to 900 mg/d of *H. perforatum* extract for 2–6 weeks. Most studies were double-blind, comparing *Hypericum* with placebo or conventional antidepressant drugs. The most common instrument used to assess depression was the Hamilton Depression Scale. For mild-to-moderate depression, *Hypericum* was equivalent to imipramine and maprotiline. Severe depression was less prone to respond.

Only 2.5% of patients complained of side effects.[58]

In a 2002 review and meta-analysis of 23 randomized studies of *Hypericum* for mild to moderately severe depression encompassing 1,757 patients, the probability that St. John's wort performed better than placebo was 2.7 (95% CI, 1.78–4.01). There were 4% dropouts for side effects in the *Hypericum* groups versus 7.7% in drug groups (OR 0.6; 95% CI, 0.27–1.38) and side effects were reported in 20% and 53%, respectively (OR 0.39; 95% CI, 0.23–0.68).[59]

The question of proper standardization and dosing of *Hypericum* remains somewhat challenging. In 10 studies using extracts prepared with 50% or 60% ethanol in water (V/V), the dosages ranged from 300 mg to 1,050 mg of extract per day. Five of the 10 studies were placebo-controlled and in all 5 cases, the *Hypericum* extract was shown to be significantly superior. Results with hypericum were as good or even better than with imipramine or fluoxetine. An additional 12 controlled studies done since 1990, have examined one particular extract prepared with 80% ethanol in water (V/V). Six of these were placebo-controlled, two compared *Hypericum* with imipramine and one each with maprotiline, amitriptyline, sertraline, or light therapy. Dosages ranged from 450 mg to 1,200 mg of extract per day. Statistical analysis of the total Hamilton scores showed significant differences between hypericum extract and placebo in four of the six placebo-controlled studies and a trend in favor of the active treatment in the other two. Of the five comparative trials against four different synthetic antidepressants, only amitriptyline was significantly superior to *Hypericum* after 6 weeks of therapy, while there were no significant differences in treatment outcome between *Hypericum* and the other drugs.

The results of the trials conducted to date show no major differences in efficacy of the alcoholic extracts. Taking all the results into account, it can be assumed that the threshold dose for efficacy against individual symptoms and complaints that occur in the course of the depressive illness could be about 300 mg/d of extract. In the medically supervised treatment of mild to moderate depression, doses of approximately 500–1,000 mg/d of extract of these preparations of St. John's wort are of comparable efficacy to synthetic antidepressants in their normally prescribed dosages.[60]

Occurring after the above review and noteworthy is a double-blind, randomized, placebo-controlled trial of a well-characterized *H. perforatum* extract (LI-160) conducted in 12 academic and community psychiatric research clinics in the United States.[61] Between December 1998 and June 2000, 340 adult outpatients with major depression and a baseline total score on the Hamilton Depression Scale (HAMD) of at least 20 were recruited. Patients were randomly assigned to receive *H. perforatum*, placebo, or sertraline (as an active comparator) for 8 weeks. Based on clinical response, the daily dose of *H. perforatum* could range from 900 mg to 1,500 mg and that of sertraline from 50 mg to 100 mg. Responders at week 8 could continue blinded treatment for another 18 weeks. Neither sertraline nor St. John's wort was significantly different from placebo. Full response occurred in 31% of the placebo-treated patients versus 23.9% of the St. John's wort-treated patients ($p = .21$) and 24.8% of sertraline-treated patients ($p = .26$). The authors concluded that the study failed to support the efficacy of St. John's wort in the treatment of moderately severe major depression, although neither did it support any efficacy for sertraline (not mentioned in the abstract). A number of letters to the editor discussed the weaknesses and implications of this study.[62–70]

In May 2002, a 12-week, double-blind, randomized, controlled, community trial in 12 offices of family physicians practicing in greater Montreal gave 87 men and women with major depression and an initial score of ≥16 on the Hamilton Rating Scale for Depression either sertraline (50–100 mg/d) or St. John's wort (900–1,800 mg/d).[71] No important differences were found in changes in mean HAMD and Beck Depression Inventory scores (using intention-to-treat analysis), with and without adjustment for baseline demographic characteristics, between the two groups at 12 weeks. Significantly more side effects were reported in the sertraline group than in the St. John's wort group at 2 and 4 weeks' follow-up. The authors concluded that the more benign side effects of St. John's wort made it a good first choice for the studied patient population.

Yet another double-blinded, placebo-controlled trial published in 2002 showed that St. John's wort (300 mg TID of hydroalcoholic *H. perforatum* extract WS 5570) was superior to placebo[72] among 375 male and female adult outpatients with mild to moderate major depression (single or recurrent episode, DSM-IV criteria). After a single-blind placebo run-in phase, the patients were randomly assigned, 186 to WS 5570 and 189 to placebo, after which they received double-blind treatment for 6 weeks. Follow-up visits were held after 1, 2, 4, and 6 weeks. The primary outcome measure was the change from baseline in the total score on the Hamilton Depression Rating Scale. In addition, analyses of responders (patients with at least a 50% reduction in Hamilton total score) and patients with remissions (patients with a total score of 6 or less on the Hamilton scale at treatment end) were carried out, and subscale/subgroup analyses were conducted. Compared to placebo, WS 5570 produced a significantly greater reduction in total score on the Hamilton depression scale and significantly more patients with treatment response or remission. It was more effective in patients with higher baseline Hamilton scores and led to global reduction of depression-related core symptoms, assessed with the melancholia subscale of the Hamilton scale. The placebo and WS 5570 groups had comparable adverse events.

St. John's wort is thought to act as a weak selective serotonin reuptake inhibitor. Recent studies also indicate that, similar to antidepressants, *Hypericum* can induce mania.[73] Quanti-tative electroencephalographic evidence exists to support the action of St. John's wort, and suggests that its mechanism of action differs from that of tricyclic antidepressants.[74] We also know that the presence of hyperforin conjugates is necessary for activity.[75]

Wagner et al.[76] used open-ended interviews with key questions to ask 22 current users (21 women; 20 white; mean age = 45 years) in a Southern city why they used St. John's wort. Four dominant decision-making themes were consistently noted: (1) personal health care values: subjects had a history of alternative medicine use and a belief in the need for personal control of health; (2) mood: all St. John's wort users reported a depressed mood and occasionally irritability, cognitive difficulties, social isolation, and hormonal mood changes; (3) perceptions of seriousness of disease and risks of treatment: St. John's wort users reported the self-diagnosis of "minor" depression, high risks of prescription drugs, and a perception of safety with herbal remedies; and (4) accessibility issues: subjects had barriers to and lack of knowledge of traditional health care providers and awareness of the ease of use and popularity of St. John's wort. Some St. John's wort users did not inform their primary care providers that they were taking the herb (6 of 22). Users reported moderate effectiveness and few side effects of St. John's wort.

While other herbs are used by traditional practitioners of numerous cultures and by naturopaths to treat depression, St. John's wort is the only non-Chinese herb to have received serious scientific attention. Most likely, investigation of other herbs is long overdue, because every culture on every continent has an herbal pharmacopeia for depression. The efficacy of a number of Chinese herbs are reviewed below in the section on "Traditional Chinese Medicine."

Exercise

Aerobic exercise is more effective than placebo or no treatment controls for the treatment of depression, and appears to be as effective as medication.[77] The effects are long-lasting. A 1990 meta-analysis of 80 studies showed that exercise decreased depression with long-lasting effects ($p <. 01$ to $p <. 001.$)[78] Generally, longer programs have greater effects than brief ones ($p < .001$). Exercise and psychotherapy together had better results ($p < .001$) than either alone. These effects are thought to be a result of enhanced endorphin production or to changes in metabolism of dopamine, norepinephrine, and serotonin.

Depression is encountered less often among those who exercise regularly. Similarly, starting regular exercise improves depression. Among 1,500 surveyed persons, 8.3% manifested depression. The odds ratio for depression in a no-exercise group was 3.1, as compared to 1.55 in an occasional-exercise group and 1.0 in a regular-exercise group.[79] Among 53 overweight, otherwise healthy men, an aerobic exercise conditioning group ($n = 24$) compared to a weight reduction group ($n = 29$) showed a significantly greater improvement in depression ($p = .05$), scores on the health scale ($p = .01$) and ego-strength of the Minnesota Multiphasic Personality Inventory.[80]

Environmental Modification

Treatment with a high-density negative ionizer appeared to act as a specific antidepressant for patients with seasonal affective disorder.[81] Twenty-five subjects with winter depression underwent a double-blind, controlled trial of negative ions at two exposure densities, 1×10^4 ions/cm^3 or 2.7×10^6 ions/cm^3, using an electronic negative ion generator with wire corona emitters. Home treatments were taken in the early morning for 30 minutes over 20 days, followed by withdrawals. The severity of depressive symptoms (prominently including the reverse neurovegetative symptoms of hypersomnia, hyperphagia, and fatigability) decreased selectively for the group receiving high-density treatment. Standard depression rating scale assessments were corroborated by clinical impressions. When a remission criterion of 50% or greater reduction in symptom frequency/severity was used, 58% of subjects responded to high-density treatment while 15% responded to low-density treatment ($p = .025$). There were no side effects attributable to the treatment, and all subjects who responded showed subsequent relapse during withdrawal. The method may be useful as an alternative or supplement to light therapy and medications.

Bright-light therapy has also been used to treat depression. In one study, subjects were randomly assigned to receive either 10,000 lux bright white light for 30 minutes between 6 and 9 AM or dim red (placebo) light at a comparable time. The group receiving bright light improved 27% in 1 week, while the group receiving placebo light did not improve, except for one outlier. The benefit of bright light was significant compared to placebo.[82]

In another study, depressed subjects were commenced on open treatment of morning light therapy, for 30 minutes daily using a fluorescent light therapy unit that produced approximately 5,000 lux at a distance of 12 inches. The treatment lasted 3 weeks, and at the end of the first and second week of treatment the duration of exposure could be increased to a maximum of 60 minutes at the discretion of the clinician. The light therapy was found to be an effective treatment for depression with a seasonal pattern. Optimal duration for the light therapy unit used in this study was 45–60 minutes daily.[83]

Traditional Chinese Medicine

While many cultural healing systems exist for depression, only traditional Chinese medicine (TCM) has been subjected to extensive research. A consideration of the various meridians of Chinese medicine and what they mean illustrates the different conceptualization of depression that TCM represents. Other indigenous healing systems are as interesting, but are not yet supported by research.

A brief review of the principles of Chinese medicine related to depression is in order to show the different conceptualization of an indigenous healing system from conventional, allopathic medicine. In Chinese medicine, the heart houses the spirit. It integrates the organs and the personality. Healthy expressions include warmth, vitality, excitement, inner peace, love, and joy. Heart deficiency signs include many of the symptoms of anxiety and depression, including sadness, absence of laughter, depression, fear, shortness of breath, cold feelings in the chest and limbs, palpitations, cold sweat, inability to speak, memory failure, and restless sleep.

The pericardium meridian is also important in depression. Its healthy expressions are joy, happiness, and healthy relationships; weakness is associated with confusion, delirium, nervousness, and psychosis.

Mental signs of triple warmer channel disorders include emotional upsets caused by breaking of friendships or family relations, depression, suspicion, anxiety, and poor elimination of harmful thoughts.

The lung meridian governs the Qi and all bodily processes. It is the home of the corporeal soul and relates to strength and sustainability. Healthy expressions are righteousness and courage. Weakness is associated with excessive grief, sadness, worry, and depression.

The spleen meridian governs digestion and manifests in the muscle tissues. Healthy expressions are fairness, openness, deep thinking, and reminiscence. Spleen deficiency signs include memory failure and, indirectly, obesity. The excessive use of the mind in thinking, studying, concentrating, and memorizing over a long period of time tends to weaken the spleen and may lead to blood stasis. This also includes excessive pensiveness and brooding. Likewise, inadequate physical exercise, overexposure to external dampness, and excess consumption of sweet and/or cold foods will deplete the spleen.

Mental signs of stomach channel disorders include depression, death wishes, instability, suicidal tendencies, being mentally overwrought, doubt, suspicions, tendency to mania, and slowness at assimilating ideas.

The liver is the home of the ethereal soul; it relates to decisiveness, control, and the principle of emergence. It stores the blood, maintains the smooth flow of Qi and blood, reflects emotional harmony and movement, and expresses itself in the nervous system. Healthy expressions include kindness and spontaneity. Stagnation is associated with frustration, irritability, tension, and feeling unable to change. With time this pattern tends to produce a gloomy emotional state of constant resentment with repressed anger or depression.

The kidney houses the will, expresses ambition and focus, provides the "fire of life," and displays the effects of aging, chronic degenerative processes, and extreme stress; likewise, any severe disturbance in the complementary relationship between the kidney and heart expresses itself in emotional distress. Healthy expressions are gentleness, groundedness, and endurance. Intense or prolonged fear depletes the kidney. Chronic anxiety may induce deficiency and then fire within the kidney. Overwork, parenting, simple aging, and a sedentary or excessively indulgent lifestyle all contribute significantly to kidney deficiency.

Some data exists to support the use of acupuncture in major depression.[84] In an open trial study of acupuncture, 68 patients with affective disorders (11 with anxiety, 8 with depression, and 49 with both) were assessed by the Hospital Anxiety and Depression Scale (range: 0–21).[85] A score of greater than 8 was accepted as a threshold value for significance. Standard individualized treatment protocols were used. At 1 month after completion of treatment, 70% of anxious patients were improved and 90% of depressed patients were improved. Mean scores pre- to posttreatment were anxiety 10.6 to 7.3 ($p < .001$) and depression 9.6 to 6.2 ($p < .001$).

A single-blind, placebo-controlled study investigated the efficacy of additional acupuncture applied to drug treatment in 70 hospitalized patients with major depression.[86] The three different treatment groups included acupuncture plus medication, placebo acupuncture plus medication, and medication alone as a control group. The acupuncture group was treated at specific points considered effective in the treatment of depression. The placebo group was treated with acupuncture at nonspecific locations. The control group received pharmacological treatment. Acupuncture was applied three times weekly over a period of 4 weeks. Psychopathology was rated by judges who were blind to patients' actual treatment group and rated patients twice a week over 8 weeks. The patients who experienced acupuncture improved more than patients treated with medication alone. No differences were detected between placebo acupuncture and intentional acupuncture, suggesting the need for a larger study or an effect of the healing interaction with the acupuncturist.

A number of Chinese herbs have been studied in animal models for the treatment of depression. A representative sample is reviewed here to show the level of research being conducted with the reader referred to Chinese texts for further examples.

The Chinese herbal medicine Kami-shoyo-san was studied in mice in the forced swimming test, with findings that it did induce antidepressive climbing behavior in the treated animals. The effective substance detected as the active agent was determined to be an O-linked glycoside with the sugar chain structure GalNAc alpha 1–3GalNAc.[87]

The antidepressant drug imipramine has been compared to liquid nutritive and tonic Chinese medicine consisting of *Ginseng radix*, *Epimedii herba*, *Holen*, and an additional 8–12 crude herbs. After preloading forced swimming, the tonic (applied orally, 0.1 mL/10 g) significantly increased the duration time of swimming and decreased the duration time of immobility, while the administration of imipramine under the same conditions and after the same treatment did not produce these positive effects. The present results indicate that the effect of Chinese medicinal tonics on fatigued subjects is different from that of imipramine, probably because of involvement of another factor in addition to the antidepressant effect.[88]

The effects of the Chinese herbal medicines Hochu-ekki-to, Yoku-kan-san, and Saiko-ka-ryukotsu-borei-to on behavioral despair and acetic acid-induced writhing in mice has been studied. The herbal medicines were administered for 14 consecutive days in the animals' drinking water. In a behavioral despair study, mice were placed in a water tank containing a water wheel from which there was no escape for 15 minutes and the number of wheel rotations was counted as escape attempts, with imipramine being used in the comparison group. All three of these herbal medicines similarly increased the number of wheel rotations and reduced the number of acetic acid-induced writhings. These results confirmed antidepressive and antinociceptive properties for these herbal medicines.[89]

Banxia Houpu decoction has been used for the treatment of depression-related diseases since ancient times, and is a traditional Chinese medicinal empirical formula consisting of *Pinellia ternata*, *Poria cocos*, *Magnolia officinalis*, *Perilla frutescens*, and *Zingiber officinale*. The effects of the total decoction extract and five derived fractions have been evaluated in mice by tail suspension and forced swimming tests. The total 90% ethanol extract of the decoction was shown to possess an antidepressant activity that was close to that of the antidepressant fluoxetine. The antidepressant effect of the water decoction of *Rhizoma acori tatarinowii* was tested using the rat forced swimming test and mouse tail suspension test models of depression. Both the water decoction of *Rhizoma acori tatarinowii* and fluoxetine significantly shortened the motionless time of rat forced swimming and the despair time of mouse tail suspension in these two animal models of depression.[90]

Innovative and Alternative Psychotherapies

Mindell's Process Therapy

Mindell, an important and original thinker in applications of psychotherapy, believes that trying to be helpful to a patient whose primary process is hopelessness is a dangerous undertaking. "Helping" polarizes the secondary process even more, creating a situation in which the helper must be resisted. If we constantly act like helpers, a vicious and dangerous cycle is possible, as the client never gets to help herself and is constantly in the position of "the depressed one." If we are unclear about the structure of the client's process, we are bound to take the unoccupied part in the client's pattern, in this case, the healer who is trying to get the client to live. Being helpful to a client who is not interested in help is a goal mismatch and is bound to isolate the client even more.[91] Mindell provides an example:

> A woman suffering from long-standing depression threatened she wanted to die. Suicide is yet another method of switching out of one state into another. I told her to do it right there with me. She closed her eyes, began to breathe deeply, and lay down on the floor. After a few minutes she opened her eyes and spoke of a vision of standing in front of the gates of heaven. A great voice yelled at her, saying, "Get the hell out of here. Go back to life and work instead of being so lazy." I then knew how to work with her depression. Instead of being sympathetic to her sad story about life, I told her to stop being so lazy and get to work. This brought immediate positive feedback from her. Altered states are full of unlived creativity. I could never have given her that vision or have helped her in any other way. Instead, I had empathized with her and felt badly for her. But for her, dying meant altering her state of consciousness, dropping out of her feelings of sadness and heaviness.
>
> From a process point of view, suicide means killing the primary process. By breathing deeply, she killed the primary experience of sadness, and a new message announced itself through vision and voice. Thus alterations in consciousness can be accomplished through accessing secondary processes. Instead of treating depression as if it were something we should overcome, we can also ask what its meaning is. If a depressed and hopeless experience is allowed to come up, then the road

is cleared for help. Instead of constantly resisting the processes in front of us, we might stop and admit their presence.[92]

Hypnosis

Hypnosis is a therapeutic intervention in which the therapist suggests meaningful images or helpful ideas to the client.[93] It produces and then uses a state of heightened awareness in the patient. A prerequisite to the use of this intervention in psychiatry is a detailed discussion regarding the wishes and hopes of the patient, and of images that are meaningful and important to them. The hypnotherapist, with the overt permission of the patient, then will use these images, and often the patients' own words, to feed back constructive suggestions that can enhance the patient's therapeutic progress. Hypnosis *itself* is not a therapy—it is an *aspect* of therapy evident in every interaction between client and psychotherapist. Like other aspects of therapy, the goal of hypnosis is to help the client overcome a debilitating disorder, such as depression. Yapko[94] has described how hypnosis can enhance therapeutic effectiveness for psychotherapy in depression. He reports that hypnosis is helpful in reducing common symptoms of depression such as agitation and rumination and thereby may decrease a client's sense of helplessness and hopelessness. Hypnosis is also effective in facilitating the learning of new skills, a core component of all empirically supported treatments for major depression. The acquisition of such skills has also been shown not only to reduce depression, but the likelihood of relapses, thus simultaneously addressing issues of risk factors and prevention. Despite its widespread use in clinical practice, the author could find no serious trials of hypnosis as a treatment for depression on MEDLINE. Such trials are long overdue.

Biofeedback/Neurofeedback

Biofeedback in conjunction with cognitive behavior therapy has been used successfully to treat depression.[95] Case studies have been presented of two depressed women who were trained with more than 34 sessions each of electroencephalogram biofeedback (neurofeedback) using an alpha asymmetry protocol. The purpose of this training was to determine if depression could be alleviated when the subjects learned to increase the activation of the left hemisphere and/or decrease the activation of the right hemisphere. The Minnesota Multiphasic Personality Inventory-2 was administered before and after training to measure changes in personality factors, including depression. The results suggested that alpha asymmetry neurofeedback training may be an effective adjunct to psychotherapy in the treatment of depression.

Cranial Electrical Stimulation

The results of stimulating human subjects with high-frequency electrical bursts (applied to the cranium) include an increase or decrease in the activities of certain neurotransmitters and neurohormones and the reduction of associated pain, insomnia, depression, and spasticity. Stimulators usually have a carrier frequency of 15,000 Hz, which uses the bulk capacitance of the body, and a 15-Hz modulating bioactive frequency. The second modulating frequency is usually 500 Hz, reducing the energy input to the patient by half. Significant increases in levels of cerebrospinal fluid serotonin and beta-endorphin have been recorded poststimulation in association with elevations of plasma serotonin, beta-endorphin, gamma-aminobutyric acid, and DHEA, together with diminished levels of cortisol and tryptophan. Concomitant with these changes were significant improvements in the symptoms of pain, insomnia, spasticity, depression, and headache.[96] On the other hand, a 1995 review[97] revealed frequent use of unreliable self-report outcome measures, insufficient description of treatment protocols, invalid double-blind and placebo conditions, and often a lack of adequate description of the electrical parameters used among existent studies. The experimental literature confirmed the capability of cranial electrical stimulation to modulate central nervous system activity. Further quality research is needed.

Overview

A systematic literature search using PubMed, PsycLit, the Cochrane Library, and previous review papers identified 37 alternative treatments used for depression.[98] Best evidence of effectiveness were for St. John's wort, exercise, cognitive behavior therapy, and light therapy (for winter depression). Some limited evidence supported the effectiveness of acupuncture, light therapy (for nonseasonal depression), massage therapy, negative air ionization (for winter depression), relaxation therapy, S-adenosylmethionine, folate, and yoga. A review of randomized, controlled trials suggested that exercise, stress reduction methods, bright-light exposure, and sleep deprivation held promise as adjuncts to conventional treatment for major depression, and that acupuncture might hold promise as a monotherapy for first episode depression.[99]

▶ Case Example 1: Depression

Conventional Medicine Treatment of Depression

Megan was a 45-year-old woman suffering from chronic pancreatitis and biliary tract disease. She also had gluten sensitivity. Her family doctor suspected depression because she was frequently irritable, had a disturbed sleep–wake cycle, had no source of pleasure in her life except for her children, and thought sometimes that death would be a desirable alternative to her life. Megan was started on venlafaxine 37.5 mg twice daily. This dose was gradually increased to 75 mg

BID. Unfortunately, the higher dose worsened her pancreatic symptoms and the dose had to be decreased. She was tried on bupropion, but had side effects at the lowest dose. Then she was tried on sertraline, which gave her intense abdominal pain at the lowest dose. Next she was given low-dose lithium carbonate 300 mg/d to augment the lower dose of venlafaxine with some improvement in her symptoms. She was willing to tolerate a slight hand tremor from the lithium. Her symptoms of depression gradually improved.

Integrative Medicine Treatment of Depression

Teresa was a 48-year-old woman whose psychotherapist had referred her for a medication consult. Paradoxically, the last thing Teresa wanted was medication. Even though she had been in psychotherapy for 6 months and was becoming more depressed instead of less, she still believed that natural remedies could work better than drugs. Exploration of her life revealed major stress at her job. She worked for the public school system, and felt used, underpaid, and unhappy. As school budget cuts continued, the size of her classroom increased and the amount of aid time decreased. She felt unable to provide quality education under the circumstances, and felt trapped in her job by her need for benefits for her family, because her husband was self-employed, and not earning as much income as they had hoped. She was frustrated, angry, and hopeless.

First, supplements were recommended. She began taking a customized multiple vitamin, along with additional B-complex, omega-3 fatty acids, alpha-lipoic acid, vitamin C, S-adenosylmethionine, mineral complex (calcium, magnesium, zinc, copper, manganese, molybdenum, selenium, germanium), and inositol. She agreed to reduce her dietary intake of simple sugars and grains. We ordered a urine screening test for *Candida* breakdown products and other nutritionally correctable disorders. She agreed to increase her intake of root and green vegetables.

Next we discussed exercise. She was interested in taking yoga and planned to start. She increased her aerobic exercise by walking to and from work instead of taking the subway. She agreed to discuss with her therapist her options for stopping work. During one of these discussions, she decided that she could file for disability for work-related stress. She began this process, and her depression began to improve.

Yeast breakdown products indicative of excess *Candida* metabolism were found in her urine, so she was started on caprylic acid, garlic, green tea extract, berberis, and undecylenic acid. These substances are well-known in the naturopathic world as treatments for *Candida*. She felt quickly better. She modified her diet to decrease fermented foods, sugars, and grains. Some intestinal complaints that she had "learned to live with," disappeared.

Over the course of 6 months, her depression cleared and she became more organized, productive, and happier. She left her job, was exercising regular, taking yoga class three times weekly, and was helping her husband in his business, which was becoming more successful. She knew that antidepressant medication was available if she wished it, but chose to treat herself nutritionally and with exercise and yoga. Changing adverse conditions in her life also contributed to her improvement.

While no research has been conducted on the treatment of *Candida* in relation to depression, it is this author's experience that a *Candida* hypersensitivity syndrome may contribute to depression in some cases. This *Candida* syndrome is seen by some as one point on the spectrum of intestinal dysbiosis described in detail by Galland in Chapter 21; it may be that the systemic inflammation resulting from chronic overstimulation of the gut-associated lymphoid tissue by *Candida* antigen may contribute in some way to the symptoms of depression. Nevertheless, the *Candida* part of this treatment could be all placebo. Serious research remains to be conducted on those treatments that many of us feel to be clinically effective.

▶ ANXIETY

Pathophysiology

A range of hypotheses attempt to explain the cause of anxiety disorders. Gamma-aminobutyric acid (GABA), serotonin (5-HT), and norepinephrine (NE) have each been implicated in the putative pathophysiology of anxiety, and patients with generalized anxiety disorder (GAD) demonstrate dysregulation of these neurotransmitters. In addition, neurobiological studies have demonstrated that these neurotransmitter systems are extensively interrelated.

Drugs that affect serotonergic systems may also, directly or indirectly, affect other neurotransmitter systems, including GABA and NE. In recent years, clinical pharmacology studies have demonstrated that pharmacotherapeutic agents that target more than one neurotransmitter system are more effective than agents that target a single system, presumably due to synergistic mechanisms. Agents that modulate more than one neurochemical have a broader spectrum of action and may facilitate the attainment of remission among patients with moderate to severe GAD, who are likely to have comorbid psychiatric illnesses such as depression. In an animal model of anxiety, the use of two nonselective 5-HT receptor antagonists released "punished responding" in pigeons with a magnitude comparable to that of benzodiazepine anxiolytics.[100] Currently, however, no one theory is sufficiently comprehensive to propose a unitary hypothesis for the development of GAD and other anxiety disorders. One of the stronger theories proposes that a genetic predisposition, coupled with early stress during the crucial phases of development may result in a phenotype that is neurobiologically vulnerable to stress and may lower an individual's threshold for developing anxiety or depression on additional stress exposure.[101]

The psychodynamic theory of psychology sees anxiety as an alerting mechanism that arises when unconscious motivations clash with the constraints of our conscious mind. This conflict is intensified in people with GAD.[102] Behavioral theory holds that anxiety results from not knowing how to behave in a given situation. The possibility of suffering negative consequences because of inappropriate behavior may result in hesitation and inaction. The anxiety may be generalized to similar situations. For example, anxiety over taking a particular test may be generalized to taking all tests in the future. Behavioral research on panic disorder suggests that panic-related fears vary across patients, and that the use of specific treatment interventions designed for that specific patient is critical for effective treatment.

Risk factors for anxiety disorders include environmental stressors (including work, school, and relationship-related), genetics, and sleep deprivation or inconsistency. Research has shown a 20% risk for GAD in blood relatives of people with the disorder and a 10% risk among relatives of people with depression. There also seems to be a correlation between GAD and other psychiatric disorders, including depression, phobia disorder, and panic disorder. Anxiety is a risk factor for sleep disorders such as insomnia. Stressful life events may precipitate gradual symptom increase, leading to the development of full-blown disorders.[104]

Incidence and Prevalence

Generalized anxiety disorder affects 4,000,000 to 5,000,000 people in the United States. The chance that any given person in the United States will develop it over a lifetime is estimated at 8–9%. More than 10% of people seen in anxiety treatment clinics are diagnosed with GAD, which affects more women (60%) than men (40%).[105] Estimates have been made of the number of patient visits to physicians for anxiety from the National Ambulatory Medical Care Surveys of office-based practices in the United States. The number of office visits with a recorded anxiety disorder diagnosis increased from 9.5 million in 1985 to 11.2 million per year in 1993–1994 and 12.3 million per year in 1997–1998, representing 1.9%, 1.6%, and 1.5% of all office visits in 1985, 1993–1994, and 1997–1998, respectively. Prescriptions for medications to treat anxiety disorders increased between 1985 and 1997–1998, while use of psychotherapy decreased over the same time period in visits to both primary care physicians and psychiatrists. Despite a large number of office visits with a recorded anxiety disorder diagnosis, underrecognition and undertreatment are a problem, especially in the primary care sector. Medication is being substituted for psychotherapy in visits to both psychiatrists and primary care physicians over time.[106]

Because perceptions and descriptions of anxiety differ among cultures, it is hard to assess the global prevalence of anxiety disorders. Many people in the United States who are diagnosed with GAD claim to have been nervous or anxious their whole lives. Eastern societies, on the other hand, perceive and treat anxiety differently, often as something associated with pain.

Conventional Treatment

Pharmacotherapy
Conventional treatment for GAD typically combines medication and psychotherapy.[107]

GAD is treated with antidepressants, benzodiazepines, beta-blockers, and buspirone.

Drug choice is determined by the patient's ability to tolerate side effects and by the drug's effectiveness in reducing symptoms. Successful treatment of anxiety disorders reduces the risk for later depression.[108] However, many patients who respond to pharmacologic treatment (defined as having a ≥50% reduction in symptoms) still exhibit subsyndromal symptoms that predispose to relapse. This is particularly true for patients with GAD who have comorbid psychiatric or medical conditions.[109]

Antidepressants commonly used include paroxetine and venlafaxine, the only antidepressants approved for use in GAD by the FDA, although it is generally believed that all antidepressant drugs significantly improve symptoms. In a representative study of venlafaxine, 61% of the patients who had responded but not remitted by week 8 showed remission by the end of 6 months. In comparison, only 39% of placebo responders who did not qualify for remission at the end of the first 8 weeks of therapy remitted by the end of the 6 months. Relapse occurred in 6% of venlafaxine-treated patients and 15% of placebo-treated patients ($p < .01$). Long-term treatment is necessary to maintain improvements with pharmacological agents.[110]

Benzodiazepines are most commonly used in the treatment of GAD and include alprazolam, chlordiazepoxide, clonazepam, diazepam, and lorazepam. Benzodiazepines increase the effectiveness of the neurotransmitter GABA, which reduces anxiety and stress and improves function, concentration, and the ability to manage an otherwise debilitating situation. Unfortunately, the short-term benefits of benzodiazepines are overshadowed by their decreased long-term effectiveness and their degradation of patient performance.[111] There are significant risks to benzodiazepine use during pregnancy, including teratogenicity and direct neonatal toxicity.[112] Benzodiazepines that work quickly tend to be abused more often, or shared with friends and family as an on-the-spot remedy for stress. Alcoholics are at greater risk for benzodiazepine abuse, because the drug's effects are similar to alcohol, including sedation and impaired physical and mental abilities. Alcohol and benzodiazepine should not be used together. Beta-blockers are used in anxiety disorders to stop the physical symptoms of anxiety. They reduce nervous tension, sweating, panic, high blood pressure, and shakiness.

Buspirone has been used for the treatment of GAD since 1986. It is not known how buspirone works to reduce symptoms of anxiety. It does not interact with alcohol, has few or no withdrawal symptoms, lacks relaxant muscular effects, lacks sedative effects, and usually works within 3–6 weeks. Protocols exist for the gradual tapering from benzodiazepines to buspirone.[113]

Psychotherapy

Psychotherapies used to treat anxiety include psychodynamic psychotherapy, which aims to identify and explore the causes of anxiety and what they mean to the patient. Behavior therapy, which aims to establish coping strategies for anxiety, teaches patients exercises for stress evaluation and reduction to be practiced during daily life. Exposure therapy helps gradually introduce the person to the anxiety producing situation while helping them manage the ensuing feelings. Behavior and cognitive therapy overlap, because new behavior is only possible after a person is able to replace irrational, anxious thoughts with healthy ones.[114] In one representative study of psychotherapeutic treatments for anxiety, clients with GAD received either (1) applied relaxation and self-control desensitization, (2) cognitive therapy, or (3) a combination of these methods. Treatment resulted in significant improvement in anxiety and depression that was maintained for 2 years. The large majority no longer met diagnostic criteria; and a minority sought further treatment during follow-up. No differences in outcome were found between conditions.[115] Other methods include biofeedback, meditation, and relaxation training.

Integrative Treatment Approaches

Dietary Therapies

No studies relating diet and anxiety were found on MEDLINE. The only available study examined the role of elimination diets in patients with both anxiety and migraine headaches.[116] Sixty patients were studied in an open trial. Each patient undertook a 5-day elimination diet, restricting their intake to pears, lamb, and spring water. Anxiety symptoms virtually disappeared in most of the patients by the fifth day, as did their migraines. Each patient then was rechallenged with potential offending foods one at a time, usually 1–3 per day. Anxiety and migraines returned with reintroduction of the offending foods. The mean number of offending foods found was 10 per patient (range: 1–30). Most common offenders were wheat, 78%; orange, 65%; eggs, 45%; coffee and tea, 40%; chocolate, 37%; milk, 37%; beef, 35%; corn, cane sugar, and yeast, 33%; mushrooms, 30%; and peas, 28%. When an average of 10 foods were completely eliminated, 100% of the 60 patients improved, 85% became headache-free, and the aggregate number of headaches in the group fell from 402 per month to 6 per month. More research on the interrelationships of diet and food allergies to anxiety is sorely needed.

Patients with anxiety and panic disorders respond differently to caffeine than do normal controls, making caffeine reduction or avoidance an important therapeutic strategy.[117] When patients with anxiety disorders were compared to normals, caffeine produced significant increases in skin conductance, systolic and diastolic blood pressure, self-rated anxiety and sweating levels, and significant decreases in alpha state brain activity, and auditory-evoked potential amplitudes ($p < .0005$ to $p < .05$).

Nutritional Therapies and Supplements
B Vitamins

Thiamine has been used successfully at doses of 250 mg/d to treat patients with anxiety disorders, including those manifesting with symptoms of chronic fatigue, insomnia, nightmares, anorexia, nausea and vomiting, diarrhea or constipation, chest and abdominal pain, depression, aggression, headache, diaphoresis, and fevers of unknown origin. Among more than 200 subjects, successful responders had deficient red blood cell transketolase, which normalized with thiamine supplementation in 73% of the subjects and led to disappearance or great clinical improvement in most of the symptoms.[118]

In a mouse model, niacinamide was found to have properties in common with benzodiazepines and barbiturates.[119] The vitamin was found to possess hypnotic and anticonvulsant activity, influence spinal cord activity, produce muscle relaxation, and have aggression-diminishing effects. Compared with controls, anxiety-disorder patients demonstrate increased flushing, anxiety, autonomic activity, and temperature after nicotinic acid (100 mg) administration, suggesting a role for nicotinic acid pathways in anxiety that could be manipulated by nutritional therapies.[120] Further controlled research is necessary to confirm and extend these pilot findings.

One hundred eighty-nine subjects with either generalized anxiety disorder, panic disorder, or obsessive-compulsive disorder were evaluated for plasma pyridoxal phosphate levels and compared with normal controls. There was no difference in plasma pyridoxal phosphate levels between the anxiety disorder groups and normal controls. Low levels of plasma pyridoxal phosphate were found in 42% of the controls. These results suggest that previous reports of low pyridoxal phosphate levels in psychiatric patients are unlikely to be significant in the etiology of the psychiatric disorders.

Inositol (12 g/d) was used to treat 21 people with panic disorder with or without agoraphobia in a double-blind, placebo-controlled, 4-week, random-assignment, crossover design.[121] The frequency and severity of panic attacks and the severity of agoraphobia declined significantly more after inositol than after placebo administration. Side effects were minimal. The authors concluded that inositol's efficacy, the absence of significant side effects, and the fact that inositol is a natural component of the human diet make it a potentially attractive therapeutic for panic disorder.

Botanical Therapies

EVENING PRIMROSE OIL

In an open trial, 18 women with premenstrual syndrome of more than 1 year's duration received 8 capsules per day of evening primrose oil in the last half of the menstrual cycles for 5 cycles.[122] Irritability ($p < .001$), depression ($p < .001$), anxiety ($p < .01$), and fatigue ($p < .01$) were significantly less when compared to baseline after the first cycle of treatment. Total premenstrual syndrome scores were significantly improved ($p < .001$). A 2000 review of evening primrose oil for premenstrual syndrome found that the results were generally favorable, although more definitive research is clearly needed.[123]

KAVA KAVA

Kava kava is an herb from the South Pacific with traditional ceremonial uses in Micronesian culture. In the West, in doses of 300 mg (containing 210 mg of kavalactone), it is used to treat anxiety. Negative effects are minimal, with possibly positive effects on reaction time and cognitive processing.[124] It decreases anxiety without loss of mental acuity. A meta-analysis of rigorous clinical trials assessing the efficacy and safety of kava kava extract versus placebo for the treatment of anxiety found seven quality studies, all of which suggested superiority of kava kava extract over placebo. Only one study found negative results, with kava kava failing to surpass placebo in a 4-week trial with generalized anxiety disorder.[130] Adverse events were mild, transient, and infrequent.[125] Two cases of hepatic failure have been associated with kava kava, although the mechanism remains mysterious, because none of the major recognized components of kava kava have demonstrated liver toxicity.[126,127] Dermatological and neurological problems are also possible and Parkinsonism can be exacerbated.[128]

Kavapyrones found in kava kava bind to many sites in the brain that are associated with addiction and craving. A preliminary study of kava kava for addiction treatment showed that its use resulted in a reduction of the desire by addicts for their drug of choice.[129] Standardized amounts of kavapyrones led to differences in abstinence from alcohol for experimental and placebo groups.

Animal studies have also demonstrated efficacy. Rex et al. compared a kava kava extract with diazepam in an animal test of anxiety (the elevated plus maze, or X-maze).[131] The kava kava extract (at doses of 120–240 mg/kg PO) performed similarly to diazepam (in doses of 15 mg/kg PO) among rats.

OTHER BOTANICALS

Valerian is used as an antianxiety agent, and is also reported to have antidepressant and sedative properties, probably related to partial agonistic activity at the A1 adenosine receptor.[132] Valerian was shown to be useful and effective in the long-term treatment of cognitively impaired children with intransigent sleep difficulties in a randomized, double-blind, placebo-controlled trial.[133] Valerian also improved the sleep of insomniacs after benzodiazepine withdrawal.[134] Stress symptoms and stress-related insomnia were ameliorated by valerian as well.[135]

Other herbs reported in the naturopathic lore as being helpful for anxiety include chamomile, skullcap, hops, and passion flower.[136] No systematic research has been conducted on these botanicals.

Energy Medicine

THERAPEUTIC TOUCH

Therapeutic touch is a form of energy healing in which the practitioner's hands are moved through the patient's bioenergy field at about 3 inches from the body. One of the first studies of this technique offered 90 hospitalized cardiovascular patients either therapeutic touch,

casual touch, or no touch. Significant decreases in state anxiety scores on the Spielberger Self-Evaluation Questionnaire occurred in the therapeutic touch group, as compared to pretreatment ($p < .01$). Therapeutic touch was also significantly better at reducing state anxiety scores, when compared to the other two groups ($p < .01$). In another randomized trial of therapeutic touch, 60 male and female subjects ages 36–81 years, hospitalized in a critical care unit, were randomly assigned to receive therapeutic touch or to a control noncontact group. All subjects completed the A-State Self-Evaluation Questionnaire before and after the intervention, which lasted 5 minutes. Postintervention anxiety scores were significantly lower in the therapeutic touch group, as compared to controls ($p = .0005$).

Exercise/Lifestyle Modification

There is little that aerobic exercise does not improve, including significant effects on reducing anxiety.[137] One representative study shows the importance of minding both the mind and the body in the treatment of anxiety disorders. Seventy-seven subjects with chronic anxiety were randomly assigned to regular exercise ($n = 44$) or meditation ($n = 33$). Those in the physical activity group reported decreased somatic symptoms and unchanged cognitive/anxiety symptoms (mental and emotional), as compared to meditators, who experienced decreases in psychological symptoms with unchanged somatic symptoms. This variance in results was significant ($p < .03$). A combination of both modalities appears to be ideal.

A study of five thousand college students taking a mental health course found that physical exercise was effective in reducing both anxiety and depression.[138] These effects persisted as long as 7 years with continuing participation in some regular exercise.

Movement Therapies

Tai chi participation reduces anxiety.[139] One study examined the effects of tai chi, walking, and relaxation therapy on 69 women and 66 men, mean age 51 years, with anxiety and/or depression, assigned to either (1) low-intensity walking; (2) low-intensity walking plus the relaxation response; (3) moderate-intensity walking; (4) a mindful exercise tai chi program; or (5) a control group. Compared to controls, women in the tai chi group experienced reductions in anxiety ($p < .01$), depression ($p < .05$), anger ($p < .008$), confusion ($p < .02$), total mood disturbance ($p < .006$), and improved general mood ($p < .04$). Men did not show a significant benefit.

Acupuncture

In a placebo-controlled, randomized, modified double-blind study the effects of acupuncture in patients with depression and patients with generalized anxiety disorders were studied. An intent-to-treat analysis was performed to compare treatment responses between true and placebo acupuncture. After completing a total of 10 acupuncture sessions, the true acupuncture group showed a significantly larger clinical improvement than did the placebo group. There were significantly more responders in the true acupuncture group than in the placebo group (60.7% versus 21.4%). In contrast, no differences in the response rates were evident after only five acupuncture sessions. The authors concluded that both the total sum of acupuncture sessions and the specific location of acupuncture needle insertions might be important factors for bringing about therapeutic success.[140]

Mind–Body Therapies
RELAXATION/MEDITATION

Relaxation training has been shown to reduce anxiety and improve depression. In one typical study, 22 participants with established diagnoses of anxiety were assessed in structured interviews. Therapist and self ratings were conducted on a weekly basis during this study of meditation-based stress reduction and relaxation and continued on a monthly basis during a 3-month follow-up. The Hamilton Panic Score, Hamilton Rating Scale for Depression and for Anxiety, and other instruments were used in assessments. The program consisted of a 2-hour weekly class for 8 weeks in training and experiencing mindfulness meditation. Also included was a one-time 7.5-hour, intensive, silent meditation retreat in the sixth week. All psychological scales significantly improved over the course of the program including anxiety, depression, and panic symptoms ($p < .001$). The accompanied ($p < .05$) and unaccompanied ($p < .01$) mobility agoraphobia indices improved . The improvements were still present when validated at a 3-year follow-up.[141]

In another study, 22 subjects seen for anxiety disorders, panic symptoms, and agoraphobia accompanying primary medical diagnoses (hypertension, chronic pain, cancer, heart disease) underwent group training sessions emphasizing nonspecific stress reduction centered on mindfulness meditation 1 hour weekly for 8 weeks. Significant improvements were seen, including reduction in Hamilton Rating Scale for Depression, Hamilton Rating Scale for Anxiety, Beck Depression, Beck Anxiety, and Fear Survey scores (all $p < .001$). Improvement in agoraphobia with fewer and less-severe panic spells and greater mobility occurred ($p = .032$). Most were still practicing their techniques at 3-year follow-up, and the improvement in Hamilton and Beck scores and the decrease in absolute numbers of panic spells were being maintained.[142]

BIOFEEDBACK

A number of studies confirm the usefulness of biofeedback in the treatment of anxiety disorders.[143] For example, anxious, hypertensive patients (10, compared to 6 normotensive patients) were treated with a comprehensive stress management program, including 9 weekly thermal biofeedback sessions and home blood pressure monitoring. Baseline systolic blood pressure ($p < .01$), diastolic blood pressure ($p < .001$), and pulse ($p < .05$) decreased significantly after participation in the program. Reactivity to a psychological stressor (oral quiz) was also significantly lower as shown in lower systolic blood pressure, diastolic blood pressure, heart rate, and cardiac output (all $p < .05$).[144]

In another study of 40 anxious, hypertensive patients, 26 (65%) met the criteria or success after biofeedback treatment. Mean diastolic pressure decreased from 107 to 96 mmHg with the initial 6 weeks of biofeedback treatment. At 1, 2, and 3 years of follow-up, 50%, 60%, and 50%, respectively, of those following up retained their criteria for successful treatment ($p = .004$, .003, and NS, respectively). Forehead electromyelogram readings, anxiety scores, and urinary cortisol and aldosterone all remained significantly reduced at the one-year follow-up in this study.[145]

▶ Case Example 2: Anxiety

Conventional Medicine Treatment

Betty was a 38-year-old woman with chronic anxiety. She worried continually about family members having accidents. She would pace about the house, looking out the window frequently, whenever anyone drove into town, even for groceries. She had lost weight because she was too anxious to eat at meals. She would startle easily, and was described as "jumpy" by family members. Her anxiety made her irritable, and sometimes she would "snap" at her children, and then apologize profusely. The anxiety was becoming too severe for her to keep her job as a cashier at a restaurant.

Betty went to a local clinic and was started on clonazepam 0.5 mg BID. The dose was gradually increased to 1 mg PO TID, and she was also started on venlafaxine 37.5 mg to reduce her anxiety. The venlafaxine dose was gradually increased until she was taking 75 mg TID with the clonazepam constant at 1 mg TID. On this regimen, she was able to continue working at her job, and was more pleasant to be around, according to her family. She still worried incessantly, but it didn't bother her or her family as much.

Integrative Medicine Treatment

Andrea was a 24-year-old graduate student referred by her psychotherapist for medication for anxiety. Andrea came reluctantly because she did not really want to take medication. Her mother had developed kidney failure, possibly related to chronic and heavy ingestion of nonsteroidal antiinflammatory drugs, so she worried about side effects. She didn't want to turn out like her mother. Nevertheless, her anxiety was disabling. She had trouble leaving her apartment unless her boyfriend accompanied her. She was missing classes. She feared being mugged in the subway. She worried about the future and about how she would support herself. She felt sure that her boyfriend would leave her imminently, even though he reassured her that he loved her and was happy with their relationship. She had many somatic symptoms of anxiety, including tremors, jitteriness, frequent sweating, cold hands and feet, headaches, shortness of breath, occasional tingling and numbness in her fingers, and feelings of disequilibrium and vertigo.

Because Andrea was opposed to medication, we discussed herbal approaches. She settled on taking kava kava 80 mg every 3 hours (with close monitoring of her liver enzymes) when she felt anxious. She would also make a strong tea of valerian root, hops, skullcap, and passion flower to take to class in a thermos and drink as needed throughout the day. We discussed decreasing her intake of caffeine and simple sugars, and increasing her intake of alkaline foods, particularly root and green vegetables. She also began drinking juices made from green and root vegetables when she felt particularly anxious. While no research has been conducted upon the use of alkaline foods and the raising of body pH to treat anxiety, it is common naturopathic practice, and appeared to work well with Andrea. Its effectiveness may relate to an inflammatory component to anxiety, as has been suggested in neurobiological research on depression reviewed in that section above.

We resolved that she would start learning meditation. Her boyfriend agreed to take her to the local Thich Nhat Hahn Buddhist sangha, where she could learn and practice mindfulness meditation. He was also interested in going with her to yoga class. She also began weekly acupuncture with the addition of Chinese herbs. She agreed to exercise in her apartment when she felt too scared to go out, and her boyfriend bought an exercise bicycle for both of them to use.

I met several times with them as a couple to explore the role that anxiety played in their relationship. I learned that they had separated for a time, and he had dated another woman. She had become quite anxious over the loss of his support, especially to someone else. In part, her anxiety showed him how much she loved him, and they reconciled. We developed other ways for her to express her love to him besides being anxious.

She continued to see her psychotherapist, who was invested in working on "childhood issues." Apparently this also helped, because the combination of therapies led to a much improved anxiety rating 6 months later. She was able to go to class alone, to complete her assignments, and even gave a speech to a medium-sized colloquium.

► SCHIZOPHRENIA AND PSYCHOTIC DISORDERS

Pathophysiology

While not the most common illness, schizophrenia is the most costly illness that psychiatrists treat.[116] The etiology of schizophrenia remains uncertain. Most research attention has focused upon the dopamine receptor, although other theories abound. Membrane phospholipid metabolic abnormalities have been proposed as the biochemical basis for the neurodevelopmental hypothesis of schizophrenia.[117] There is substantial evidence of phospholipid and polyunsaturated fatty acid abnormalities in schizophrenia.[118] Patients with schizophrenia often have low levels of poly-unsaturated fatty acids (PUFAs) in their red blood cells[119–151] and in the brain.[152] Skin fibroblasts have shown reduced levels of certain phospholipid subtypes (phosphatidylcholine and phosphatidylethanolamine) in schizophrenic patients.[153] It has been proposed that abnormal membrane PUFA metabolism (i.e., reduced incorporation into phospholipids and increased breakdown) may contribute to the etiology of schizophrenia.

Epidemiologic data in support of this theory comes from studies showing that the ratio of saturated fatty acid to PUFA in a country's national diet correlates with outcome figures by country for schizophrenia published by the World Health Organization. Those countries that obtained most of their dietary fat from land animals and birds (mostly saturated fatty acids) and relatively less of their fat from vegetable, fish, and seafood sources (mostly PUFAs) had worse outcomes for schizophrenia.[151] Similar relationships have been seen within groups of schizophrenic patients.

Because the PUFA metabolism can be altered by years of untreated illness or differentially altered by various antipsychotics, the significance of PUFA membrane status to the etiology of schizophrenia psychopathophysiology is unclear. Most of the published studies have reported changes in the levels of membrane PUFA in chronically medicated patients or in drug-naive patients long after the onset of illness (1–2 years). One study did examine the erythrocyte membrane PUFA levels in drug-naive patients within ±4.5 days of onset of psychosis from an Army Medical Center, as well as in patients treated for 1–5 years with antipsychotics from a Veterans Affairs Medical Center. The levels of plasma lipid peroxides (thiobarbituric acid reactive substances), products of damaged PUFAs, were also determined. The levels of PUFAs, particularly arachidonic acid and docosahexaenoic acid were significantly lower ($p < .001$) in drug-naive patients at the onset of psychosis than in matched normal controls. These lower PUFA levels were associated with significantly higher levels of thiobarbituric acid reactive substances in patients ($p < .001$). The levels of arachidonic acid and docosahexaenoic acid were also lower ($p < .001$) and thiobarbituric acid reactive substances higher in chronic medicated patients than in normal controls. However, the PUFA levels were higher in chronic medicated patients than in drug-naive first-episode patients. These data indicated that lower membrane arachidonic acid and docosahexaenoic acid may in fact contribute to the onset of illness, and suggest that treatment with some antipsychotics may increase the levels of PUFAs. The lipid peroxidation data suggested that possible increased oxidative stress, either as a part of the illness and/or its treatment with antipsychotics, may be one of the mechanisms of reduced membrane PUFAs. These findings could have a significant impact on improving strategies for supplementation of PUFAs and antioxidants to improve the outcome of schizophrenia.[155]

An important concept in the theory of a number of psychiatric diseases that explains the tremendous overlap of therapies between conditions is that of the bioelectric modulator. The term specifically applies to anticonvulsant drugs and mood stabilizers; however, it also embodies the larger more generic concept that bioelectrical modulators can mitigate any pathological condition caused by a dysregulation of the mechanisms that control cellular excitability, especially the excitability of neurons. The beneficial effects of these agents occur primarily as a result of modulatory influences on the bioelectrical properties of the cellular plasma membrane. Channels, transporters, and most other membrane proteins directly or indirectly involved in excitatory or inhibitory synaptic potentials and action potentials are regulated by protein phosphorylation. These proteins are phosphorylated by a class of enzymes termed protein kinases. The overlapping beneficial effects of antipsychotics, antidepressants, anticonvulsants, omega-3 fatty acids, and nonpsychoactive cannabinoids may relate to their common effects on protein kinases, thus affecting the structure and function of the cell membrane and the cell. These changes should help the cell operate within an optimal level of excitation, which may be related to emerging evidence that these therapeutic agents have neuroprotective value. These concepts are important in guiding potential nutritional therapies for schizophrenia.[156]

Conventional Therapies

The conventional therapy of schizophrenia focuses upon modulating neurotransmitters and their receptors, despite the relative lack of evidence of a primary abnormality in these systems. Treatments focus on the dopamine receptor. Common medications include risperidone and quetiapine (novel antipsychotics), as well as older compounds like haloperidol. The most important problems of existing medications are their limited efficacy, their often prohibitive expense,[157] and their propensity to induce extrapyramidal side effects. Beyond extrapyramidal side effects comes the potential for persistent, abnormal, involuntary movements (tardive dyskinesia), and the toxic neuroleptic malignant syndrome, consisting of hypertension, extreme fever, and, occasionally, death. Weight gain is also common with neuroleptics, including an increased predisposition to diabetes.

Integrative Treatment Approaches

Dietary Therapies

Dohan proposed that schizophrenia is caused by a genetic predisposition that interacts with an overload of dietary proteins such as casein and gluten or gliadin to produce symptoms.[158,159] Evidence to support the role of gluten- and casein-free diets in the treatment of schizophrenia emerged as early as 1973 in mainstream psychiatry, but has been largely ignored since.[160] Hospitalized schizophrenic patients were randomized to either a grain-free, milk-free diet or to a high-grain, unrestricted-milk diet. The grain- and dairy-free group had a mean day of discharge on the 65th day as compared to a mean of the 102nd day in the high-grain, unrestricted-dairy group ($p < .01$). Significantly more patients were discharged within 30 days in the grain-free group as compared to the high-grain group. In a later, double-blind, control trial of a gluten-free versus a gluten-containing diet carried out in a ward of a maximum security hospital for 14 weeks among schizophrenics, beneficial changes were found in the whole group of patients between pretrial and gluten-free period in five dimensions of the Psychotic In-Patient Profile, maintained during the gluten-challenge period. Two patients, who improved during the gluten-free period, relapsed when the gluten diet was reintroduced.[161]

A related case report suggests that a subset of patients diagnosed as schizophrenic could respond to a celiac diet (gluten and casein free). A 33-year-old patient, with a preexisting diagnosis of schizophreniform disorder, came to clinical attention for severe diarrhea and weight loss. Use of ^{99m}Tc hexamethylpropylene amine oxime single-photon emission computed tomography (SPECT) demonstrated hypoperfusion of the left frontal brain area, without evidence of structural cerebral abnormalities. Jejunal biopsy showed villous atrophy. Antiendomysial antibodies were present. A gluten-free diet was started, resulting in a disappearance of psychiatric symptoms, and normalization of histological duodenal findings and of SPECT pattern.[162] A second case study also demonstrated the disappearance of schizophrenic symptoms when the patient was placed on a gluten- and casein-free diet.[163]

Nutritional Supplements

B VITAMINS

Folic acid has been shown helpful among schizophrenics (as well as depressed patients).[164] Hospitalized patients with schizophrenia had low or low-borderline red blood cell folate levels (below 200 μg/L). They were given methylfolate 15 mg/d or placebo for 6 months in a double-blind fashion, in addition to psychotropic medications. The methyl derivative was chosen because it is found in the cerebrospinal fluid in three times the concentrations found in serum. Active treatment significantly outscored placebo in social and clinical recovery at 6 months ($p < .05$). The disparity between folate and placebo widened with time.

A review of folic acid in psychiatric illness[165] found that 10–30% of psychiatric patients are deficient in folic acid. The review documents a number of studies showing deficiencies in B_2, B_6, B_{12}, and folic acid among schizophrenics. Medications commonly used for schizophrenic and bipolar patients can further reduce the levels of these vitamins (psychotropics and anticonvulsants). In one study, 25% of 423 psychiatric inpatients had B-vitamin levels lower than 2 ng/mL as compared to only 6 of 62 normal controls ($p < .001$). In a study of 39 patients who had been deficient in folate and B_{12}, those taking supplements of both had a shorter length of hospital stay and were in a better state at discharge compared to 62 unsupplemented controls ($p < .01$).

An open Italian study of 15 chronic schizophrenic patients showed that pyridoxine augmented the effectiveness of neuroleptic medication. When 150 mg/d of pyridoxine was added, 8 of the 15 patients showed gradual objective and subjective evidence of improvement over 60–90 days, with decreased flat affect and increased motivation and drive to actively participate in an occupational and vocational rehabilitation programs.[166] This effect may be explained by the fact that B_6 is essential in the synthesis of some of the neurotransmitters that take part in the development of psychotic states.

Lerner et al.[167] studied the effects of vitamin B_6 supplementation on positive and negative symptoms in schizophrenic patients in a double-blind, placebo-controlled, crossover study spanning 9 weeks. All patients had stable psychopathology for at least 1 month before entry into the study and were maintained on treatment with their prestudy psychoactive and antiparkinsonian medications throughout the study. All patients were assessed using the Positive and Negative Syndrome Scale for schizophrenia on a weekly basis. Patients randomly received placebo or vitamin B_6, starting at 100 mg/d in the first week and increasing to 400 mg/d in the fourth week by 100-mg increments each week. Positive and Negative Syndrome Scale scores revealed no differences between vitamin B_6- and placebo-treated patients in amelioration of their mental state. Questions remain as to whether the dosage was high enough or long enough, whether the number of subjects was too low to demonstrate power, and whether the Positive and Negative Syndrome Scale is the proper instrument to identify change.

Thiamine and acetazolamide (Diamox) showed benefit among schizophrenics in one study. Sixteen schizophrenics were given up to 2 g/d of acetazolamide and 1.5 g/d of thiamine. Diamox and thiamine are both effective in treating pyruvate dehydrogenase deficiency. Most patients showed marked clinical improvement, with disappearance of hallucinations and decreased delusional thought and behavior. Four of 9 older patients improved noticeably in communication and sociability when 1.5 g/d each of Diamox and thiamine were used. Results were confirmed in a double-blind trial on these same patients. All patients relapsed within a few months following cessation of treatment.[168]

OMEGA-3 FATTY ACIDS

The administration of omega-3 fatty acids may improve both schizophrenia and its accompanying membrane abnormalities.[169] Two literature reviews of the use of fish oils found the data to be encouraging but preliminary.[170] In one study, twenty hospitalized schizophrenic patients were given eicosapentaenoic acid (EPA) 10 g daily for 6 weeks resulting in significant improvement in both tardive dyskinesia and psychopathological symptoms.[171] Red blood cell membrane levels of omega-3 fatty acids also increased, suggestive of a cell membrane abnormality in schizophrenics.

A group from Sheffield, UK,[172] treated 45 schizophrenics who were still symptomatic despite stable antipsychotic medication, with EPA, docosahexaenoic acid (DHA), or placebo for 3 months. Improvement on EPA was statistically significantly superior to DHA or placebo using changes in symptom score on the Positive and Negative Syndrome Scale. In a second study, these investigators used EPA as a sole treatment, although the use of antipsychotic drugs was still permitted if clinically imperative. By the end of the study, all 12 patients on placebo were still taking antipsychotic drugs, compared to 8 of 14 taking EPA. Patients on EPA again had significantly lower scores on the Positive and Negative Syndrome Scale at the end of the study. Another group from the University of Stellenbosch (South Africa)[173] treated 40 patients with persistent symptoms after 6 months of antipsychotic medication with either 3 g/d of ethyl-EPA or placebo, in addition to their usual treatment in a randomized, double-blinded, placebo-controlled study conducted over 12 weeks. The EPA group had significant reductions in Positive and Negative Syndrome Scale scores as well as Extrapyramidal Symptom Rating Scale dyskinesia scores. The FDA has affirmed the status of fish oil in doses inclusive of 3 g/d as generally recognized as safe.[174]

Vitamin C

The use of vitamin C for schizophrenia was popularized by Abram Hoffer, a Canadian psychiatrist who, with his colleagues in the 1950s, introduced the adrenochrome hypothesis of schizophrenia. They postulated that a toxic epinephrine metabolite called adrenochrome acts as a hallucinogen that causes schizophrenic disorders. They used large doses of niacin and vitamin C to inhibit the formation of adrenochrome, in the treatment of schizophrenia. In 1965, Linus Pauling came across Hoffer's book *Niacin Therapy in Psychiatry,* and was astonished to learn that certain vitamins could be used therapeutically in large doses with little if any toxicity. This discovery stimulated Pauling's introduction of orthomolecular medicine (the right molecules in the right amount) in his seminal 1968 paper, "Orthomolecular Psychiatry."[175]

Vitamin C has been used successfully with schizophrenics who fail to respond to psychotropic drugs.[176] Twenty-one schizophrenic patients who had not responded to neuroleptics received 2–6 g/d of vitamin C in addition to their medication for more than 1 month in an open trial. Seven of the 21 patients made marked clinical improvement. One floridly psychotic patient achieved full remission within 2 weeks of starting vitamin C. All responding patients maintained their progress. Only one

patient exhibited side effects, experiencing akathisia at the 6 g/d dose.

Combined Vitamin Therapy

Vaughan and McConaghy[177] assessed the efficacy of adjunctive vitamin and dietary treatment in schizophrenia. They used a random allocation, double-blind, controlled comparison of vitamin treatment for 5 months to 19 outpatients with a diagnosis of schizophrenia. The experimental group received amounts of vitamins based on their individual serum vitamin levels plus dietary restriction based on radioallergosorbent tests. The control group received vitamin C 25 mg and were prescribed substances considered allergenic from the radioallergosorbent test. Five months of treatment showed marked differences in serum levels of vitamins but no consistent self-reported symptomatic or behavioral differences between groups. Either the vitamins were unhelpful, or the doses were too small, or other factors intervened to vitiate potential therapeutic effects.

Electroacupuncture

A combination of electroacupuncture and Chinese herbs was found to provide a twofold greater effectiveness with 182 schizophrenic patients when compared to either electroacupuncture or Chinese herbs alone, or to neuroleptic alone ($p < .01$).[178] Of interest was the equivalence of acupuncture alone, herbs alone, and neuroleptics alone. In another study, sixty schizophrenic patients were treated with electroacupuncture and chlorpromazine therapy or with chlorpromazine therapy alone, 30 patients for each group, and their curative effects evaluated according to the Brief Psychiatric Rating Scale. The result showed the total curative effects of the two groups were similar. However, the marked effects appeared earlier in time for combined therapy than those when using chlorpromazine alone. Less chlorpromazine was needed in the combined therapy group, which also displayed fewer side effects.[179]

▶ Case Example 3: Schizophrenia

Conventional Medicine Treatment

Robert's parents brought him for consultation because he wouldn't leave the house. He spent hours on the Internet accomplishing nothing, appeared to have no interests in anything particular, and would doodle for hours. He had stopped producing art, which had been his passion during high school. He had stopped going to work, and sometimes sat alone for hours in a dark room talking to himself. They had to monitor his activities in the house, because he had almost set the kitchen on fire while cooking. Robert would start activities and then forget about them, wandering from room to room. He would leave food cooking on the stove until it burned. He would forget to turn off the shower, and would let the sink fill up with water and overflow.

On meeting, Robert was a pleasant, talkative 20-year-old male. He had long, rambling explanations for all of his parents concerns, which actually made no sense once they were completed, but fully occupied the listener. He insisted that he was perfectly normal and this was a phase he was going through. He insisted he could hold a job if he wanted to, but that he was trying to find his higher purpose, and couldn't work until that was discovered. He occasionally heard voices giving him simple instructions to cook various foods, or to go to particular websites, or to try various keyboard combinations of letters and numbers. He was fascinated by the occult and was trying unsuccessfully to write a Tarot card computer program. He had been able to program during high school, but now felt befuddled by the simplest loop routine.

Robert was started on Risperdal (risperidone) 2 mg twice daily. The dose was gradually increased to a total of 10 mg daily.

He began to have mild extrapyramidal symptoms, which were controlled with Cogentin (benzatropine) 2 mg daily. He began to make more sense and to talk about more mundane concerns, but he was not able to get a job. He no longer searched for a higher purpose, was safer in the kitchen and the remainder of the house, did not overflow the bathroom, and spent most of his time playing various computer games.

Integrative Medicine Treatment

Tim was an 18-year-old male who was brought to a weekend workshop by his father and stepmother. They were concerned because Tim was disrupting all semblance of order in the house. The family lived in a rural area, but when they wanted to drive to town, it could take 2–3 hours to convince Tim to get in the car. He would walk back and forth in the driveway until finally he could be coaxed inside. Once in the car, he would moan repeatedly until the car had stopped. Then the same amount of time was required to get him back in the car to make the journey home. He could roll around in the parking lot or cry loudly, causing embarrassment to the family. At home, he would moan all night long, keeping the adults and their other three children awake. Tim had been a talented artist, but had stopped all art work. He spent his time drawing squares and circles and walking in squares and circles outside. He would repeat phrases said to him over and over. He interrupted conversations with bizarre and embarrassing questions. The family wondered what was wrong. Did he need Prozac?

Tim was clearly schizophrenic on mental status examination. During the weekend workshop he stood off by himself and was very anxious about being around people. He wandered into the desert and was briefly lost until his father went to find him. He was highly disorganized, and had lost all semblance of executive functioning ability.

The weekend workshop included two sweat lodge ceremonies. Tim participated in both of them—first with his father, then with his stepmother. Amazingly, during the ceremony, Tim was lucid and communicative, talking about painful areas in his life and his severe distress. Upon leaving the sweat lodge he became disorganized again.

The idea emerged of giving him a structure of ceremony and ritual. He was started on risperidone 1 mg at bedtime, and was taught a ceremony to conduct as an alternative to moaning. In this ceremony, he was to go outside to the tepee that his parents had raised behind the house. He was to go inside and to beat on a drum over and over, as hard as he could, until his discomfort improved, or he broke the drum. He was taught a prayer song to sing, and was shown how to conduct a basic ceremony. Family therapy was conducted with all present (including his two younger and one older siblings). During these meetings, we discussed how anyone could recognize that Tim was improving and what the grades of improvement would be. We also wondered how long it would take Tim to reach each level of improvement. Family members unanimously agreed that the first grade of improvement would occur when Tim could go the entire night without moaning or waking anyone up. The second grade of improvement would occur when he could take himself out of the house and to the tepee when he needed to perform his ceremony. The third grade of improvement would occur when he could

get into the car, at home or in town, within 20 minutes no matter how uncomfortable he felt.

Tim was started on a grain-, dairy-, and soy-free diet. He was also started on vitamin supplements, including a multivitamin; B-complex 150; omega-3 fatty acids; omega-6 fatty acids; extra folic acid, B_6, B_{12}, and niacin; a comprehensive antioxidant supplement (Thorn Antioxidant); inositol; phosphatidylserine; taurine; SAMe; and a trace mineral complex.

Tim was referred to a homeopath in his own area, as well as a spiritually oriented psychotherapist, who would help him practice and refine his ceremony and practices.

I was in contact with Tim approximately every 6 months for the next 5 years. The psychotherapy continued. Tim improved one grade approximately every 4–6 months. After 2 years, he started drawing and painting again. After 4 years, he started attending junior college. After 5 years, he had a new girlfriend, felt very excited about his future, had paintings hanging in local galleries in the nearest big city, and was soon to graduate from junior college with a degree in art. He planned to transfer to the local 4-year college and earn a BFA in painting. He hoped that his girlfriend would fall in love with him. This was his first relationship, and his girlfriend, whom I met, was shy, but clearly not schizophrenic or seriously disabled in any way. Tim still showed some signs of obsessive–compulsive behavior but did not appear to be psychotic in any way. He continued on risperidone 1 mg at bedtime without side effects. He felt that it helped contain his fears and worries and allowed him to keep his compulsions in check. His vitamin program has been modified over the years, and continues to change as he does.

► BIPOLAR DISORDER (MANIC-DEPRESSIVE DISORDER)

Pathophysiology

Bipolar disorder is one of the earliest described mental maladies. In 1921, when Kraepelin applied the term manic-depressant insanity to cyclic episodes of mania alternating with depression, the syndrome had already been recognized for more than 2,000 years.[180] The term *bipolar disorder* was introduced in the mid-1970s in a largely unsuccessful attempt to lessen confusion between this condition and schizophrenia. The core features are a pathological disturbance in mood, ranging from extreme elation, or mania, to severe depression, usually accompanied by disturbances in thinking and behavior, which can be psychotic.

Genetic factors play a role in bipolar disorder,[181] with monozygotic twins having a risk of contracting the disease as much as 75 times greater than that for the general population. In addition, adoption studies demonstrate that biological relatives of bipolar patients are substantially more likely to have the disorder than are adoptive relatives. The approximate lifetime risk of acquiring bipolar disorder for relatives of an affected person are monozygotic co-twin, 40–70%; first-degree relative, 5–10%; unrelated person, 0.5–1.5%.[182]

Studies comparing urinary norepinephrine (NE) and its metabolites in unipolar or bipolar depressed patients and healthy volunteers have not yielded consistent findings. However, in unipolar depressed patients, most studies in nonelderly populations consistently report elevated concentrations of plasma norepinephrine, at least following an orthostatic challenge. Some have suggested that unmedicated unipolar and bipolar depressed patients have a "hyperresponsive" noradrenergic system.[183]

Chronic stress early in life in vulnerable persons predisposes them to both bipolar and unipolar depression, which is also compatible with the hyperresponsive noradrenergic hypothesis. Approximately 1.6% of the US population has bipolar disease,[181] and the prevalence seems to be rising. The recognized incidence is probably an underestimate because of underreporting and underrecognition of manic and hypomanic episodes.

Conventional Therapies

Lithium is the mainstay of conventional treatment for this illness, with robust acute antimanic and long-term prophylactic effects. Over the past decade, in double-blind controlled trials, valproate has been another medication shown possibly to have mood-stabilizing properties similar to lithium. Nonetheless, among patients suffering from bipolar disorder, a substantial percentage appears to respond poorly to currently available pharmacological therapies, including lithium, valproate, carbamazepine, and other newer compounds, clearly demonstrating that there is a substantial need for improved therapeutic agents. The available evidence points to a modulatory action of lithium and valproate over multiple neural biochemical pathways, and most investigations have found relevant actions of mood stabilizers on intracellular signal transduction mechanisms. Moreover, it has been shown in recent years that lithium and valproate lead to long-term changes in neural plasticity, with eventual neurotrophic and neuroprotective effects. Although these actions are not fully understood, stimulation of transcription factors and effects on gene expression are potentially involved.[185]

Psychological treatments include schema-focused cognitive therapy as an approach to help patients reduce cognitive vulnerability to relapse in addition to adopting effective mood management strategies. This therapy targets the temperament, developmental experiences, and cognitive vulnerabilities that determine adjustment to illness.[186]

Integrative Treatment Approaches

Nutritional Therapies

INOSITOL
Among 28 patients with either severe major depression or bipolar disorder, all of whom had failed a standard course of antidepressants, cerebrospinal fluid levels of inositol were consistently low.[187] These patients were randomized to take either inositol 12 g/d or a comparable D-glucose placebo for 4 weeks in a double-blind trial. The Hamilton Depression Scale scores showed no significant differences at 2 weeks, but decreased from 32 to 29 with placebo and 32 to 19 with inositol at 4 weeks ($p = .05$). Inositol was equivalently effective to single-drug therapy. The authors proposed that one action of lithium may be to treat bipolar depression by modifying inositol levels.

PHENYLALANINE PLUS PYRIDOXINE
A combination of L-phenylalanine in doses of 1–14 g/d with pyridoxine 100 mg BID was found to improve mood by clinical assessment among patients with bipolar depression and bipolar mania.[188] Mean serum 2-phenylethyl-amine (converted from D- or L-phenylalanine) levels were reduced in all these patients as compared to healthy controls (300 ng/mL versus 492 ng/mL for nonbipolar controls; $p < .02$). Phenylalanine's principal metabolite, phenylacetic acid, was measured in the urine and was also significantly lower among the patients compared to controls.

COMPREHENSIVE PROGRAMS
Kaplan et al.[189] reported an open trial of the therapeutic benefit of a comprehensive nutritional supplement for bipolar disorder. Those investigators studied 11 patients with bipolar disorder, aged 19–46 years, who were taking a mean of 2.7 psychotropic medications each at study entry. The supplement was a broad-based mixture of chelated trace minerals and vitamins administered in high doses. At study entry and at periodic intervals, patients were assessed with the Hamilton Rating Scale for Depression, the Brief Psychiatric Rating Scale, and the Young Mania Rating Scale. Patients who completed the minimum 6-month open trial experienced symptom reduction ranging from 55% to 66% on the outcome measures. Their need for psychotropic medication decreased by more than 50%. Paired t-tests revealed significant treatment benefit on all measures for patients completing the trial. The effect size for the intervention was large (> 0.80) for each measure. The number of psychotropic medications decreased significantly to a mean of 1.0 + 1.1. In some cases, the supplement replaced psychotropic medications and the patients remained well. The only reported side effect (nausea) was infrequent, minor, and transitory. A randomized, placebo-controlled trial in adults with bipolar I disorder is currently underway, as well as open trials in children.

Light Therapy
Bipolar patients with a seasonal pattern to their depression have been treated with bright, full-spectrum light.[190] Among 29 symptomatic patients (insomnia, overeating, carbohydrate craving), the Hamilton Depression Scale scores dropped from 19 to 7 ($p < .001$) during bright-light treatment. Relapse occurred 3–4 days following crossover to dim yellow light treatment.

► Case Example 4: Bipolar Disorder

Conventional Medicine Treatment
Samantha was a 19-year-old woman who had just completed her freshman year of college. She came home briefly and left for a summer abroad program in Madrid, Spain. Her housing turned out to have been poorly arranged, and she was shunted frequently from various dorms and private houses to

hotels and hostels. The program was quite chaotic for her, and she returned home in moderate distress. She had not slept well for the last 3 weeks of the program, and was becoming progressively more agitated and anxious. In the 3 days before her hospitalization she was wandering through the streets of Manhattan at all hours, and was finally taken to the hospital by the police when she refused to leave an office building that she thought was her home. She was diagnosed with bipolar disorder, treated with valproic acid (Depakote), and her symptoms resolved. She was maintained on Depakote until she returned to college in Ohio, where she stopped taking her medication because of excessive weight gain. She began to sleep progressively less until she was not sleeping at all, became paranoid, and was eventually taken by her dormitory roommates to the Student Health Center. She was again diagnosed as manic and was sent to the University Medical Center. Again, her mania resolved with Depakote. This time she agreed to continue the medication. She was discharged with monthly psychotherapy and a prescription for Depakote. She continued to have excessive weight gain, and had three further hospitalizations for mania during her college career related to her stopping medication because of weight gain. She had been a model and a dancer prior to her diagnosis, which related to her objection to putting on weight.

Integrative Medicine Treatment

Tanya was a 32-year-old female who had been diagnosed with bipolar disease at the psychiatric clinic of New York University. She was born in New Orleans, where she lived until going to college. During college she had a string of difficulties with alcohol, drugs, tumultuous relationships, and minor legal skirmishes. She graduated finally with a degree in sociology from Boston University. After college, she returned to attempt to work in the family business in New Orleans but was unsuccessful there. She left New Orleans for New York City where she worked in a string of jobs. Her bipolar disorder manifested as fairly rapid cycling between periods of extreme irritability with periods of severe depression. Her irritability would peak alongside a sense that she could do anything. During these times she would commit to seemingly impossible projects that she couldn't complete, ostensibly because of her descent into depression, but also because of their extreme difficulty. This string of failures further demoralized her.

On presentation to the author, she was on five different medications: Depakote, lithium, Restoril (temazepam), Klonopin (clonazepam), and Zyprexa (olanzapine). She complained of tremor and weight gain from the Depakote, excessive nervousness, muscle spasms, and lack of sleep despite her sleeping medications. Over the course of the next 6 months, we were able to wean her off all medications.

Tanya began with a dietary program which consisted of the ketogenic diet. This diet has been used extensively for pediatric seizures with good results. While less explored, I have used the diet with patients with bipolar disorder, Tourette syndrome, and obsessive-compulsive disorder with good results. All of these disorders have an element of runaway, rekindling type neural activity that could theoretically benefit similarly to seizures. Tanya also reduced her intake of grains and dairy products, and we began an elimination/rotation diet program to determine what other food allergies might exist.

A supplement program was designed with a complete multivitamin, extra B-complex, omega-3 and omega-6 fatty acids, minerals, antioxidants, and vitamin C. Intensive psychotherapy was started, consisting of journaling, internal family systems therapy, hypnosis, guided imagery/visualization, and cognitive-behavioral experiential therapy. Energy medicine and body therapies were included through the use of a team of prac-

titioners. Acupuncture was used periodically when symptoms worsened.

Over the course of 2 years, Tanya began to work reliability. She had stabilized on no medications, using therapy, journaling, massage, energy medicine, nutrition, and vitamins. She felt she had good results from her treatment approach and suffered no side effects.

▶ CONCLUSIONS

Integrative psychiatry is an exciting area, still in its infancy, but providing exciting options to the pharmaceutical-only approach so prominent in psychiatry today. Much more work remains to be done to determine what works for specific reasons, what works for nonspecific reasons, and what does not work at all. An approach to psychiatry that is more effective with fewer side effects would be beneficial to all.

REFERENCES

1. Murray CJ, Lopez AD. Global mortality, disability, and the contribution of risk factors: Global Burden of Disease Study. *Lancet.* 1997;349(9063): 1436–1442.
2. Banerjee S, Shamash K, Macdonald AJ, Mann AH. Randomised controlled trial of effect of intervention by psychogeriatric team on depression in frail elderly people at home. *BMJ.* 1996;313(7064):1058–1061.
3. Goldman W, McCulloch J, Cuffel B, Zarin DA, Suarez A, Burns BJ. Outpatient utilization patterns of integrated and split psychotherapy and pharmacotherapy for depression. *Psychiatric Services.* 1998;49(4):477–482.
4. Von Korff M, Katon W, Bush T, et al. Treatment costs, cost offset, and cost-effectiveness of collaborative management of depression. *Psychosom Med.* 1998;60(2):143–149.
5. Thase ME. Psychotherapy of refractory depressions. *Depress Anxiety.* 1997;5(4):190–201.
6. Uhlenhuth EH, Rickels K, Fisher S, Park LC, Lipman RS, Mock J. Drug, doctor's verbal attitude, and clinic setting in the symptomatic response to pharmacotherapy. *Psychopharmacologia.* 1966;9: 392–418.
7. Kast EC, Loesch J. A contribution to the methodology of clinic appraisal of drug action. *Psychosom Med.* 1959;21:228–234.
8. Uhlenhuth EH, Canter A, Neustadt OJ, Payson HE. The symptomatic relief of anxiety with meprobamate, phenobarbital, and placebo. *Am J Psychiatry.* 1959;115:905–910.
9. Saddock B, Saddock R. *Kaplan and Saddock's Comprehensive Textbook of Psychiatry.* 8th ed. New York: WB Saunders; 1996; also see Murray CJ, Lopez AD. Global mortality, disability, and the contribution of risk factors: Global Burden of Disease Study. *Lancet.* 1997;349(9063): 1436–1442.
10. The National Mental Health Association. Depression and Co-occurring Illnesses. Available at: http://www.nmha.org/ccd/support/symptoms. cfm. Accessed July 7, 2002.
11. Loo H, Scatton B, Dennis T, Johre MS, et al. Study of noradrenaline metabolism in depressed patients by the determination of plasma dihydroxyphenylethylene glycol. *Encephale.* 1983;9(4):297–316. See also *Int Clin Nutr Rev.* 1983;3(2):1–3.
12. *Science Today.* Current Research Pages. Accessed at: http://www.ucop.edu/sciencetoday/pages/ archive/transcripts/2000/sci656.html#E. Accessed July 8, 2002.
13. Brown GW, Harris T. *Social Origins of Depression: A Study of Psychiatric Disorder in Women.* London: Tavistock Publications; 1978.
14. Royal College of General Practitioners Birmingham Research Unit. *Annual Report of the Weekly Returns Service for 1998.* Birmingham: RCGP BRU; 1998.
15. Office for National Statistics. *Key Health Statistics from General Practice 1996.* London: Her Majesty's Stationery Office; 1998:28–29.

16. The Mental Health Channel. Major Depressive Disorder. Available at: http://www.mentalhealth-channel. net/depression/. Accessed July 5, 2002.

17. Bebbington P. The origins of sex differences in depressive disorder: bridging the gap. *Int Rev Psychiatry.* 1996;8(4):295–332.

18. Nolen-Hoeksema S. Sex differences in unipolar depression: evidence and theory. *Psychol Bull.* 1987;101(2):259–282.

19. Kessler RC, McLeod JD. Sex differences in vulnerability to undesirable life events. *Am Sociol Rev.* 1994;49:620–631.

20. Meltzer H, Gill B, Petticrew M, Hinds K. *OCPS Surveys of Psychiatric Morbidity in Great Britain, Report 1: The Prevalence of Psychiatric Morbidity Among Adults Living in Private Households.* London: Her Majesty's Stationery Office; 1995.

21. DasGupta K. Treatment of depression in elderly patients: recent advances. *Arch Fam Med.* 1998; 7(3):274–280.

22. Banerjee S, Shamash K, Macdonald AJ, Mann AH. Randomised controlled trial of effect of intervention by psychogeriatric team on depression in frail elderly people at home. *BMJ.* 1996;313(7064):1058–1061.

23. Lynch DJ, Tamburrino MB, Nagel R. Telephone counseling for patients with minor depression: preliminary findings in a family practice setting. *J Fam Pract.* 1997;44(3):293–298.

24. Gloaguen V, Cottraux J, Cucherat M, Blackburn IM. A meta-analysis of the effects of cognitive therapy in depressed patients. *J Affect Disord.* 1998;49(1):59–72.

25. Wang JL, Patten SB, Russell ML. Alternative medicine use by individuals with major depression. *Can J Psychiatry.* 2001;46(6):528–533.

26. Kessler RC, Soukup J, Davis RB, et al. The use of complementary and alternative therapies to treat anxiety and depression in the United States. *Am J Psychiatry.* 2001;158(2):289–294.

27. Unutzer J, Klap R, Sturm R, et al. Mental disorders and the use of alternative medicine: results from a national survey. *Am J Psychiatry.* 2000; 157(11):1851–1857.

28. Rodriguez Jimenez J, Rodriguez JR, Gonzalez MJ. Indicators of anxiety and depression in subjects with different kinds of diet: vegetarians and omnivores. *Bol Asoc Med P R.* 1998;90(4–6):58–68.

29. Lombard CB. What is the role of food in preventing depression and improving mood, performance and cognitive function? *Med J Aust.* 2000 6;173(suppl):S104–S105.

30. Tanskanen A, Hibbeln JR, Hintikka J, Haatainen K, Honkalampi K, Viinamaki H. Fish consumption, depression, and suicidality in a general population. *Arch Gen Psychiatry.* 2001; 58(5):512–513.

31. Mischoulon D, Fava M. Docosahexanoic acid and omega-3 fatty acids in depression. *Psychiatr Clin North Am.* 2000;23(4):785–794.

32. Cogan E. DHEA: orthodox or alternative medicine? *Rev Med Brux.* 2001;22(4):A381–A386.

33. Morelli V, Zoorob RJ. Alternative therapies: part I. Depression, diabetes, obesity. *Am Fam Physician.* 2000;62(5):1051–1060.

34. Fetrow CW, Avila JR. Efficacy of the dietary supplement S-adenosyl-L-methionine. *Ann Pharmacother.* 2001;35(11):1414–1425.

35. Di Rocco A, Rogers JD, Brown R, Werner P, Bottiglieri T. S-adenosyl-methionine improves depression in patients with Parkinson's disease in an open-label clinical trial. *Mov Disord.* 2000;15(6):1225–1229.

36. Leeton J. Depression induced by oral contraception and the role of vitamin B_6 in its management. *Aust N Z J Psychiatry.* 1974;8(2):85–8.

37. Howard JS 3rd. Folate deficiency in psychiatric practice. *Psychosomatics.* 1975;16(3):112–115.

38. Mischoulon D, Burger JK, Spillmann MK, Worthington JJ, Fava M, Alpert JE. Anemia and macrocytosis in the prediction of serum folate and vitamin B_{12} status, and treatment outcome in major depression. *J Psychosom Res.* 2000;49(3): 183–187.

39. Coppen A, Bailey J. Enhancement of the antidepressant action of fluoxetine by folic acid: a randomised, placebo-controlled trial. *J Affect Disord.* 2000;60(2):121–130.

40. Bottiglieri T, Laundy M, Crellin R, Toone BK, Carney MW, Reynolds EH. Homocysteine, folate, methylation, and monoamine metabolism in depression. *J Neurol Neurosurg Psychiatry.* 2000;69(2):228–232.

41. Fava M, Borus JS, Alpert JE, Nierenberg AA, Rosenbaum JF, Bottiglieri T. Folate, vitamin B_{12}, and homocysteine in major depressive disorder. *Am J Psychiatry.* 1997;154(3):426–428.

42. National Health Consultants, Inositol. Accessed at: http://www.naturalhealthconsult.com/Monographs/Inositol.html. Accessed July 5, 2002.

43. Benjamin J, Agam G, Levine J, Bersudsky Y, Kofman O, Belmaker RH. Inositol treatment in psy-

chiatry. *Psychopharmacol Bull.* 1995;31(1): 167–175.

44. Levine J, Barak Y, Kofman O, Belmaker RH. Follow-up and relapse analysis of an inositol study of depression. *Isr J Psychiatry Relat Sci.* 1995;32(1):14–21.

45. Shealy CN. *Neurochemical Substrates of Depression and Their Relation to Cardiac Disease. Clinically Relevant Risk Factor Management of Cardiac Disease.* Springfield, MO: Holos Institute of Health; Feb 15–16 1991.

46. Eby G. Rapid Recovery from Depression using Magnesium Treatment. Accessed at: http://coldcure.com/html/dep.html. Accessed July 5, 2002.

47. Ferenczi M. The National Institute for Medical Research. 1997: Seasonal Depression and Light Therapy. Accessed at: http://www.nimr.mrc.ac. uk/MillHillEssays/1997/sad.htm. Accessed July 5, 2002.

48. Mauri MC, Ferrara A, Boscati L, et al. Plasma and platelet amino acid concentrations in patients affected by major depression and under fluvoxamine treatment. *Neuropsychobiology.* 1998;37(3): 124–129. See also *Stress Med.* 1995;11:75–77.

49. Young SN, Chouinard G, Annable L. Tryptophan in the treatment of depression. *Adv Exper Med Biol.* 1981;133:727–737.

50. Thomson J, Rankin H, Ashcroft GW, Yates CM, McQueen JK, Cummings SW. The treatment of depression in general practice: a comparison of L-tryptophan, amitriptyline and a combination of L-tryptophan and amitriptyline with placebo. *Psychol Med.* 1982;12(4):741–751.

51. Benkelfat C, Ellenbogen MA, Dean P, Palmour RM, Young SN. Mood-lowering effect of tryptophan depletion. Enhanced susceptibility in young men at genetic risk for major affective disorders. *Arch Gen Psychiatry.* 1994;51(9):687–697.

52. Peet M, Murphy B, Shay J, Horrobin D. Depletion of omega-3 fatty acid levels in red blood cell membranes of depressive patients. *Biol Psychiatry.* 1998;43(5):315–319.

53. Horrobin DF. Phospholipid metabolism and depression: the possible roles of phospholipase A_2 and coenzyme A-independent transacylase. *Hum Psychopharmacol.* 2001;16(1):45–52.

54. Maidment ID. Are fish oils an effective therapy in mental illness—an analysis of the data. *Acta Psychiatr Scand.* 2000;102(1):3–11.

55. Maes M, Christophe A, Delanghe J, Altamura C, Neels H, Meltzer HY. Lowered omega-3 polyunsaturated fatty acids in serum phospholipids and cholesteryl esters of depressed patients. *Psychiatry Res.* 1999 22;85(3):275–291.

56. Josey ES, Tackett RL. St. John's wort: a new alternative for depression? *Int J Clin Pharmacol Ther.* 1999;37(3):111–9.

57. Harrer G, Schultz V. Clinical investigation of the antidepressant effectiveness of hypericum. *J Gen Psychiatry Neurol.* 1994;7(suppl 1):S6–S8.

58. Bottiglieri T, Laundy M, Crellin R, Toone BK, Carney MW, Reynolds EH. Homocysteine, folate, methylation, and monoamine metabolism in depression. *J Neurol Neurosurg Psychiatry.* 2000; 69(2):228–232.

59. Linde K, Ramirez G, Mulrow CD, Pauls A, Weidenhammer W, Melchart D. St. John's wort for depression—an overview and meta-analysis of randomized clinical trials. *BMJ.* 1996;313(7052):253–258.

60. Schulz V. Clinical trials with hypericum extracts in patients with depression—results, comparisons, conclusions for therapy with antidepressant drugs. *Phytomedicine.* 2002;9(5):168–174.

61. Hypericum Depression Trial Study Group. Effect of *Hypericum perforatum* (St. John's wort) in major depressive disorder: a randomized controlled trial. *JAMA.* 2002;287(14):1807–14.

62. Kupfer DJ, Frank E. Placebo in clinical trials for depression: complexity and necessity. *JAMA.* 2002;287(14):1853–1854.

63. No author. Study shows St. John's wort ineffective for major depression. *FDA Consum.* 2002; 36(3):8.

64. Jonas W. St. John's wort and depression. *JAMA.* 2002;288(4):446, discussion 448–449.

65. Wheatley D. St. John's wort and depression. *JAMA.* 2002;288(4):446, discussion 448–449.

66. Spielmans GI. St. John's wort and depression. *JAMA.* 2002;288(4):446–447, discussion 448–449.

67. Volp A. St. John's wort and depression. *JAMA.* 2002;288(4):447, discussion 448–449.

68. Linde K, Melchart D, Mulrow CD, Berner M. St. John's wort and depression. *JAMA.* 2002;288(4): 447–448, discussion 448–449.

69. Gott J, Wisner KL. St. John's wort and depression. *JAMA.* 2002;288(4):448, discussion 448–449.

70. Hawley C, Dale T. St. John's wort was not better than placebo for reducing depression scores. *Evid Based Ment Health.* 2002;5(1):24.

71. van Gurp G, Meterissian GB, Haiek LN, McCusker J, Bellavance F. St. John's wort or

sertraline? Randomized controlled trial in primary care. *Can Fam Physician*. 2002;48:905–912.

72. Lecrubier Y, Clerc G, Didi R, Kieser M. Efficacy of St. John's wort extract WS 5570 in major depression: a double-blind, placebo-controlled trial. *Am J Psychiatry*. 2002;159(8):1361–1366.

73. Boniel T, Dannon P. The safety of herbal medicines in the psychiatric practice. *Harefuah*. 2001;140(8):780–783, 805.

74. Siepmann M, Krause S, Joraschky P, Muck-Weymann M, Kirch W. The effects of St John's wort extract on heart rate variability, cognitive function and quantitative EEG: a comparison with amitriptyline and placebo in healthy men. *Br J Clin Pharmacol*. 2002;54(3):277–282.

75. Muruganandam AV, Bhattacharya SK, Ghosal S. Antidepressant activity of hyperforin conjugates of the St. John's wort, *Hypericum perforatum* Linn: an experimental study. *Indian J Exp Biol*. 2001;39(12):1302–1304.

76. Wagner PJ, Jester D, LeClair B, Taylor AT, Woodward L, Lambert J. Taking the edge off: why patients choose St. John's wort. *J Fam Pract*. 1999;48(8):615–619.

77. Moore KA, Blumenthal JA. Exercise training as an alternative treatment for depression among older adults. *Altern Ther Health Med*. 1998;4(1):48–56.

78. North TC, McCullagh P, Tran ZV. Effect of exercise on depression. *Exerc Sport Sci Rev*. 1990;18:379–415.

79. Weyerer S. Physical inactivity and depression in the community. Evidence from the Upper Bavarian Field Study. *Int J Sports Med*. 1992;13(6):492–496.

80. Koeppl PM, Heller J, Bleecker ER, Meyers DA, Goldberg AP, Bleecker ML. The influence of weight reduction and exercise regimes upon the personality profiles of overweight males. *J Clin Psychol*. 1992;48(4):463–471.

81. Terman M, Terman JS. Treatment of seasonal affective disorder with a high-output negative ionizer. *J Altern Complement Med*. 1995;1(1):87–92.

82. Loving RT, Kripke DF, Shuchter SR. Bright light augments antidepressant effects of medication and wake therapy. *Depress Anxiety*. 2002;16(1):1–3.

83. Levitt AJ, Lam RW, Levitan R. A comparison of open treatment of seasonal major and minor depression with light therapy. *J Affect Disord*. 2002 Sep;71(1–3):243–8.

84. Ernst E, Rand JI, Stevinson C. Complementary therapies for depression: an overview. *Arch Gen Psychiatry*. 1998;55(11):1026–1032.

85. Luo H, Meng F, Jia Y, Zhao X. Clinical research on the therapeutic effect of the electro-acupuncture treatment in patients with depression. *Psychiatry Clin Neurosci*. 1998;52(suppl):S338–S340. See also *Am J Acupunct*. 1993;21(4):327–329.

86. Roschke J, Wolf C, Muller MJ, et al. The benefit from whole body acupuncture in major depression. *J Affect Disord*. 2000;57(1–3):73–81.

87. Masuda Y, Ohnuma S, Sugawara J, Kawarada Y, Sugiyama T. Behavioral effect of herbal glycoside in the forced swimming test. *Methods Find Exp Clin Pharmacol*. 2002;24(1):19–21.

88. Tadano T, Nakagawasai O, Niijima F, Tan-No K, Kisara K. The effects of traditional tonics on fatigue in mice differ from those of the antidepressant imipramine: a pharmacological and behavioral study. *Am J Chin Med*. 2000;28(1):97–104.

89. Koshikawa N, Imai T, Takahashi I, Yamauchi M, Sawada S, Kansaku A. Effects of Hochu-ekki-to, Yoku-kan-san and Saiko-ka-ryukotsu-borei-to on behavioral despair and acetic acid-induced writhing in mice. *Methods Find Exp Clin Pharmacol*. 1998;20(1):47–51.

90. Li M, Chen H. Antidepressant effect of water decoction of Rhizoma acori tatarinowii in the behavioural despair animal models of depression. *Zhong Yao Cai*. 2001;24(1):40–41.

91. Mindel A. *Quantum Mind: The Edge Between Physics and Psychology*. New York: Lao Tse Press; 2000.

92. Roschke J, Wolf C, Muller MJ, et al. The benefit from whole body acupuncture in major depression. *J Affect Disord*. 2000;57(1–3):73–81.

93. Managing Depression Intelligently. Treatments: Clinical Hypnosis. Accessed at: http://www.managing-depression-intelligently.com/html/hypnosis.html. Accessed July 5, 2002.

94. Yapko M. Hypnosis in treating symptoms and risk factors of major depression. *Am J Clin Hypn*. 2001;44(2):97–108.

95. Elemaya Biofeedback Instruments for psychophysical biofeedback and brain electrostimulation. Accessed at: http://www.elemaya2.com/Rosenfel.htm. Accessed July 5, 2002.

96. Liss S, Liss B. Physiological and therapeutic effects of high frequency electrical pulses. *Integr Physiol Behav Sci*. 1996;31(2):88–95.

97. Taylor DN. Clinical and experimental evaluation of cranial TENS in the US: a review *Acupunct Electrother Res.* 1995;20(2):117–132.

98. Jorm AF, Christensen H, Griffiths KM, Rodgers B. Effectiveness of complementary and self-help treatments for depression. *Med J Aust.* 2002; 176(suppl):S84–S96.

99. Manber R, Allen JJ, Morris MM. Alternative treatments for depression: empirical support and relevance to women. *J Clin Psychiatry.* 2002;63(7): 628–640.

100. Graeff FG. On serotonin and experimental anxiety. *Psychopharmacology (Berl).* 2002;163(3–4): 467–476.

101. Jetty PV, Charney DS, Goddard AW. Neurobiology of generalized anxiety disorder. *Psychiatr Clin North Am.* 2001;24(1):75–97.

102. The Mental Health Channel. General Anxiety Disorder. Accessed at: http://www.mentalhealthchannel. net/gad/. Accessed on January 5, 2003.

103. Chambless DL, Beck AT, Gracely EJ, Grisham JR. Relationship of cognitions to fear of somatic symptoms: a test of the cognitive theory of panic. *Depress Anxiety.* 2000;11(1):1–9.

104. Rueter MA, Scaramella L, Wallace LE, Conger RD. First onset of depressive or anxiety disorders predicted by the longitudinal course of internalizing symptoms and parent-adolescent disagreements. *Arch Gen Psychiatry.* 1999;56(8):726–732.

105. Wittchen HU, Kessler RC, Beesdo K, Krause P, Hofler M, Hoyer J. Generalized anxiety and depression in primary care: prevalence, recognition, and management. *J Clin Psychiatry.* 2002; 63(suppl 8):24–34.

106. Harman JS, Rollman BL, Hanusa BH, Lenze EJ, Shear MK. Physician office visits of adults for anxiety disorders in the United States, 1985–1998. *J Gen Intern Med.* 2002;17(3):165–172.

107. The Mental Health Channel. General Anxiety Disorder. Accessed at: http://www.mentalhealthchannel.net/gad/treatment.shtml. Accessed on January 5, 2003.

108. Goodwin RD, Gorman JM. Psychopharmacologic treatment of generalized anxiety disorder and the risk of major depression. *Am J Psychiatry.* 2002;159(11):1935–1937.

109. Ninan PT. New insights into the diagnosis and pharmacologic management of generalized anxiety disorder. *Psychopharmacol Bull.* 2002;36(2): 105–122.

110. Montgomery SA, Sheehan DV, Meoni P, Haudiquet V, Hackett D. Characterization of the longitudinal course of improvement in generalized anxiety disorder during long-term treatment with venlafaxine XR. *J Psychiatr Res.* 2002;36(4): 209–217.

111. Culpepper L. Generalized anxiety disorder in primary care: emerging issues in management and treatment. *J Clin Psychiatry.* 2002;63(suppl 8): 35–42.

112. Iqbal MM, Sobhan T, Aftab SR, Mahmud SZ. Diazepam use during pregnancy: a review of the literature. *Del Med J.* 2002;74(3):127–135.

113. Arato M. Switching from benzodiazepines to buspirone using a tapered overlap method in generalized anxiety disorder. *J Clin Psychiatry.* 2001; 62(8):657–658.

114. Bandelow B. Behavior therapy and antidepressive drugs. What helps with anxiety? *MMW Fortschr Med.* 2002;(suppl 2):50:60–62, 64–65.

115. Borkovec TD, Newman MG, Pincus AL, Lytle R. A component analysis of cognitive-behavioral therapy for generalized anxiety disorder and the role of interpersonal problems. *J Consult Clin Psychol.* 2002;70(2):288–298.

116. Grant EC. Food allergies and migraine. *Lancet.* 1979;1(8123):966–968.

117. Bruce M, Scott N, Shine P, Lader M. Anxiogenic effects of caffeine in patients with anxiety disorders. *Arch Gen Psychiatry.* 1992;49(11):867–869.

118. Lonsdale D, Shamberger RJ. Red cell transketolase as an indicator of nutritional deficiency. *Am J Clin Nutr.* 1980;33(2):205–211.

119. Voronina TA. Pharmacological properties of nicotinamide—possible ligand of benzodiazepine receptors. *Farmakol Toksikol.* 1981;44(6): 680–683.

120. Bouwer C, Stein DJ. Hyperresponsivity to nicotinic acid challenge in generalized social phobia: a pilot study. *Eur Neuropsychopharmacol.* 1998;8(4):311–313.

121. Benjamin J, Levine J, Fux M, Aviv A, Levy D, Belmaker RH. Double-blind, placebo-controlled, crossover trial of inositol treatment for panic disorder. *Am J Psychiatry.* 1995;152(7):1084–1086.

122. Khoo SK, Munro C, Battistutta D. Evening primrose oil and treatment of premenstrual syndrome. *Med J Aust.* 1990;153(4):189–192.

123. Hardy ML. Herbs of special interest to women. *J Am Pharm Assoc (Wash).* 2000;40(2):234–242, quiz 327–329.

124. Bilia AR, Gallon S, Vincieri FF. Kava kava and

anxiety: growing knowledge about the efficacy and safety. *Life Sci.* 2002;70(22):2581–2597.

125. Pittler MH, Ernst E. O. Kava extract for treating anxiety. *Cochrane Database Syst Rev.* 2002;2: CD003383.

126. Campo JV, McNabb J, Perel JM, Mazariegos GV, Hasegawa SL, Reyes J. Kava-induced fulminant hepatic failure. *J Am Acad Child Adolesc Psychiatry.* 2002;41(6):631–632.

127. Stevinson C, Huntley A, Ernst E. A systematic review of the studies of the safety of kava extract in the treatment of anxiety. *Drug Saf.* 2002;25(4): 251–261.

128. Meseguer E, Taboada R, Sanchez V, Mena MA, Campos V, Garcia de Yabenes J. Life-threatening parkinsonism induced by kava kava. *Mov Disord.* 2002;17(1):195–6.

129. Steiner GG. Kava as an anticraving agent: preliminary data. *Pac Health Dialog.* 2001;8(2): 335–9.

130. Connor KM, Davidson JR. A placebo-controlled study of kava kava in generalized anxiety disorder. *Int Clin Psychopharmacol.* 2002;17(4): 185–188.

131. Rex A, Morgenstern E, Fink H. Anxiolytic-like effects of kava kava in the elevated plus maze test—a comparison with diazepam. *Prog Neuropsychopharmacol Biol Psychiatry.* 2002;26(5): 855–860.

132. Maller CE, Schumacher B, Brattstram A, Abourashed EA, Koetter U. Interactions of valerian extracts and a fixed valerian-hop extract combination with adenosine receptors. *Life Sci.* 2002;71(16):1939–1949.

133. Francis AJP, Dempster RJW. Effect of valerian, *Valeriana edulis,* on sleep difficulties in children with intellectual deficits: randomized trial. *Phytomedicine.* 2002;9(4):273–279.

134. Poyares DR, Guilleminault C, Ohayon MM, Tufik S. Can valerian improve the sleep of insomniacs after benzodiazepine withdrawal? *Prog Neuropsychopharmacol Biol Psychiatry.* 2002; 26(3):539–45.

135. Wheatley D. Kava and valerian in the treatment of stress-induced insomnia. *Psychother Res.* 2001; 15(6):549–551.

136. Volz HP. Phytochemicals as a means to induce sleep. *Z Arztl Forthild Qualitatssich.* 2001;95(1): 33–34.

137. Lavie CJ, Milani RV, Squires RW, Boykin C. Exercise and the heart. Good, benign or evil? *Postgrad Med.* 1992;91(2):130–148.

138. Brown DR, Wang Y, Ward A, et al. Chronic psychological effects of exercise and exercise plus cognitive strategies. *Phys Sports Med.* 1995; 23(9):44–56.

139. Wanning T. Healing and the mind/body arts: massage, acupuncture, yoga, t'ai chi, and Feldenkrais. *AAOHN J.* 1993;41(7):349–51.

140. Eich H, Agelink MW, Lehmann E, Lemmer W, Klieser E. Acupuncture in patients with minor depressive episodes and generalized anxiety. Results of an experimental study. *Fortschr Neurol Psychiatr.* 2000;68(3):137–144.

141. Domar AD, Seibel MM, Benson H. The mind/body program for infertility: a new behavioral treatment approach for women with infertility. *Fertil Steril.* 1990;53(2)246–249.

142. Kabat-Zinn J, Massion AO, Kristeller J, et al. Effectiveness of a meditation-based stress reduction program in the treatment of anxiety disorders. *Am J Psychiatry.* 1992;149(7):936–943.

143. Miller NE. Biofeedback and visceral learning. *Ann Rev Psychol.* 1978;29:373–404.

144. Albright GL, Andreassi JL, Brockwell AL. Effects of stress management on blood pressure and other cardiovascular variables. *Int J Psychophysiol.* 1991;11(2):213–217.

145. McGrady A, Nadsady PA, Schumann, Brzezinski C. Sustained effects of biofeedback-assisted relaxation therapy in essential hypertension. *Biofeedback Self Reg.* 1991;16(4):399–411.

146. Andreasen NC. Assessment issues and the cost of schizophrenia. *Schizophr Bull.* 1991;17:408–410.

147. Horrobin DF. The membrane phospholipids hypothesis as a biochemical basis for the neurodevelopmental concept of schizophrenia. *Schizophr Res.* 1998;30:193–208.

148. Peet M, Glen I, Horrobin DF, eds. *Phospholipid Spectrum Disorder in Schizophrenia.* Carnforth, UK: Marius Press; 1999.

149. Glen A, Glen EM, Horrobin DF, et al. A red cell membrane abnormality in a subgroup of schizophrenic patients: evidence for two diseases. *Schizophr Res.* 1994;12:53–61.

150. Yao JK, van Kammen DP, Welker JA. Red blood cell membrane dynamics in schizophrenia II: fatty acid composition. *Schizophr Res.* 1994;13: 217–226.

151. Peet M, Laugharne JDE, Rangarajan N, Horrobin DF, Reynolds G. Depleted red cell membrane essential fatty acids in drug-treated schizophrenia patients. *J Psychiatr Res.* 1995;29:227–232.

152. Horrobin DF, Manku MS, Hillman S, Glen AI. Fatty acid levels in the brains of schizophrenics and normal controls. *Biol Psychiatry.* 1991;30: 795–805.

153. Hitzemann RJ, Mark C, Hirschowitz J, Garver DL. Characteristics of phospholipid methylation in human erythrocyte ghosts: relationship to the psychoses and affective disorders. *Biol Psychiatry.* 1985;20:297–307.

154. Christiansen O, Christiansen E. Fat consumption and schizophrenia. *Acta Psychiatr Scand.* 1998; 78:587–591.

155. Khan MM, Evans DR, Gunna V, Scheffer RE, Parikh VV, Mahadik SP. Reduced erythrocyte membrane essential fatty acids and increased lipid peroxides in schizophrenia at the never-medicated first-episode of psychosis and after years of treatment with antipsychotics. *Schizophr Res.* 2002 ;58(1):1–10.

156. Ryback R. Bioelectrical modulators and the cell membrane in psychiatric medicine. *Psychopharmacol Bull.* 2001;35(4):5–44.

157. Emsley RA, Oosthuizedn PP, Joubert AF, Hawkridge SM, Stein DJ. Treatment of schizophrenia in low-income countries. *Int J Neuropsychopharmacol.* 1999;2:321–325.

158. Reichelt KL, Seim AR, Reichelt WH. Could schizophrenia be reasonably explained by Dohan's hypothesis on genetic interaction with a dietary peptide overload? *Prog Neuropsychopharmacol Biol Psychiatry.* 1996;20(7):1083–114.

159. Jenner FA, Vlissides DN. Gluten sensitivity in schizophrenia. *Br J Psychiatry.* 1987;150:559.

160. Dohan, FC, Grasberger JC. Relapsed schizophrenics: earlier discharge from the hospital after cereal-free, milk-free diet. *Am J Psychiatry.* 1973;130(6):685–688.

161. Vlissides DN, Venulet A, Jenner FA. A double-blind gluten-free/gluten-load controlled trial in a secure ward population. *Br J Psychiatry.* 1986; 148:447–452.

162. De Santis A, Addolorato G, Romito A, et al. Schizophrenic symptoms and SPECT abnormalities in a coeliac patient: regression after a gluten-free diet. *J Intern Med.* 1997;242(5):421–423.

163. Jansson B, Kristjansson E, Nilsson L. Schizophrenic psychosis disappearing after patient is given gluten-free diet. *Lakartidningen.* 1984; 81(6):448–449.

164. Godfrey PS, Toone BK, Carney MW, et al. Enhancement of recovery from psychiatric illness by methylfolate. *Lancet.* 1990;336(8712): 392–395.

165. Carney MW. Vitamins and mental health. *Br J Hosp Med.* 1992;48(8):451–452.

166. Bucci L. Pyridoxine and schizophrenia [letter]. *Br J Psychiatry.* 1973;122(567):240.

167. Miodownik C, Kaptsan A, Cohen H, Loewenthal U, Kotler M. Vitamin B6 as add-on treatment in chronic schizophrenic and schizoaffective patients: a double-blind, placebo Lerner-controlled study. *J Clin Psychiatry.* 2002;63(1):54–58.

168. Sacks W, Cowen MA, Green MR, Esser AH, Talarico P, Cankosyan G. Acetazolamide and thiamine (A + T): a preliminary report of an ancillary therapy for chronic mental illness. *J Clin Psychopharmacol.* 1988;8(1):70.

169. Puri BK, Richardson AJ, Horrobin DF, et al. Eicosapentaenoic acid treatment in schizophrenia associated with symptom remission, normalisation of blood fatty acids, reduced neuronal membrane phospholipid turnover and structural brain changes. *Int J Clin Pract.* 2000;54(1):57–63.

170. Joy CB, Mumby-Croft R, Joy LA. Polyunsaturated fatty acid (fish or evening primrose oil) for schizophrenia. *Cochrane Database Syst Rev.* 2000;2: CD001257.

171. Laugharne JD, Mellor JE, Peet M. Fatty acids and schizophrenia. *Lipids.* 1996;31(suppl):S163–S165.

172. Peet M, Brind J, Ramchand CN, Shah S, Vankar GK. Two double-blind, placebo-controlled pilot studies of eicosapentaenoic acid in the treatment of schizophrenia. *Schizophr Res.* 2001;49:243–251.

173. Emsley RA, Myburgh CC, Oosthuizen PP, van Rensburg SJ. Randomized placebo-controlled study of ethyl-eicosapentaenoic acid as supplemental treatment in schizophrenia. *Am J Psychiatry.* 2002;159(9):1596–1598.

174. Department of Health and Human Services, Food and Drug Administration. 21 CFR Part 184 (Docket No. 86G-0289). Thursday, June 5, 1997. Rules and Regulations. *Fed Reg.* 62;108; 30751–30757.

175. The Linus Pauling Institute. Recent Noteworthy Books. Accessed at: http://www.orst.edu/dept/lpi/ss01/books.html. Accessed July 5, 2002.

176. Sandyk R, Kanofsky JD. Vitamin C in the treatment of schizophrenia. *Int J Neurosci.* 1993; 68(1–2):67–71. See also [abstract 7]. *J Am Coll Nutr.* 1989;8(5):425.

177. Vaughan K, McConaghy N. Megavitamin and dietary treatment in schizophrenia: a randomised,

controlled trial. *Aust N Z J Psychiatry*. 1999; 33(1):84–88.

178. Zhang LD, Tang YH, Zhu WB, Xu SH. Comparative study of schizophrenia treatment with electroacupuncture, herbs and chlorpromazine. *Chin Med J*. 1987;100(2):152–157.

179. Zhuge DY, Chen JK. Comparison between electro-acupuncture with chlorpromazine and chlorpromazine alone in 60 schizophrenic patients. *Zhongguo Zhong Xi Yi Jie He Za Zhi*. 1993;13(7): 408–409, 388.

180. Robertson GM, (ed. *Manic-Depressive Insanity and Paranoia*. Barclay RM, trans. Edinburgh: E & S Livingstone; 1921.

181. Taylor L, Faraone SV, Tsuang MT. Family, twin, and adoption studies of bipolar disease. *Curr Psychiatry Rep*. 2002;4(2):130–133.

182. Craddock N, Jones I. Genetics of bipolar disorder. *J Med Genet*. 1999;36(8):585–594.

183. Grossman F, Potter WZ. Catecholamines in depression: a cumulative study of urinary norepinephrine and its major metabolites in unipolar and bipolar depressed patients versus healthy volunteers at the NIMH. *Psychiatry Res*. 1999; 87(1):21–27.

184. Kessler RC, McGonagle KA, Zhao S, et al. Lifetime and 12-month prevalence of DSM-III-R psychiatric disorders in the United States. *Arch Gen Psychiatry*. 1994;51:8–19.

185. Sassi RB, Soares JC. Emerging therapeutic targets in bipolar mood disorder. *Expert Opin Ther Targets*. 2001;5(5):587–599.

186. Ball J, Mitchell P, Malhi G, Skillecorn A, Smith M. Schema-focused cognitive therapy for bipolar disorder: reducing vulnerability to relapse through attitudinal change. *Aust N Z J Psychiatry*. 2003;37(1):41–48.

187. Levine J, Barak Y, Kofman O, Belmaker RH. Follow-up and relapse analysis of an inositol study of depression. *Isr J Psychiatry*. 1995;32(1):14–21.

188. Simonson M. L-phenylalanine. *J Clin Psychiatry*. 1985;46(8):355.

189. Kaplan BJ, Simpson JS, Ferre RC, Gorman CP, McMullen DM, Crawford SG. Effective mood stabilization with a chelated mineral supplement: an open-label trial in bipolar disorder. *J Clin Psychiatry*. 2001;62(12):936–944.

190. Rosenthal NE, Sack DA, Gillin JC, et al. Seasonal affective disorder. A description of the syndrome and preliminary findings with light therapy. *Arch Gen Psychiatry*. 1984;41(1):72–80.

CHAPTER 29

Integrative Approach to Rheumatology

DAVID RAKEL AND DANIEL MULLER

Many autoimmune and rheumatologic processes can be impacted not only by the pharmaceutical regimens that we have traditionally relied upon, but by other modalities as well, including proper nutrition, botanicals, mind–body therapies, and acupuncture among others. Applying the integrative approach to this area of chronic illness may help to reduce the need for therapies that may be associated with more side effects and cost, while empowering the individual to take a more active role in their health management. This chapter explores the evidence behind a number of these therapies for treatment of rheumatoid arthritis, gout, osteoarthritis, and fibromyalgia.

▶ RHEUMATOID ARTHRITIS

Pathophysiology and Prevalence

Rheumatoid arthritis (RA) is a chronic inflammatory disorder that generally presents with symmetric peripheral arthritis and associated synovial swelling. There is a genetic predisposition, although no specific gene has been identified to date. The diagnosis of RA requires arthritis lasting at least 6 weeks with a positive rheumatoid factor and evidence of erosive articular changes on radiograph. Cortisol and corticotropin-releasing factor, and the function of the hypothalamic–pituitary–adrenal axis are linked to disease activity in RA,[1] and may be important in the systemic presentations of RA outside of the joints, which can include severe fatigue and pulmonary symptoms, among others. Stress and psychological factors have been linked to both the etiology and to exacerbations of RA disease.[2] In one study, psychological factors and depression accounted for at least 20% of disability in patients with RA, compared with the 14% of disability explained by articular signs and symptoms.[3] In another study, helplessness had a direct effect on disease activity.[4]

Rheumatoid arthritis can be seen in 0.5–1.5% of the population in industrialized countries, and is more common in women than in men, with a ratio of 2.5:1.

▶ Case Example 1: Rheumatoid Arthritis

A 38-year-old Asian American female comes into your office and gives a general impression of being friendly but slightly withdrawn. She was diagnosed with rheumatoid arthritis when she was 22 years old. When asked what she believed brought her disease on, she states that she thought it was directly related to being rejected from a bible study group she was deeply involved with in college. She reports that stress and depression had a tendency to worsen her symptoms and that her symptoms improved when she became in-volved in a different religious group. She was unable to tolerate methotrexate and is currently taking gold injections and a multivitamin. Her diet consists of fast foods, cold cut sandwiches, pizza, and limited fruits and vegetables. She has reported some improvement in her symptoms when she fasts. Her main stress at this time is her struggle between her sexual orientation and her religious beliefs. Her passions include travel and exotic birds. For exercise she enjoys swimming but does not exercise on a regular basis.

Conventional Treatment Approach

Conventional treatment of RA has generally focused on pharmaceutical agents that block the inflammatory cascade that can lead to synovial proliferation and joint erosion. There are four classes of drugs that have been traditionally used for treating rheumatoid arthritis: non-steroidal antiinflammatory drugs (NSAIDs), corticosteroids, analgesics, and disease-modifying antirheumatic drugs (DMARDs). The majority of pharmaceutical research is now targeted toward biologic agents that modify the inflammatory response by blocking receptors to cytokines that have been found to worsen joint inflammation, such as tumor necrosis factor and interleukin-1. If patients do not respond well to a DMARD such as methotrexate, the addition of one of these biologics may be indicated. The goal in therapy is to reduce inflammation early in the disease process before joint erosion and other secondary complications occur; current conventional thinking holds that early aggressive pharmaceutical intervention will improve long-term prognosis in patients with RA.

Once joint erosion and deformity occurs, surgery is often useful to help restore joint function and mobility.

Integrative Treatment Approach

Nutritional Therapies

FASTING

Although the exact mechanism of action of fasting remains unclear, some patients with RA experience great benefit from this strategy. This benefit may be simply a result of a food intolerance that has been contributing to the inflammatory response, which is eliminated by fasting, or may be mediated by a different mechanism. Water-only fasting has been found to improve symptoms, and in some incidences, result in a remission of autoimmune disease.[5] A systematic review of 31 studies, of which 4 were controlled, showed a statistically significant beneficial long-term effect of fasting followed by a vegetarian diet for at least 3 months in patients with rheumatoid arthritis.[6] Fasting also appears to have a beneficial effect on inflammatory markers such as C-reactive protein and interleukin-6 in patients with RA.[7] A small case series describes a group of patients with rheumatologic diseases (RA, lupus, mixed connective-tissue disease, and fibromyalgia) who were tapered off their medications and underwent a 1–3-week water fast. This was then followed by a vegetarian diet consisting of fresh vegetables, fruits, beans, and nuts. Six cases of prolonged remission were seen. Maintaining the vegetarian diet was important to prevent recurrence.[8]

ELIMINATION DIET

In RA, as in many other conditions discussed in this text, an elimination diet can be both diagnostic and therapeutic. Hafstrom and colleagues took 66 patients with RA and divided them into two groups after testing them for antibodies for wheat (antigliadin) and dairy (anti–beta-lactoglobulin). Thirty-eight patients were placed on a vegan, wheat- and dairy-free diet, and 28 were placed on a regular, nonvegan diet that included wheat and dairy for 1 year. The groups were evaluated for response by using American College of Rheumatology criteria at baseline, 3 months, 6 months, and 1 year. There was a 40.5% significant improvement in symptoms in the study group versus 4% improvement in the control group. All of the patients that responded in the study group had resolution of the antibodies to gliadin (wheat) and lactoglobulin (dairy). Although this diet can be very effective, long-term adherence is a challenge: only 22 of the 38 patients in the vegan group maintained the diet for 9 months.[9] Strategies for implementing an elimination diet are discussed in Chapters 7 and 17.

ESSENTIAL FATTY ACIDS

Essential fatty acid (EFA) balance may play an important role in control of symptoms in some patients with RA. As discussed in Chapter 26, omega-6 fatty acids—found in many vegetables oils and in most processed foods—are a source of arachidonic acid (AA), which fuels the fire of inflammation. Omega-3 fatty acids—found in cold-water fish, flax seed, dark green leafy vegetables, seeds and nuts—can reduce inflammation through a downregulation of the mediators of inflammation. It may be that the reason vegetarian diets seem to be associated with less inflammation in RA is related to the change in EFA balance generated by avoiding animal products, which are rich in saturated fats and arachidonic acid. Kjeldsen-Kragh et al., for example, found that 13 months of a vegan diet resulted in significant improvement in all clinical measures.[10] In recommending a vegan-based diet, it is important to note that it can take as long as 6 months for the individual to notice a positive effect.

Kremer et al. found that supplementing with eicosapentaenoic acid (EPA) 1.8 g/d (an omega-3 fatty acid in fish oil) resulted in less morning stiffness and tender joints in patients with RA.[11] A review of randomized controlled trials also showed that fish oil leads to a significant reduction in long-term use of nonsteroidal antiinflammatory drugs in RA.[12] Cooked vegetables and olive oil (omega-9) have also been found to be independently protective for the development of RA and may have anti-RA activity.[13]

The most important nutritional recommendations in RA are summarized below:

- Encourage a more vegan-based diet with less red meat and dairy.
- Reduce foods rich in omega-6 essential fatty acids and those rich in *trans*-fatty acids, including partially hydrogenated vegetable oils.
- Increase intake of foods rich in omega-3 fatty acids, such as cold-water fish, flax, green vegetables, and nuts.
- Use monounsaturated oils (olive and canola) for cooking.
- Consider supplementing with 2 g of an omega-3–rich fish oil daily.
- Consider a modified water fast or an elimination diet to see if certain foods may be exacerbating symptoms.
- Limit coffee intake. Amounts more than 4 cups a day increase the risk of RA.[11]

SUPPLEMENTS AND BOTANICALS

A number of botanicals with antiinflammatory properties are frequently used by patients with RA. These include ginger, turmeric (curcumin), *Boswellia serrata*, feverfew (*Tanacetum parthenium* Schultz-Bip.), red pepper (capsaicin), onions/apples (as sources of quercetin) and rosemary (*Rosmarinus officinulis* L.) Although most of these substances have not been studied specifically for RA, there is some preliminary evidence showing benefit. For example, a study of 28 patients with RA treated with ginger resulted in 75% of patients showing reduced pain and joint swelling.[15] The dose of ginger is 1 g of the dried root two to three times daily. The dose can be increased to 4 g daily if needed.

ANTIOXIDANTS

Antioxidant supplements are often used in RA, and here, as well, there is some preliminary evidence of benefit. Synovial swelling around an involved joint is in part triggered by free radicals and nitric oxide synthetase. Suppression of this enzyme occurs with aspirin, tetracycline, steroids, and methotrexate, and with several antioxidants including vitamin E, selenium, ascorbate, and beta-carotene in high doses.[16] Vitamin E not only has an inhibitory influence on nitric oxide synthetase, but it also reduces lipid peroxidation. Studies show that the amount of lipid oxidation in tissue is correlated with the erythrocyte sedimentation rate,[17] and possibly with the level of inflammation in the joints. Vitamin E reduced joint inflammation and bone destruction in a mouse model of rheumatoid arthritis, although it did not have an influence on clinical features.[18] When vitamin E was combined with selenium, inflammatory mediators were reduced by 80% in vitro. A pilot study of 20 patients with RA who were treated with selenium for 4 weeks showed improvement in clinical and immunological outcomes.[19] Although these studies are not at all definitive, the wide safety margin and affordability of vitamin E and selenium may make the use of these supplements worthwhile as part of an integrative approach to RA.

Vitamin E is fat soluble and is better absorbed with food. Vitamin E also enhances the absorption of selenium. The standard dose of vitamin E in the form of mixed tocopherols (alpha, gamma, and delta) is 800 IU daily. The dose of selenium is 200 μg daily.

Mind–Body Therapies

As discussed in Chapter 3, there is now ample evidence that chronic daily stress can worsen inflammation. It also seems that long-term stress can lead to a loss of proper feedback function in the hypothalamic–pituitary–adrenal axis, resulting in less endogenous corticosteroid production to inhibit the inflammatory cascade.[20] As a result, inflammation becomes more chronically activated.

One interesting study which examined the relationship between nutrition and mind–body influences on inflammation measured the baseline ratio of omega-3 to omega-6 fatty acids in 27 university students. These students were then divided into two groups: those with a high omega-3 to omega-6 ratio and those with a low omega-3 to omega-6 ratio. The students then went through a stressful exam, after which the researchers measured the students' levels of inflammatory cytokines such as interleukin-6, tumor necrosis factor, and interleukin-10. This study found that those students who had a low ratio of omega-3 to omega-6 fatty acids at baseline had a much higher release of inflammatory cytokines than those students who had a high ratio.[21] This study had two important conclusions: first, that stress triggers the release of inflammatory cytokines; and second, that our underlying nutritional status—in particular, the EFA balance—can have an influence on how much these inflammatory cytokines are stimulated after a stressful event.

A systematic review of the literature examining psychological interventions (relaxation, biofeedback, and cognitive behavior therapy) in people with RA found 25 trials that met inclusion criteria. The overall conclusion of this review found a significant postintervention benefit for pain, functional disability, psychological status, coping and self-efficacy. At follow-up (averaging 8.5 months), benefit in tenderness of joints, psychological status, and coping persisted.[22]

It is important to recommend a relaxation technique that matches the patient's lifestyle. For a driven, "type A" individual, recommending a mantra meditation may worsen stress. A form of relaxation that involves more physical activity such as tai chi, a walking meditation, or progressive muscle relaxation may be more appropriate. The range of mind–body therapies that may be appropriate for patients with RA is reviewed in Chapters 3 and 11.

Journaling

"The sorrow that hath no vent in tears may make other organs weep."

William Boyd, M.D.

Unresolved stressful or traumatic events can be major contributors to inflammation and to the subjective experience of pain. Smyth et al. studied 107 patients with either RA or asthma to assess the influence of journaling about an emotional event on these conditions. Half of each disease group wrote about daily events, while the other half wrote about an emotional event that they felt had not been dealt with

completely and they still had strong feelings about. Both groups wrote for just 20 minutes a day for 3 days. Follow-up evaluation showed that of the group that wrote about the emotional event, the asthma patients averaged a 20% improvement in lung function versus no improvement in the controls. The RA patients showed a 28% improvement in disease severity, as compared to no improvement in the controls. This positive effect persisted into the 6-month follow-up evaluation.[23]

Journaling is an inexpensive therapy that individuals can do in the privacy of their own home. The therapeutic benefit of this technique is thought to stem from organizing the stressful event in a way that brings it under conscious understanding and control. If the symptoms are related to repressed emotions, once the mind develops insight into this relationship, the body no longer needs to ask for attention and symptoms improve. Psychotherapy may provide a benefit through a similar mechanism.

It is important to recommend journaling only if the patient is prepared and ready to explore these issues. Referral for counseling should be available if this process brings out emotions that require further exploration. Table 29–1 provides directions on how to recommend journaling.

▶ **TABLE 29-1** RECOMMENDING JOURNALING TO YOUR PATIENTS

- Write about the most upsetting or troubling experience in your life, something that has affected you deeply and that you have not discussed with others.
- First describe the event in detail, the situation, surroundings, and sensations that you remember.
- Then describe your deepest feeling regarding the event. Let go and allow the emotions to run freely in your writing. Describe how you felt about the event then and now.
- Write continuously. Do not worry about grammar, spelling, or sentence structure. If you come to a block, simply repeat what you have already written.
- Think of how you may have grown or what you may have learned from the event.
- Write for 20 minutes for at least 4 days. You can write about different traumas or reflect on the same trauma each day.
- Consider keeping a regular journal if the process proves helpful.

Adapted from Rakel DP, Shapiro D. Mind–body medicine. In: Rakel RE. The Textbook of Family Practice. 6th ed. Philadelphia: WB Saunders; 2002:56.

Acupuncture

Although acupuncture is often recommended for RA, to date there is limited evidence demonstrating efficacy for this condition. A systematic review of eight trials concluded that five of the trials found a positive effect on pain control, with one study claiming antiinflammatory effects. There were many design flaws and the review concluded that further research is needed.[24]

Spirituality

As with many chronic conditions, the impact of an exploration of a patient's "spirituality" on symptoms and well-being may be significant. For many patients in whom chronic disease has limited the experiences they would have hoped to have during their lives, spirituality can provide the sense of a connection in life that gives a feeling of meaning and purpose. In some cases, if we can help our patients direct energy toward increasing this sense of connectedness, the body often responds with improved health.

▶ Case Example 1: Rheumatoid Arthritis Conclusion

This patient's major stressor was the internal conflict between her religious beliefs and her sexual orientation. These emotions can have a significant effect on the severity of RA and if resolved, can result in significant benefit related to the psychoneuroimmunological stimuli of inflammation. The patient was referred to a spiritual advisor that matched her belief system to further find an acceptable balance for this conflict.

Her diet consisted of products high in saturated fat and processed foods. She was placed on a 5-day modified water fast while using a hypoallergenic "medical food" supplement designed to provide adequate nutrient intake during a fast. This was followed by a hypoallergenic diet for 7 days. She noticed significant improvement in pain and morning stiffness during this time. A food challenge with individual food groups reintroduced every 3 days demonstrated that her symptoms were exacerbated by dairy products. These were then eliminated from her diet. Journaling was recommended to explore and express emotions related to the trauma of being rejected from the bible study group in college. A simple breathing exercise was also taught for her to use when needed to induce relaxation. She also added fish oil 2 g, vitamin E 800 IU, and selenium 200 μg daily to her current regimen of gold therapy. To provide the increased sense of control that often comes to patients with the recognition that there are many choices open to them for treatment, the patient was also educated regarding the new tumor necrosis factor inhibitors (infliximab, etanercept, and adalimumab).

▶ FIBROMYALGIA SYNDROME

Pathophysiology

The fibromyalgia syndrome (FMS) is classically diagnosed by finding (1) widespread pain and (2) tenderness in at least 11 of 18 defined points.[25] In clinical practice, patients with a diagnosis of FMS commonly present with fewer tender points or tender points in other muscle groups. Additional characteristic complaints include nonrestorative sleep, stiffness, headache, cognitive difficulties, irritable bowel syndrome, and temporomandibular joint syndrome.[25,26] Fatigue is usually a prominent feature of FMS and is similar to that seen in chronic fatigue syndrome.[27] Some studies have found physiologic differences in cortisol responses for subjects with FMS or chronic fatigue syndrome, but the significance of these findings is not clear.[28] Studies find little abnormality in the peripheral musculature, but point to increased central nervous system sensitivity to pain as the likely mechanism in fibromyalgia.

There are known to be a number of other subtle alterations of the endocrine system in FMS. While some physiologic abnormalities, such as lower growth hormone and somatomedin levels, do not appear to be critical in the etiology of FMS, they may participate in sustaining symptoms and increasing central pain sensitivity.[29] Cerebrospinal fluid levels of substance P are elevated, and there are additional abnormalities in the regulation of cortisol and in the adrenergic and serotonin systems.[30,31] Alterations in the pituitary–adrenal axis in FMS appear to be quite different from those seen in clinical depression.[32]

The affinity of corticosteroid receptors on mononuclear cells appears to be decreased in FMS, but there is an overall increase in the cellular response of the lymphocytes to stimulation with the mitogen phytohemagglutinin, suggesting that this decreased affinity may actually represent an increased feedback resistance to cortisol.[33] Studies also show decreased numbers of T cells expressing activation markers and a deficiency of interleukin-2 release.[34] These immune changes in FMS do not meet criteria for an immunodeficiency or autoimmune disease. However, the immune changes and altered patterns of cytokine release could contribute to the fatigue and inflammatory-like symptoms seen in this condition.

The degree to which psychological components contribute to pain sensitivity and symptom expression remains controversial. At least 25% of patients with FMS show no current or past history of depression.[35] Some have noted a high occurrence of FMS in patients with post-traumatic stress disorder.[36] One possible explanation for the variable symptom spectrum of chronic pain, fatigue, headache, irritable bowel and bladder, and affective disorders seen in FMS might be an underlying higher than average sensitivity to both emotional and physical stressors, with subsequent expression according to other genetic and environmental factors.

▶ **TABLE 29–2** MINIMUM BASELINE LABORATORY EXAM FOR FIBROMYALGIA

Laboratory Assay	Differential Diagnosis
Complete blood count	Leukemia, occult infection
Thyroid stimulating hormone	Thyroid disease
Westergren sedimentation rate	Neoplasia, occult infection, rheumatic disease
Electrolytes	Adrenal disease*
Calcium	Parathyroid disease†
Alanine aminotransferase	Hepatic disease
Creatinine, urinalysis	Renal disease
Antihepatitis C antibody	Chronic hepatitis C‡
HIV serology	Acquired immunodeficiency syndrome

*If abnormal potassium, check a 24-hour urine cortisol.
†If abnormal calcium, check parathyroid hormone.

▶ **TABLE 29-3** POSSIBLE ADDITIONAL LABORATORY TESTS IN FIBROMYALGIA

Clinical Finding	Laboratory Test	Disease
Joint swelling, skin changes abnormal sedimentation rate, or urinalysis	Antinuclear antibody; rheumatoid factor; anticytoplasmic antibody; complement factors 3 and 4; Lyme serology[†]	Autoimmune or infectious*
Muscle weakness	Creatine kinase	Polymyositis
Low thyroid-stimulating hormone and cortisol	Prolactin	Panhypopituitarism

*Rheumatoid arthritis, systemic lupus erythematosus, scleroderma, polymyalgia rheumatica, vasculitis, Lyme disease
[†]Screening using enzyme-linked immunosorbent assay (ELISA); if positive, confirm using Western blot.

Prevalence

FMS has been documented in 2% of the general population and has a female to male ratio of about 8:1.[37] This increased prevalence in females may point to a hormonal influence. FMS also can coexist with a variety of autoimmune diseases, and often presents after a severe flu-like syndrome, a defined infection (i.e., Lyme disease), or physical trauma such as a motor vehicle accident.

Because many other diseases or syndromes may either mimic or commonly coexist with FMS (e.g., rheumatoid arthritis and systemic lupus), a thorough history and physical examination, and laboratory testing, are important in making a proper diagnosis. Baseline laboratory tests should all be normal and will rule out most cases of underlying neoplastic, chronic infectious, hepatic, adrenal, thyroid, and parathyroid diseases (Table 29-2). Additional testing should be based on clinical and laboratory findings (Table 29-3).

Sleep apnea syndrome and neurally mediated hypotension may be treatable contributors to the FMS syndrome; a sleep study and a tilt-table test, respectively, may be required for proper diagnosis. No other psychological testing or immune function tests have been shown to be helpful in diagnosis or treatment outside of research studies. Once laboratory tests are shown to be normal, the practitioner should refrain from frequent retesting unless there are significant changes in symptoms or signs.

Conventional Treatment Approach

Patients with a new diagnosis of FMS are usually started on treatment including a sedating tricyclic antidepressant at night, often with an activating antidepressant in the morning, as well as low-level aerobic exercise and physical therapy. The antidepressants are tailored to minimize side effects and balance the fatigue and sleep problems for each patient. Therapeutic benefit is associated with improvements in sleep.[38,39] If the dosage of tricyclic antidepressants required to reduce FMS symptoms produces excessive sedation, sertraline (Zoloft) 25 mg in the morning is often used, or another of the more activating antidepressants such as fluoxetine (Prozac). Other less-sedating tricyclic antidepressants can be substituted for amitriptyline in the evening, including nortriptyline. Doxepin (Sinequan), a nontricyclic antidepressant, can be particularly useful in liquid form to titrate at low doses, 2–5 mg, for sedation at night. Trazodone 25–300 mg also can be helpful for promoting sleep. Cyclobenzaprine (Flexeril), 2.5–40 mg in divided doses, has muscle relaxant and sedative effects.

▶ Case Example 2: Fibromyalgia Syndrome

A 45-year-old woman with a 2-year history of fibromyalgia presents to your clinic because she heard "you know something about alternative medicine." She complains of pain all over, all joints and muscles, with particularly severe neck, shoulder, and low back pain. She states she does not sleep more than 3 hours per night because of pain and restless legs. She has chronic migraine headaches and abdominal pain with alternating diarrhea and constipation. She also complains of severe memory difficulties. She has been frustrated first by a year of missed diagnosis and then by visits to multiple physicians who have been unable to help her. She has tried guaifenesin and multiple other over-the-counter supplements.

Prior to the onset of this condition she was healthy, working in advertising 50 plus hours per week, taking care of her two children in their early teens, and helping her elderly mother living across town. Additional stressors include a hardworking architect husband and one child doing poorly in school. Onset was with a flu-like syndrome lasting 2 weeks from which she never fully recovered. She decreased her work by approximately 50% in the past year. Her work partners are flexible and understanding. She is taking amitriptyline 5 mg each evening to help her sleep, citalopram (Celexa) in the morning for depression, and tizanidine (Zanaflex) for restless leg syndrome. She has been tried on hydromorphone and then OxyContin (oxycodone) for her pain, but she was unable to tolerate these because of nausea and drowsiness. She had exercised regularly doing aerobics before having children and continued after her first child was born. She stopped most aerobic exercise after having her second child. She is about 25 pounds over her weight in college; 15 pounds were gained in the past 1 year. She eats a diet mostly of salads, fresh fruits, and chicken. A review of systems is diffusely positive with complaints of blurry vision, dry eyes and mouth, sharp chest pain and palpitations, dyspnea on exertion, chronic nausea without vomiting, getting up at night to pass urine, dyspareunia, swollen glands, and anxiety.

On physical examination she has 18 of 18 defined fibromyalgia tender points and tenderness over all joints and between joints, but no swelling, synovitis, increased warmth, or redness of any joint. She is tender in all large muscle groups of the upper and lower extremities. She has mild shotty anterior cervical adenopathy. The rest of the physical exam is completely normal.

Recently, some physicians have been using the antispasticity and sedating medication tizanidine (Zanaflex) 4–8 mg three times per day both for pain and for sleep problems in FMS patients. Antiseizure medications, particularly gabapentin, are also commonly used for neuropathic pain and the pain associated with FMS. NSAIDs are not effective for FMS pain.[40] Preliminary reports on two new medications for fibromyalgia show that some upcoming treatments may have promise: Pregabalin (Pfizer) is an anxiolytic and antiepileptic that showed a 50% reduction in pain in 29% of treated subjects, as compared to 13% of those receiving placebo (n = 529)[41]; Milnacipran (Cypress Bioscience) is a new norepinephrine and serotonin reuptake inhibitor antidepressant that in a Phase II study showed a 50% reduction in pain in 36% of treated subjects, as compared to 9% of those receiving placebo (n = 95).

Soft Tissue (Tender Point) Injection

The injection of subcutaneous tender points may be helpful particularly if given into palpable areas of muscle spasm. These are often given as 1% lidocaine 0.5–1.0 mL per site, although dry needling or saline may work as well. Corticosteroids do not have a significant role as there is no advantage except in documented clear inflammatory bursitis syndromes without infection.

Physical Therapy

Physical therapy, including stretching, heat, and cold, can be helpful in restoring muscle balance and controlling pain in FMS. However, approaches that are too aggressive or vigorous can exacerbate symptoms. Physical therapy is best used along with other therapies and by a therapist with experience in working with patients with FMS.

Integrative Treatment Approach

Nutritional Approaches

No specific diet has been shown to be effective in FMS. An omega-3 essential fatty acid-rich diet may be helpful because of the tendency of these substances to reduce inflammatory activity. Doses of omega-3 EFAs generally recommended for this antiinflammatory effect are on the order of eicosapentaenoic acid at 30 mg/kg/d and docosahexaenoic acid at 50 mg/kg/d. Gamma linolenic acid, 1.4–2.8 g/d—the equivalent of 6–11 g of borage oil—may have similar effects. These doses can be consumed either in foods or via supplementation.

Chlorella pyrenoidosa (freshwater green alga) is a source of many nutrients, including protein, omega-3 fatty acids, vitamins, and minerals. A double-blind, crossover study has shown significant reduction in FMS tender points after 3 months of supplementation with this nutrient.[42] *Chlorella* contains iodine and allergic reactions have been reported; as a significant source of vitamin K, it can also antagonize the anticoagulant activity of Coumadin.

Chlorella is typically used in a dose of approximately 10 g or equivalent daily.[12]

S-adenosylmethionine (SAMe) has mild antidepressant analgesic effects. A randomized, placebo-controlled 6-week trial of SAMe in patients with FMS showed modest but statistically significant changes in morning stiffness, pain at rest, fatigue, and mood ($n = 44$).[13] However, no statistically significant changes were seen in tender points, pain with activity, sleep quality, or overall well-being. A dose of 400 mg two or three times per day 30 minutes before meals can be tried.[43]

Botanical Medicines

There are no adequate controlled trials of botanical treatments for treatment of FMS.

Many patients do take herbs such as valerian and St. John's wort for symptoms of FMS, but none have been seriously studied to date in clinical trials. Ginger and turmeric (curcumin) have not been tested in FMS, but are being used in other inflammatory pain syndromes to inhibit production of proinflammatory prostaglandins.

Exercise and Movement Therapies

Exercise can be helpful in decreasing the symptoms of FMS.[44] However, overuse can result in increased symptoms, often severe, and can lead to a cycle of muscle disuse. In one study, 9 of 16 subjects were worse or unchanged after a 14-week aerobic training intervention. However, 3 of the 16 subjects able to maintain a program of aerobic exercise no longer fulfilled criteria for FMS diagnosis 4 years later.[44] In a 21-week study of strength training in FMS patients, neck pain, fatigue, and depression decreased.[45] Warm water pool aerobic therapy may be helpful, particularly for severe cases.[46] Eastern forms of exercise such as tai chi and yoga can also be beneficial. A form of tai chi called the range-of-motion dance is particularly suited to persons with disabilities.

A study that compared massage therapy, transcutaneous electrical nerve stimulation (TENS) treatment, and sham TENS, found that massage therapy was more useful than TENS in reducing pain for FMS patients. TENS was better than sham TENS and also may be helpful in some cases.[17]

Mind–Body Therapy

Mindfulness meditation is helpful in FMS.[18,19] By increasing the patient's ability to live in the present moment, meditation can lessen the anxiety and fear of future pain, and, with practice, can transform the sensation of pain. In one study, 10 of 15 subjects responded to a 14-week cognitive-behavioral and relaxation training intervention.[50] However, none remained improved at 4-year follow-up.

Electromyelogram (EMG) biofeedback was studied in a small open study (n = 15) followed by a randomized controlled blinded study (n = 12).[51] In the open study, after 15 twice-per-week sessions, there were statistically significant decreases in tender points, morning stiffness, and pain. This improvement was maintained at 6 months. However, only 9 of 15 patients had a 50% improvement. Of the six patients with no benefit, three were depressed, two had high hypochondriasis scores on the Minnesota Multiphasic Personality Inventory, and one had a normal Minnesota Multiphasic Personality Inventory. In the controlled study, statistically significant improvements were seen in tender points, morning stiffness, pain, and overall clinical symptoms for patients undergoing "true EMG-biofeedback." Minor statistically significant improvements were seen only in tender points, but not morning stiffness, pain, and overall clinical symptoms for patients undergoing "false EMG-biofeedback." Hypnotherapy was helpful in a single controlled trial.[52] Hypnotherapy was compared to physical therapy in a 12-week trial and had a better outcome as measured by pain, fatigue, and sleep at 12 and 24 weeks (n = 40).

Dr. John Sarno labels FMS a tension-myositis syndrome.[53] His work is based on the premise that patients substitute physical pain for emotional pain. This simple realization can often relieve pain. A discussion with the patient outlining how certain individuals may have increased sensitivity to stressful events, physical and emotional trauma, and even infections or chemical exposure may be helpful. Outlining how stress may directly affect hormones and immune mediators may help the patient understand the connections between mind and body. This can reinforce the importance of introspection and identifying those events causing the most distress.

Homeopathy

A double-blind, placebo-controlled trial of a homeopathic treatment (R toxicodendron 6c) in 30 subjects with FMS showed statistically significant improvements in pain and sleep.[51] Tender points averaged 14.1 for the placebo versus 10.6 with the homeopathic preparation, a statistically significant decrease.

Acupuncture

One high-quality trial of electroacupuncture for FMS showed almost complete remissions in 20%, satisfactory benefit in 40%, and no effects in 40% of subjects in a short-term study.[55] A review of several trials concluded that benefits were reduced with time.[56] Nonetheless, acupuncture may be beneficial as part of an initial program to get patients started on increasing physical activity.

Summary

There is no documented "cure" for FMS. Prior studies have reported a spontaneous improvement in 5–53% of patients, although 47–100% continue to meet criteria for FMS 2–5 years after diagnosis.[27,57] Only a small minority of patients have complete resolution of symptoms. In our clinic, approximately 75% of patients report "some" relief of symptoms with treatment. Better response to treatment is seen in patients of younger age, with continued employment, supportive families, and an absence of litigation and of affective disorders.[27,58]

▶ **Case Example 2: Fibromyalgia Snydrome Conclusion**

This patient presents with a classic middle-aged muscle disuse syndrome. She exercised prior to having children, and central to any therapy will be for her to return slowly to 30–60 minutes of aerobic exercise three to five times per week. Warm-water pool aerobics may help her to start exercising in a gentle manner. She has been receiving adequate conventional therapy and her diet is fairly good. Dietary recommendations should include adding more cold-water fish for increased omega-3 fatty acid intake, and supplements including multivitamins, calcium, magnesium, vitamin E, and selenium. The use of the botanicals turmeric and ginger may be helpful for their antiinflammatory analgesic activity as may a trial of acupuncture.

We would also explore with the patient the possible use of journaling, meditation, and psychotherapy. We would recommend she read the books by Drs. John Sarno and Nancy Selfridge,[53,59] and discuss in depth the theory that persons with FMS may have an underlying higher-than-average sensitivity to both emotional and physical stressors, with expression according to genetic predisposition and environmental factors in her current and past experiences. Thus, she may be the "canary in the coal mine," showing us the consequences of a sensitive individual living with the high emotional and physical stresses in our Western lifestyle. We would encourage this patient to keep working at a reduced level and to focus on what is "right" in her life, and explain that although there are no magic bullet "cures" for FMS, many people learn to adjust to intermittent pain and fatigue with compassion and understanding of their own needs.

▶ **OSTEOARTHRITIS**

Pathophysiology and Prevalence

In osteoarthritis (OA) the hyaline cartilage of the joint becomes irregular and irritated. This leads to an inflammatory process that causes remodeling of the bone and synovium resulting in joint space narrowing, osteophyte development, and chronic synovitis. These changes cause the classic symptoms of pain, crepitus, restricted movement, and even muscle wasting seen in advanced OA. The most commonly involved joints include the knees, hips, carpometacarpal joint of the thumb, distal interphalangeal joints (with Heberden nodes), and the proximal interphalangeal joints (with Bouchard nodes), as well as the cervical and lumbosacral joints of the spine.

That some people develop these changes much more readily than others who have been exposed to similar amounts of overuse suggests that there may also be a genetic influence in regard to the incidence of OA.[60] Also of interest regarding the pathophysiology of this pain syndrome is that changes on radiograph do not necessarily correlate with severity of symptoms: some patients with very severe OA changes can be asymptomatic, while some of those with what would appear to be minor changes are severely impaired. One study showed that only 50% of patients with radiographic changes of OA of the knee complained of pain.[61] This observation helps us realize that the subjective experience of pain and disability in this, as in almost every chronic condition, is much more complicated than simple mechanics.

Osteoarthritis is the most common cause of disability in the United States and accounts for 2% of all visits to family physicians. It is the tenth most common complaint seen in the primary care setting,[62] being found in 60% of all people older than 60 years of age.[63]

▶ Case Example 3: Osteoarthritis

Martin is a 63-year-old ex-college basketball player who is 6'4″ and weighs 268 lb with truncal obesity. He has complained of gradually progressing bilateral knee pain with the right worse than the left. He also suffers from hypertension and prediabetes with an elevated triglyceride level, low high-density lipoprotein level and a fasting blood sugar of 122. He had standing anteroposterior radiographic views of both knees, which showed medial joint space narrowing, with the right being more severe. His medical history is significant for a bleeding peptic ulcer, which he attributed to job stress. He works in public office as a city manager. He does not tolerate NSAIDs or cyclooxygenase-2 inhibitors because of gastrointestinal upset and elevation of blood pressure. He wants to do all he can to delay his surgery and to help reduce pain so as to increase his ability to exercise, which he realizes he needs to do to help prevent overt diabetes.

Conventional Treatment Approach

Treatment of OA has focused on pain control, exercise, and physical therapy to increase strength and range of motion of the affected joints. Care may be taken to release pressure on the involved joint with the use of a cane or through weight loss. Analgesics in the form of aspirin or nonsteroidal antiinflammatory drugs are often used. Intraarticular therapy with steroids or hyaluronic acid can give some short-term relief. If joint destruction progresses to the point of severe pain and disability, surgical replacement can result in significant improvement in symptoms.

Integrative Treatment Approach

Lifestyle Measures
A review of 12 randomized controlled studies showed that regular exercise (aerobic, strength training, and range of motion) improved pain, walking tolerance, patient-rated disability, and global assessment of symptoms in those with mild to moderate OA. The results were better for those with OA of the knee versus the hip.[64] Weight management is very important in prevention, in part to reduce the amount of joint pressure. Weight loss can also reduce the amount of pain and slow the progression of OA in those who already have the disease.[65]

There may be a metabolic component to OA as well, which may add to the efficacy of weight loss as a treatment, particularly in patients with coexisting diabetes. OA of non–weight-bearing joints such as the hands is much more prevalent in those with a higher body mass index.[66] This metabolic effect may be mediated by growth hormone and somatomedin levels: insulin resistance (as seen in type 2 diabetes) leads to increased growth hormone levels and a decrease in somatomedins. Growth hormones worsen OA and somatomedins have a beneficial influence on chondrocyte activity. Those with diabetes thus have a greater incidence of a more severe form of OA than do nondiabetics.[67]

Nutritional Approaches

DIETARY MANIPULATION
As discussed earlier in the section on rheumatoid arthritis, reducing foods rich in saturated fats (red meat, dairy, fried foods) may help reduce inflammation by modulating the arachidonic acid component of the inflammatory cascade. A diet rich in omega-3 fatty acids may also be of benefit to patients with OA.

Although an elimination diet is not commonly recommended in a degenerative type of arthritis such as OA, there is some limited evidence that nightshade vegetables may worsen symptoms. Nightshades, such as, tomatoes, potatoes, eggplant, peppers, and tobacco, contain solanum alkaloids, which inhibit normal collagen repair and promote inflammatory changes in the joint.[68] It may be worthwhile to eliminate nightshades for 2 weeks to see if symptoms improve.

GLUCOSAMINE SULFATE

Glucosamine is a simple molecule that occurs naturally in cartilage. It increases mucopolysaccharide and collagen production in fibroblasts and inhibits the enzyme (elastase) that breaks down cartilage. It may be that as we age, we do not produce as much glucosamine, and consequently our cartilage loses some of its "gel-like" shock-absorbing properties.

Several randomized controlled studies have shown benefit with the use of glucosamine in OA. Although there is arguably publication bias with many of these studies, the evidence nevertheless appears to support the use of glucosamine. In one study (n = 200), for example, when glucosamine 500 mg TID was compared to ibuprofen 400 mg TID, the clinical outcome was similar in both groups and more side effects were noted in those taking ibuprofen.[69] A systematic Cochrane review of controlled studies found that glucosamine worked as well or better than NSAIDs for treatment of OA.[70]

There is some preliminary evidence that glucosamine may not only be effective in pain relief, but may also be a disease-modifying agent in OA. In a double-blind, randomized, controlled trial, 212 patients were assigned to either placebo or glucosamine 1,500 mg daily for 3 years. Those taking glucosamine had no radiographic evidence of joint space narrowing versus progressive narrowing in the placebo group.[71] More research is needed to clarify whether glucosamine in fact can slow progression of arthritis.

In patients with diabetes, there may be concern about giving a product that contains glucose over a prolonged period of time. This needs further study, but one report showed that 4 weeks of supplementation with glucosamine did not have a negative effect on insulin sensitivity or increase fasting glucose levels.[72] The standard dose of glucosamine used in clinical trials has been 500 mg TID, but in clinical practice, it appears that taking 750 mg twice daily works as well and is more convenient. Those who have seafood allergies should avoid glucosamine, which is derived from chitin in crustacean shells.

CHONDROITIN SULFATE

This supplement, which is obtained from bovine tracheal cartilage, has not been as well studied as glucosamine, but appears to also be beneficial in OA. Chondroitin is thought to have its effects by stimulating hyaluronic acid in synovial cells, increasing viscosity in the joint space. Like glucosamine, chondroitin also inhibits enzymes (elastase and hyaluronidase) that break down cartilage. Questions have been raised regarding whether chondroitin, which is a much larger molecule than glucosamine, can be absorbed into the cartilage in quantities sufficient to have a positive effect. Despite this, a meta-analysis of seven randomized controlled studies showed benefit for patients taking this supplement in terms of reduced pain and improved mobility.[73] A second meta-analysis of both chondroitin and glucosamine confirmed this positive overall conclusion with moderate to large effects.[74] The typical dose of chondroitin is 400 mg BID or TID. It is often used in combination with glucosamine, although the benefit of using both together in OA has not been established.

S-ADENOSYLMETHIONINE

This naturally occurring molecule is distributed throughout virtually all body tissues and fluids. It transports and donates methyl groups that are involved in the synthesis of hormones, neurotransmitters, proteins, and phospholipids. It has been found to stimulate cartilage growth and repair, possibly by enhancing the production of proteoglycans in cartilage in those with OA.[75] As with glucosamine, it is believed that a deficiency of SAMe in the joint may contribute to the loss of the gel-like, shock-absorbing qualities of the cartilage.

Although more research needs to be done in regard to its mechanism of action, the evidence supports its analgesic and antiinflammatory effects. SAMe at a dose of 1,200 mg daily has been compared to both ibuprofen 1,200 mg[76] and indomethacin 150 mg[77] daily. In both cases, SAMe showed similar benefit for the symptoms of OA and was better tolerated. A recent meta-analysis came to a similar conclusion, finding that SAMe was as effective as NSAIDs in improving pain and functional limitations for OA without the gastrointestinal side effects.[78] The dose of SAMe is 600–1,200 mg daily; it is generally very well tolerated, with gastrointestinal distress as its most common side effect. SAMe does not work as quickly as NSAIDs, and at least 4 weeks of treatment are needed to determine efficacy.

METHYL SULFONYL METHANE

This supplement is commonly used for pain and musculoskeletal conditions. It is a rich source of sulfur, which is used for the synthesis of connective tissue and is commonly found in green vegetables (asparagus), garlic, onions, fruits, grains, algae, and milk. Methyl sulfonyl methane can be used to increase the synthesis of SAMe, and this may be why it has been found to have some benefit in the treatment of OA. Although animal studies appear promising, there is limited human research and until more is known, simply taking SAMe may provide the same benefit without having to increase the number of supplements for the patient.

Patients currently taking NSAIDs may benefit from adding or substituting these agents that have a different mechanism of action and potentially disease-modifying properties.[79]

Botanical Medicines

PHYTODOLOR

This combination botanical product has been studied quite extensively and is commonly used in Europe. It contains three ingredients that are high in salicylates: common ash *(Fraxinus excelsior)* bark extract, aspen *(Populus tremula)* leaf and bark extract, and goldenrod *(Solidago virgaurea)* aerial part extract. The mechanism of action is thought to be related to its ability to inhibit arachidonic acid metabolism and prostaglandin E_2 production via the lipoxygenase and cyclooxygenase pathways. A systematic review of 10 randomized placebo-controlled trials with a total sample size of 1,035 patients showed Phytodolor to work as well as NSAIDs at reducing pain and restoring function without the gastrointestinal side effects.[80] The dose is 20–40 drops TID mixed in water or juice.

AVOCADO/SOYBEAN UNSAPONIFIABLES

An extract of avocado and soybeans, ASU is made of unsaponifiable fractions of avocado and soybean oils. This botanical has been studied for OA and appears to have a positive effect, particularly for OA of the hip. Two randomized controlled trials showed that ASU significantly improved OA symptoms of the hip and knee while reducing the need for NSAIDs.[81,82] This product appears to be slow acting and generally takes at least 2 months to have an effect. Unlike other botanicals, ASU may also have a positive effect on the preservation of the cartilage by stimulating collagen synthesis and deposition and repair of extracellular matrix components.[83] Although the active ingredient remains unknown, ASU has inhibitory effects on prostaglandin E_2 production, interleukins, and enzymes that degrade collagen (collagenase).[81] The dose used in the randomized studies above was ASU 300 mg daily. At this point, this product is still difficult to find commercially in the United States, although it may become more widely available in the future.

CAPSAICIN

A derivative of hot chili pepper, capsaicin (*trans*-8-methyl-N-vanillyl-6-nonenamide) is well established as a topical treatment for pain, including the pain of OA. Capsaicin has its effect by depleting levels of substance P, thereby reducing the sensitivity of nociceptive neurons to pain. A meta-analysis of topical capsaicin for OA showed benefit for reducing pain and articular tenderness when compared to placebo.[85] The dose used in the study was 0.025% capsaicin cream applied to the joint four times daily. Capsaicin is also available in a stronger 0.075%, but patients should be warned that this stronger formulation often stings with the first few applications.

BOSWELLIA, CURCUMIN, AND GINGER

Three Ayurvedic herbs, boswellia *(Boswellia serrata)*, curcumin *(Curcuma longa)*, and ginger *(Zingiber officinale* Rescoe), appear to have antiinflammatory properties that may be mediated, at least in part, by inhibition of leukotriene synthesis. A combination of boswellia, curcumin, and zinc was found to improve pain and disability in a double-blinded crossover study of patients with OA.[86] In another study (n = 67) of OA of the hip and knee, patients were randomized to receive either ginger 170 mg capsules TID, ibuprofen 400 mg TID, or placebo. Ibuprofen had the best response, and there was little difference between ginger and placebo.[87]

There is currently a major National Institutes of Health-funded study underway at the University of Arizona to study the antiinflammatory properties of these three herbs, which should bring more insight into their use for OA and other inflammatory conditions. Table 29–4 reviews the literature on botanicals for OA.

▶ **TABLE 29-4** REVIEW OF BOTANICALS FOR OSTEOARTHRITIS

Botanical	Evidence for Effectiveness X to XXXX	Dosage	Effect
Phytodolor	XXXX	20–40 drops TID	As effective as NSAID without the side effects
Capsaicin	XXXX	0.025–0.075% topically QID	Reduced tenderness and pain
Avocado/soybean unsaponifiables	XXX	300 mg daily	Improved pain and function; may help protect cartilage from degeneration
Devil's claw	XXX	Two 400 mg (*Harpagophytum* extract) capsules TID	Reduced pain and improved joint mobility
Willow bark	XX	Equivalent of 240 mg of salicin daily	Moderate analgesic effect
Stinging nettle	XX	Topical application of leaf applied daily	Pain and disability improved after 1 week of treatment
Ginger	X	170 mg TID	Less effective than ibuprofen when used alone

Adapted from Long L, Soeken K, Ernst E. Herbal medicines for the treatment of osteoarthritis: a systematic review. Rheumatology. 2001;40:Table 1.

Mind–Body Therapies

The importance of the distinction between the experience of pain and the experience of suffering is critical in understanding the integrative approach to the patient with a chronic pain condition such as OA. An example of how social support can reduce pain through improving suffering can be seen in studies that show that even regular monthly phone calls from health care workers can have significant benefit on health care costs, pain, and functional status.[88] Education of family members has also been found to reduce OA pain,[89] as has regular social support.[90]

There are numerous studies showing the benefits of hypnosis and relaxation on perceived pain levels for other conditions, but few specifically for OA. One study compared hypnosis/imagery versus relaxation therapy versus a waiting list control group for patients with OA of the hip or knee. The hypnosis consisted of eight 30-minute sessions that involved a relaxation induction and suggestion that encouraged regression to childhood when they had good joint mobility, movement, and posture adaptation. No suggestions were specifically made for analgesia. The relaxation sessions consisted of eight 30-minute sessions of Jacobson progressive muscle relaxation where muscles were tensed and then relaxed. The wait list control did not receive any mind–body therapy. After 4 weeks of therapy, hypnosis/imagery was associated with a 50% reduction in pain, whereas there was no improvement in either the relaxation or the control groups. This 50% reduction persisted until the 6-month follow-up evaluation, 4 months after the therapy was completed. The relaxation group in this study also ultimately showed improvement versus control, but this effect took longer (8 weeks) to appear, and provided a 31% improvement in pain. Both hypnosis and relaxation also significantly reduced the amount of pain medication taken by the participants. A limitation of this study was the small number of participants (n = 36).[91]. Table 29–5 summarizes the findings from this trial.

Acupuncture

A systematic review of acupuncture for osteoarthritis of the knee showed that there was strong evidence to support its use in treating the pain of OA, but did not show a change in knee function with this approach. This study concluded that there was not enough evidence to evaluate the effect of acupuncture as compared to other treatments for OA.[92] When acupuncture was compared to the NSAID piroxicam (Feldene), the degree of improvement was equal after 2 weeks of therapy, but acupuncture had a better effect with use after 4, 6, 12, and 16 weeks of weekly therapy.[93] At this time, it appears reasonable to conclude that acupuncture is a useful tool to help reduce pain of OA and thus reduce the need for NSAID therapy.

▶ **TABLE 29-5** MIND–BODY THERAPIES FOR OSTEOARTHRITIS

	Hypnosis	Relaxation	Control
After 4 weeks of treatment	−52%	+2%	+15%
After 8 weeks of treatment	−56%	−31%	−4%
3-month follow-up	−60%	−22%	−2%
6-month follow-up	−51%	−23%	−2%

Percentage change in pain experienced from osteoarthritis when treated with hypnosis, relaxation and a wait list control. *From Gay MC, Philippot P, Luminet O. Differential effectiveness of psychological interventions for reducing osteoarthritis pain: a comparison of Erickson hypnosis and Jacobson relaxation. Eur J Pain. 2002;6:1–16.*

Manual Physical Therapy

In one study of the role of manual manipulation for OA, physical therapists with formal training in manual therapy treated patients with OA of the knee with manual therapy and exercise versus a control that consisted of subtherapeutic ultrasound treatment. There was significant functional benefit (distance walked in 6 minutes) in the treatment group, as compared to the control that lasted for a year after treatment.[94] It is difficult to say if this benefit was related to the manual therapy or the exercise.

▶ Case Example 3: Osteoarthritis Conclusion

This patient is at risk for more than just his arthritis. If he is unable to exercise, he will be at greater risk for developing overt diabetes and the complications associated with this disease. Reducing foods rich in saturated fats and increasing those high in omega-3 fatty acids will have a beneficial influence on inflammation seen with OA. Reducing calories will also help with weight loss; this will help prevent both OA and diabetes.

Before we can recommend an exercise routine, we need to reduce arthritic pain. Because he is not able to tolerate NSAIDs, we can look at other measures that may help reduce his pain. Botanical products that improve pain but do not increase the risk of gastrointestinal side effects include Phytodolor, capsaicin, and ASU. Products that may help with both pain and the prevention of disease progression include glucosamine, chondroitin, SAMe, and ASU. Combining one or more of the potentially structure-modifying agents with a symptom-modifying agent for pain will have a positive effect in helping this individual get started with his exercise routine. We need to be patient and give these agents 6–8 weeks to reach therapeutic efficacy. Adjunctive therapies that will enhance symptom relief include hypnosis/imagery, relaxation therapy, acupuncture, and manual physical therapy. We recommend the one that best matches this patient's belief system.

▶ GOUT

Pathophysiology and Prevalence

Gout is a metabolic disease characterized by the overproduction and/or the underexcretion of uric acid. The limit of solubility of uric acid in plasma is approximately 7 mg/dL. Above this level, crystals of monosodium urate may precipitate out of solution often inciting local inflammation. Hyperuricemia has been shown to result from an interaction of environmental and genetic factors.[95,96] Uric acid is a building block for the purine nucleotides guanine and adenine (Figure 29–1). Genes control levels and activities of the enzymes in the purine pathway of nucleotide synthesis and degradation. Environmental factors such as diet, water intake, alcohol use, and body weight all influence levels and solubility of uric acid. The majority of uric acid is excreted through the kidney.

Severe deficiency of the hypoxanthine-guanine phosphoribosyltransferase (see Figure 29–1) salvage enzyme leads to extremely high uric acid levels and the subsequent self-mutilation seen in the Lesch-Nyhan syndrome. Milder forms of enzyme deficiencies can lead to early-onset familial gout. Overproduction of

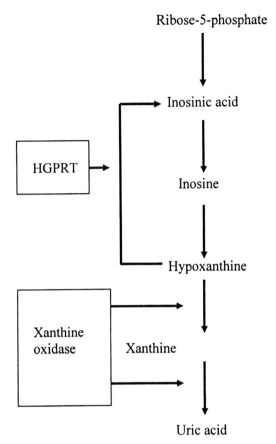

Ribose-5-phosphate

Inosinic acid

HGPRT

Inosine

Hypoxanthine

Xanthine
oxidase

Xanthine

Uric acid

Figure 29–1. Purine metabolism. HGPRT = hypoxanthine-guanine phosphoribosyltransferase.

phagocytosis and release of inflammatory mediators are believed to be responsible for the initial inflammation in acute gout. Systemic manifestations such as fever and leukocytosis are likely secondary to leaking of cytokines from the inflamed joint into the bloodstream.

The prevalence of gout in the United States is approximately 1.4% for men and 0.6% for women.[97] Disease peaks for men in their fifties and for women in their sixties.

Clinical presentations include asymptomatic hyperuricemia, acute monoarticular gout, recurrent acute gout, and chronic tophaceous gout.[98] Polyarticular gout, recurrent or chronic, can mimic rheumatoid arthritis. Podagra, involvement of the great toe, is the most common presentation, followed by the ankle and knee. However, any joint in the body can be affected including the sternal and cricoarytenoid joints. Bursitis and tendonitis are common, with involvement of the olecranon bursa being most common. The kidney is commonly affected, and uric acid nephropathy can lead to renal failure. Large deposits of solid uric acid, tophi, can be found in subcutaneous tissues, can erode into joints, or can be found in various organs, including the heart. Diagnosis is usually made by arthrocentesis of an affected joint. Finding uric acid crystals is diagnostic and also allows the practitioner to rule out infection or other causes of arthritis.[99]

uric acid can also occur secondary to excessive nucleic acid turnover associated with neoplasia, hemolysis, and psoriasis. Underexcretion can occur with renal disease and dehydration. Diuretics, cyclosporine, low-dose salicylates, and lead exposure can all increase the risk for gout. Ethanol use and abuse can contribute to both overproduction and underexcretion of uric acid. Injection of monosodium urate crystals can induce inflammation, but these crystals also can be found in asymptomatic joints. Therefore, crystals can directly cause inflammation, yet are not sufficient to cause gout. Neutrophil

Conventional Treatment Approach

Conventional treatment often involves pharmaceutical agents to block the production of uric acid and to inhibit the inflammatory response that it creates. Termination of an acute attack often involves the use of NSAIDs, such as ibuprofen (Motrin, Advil), naproxen sodium (Aleve), or indomethacin (Indocin), at maximum doses. These drugs should be used with caution in patients with preexisting renal impairment or peptic ulcer disease. Alternatively, oral or intravenous colchicine can be used.

▶ Case Example 4: Gout

A 55-year-old African American gentleman with a long history of hypertension presents to your clinic with complaints of swelling, tenderness, and redness of the left great toe. He reports that over the past 5 years he suffered thrice-yearly episodes of pain and swelling of various joints including the ankles, knees, elbows, and great toes. All previous episodes were mild and self-treated with over-the-counter ibuprofen. This episode has lasted a week despite treatment with 3 tablets of ibuprofen 4 times per day. He reports that he had fever and chills yesterday. He is using a friend's crutches, because he is unable to step on that foot because of pain. He reports that even the breeze from a fan blowing on his toe is painful. Physical examination reveals moderate truncal obesity, elevated blood pressure, a new heart murmur, and the red, swollen, tender great toe. A radiograph shows a 1-cm (0.4-inch) tophus eroded into left first metatarsal–phalangeal joint. Arthrocentesis reveals negatively birefringent crystals under polarizing microscopy. Your initial laboratory work-up shows a normal uric acid and an elevated serum creatinine of 2.3 mg/dL. You successfully treat him with oral colchicine and bring him back to clinic 2 months later. His repeat uric acid is very elevated at 11 mg/dL and his creatinine is unchanged.

Acute attacks are often treated with colchicine 0.6 mg tablets, 1 tablet each hour, until 4–8 mg total is taken per 24 hours. Treatment is usually stopped by intolerable nausea, vomiting, or diarrhea. Intravenous colchicine can be given to hospitalized patients unable to take oral medications and must be given with care because of high toxicity. Systemic corticosteroids can also be used to terminate an acute attack. Long-acting triamcinolone (Kenalog) can be given intramuscularly 40–80 mg as a single dose. Oral prednisone can be given at 40–60 mg once per day on the first day and tapered rapidly over 7–10 days. Long-acting triamcinolone (Kenalog) can also be used interarticularly by injection for monoarthritis, after arthrocentesis to rule out infection. Recurrent episodes of gout, more than twice per year, should be treated with prophylaxis. Low-dose NSAIDs or colchicine 0.6 mg twice per day can be used. Lower doses of colchicine (0.6 mg daily or 3 times per week) can used for patients with nausea or diarrhea. In cases of renal insufficiency or failure, avoid NSAIDs and use colchicine 0.6 mg once per day. Serious adverse reactions for colchicine include cytopenias and myoneuropathies.

The presence of tophi, renal disease, or repeated attacks despite prophylaxis, indicates the need for life-long therapy to reduce hyperuricemia. Reducing hyperuricemia will decrease attacks of gout and may slowly dissolve tophi and possibly decrease early renal disease. Uricosuric drugs, such as probenecid and sulfinpyrazone, decrease uric acid in the blood by increasing renal excretion. These drugs may also promote the formation of kidney stones, and so are contraindicated in renal insufficiency or failure. A 24-hour urine for creatine clearance and uric acid can identify "undersecretors." In practice, few patients can take the uricosuric drugs, particularly the elderly; therefore, allopurinol is used.[100] Allopurinol is an inhibitor of the uric acid synthesizing enzyme xanthine oxidase, which effectively blocks production of uric acid (see Figure 29–1). However, because of large uric acid loads in the body, it can take many years after normalizing serum uric acid levels for tophi to dissolve. Allopurinol should not be started until 2 months after the last attack, and prophylactic NSAIDs or colchicines must be given before starting the allopurinol and during the initial 2–3 months to avoid precipitating an acute gout attack. Serious adverse reactions for allopurinol include cytopenias, hepatitis, and severe life-threatening skin reactions. Allopurinol can increase the toxicity of azathioprine. In cases where immunosuppression must be continued, consider switching the azathioprine to mycophenolate mofetil.

Integrative Treatment Approach

Although asymptomatic hyperuricemia requires no treatment, dietary and other lifestyle changes should be encouraged. Acute monoarticular gout will often resolve without treatment within 1 week. Recurrent episodes occur in at least 90% of patients unless preventive measures are taken. The presence of tophi or renal disease indicates the need for long-term therapy to reduce hyperuricemia.

Nutrition and Lifestyle
Foods high in purines should be avoided, especially red meat and organ foods such as liver, brains, kidneys, and sweetbreads. Avoid sardines, anchovies, herring, and shellfish as these can also be high in purines. Limited portions of chicken and fish are acceptable. A vegetarian diet might be helpful; particularly with an increased intake of raw fruits and vegetables. However, intake of cooked spinach, rhubarb, cauliflower, asparagus, peas, beans, and mushrooms should be limited. Replacing simple carbohydrates with more complex whole grains will increase dietary fiber.

Dehydration increases the risk of gout, likely by decreasing the solubility of uric acid in the tissues, and is particularly a problem in the elderly.[100] Intake of water and dilute fruit juices should be increased to at least six to eight 8-ounce glasses per day. Carrot juice may be beneficial, as may be dark berries. Berries, such as cherries, blueberries, blackberries, raspberries, hawthorn berries, and elderberries, are good sources of flavonoid compounds. Fresh, frozen, dried, canned, juiced, or extracted berries, 1 cup fresh or about half a pound, should be consumed daily.

Weight loss may be helpful but patients should avoid "crash diets" that may affect uric acid solubility and precipitate gout attacks. Increasing aerobic exercise and muscle strengthening around affected joints can be beneficial as can limiting caffeine and especially alcohol. Moonshine liquor prepared using old car radiators carries an especially high risk of both gout and nephropathy as a consequence of lead contamination (saturnine gout).[101,102] Medications that can increase plasma uric acid levels such as diuretics, cyclosporine, tacrolimus, and low-dose aspirin or other salicylates should be discontinued.

Supplements
A high-potency multivitamin with minerals and extra B vitamins is recommended. Vitamin E has antiinflammatory activity and should be taken at 800–1,600 IU daily. High doses of vitamin C may decrease renal excretion of uric acid, therefore, excessive supplemental vitamin C should be avoided and patients should obtain vitamin C from fresh fruit and juices. Selenium also may be helpful; intake should be at least 100 μg daily, but not to exceed 400 μg daily.

Botanicals
Many botanicals can inhibit xanthine-oxidase, the processing enzyme for uric

acid.[103–107] However, none of the usual recommended botanicals have been studied in a substantial clinical trial. The traditional Chinese antirheumatic herb Danggui-Nian-Tong-Tang (DGNTT) *(Angelica sirensis)* was compared to indomethacin and allopurinol for antiinflammatory and antihyperuricemic effects in patients with gout. There was no significant reduction in the total number of painful and swollen joints, articular index, or pain score, and DGNTT did not lower the serum level of uric acid.[108]

Devil's claw has been used for both arthritis and gout. However, it can have adverse cardiovascular effects including hypertension, and it can also antagonize the effects of peptic acid inhibitors, and adversely affect diabetic control. There are safer botanicals, such as ginger, tumeric (circumin) and boswellia. Autumn crocus *(Colchicum autumnale)* is the original source for colchicine; however, this botanical is highly toxic. Only standardized, FDA-approved, colchicine should be used for treatment.

▶ Case Example 4: Gout Conclusion

Podagra, gout of the great toe, is unlikely to be infectious. A similar presentation in any other joint is presumed to be infected until proven otherwise. This would require arthrocentesis and culture, with possible overnight hospitalization and intravenous antibiotics until the culture comes back negative. Infection and gout rarely coexist except in immunosuppressed individuals. Often uric acid is normal during a flare of gout; hence, the patient's normal uric acid level on presentation. The diagnosis of tophaceous gout indicates the need for lowering systemic uric acid. This patient's renal insufficiency rules out the use of uricosuric agents and, therefore, we must use allopurinol in the future. If no tophi were found we could treat intermittently with colchicine. We also would avoid NSAIDs because of re-

nal insufficiency. We will need to treat with colchicine until there are no symptoms for 2 months, and then start allopurinol. We would also continue the colchicine for at least another 2 months. This avoids a flare secondary to starting allopurinol. The renal insufficiency may be combination of uric acid nephropathy and hypertension. Conversely, the increased uric acid level might be secondary to hypertension-induced renal insufficiency. The heart murmur is likely a result of mild aortic sclerosis, not cardiac tophi involving the valve. Although pharmaceuticals are indicated, we would also council this patient in proper diet, fluid intake, supplements, and possibly a trial of botanical therapy to reduce the use of colchicine.

REFERENCES

1. Straub RH, Cutolo M. Involvement of the hypothalamic-pituitary-adrenal/gonadal axis and the peripheral nervous system in rheumatoid arthritis. *Arthritis Rheum.* 2001;44:493–507.

2. Huyser B, Parker JC. Stress and rheumatoid arthritis: an integrated review. *Arthritis Care Res.* 1998;11:135–145.

3. Escalante A, Del Rincon I. How much disability in rheumatoid arthritis is explained by rheumatoid arthritis? *Arthritis Rheum.* 1999;42:1712–1721.

4. Parker JC, Smarr KL, Angelone EO, et al. Psychological factors, immunologic activation, and disease activity in rheumatoid arthritis. *Arthritis Care Res.* 1992;5:196–201.

5. Palmblad J, Hafstrom I, Ringertz B. Antirheumatic effects of fasting. *Rheum Dis Clin North Am.* 1991;17(2):351–362.

6. Muller H, de Toledo FW, Resch K-L. Fasting followed by vegetarian diet in patients with rheumatoid arthritis: a systematic review. *Scand J Rheumatol.* 2001;30(1):1–10.

7. Fraser DA, Thoen J, Djoseland O, et al. Serum levels of interleukin-6 and dehydroepiandrosterone sulphate in response to either fasting or a ketogenic diet in rheumatoid arthritis patients. *Clin Exp Rheumatol.* 2000;18(3):357–362.

8. Fuhrman J, Sarter B, Calabro DJ. Brief case reports of medically supervised, water-only fasting associated with remission of autoimmune disease. *Alt Ther.* 2002;8(4):110–112.

9. Hastrom I, Ringertz B, Spangberg A, et al. A vegan diet free of gluten improves the signs and symptoms of rheumatoid arthritis: the effects on arthritis correlate with a reduction in antibodies to food antigens. *Rheumatology.* 2001;40(10):1175–1179.

10. Kjeldsen-Kragh J. Rheumatoid arthritis treated with vegetarian diets. *Am J Clin Nutr.* 1999;70(suppl 3):594S–600S.

11. Kremer JM. n-3 fatty acid supplements in rheumatoid arthritis. *Am J Clin Nutr.* 2000;71(1 suppl):349S–351S.

12. Ariza-Ariza R, Mestanza-Peralta M, Cardiel MH. Omega-3 fatty acids in rheumatoid arthritis: an overview. *Semin Arthritis Rheum.* 1998;27(6):366–370.

13. Linos A, Kaklamani VG, Kaklamani E, et al. Dietary factors in relation to rheumatoid arthritis: a role for olive oil and cooked vegetables? *Am J Clin Nutr.* 1999;70:1077–1082.

14. Heliovaara M, Aho K, Knekt P, et al. Coffee consumption, rheumatoid factor, and the risk of rheumatoid arthritis. *Ann Rheum Dis.* 2000;59:631–635.

15. Srivastava KC, Mustafa T. Ginger in rheumatism and musculoskeletal disorders. *Med Hypotheses.* 1992;39:342–348.

16. Darlington LG, Stone TW. Antioxidants and fatty acids in the amelioration of rheumatoid arthritis and related disorders. *Br J Nutr.* 2001;85(3):251–269.

17. Deaney CL, Feyi K, Forrest CM, et al. Levels of lipid peroxidation products in a chronic inflammatory disorder. *Res Commun Mol Pathol Pharmacol.* 2001;110(1–2):87–95.

18. Bandt MD, Grossin M, Driss F, et al. Vitamin E uncouples joint destruction and clinical inflammation in a transgenic mouse model of rheumatoid arthritis. *Arthritis Rheum.* 2002;46(2):522–532.

19. Treatment of RA with Selenium. *Therapiewoche.* 1996;46:1529–1532.

20. Strausbaugh HJ, Dallman ME, Levine JD. Repeated, but not acute, stress suppresses inflammatory plasma extravasation. *Proc Natl Acad Sci U S A.* 1999;96(25):14629–14634.

21. Maes M, Christophe A, Bosmans E, et al. In humans, serum polyunsaturated fatty acid levels predict the response of proinflammatory cytokines to psychologic stress. *Biol Psychiatry.* 2000;47(10):910–920.

22. Astin JA, Beckner W, Soeken K, et al. Psychological interventions for rheumatoid arthritis: a meta-analysis of randomized controlled trials. *Arthritis Rheum.* 2002;47(3):291–302.

23. Smyth JM, Stone AA, Hurewitz A, et al. Effects of writing about stressful experiences on symptom reduction in patients with asthma and rheumatoid arthritis. *JAMA.* 1999;281:1304–1309.

24. Bhatt-Sanders D. Acupuncture for rheumatoid arthritis: an analysis of the literature. *Semin Arthritis Rheum.* 1985;14:225–231.

25. Wolfe F, Smythe H, Yunus M, et al. The American College of Rheumatology 1990 criteria for the classification of fibromyalgia. *Arthritis Rheum.* 1990;33:160–172.

26. Yunus M, Masai A, Calabro J, et al. Primary fibromyalgia (fibrositis): clinical study of 50 patients with matched normal controls. *Semin Arthritis Rheum.* 1981;11:151–171.

27. Buchwald D. Fibromyalgia and chronic fatigue syndrome. Similarities and differences. *Rheum Dis Clin North Am.* 1996;22:219–243.

28. Crofford LJ, Demitrack MA. Evidence that abnormalities of central neurohormonal systems are key to understanding fibromyalgia and chronic fatigue syndrome. *Rheum Dis Clin North Am.* 1996;22:267–284.

29. Neeck G. Pathogenic mechanisms of fibromyalgia. *Ageing Res Rev.* 2002;1:243–255.

30. Russell IJ, Orr MD, Littman B, Viprano GA, Alboureck D, et al. Elevated cerebrospinal fluid levels of substance P in patients with fibromyalgia syndrome. *Arthritis Rheum.* 1994;37:1593–1601.

31. Neeck G, Crofford LJ. Neuroendocrine pertubations in fibromyalgia and chronic fatigue syndrome. *Rheum Dis Clin North Am.* 2000;26:989–1002.

32. Hudson J, Pope H. The relationship between fibromyalgia and major depressive disorder. *Rheum Dis Clin North Am.* 1996;22:285–303.

33. Lentjes E, Griep E, Boersma J, et al. Glucocorticoid receptors, fibromyalgia and low back pain. *Psychoneuroendocrinol.* 1997;22:603–614.

34. Hader N, Rimon D, Kinarty A, Lahat N. Altered interleukin-2 secretion in patients with primary fibromyalgia syndrome. *Arthritis Rheum.* 1991;34:866–872.

35. Hudson J, Pope H. The relationship between fibromyalgia and major depressive disorder. *Rheum Dis Clin North Am.* 1996;22:285–303.

36. Amir M, Kaplan Z, Neumann L, et al. Posttraumatic stress disorder, tenderness, and fibromyalgia. *J Psychosom Res.* 1997;42:607–613.

37. Wolfe F, Ross K, Anderson J, Russell IJ, Herbert L. The prevalence and general characteristics of fibromyalgia in the general population. *Arthritis Rheum.* 1995;38:19–28.

38. Simms R. Fibromyalgia syndrome: current concepts in pathophysiology, clinical features, and management. *Arthritis Care Res.* 1996;9:315–328.

39. McCain G. A cost-effective approach to the diagnosis and treatment of fibromyalgia. *Rheum Dis Clin North Am.* 1996;22:323–349.

40. Goldenberg D, Felson D, Dinerman H. A randomized, controlled trial of amitriptyline and naproxen in the treatment of patients with fibromyalgia. *Arthritis Rheum.* 1986;29:655–659.

41. Crofford L, Russell IJ, Mease P, et al. Pregabalin improves pain associated with fibromyalgia syndrome in a multicenter, randomized, placebo-controlled monotherapy trial. *Arthritis Rheum.* 2002;46(suppl):S613.

42. Merchant RE, Carmack CA, Wise CM. Nutritional supplementation with Chlorella pyrenoidosa for patients with fibromyalgia syndrome: a pilot study. *Phytother Res.* 2000;14:167–173.

43. Jacobsen S, Danneskiold-Samose B, Anderson RB. Oral S-adenosylmethionine in primary fibromyalgia. Double-blind clinical evaluation. *Scand J Rheumatol.* 1991;20:294–302.

44. Wigers SH, Stiles TC, Vogel PA. Effects of aerobic exercise versus stress management treatment in fibromyalgia. *Scand J Rheum.* 1996;25:77–86.

45. Hakkinen A, Hakkinen K, Hannonen P, Alen M. Strength training induced adaptations in neuromuscular function of premenopausal women with fibromyalgia: comparisons with healthy women. *Ann Rheum Dis.* 2001;60:21–26.

46. Jentoft ES, Kvalvik AG, Mengshoel AM. Effects of pool-based and land-based aerobic exercise on women with fibromyalgia/chronic widespread muscle pain. *Arthritis Care Res.* 2001;45:42–47.

47. Sunshine W, Field TM, Quintino O, et al. Fibromyalgia benefits from massage therapy and transcutaneous electrical stimulation. *J Clin Rheumatol.* 1996;2:18–22.

48. Kaplan KH, Goldenberg DL, Galvin-Nadeau M. The impact of a meditation-based stress reduction program on fibromyalgia. *Gen Hosp Psych.* 1993;15:284–289.

49. Kabat-Zinn J. *Full Catastrophe Living: Using the Wisdom of Your Body and Mind to Face Stress, Pain, Illness.* New York: Bantam Doubleday Dell; 1990.

50. Wigers SH, Stiles TC, Vogel PA. Effects of aerobic exercise versus stress management treatment in fibromyalgia. *Scand J Rheum.* 1996;25:77–86.

51. Ferraccioli G, Ghirelli L, Scita F, et al. EMG-biofeedback training in fibromyalgia syndrome. *J Rheumatol.* 1987;14:820–825.

52. Haanen HCM, Hoenderdos HTW, van Romunde

LKJ, et al. Controlled trial of hypnotherapy in the treatment of refractory fibromyalgia. *J Rheumatol.* 1991;18:72–75.

53. Sarno JE. *The Mind Body Prescription.* New York: Warner Books; 1998.

54. Fisher P, Greenwood A, Huskisson EC, et al. Effect of homeopathic treatment on fibrositis (primary fibromyalgia). *BMJ.* 1989;299:365–366.

55. Deluze C, Bosia L, Zirbs A, et al. Electroacupuncture in fibromyalgia: results of a controlled trial. *BMJ.* 1992;305:1249–1252.

56. Berman BM, Ezzo J, Hadhazy V, Swyers JP. Is acupuncture effective in the treatment of fibromyalgia. *J Fam Pract.* 1999;48:213–218.

57. Yunus M, Bennett R, Romano T, et al. Fibromyalgia consensus report: additional comments. *J Clin Rheum.* 1997;3:324–327.

58. Turk DC, Okifuji A, Sinclair JD, Starz T. Pain, disability, and physical functioning in subgroups of patients with fibromyalgia. *J Rheumatol.* 1996;23:1255–1262.

59. Selfridge N, Peterson F. *Freedom from Fibromyalgia. The 5-Week Program Proven to Conquer Pain.* New York: Three Rivers Press; 2001.

60. Lanyon P, Muir K, Doherty S. Assessment of a genetic contribution to osteoarthritis of the hip: sibling study. *BMJ.* 2000;321:1179–1183.

61. Lawrence RD, Everett D, Hochberg MC. Arthritis. In: Huntley R, Comoni-Huntley J, eds. *Health Status and Well-being of the Elderly: National Health and Nutrition Examination-I Epidemiologic Follow-up Survey.* Oxford, England: Oxford University Press; 1990.

62. Stange KC, Zyzanski JS, Jaen CR, et al. Illuminating the "black box": a description of 4454 patient visits to 138 family physicians. *J Fam Pract.* 1998;46:377–389.

63. Centers for Disease Control and Prevention. Prevalence of disabilities and associated health conditions—United States, 1991–1992. *JAMA.* 1994;272:735–736.

64. Van Baar ME, Assendelft WJJ, Dekker J, et al. Effectiveness of exercise therapy in patients with osteoarthritis of the hip or knee: a systematic review of randomized clinical trials. *Arthritis Rheum.* 1999;42;1361–1369.

65. McGoey BV, Deitel M, Saplys RJ, et al. Effect of weight loss on musculoskeletal pain in the morbidly obese. *J Bone Joint Surg.* 1990;72B:322–323.

66. Oliveria SA, Felson DT, Cirillo PA, Reed JI, Walker AM. Body weight, body mass index, and incident symptomatic osteoarthritis of the hand, hip, and knee. *Epidemiology.* 1999;10:161–166.

67. Bland JH, Cooper SM. Osteoarthritis: a review of the cell biology involved and evidence for reversibility. Management rationally related to known genesis and pathophysiology. *Semin Arthritis Rheum.* 1984;14:106–133.

68. Pizzonro JE, Murray MT. *Textbook of Natural Medicine: Osteoarthritis.* Edinburgh: Churchhill Livingstone; 1999:1444.

69. Miller-Fabbender H, Bach GL, Haase W, et al. Glucosamine sulfate compared to Ibuprofen in osteoarthritis of the knee. *Osteoarthritis Cartilage.* 1994;2:61–69.

70. Towheed TE, Anastassiades TP, Shea B, et al. Glucosamine therapy for treating osteoarthritis. *The Cochrane Library.* Oxford, England: Update Software; 2001.

71. Reginster JY, Deroisy R, Rovati LC, et al. Long-term effects of glucosamine sulfate on osteoarthritis progression: a randomized, placebo-controlled clinical trial. *Lancet.* 2001;357:251–256.

72. Russell AI, McCarty MF. Glucosamine in osteoarthritis. *Lancet.* 1999;354(9190):1640–1641.

73. Leeb BF, Scweitzer H, Montag K, et al. A meta-analysis of chondroitin sulfate in the treatment of osteoarthritis. *J Rheumatol.* 2000;27:1.

74. McAlindon TE, LaValley MP, Gulin JP, et al. Glucosamine and chondroitin for the treatment of osteoarthritis. A systematic quality assessment and meta-analysis. *JAMA.* 2000;283:1469–1475.

75. Di Padavoa D. S-adenosylmethionine in the treatment of osteoarthritis. Review of the clinical studies. *Am J Med.* 1987;83(5A):60–65.

76. Muller-Fassbender H. Double-blind clinical trial of S-adenosylmethionine versus ibuprofen in the treatment of osteoarthritis. *Am J Med.* 1987;83(suppl 5A):S89–S94.

77. Vetter G. Double-blind clinical trial with S-adenosylmethionine and indomethacin in the treatment of osteoarthritis. *Am J Med.* 1987;83(suppl 5A):S78–S80.

78. Soeken KL, Lee WL, Bausell RB, et al. Safety and efficacy of S-adenosylmethionine (SAMe) for osteoarthritis. *J Fam Pract.* 2002;51(5):425–430.

79. Perlman AI, Spierer MM. Osteoarthritis. In: Rakel DP, ed. *Integrative Medicine.* Philadelphia: WB Saunders; 2002:414–422.

80. Ernst E. The efficacy of Phytodolor for the treatment of musculoskeletal pain—a systematic review of randomized clinical trials. *Nat Med J.* 1999;2:14–16.

81. Blotman F, Maheu E, Wulwik A, et al. Efficacy and safety of avocado/soybean unsaponifiables in the treatment of symptomatic osteoarthritis of the knee and hip. A prospective, multicenter, three-month, randomized, double-blind, placebo-controlled trial. *Rev Rhum Engl Ed.* 1997;64: 825–834.

82. Maheu E, Mazieres B, Valat JP, et al. Symptomatic efficacy of avocado/soybean unsaponifiables in the treatment of osteoarthritis of the knee and hip: a prospective, randomized, double-blind, placebo-controlled, multicenter clinical trial with a six-month treatment period and two-month follow-up demonstrating a persistent effect. *Arthritis Rheum.* 1998;41:81–91.

83. Henrotin Y, Labasse A, Zheng SX, et al. Effects of three avocado/soybean unsaponifiable mixtures on human articular chondrocyte metabolism. *Clin Rheumatol* 1998;17(1):31–39.

84. Long L, Soeken K, Ernst E. Herbal medicines for the treatment of osteoarthritis: a systematic review. *Rheumatology.* 2001;40:779–793.

85. Zhang WY, Li Wan Po A. The effectiveness of topically applied capsaicin. A meta-analysis. *Eur J Clin Pharmacol.* 1994;46:517–522.

86. Kulkarni RR, Patki PS, Jog VP, et al. Treatment of osteoarthritis with a herbomineral formulation: a double-blind, placebo controlled, cross-over study. *J Ethnopharmacol.* 1991;33:91–95.

87. Bliddal H, Rosetzky A, Schlichting P, et al. A randomized, placebo-controlled, cross-over study of ginger extracts and ibuprofen in osteoarthritis. *Osteoarthritis Cartilage.* 2000;8:9–12.

88. Rene J, Weinberger M, Mazzuca SA, Brandt KD, Katz BP. Reduction of joint pain in patients with knee osteoarthritis who have received monthly telephone calls from lay personnel and whose medical treatment regimes have remained stable. *Arthritis Rheum.* 1992;35:511–515.

89. Keefe FJ, Caldwell DS, Baucom D, et al. Spouse-assisted coping skills training in the management of osteoarthritic knee pain. *Arthritis Care Res.* 1996;9.279–291.

90. Weinberger M, Hiner SL, Tierney WM. Improving functional status in arthritis: the effect of social support. *Soc Sci Med.* 1986;23:899–904.

91. Gay MC, Philippot P, Luminet O. Differential effectiveness of psychological interventions for reducing osteoarthritis pain: a comparison of Erickson hypnosis and Jacobson relaxation. *Eur J Pain.* 2002;6:1–16.

92. Ezzo J, Hadhazy V, Birch S, et al. Acupuncture for osteoarthritis of the knee: a systematic review. *Arthritis Rheum.* 2001;44(4):819–825.

93. Junnila SYT. Acupuncture is superior to piroxicam for the treatment of osteoarthritis. *Am J Acupunct.* 1982;10:341–345.

94. Deyle GD, Henderson NE, Matekel RL, et al. Effectiveness of manual physical therapy and exercise in osteoarthritis of the knee. A randomized, controlled trial. *Ann Intern Med.* 2000; 132(3):173–181.

95. Hauge M, Harvald B. Heredity in gout and hyperuricemia. *Acta Med Scand.* 1955;152: 247–257.

96. Emmerson BT. Heredity in primary gout. *Aust Ann Med.* 1960;9:168–175.

97. Roubenoff R. Gout and hyperuricemia. *Rheum Dis Clin North Am.* 1990;16:539–550.

98. Emmerson BT. The management of gout. *N Engl J Med.* 1996;334(7):445–451.

99. Wild JH, Zvaifler NJ. An office technique for identifying crystal in synovial fluid. *Am Fam Physician.* 1975;12:72–81.

100. Agudelo CA, Wise CM. Crystal-associated arthritis in the elderly. *Rheum Dis Clin North Am.* 2000;26:527–546.

101. Reynolds PP, Knapp MJ, Baraf HS, Holmes EW. Moonshine and lead. Relationship to the pathogenesis of hyperuricemia in gout. *Arthritis Rheum.* 1983;26:1057–1064.

102. Loghman-Adham M. Renal effects of environmental and occupational lead exposure. *Environ Health Perspect.* 1997;105:928–939.

103. Schmeda-Hirschmann G, Theoduloz C, Franco L, Ferro E, de Arias AR. Preliminary pharmacological studies on *Eugenia uniflora* leaves: xanthine oxidase inhibitory activity. *J Ethnopharmacol.* 1987;21:183–186.

104. Theoduloz C, Franco L, Ferro E, Hirschmann GS. Xanthine oxidase inhibitory activity of Para-

guayan Myrtaceae. *J Ethnopharmacol.* 1988; 24:179–183.

105. Theoduloz C, Pacheco P, Schmeda-Hirschmann G. Xanthine oxidase inhibitory activity of Chilean Myrtaceae. *J Ethnopharmacol.* 1991;33:253–255.

106. Chiang HC, Lo YJ, Lu FJ. Xanthine oxidase inhibitors from the leaves of Alsophila spinulosa (Hook) Tryon. *J Enzyme Inhib.* 1994;8:61–71.

107. Guerrero RO, Guzman AL. Inhibition of xanthine oxidase by Puerto Rican plant extracts. *PR Health Sci J.* 1998;17:359–364.

108. Chou CT, Kuo SC. The anti-inflammatory and anti-hyperuricemic effects of Chinese herbal formula danggui-nian-tong-tang on acute gouty arthritis: a comparative study with indomethacin and allopurinol. *Am J Chin Med.* 1995;23:261–271.

PART IV

Integrative Approaches Through the Life Cycle

CHAPTER 30

Integrative Approach to the Care of Children: Well-Child Care

Benjamin Kligler

There are many ways in which the integrative medicine approach to pediatrics and well-child care is very similar to that of conventional pediatrics. Both encourage a preventive approach to long term health. The important tasks of monitoring for normal growth and development and of providing anticipatory guidance to parents regarding safety issues, inform the practice of integrative pediatrics as they do conventional pediatrics. In addition, emphasis on the child as part of the family with attention to the role of the family in determining that child's health and well-being is important in both approaches.

This chapter focuses on the areas in which the integrative approach to well-child care may differ somewhat from the conventional approach. These differences arise from two sources: first, a strong conviction in integrative medicine that the patient—or in this case, the child and the parents—not the physician, is the most important decision maker in the therapeutic relationship; and second, a heightened awareness of and attention to the more natural approach to health and illness. These two core beliefs lead to a different approach to some of the controversial questions in well-child care than that taken by conventional pediatrics, an approach in which the practitioner's role is to assist the parent in gathering the available information, and in coming to an informed decision, rather than to act as the decision maker. This difference is particularly evident in discussing the issues of home birth versus hospital birth, co-sleeping or family bed, choices regarding childhood immunizations, fluoride supplementation, the place of television watching in a healthy child's life, and the discussion of environmental health as it applies to children.

► HOME BIRTH VERSUS HOSPITAL BIRTH

Although the decision regarding where to deliver a child is not typically considered part of the domain of the pediatrician, it often does arise in the context of a family with a child in a physician's care now planning to deliver their second or third child. Many families committed to a more natural approach to health care develop an interest in out-of-hospital birthing options and approach their child's physician for advice on the safety of this choice. Out-of-hospital birthing options include home birth, generally with the assistance of a midwife or a physician, or delivery at a birthing center. Women who choose these options typically cite a wish for more self-determination regarding the course of their labor, as well as a view of birthing not as a medical experience but as an empowering, personal spiritual experience not consistent with the typical hospital environment.[1]

Of the two out-of-hospital options, home birth is obviously the less conventional and more controversial, at least from the point of view of mainstream medicine. Many physicians believe that there are increased risks to mother and infant in a home birth that make it an unacceptable option. The American College of Obstetricians and Gynecologists explicitly opposes home birth based on safety concerns.[2] In fact, a close examination of the data regarding home birth calls into question these concerns regarding safety.

Generally, home birth statistics combine planned home births with unintentional out-of-hospital births. This can generate high perinatal mortality rates for home birth as a whole, which disappear when the unplanned out-of-hospital births are excluded. For example a study of home births from Kentucky[3] and North Carolina[4] found a neonatal mortality rate 18 to 20 times greater in the unplanned out-of-hospital birth category than in the planned home birth group. Other studies from Washington[5] and Missouri[6] confirm statistics showing an increased infant mortality rate when all out-of-hospital births are evaluated as a group. Likewise, the rates of infant mortality drop significantly when the unplanned out-of-hospital births are removed from analysis.

The most recent US data estimates a home birth rate of 0.6%, or roughly 26,000 births per year nationally.[7] In Holland, a nation with a perinatal mortality rate lower than that of the United States, 35% of births take place at home, with a perinatal mortality rate of 9.4 per 1,000 births (unadjusted for "planned" status").[8] A United Kingdom study found perinatal mortality rates of 7.8 per 1,000 for home births, which dropped to 4.1 per 1,000 when only planned home births were included.[9] The largest study to date of planned home births in the United States, which included more than 11,000 deliveries attended by a nurse midwife, found a perinatal mortality rate of 4.2 per 1,000.[10] These rates are very similar to the commonly cited rates for low-risk in-hospital births.

The importance of an adequately trained birth attendant and of adequate screening for conditions such as breech presentation, postdates delivery, and twin gestation—factors that can increase peripartum risk—cannot be overemphasized, and should be an important factor in counseling the family deciding on home versus hospital birth. For example, a study of midwife-attended planned home births in California and Wisconsin found that a higher-than-expected perinatal mortality rate of 14 per 1,000 births disappeared when breech deliveries, twins, and postdate pregnancies were excluded.[11] Clearly, an important part of advising the family on this choice is to counsel specifically that they inquire what the home birth practitioner's position is on breech, twins, and postdate situations.

The alternative perspective argues that many of the interventions that accompany conventional hospital birth—continuous fetal monitoring, for example—have not been shown to improve outcomes when studied in a systematic fashion. Although physicians in general believe that continuous monitoring is the safest possible approach to labor and delivery, studies show that this practice leads to higher rates of cesarian section and possibly to higher rates of birth-related neurological deficits.[12] The mounting evidence that technological intervention in the natural process of birthing is not always a positive influence is leading more parents to consider out-of-hospital birth an option.

There is no correct position on this question; however, the integrative approach to counseling parents on this decision is to assist them in gathering all the information relevant to their choice, and then to help them in processing the potential risks and benefits of each option.

▶ CO-SLEEPING/ "THE FAMILY BED"

In the 1990s, the popularity of the "attachment parenting" or "child-centered parenting" approach led many families to make a number of unconventional choices, including that of having young children sleep in the parental bed for an extended period. This would often extend up to several years of age. The rationale for this choice was derived from anthropological studies showing that humans in most traditional cultures co-sleep with their children during the first several years of life, suggesting that this may be a more "natural" way to sleep.[13] Despite the recent backlash against this parenting approach, many families continue to make this choice.

Several major objections have been raised to the family bed by conventional authorities in pediatrics. First, is the issue of safety: the question has been raised regarding whether there are cases of sudden infant death syndrome (SIDS), or otherwise unexplained infant deaths, that result from "overlying." Overlying is the asphyxiation of a child caused by a parent who accidentally rolls on top of the young child during the night. Second, the issue of whether co-sleeping somehow interferes with the development of proper sleep habits in the young child, and/or with the development of the proper sense of self-reliance and independence regarding sleep has been raised. Third, the issue of whether co-sleeping interferes with parental sexual intimacy, by discouraging sexual contact because of the child's presence in the parental bed, has been a concern.

Much of the recent concern about the safety of co-sleeping stems from a study by Nakamura et al. of 515 deaths reported between 1990 and 1997 in children younger than 2 years of age who were asleep in adult beds at the time of death.[14] This study found that 121 of these deaths were attributable to overlying. The authors concluded from this finding that co-sleeping with children younger than age 2 years is not a safe practice. Subsequent authors, although acknowledging the possibility of overlying as a real concern, have critiqued Nakamura's conclusions on the grounds that overlying is not readily distinguishable from SIDS as a cause of death. Without denominator data on how many children younger than age 2 years regularly sleep in adult beds, it is impossible to conclude whether or not these 121 deaths represent a higher-than-expected rate of SIDS. Thus, it is impossible to conclude from this data whether in fact children younger than age 2 years die more or less frequently in adult beds than when sleeping alone.

To date, there have been four large studies specifically designed to examine whether co-sleeping confers an increased risk of SIDS. One of these, a case control study of 200 SIDS deaths in California, found no increased risk with bed sharing.[15] Two other case-control studies, one of 393 cases from New Zealand[16] and one of 195 cases in England,[17] did find an increased risk in infants who shared a bed with parents, but only in families in which the mother smoked; in the New Zealand study, the risk of SIDS in co-sleeping infants of mothers who smoked was 4.5 times that of co-sleeping infants whose mother did not smoke. Finally a prospective study of 127 cases of SIDS, also done in New Zealand, found that bed sharing was a risk factor for SIDS only if the mother smoked.[18] The reason for this association with smoking is not clear, although it has been suggested that proximity to maternal smoking could impair the newborn's arousal response to hypoxia and by so doing increase the risk of asphyxiation and SIDS.[19] There has been absolutely no association found in any of the studies between co-sleeping and SIDS in families with nonsmoking parents. Clearly, this is not a safe practice in families with a mother who smokes.

There are a number of caveats that should qualify this statement, however, based on the data of Nakamura and others regarding other potential hazards for infants in adult beds. Water beds are clearly unsafe for young infants. Likewise, soft bedding probably increases asphyxiation risk. Bed rails may pose a risk as well, as an infant's head can become trapped between the rails if the item is not of proper dimensions. Parents should be cautioned that if they are choosing the family bed, the sleeping space must be made safe for the young infant. These hazards aside, it is reasonable to conclude on the question of safety that "except for infants whose mothers smoked during pregnancy, there is insufficient evidence to either support or reject infant co-sleeping."[20]

Some researchers have posited that co-sleeping, because of its influence on infant sleep patterning, may in fact reduce the incidence of SIDS. McKenna et al.[21] have found that co-sleeping mother–infant pairs experience more frequent infant arousals and a synchronization of mother's and infant's periods of arousal during the night. These investigators hypothesize that this "sensory-rich" environment is more consistent with normal infant growth and development as an evolutionary phenomenon than the practice of solitary infant sleep. They hypothesize as well—although this has not been shown to date—that this increased nighttime communication between mother and child may in fact reduce the risk of SIDS. Clearly more research on this is needed.

Conversely, other studies have alluded to potential problems with the family bed approach for many families. There is evidence that co-sleeping infants do wake more frequently, and also breast-feed more frequently than do infants sleeping alone. There is certainly decreased privacy for the parents and for most couples, and a decrease in the frequency of sexual relations as consequence of the co-sleeping choice. The impact of these facts on the family seeking advice from the integrative practitioner should not be underestimated.

Finally, conventional authorities often raise concerns regarding the question of whether children raised in the family bed have a higher incidence of ongoing sleep problems or of separation or independence problems later in childhood. There is no evidence to date of either of these being an issue. Child-rearing entails an ongoing and delicate balance between fostering independence and autonomy, and promoting a sense of family coherence, interdependence, and togetherness. The pendulum of pediatric advice continues to swing back and forth between these poles as it has for the past 50 or more years, and there is no clear evidence on the sleep question to point either toward or away from the family bed regarding development of a healthy, independent and connected child.

Once again, there is no right answer to the questions parents raise regarding sleep. However, an integrative management strategy should be one that fosters an atmosphere of open discussion to unconventional choices that may be appropriate for that particular family's situation. There should be the sense that it is really the parents who have the authority to make the right decisions regarding sleep for the infant and child. Thus the role of the physician is to serve as an advisor who helps them integrate the available information.

▶ FLUORIDE SUPPLEMENTATION

Since the 1940s, our society has relied on fluoride supplementation to reduce the risk of dental caries. This supplementation has been in the form of fluoridated water supplies, of oral fluoride supplements administered to young children, and of fluoridated dental products such as toothpaste and mouthwash. The data does clearly show that fluoride supplementation reduces the incidence of caries.[22]

However, over the years it has become clear that excessive fluoride poses certain risks, in particular the risk of dental fluorosis, a discoloration of the teeth. Additional concerns raised over the years have included bone health, mutagenic potential, and possible neurodevelopmental toxicity.

The possible role of fluoride in increased incidence of hip fractures has now been fairly extensively studied. There is an increased incidence of hip fractures and fractures overall in populations exposed to fluoride from drinking water at a level above 4.3 parts per million (ppm).[23] No increased risk has been shown in those ingesting water fluoridated at a level of 1 ppm, which is much more in the typical range for fluoridated water supplies. In fact, at this level it appears there may be a decreased fracture risk as compared to populations with no fluoride in their water.[23,24]

The issue of possible carcinogenicity or mutagenicity, which has concerned many parents, also seems to have been resolved by recent studies. Although there was initially found to be an increased incidence of osteogenic sarcoma in males in areas with fluoridated water supplies over the period from 1973 to 1987, the National Cancer Institute analysis of fluoridation concluded that this increased incidence was "unrelated to either the introduction or duration of fluoridation."[23] No other evidence has emerged to date of a mutagenic or carcinogenic effect of fluoride in humans.

Based on animal studies, there is some concern regarding an increased risk of hyperactivity in offspring of rats exposed to fluoride at only moderate levels during a critical stage of pregnancy for neurological development.[25] The implications of this for exposure during human pregnancy are not known; however, because there is no evidence to suggest that pregnant women need fluoridated water, it may be wise to counsel the use of nonfluoridated water sources during pregnancy. A population-based study from China found lower IQ levels in a community with fluoride levels over 4 ppm when compared to a community with a level under 1 ppm, even when other variables such as parental education level were controlled for.[26] This, again, suggests that fluoride levels should be maintained at or below 1.0–1.5 ppm in drinking water to reduce the risk of neurotoxicity.

In summary, it is safe to say that to date no major health problems are associated with consumption of fluoridated water at the relatively low levels that are used in most communities. It may be safest to avoid any fluoride during pregnancy if possible. It is also clear that excessive fluoride consumption does have significant potential health risks, and should be avoided.

What has also become clear recently, however, which most conventional pediatricians and family practitioners remain unaware of, is that the role of fluoride in caries prevention is not, as was originally thought, in the preeruptive phase, but rather in the disruption of plaque development on already erupted teeth.[27] What this means is that the previous recommendation for oral fluoride supplements in breast-fed babies who are not taking any fluoridated water is now completely incorrect. Some dental authorities have even proposed that fluoride supplementation will ultimately prove to be only beneficial in certain high-risk groups, and potentially should be used only in groups that are demonstrably at higher risk for caries.[28]

Thus, the parent of a breast-fed child who is drinking only nonfluoridated water can now be advised that although there is certainly a benefit from fluoride use, this benefit is not in the first 6 months of life. Although the current American Academy of Pediatrics guidelines recommend fluoridated water starting at 6 months,[29] it may be prudent to limit fluoride exposure even until 12–18 months, when dietary intake is fairly controlled and the number of foods somewhat limited. Fluoride supplementation is recommended now only for children who have no exposure to a fluoridated water supply. Thus there is no role for fluoride supplementation at all for many children, and

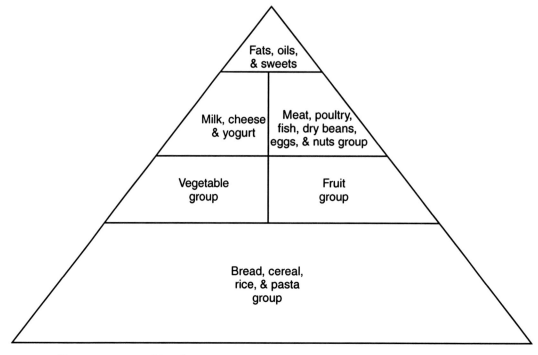

Figure 30–1.   USDA food guide pyramid.

perhaps none in anyone until 12–18 months of age when dental eruption has occurred and dietary exposure is such that risk of plaque development and cary formation becomes substantial.

Finally, given the known risks of excessive exposure, it is important to remind parents that there is no role for fluoride-containing toothpastes until the child is at least 2 years of age, as prior to that time toothpaste is generally ingested rather than expelled and this can put a child at risk for elevated fluoride levels and the attendant complications described above.[30]

However, equally important is to ensure that parents oriented toward the "natural" approach and suspicious of any intervention have adequate information about the importance of fluoride in caries prevention. The trust that has been lost because of overuse of this approach need not lead parents to reject an intervention that, if done in a more cautious and gentle way, can actually be very important in promoting dental health.

▶ TELEVISION

In every domain of integrative medicine, attention to the intimate connection between mind and body, both in terms of present-day health status and in terms of prevention, is a critical part of the practitioner's approach to the patient. Nowhere is this attention more critical than in advising patients on the risks of excessive television watching in childhood. Despite extensive research on this issue, conventional physicians have yet to take this on as a major focus of their work with their pediatric patients; unfortunately, because of the pervasive influence of commercial television and advertising in our culture, health care practitioners must take the lead in speaking up regarding

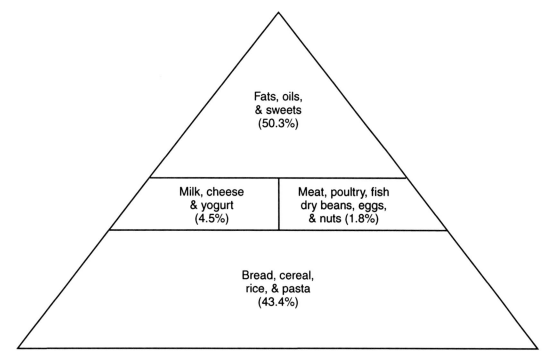

Figure 30-2. Foods recommended to children by television advertisments on Saturday morning. *Reproduced with permission from Kotz K, Story M. Food advertisements during children's Saturday morning television programming: are they consistent with dietary recommendations? J Am Diet Assoc. 1994;94:1296–1300.*

this problem. Furthermore, although the evidence to date has emerged from studies of television watching and not of video game use or extensive computer use in young children, it is likely that many of the same risks will apply to these behaviors as well because they all share many similar qualities.

The best-studied risk associated with excessive television watching is childhood obesity. Obesity is perhaps the leading health problem confronting us in America, and once established is extremely difficult to treat. Childhood obesity has been correlated with obesity in adulthood and its attendant increased morbidity and mortality.[31] Using data from the National Health and Nutrition Examination Survey (NHANES II), Andersen et al. found that chil-

dren aged 8 to 16 years who watched 4 or more hours of television daily had a significantly greater percentage of body fat and significantly greater body mass index (BMI) than did children who watch less than 2 hours per day.[32] Using a different database, Gortmaker et al. found similarly that in youths aged 10 to 15 years, watching more than 5 hours of television daily was associated with a greater than eightfold risk in the incidence of obesity as compared to watching 2 hours or less per day.[33]

The reason for the association between television-watching and obesity is thought to stem from the reduced physical activity associated with television, combined with the increased consumption of calories associated with snacking while watching. An interesting study by two nutritionists examined the nature of advertising during children's programming, and found what may be yet another important part of this connection. Of the 564 food advertisements studied from a Saturday morning selection of children's television programming, more than half were for food, such that roughly every 5 minutes a child was exposed to a food commercial. Of these, 33% were for high-sugar cereals and 11% were for fast-food restaurants.[34] Viewed differently, 50.3% of the food commercials were for foods classified as high in fats, oils, and sweets by USDA food pyramid criteria (Figures 30–1 and 30–2). Thus, not only are children not physically active while watching television, they are being advised by advertisers to eat the food most likely to lead to unhealthy weight gain.

On average, "screen time" for most American children—which includes computer and video games, as well as television watching—has most likely increased over the past decade with the advent of Internet for children. It is not known if these activities, which are somewhat less passive than standard television watching and not subject to the same advertising barrage, will lead to the same degree of overeating and obesity that is associated with television watching. If so, we may see an even more dramatic rise in childhood obesity as a function of the 'Internet age.'

Although the data is clear, the strategy for parents is not always so. Counseling no television and no other "screen time" is perhaps not a reasonable strategy in our society if children are to be allowed to engage in normal social discourse. Based on the data, however, it does seem that advising parents to restrict overall screen time to less than 2 hours daily will probably prevent most of the obesity risk associated with excessive television watching. Many parents may choose to go beyond this because of concerns regarding the influence of mass media and culture on the developing mind of their young children; this is much more difficult to study objectively and will remain a personal choice for parents.

► CHILDHOOD IMMUNIZATIONS

The conventional approach to advising parents regarding childhood immunization has been to consider it a nonnegotiable area, with the only acceptable choice being to follow the standard vaccination schedule as defined by the Advisory Committee on Immunization Practices, the American Academy of Pediatrics, and the American Academy of Family Physicians. Many pediatricians and family practitioners carry this to the extreme of refusing to continue to care for unvaccinated children in their practices.

The problem with this approach is that for the parent who is questioning some of the standard recommendations regarding well-child care, including the sanctity of the conventional vaccination schedule, it leaves no room for discussion or dialogue. In fact, it can often force parents who are confused and potentially open to discussion on the subject into a more radical position of refusing all vaccinations, because of the mistrust engendered by the authoritarian, "doctor knows best" approach. A more open, patient/parent-centered, "common ground" approach to this problem—which is what is dictated here by the philosophy of integrative medicine as it is in all situations—is often successful in not only keeping these families in the care of reasonable physicians, but in helping them embrace at least some of the childhood immunizations.

The best way to approach this subject is to look at the most pressing concerns on both sides of the discussion. Physicians are concerned with the public health mandate to continue vaccination, an understandable concern given the degree to which mandatory immunization has been successful in reducing a number of serious childhood illnesses. The decision of an individual family to forego vaccination for their child clearly poses a threat to this mandate and opens the door to resurgence of a number of childhood diseases. For most physicians, the other primary concern is the health of the individual child, and the risk of that particular child contracting a vaccine-preventable disease and having a bad outcome. These are both completely valid concerns, and must be taken seriously by the parents if there is to be an open and serious discussion of the options. The physician, however, must also be open to questioning some of his or her assumptions; for example, is the public health mandate regarding vaccination against varicella as compelling as those regarding rubella or polio?

The parent's primary concerns are as follows:

1. Are the vaccines absolutely necessary? What are the risks to my child of not vaccinating against each of the diseases in question? Are all the vaccines recommended in the conventional schedule absolutely necessary for my child?
2. Are the vaccines safe? What are the short-term side effects? What are the long-term side effects?
3. Are there more natural alternatives that are effective in preventing these diseases?

The third question is the simplest to address: There are no alternative strategies for preventing pertussis, tetanus, diphtheria, polio, *Haemophilus influenzae* Type b meningitis, measles, or any of the other common childhood illnesses that have been tested adequately for the physician to be able to recommend them with confidence. There are homeopathic vaccination protocols for a number of these diseases, but the efficacy of these has not been systematically examined. Many parents feel that if they maintain a state of "healthy immune function" in their child through diet, supplements, herbs, or other approaches, the child will be more resistant to these illnesses. This approach also has not been adequately studied.

The first and second questions are much more difficult to address definitively, as they require that each vaccine in the schedule be considered individually. The continuing expansion of the recommended schedule to include more of the typically non–life-threaten-ing illnesses, such as chicken pox, make this effort even more challenging. Many parents, for example, question the inclusion of hepatitis B in the childhood vaccination schedule. Although from a public health perspective the decision to administer this vaccine to infants may be correct, from the point of view of a parent seeking a more natural approach to child rearing, it makes little sense. Thus, to proceed with this type of approach to the discussion of vaccination with parents, the physician must be open to the idea of a modified vaccination schedule decided upon in a partnership between physician and parent. Options might include starting somewhat later than the recommended 2 months of age; in fact the immunization schedules in many other highly developed countries do start later than we do in the United States. A second option might be to forgo vaccines for certain conditions for which the newborn is not at risk until the second or third year of life. These might include hepatitis B, as mentioned above, and polio, for the child whose family is not planning to travel outside the United States, where polio is no longer endemic. The ability to offer a family options—and to give the greater sense of control over the risk that comes with having options—is an invaluable tool for the physician working to help a family apprehensive regarding vaccination to make the right choices. Study of risk communication clearly shows that a patient with more perceived control in a given situation is much more likely to be willing to assume a risk than is a patient offered no choices or control.[35]

The questions regarding safety are very difficult to answer. Two widely cited Institute of Medicine committee reports from 1991 and 1994 concluded that there was either no or inadequate research to draw conclusions regarding 66% of the 76 vaccine adverse reactions they reviewed.[36] Although ongoing efforts to gather more information regarding adverse effects are significant—including the Vaccine Safety Datalink project, a CDC-sponsored project using active surveillance on a population of

500,000 children to assess for causality in adverse vaccine effects—there remains a great deal of uncertainty regarding the potential for extremely rare but serious short-term complications of vaccinations such as encephalopathy, Guillain-Barré syndrome, and others.[37]

A more significant problem for the physician counseling the "natural health"-oriented parent, which is of even greater concern to these parents than the short-term adverse effects, is the potential for long-term health effects from vaccination. This area has even less-reliable data at hand than that of short-term effects. Parent concerns generally focus around two questions: first, the possible long-term toxicity, neurological and otherwise, from the preservatives used in vaccine manufacture. This concern reached a peak around the use of thimerosal, a mercury-based preservative agent, in many childhood vaccines. As more information has become available regarding the potential long-term neurotoxicity of mercury, it has become clear that this is not an appropriate agent for use in vaccines. The FDA mandated removal of this agent from all single-dose vaccine preparations as of March 2002; however, thimerosal is still in use in multidose vials of the common childhood vaccines. Furthermore, other potentially toxic agents, such as formaldehyde, are still in wide use, and little is known about the potential health risks of these agents.

The second major area of concern for most parents concerns the fear of an increased risk of autism in children who are vaccinated, particularly as a consequence of the measles-mumps-rubella vaccine. This fear stems from a case series of several children with autism and chronic diarrhea who were found to have measles antibodies in the lining of their gastrointestinal tract.[38] The authors of this study concluded that the presence of such antibodies was potentially linked to the development of autism in these children. Subsequent population-based studies, including a large Danish study of more than 500,000 children published

in 2002, have failed to demonstrate a link of a magnitude large enough to be measured; however, the possibility that a causal connection could exist is virtually impossible to rule out definitively.[39,40] Even if the risk of such an outcome is 1 in 1 million, many parents feel that where the outcome is so negative, there is no level of risk that is tolerable. Table 30–1 outlines factors influencing perception of risk.

The administration of measles-mumps-rubella vaccine as three separate shots has been advocated by some as a way to reduce the potential risk of autism following measles-mumps-rubella vaccination. The rationale for this approach is that prevaccination studies show that children who developed measles and mumps simultaneously had a much higher likelihood of developing a chronic diarrhea. If, in fact, this diarrhea is related to the development of autism as the case series cited above posits, then the risk of diarrhea might be decreased by administering the vaccines separately. This approach has not been studied, and requires a number of assumptions regarding connection and causality that might not be correct. However, because the decision to administer the vaccines separately has little downside, many parents are making this choice. Being open to accepting this strategy is another way for the integrative physician to help the parents attain a level of control in the decision-making process, which may make the perceived risks of vaccination acceptable to the concerned parent.

▶ **TABLE 30–1** FACTORS IN RISK PERCEPTION

High Risk	Low Risk
Unfamiliar	Familiar
Mandatory	Voluntary
Synthetic	Natural
Unknown	Known
System control	Individual control
Commission	Omission

Adapted from Chen R, Hibbs B. Vaccine safety: current and future challenges. Pediatr Ann. 1998;27(7):453.

Effective communication on the subject of vaccinations poses one of the greatest challenges to the integrative practitioner committed to natural methods and family-centered care who is also committed to the importance of childhood immunization. Skills in negotiation and an understanding of risk communication, as well as a familiarity with the real facts where they are available, are essential to successful communication with parents on this subject.

▶ ENVIRONMENTAL HEALTH

Counseling on environmental health issues is particularly critical to the health of children. Although conventional pediatrics has emphasized the dangers of certain environmental hazards—in particular exposure to lead, tobacco smoke, and ethanol (in utero)—and has instituted routine screening for exposures to these toxins, there are other potential toxic exposures that, to date, have not been adequately attended to. In particular, exposure of children to pesticides, mercury, organic solvents, dioxins and polychlorinated biphenyls (PCBs), and certain plastics can pose significant risks to normal brain development. As with the damaging role of television for many children discussed above, a true commitment to the preventive approach requires a heightened awareness of and commitment to screening and counseling about these environmental threats to our young patients.

Not surprisingly, children in poor communities and children of color bear a disproportionate burden of the risk of exposure to many of these hazards. Lead paint exposure in deteriorated houses is the most commonly cited example of this, and African American children have rates of lead poisoning more than double those of non-Hispanic white children.[41] Less well known is the fact that toxic waste sites, which may be sources of dioxin and PCB exposure, are more likely to be located in areas with a higher concentration of racial and ethnic minorities, and that African American, Hispanic, and Native American children are disproportionately represented in communities with a toxic waste site.[42] Although this may simply be a function of socioeconomic status rather than race, it is clear that practitioners caring for children of poor families and children of color must be especially alert for possible environmental exposures.

There are several reasons why exposure of young children to environmental toxins is an even more serious problem than exposure of adults. First, the brain and nervous system are still actively developing in the first few years of life. Exposure to a neurotoxin during this crucial period of brain development can have consequences far exceeding that of exposure after brain development is completed. For example, exposure to PCBs while in utero (studied in women who ate Lake Michigan fish during pregnancy and lactation) has been linked to significantly lower IQ scores and reading comprehension at age 11 years.[43] Interestingly, this study found that although larger concentrations of PCBs were transferred in breast milk than in utero, there was no impairment associated with only breast-feeding; this suggests that the fetal brain may be uniquely sensitive to this neurotoxin.

The second reason that fetal or childhood exposure is uniquely dangerous is that many neurotoxins act via cumulative exposure over time. A child exposed repeatedly to a toxin at an early age has a greater probability of developing a problem associated with that exposure over the course of his or her lifetime than someone exposed later in life. For example, many of the commonly used pesticides are known to be neurotoxic. Children are frequently exposed to herbicides, insecticides, and fungicides via careless home use. If exposure to home pesticide use is a lifetime risk factor for Parkinson's disease, as recent studies seem to indicate,[44] it is likely that exposure in childhood will pose an even more significant risk than exposure in adulthood. This "duration of exposure" issue is equally pertinent for exposure to solvents and other possible mutagens. Finally, because children have a faster metabolic rate than adults and tend to eat more fruits and vegetables and drink more milk per body weight than adults, the ratio of toxic intake to body mass in children can be much greater for certain toxins, particularly for pesticides.[45]

Because there are no established treatments for toxic injury after the fact, screening and prevention are the cornerstones of the approach to environmental medicine in children. Just as we currently screen every child for exposure to lead and tobacco smoke, we must begin to inquire regarding exposure to pesticides via home use or via diet, to mercury via excessive fish consumption or defective mercury thermometers, to dioxins and PCBs, and to commonly used solvents. Parents' occupations and hobbies are critical—certain toxins can be brought home on clothing, or from a home workshop or studio. Sources of solvent exposure near the home, such as dry cleaners, gas stations, auto repair shops, and industrial sites, should be identified. Safety of the drinking water is important as well.

A number of simple strategies can dramatically reduce the exposure of our children to certain toxins. Installing a water filter for drinking water, making sure parents with potential toxic exposures at work change clothes before entering common areas of the house, and disposing of mercury thermometers are just a few of the obvious steps parents can take. Avoiding products such as toxic home pesticides or insecticides, cleaning solutions containing strong solvents, and conventional glues and adhesives are other simple steps. Plastic wraps on foods should be avoided as certain chemicals from the plastic, which may be subtle endocrine disrupters, may be unintentionally absorbed into food; in particular, food should not be microwaved or stored in plastic containers if possible.

Avoidance of these environmental hazards is particularly important during pregnancy. Just as the impact of one glass of alcohol daily during pregnancy can be substantial, so might that of a relatively small exposure to other solvents. Installing new carpets or doing extensive painting or home renovation during pregnancy should probably be avoided. Dry-cleaned clothes should be removed from their wrappers and placed in a well-ventilated area to reduce exposure to perchloroethylene, a toxic solvent used in dry cleaning. Likewise, home use of pesticides during pregnancy should be avoided if at all possible.

Perhaps the single most important way in which a parent can have an impact on the exposure of their child to environmental toxins is in the type of diet they choose. Dioxins and PCBs, produced by waste incineration, paper manufacture, and a variety of other industrial processes, are now ubiquitous in the environment and in our foods. Because these substances—like many other neurotoxins—concentrate in fat, they are present in much greater concentrations in animal products; in fact, meats and dairy products are thought to account for at least 95% of current human exposure to dioxins and PCBs.[21] Choosing a more plant-based diet and emphasizing organic foods, particularly if a family is consuming animal products, can significantly reduce exposure to this highly toxic class of chemicals. When animal products are eaten, low-fat meats and dairy products should be chosen as they will contain lower concentrations by weight of dioxins. Highly processed meats, such as hot dogs and lunch meats, are extremely high in fat, and should probably be totally avoided if possible.

Pesticide consumption can be largely eliminated by choosing organic produce. If this is not possible, peeling or washing may reduce or eliminate some of the residues, but in many cases, the pesticide residue is concentrated in the actual fruit or vegetable and peeling is not an effective strategy. The FDA has published lists describing which fruits and vegetables generally contain the greatest pesticide residues and parents may choose to avoid, or at least limit, these foods if organic products are not available.

The major avoidable source of mercury in our environment is in fish. Freshwater fish from many areas are now contaminated and should be avoided, particularly by pregnant and lactating women. Ocean fish, such as swordfish and fresh tuna that have high mercury levels should also be avoided. Canned tuna is considered by the EPA to have "moderate" mercury levels, meaning that consumption of one can per week by a pregnant woman is considered safe. However, given that no safe level of mercury consumption has been conclusively established, even this should probably be avoided if possible. The safety of fish consumption in young children has not been adequately evaluated; however, given that mercury is potentially neurotoxic and that the potential impact on the developing brain of even a modest exposure could be significant, it is probably wise to restrict the consumption of any fish with moderate or high mercury levels by young children.

As with all the areas discussed in this chapter, there are few "right or wrong" answers regarding protecting our children from environmental hazards. We live in a complex world, and exposures are inevitable. Active screening and counseling on this subject, however, can help put parents in a well-informed enough position to make the choices that are best for their particular family.

REFERENCES

1. Jackson ME, Bailer AJ. Home birth with certified nurse-midwife attended in the United States an overview. *J Nurse Midwifery.* 1995;40:6493–6506.
2. *Statement of Home Delivery. Statement of Policy issued by the Executive Board of the American Board of Obstetricians and Gynecologists.* Washington, DC: American Board of Obstetricians and Gynecologists; March 1999.
3. Hinds MW, Bergeisen GH, Allen DT. Neonatal outcomes in planned v unplanned out-of-hospital births in Kentucky. *JAMA.* 1985;253(11):1578–1582.
4. Burnett CA, Jones JA, Rooks J, et al. Home delivery and neonatal mortality in North Carolina. *JAMA.* 1980;244:2741–2745.
5. Janssen PA, Holt VL, Myers SJ. Licensed midwife attended, out-of-hospital births in Washington state: are they safe? *Birth.* 1994;21:141–148.
6. Schramm WF, Barnes DE, Bakewell JM. Neonatal mortality in Missouri home births, 1978–84. *Am J Public Health.* 1987;77:930–935.
7. Ventura SJ, Martin JA, Taffel SM, et al. Report of final natality statistics. 1996. *Mon Vital Stat Rep.* 1998;46(225):1–99.
8. Van Alten D, Eskes M, Treffers PE. Midwifery in the Netherlands; the Wormerveer study: selection, mode of delivery, perinatal mortality, and infant morbidity. *Br J Obstet Gynaecol.* 1989;96:656–662.
9. Hosmer L. Home birth. *Clin Obstet Gynecol.* 2001; 44(4):671–680.
10. Anderson RE, Murphy PA. Outcomes of 11,788 planned home births attended by certified nurse-midwives: a retrospective, descriptive study. *J Nurse Midwifery.* 1995;40:483–492.
11. Mehl-Madrona L, Madrona MM. Physician and midwife attended home births effects of breech, twin and postdates; outcome data on mortality rates. *J Nurse Midwifery.* 1997;42(2):91–103.
12. Nelson KB, Dambrosia JM, Ting TY, Grether JK. Uncertain value of electronic fetal monitoring in predicting cerebral palsy. *N Engl J Med.* 1996; 334(10):613–618.
13. McKenna JJ, Mosko SS. Sleep and arousal, synchrony and independence among mothers and infants sleeping apart and together: an experiment in evolutionary medicine. *Acta Paediatr Suppl.* 1994;397:94–102.
14. Nakamura S, Wind M, Danello MA. Review of hazards associated with children placed in adult beds. *Arch Pediatr Adolesc Med.* 1999;153: 1019–1023.
15. Klonoff-Cohen H, Edelstein SL. Bed sharing and the sudden infant death syndrome. *BMJ.* 1995;311:1269–1272.
16. Scragg R, Mitchell EA, Taylor BJ, et al. Bed sharing, smoking, and alcohol in the sudden infant death syndrome: New Zealand Cot Death Study Group. *BMJ.* 1993;307:1312–1318.
17. Fleming PJ, Blair PS, Bacon C, et al. Environment of infants during sleep and risk of the sudden infant death syndrome: results of 1993–1995 case-control study for confidential inquiry into stillbirths and deaths in infancy. *BMJ.* 1996;313: 191–195.

18. Mitchell EA, Tuohy PG, Brunt JM, et al. Risk factors for sudden infant death syndrome following the prevention campaign in New Zealand: a prospective study. *Pediatrics.* 1997;100:835–840.

19. Lewis KW, Bosque EM. Deficient hypoxia awakening response in infants of smoking mothers: possible relationship to sudden infant death syndrome. *J Pediatr.* 1995;127:691–699.

20. Rosenberg KD. Sudden infant death syndrome and co-sleeping. *Arch Pediatr Adolesc Med.* 2000;154(5):529–530.

21. McKenna J, Mosko S, Richar C, et al. Experimental studies of infant-parent co-sleeping: mutual physiological and behavioral influences and their relevance to SIDS. *Early Hum Dev.* 1994;38(3): 187–201.

22. CDC. Public health service report on fluoride benefits and risks. MMWR *Morb Mortal Wkly Rep.* 1991;40(RR-7):1–8.

23. Li Y, Liang C, Slemenda CW, et al. Effect of Long-term exposure to fluoride in drinking water on risks of bone fractures. *J Bone Miner Res.* 2001; 16(5):932–939.

24. Cauley JA, Murphy PA, Riley TJ, Buhari AM. Effects of fluoridated drinking water on bone mass and fractures: the study of osteoporotic fractures. *J Bone Miner Res.* 1995;10(7):1076–1086.

25. Mulleinix PJ, Denbesten PK, Schunior A, et al. Neurotoxicity of sodium fluoride in rats. *Neurotoxicol Teratol.* 1995;17(2):169–177.

26. Greater Boston Physicians for Social Responsibility. *In Harm's Way: Toxic Threats to Child Development.* Boston, MA. 2000:1–140.

27. Burt BA. The case for eliminating the use of dietary fluoride supplements for young children. *J Public Health Dent.* 1999;59(4):269–74.

28. Riordan PJ. The place of fluoride supplements in caries prevention today. *Aust Dent J.* 1996;41(5): 335–342.

29. American Academy of Pediatrics Committee on Nutrition. Fluoride supplementation for children: interim policy recommendations. *Pediatrics.* 1995; 95(5):777.

30. Record S, Montgomery DF, Milano M. Practice guidelines: fluoride supplementation and caries prevention. *J Pediatr Health Care.* 2000;14: 247–249.

31. Nieto FJ, Szklo M, Comstock GW. Childhood weight and growth rate as predictors of adult mortality. *Am J Epidemiology.* 1992;136:201–213.

32. Andersen RE, Crespo CJ, Bartlett SJ, et al. Relationship of physical activity and television watching with body weight and level of fatness among children: results from the Third National Health and Nutrition Examination Survey. *JAMA.* 1998; 279(12):938–942.

33. Gortmaker SL, Must A, Sobol A, et al. Television viewing as a cause of increasing obesity among children in the United States, 1986–1990. *Arch Pediatr Adolesc Med.* 1996;150(4):356–362.

34. Kotz K, Story M. Food advertisements during children's Saturday morning television programming: are they consistent with dietary recommendations? *J Am Diet Assoc.* 1994;94:1296–1300.

35. Ball LK, Evans G, Bostrom A. Risky business: challenges in vaccine risk communication. *Pediatrics.* 1998;101(3):453–458.

36. Chen RT, Hibbs B. Vaccine safety: current and future challenges. *Pediatr Ann.* 1998;27(7):445–455.

37. Shoenfeld Y, Aron-Maor A. Vaccination and autoimmunity—"vaccinosis": a dangerous liaison? *Journal of Autoimmunity.* 2000;14(1):1–10.

38. Wakefield AJ, Murch SH, Anthony A, et al. Ileal-lymphoid-nodular hyperplasia, non-specific colitis, and pervasive developmental disorder in children. *Lancet.* 1998;351:637–641.

39. Madsen KM, Hviid A, Vestergarrd M, et al. A population-based study of measles, mumps, and rubella vaccination and autism. *N Engl J Med.* 2002; 347:1477–1482.

40. Taylor B, Miller E, Farrington CP, et al. Autism and measles, mumps, and rubella vaccine: no epidemiological evidence for a causal association. *Lancet.* 1999;353:2026–2029.

41. CDC. Update: blood lead levels United States, 1991–1994. *MMWR Morb Mortal Wkly Rep.* 1997; 46(7):141–146.

42. Children's Environmental Health Network. An introduction to children's environmental health. Available at: http://www.cehn.org/cehn/Whatis PEH.html. Accessed: February 20, 2003.

43. Jacobson JL, Jacobson SW. Intellectual impairment in children exposed to polychlorinated biphenyls in utero. *N Engl J Med.* 1996;335(11):783–789.

44. Stephenson J. Exposure to home pesticides linked to Parkinson's disease. *JAMA.* 2000;283(23): 3055–3056.

45. National Research Council. *Pesticides in the Diets of Infants and Children.* Washington, DC: National Academy Press; 1993.

CHAPTER 31

Integrative Approach to Common Pediatric Conditions

BENJAMIN KLIGLER, SANFORD NEWMARK, LEWIS MEHL-MADRONA,
JAMAL ISLAM, AND SUSAN GERIK

The integrative approach to pediatric care poses two unique challenges. First, the logistical and ethical challenges of clinical research are particularly difficult in children. Thus, there exists significantly less research on the applications of unconventional approaches to health problems in this population of patients. Even for conventional treatments, there is often much less hard evidence of efficacy in children, and clinicians tend to extrapolate liberally from clinical research on adults. Second, many of the tools commonly used in integrative practice—dietary manipulation, herbals, and acupuncture, for example—are difficult to implement with children. Yet, this is a population of patients most in need of the nontoxic, more gentle treatment options—many of which are available in the integrative approach.

This chapter describes the integrative approach to the treatment of four common childhood conditions: infantile colic, atopic dermatitis, autism-spectrum disorders, and acne. Other common conditions in pediatric medicine, such as asthma, allergy, and recurrent otitis, are covered elsewhere in this text.

▶ INFANTILE COLIC

Pathophysiology

Infantile colic is a poorly understood condition defined as "excessive crying in an otherwise healthy baby." The most commonly used definition of colic defines excessive crying as lasting at least 3 hours a day on at least 3 days per week, for at least 3 weeks.[1] Many investigators in recent years, however, have questioned the validity of this definition; some have proposed that colic may represent simply an extreme point on the normal continuum of infant crying patterns. Among those who view colic as a pathological state, there are two prevailing theories on etiology, neither of which has yet been proven correct: (1) colic represents a dysfunction of the gastrointestinal tract, related either to milk intolerance or to excess gas production; and (2) colic is a "behavioral" problem in which the difficult constitutional temperament of an infant leads to disordered parent–infant interaction, which leads, in turn, to maladaptive parental reactions to the crying and thus to further symptoms.

Incidence

Depending on the definition used and the study population, the incidence of colic varies from 3–40%; prospective studies tend to identify a lower rate, in the range of 5–19%.[2] There are no consistently reported differences in incidence based on sex of the infant, on socioeconomic status, type of feeding (breast versus formula), parental smoking, or family history of atopic conditions.[3]

Conventional Treatment Approach

Three pharmacological agents have been studied for the treatment of colic: simethicone, dicyclomine, and methylscopolamine. Simethicone, although still widely used, was found to be without adverse effects but also without significant benefits in two of three randomized controlled trials (RCTs).[4] Dicyclomine, an anticholinergic agent, was found to be effective but had such frequent side effects (drowsiness and constipation being the most common) that the manufacturer now no longer recommends its use in children younger than 6 months of age.[4] Methylscopolamine was found to be neither safe nor effective.[4] Dietary manipulation as described below has also been part of the standard approach to colic.

Integrative Treatment Approach

Nutritional Approaches

The most extensively studied strategy for treating colic is the use of a hypoallergenic diet either in the mother, in the case of the breast-fed infant, or in the infant formula, in the case of the bottle-fed infant. Hill et al. randomized breast-feeding mothers to a diet free of milk, wheat, eggs, and nuts, and found a reduction of greater than 25% in colic symptoms over an 8-day period in 61% of infants.[5] Of those in the control group in this study, who remained on a maternal diet including all of the above food

groups, 43% demonstrated improvement, and the difference between the groups was statistically significant. The same authors randomized formula-fed babies to a hypoallergenic formula and again found significantly greater improvement in colic scores in the treatment group as compared to placebo. Interestingly, although cow's milk is commonly identified as the likely culprit for food sensitivity in infants with colic, neither of the two RCTs that studied the use of lactase in formula demonstrated any benefit.[6,7] Thus, if cow's milk is implicated, it is almost certainly the milk protein as opposed to the lactose fraction that is responsible for the colic symptoms. It is also possible that the response to hypoallergenic diet in the breast-fed population may represent a food sensitivity to something other than milk. This question needs to be clarified in further research studies.

The substitution of a soy-based formula has been examined in one trial using a crossover design.[8] This trial found that infants had significantly fewer hours of crying during the soy formula periods as compared to the control formula periods. This study has been criticized for inadequate blinding of the parents to the type of formula used during each study period, which could have introduced bias in reporting.

Two RCTs recently found that the use of sucrose solution was associated with a short-term decrease in crying. One of these trials defined this decrease as less than 3 minutes in duration[9] and the other as less than 30 minutes,[10] but both found the effect significantly greater than that of a placebo solution. In one of these studies, 89% of infants were reported to respond to the sucrose, as compared to 32% responding to placebo.[33] Although this strategy provides only short-term relief, and although extensive use of sucrose in a young child would seem intuitively to have other potential drawbacks, the use of sucrose solution should be considered on an occasional basis if the family stress warrants an intervention that is simple and likely to be effective.

One approach that has not been studied to date but is intuitively appealing is the use of probiotics for colic. Probiotics are the class of intestinal microbes including *Lactobacillus, Saccharomyces, Bifidobacterium,* and others felt to be essential to the maintenance of a healthy balance of flora in the gut. If, in fact, the crying of colic is related to gastrointestinal dysfunction of some kind, it seems plausible that this dysfunction could be related to an imbalance in the gut flora. The fetal gut is colonized with flora ingested during the passage through the birth canal. If maternal fecal flora are not in a healthy balance, why wouldn't the infant manifest with a symptom stemming from the proliferation of this disordered flora? The use of probiotics in pediatric populations has been studied to date in the treatment of antibiotic-associated diarrhea, infectious diarrhea, and intestinal allergy with promising results for all.[11] There are no known or reported adverse effects of probiotic supplementation. Given the possible link with food allergy discussed above and the lack of adverse effects, the use of probiotics would seem a potentially promising strategy for treatment of infantile colic.

Herbal Medicine

Various herbal remedies are often recommended to parents for treatment of colic. Weizman et al. compared an herbal tea preparation containing chamomile, vervain, licorice, balm mint, and fennel to placebo in a randomized controlled trial in 1993.[12] Infants were given up to 150 mL of this tea three times daily; after 1 week, 57% of the children in the treatment group were significantly improved, as compared to 26% of those in the placebo group. All of these herbs are traditional digestive aids, and the possibility that a simpler preparation containing fewer herbs might be effective has not yet been studied.

Manipulative Medicine

Chiropractic manipulation for colic has been popular in the Scandinavian countries for many years and has recently begun to gain in popularity in the United States. The manipulation strategy most commonly used involves palpa-

tion of the infant's spinal articulations and mobilization of misaligned areas using fingertip pressure; the rationale for this approach is that dysfunctional spinal segments may cause visceral pain via the effect on the parasympathetic nervous system. Three trials to date have shown conflicting results. The first, a large prospective trial by Klougart, in 1989, showed a positive effect of manipulation but lacked a control group.[13] The second, a randomized trial by Wiberg with a blinded observer, showed a positive short-term effect of manipulation when compared to dimethicone, the control intervention.[11] Treated infants cried 2.7 hours less per day from pretreatment levels to days 8–11; control group babies cried 1 hour less per day over the same interval. Infants in this study received three to five sessions over a 14-day period. Furthermore, this study had nine dropouts from the control group (all as a result of worsening of symptoms) and none from the manipulation group, suggesting perhaps an even more significant benefit to manipulation than the authors reported in their analysis.[15] This study did fail to blind the parents, introducing the possibility of bias in parental reporting of response to treatment. Finally, a recent study in Norway of 86 infants randomized either to active manipulation or to gentle holding, in which parents were blinded and again a blinded observer was used, found no significant benefit to manipulation.[16] Some degree of improvement occurred in both treatment (69.9%) and control (60%) groups, but the difference between the two was not significant.

Although efficacy has not been conclusively proven, Hughes[15] points out that what has been proven is that parents perceive chiropractic care to be helpful in reducing the number of hours of crying per day. Given the stress that colic can create for a family and the dearth of proven treatments, chiropractic remains a reasonable option for the parent of a child with colic.

Behavioral Strategies

A number of behavioral interventions have been recommended as strategies for dealing with an infant with colic. Two RCTs have shown that frequent carrying, which is often recommended and which many parents' instincts lead them to try, does not result in any reduction of colic symptoms.[17,18] Likewise, the use of a "car ride simulator" has not been shown to have any impact on symptoms.[18]

The two behavioral interventions that seem most promising based on trials to date are "intensive parent training" in parent-infant communication skills, and decreasing infant stimulation. The first strategy, which is based on the notion that colic is a function of disordered parent response to an infant who cries more than the norm, has been shown in two small RCTs to result in a statistically significant decrease in number of hours crying per day.[19,20] Neither of these trials was blinded, and in one trial, the investigators who analyzed the parental journals were the same ones who provided the training, introducing substantial possibility of investigator bias. Furthermore, the resources needed to provide daily counseling for parents may be beyond the means of most clinicians outside of a research context. The study which examined decreased infant stimulation as a strategy found that 93% of infants in the treatment group improved compared to 50% in the control group.[21] Here again, the trial was not blinded and parental diaries in this circumstance may not represent a valid strategy for assessing a real impact of the treatment strategy.

▶ ATOPIC DERMATITIS

Atopic dermatitis (AD) is a common, chronic dermatitis, that usually begins during the first year of life and is usually associated with intense itching. It is characterized by pruritic, erythematous papules, plaques, and vesicles that are excoriated by scratching and often become lichenified. In infancy, the disease tends to occur primarily on the face but can generalize to the trunk and extensor surfaces of the extremities. In childhood, and in those cases that persist to adulthood, the disease tends to occur in the flexural areas, especially the antecubital and popliteal fossae.

Atopic dermatitis is the most common skin disease of children, with a prevalence of around 20%, although prevalence estimates can vary significantly, depending on diagnostic criteria and geographical area.[22–24] Numerous studies indicate that there is an increasing prevalence of AD in the developed world.[25] It has been common wisdom that most cases of atopic dermatitis resolve by adulthood, but two recent studies contradict that assertion, showing that at least half of children with AD may continue to have AD as adults.[26,27]

Pathophysiology

The exact cause of AD is unknown. It can be characterized as a chronic inflammatory skin disease with a strong hereditary predisposition. The concordance rate for monozygotic twins is 77% and for dizygotic twins it is 15%, demonstrating that there is a strong genetic component influenced significantly by environmental factors.[28] The eczematous lesions themselves have an inflammatory character, with prominent lymphocytic infiltration of the dermis. These are mainly activated T cells, but Langerhans and mast cells are also present. This infiltrate, the elevated levels of immunoglobulin (Ig) E in most patients with eczema, and the strong association of eczema with asthma and allergic rhinitis point to an abnormality of immune regulation as the primary cause. One recent study demonstrated that patients with atopic dermatitis and cow's milk allergy had abnormal T-cell reactivity, with an elevated level of T-helper (Th) 2 cytokines, again indicating an abnormality of immune regulation.[29] There has also been research suggesting that there is a defect in delta-6-desaturase activity, which is responsible for the conversion of linoleic to gamma-linoleic acid.[30] This leads to specific treatment possibilities, which are discussed later in the section on herbal approaches to AD.

Many dermatologists refer to eczema as "the itch that scratches." This emphasizes the view that the lesions of eczema are caused by the actual scratching that results from abnormally dry skin with a lowered threshold for itching. This view would also have significant implications for the treatment of AD.

A more recent and interesting explanation for the increased incidence of AD and allergies in general is the "hygiene hypothesis."[31,32] It is known that children from large families and children raised on farms have a decreased incidence of AD. It is suspected that these children have an increased incidence of viral or bacterial infection in the first year of life. This would cause the activation of the Th1 immune response that is associated with infection, which would then suppress the Th2 cell types that are associated with the allergic response, thus decreasing the likelihood of allergic disease. This concept has not been entirely proven, and it is not yet clear what the importance of this factor may be in the pathogenesis of AD and allergies.

The Role of Food Allergy

The role of food allergy in the pathogenesis and clinical course of AD remains controversial. Most dermatologists dismiss the role of food allergy as having little or no clinical importance. However, several recent studies demonstrate that food allergies play a significant role in many patients with AD. From a research perspective, the gold standard for establishing food allergy is the double-blind, placebo-controlled food challenge. In this procedure, usually done as an inpatient, a patient is given identical capsules of suspected foods or placebo and observed for any reaction. This test has very good specificity and reproducibility, but it is likely to have poor sensitivity, especially in the case of nonimmediate food sensitivity.[33] Food allergy tests, such as skin prick testing, food-specific IgE (such as radioallergosorbent test or cholesteric analysis profile test), and the atopy patch tests, have varying degrees of specificity and sensitivity and cannot be relied upon as a sole method of diagnosing food allergy. Nevertheless, using

the double-blind, placebo-controlled, food challenge as a standard, recent studies have shown the presence of food allergy in 27%, 56%, and 40% of children with AD.[34,35] The most common food allergens are egg, milk, soy, wheat, peanut, and fish.[36] Recent research has also shown that treatment of AD based on food avoidance can be successful. A 1999 review by Wahn et al. stated that "at least one-third of children with atopic eczema during the first year suffer from clinically relevant food allergy requiring elimination diets for at least 1 or 2 years."[37] In another study of 91 children with atopic eczema, 74% improved on an elimination diet. In that study, skin prick testing and food-specific IgE were of no help in predicting responders.[38] It should be kept in mind that food allergies are most prevalent in the first 2 years of life and do tend to decrease over time, so eliminated foods can often be successfully reintroduced at a later date.

The Role of Stress

It seems intuitively clear to patients, parents, and practitioners that psychological stress has a significant role in the clinical course of eczema, and a recent review by Buske-Kirschbaum reports that several investigators have confirmed this relationship.[39] Recent studies in psycho-neuroimmunology, the study of behavioral, neural, and immune interactions, have elicited some of the pathophysiological mechanisms by which stress and atopic dermatitis may be related. One study demonstrated that, in response to mental stress, patients with atopic dermatitis had a significantly higher increase of cutaneous lymphocytes and T-helper cell stimulation than did healthy controls, indicating the possibility that these patients had an increased tendency for immune cells to migrate to the skin during this stress.[40] In a study by Garg et al., patients with atopic dermatitis were found to have a de-creased skin permeability barrier during periods of stress.[41] Finally, a study by Buske-Kirschbaum et al. indicated that patients with atopic dermatitis had a blunted hypothalamic–pituitary axis response to stress with a concurrent overreactivity of the sympathetic adrenomedullary system.[12] It should also be kept in mind that the relationship of stress and atopic dermatitis can be bidirectional. A recent review noted that there have been a number of studies indicating that atopic dermatitis and other skin diseases can themselves have significant psychosocial effects, leading to increases in psychological stress and other problems.[13]

▶ Case Example 1: Atopic Dermatitis

Jenny is a 3-year-old girl with the diagnosis of atopic dermatitis or eczema since the age of 3 months. She has chronic widespread erythematous papules and plaques on her cheeks, neck, chest, antecubital and popliteal fossae, wrists, and ankles. She is constantly scratching, especially at night, and usually awakens several times per night. She is often cranky and irritable. Her parents report a high level of anxiety and stress relative to this condition.

Jenny has seen her pediatrician and dermatologist frequently. Treatment has mainly consisted of topical steroids of various strengths, emollients, and the use of diphenhydramine at bedtime. She had one course of oral steroids when the rash was particularly bad; this was effective, but only for a short time.

She has no other medical problems. Family history is positive for asthma and allergic rhinitis in the father, and mild eczema and allergic rhinitis in the mother. She has a typical toddler's diet, including cow's milk. Mom is frustrated with the difficulty and ineffectiveness of the treatments prescribed so far and wants to know if there are some alternative treatments that could be helpful.

Conventional Treatment Approach

The conventional treatment of AD is directed at optimizing skin hydration and decreasing itching and inflammation. Mainstays of therapy are the use of moisturizing agents, avoidance of triggering factors, and the use of topical steroids, with the more recent introduction of nonsteroidal topical immune modulators such as tacrolimus and pimecrolimus. Antihistamines are often prescribed for nighttime use to prevent scratching. Antibiotics are employed for the treatment of staphylococcal superinfections, which are relatively common. Ultraviolet light therapy (UVA and UVB) is employed in some difficult cases. Oral immunosuppressants such as prednisone (most commonly), cyclosporine, and methotrexate are sometimes used in moderate to severe disease.

Triggering factors in AD are extremely important and basically refer to any condition that tends to promote dryness or itching. The most common conditions are temperature changes, sweating, use of harsh soaps or detergents, decreased humidity, excessive washing, and contact with any irritating substances. Aeroallergens, especially the house dust mite, are felt to have a significant effect in some patients with AD, with some studies indicating a beneficial effect to standard allergy avoidance measures such as occlusive bedding.[14,15]

Psychological or emotional stress was discussed above as a significant triggering factor that also has implications for the integrative treatment of AD.

Topical steroids are the mainstay of conventional AD treatment. Used correctly, they are usually effective in most mild to moderate cases. For moderate to severe AD in children, they are labor intensive and with high potencies, pose some risk of side effects, both locally and as a consequence of systemic absorption. The nonsteroidal immune modulators do not have this risk but at present are expensive and often not covered by health insurance. As they become more widely available, their use as a first-line treatment should become more common.

It should be noted that antihistamines such as Benadryl (diphenhydramine) or chlorpheniramine can reduce itching, but can also interfere with rapid eye movement sleep, probably not an insignificant problem if antihistamines are used on a daily basis.[16] The risks of oral prednisone and the more potent immunosuppressants are obvious and need not be further discussed here.

Integrative Approach to Treatment

The integrative approach relies first on assessing a whole person, with an entire set of physical, mental, and emotional characteristics and qualities, rather than simply a case of eczema. This also includes the patient's relationship to family and community. Once this initial assessment is made, an integrative treatment approach focuses on the prevention and treatment of further episodes by using the most effective and least toxic means available. These could be conventional medical treatments, nutritional interventions, or the use of a wide variety of complementary or alternative medical approaches, such as traditional Chinese medicine, homeopathy, or mind–body medicine.

Prevention

Ideally, the prevention of any disease state would be of great importance in an integrative or conventional medical approach, and there has been some interesting research concerning the prevention of atopic dermatitis in high-risk children, mainly those with a family history of atopy.

There have been several intriguing studies on the possible role of probiotics in the prevention of atopic dermatitis. In one randomized study, probiotics or placebo were given to mothers with a family history of atopy during the pregnancy and to infants for 6 months postnatally. At age 2 years, those in the treatment group had half the incidence of eczema of those

in the placebo group.[17] A similar study supplementing breast-feeding mothers with probiotics showed an even greater reduction in the incidence of AD by age 2 years.[18] In both of the above studies, a dose of 20 billion live *Lactobacillus* per day was used, either given to nursing mothers or directly to bottle-feeding infants. The presumed mechanism of this action would be increased immunoprotection through alteration of gastrointestinal flora. This could cause decreased gut permeability, as well as other immunological changes. Given this data, and the extremely low risk of adverse effects, it would seem reasonable to recommend probiotics for pregnant and nursing mothers with a strong family history of atopy. For non–breast-feeding infants, probiotics can be given directly with safety.[19] In fact, a recent study showed that infants with AD of a mean age of 4–5 months who were weaned to a probiotic-supplemented formula had significantly decreased eczema severity as compared to controls.[50]

The question of whether breast-feeding itself prevents atopic dermatitis and other allergic disease has been long debated. Numerous studies of this issue have yielded conflicting results. A 2001 systemic review and meta-analysis of 18 studies concluded that breast-feeding had a significant effect in preventing AD, but only in children with a first-degree relative with atopy.[51] Part of the reason for this variation in results is that such factors as duration of exclusive breast-feeding, timing and variety of introduction of solids, and whether maternal diet was limited were not standardized across studies.

From a practical point of view, most pediatricians encourage breast-feeding for all infants, but exclusive breast-feeding for 6 months would be more strongly recommended for all infants with a strong family history of atopy. Decisions about whether to restrict maternal diet to avoid common food antigens would have to be made on an individualized basis. If breast-feeding were not possible, it would make sense to avoid milk-based infant formula and consider instead a hydrolyzed formula. A recent review described several prospective studies demonstrating that using hydrolyzed formula for infants at high risk of atopy who could not exclusively breast-feed had a protective effect on the prevalence of food allergy and atopic dermatitis during the first 2–4 years of life.[52] Probiotic supplementation for high-risk infants may also help to prevent or lessen the severity of AD. A reasonable case could be made for restricting the high-risk infant's diet during the first year of life to avoid the most common food allergens, including milk, eggs, wheat, nuts, fish, and soy. Certainly, none of these foods is necessary for infant nutrition during the first year of life.

For any child, but especially one with atopic dermatitis, making sure the diet provides optimal nutrition is important. The diet should contain adequate amounts of fresh fruits and vegetables and avoid food additives and preservatives. Adequate protein and fat intake is necessary, but the diet should provide a preponderance of mono-unsaturated fats and avoid *trans* fats completely. An adequate intake of omega-3 fatty acids should be provided, either by diet or supplementation. The most common food sources of omega-3 fatty acids are cold-water fish (e.g., salmon, cod, and sardines), flaxseed, and walnuts. A complete multi-vitamin with antioxidants and minerals will ensure against any vitamin or mineral deficiencies.

Nutritional Approaches: Food Allergies

In any child or adult with significant atopic dermatitis, the presence of food allergies as a contributing factor should be considered. How that should be evaluated is not entirely clear. For food allergy testing, the three main tests—skin prick, food-specific IgE (i.e., radioallergosorbent tests), and the newer atopic patch tests—have all been used to try and predict which children are likely to have food allergies. There is great variability in results. Although some studies have shown a greater than 95% sensitivity for some single test or a combination of tests, other studies do not confirm this. Specificity is often poor, so a positive test does not necessarily prove true food allergy. Many alternative practitioners recommend food-specific IgG testing. However, although it is well known that patients with atopic disease have food-specific IgG antibodies, the complete lack of data as to specificity, sensitivity, and cross-reactivity make it hard to evaluate their clinical utility.

A trial of avoidance of one or more foods is necessary to establish clinically significant food sensitivity. Although the double-blind, placebo-controlled food challenge is a good research tool, it is usually impractical for clinical practice. The more practical choices are to remove either one food at a time and observe clinical response, or to use a modified elimination diet, in which the four or five most common food allergens are avoided. These would be added back to the diet one at a time if there were a good response. Some practitioners would use some kind of food allergy testing first, to see if any single food or foods seemed more likely to be involved; this is not unreasonable. Careful clinical observation and follow-up are very important to ensure that patients are not unnecessarily restricting intake and that nutritional status is not compromised.

Herbal Approaches

EVENING PRIMROSE OIL

Because of the above-mentioned biochemical defect in delta-6-desaturase, it was postulated that treatment with evening primrose oil, which contains gamma-linoleic acid, would improve atopic eczema. A number of studies have addressed this question. Most recently, a 2002 study showed significant improvement in 14 patients with AD, and also demonstrated that serum levels of interferon gamma, which were initially reduced in these patients, returned to normal with evening primrose oil treatment.[53] However, other recent controlled studies have failed to show a difference between evening primrose oil and placebo treatment.[54,55] A 1989 meta-analysis of nine controlled trials did show a significant positive effect of evening primrose oil as compared to placebo.[56]

Evening primrose oil is generally considered safe and is well tolerated in children. A trial of evening primrose oil would be reasonable in most children. It should be noted that it could take several weeks before a maximum effect is seen. Black currant oil also contains gamma-linoleic acid and has been used for eczema, but there is less research available for this product. There has also been little research on fish oil or omega-3 fatty acid supplementation for atopic dermatitis, and the results have been equivocal.

OTHER BOTANICALS

Various herbs such as aloe vera, calendula, chamomile, and licorice have been used as topical treatments. There are no good studies about their efficacy, but it is possible that they are as good or better than more conventional moisturizers. Oregon grape tincture and aloe vera have been recommended orally. There is no scientific evidence concerning the efficacy of either of these products.

Mind–Body Approaches

It is clear that increased stress can result in increased itching and thus worsening of AD symptoms. That is one reason an integrative approach is so important. In children, examining the family dynamics and behavioral response to the child's condition can be very helpful. As an example, some children may receive secondary gain from parents' reaction to scratching, or conversely, parental emotional issues can come into play and exacerbate the existing problem. An interesting article by Koblenzer described relatively simple stress-reducing family interventions that were extremely helpful in certain situations.[57] If severe symptoms are disrupting family relationships, counseling may be indicated.

Mind–body modalities such as hypnosis, biofeedback, relaxation training, and guided imagery may be very helpful for the treatment of atopic dermatitis. They may be used simply to decrease stress or anxiety, with a resulting decrease in scratching and improvement in symptoms. However, as mentioned, recent developments in psychoneuroimmunology have described some of the physiological mechanisms by which neurological and endocrine responses can directly impact atopic dermatitis.[39] Hypnosis, or other mind–body therapies may operate by influencing the autonomic nervous system, resulting in endocrine and immune responses that would directly effect the underlying pathophysiology of the disease.

The research on mind–body therapy of atopic dermatitis is mainly limited to case reports or case series. However, in one randomized study comparing standard dermatological treatment, dermatological education, cognitive therapy, and autogenics, it was shown that the psychological therapies, either alone or in combination with dermatological education, were significantly more successful than standard dermatology care or dermatological education alone.[58]

In another study, 20 adults and 18 children with severe, resistant AD were treated with hypnosis. Both groups showed significant responses, which were maintained over time.[59] Another study using electromyographic (EMG) biofeedback showed clinically meaningful improvements in all five treated patients.[60] Biofeedback has been used successfully for patients with atopic dermatitis but again there are no well-controlled trials.

In summary, although controlled trials are lacking, the noncontrolled studies have shown significant positive effects, there are reasonable biological mechanisms that would explain their efficacy, and the risk of negative side effects is negligible. Therefore, it seems reasonable to recommend mind–body modalities as useful adjunctive therapy for children or adults with moderate to severe AD.

Traditional Chinese Medicine

Traditional Chinese medicine is generally divided into the areas of acupuncture and Chinese herbal medicine. There is little evidence for the efficacy of acupuncture in atopic dermatitis; however, the evidence for traditional Chinese herbal medicine is more robust. Sheehan and colleagues performed two successful randomized controlled trials that demonstrated significant improvement using a traditional Chinese herbal medicine formulation in both children and adults. In the first study, 37 children were treated using a formula of 10 herbs. The decrease in erythema scores and surface damage scores were 51% and 63%, respectively, as compared to 6.1% and 6.2%, respectively, in the placebo group.[61] A 1-year follow-up of these children showed that almost half had maintained a greater than 90% improvement in eczema scores.[62] Temporary, asymptomatic, elevation of aspartate aminotransferases was shown in two of those children. A second study of 40 adults showed similarly positive results, although the unpalatability of the herbal mixture was a problem.[63] Another noncontrolled study, using a freeze-dried preparation (Zemaphyte), demonstrated clinical improvement and significant beneficial changes in the immune expression of T cells in the skin of patients with AD.[64] On the other hand, Fung and colleagues reported a double-blind study using Zemaphyte with 40 patients with "recalcitrant" atopic dermatitis in which there was no statistically significant difference between active and control groups except for lichenification.[65]

It should be noted that there have been reports of adulteration of some Chinese herbal medicine preparations with cortico-steroids, and of contamination of others with heavy metals.[66] There have also been reports of liver damage strongly associated with the use of Chinese herbal medicines for skin conditions.[67] The frequency of these problems is not known, especially as compared to the overall number of people using Chinese herbal medicines. In sum, traditional Chinese herbal medicine has shown excellent potential for the treatment of atopic dermatitis, but some caution must be exercised in view of possible contamination and side effects.

Homeopathy

From a homeopathic viewpoint, a skin disease like AD would reflect an imbalance at its early, or less-severe stage, and any therapy that successfully suppressed the eczema, would likely cause deeper problems in another organ or system at some later date. There are many case reports of successful homeopathic treatment of atopic dermatitis in both children and adults. However, there are no randomized clinical trials and no formal case series. The lack of any known negative effects from homeopathic treatment certainly increases the risk: benefit ratio of this modality.

▶ Case Example 1: Atopic Dermatitis Conclusion

Because Jenny's eczema is moderately severe and has not responded adequately to conventional therapy, it would be worthwhile to explore the possibility of food allergy as a contributing factor. This could be done through a modified elimination diet, with the elimination of dairy, eggs, wheat, soy, and nuts for at least 1 month, if necessary. It would be necessary to assure adequate protein and calcium once dairy products were eliminated, and nutritional recommendations as noted earlier should be instituted, including a multivitamin with minerals and antioxidants. If there was improvement, this could be followed by reintroduction of each food separately, observing clinical response. Radioallergosorbent tests, skin prick tests, or atopy patch tests could be used adjunctively, if desired.

It is important to not institute other therapies while investigating for food allergies, so as not to confuse the situation. After the food allergy issue is resolved, a trial of evening primrose oil 1 g/d for at least 3 to 4 months, along with a probiotic supplement, could be instituted.

It is also important to evaluate the family dynamics with respect the child's symptoms. If these were felt to be problematic, intervention could range from relatively simple suggestions for behavior modification to recommending family counseling.

Other modalities that could be considered in the future include some form of mind–body therapy, traditional Chinese medicine, and homeopathy.

▶ AUTISM AND DEVELOPMENTAL DISORDERS

The diagnosis of autism first appeared in 1943, in a description of 11 children who presented with what are now recognized as its characteristic features: an inability to develop relationships with other people; extreme aloofness; delayed speech development; noncommunicative use of speech; repeated, stereotypical, simple patterns of play activities; and specific areas of unusual ability. The two most prominent features were recognized as aloneness and an obsessive insistence on sameness. Today's definition of autism includes the above, along with restricted, repetitive, and stereotypical patterns of behavior, interests, and activities; a recognition that nonverbal communication may be as impaired as verbal communication; and an awareness that some children suffer from involuntary, violent outbursts. Abnormal movements, problems with coordination and fine motor movements, and sensory impairments are also part of the disorder.[68]

Research during the past five decades has changed this original concept of a single disorder (called infantile autism in 1943) to the current concept of a spectrum of disorders with multiple subtypes. Although this spectrum contains a variety of named conditions, all are descriptive, and none represent actual biochemical or metabolic conditions. The various names are readily recognizable by parents and include autism itself, Rett's disorder, childhood disintegrative disorder, Asperger syndrome, pervasive developmental disorder, Landau-Kleffner syndrome, and atypical autism. While these names represent different patterns of clustering of symptoms, they do not reflect a true understanding of the causes of these conditions. Because what can be said about autism is relevant to all the other conditions, the term *autism* will be used here to refer to all related developmental disorders.

The alternative therapies for these disorders are not all that different, and what is said here about developmental disorders, is generally relevant to attention deficit hyperactivity disorder, Tourette syndrome, and other psychiatric disorders of childhood as well. While some specifics may differ, the overall principles remain the same.

In addition to the attributes used to define autism, symptoms related to other conditions are frequently found among these children. Approximately 60% of these children have poor attention and concentration; 40% are hyperactive; 43–88% exhibit morbid or unusual preoccupations; 37% have obsessions; 16–86% show compulsions or rituals; 50–89% demonstrate stereotypical speech; 70% exhibit stereotypical behaviors; 17–74% have anxiety or fears; 9–44% show depressive mood, irritability, agitation, and inappropriate affect; 11% have sleep problems; 24–43% have a history of self-injury; and 8% have tics.[69]

Pathophysiology

Several potential genes may contribute to autism, but no clear genetic linkage has been established. For this reason, it has been suggested that autism may have multiple causes, some environmental. While autism was once thought to affect only 1 in 500 children, recent trends indicate that its incidence is increasing, and that it may be as common as 1 in every 150 US children. Studies in both California and New Jersey show a dramatic, unexplained increase in the numbers of children diagnosed with developmental disorders in the past 10 years. This dramatic increase argues against a purely genetic cause, and more in favor of environmental factors (increasing pollution, increasing vaccination, increasing toxic metal exposure during development) playing a role in its development.

Using electrophysiology (recordings of brain electrical activity, heart rate, blood pressure, breathing rates, and skin conductance) two subtypes were identified among 145 children with developmental disorders.[70] These different profiles were thought to reflect different types of brain dysfunction. One type was associated with intellectual impairment and excessive reactivity of the central, parietal part of the brain, while the other subtype linked typical autistic behavior with excessive reactivity of the temporal part of the brain (the part of the brain that is also involved with language processing). In an earlier study of 222 children, these same researchers had identified four subtypes of developmentally disabled children based on information from clinical assessments.[71] They used the type of communication disorder, type of abnormal findings on the neurological examination, type of impairment of intelligence, and types of autistic behaviors to separate out four different groups of children. These subtypes correlated with different urinary levels of dopamine and homovanillic acid levels, two brain neurotransmitter metabolites.

Another approach to formulating a biological basis for developmental disorders involves single-photon emission computed tomography (SPECT) scans of the brain.[72] SPECT scanning is being used to find underfunctioning and overfunctioning parts of the brain in a number of childhood neurological disorders.[73] SPECT scans have shown differences among children with attention deficit hyperactivity disorder from "normal" controls, particularly decreased activity of the striatal and periventricular brain areas, along with increased activity in the part of the brain that handles sensation and movement (the sensorimotor cortex). Other specific abnormalities have been found among children with cerebral palsy and in brain conditions manifesting as problems with behavior (phenylketonuria, mitochondrial disorders, Wilson disease, and others).[74] Eventually these biological approaches will allow us to clearly understand the different subtypes of developmental disorders and how each one may respond similarly or differently to treatment.

The symptoms of people with autism change with age. In early childhood, hyperac-

tivity, stereotypical behaviors, irritability, and temper tantrums predominate. Tics, aggressiveness, and self-injurious behaviors appear in older children. In adolescence and adulthood, particularly in higher functioning individuals, depression or obsessive–compulsive phenomena can appear and restrict the person's ability to function and his or her quality of life.[75]

Conventional Treatment Approach

Despite tremendous efforts, we are far from a biochemical, metabolic understanding of autism. No treatments have been developed that address the underlying cause, because it is not known. In fact, autism may have many causes, all culminating in the cluster of symptoms that present as a developmental disorder. Conventional medicine approaches autism with parental counseling, behavior modification, special education in a highly structured environment, sensory integration training, speech therapy, social skills training, and medication. The results of these comprehensive suites of therapies have not been sufficiently satisfying to prevent many parents from seeking alternative therapies for the benefit of their children.

Findings from preliminary studies of major neurotransmitters and other neurochemical agents strongly suggest that neurochemical factors play a major role in autism. The findings also provide the rationale for drug treatment. Some of the more common medications include serotonin reuptake inhibitors (Prozac [fluoxetine], Zoloft [sertraline], Paxil [paroxetine]), risperidone, and donepezil. Most of these medications are of marginal efficacy in the treatment of autism.

Pygmalion Effect

A major problem in autism treatment is separating what could be called the Pygmalion effect from true biological efficacy. The Pygmalion effect is named after George Bernard Shaw's play in which a lower class, "uncultured" woman from the slums of London is trained to be a "lady." She becomes every bit as cultured and sophisticated as a woman born to this social class.

The Pygmalion effect has been demonstrated in elementary school classrooms. In the classic experiment, children's IQs were measured and the children were ranked as higher or lower IQ. Teachers were told the opposite from what was found. Higher IQ children were presented to teachers as lower IQ. Lower IQ children were presented as higher. One year later, the teachers' expectations were much more important in predicting children's actual classroom performance than the children's measured IQs. We could never ethically repeat this experiment. Knowing that the teachers' expectations for how the students would perform were more important than the students' actual abilities, we could not consign students to an experiment that might track them for life to lower achievement. We have yet to realize that conventional medicine may be doing just this when a diagnosis like autism is made. When we believe that treatment is useless, how can we expect results? Parents who refuse to accept hopelessness may demonstrate how the expectation of improvement actually produces it.

Until sophisticated clinical trials are completed, it is true that we cannot determine whether or not the benefit of many alternative therapies could be explained partially or completely by the Pygmalion effect. What is exciting about this is the realization that expectations can alter behavior. If parents expect strongly that their autistic child will improve, the child may. We should not be afraid to try safe therapies that could only work because they activate this Pygmalion effect. This type of healing is just as real as that produced by drugs, and probably much safer. While we struggle to find biologically active treatments, we cannot err too greatly by supporting parents' enthusiasm for safe, new treatments. We know from research on the placebo effect that an enthusiastic doctor whose patients believe in her or him has a 70% success rate regardless of the biological effectiveness of the treatment.[76] An unenthusiastic doctor has only a 17–33% success rate with an ineffective treatment.[77]

Integrative Treatment Approach

Nutritional Therapy

DIETARY MANIPULATION

Nutritional manipulation is a common strategy in the integrative approach to autism. The most common offenders for food allergies and sensitivities are gluten, casein, and soy. The basis for the gluten/casein-free diet is the opioid theory of autism. In the early 1980s, similarities were noted between the behavioral effects on animals of opioids, such as morphine, and the symptoms of autism. People with autism were thought to have elevated opioids in their nervous system, the best known being beta-endorphin. To support this hypothesis, elevated levels of "endorphin-like substances" were found in the cerebrospinal fluid of some people with autism, especially among those children who appeared pain insensitive and also exhibited self-injurious behavior. In the urine of approximately 50% of people with autism there appeared to be elevated levels of substances with properties similar to those expected from opioid peptides.[78]

The quantities of these opioid compounds in the urine are too large to come from the nervous system and could only have come from the incomplete breakdown of food. Normal proteins are digested by enzymes in the intestines and are broken down into these units. Incomplete digestion of proteins results in short chains of amino acids known as peptides. Some of these peptides are biologically active, and thought to potentially contribute to the symptoms of autism. Among those found in urine, a small proportion cross the blood-brain barrier and interfere with nervous signal transmission in such a way that normal activity is altered or disrupted.

Glutens are proteins found in members of the grass family of wheat, oats, barley, rye, and triticale, and their derivatives, including malt, grain starches, hydrolyzed vegetable/plant proteins, textured vegetable protein, grain vinegar, soy sauce, grain alcohol, flavorings, and the binders and fillers found in vitamins and medications.

Casein is a milk protein, with a molecular structure similar to that of gluten. Casein (from human or cow's milk) breaks down in the stomach into a peptide known as casomorphine, which has opioid activities.

Defective intestinal enzymes (especially dipeptidyl-dipeptidase IV) allow incompletely digested gluten and casein (with opioid properties) to "leak" across the gut and into the bloodstream. While we do not know why these defective enzymes create opioid peptides, their presence and effect is clearly demonstrable. In larger doses, these molecules can cause hallucinations. Those who cannot metabolize gluten produce alpha-gliadin and gliadinomorphins, compounds that bind to the opioid receptors that are associated with mood and behavior disturbances.

A single blind study evaluated the effect of a gluten- and casein-free diet on children with autistic syndromes and urinary peptide abnormalities.[79] Observations and tests were done before and after a period of 1 year. The development of the group of children on the diet was significantly better than of the controls. A strict gluten- and casein-free diet appears to reduce the level of opioid peptides and improve autism in some people. The younger the child is when the diet is implemented, the better are the results.

The initial response to the diet may be negative, consisting of an upset stomach, anxiety, clinginess, and slight ill temper. Experience suggests that these are good signs that a positive response will follow. While the diet is difficult, 1 month is usually sufficient to determine if following it will help. After 1 month, if any question exists, challenging the child with a gluten- and casein-containing meal helps to determine whether symptoms will worsen after exposure to gluten or casein. Sensitive children become worse after this meal. Outcomes during the grain- and dairy-free month are best tracked by counting behaviors of interest in the same 30–60-minute time slot every day. These could include self-stimulation behaviors, the number of times the child initiates eye contact in a 30-minute frame, and amount of time interacting with an adult versus playing alone, to name a few. Gastrointestinal complaints made per day are also important to record. Objective scales like the Autism Child Behavior Checklist and the Achenbach Child Behavior Checklist are also helpful.

Nutritional Supplements

Because several metabolic (genetic) defects are associated with autistic-like symptoms (e.g., phenylketonuria, histidine disorders), it stands to reason that milder versions of these more severe disorders could exist on the autism spectrum. When the metabolic consequences of an enzyme defect are well defined, treatment with diet, drugs, or nutritional supplements may bring about a dramatic reduction in autistic symptoms.[80] A number of vitamins have research to support their use among children with developmental disorders. Others are used based upon theory or case reports of benefit.

MAGNESIUM

Magnesium deficiency is involved in a number of children's developmental disorders, as well as other conditions found among developmentally disabled children (Tourette syndrome, allergy, asthma, attention deficit hyperactivity disorder, obsessive–compulsive disorder, and others).[81–83] While we do not know if its deficiency causes any of these problems or merely facilitates their appearance, magnesium has been linked to multiple biochemical effects, including those upon substance P, kynurenine, N-methyl-D-aspartate receptors, and vitamin B_6, all substances involved in the neurochemistry of autism. A number of studies have reported improvement with magnesium supplementation, although usually in conjunction with vitamin B_6. Doses of magnesium have ranged from 10 to 15 mg/kg of body weight per day (380–500 mg/d). It is possible that the benefits of magnesium in autism may only come from its calming effects and its effects on relaxing smooth muscles.[84]

MINERALS

Zinc has crucial functions in the proper development and function of the brain cortex and adrenal glands. For example, the synthesis of serotonin involves zinc-requiring enzymes. Serotonin, in turn, is essential for melatonin synthesis. A zinc deficiency may therefore result in low levels of both serotonin and melatonin. Zinc levels tend to be low when levels of copper and cadmium are elevated. Exposure to second-hand smoke and eating foods contaminated with cadmium both decrease zinc levels. Increased copper levels (and therefore low zinc) are found in people with Wilson disease, which is rare. However, partial forms of Wilson disease (only one faulty copy of the gene) are not so rare. Therefore, the fetal brain could develop abnormally in a mother who has low zinc and high copper levels. The ensuing problems in brain development could later manifest as autism. Similarly, a person who gradually accumulates copper will lose zinc, with a corresponding increase in oxidative damage, worsening autistic symptoms.

Although controversial, analysis of the mineral content in hair has provided some potentially important information about the possible importance of minerals and micronutrients in the pathogenesis of autism. In one study, children with autism had significantly lower levels of calcium, magnesium, copper, manganese, and chromium with higher levels of lithium and mercury, as compared to children without de-

velopmental disorders who were the same sex and age. Children with autistic spectrum disorders (e.g., pervasive development disorder) had lower levels of magnesium, cadmium, cobalt, and manganese, as compared to these same controls. Statistical methods using the values of the 14 trace elements correctly identified 90% of the children without developmental disorders and 100% of the children with developmental disorders.[85] The five elements that best predicted autism were calcium, copper, zinc, chromium, and lithium. Affected children may need supplementation with calcium, magnesium, copper, manganese, zinc, chromium, cobalt, and other trace minerals. They may benefit from reducing mercury and lithium levels. Mineral and trace mineral supplements are frequently prescribed to children with developmental disabilities with reports of good results.[86]

Nevertheless, these findings are only suggestive, since hair analysis has large variability. Hair concentrations of elements are affected by different factors that are also specific to certain regions and subjects. Comparison of the results of element levels in hair for certain factors shows different trends because of regional variation. Regarding certain factors (e.g., age, sex, health, occupation), the influence causing the change in element levels is obvious, whereas the influence of other factors (e.g., structure of hair, height and weight of the subject) is obscure. It is very important to consider all the factors at the time of investigation for effective interpretation, validity, and application of results of hair analysis.[87]

VITAMIN A

A currently popular theory of autism links its symptoms to the separation of an important protein (the G-alpha protein) from retinoid receptors in the brain by the pertussis toxin found in the diphtheria, pertussis, and tetanus vaccine, occurring among already genetically susceptible children.[88] Natural vitamin A is thought to provide the material necessary to reconnect these G proteins to the retinoid receptors that are critical for vision, sensory perception, language processing, and attention. Children at highest risk for this way of developing autism have a family history of at least one parent with a preexisting G-alpha protein defect, manifesting as night blindness, pseudohypoparathyroidism (a disorder of calcium metabolism), or benign tumors of the thyroid and pituitary gland.

An example of the type of children who benefit from vitamin A would be an 8-year-old boy with autism who developed a limp and swelling around his eyes. His calcium was low and he appeared to have rickets from vitamin D deficiency. His eye examination was abnormal. No vitamin A could be detected in his bloodstream, and his vitamin D levels (25-hydroxyvitamin D) were low. His diet had consisted of mainly French fries and water for several years. His biochemical and physical abnormalities reversed with vitamin A supplementation.[89]

PYRIDOXINE (VITAMIN B6)

Vitamin B6, or pyridoxine, plays a key role in the synthesis of certain neurotransmitters. When children with autism respond to high-dose vitamin B6 and magnesium, physical aggression decreases and social responsiveness improves. Doses of B6 range from 15 to 30 mg/kg of body weight per day (700–1000 mg/d). The majority of studies of B6 in combination with magnesium, although not all, show a positive effect. The treatment periods in these studies were short (2 weeks to 30 days), but no side effects occurred.[90–93]

A typical case report describes a 15-year-old boy with autism, seizures, mental retardation, frequent belching, breath holding, and self-injurious activities.[94] Giving vitamin B6 dramatically reduced his seizures and also improved his other symptoms. Some researchers think that the variations in the effectiveness of vitamin B6, seen among studies and between individual patients, relate to the degree to which individuals have a partial or complete

genetic disorder affecting the binding of B6 to the enzyme glutamic acid decarboxylase-1. Lower activity of this enzyme leads to reduced levels of gamma-aminobutyric acid, an important neurotransmitter affecting autism, seizures, and other conditions. The condition is genetic (autosomal recessive) with a wide range of expression from minimal to severe. Severely affected children have seizures appearing before birth.

VITAMIN B12 AND FOLIC ACID

Some children with fragile X syndrome (a genetic condition producing autistic-like symptoms) respond to folic acid (with B12) 10 mg/d. Other studies have shown positive effects among children with autism itself, although there has been at least one study showing no effect.[95–98]

MELATONIN

Abnormal daily rhythms of melatonin occur in people with autism. Melatonin, at a dose ranging from 1 to 10 mg per night, has been effective for sleep problems in some autistic children without significant side effects. In one study, researchers examined the use of melatonin in the treatment of chronic sleep disorders among children with disabilities. Their first 100 patients, half of whom were visually impaired or blind, had chronic sleep disturbances, which children with neurological, neuropsychiatric, and developmental disabilities are prone to have. Blindness, deafness-blindness, mental retardation, autism, and other brain diseases diminish the person's ability to perceive and interpret the necessary cues others use to synchronize sleep with the environment. Melatonin normalized the sleep–wake cycle of more than 80% of their patients, without side effects and at minimal cost. The dose of fast-release melatonin taken at bed time ranged from 2.5 mg to 10.0 mg.[99–101]

FATTY ACIDS

A number of disorders of neurodevelopment, including attention deficit hyperactivity disorder, dyspraxia, dyslexia, and autism, are linked to fatty acid abnormalities, ranging from genetic defects in the enzymes involved in phospholipid metabolism to symptoms improving following dietary supplementation with long-chain fatty acids.[102] Supplementation with specific fatty acids (especially omega-3 and omega-6) can alter proinflammatory tendencies toward antiinflammatory and may benefit some children with these disorders.

Environmental Toxins, Detoxification Approaches, and Chelation

The argument that links autism to environmental toxins draws upon extensive studies of the role of environmental toxins, including pesticides and herbicides, in the pathogenesis of Parkinson's disease, an adult neurodegenerative disorder. Proponents of the environmental toxin theory argue that early exposure to synthetic chemicals is one suspect for the dramatic, recent increase in the incidence of autism. Impaired detoxification of environmental chemicals is thought to be common to both autism and neurodegenerative diseases like Parkinson's disease.

A small pilot study of 20 children with autism, ages 3–12 years, investigated the possible role of toxins coupled with impaired liver detoxification. Measures included (1) glucaric acid analysis, (2) blood analyses for identification of specific environmental (or xenobiotic) agents, and (3) comprehensive liver detoxification evaluation.

Children with autism differed significantly from children without developmental disorders ($p < .01$). All 20 children showed impaired liver detoxication profiles. Blood analyses conducted for 18 of the children showed increased levels of toxic chemicals, exceeding adult maximum tolerance in 16 children. In the two cases where elevated levels of toxic chemical were not found, the abnormal D-glucaric acid findings suggested that environmental toxins had adversely influenced liver detoxification. The authors proposed that the interaction of environmental toxins with immune system dysfunc-

tion and continuous or progressive endogenous toxicity leads to the development of behaviors found in the autistic spectrum.[103,104]

Closely related to theories of excessive toxic exposure coupled with impaired liver detoxification is the impaired sulfate theory of autism. Sulfation is an important method of detoxification, and its impairment has been found in a number of degenerative neurological and immunological conditions, including Alzheimer's disease, Parkinson's disease, motor neuron disease, rheumatoid arthritis, delayed food sensitivity, and drug intolerances.[105,106] Attachment of sulfur-based molecules to toxins renders them inactive and more capable of being eliminated by the body. Preliminary data suggests that impaired sulfation may also be important in multiple chemical sensitivities and diet responsive autism.

Reduced activity of the enzymes involved in sulfur-dependent detoxification has been found in some autistic children, as well as in the other conditions described above. Impairment in sulfation can be demonstrated by measuring the speed with which acetaminophen is metabolized and eliminated. A typical test gives one acetaminophen tablet and then follows the appearance of acetaminophen in urine and its disappearance from blood. Delayed processing is thought to be a result of starvation of the detoxification enzymes (transferases) for sulfur. The Feingold diet (e.g., no sugar, preservatives, dyes, salicylates) may be especially helpful for children with impaired sulfation (who are intolerant of phenol, tyramine, and phenylic food constituents). Compensation for impaired sulfation may be one explanation for the success of the Feingold diet.[107]

Another popular environmental theory of autism is that it is caused by environmentally acquired mercury, either through casual contact or through vaccination. Mercury exposure causes immune, sensory, neurological, motor, and behavioral dysfunctions similar to what is observed in autism. Abnormalities in neuroanatomy, neurotransmitters, and biochemistry of individuals with autism closely resemble what is seen in mercury poisoning. Nevertheless, resemblance does not prove cause.

Thimerosal, a preservative added to many vaccines, is argued to be the major source of mercury in children. Prior to the removal of thimerosal from childhood immunizations in 2002, many children during their first 2 years of life may have received via vaccination a quantity of mercury that exceeds safety guidelines. Proponents of the mercury theory suggest that (1) many cases of idiopathic autism are induced by early mercury exposure from thimerosal; (2) this type of autism represents an unrecognized mercurial syndrome; and (3) genetic and nongenetic factors establish a predisposition whereby thimerosal's adverse effects occur only in some children.[108]

Important to the environmental toxin theory is the reality that the developing nervous system is exquisitely sensitive to toxic insult during certain critical periods. Brain development extends from the embryonic period all the way through adolescence. Developmental exposure of animals or humans to toxic agents (for example, x-ray irradiation, methylazoxymethanol, ethanol, lead, methylmercury, or cadmium) demonstrates that interference with developmental processes can lead to developmental neurotoxicity. What this means is that development is impaired by subtle interference from levels of toxins that would not cause damage in the fully developed adult organism.

This concern is compounded by amplification of subtle damaging effects as development proceeds, producing much larger effects later in life when the full impact of disrupted, earlier processes become apparent. The argument here is that amounts of mercury and other environmental toxins that would be inconsequential to the adult brain may have profound impacts if encountered during critical phases of development.

Toxic chemicals in the environment—lead, polychlorinated biphenyls, mercury, and certain pesticides—are known to cause some fraction of neurodevelopmental disabilities, although how much is vigorously debated.

Unfortunately, too few chemicals are tested for toxicity to early brain development, knowledge of infants' and children's special vulnerabilities and unique exposures is scant, and paradigms for environmental risk assessment have only begun to address the hazards confronting infants and children.[109–111]

Treatment for autism under this theory is to apply chelating agents to extricate the toxic agents, including mercury. Utilization of the body's own detoxification mechanisms is also important. Endogenous enteric bacteria are argued to be the largest detoxification component of the body, providing an enormous detoxification reservoir, which can be constantly and safely replenished. *Lactobacillus* is one of the agents used to accomplish this, and is frequently and safely given to autistic children. High-dose probiotics have been used as an adjuvant for detoxification protocols among individuals with autism, whatever the toxic cause may be.

Secretin

Secretin is a protein-based hormone, produced in the intestines, and commercially marketed to help with gastrointestinal procedures. The interest in secretin for treatment of autism spectrum disorders began in 1996, when Dr. Karoly S. Horvath, director of the Pediatric Gastrointestinal and Nutrition Laboratory at the University of Maryland, Baltimore, administered intravenous secretin during a procedure with an autistic child who had chronic diarrhea. Several weeks later, the child's mother, Victoria Beck, called with surprising news: her 3-year-old son, Parker, had started to talk. His eye contact had greatly improved. Subsequent intravenous infusions of secretin, obtained by the parents against medical advice, led to further gains in development.

Dr. Horvath and associates gave secretin while assessing intestinal complaints in two other autistic children, and reported "a dramatic improvement in their behavior, manifested by improved eye contact, alertness, and expansion of expressive language," in the next several weeks along with relief of gastrointestinal symptoms.[111a] In a subsequent study, Rimland reported that 50 of 100 children with autism treated with secretin improved in behavior, sleep, and/or digestive symptoms—based on questionnaires returned by self-selected parents.[112] In another series, 70% of 200 children responded positively, according to the treating physician, with dramatic effect among 10%.[113,114] These reports did not control for concurrent treatment, nor was diagnosis rigorously established.

The results of a randomized, controlled trial of one dose of secretin were reported by Sandlin in the *New England Journal of Medicine* in 1999.[111a] Children were randomized to receive either secretin in an appropriate dose or placebo. Change was measured on the Autism Behavior Checklist. Both placebo and treatment groups improved equally over the course of 1 month. Opponents of secretin have used this study to argue that secretin is ineffective in autism. Secretin advocates say the study was not long enough to draw serious conclusions and that important variables that change in response to secretin were not included in this study. The Autism Behavior Checklist, for example, typically does not show change in 1 month's time. This study showed no adverse reactions to secretin; in this author's experience, approximately 15% of children treated with secretin react with increased hyperactivity and/or aggressiveness.

One of the authors (LM-M) has presented a case series of secretin infusions lasting more than 1 year among 35 patients.[115] Approximately 70% of patients improved, some quite dramatically—again, a figure within the range of what could be expected with enthusiastic placebo. More importantly, when the children who improved were compared to those who did not, several important differences emerged. Children who improved were receiving more therapy, their autism or pervasive developmental disorder was no more than moderately severe, and their parents refused to accept the diagnosis and believed that they would find a cure more than the parents of children who did not respond. None of the children who responded was taking psychiatrically active medications. A substantial number of the children who did not respond were taking a selective serotonin reuptake inhibitor.

If the improvement seen in both the Sandlin study over the course of 1 month and in one of the author's (LM-M) study[111] over the course of 1 year is only a result of placebo and parent expectation (Pygmalion effect), this is still remarkable. Such a finding could open a new awareness for the need to expect more from autistic children. If secretin is not biologically active, then what do parents do who believe in secretin to foster such dramatic improvements in their child? Knowing this and being able to train parents in how to influence the course of autism would be as significant as finding an active biological agent.

Secretin may open the pathway for searching for other neurohormonal therapies that activate brain receptors. We know that secretin receptors are found in the brain, especially in the temporal lobe speech areas. Brain-imaging studies in one of Horvath's original cases showed a "marked" postinfusion increase in cerebral blood flow to these areas.[111a] Secretin may also activate receptors for a related hormone, vasoactive intestinal polypeptide, which is more widely distributed in the brain. Secretin also stimulates pituitary adenylate cyclase, which increases intracellular cyclic adenosine monophosphate (cAMP), a messenger molecule for brain biochemical reactions. Opioid-like peptides are known to lower levels of cAMP. Perhaps secretin prevents this or replenishes the missing cAMP.

Lectins may also be important in explaining the mechanism of action of secretin. Lectins are molecules that bind to cholecystokinin (CCK) receptors and other glycosylated (meaning attached to long-chain sugars) membrane proteins. CCK is another gut hormone with receptors in the brain. Lectins inhibit CCK-8–induced alpha-amylase secretion by the pancreas. This inhibition does not occur after administration of secretin.

Body Therapy and Manipulative Therapies

In a study from the University of Miami, 20 children with autism, ages 3 to 6 years, were randomly assigned to massage therapy or to a reading attention control group. Parents in the massage therapy group were trained by a massage therapist to massage their children for 15 minutes prior to bedtime every night for 1 month, and the parents of the attention control group read Dr. Seuss stories to their children on the same time schedule. Conners Teacher and Parent scales, classroom and playground observations, and sleep diaries were used to assess the effects of therapy on various behaviors, including hyperactivity, stereotypical and off-task behavior, and sleep problems. Results suggested that the children in the massage group exhibited less stereotypic behavior and showed more on-task and social relatedness behavior during play observations at school, and they experienced fewer sleep problems at home.[116]

Other studies have also reported positive results for massage therapy for autism and developmental delays.[117] Generally, the massage therapy has resulted in lower anxiety and stress hormones and improved clinical course. Having grandparent volunteers and parents give the therapy enhances their own wellness and provides a cost-effective treatment for the children.[118]

One popular form of touch therapy is craniosacral therapy, in which the bones of the skull are adjusted along with subtle adjustments of the spine all the way to the sacrum. Craniosacral therapy is different from chiropractic manipulation in that the adjustments are very subtle and are aimed at improving the flow of cerebrospinal fluid down the spinal canal. One study showed improved concentration, socialization, and less self-stimulation behavior after a course of craniosacral therapy.[119]

Holding children with autism, even when they resist, has been reported effective in improving social interaction and responsivity. In one study, 7 autistic children were selected at random from a group of 14 and treated with modified holding therapy for 4 weeks. The remaining seven children (control group) were not treated during this 4-week waiting period. Four of these children were then treated with modified holding therapy. The children's parents assessed positive behavior changes (increases in desirable behavior and decreases in undesirable behavior) and negative changes on a behavior rating scale. Significantly more positive changes in behavior problems were reported for the treatment group than for the untreated group in each of the four symptom categories assessed (disturbances in perception, speech, social interaction, and obsessive–compulsive or ritualistic behavior). The four children in the control group who were later treated with modified holding therapy showed behavior changes that correlated highly with those reported for the experimental group.[120]

It is important to remember with healing methods that are nonpharmacological that their effectiveness is a complex mixture of technique, therapist, expectation, and communication.[121–125]

Psychological Therapies, Including Behavior Therapy

A tactile prompting device (the gentle reminder) has been studied as a means for prompting children with autism to make verbal initiations about play activities. The device served as an effective, unobtrusive prompt for verbal initiations during play contexts and during cooperative learning activities. More importantly, it showed that learning received from the use of the device would generalize to other contexts and activities.[126]

Seeing adults imitate the behaviors of children with autism leads to increased social behavior in the children. Twenty children were recruited from a school for children with autism to attend three sessions during which an adult either imitated all of the children's behaviors or simply played with the child. During the second session the children in the imitation group spent a greater proportion of time showing distal social behaviors toward the adult, including (1) looking, (2) vocalizing, (3) smiling, and (4) engaging in reciprocal play. During the third

---

▶ Case Example 2: Autism

Michael is an example of a child treated with an integrative approach for autism. Michael presented on multiple medications, of questionable value, according to his parents. His development was moderately impaired. He was in a special school for developmentally disabled children. We began with the implementation of a gluten- and casein-free diet, which improved his functioning and ratings on the Achenbach Child Behavior Checklist over 3 months. Then we implemented a number of supplements, including vitamin C, B-complex vitamins, omega-3 fatty acids, magnesium, zinc, and vitamin A. Further improvement occurred. Secretin was implemented next. Michael appeared to benefit enormously from secretin, although other therapies began at the same time, including craniosacral therapy, Reiki therapy (a Japanese energy-healing method), and ongoing extensive applied behavior therapy. Over the course of 1 year, Michael was transferred to a mainstream school and was participating with an aide. Consultation was provided to the teachers on how to implement naturalistic behavior therapy. Older, popular girls were paid to help Michael learn how to interact with other children. Then neurofeedback was implemented and Michael learned to control his brain waves to play a Pac Man-like game. By the second year of treatment, he was in a mainstream class without an aide. His teacher periodically forgot that he had been autistic. By the third year of treatment, he was mainstreamed. He changed schools. The new teacher did not know of his autistic background and did not inquire. Michael was near normal, although still exhibiting some minor stereotypies and a tendency to play alone. His therapies continued, although at a reduced frequency.

---

session, the children in the imitation group spent a greater proportion of time showing proximal social behaviors toward the adult including (1) being close to the adult, (2) sitting next to the adult, and (3) touching the adult. These data suggested the potential usefulness of adult imitative behavior as an early intervention.[127]

MUSIC THERAPY

Music has been an element in medical practice throughout history. There is growing interest in music as a therapeutic tool. There is no generally accepted standard for how, when, and where music should be applied within a medical framework. Traditionally, music has been linked to the treatment of mental illness, and has been used successfully to treat anxiety and depression and improve function in schizophrenia and autism. The role of music in medicine is primarily supportive and palliative. Mu-sic is well tolerated, inexpensive, with good compliance and few side effects.[128]

NATURALISTIC BEHAVIOR THERAPY

Most practitioners in the autism world have heard of Lovass' technique of applied behavioral analysis. This approach is based upon teaching the child skills through interaction in discrete trials in which the child is rewarded for the correct response. Rewards often include food: sometimes, unfortunately, foods to which the child may be allergic such as nut-containing candies. Studies from the Autism Research Center at the School of Education, at the University of California at Santa Barbara, have shown that naturalistic behavior therapies are better than applied behavioral analysis at changing autistic behaviors. This approach incorporates natural situations in which the child is already interacting and rewards the child through creating opportunities to do more of what the child already enjoys doing. Nonautistic children may be recruited to be part of the therapeutic process. Examples of therapies in the classroom include a teacher developing a game for the entire class when her autistic student was obsessed with maps. The game consisted of the children dividing into teams and drawing states on sidewalks with chalk as fast as possible, including locating the capitol of the state. The autistic student was excellent at this game and was soon desired as a team member, thereby improving his opportunities for interaction with other children.

▶ ACNE

Pathophysiology

There are several important factors in the evolution of acne. First, the squamous epithelial lining of the hair follicle is not appropriately sloughed, leading to the formation of a plug.[129] The follicular canal is blocked causing a lesion called a microcomedone. The next important factor is the overproduction of sebum as a consequence of the influence of androgenic hormones. Hyperandrogenic states such as adrenal androgen excess, 21-hydroxylase deficiency, and polycystic ovary syndrome contribute to acne. Dihydrotestosterone is a powerful stimulus for production of sebum. Patients who suffer from acne have a 30-fold increase in their conversion of testosterone to dihydrotestosterone in their sebaceous glands.

Eventually, the hair follicle enlarges because of sebum and keratinous materials trapped below the plug. A cystic lesion is formed called a closed comedone (whitehead). The pore then enlarges, and sebum protrudes and becomes oxidized. The protruding sebum appears black, forming the so-called open comedone (blackhead). Another important contributor to the evolution of acne is proliferation of *Propionibacterium acne*, a gram-negative anaerobic diphtheroid that is normally found in hair follicles. The final factor is the release of chemotactic factors and proinflammatory mediators, which cause damage, and rupture of hair follicles. Pustules, papules and nodules are formed when the follicular contents spill into surrounding tissues causing inflammation.

Acne can be classified into three different categories. Table 31–1 outlines the classification of acne.

Prevalence

Acne vulgaris is the most common skin condition evaluated and treated by physicians. It affects almost 45 million people in the United States.[130] The prevalence rate of acne increases

▶ TABLE 31–1 TYPES OF ACNE

Type	Description	Treatment
Comedonal acne	Open or closed comedones with almost no inflammatory lesions	Comedonolytic agents
Inflammatory acne	Comedonal lesions plus inflammatory lesions such as erythematous papules and pustules	A topical agent and a systemic antibiotic
Nodulocystic acne	Comedonal and inflammatory lesions plus nodule	May require isotretnoin when it fails to respond with an 8-week course of systemic antibiotic treatment

at puberty and usually decreases by 30 years of age. It affects 80% of people between the ages of 15 and 24 years. The prevalence of acne decreases with advancing age after adolescence, falling to 8% in the 25–34 years age range and 3% in the 35–44 years age range.[131] The duration of acne is on an average 8 to 12 years.[132]

Psychological Impact

The psychological impact of acne can be devastating. Adolescence is a time of low self-esteem, high peer pressure, rebellion against authority, and struggles to establish independence. The young person who has concerns about appearance will frequently miss school, work, or social events, thus increasing feelings of depression and isolation.[133] Kellett found that patients with acne reported similar levels of social, psychological, and emotional problems when compared to reports of patients with chronic disabling asthma, epilepsy, diabetes, back pain, or arthritis.[134] A recent survey of English teenagers suffering from acne found that there was a strong relationship between acne and poor emotional health.[135]

Conventional Medicine Approach

The spectrum of antiacne agents found on the market targets the four pathogenic factors for acne: overproduction of sebum, hyperkeratinization of follicular cells, proliferation of *P. acne*, and inflammation. Choice of medication should be tailored to act on the predominant type of lesion. The topical tretinoins (all-*trans*-retinoic acid) are very effective comedolytic agents. They normalize follicular keratinization, help drain comedones, and also inhibit the formation of new comedones.[136] Combination therapy with topical or systemic antibiotics is also effective because the retinoids increase the penetration and enhance efficacy of other agents.[137]

Adapalene, derived from synthetic naphthalic acid, modulates keratinization and inflammation. A recent meta-analysis, comparing adapalene and tretinoins, showed that adapalene 0.1% gel provides equivalent efficacy and superior local tolerability compared to that of tretinoin 0.025% gel.[138] Tazarotene is a synthetic acetylcholine retinoid. This agent can be used overnight everyday or every other day.[139]

Oral isotretinoin is the only systemic agent that affects all four factors that cause acne.[140] It is very effective in treatment of nodulocystic or severe inflammatory acne.[141] However, there are significant side effects, and the medication is teratogenic. Side effects of oral isotretinions include elevation of triglycerides and liver enzymes and dryness of skin and mucous membranes, which can lead to epistaxis.

The first-line acne medication, benzoyl peroxide, was introduced in the 1950s. Benzoyl peroxide is a potent topical bactericidal and is effective against *P. acne*. The most frequent side effect is skin irritation. Benzoyl peroxide may bleach clothing and bed linens.

Topical antibiotics that are available include erythromycin, clindamycin, sodium sulfacetamide, and salicylic acid. Erythromycin and clindamycin have equivalent efficacy for treatment of moderate acne. These products can be used in combination with benzoyl peroxide or tretinoin to increase efficacy. Resistant strains of *P. acne* are becoming more prevalent.[142] Resistance to erythromycin may be reduced if it is used in combination with benzoyl peroxide.[143] The combination of clindamycin with benzoyl peroxide gel has demonstrated efficacy and good overall tolerability in several well-designed clinical studies in the topical treatment of patients with mild to moderately severe acne vulgaris.[144]

Systemic antibiotics used for acne include erythromycin and tetracycline or its derivatives, doxycycline, and minocycline. Systemic antibiotics are needed for moderate to severe inflammatory acne that has not responded to topical combinations. Erythromycin and tetracycline also possess intrinsic antiinflammatory activity. Minocycline is the most effective and is least likely to be resistant to *Propionibacterium.*

Estrogens, antiandrogens such as spironolactone, and the retinoid isotretinoin can influence the production of sebum. The sebaceous gland is androgen dependent, thus estrogen and antiandrogens are useful in acne therapy for women who have new-onset or worsening acne in their adult lives, premenstrual flare-ups, or who have failed to respond to other systemic antiacne medication.[145] Results are noted after 2 to 3 months of use. Antiandrogens can cause feminizing effects on a male fetus. Side effects include irregular vaginal bleeding and breast tenderness. Spironolactone has not been approved by FDA for treatment of acne.

Integrative Medicine Approach

The goal of treatment of acne is to decrease inflammation and prevent scarring. Patients should be advised to gently hand wash the face twice a day with lukewarm water using a non–soap-based cleanser. Patients should also be encouraged not to squeeze comedones indiscriminately. Use of thick, oily facial makeup and greasy hair products has the propensity to plug up sebaceous glands and should be avoided.

NUTRITIONAL APPROACHES

Diet has not been specifically associated with acne formation; however, because inflammation is an important contributor to the pathophysiology of acne, it may be helpful to cut down on foods that can increase the inflammatory process. Diets containing high omega-3 fatty acids may reduce prostaglandins and leukotrienes and thus reduce inflammation.[146]

Vitamin A reduces sebum and follicular hyperkeratosis. A high dose of vitamin A is required to attain results, which precludes everyday use because of the probability of hypervitaminosis A. In one study, a high dose of vitamin A was used to treat severe acne in teenagers. There was an initial improvement

of the acne lesions, but the effect was not sustained when therapy was discontinued.[147] Side effects include headache, myalgia, fatigue, and abnormal liver enzymes. Toxicity can cause nausea, anorexia, dry skin, hair loss, and hepatitis.

Women with premenstrual acne may find benefit with vitamin B_6. One small trial found that vitamin B_6 (pyridoxine) 50 mg/d alleviated flare-ups of acne before the onset of the menstrual cycle.[148] No large clinical trials have substantiated these findings.

Zinc is required in wound healing. Mixed results have been found on oral zinc supplements in double-blinded trials. Michaelsson[149] found a benefit of zinc but Cunliffe[150] failed to show any benefit of zinc on acne. A trial of zinc supplementation may be helpful to determine efficacy. The patient is counseled to take zinc 30 mg two to three times a day for a few months, then once a day thereafter. Zinc picolinate is best for its bioavailability compared to other preparations. If no improvement is noted after 12 weeks of therapy, most likely no benefit will occur. Prolonged intake of zinc can cause copper deficiency.

BOTANICAL MEDICINES
TANNINS

There are some reports of success using tannin-containing herbs such as witch hazel and oak bark as topical astringents for acne, but no controlled studies showing efficacy are available in the literature. Witch hazel (*Hamamelis virginiana)* bark extract can be prepared from its decoction. It is quite safe for topical use. Commercially available preparations may not be suitable as tannins are lost in the distillation process.[151] Astringents do not change the prognosis of acne, but can be used in patients with very oily skin, and they may offer a soothing effect on inflamed skin.

Fruit acids, such as citric, gluconic, gluconolactone, glycolic, malic, and tartaric acids, have been used topically to control acne with some success because of their exfoliative properties. In one study, gluconolactone was as effective as 5% benzoyl peroxide in clearing inflamed and noninflamed acne lesions. Gluconolactone was also found to be more effective than placebo.[152] The main side effect of fruit acids is skin irritation, especially with higher concentrations.

Tea tree oil may play a role in acne treatment, when applied to the skin directly, through its antimicrobial properties. It is an essential oil extracted from the leaves of a tree, *Melaleuca alternifolia,* found in Australia. The oil is composed of several compounds, mainly plant terpenes and their corresponding alcohols.[153] In 1990, a study of 124 patients compared 5% tea tree oil in a water-based gel with 5% benzoyl peroxide. There was a statistically significant improvement in the number of acne lesions at the end of 3 months.[154] There was also significant lower incidence of adverse effects such as dryness, irritation, itching, and burning with the tea tree oil as compared to benzoyl peroxide. A recent systematic review of randomized clinical trials found tea tree oil to be effective as a treatment for acne; the evidence appears to be compelling but requires further study.[155] Patients should be warned about possible development of allergic dermatitis with the use of tea tree oil.[156]

Brewers yeast, a medicinal yeast consisting of fresh or dried cells of *Saccharomyces cerevisiae* has been used for acne. It has high chromium content and has antibacterial action.[157]

Azelaic acid is a naturally occurring dicarboxylic acid found in wheat, rye, and barley. The Food and Drug Administration has approved the use of azelaic acid as a 20% concentration. Azelaic acid contains both bacteriostatic and bactericidal properties against a variety of aerobic and anaerobic microorganisms present on the skin of patients suffering from acne. It also has an antikeratinization effect. Most likely the antiproliferative/cytotoxic effects of azelaic acid are mediated primarily via disruption of mitochondrial respiration and/or cellular DNA synthesis. Topical application of azelaic acid has similar efficacy to

topical benzoyl peroxide gel 5%, tretinoin cream 0.05%, erythromycin cream 2%, and oral tetracycline 0.5–1.0 g/d in treating comedonal and mild to moderate inflammatory acne.[158,159] Side effects of azelaic acid include mild transient erythema and cutaneous irritation that usually subsides after 2–4 weeks of treatment. Hypopigmentation and photosensitization may also occur but these are rare.[160]

Azelaic acid cream 20% should be applied twice daily for at least 2–3 months and can be used for up to 1 year. Improvement is noticed within 1–2 months. Cream should be rubbed thoroughly (but not too vigorously) into cleansed skin for 2–3 minutes.

Vitex (Vitex agnus-castus) taken orally is effective in treating premenstrual acne. For medicinal activity, the whole-fruit extract is to be taken.[161] The whole-fruit extract is thought to act on follicle-stimulating hormone and luteinizing hormone levels in the pituitary to increase progesterone levels and reduce estrogen levels. The main adverse effects reported are gastrointestinal tract upset and rash. It is contraindicated for pregnant or nursing women.

Guggul (Commiphora mukul) has been used mostly for lowering cholesterol. A small clinical trial found positive results when guggulipid was compared to tetracycline in patients with nodulocystic acne. It was also observed that patients with oily faces responded better.[162]

BURDOCK ROOT

Historically, alterative ("blood cleansing") herbs such as burdock root (*Arctium lappa*) have been recommended by traditional herbalists as an internal approach to acne, eczema, and psoriasis.[163] The proposed mechanism of action of burdock root is the underlying belief that the skin becomes diseased when the input of toxins exceeds that which the liver, kidneys, and immune system can handle.

KAMPO

Kampo medicine's origin is traced back to the Chinese herbal tradition; it was introduced to

Japan over a millennium ago and was gradually adapted there. Several Kampo formulations have proven to be bactericidal to *P. acnes, Staphylococcus aureus,* and *S. epidermidis.* A study on susceptibility of *P. acnes, S. aureus,* and *S. epidermis* to 10 Kampo formulations was done. *P. acne* was most susceptible to Keigai-rengyo-to.[164]

LIGHT THERAPY

Irradiation of *P. acne* colonies with blue visible light leads to bacterial destruction.[165] Acne may be treated successfully with blue visible light phototherapy in vivo.[166] Light therapy can be prescribed for moderately inflamed acne. The FDA has recently approved the use of Clear Light in the United States.

AYURVEDA

The 5,000-year-old Indian traditional system of medicine has formulations that have been used for acne. Most of these formulas are compounded from plant extracts and minerals. In Ayurveda, acne is believed to arise from an aggravation of the Pitta dosha.

Various combinations of approaches have been recommended for treating acne. The combinations are based on thousands of years of tradition, but are not presently supported in the Western conventional medical literature. Such combinations may include herbs such as cinnamon, sandalwood, tumeric, neem, and giloy, and supplements such as Neem Guard capsule, Surakta syrup, Mahamanjisthadyarishta, and Haridra Khand, coupled with dietary recommendations to avoid excess meat, sugar, tea or coffee, pickles, soft drinks, and processed foods, and lifestyle recommendations such as yoga.[167] Other treatments include Dispirin in a glass of water used as a face wash and drinking herbal water to promote the body's self-cleansing, self-purifying system. In one popular folk treatment, an herbal water is prepared by boiling the corn silk of one ear of corn with 1–2 methi seeds in a glass full of water.

A number of herbal formulas have been used for acne such as Sookshama Triphala, Thisotanin, Amalakimashi Vati, Shankhbhasama Vati, and Sunder Vati.[168] Four ayurvedic formulations were studied in a double-blind, randomized, placebo-controlled clinical trial. Sunder Vati 250 mg (composition *Holarrhena antidysnterica* Linn, *Emblica officinalis, Embelia ribes* Burm, and *Zingiber officinale* Roscoe) significantly decreased the acne lesion count posttreatment when compared to placebo.[169] Sunder Vati is apparently quite safe with no side effects reported by the authors of the study.

MIND–BODY MEDICINE

Psychological stress can worsen acne.[170–172] It is therefore possible that relaxation therapies such as biofeedback, together with guided imagery, may improve acne symptoms. In a study of 30 individuals with acne, those who participated in electromyographic feedback and guided imagery demonstrated a significant improvement in acne symptoms compared to those who did not receive these treatments.[173]

Hypnosis has been used in several different types of dermatological diseases. A recent review by Shenefelt provides evidence that acne is one of the skin diseases that can be improved or cured by hypnosis.[174] Hypnosis enables the individual to relax and may influence the activity of hormones and the immune system to reduce inflammation.

CHINESE MEDICINE

Based on principles of traditional Chinese medicine, acne is treated by clearing the heart, dispelling wind and damp, detoxification, cooling the blood, and reducing stagnation. Both the body and auricular points have been used for acupuncture. To date, a number of case series do suggest that acupuncture may be effective in treating acne, but further research is needed before we can draw definite conclusions.[175]

► Case Example 3: Acne

AI is a 19-year-old adolescent male who has been suffering with acne since he was 15 years old. He is now a college sophomore, and his lifestyle includes eating fast food on a regular basis. He goes to the gymnasium to build his muscles and is trying to keep a steady relationship with his girlfriend. His acne has been mild for several years. He sought treatment intermittently from his primary care physician, but has not been able to control the flare-ups of inflammation and formation of pustular nodules with over-the-counter and prescribed medications, including benzoyl peroxide, topical antibiotic, oral antibiotic, and topical retinoid. During the last year, his acne became more severe resulting in scarring of his face, thus affecting his self-esteem and self-confidence. He finally sought a consultation with a dermatologist. He was advised to start an oral retinoid. He agreed to start the treatment but is planning to return to his primary care physician to obtain advice on alternative therapies because of his concern about long-term side effects of the oral retinoids.

Conclusion

AI saw a primary care physician who after a thorough history and physical exam obtained important information that would help in the management of his acne. The patient apparently had been taking steroids for bodybuilding and admitted noticing a flare-up of his acne within a month of starting. He stated that his face got sweaty, so he wiped his face with a towel when exercising in the gymna-sium. He had also been washing his face vigorously three times a day with a pad that was abrasive. He had two incidents of epistaxis, which stopped after putting pressure over his nose. The patient also complained that he felt very anxious, which has affected his relationship with his girlfriend. His anxiety was fueled by the thought of having a scarred face and becoming ugly. The examination of his face showed few nodular and several pustular lesions around his chin, cheek and chest. His facial skin was dry and his lips were quite dry and peeling.

AI was advised to stop taking the steroid and to stop washing his face vigorously, and to wash with lukewarm water and pat dry with a soft towel. He agreed to start jogging and exercise outside instead of inside the gymnasium. For epistaxis, he was advised to use synephrine if it recurred and use nasal saline spray frequently. He agreed to change his dietary habits by drinking more water instead of carbonated drinks, to decrease the amount of food he ate that was prepared with refined sugar, and to start a supplement of zinc daily. He also considered consulting with a biofeedback specialist to control his anxiety. He agreed to continue with isoretinoin. After a month, AI returned to the primary care office to report that his acne was much better. His skin had stopped peeling, and he had not had any further epistaxis. He also learned how to perform biofeedback for relaxation; he now feels much better about himself. AI was encouraged to continue with his present management and follow-up with his dermatologist.

REFERENCES

1. Wessel MA, Cobb SC, Jackson EB, et al. Paroxysmal fussing in infancy: sometimes called "colic." *Pediatrics.* 1954;14:421–424.

2. Wade S, Kilgour T. Infantile colic. *BMJ.* 2001;323(7310):437–440.

3. Lucassen PL, Assendelft WJ, van Eijk J, et al. Systematic review of the occurrence of infantile colic in the community. *Arch Dis Child.* 2001;84(5):398–403.

4. Garrison M, Christakis D. A systematic review of treatments for infant colic. *Pediatrics.* 2000;106 (1):184–190.

5. Hill DJ, Hudson IL, Sheffield LJ, Shelton MJ, Hosking CS. A low allergen diet is a significant intervention in infantile colic: results of a community-based study. *J Allergy Clin Immunol.* 1995;96:886–892.

6. Miller JJ, McVeagh P, Fleet GH, Petocz P, Brand JC. Effect of yeast lactase enzyme on "colic" in infants fed human milk. *J Pediatr.* 1990;117: 261–263.

7. Stahlberg MR, Savilahti E. Infantile colic and feeding. *Arch Dis Child.* 1986;61:1232–1233.

8. Campbell JPM. Dietary treatment of infant colic: a double-blind study. *J R Coll Gen Pract.* 1989; 39:11–14.

9. Barr RG, Young SN, Wright JH, et al. Differential calming responses to sucrose taste in crying infants with and without colic. *Pediatrics.* 1999;103(5).

10. Markestad T. Use of sucrose as a treatment for infant colic. *Arch Dis Child.* 1997;76:356–357.

11. Vanderhoof JA, Young RJ. Use of probiotics in childhood gastrointestinal disorders. *J Pediatr Gastroenterol Nutr.* 1998;27(3):323–332.

12. Weizman Z, Alkrinawi S, Goldfarb D, Bitran C. Herbal teas for infantile colic. *J Pediatr.* 1993; 123:670–671.

13. Klougart N, Nilsson N, Jacobsen J. Infantile colic treated by chiropractors: a prospective study of 316 cases. *J Manipulative Physiol Ther.* 1989; 12:281–288.

14. Wiberg JMM, Nordsteen N, Nilsson N. the short-term effect of spinal manipulation in the treatment of infantile colic: a randomized controlled trial with a blinded observer. *J Manipulative Physiol Ther.* 1999;22:517–522.

15. Hughes S, Bolton J. Is chiropractic an effective treatment in infantile colic? *Arch Dis Child.* 2002;86(5):382–384.

16. Olafsdottir E, Forshei S, Fluge G, Markestad T. Randomised controlled trial of infantile colic treated with chiropractic spinal manipulation. *Arch Dis Child.* 2001;84 (2):138–141.

17. Barr RG, McMullan SJ, Speiss H, et al. Carrying as colic "therapy": a randomized control trial. *Pediatrics.* 1991;87:623–630.

18. Parkin PC, Schwartz CJ, Manuel BA. Randomized controlled trial of three interventions in the management of persistent crying of infancy. *Pediatrics.* 1993;92:197–201.

19. Taubman B. Parental counselling compared with elimination of cow's milk or soy milk protein for the treatment of infantile colic: a randomised trial. *Pediatrics.* 1988;81:756–761.

20. Dihigo SK. New strategies for the treatment of colic: modifying the parent/infant interaction. *J Pediatr Health Care.* 1998;12:256–262.

21. McKenzie S. Troublesome crying in infants: effect of advice to reduce stimulation. *Arch Dis Child.* 1991;66:1416–1420.

22. Kay, J. Gawkrodger DJ, et al. The prevalence of childhood atopic eczema in a general population. *J Am Acad Dermatol.* 1994;30:35–39.

23. Tay YK, Kong KH, Khoo L, Goh CL, Giam YC. The prevalence and descriptive epidemiology of atopic dermatitis in Singapore school children. *Br J Dermatol.* 2002;146(1):101–106.

24. Mortz CG, Lauritsen JM, Bindslev-Jensen C, Andersen KE. Prevalence of atopic dermatitis, asthma, allergic rhinitis, and hand and contact dermatitis in adolescents. The Odense Adolescence Cohort Study on Atopic Diseases and Dermatitis. 2001;144(3):523–532.

25. Laughter D, Istvan JA, Tofte SJ, Hanifin JM. The prevalence of atopic dermatitis in Oregon schoolchildren. *J Am Acad Dermatol.* 2000;43(4): 649–655.

26. Williams HC, Strachan DP. The natural history of childhood eczema: observations from the British 1958 birth cohort study. *Br J Dermatol.* 1998; 139(5):834–839.

27. Hirai S, Shin Y, Kageshita T, Syono M, Maekawa Y, Ono T. Clinical course of atopic dermatitis in Japanese patients. *J Dermatol Sci.* 1998;18(2): 128–131.

28. Larsen FS, Holm NV, Henning K. Atopic dermatitis: a genetic-epidemiological study in a population based twin sample. *J Am Acad Dermatol.* 1993;28:719–723.

29. Schade RP, Van Ieperen-Van Dijk AG, Van Reijsen FC, et al. Differences in antigen-specific T-cell responses between infants with atopic dermatitis with and without cow's milk allergy: relevance of Th2 cytokines. *J Allergy Clin Immunol.* 2000;106(6):1155–1162.

30. Manku MS, Horrobin DF, Morse N, et al. Reduced levels of prostaglandin precursors in the blood of atopic patients: defective delta-6-desaturase function as a biochemical basis for atopy. *Prostaglandins Leukot Med.* 1982;9(6):615–628.

31. Strachan DP, Taylor EM, Carpenter RG. Family

size, neonatal infection, and hay fever in adolescence. *Arch Dis Child.* 1996;74:422–426.

32. Strachan DP. Allergy and family size: a riddle worth solving. *Clin Exp Allergy.* 1997;27:235–236.

33. Brostoff J, Challacombe S. *Food Allergy and Intolerance.* Philadelphia: WB Saunders; 2002: 818–819.

34. Eigenmann PA, Calza AM. Diagnosis of IgE-mediated food allergy among Swiss children with atopic dermatitis. *Pediatr Allergy Immunol.* 2000; 11(2):95–100.

35. Majamaa H, Moisio P, Holm K, Turjanmaa K. Wheat allergy: diagnostic accuracy of skin prick and patch tests and specific IgE. *Allergy.* 1999; 54(8):851–856.

36. Sicherer SH, Sampson HA. Food hypersensitivity and atopic dermatitis: pathophysiology, epidemiology, diagnosis, and management. *J Allergy Clin Immunol.* 1999;104(3 pt 2):S114–S122.

37. Wahn U, Staab D, Nilsson L. Atopic eczema: how to tackle the most common atopic symptom. *Pediatr Allergy Immunol.* 1999;10(12 suppl):19–23.

38. Sloper KS, Wadsworth J, Brostoff J. Children with atopic eczema. I: clinical response to food elimination and subsequent double-blind food challenge. *QJM.* 1991;80(292):677–693.

39. Buske-Kirschbaum A, Geiben A, Hellhammer D. Psychobiological aspects of atopic dermatitis: an overview. *Psychother Psychosom.* 2001;70(1): 6–16.

40. Schmid-Ott G, Jaeger B, Meyer S, Stephan E, Kapp A, Werfel T. Different expression of cytokine and membrane molecules by circulating lymphocytes on acute mental stress in patients with atopic dermatitis in comparison with healthy controls. *J Allergy Clin Immunol.* 2001;108(3): 455–462.

41. Garg A, Chren MM, Sands LP, et al. Psychological stress perturbs epidermal permeability barrier homeostasis: implications for the pathogenesis of stress-associated skin disorders. *Arch Dermatol.* 2001;137(1):53–59.

42. Buske-Kirschbaum A, Geiben A, Hollig H, Morschhauser E, Hellhammer D. Altered responsiveness of the hypothalamus-pituitary-adrenal axis and the sympathetic adrenomedullary system to stress in patients with atopic dermatitis. *J Clin Endocrinol Metab.* 2002;87(9):4245–4251.

43. Barankin B, DeKoven J. Psychosocial effect of common skin diseases. *Can Fam Physician.* 2002;48:712–716.

44. Holm L, Bengtsson A, van Hage-Hamsten M, Ohman S, Scheynius A. Effectiveness of occlusive bedding in the treatment of atopic dermatitis—a placebo-controlled trial of 12 months' duration. *Allergy.* 2001;56(2):152–158.

45. Sanda T, Yasue T, Oohashi M, Yasue A. Effectiveness of house dust-mite allergen avoidance through clean room therapy in patients with atopic dermatitis *J Allergy Clin Immunol.* 1992;89(3):653–657.

46. Kales A. *The Pharmacology of Sleep.* Berlin: Springer-Verlag; 1995:451.

47. Kalliomaki M, Salminen S, Arvilommi H, Kero P, Koskinen P, Isolauri E. Probiotics in primary prevention of atopic disease: a randomised placebo-controlled trial. *Lancet.* 2001;357(9262): 1076–1079.

48. Rautava S, Kalliomaki M, Isolauri E. Probiotics during pregnancy and breast-feeding might confer immunomodulatory protection against atopic disease in the infant. *J Allergy Clin Immunol.* 2002;109(1):119–121.

49. Duggan C, Gannon J, Walker WA. Protective nutrients and functional foods for the gastrointestinal tract. *Am J Clin Nutr.* 2002;75(5):789–808.

50. Isolauri E, Arvola T, Sutas Y, Moilanen E, Salminen S. Probiotics in the management of atopic eczema. *Clin Exp Allergy.* 2000;30(11): 1604–1610.

51. Gdalevich M, Mimouni D, David M, Mimouni M. Breast-feeding and the onset of atopic dermatitis in childhood: a systematic review and meta-analysis of prospective studies. *J Am Acad Dermatol.* 2001;45(4):520–527.

52. Halken S, Jacobsen HP, Host A, Holmenlund D. The effect of hypo-allergenic formulas in infants at risk of allergic disease. *Eur J Clin Nutr.* 1995;49(suppl 1):S77–S83.

53. Yoon S, Lee J, Lee S. The therapeutic effect of evening primrose oil in atopic dermatitis patients with dry scaly skin lesions is associated with the normalization of serum gamma-interferon levels. *Skin Pharmacol Appl Skin Physiol.* 2002;15(1): 20–25.

54. Henz BM, Jablonska S, van de Kerkhof PC, et al. Double-blind, multicentre analysis of the efficacy of borage oil in patients with atopic eczema. *Br J Dermatol.* 1999;140(4):685–688.

55. Hederos CA, Berg A. Epogam evening primrose oil treatment in atopic dermatitis and asthma. *Arch Dis Child.* 1996;75(6):494–497.

56. Morse PF, Horrobin DF, Manku MS, et al. Meta-analysis of placebo-controlled studies of the efficacy of Epogam in the treatment of atopic eczema. Relationship between plasma essential fatty acid changes and clinical response. *Br J Dermatol.* 1989;121(1):75–90.

57. Koblenzer PJ. Parental issues in the treatment of chronic infantile eczema. *Dermatol Clin.* 1996;14(3):423–427.

58. Ehlers A, Stangier U, Gieler U. Treatment of atopic dermatitis: a comparison of psychological and dermatological approaches to relapse prevention. *J Consult Clin Psychol.* 1995;63(4): 624–635.

59. Stewart A, Thomas SE. Hypnotherapy as a treatment for atopic eczema in adults and children. *Hypnosis.* 1996;23(1):48–55.

60. McMenamy CJ, Katz RC, Gipson M. Treatment of eczema by EMG biofeedback and relaxation training: a multiple baseline analysis. *J Behav Ther Exp Psychiatry.* 1988;19(3):221–227.

61. Sheehan MP, Atherton DJ. A controlled trial of traditional Chinese medicinal plants in widespread non-exudative atopic eczema. *Br J Dermatol.* 1992;126(2):179–184.

62. Sheehan MP, Atherton DJ. One-year follow up of children treated with Chinese medicinal herbs for atopic eczema. *Br J Dermatol.* 1994;130(4): 488–493.

63. Sheehan MP, Rustin MH, Atherton DJ, et al. Efficacy of traditional Chinese herbal therapy in adult atopic dermatitis. *Lancet.* 1992;340(8810): 13–17.

64. Latchman Y, Banerjee P, Poulter LW, Rustin M, Brostoff J. Association of immunological changes with clinical efficacy in atopic eczema patients treated with traditional Chinese herbal therapy (Zemaphyte). *Int Arch Allergy Immunol.* 1996;109(3):243–249.

65. Fung AY, Look PC, Chong LY, But PP, Wong E. A controlled trial of traditional Chinese herbal medicine in Chinese patients with recalcitrant atopic dermatitis. *Int J Dermatol.* 1999;38(5): 387–392.

66. Ernst E. Adulteration of Chinese herbal medicines with synthetic drugs: a systematic review. *J Intern Med.* 2002;252(2):107–113.

67. Perharic L, Shaw D, Leon C, De Smet PA, Murray VS. Possible association of liver damage with the use of Chinese herbal medicine for skin disease. *Vet Hum Toxicol.* 1995;37(6):562–566.

68. Kanner L. (1943). Autistic disturbances of affective contact. *J Nerv Dis Child.* 1943;2:217–250.

69. Tsai LY, Ghaziuddin M. Autistic disorder. In: Weiner J, ed. *The Comprehensive Textbook of Child and Adolescent Psychiatry.* 2nd ed. Washington, DC: American Psychiatric Press; 1996: 219–254.

70. Hameury L, Roux S, Barthelemy C, et al. Quantified multidimensional assessment of autism and other pervasive developmental disorders. Application for bioclinical research. *Eur Child Adolesc Psychiatry.* 1995;4(2):123–135.

71. Hameury L, Roux S, Barthelemy C, et al. Quantified multidimensional assessment of autism and other pervasive developmental disorders. Application for bioclinical research. *Eur Child Adolesc Psychiatry.* 1995;4(2):123–135.

72. Roux S, Bruneau N, Garreau B, et al. Bioclinical profiles of autism and other developmental disorders using a multivariate statistical approach. *Biol Psychiatry.* 1997;42(12):1148–1156.

73. O'Tuama LA, Treves ST. Brain single-photon emission computed tomography for behavior disorders in children. *Semin Nucl Med.* 1993;23(3): 255–264.

74. Hameury L, Roux S, Barthelemy C, et al. Quantified multidimensional assessment of autism and other pervasive developmental disorders. Application for bioclinical research. *Eur Child Adolesc Psychiatry.* 1995;4(2):123–35.

75. Wing L. Social and interpersonal needs. In: Schopler E, Mesibov GB, eds. *Autism in Adolescents and Adults.* New York: Plenum Press; 1983:337–353.

76. Roberts AH, Kewman DG, Mercier L, Hovell M. The power of non-specific effects in healing: implications for psychosocial and biological treatments. *Clin Psychol Rev.* 1993;12:375–391.

77. Roberts AH. The powerful placebo revisited: magnitude of nonspecific effects. *Mind Body Med.* 1995;1(1):35–43.

78. Knivsberg AM, Reichelt KL, Hoien T, Nodland M. A randomised, controlled study of dietary intervention in autistic syndromes. *Nutr Neurosci.* 2002;5(4):251–261.

79. Knivsberg AM, Reichelt KL, Hoien T, Nodland M. A randomised, controlled study of dietary intervention in autistic syndromes. *Nutr Neurosci.* 2002;5(4):251–261.

80. Page T. Metabolic approaches to the treatment of autism spectrum disorders. *J Autism Dev Disord.* 2000;30(5):463–469.

81. Johnson S. Micronutrient accumulation and depletion in schizophrenia, epilepsy, autism and Parkinson's disease? *Med Hypotheses*. 2001;56(5): 641–645.

82. Galland L. Magnesium, stress and neuropsychiatric disorders. *Magnes Trace Elem*. 1991–92; 10(2–4):287–301.

83. Shearer TR, Larson K, Neuschwander J, Gedney B. Minerals in the hair and nutrient intake of autistic children. *J Autism Dev Disord*. 1982;12(1): 25–34.

84. Grimaldi BL. The central role of magnesium deficiency in Tourette's syndrome: causal relationships between magnesium deficiency, altered biochemical pathways and symptoms relating to Tourette's syndrome and several reported comorbid conditions. *Med Hypotheses*. 2002;58(1): 47–60.

85. Wecker L, Miller SB, Cochran SR, Dugger DL, Johnson WD. Trace element concentrations in hair from autistic children. *J Ment Defic Res*. 1985;29(pt 1):15–22.

86. Henderson GI, Patwardhan RV, Hoyumpa AM Jr, Schenker S. Fetal alcohol syndrome: overview of pathogenesis. *Neurobehav Toxicol Teratol*. 1981;3(2):73–80.

87. Sukumar A. Factors influencing levels of trace elements in human hair. *Rev Environ Contam Toxicol*. 2002;175:47–78.

88. Megson MN. Is autism a G-alpha protein defect reversible with natural vitamin A? *Med Hypotheses*. 2000;54(6):979–983.

89. Clark JH, Rhoden DK, Turner DS. Symptomatic vitamin A and D deficiencies in an eight-year-old with autism. *J Parenter Enteral Nutr*. 1993;17(3): 284–286.

90. Lerner V, Miodownik C, Kaptsan A, Cohen H, Loewenthal U, Kotler M. Vitamin B6 as add-on treatment in chronic schizophrenic and schizoaffective patients: a double-blind, placebo-controlled study. *J Clin Psychiatry*. 2002;63(1):54–58.

91. Rimland B. High dose vitamin B6 and magnesium in treating autism: response to study by Findling et al. *J Autism Dev Disord*. 1998;28(6): 581–582.

92. Pfeiffer SI, Norton J, Nelson L, Shott S. Efficacy of vitamin B6 and magnesium treatment of autism: a methodology review and summary of outcomes. *J Autism Dev Disord*. 1995;25:481–493.

93. Findling RL, Maxwell K, Scotese-Wojtila L, Huang J, Yamashita T, Wiznitzer M. High-dose pyridoxine and magnesium administration in children

with autistic disorder: an absence of salutary effects in a double-blind, placebo-controlled study. *J Autism Dev Disord*. 1997;27(4):467–478.

94. Burd L, Stenehjem A, Franceschini LA, Kerbeshian J. A 15-year follow-up of a boy with pyridoxine (vitamin B6)-dependent seizures with autism, breath holding, and severe mental retardation. *J Child Neurol*. 2000;15(11):763–765.

95. Lowe TL, Cohen DJ, Miller S, Young JG. Folic acid and B12 in autism and neuropsychiatric disturbances of childhood. *J Am Acad Child Psychiatry*. 1981;20:104–111.

96. Hagerman RJ, Jackson AW, Levitas A, et al. Oral folic acid versus placebo in the treatment of males with the fragile X syndrome. *Am J Med Genet*. 1986;23:241–246.

97. Gillberg C, Whalstrom L, Johansson R, Tornblom M, Albertson-Wikland K. Folic acid as an adjunct in the treatment of children with the autism fragile X syndrome (AFRAX). *Dev Med Child Neurol*. 1986;28:624–627.

98. Brown WT, Jenkins EC, Cohen IL, et al. Fragile X and autism: a multicenter survey. *Am J Med Genet*. 1986;23:341–352.

99. For Nir I, Meir D, Zilber N, Knobler H, Hadjez J, Lerner Y. Brief report: circadian melatonin, thyroid-stimulating hormone, prolactin, and cortisol levels in serum of young adults with autism. *J Autism Dev Disord*. 1995;25:641–654.

100. Jan JE, O'Donnell ME. Use of melatonin in the treatment of paediatric sleep disorders. *J Pineal Res*. 1996;21:193–199.

101. Tsai LY. Medical treatment. In: Berkell Zager DE, ed. *Autism: Identification, Education, and Treatment*. 2nd ed. Mahweh, NJ: Lawrence Erlbaum; 1999:199–257.

102. Ward PE. Potential diagnostic aids for abnormal fatty acid metabolism in a range of neurodevelopmental disorders. *Prostaglandins Leukot Essent Fatty Acids*. 2000;63(1–2):65–68.

103. Woodward G. Autism and Parkinson's disease. *Med Hypotheses*. 2001;56(2):246–249.

104. Edelson SB, Cantor DS. Autism: xenobiotic influences. *Toxicol Ind Health*. 1998;14(6):799–811.

105. McFadden SA. Phenotypic variation in xenobiotic metabolism and adverse environmental response: focus on sulfur-dependent detoxification pathways. *Toxicology*. 1996;111(1–3):43–65.

106. Horvath K, Perman JA. Autism and gastrointestinal symptoms. *Curr Gastroenterol Rep*. 2002;4(3): 251–258.

107. McFadden SA. Phenotypic variation in xenobiotic metabolism and adverse environmental response: focus on sulfur-dependent detoxification pathways. *Toxicology.* 1996;111(1–3):43–65.

108. Brudnak MA. Probiotics as an adjuvant to detoxification protocols. *Med Hypotheses.* 2002;58(5): 382–385.

109. National Research Council. *Pesticides in the Diets of Infants and Children.* Washington, DC : National Academy Press; 1993.

110. Rice D, Barone S Jr. Critical periods of vulnerability for the developing nervous system: evidence from humans and animal models. *Environ Health Perspect.* 2000;108(suppl 3):511–533.

111. NIEHS. A research-oriented framework for risk assessment and prevention of children's exposure to environmental toxicants. *Environ Health Perspect.* 1999;107(6):510.

111a. Horvath K, Perman JA. Autism and gastrointestinal symptoms. *Curr Gastroenterol Rep* 2002; 4(3):251–258.

112. Rimland B. Secretin: real therapeutic potential [response]. *J Pediatr Gastroenterol Nutr.* 2000; 30(2):113.

113. Rimland B. Secretin treatment for autism. *N Engl J Med.* 2000;342(16):1216–1217.

114. Kern JK, Van Miller S, Evans PA, Trivedi MH. Efficacy of porcine secretin in children with autism and pervasive developmental disorder. *J Autism Dev Disord.* 2002;32(3):153–160.

114a. Sandler AD, Sutton KA, DeWeese J, Girardi MA, Sheppard V, Bodfish JW. Lack of benefit of a single dose of synthetic human secretin in the treatment of autism and pervasive developmental disorder. *New Engl J Med* 1999; 341(24): 1801–1806.

115. Mehl-Madrona L. Longitudinal study of secretin. Manuscript under editorial review, 2003.

116. Escalona A, Field T, Singer-Strunck R, Cullen C, Hartshorn K. Brief report: improvements in the behavior of children with autism following massage therapy. *J Autism Dev Disord.* 2001;31(5): 513–516.

117. Field T. Massage therapy for infants and children. *J Dev Behav Pediatr.* 1995;16(2):105–111.

118. Cullen L, Barlow J. "Kiss, cuddle, squeeze": the experiences and meaning of touch among parents of children with autism attending a touch therapy programme. *J Child Health Care.* 2002; 6(3):171–181.

119. Upledger JE. Infants, children, and brain dysfunction [videorecording] / with John E. Upledger. Palm Beach Gardens, FL: Upledger Institute; 1999.

120. Burchard F. Follow-up study of holding therapy—initial results in 85 children. *Prax Kinderpsychol Kinderpsychiatr.* 1988;37(3):89–98.

121. Field T, Lasko D, Mundy P, et al. Brief report: autistic children's attentiveness and responsivity improve after touch therapy. *J Autism Dev Disord.* 1997;27(3):333–338.

122. Escalona A, Field T, Singer-Strunck R, Cullen C, Hartshorn K. Brief report: improvement in the behavior of children with autism following massage therapy. *J Autism Dev Disord.* 2001;31(5): 513–516.

123. Stades-Veth J. Holding. 2. Prevention of autistiform behavior. *TVZ.* 1988;42(5):150–153.

124. Rohmann UH, Hartmann H. Modified holding therapy. A basic therapy in the treatment of autistic children. *Z Kinder Jugendpsychiatr.* 1985; 13(3):182–198.

125. Field T. Massage therapy for infants and children. *J Dev Behav Pediatr.* 1995;16(2):105–111.

126. Taylor BA, Levin L. Teaching a student with autism to make verbal initiations: effects of a tactile prompt. *J Appl Behav Anal.* 1998;31(4): 651–654.

127. Field T, Field T, Sanders C, Nadel J. Children with autism display more social behaviors after repeated imitation sessions. *Autism.* 2001;5(3): 317–323.

128. Myskja A, Lindbaek M. Examples of the use of music in clinical medicine. *Tidsskr Nor Laegeforen.* 2000;120(10):1186–1190.

129. Cunliffe W. *Acne.* London: Martin Dunitz; 1989.

130. White G. Recent findings in the epidemiologic evidence, classification, and subtypes of acne vulgaris. *J Am Acad Dermatol.* 1998;39:S34–S37.

131. Kraning K, Odland G. Prevalence, morbidity, and cost of dermatological diseases. *J Invest Dermatol.* 1979;73(suppl):395–401.

132. Cunliffe W. *Acne.* London: Martin Dunitz; 1989.

133. Mallon E, Newton J, Klassen A. The quality of life in acne: a comparison with general medical conditions using generic questionnaires. *Br J Dermatol.* 1999;140:672–676.

134. Kellett S, Gawkrodger D. The psychological and emotional impact of acne: the effect of treatment with isotretinoin. *Br J Dermatol.* 1999;140: 273–282.

135. Smithard A, Glazebrook C, Williams H. Acne

prevalence, knowledge about acne and psychological morbidity in mid-adolescence: a community-based study. *Br J Dermatol.* 2001;145(2): 274–279.

136. Bergefeld W. Topical retinoids in the management of acne vulgaris. *J Drug Dev Clin Pract.* 1996;8:151–160.

137. Gibson J. Rationale for the development of new topical treatments of acne vulgaris. *Cutis.* 1996; 57:13–19.

138. Cunliffe W, Poncet M, Loesche C. A comparison of the efficacy and tolerability of adapalene 0.1% gel versus tretinoin 0.025% gel in patients with acne vulgaris: a meta-analysis of five randomized trials. *Br J Dermatol.* 1998;139(S52): 48–56.

139. Leyden J, Lowe N, Kakita L, Draelos Z. Comparison of treatment of acne vulgaris with alternate-day applications of tazarotene 0.1% gel and once-daily applications of adapalene gel: a randomized trial. *Cutis.* 2001;67(suppl 6): 10–16.

140. Cunliffe W. Acne. In: Arndt K, Le-Boit P, Robinson J, Wintraub B, eds. *Cutaneous Medicine and Surgery*. Philadelphia: WB Saunders; 1996: 461–480.

141. Sykes N, Webster G. Acne: a review of optimum treatment. *Drugs.* 1994;48:59–70.

142. Eady E, Jones C, Tipper J. Antibiotic-resistant propionibacteria in antibiotic-treated acne patients: need for policies to modify antibiotic usage. *BMJ.* 1993;306:555–556.

143. Bearson D, Shalita A. The treatment of acne: the role of combination therapies. *J Am Acad Dermatol.* 1995;32:531–541.

144. Warner GT, Plosker G. Clindamycin/benzoyl peroxide gel: a review of its use in the management of acne. *Am J Clin Dermatol.* 2002;3(5): 349–360.

145. Shaw J. Spironolactone in dermatologic therapy. *J Am Acad Dermatol.* 1991;24:236–243.

146. Berbis P, Hesse S, Privat Y. Essential fatty acids and the skin. *Allergy Immunol.* 1990;22:225–231.

147. Kligman A, Mills O, Leyden. Oral vitamin in acne vulgaris. Preliminary report. *Int J Dermatol.* 1981; 20:278–285.

148. Snider B, Dietman D. Pyridoxine therapy for premenstrual acne flare. *Arch Dermatol.* 1974; 110:130–131.

149. Michaelsson G, Juhlin L, Ljunghall K. A double-blind study of the effect of zinc and oxytetracycline in acne vulgaris. *Br J Dermatol.* 1977;97: 561–566.

150. Cunliffe W, Burke B, Dodman B, Gould D. A double-blind trial of a zinc sulphate/citrate complex and tetracycline in the treatment of acne vulgaris. *Br J Dermatol.* 1979;101: 321–325.

151. Blumenthal M. Witch Hazel Leaf and Bark. In: *Herbal Medicine: Expanded Commission E Monographs*. Blumenthal M, Goldberg A, Brinckmann J. Eds. Newton, MA: Integrative Medicine Communications. 2000;231.

152. Hunt M, Barnston R. A comparative study of gluconolactone versus benzoyl peroxide in the treatment of acne. *Australas J Dermatol.* 1992;33: 131–134.

153. Swords G, Hunter G. Composition of Australian tea tree oil. *J Agric Food Chem.* 1978;26:734–737.

154. Bassett I, Pannowitz D, Barnston R. A comparative study of tea-tree oil versus benzoyl peroxide in the treatment of acne. *Med J Aust.* 1990; 153(8):455–488.

155. Ernst E, Huntley A. Tea tree oil: a systematic review of randomized clinical trials. *Forsch Komplementarmed Klass Naturheilkd.* 2000;7(1): 17–20.

156. Knight T, Hansen B. Melaleuca oil (tea tree oil) dermatis. *J Am Acad Dermatol.* 1994;30:423–427.

157. Blumenthal M, Yeast. In: Blumenthal M, Goldberg A, Brinckmann J, eds. *Herbal Medicine: Expanded German Commission E Monographs*. Newton, MA: Integrative Medicine Communication; 2000:424–428.

158. Nguyen Q, Bui T. Azelaic acid: pharmacokinetic and pharmacodynamic properties and its therapeutic role in hyperpigmentary disorders and acne. *Int J Dermatol.* 1995;34:75–84.

159. Fitton A, Goa K. Azelaic acid: a review of its pharmacological properties and therapeutic efficacy in acne and hyperpigmentary skin disorders. *Drugs.* 1991;41:780–798.

160. *Azelaic acid*—a new topical treatment for acne. *Drug Ther Bull.* 1993;31:50–52.

161. Blumenthal M. Witch Hazel Leaf and Bark. In: *Herbal Medicine: Expanded Commission E Monographs*. Blumenthal M, Goldberg A, Brinckmann J. eds. Newton, MA: Integrative Medicine Communications. 2000;108.

162. Thappa D, Dogra J. Nodulocystic acne: Oral guggulipid versus tetracycline. *J Dermatol.* 1994; 21(10):729–731.

163. Leung A, Foster S. *Encyclopedia of Common Natural Ingredients Used in Food, Drugs, and*

Cosmetics. New York: John Wiley & Sons; 1996.

164. Higaki S, Morimatsu S, Morohashi M. Susceptibility of *P. acne, Staphylococcus aureus* and *epidermis* to 10 Kampo formulations. *J Intern Med Res*. 1997;25:318–324.

165. Arakane K, Ryu A, Hayashi C. Singlet oxygen (1 delta g) generation from coproporphyrin in *Propionibacterium* acnes on irradiation. *Biochem Biophys Res Commun*. 1996;223: 578–582.

166. Papageorgiou P, Katsambas A, Chu A. Phototherapy with blue (415 nm) and red (660 nm) light in the treatment of acne vulgaris. *Br J Dermatol*. 2000;142:973–978.

167. Magic of Ayurveda.com Natural Treatments. Netbusmodel, Inc. Available at: http://www.magicofayurveda.com. Accessed January 14, 2003.

168. Sharangdhar S. In: Sharangdhar S, ed. *Chaukhamaha Orientia*. Varanasi, India; 1984:82–85.

169. Paranjpe P, Kulkarni P. Comparative efficacy of four ayurvedic formulations in the treatment of acne vulgaris: a double-blind randomized placebo-controlled clinical evaluation. *J Ethnopharmacol*. 1995;49:127–132.

170. Kenyon F. Psychosomatic aspects of acne. *Transact St John's Dermat Soc*. 1966;52(1): 71–78.

171. Kraus S. Stress, acne and skin surface free fatty acids. *Psychosom Med*. 1970;32:503–508.

172. Lorenz T, Graham D, Wolf S. The relation of life stress and emotions to human sebum secretion and to the mechanism of acne vulgaris. *J Lab Clin Med*. 1953;41:11–28.

173. Hughes H, Brown B, Lawlis G. Treatment of acne vulgaris by biofeedback relaxation and cognitive imagery. *J Psychosom Res*. 1983;27(3): 185–191.

174. Shenefelt P. Hypnosis in dermatology. *Arch Dermatol*. 2000;136(3):393–399.

175. Guoqing D. Advances in the acupuncture treatment of acne. *J Tradit Chin Med*. 1997;17(1): 65–72.

CHAPTER 32

Integrative Approach to Pregnancy

Aviva Romm

The use of the integrative approach during the childbearing cycle presents a significant dilemma for both the childbearing woman and the conscientious health practitioner. On the one hand, childbearing women are prone to a number of minor common complaints ranging from nausea during pregnancy to pain during labor to hemorrhoids in the postnatal period, for which the use of simple, effective, and safe natural remedies is frequently preferable to many over-the-counter and prescription pharmaceutical preparations. On the other hand, during the childbearing cycle, perhaps more than at any other time, there is a need for reassurance—even certainty—of the safety of the therapies that a childbearing woman is considering using. Unfortunately, that certainty is not always available, and patients and professionals must make difficult choices.

▶ SAFETY ISSUES

Safety issues need to be considered for all of the complementary therapies that a childbearing woman might choose or that the practitioner might prescribe. Hazards range from the possible physical consequences that can result from inappropriately applied massage or acupuncture techniques to teratogenic, mutagenic, or abortifacient qualities of botanical medicines. Even seemingly benign therapies, for example various "nonphysical" or "spiritual" interventions, such as sound therapy, color therapy, or faith healing, can pose harm to a childbearing woman if they are used in lieu of efficacious alternative therapies or necessary medical treatments. Mazotta et al. state this clearly, ". . . effectiveness must be ensured, given that ineffective treatment, when it results in a delay in administration of effective therapy, may be dangerous for the mother. That is, . . . therapies may be considered harmful if they are advocated as first-line therapies but are not effective."[1]

For practitioners caring for parturient women, a major dilemma is posed by the fact that so much is still unknown about the physiological effects of substances the mother might be exposed to or consume on the pregnancy and on the embryo and fetus. Most practitioners, therefore, take an extremely cautious approach to alternative therapies in pregnancy. Unfortunately, however, when practitioners—even with the best of intentions—invalidate their client's desire to try alternative therapies, the result might be to drive the client to use the therapy without informing the practitioner.

This situation may further jeopardize the patient's safety and interfere with other therapies the practitioner might be prescribing. Practitioners who are willing to be open minded and accurately informed may provide their patients with the broadest health options with the greatest safety margin.

Few alternative disciplines offer an additional credential for obstetric care as a specialty, with the exception of massage therapists who offer certification for prenatal massage and naturopathic physicians who specialize in midwifery. While one may be a highly experienced, licensed acupuncturist or naturopathic doctor, for example, this does not mean that one possesses the specialized knowledge needed for the care of pregnant women. This lack of specific credentialing can make it difficult for the primary medical practitioner and patient to determine the competence of any given complementary care practitioner for the special needs of pregnant women. Yet this is critical to the well-being of both patients involved in the prenatal dyad. Therefore, it is necessary to carefully interview potential practitioners for their experience specifically in the treatment of pregnant and parturient women and to contact professional organizations to determine whether such specialty training is available in that discipline. It may also be necessary for the patient or the primary physician to do some independent research on the safety of any therapies recommended by such practitioners before complying with those suggestions.

▶ OVERVIEW OF ALTERNATIVE THERAPIES IN PREGNANCY

This chapter reviews historical information, clinical applications, and known or available safety information for five major and commonly used complementary therapies: acupuncture (and Chinese medicine), massage therapy, aromatherapy, homeopathy, and herbal medicine. Because of the limited amount of research and evidence-based literature available on the therapeutic use of alternative therapies during pregnancy, the information presented below is necessarily more cautionary than prescriptive.

Chinese Medicine

Gynecology has been a medical subspecialty of traditional Chinese medicine (TCM) for 3,000 years.[2] TCM gynecology has within its domain five categories: menstruation, leukorrhea, pregnancy, parturition, and miscellaneous conditions. TCM philosophies and terminology are vastly different from those of Western medicine, relying on ancient cosmological and social viewpoints, which may at times seem archaic to the modern practitioner. Such beliefs and language are reflected in some of the major prescriptions for prenatal care and fetal education. For example, "For reproductive health, the physician should pay particular attention to the kidney channel in the early years of life, the liver channel in her prime, and the spleen in old age" (Li Dong Yuan, thirteenth century), and "If a mother wants the child to possess a dignified and elegant stature, the mother should think, speak, and act discreetly at this time; if a handsome child is desired, the mother should wear a piece of jade; if the desire is to have a witty baby, the mother should read verses and poems" (Huangdi Neijing, first century).

In spite of such archaic prescriptions, the TCM medical recommendations for health during the prenatal period consist of extremely practical advice: observe moderate living, practice meditation, get exercise (Tai Chi, Qigong), get adequate rest, and take good nourishment. In addition, the pregnant woman should "nourish the blood and yin" (the material and fluid aspects of the body), and "preserve and nourish the kidney essence," thought to govern reproduction and fetal development. Both nourishing the blood and yin and preserving and nourishing the kidney would primarily be accomplished with the use of diet and herbs appropriate to pregnancy and directed to these purposes.

Interestingly, among the traditional fetal care cautions in Chinese medicine are prescriptions to avoid lifting (presumably heavy objects) and the consumption of alcohol, as well as any disturbance in emotions that can "disrupt blood or Qi flow to baby causing injury." In addition, there is a traditional precaution against the use of acupuncture. In spite of this ancient precaution, however, acupuncture has been extensively used therapeutically during pregnancy both in China and in the West with beneficial outcomes, and modern clinical research has begun to support and validate such use. In modern clinical practice, acupuncture is routinely applied for a number of pregnancy-related conditions as detailed in Table 32–1.

Some of these applications have been studied in clinical trials specifically for the treatment of these conditions in pregnancy; for others there is no specific data regarding pregnancy, but there are studies demonstrating efficacy and safety of acupuncture outside of pregnancy.

A number of studies have been published demonstrating the effectiveness of acupuncture for the suppression and relief of nausea and vomiting of pregnancy (NVP) through the use of acupuncture or acupressure stimulation of what is referred to in TCM as the Neiguan, or pericardium 6 (P-6), an acupuncture point on the underside of the wrist.[3–7] Stimulation of the P-6 point, three fingers above the wrist on the palmar aspect of the forearm, has been shown to alleviate NVP by at least 50%.[1] P-6 stimulation for 5 minutes four times daily, or as continuously as possible, may be administered by acupuncture, acupressure, manual pressure, Seabands, or by a small transcutaneous electrical nerve stimulation unit.

In one study,[3] researchers randomly assigned 33 women with hyperemesis gravidarum (severe NVP) to acupuncture treatments on P-6 or to mock treatments at a different location. After 2 days, all treatments were stopped for an additional 2 days to allow any effects to dissipate. The groups were then reversed for 2 additional days of treatment. Before treatment all women were vomiting. On day 3, only 7 of 17 women (41%) receiving active acupuncture were still vomiting, as compared with 12 of 16 (75%) receiving mock treatment. After the active and mock treatment groups were switched, more of the women in the active treatment group ceased vomiting. The women in the active treatment group also reported decreased nausea.

In a study by Slotnick,[8] 41 patients were treated with acustimulation of P-6 with an acustimulation device at the Department of Maternal–Fetal Medicine at Eastern Virginia Medical School. Prior to treatment, patients averaged a score of 4.2 on a nausea severity scale, with 5 being completely debilitating nausea. Posttreatment device effectiveness averaged 4.2, with significant or complete relief rated 5. All neonates were evaluated for congenital abnormalities and all neonates were found to be normal. Slotnick concluded, "Because current pharmacological treatments for nausea in early pregnancy are not consistent, efficacious or without unwanted side effects or increased teratogenic risks, acustimulation of P-6 in pregnancy may prove to be a significant therapeutic alternative." The acupuncture principles and practices for the treatment of nausea and vomiting using P-6 and for the alleviation of pain have also been effectively and successfully extended to the treatment of postsurgical nausea and postsurgical pain relief, including postcesarean section.[9]

▶ **TABLE 32–1** COMMON APPLICATIONS OF ACUPUNCTURE DURING PREGNANCY

Nausea and vomiting of pregnancy	Hyperemesis gravidarum
Carpal tunnel syndrome	Heartburn
Varicose veins	Constipation
Hemorrhoids	Backache/sciatica
Drug addiction	Breech presentation
Smoking	Skin problems
Sinusitis	Induction of labor

In addition to the benefits from acupuncture for the treatment of NVP, acupuncture reduces the pain and duration of labor and birth. A study by Hyodo and Gega[10] demonstrated the effectiveness of acupuncture anesthesia for normal delivery. Definite subjective and objective relief of labor pain, as well as objective reporting of shortened second and third stages of labor by both primiparous and multiparous women was documented. There were no adverse effects to mother or child. These researchers concluded, "acupuncture anesthesia is useful for delivery, especially because of its safety, despite more erratic and less potent results than conventional anesthetic techniques." Wang et al.[11] conducted a survey between 1981 and 1987, and analyzed a collection of 16,649 cases involving the use of acupuncture anesthesia for cesarean sections conducted throughout 5 Chinese provinces. Not only did the researchers find a success rate of 99.9%, but also blood loss was found to be less than in cesareans in which epidural or local anesthesia were used. There were also no complications or anesthetic accidents when acupuncture anesthesia was conducted.

Another area in which TCM has shown some promise in the care of childbearing women is the use of the TCM practice of moxibustion to turn breech babies. A study by Cardini and Weixin of this technique, which involves the lighting of a cigar-like stick of *Artemesia vulgaris* over an acupuncture point on the little toe—beginning at 34 weeks' gestation—found increased fetal activity during the treatment period and increased cephalic presentation after the treatment period and at the time of birth. Of fetuses whose mothers used moxibustion, 75% rotated to a head-down position versus 48% in the control group.[12] A study published in 1998 in the *Journal of the American Medical Association* corroborated these findings.[12]

From a Western medical perspective, the mechanism of action is entirely unknown.[13] One proposed mechanism is an adrenocortical stimulation from the moxibustion leading to changes in prostaglandin level and thus increased uterine myometrial activity as a result of treatment.[12] The treatment appears to be entirely safe and inexpensive, is applied externally only, and is certainly a preferable alternative to external cephalic version or caesarean section for the management of persistent breech presentation. Because it is advised to be done from 34 weeks onward, treatment does not preclude the decision to perform external version or surgical delivery.

One further application of acupuncture is for cervical maturation at term.[11] Researchers organized 98 patients in the beginning of the ninth month of gestation into one control, two "placebo," and three acupuncture treatments groups. Cervical maturation was evaluated at 10-day intervals by using a Bishop score. The Bishop scores in the three treatment groups showed significant progression of 2.61 points versus 0.89 and 1.08 points, respectively, in the placebo and control groups. Tiran and Mack report on the findings of 12 separate clinical trials for the induction of labor, citing that none of the studies demonstrated negative side effects, although "some researchers found a disadvantage in that the strength and frequency of contractions cannot be controlled, although the contractions stimulated by acupuncture resembled those of spontaneous labor."[15]

Chinese herbs should be used with caution during pregnancy, particularly patent products, as they are well known to contain contaminants including botanical substitutions with toxic plant species, adulterants, heavy metals, and added pharmaceutical medications frequently not listed on the label, all of which can pose a threat to the safety of the pregnant woman and fetus. It is important that any pregnant or lactating women planning to use Chinese herbs research the source of the products and know with certainty that what she is getting is a botanically authenticated, high-quality herbal product.

Massage Therapy

There is a long tradition of providing pregnant women with massage to alleviate their physical discomforts, to prevent stretch marks, and to ensure that the baby is in the proper position. In one cultural anthropological book on birth, *Mamatoto*, massage during pregnancy is described as such:

> A Mayan Mexican woman is given an abdominal massage by the midwife as they chat about how she feels, how the baby is doing, when it might be born. The midwife, stroking oil . . . into the woman's belly, can feel from one visit to the next how the fetus is growing and in what position it's lying. Massage is a way of keeping in touch with the growing fetus, besides giving the expectant mother time to relax and feel at one with her body.[16]

The practice of prenatal, intranatal, and postnatal massage can be found ubiquitously worldwide in cultures from Japan to Jamaica.[17,18]

Prenatal massage therapy has gained such popularity in the past several years in the United States that there are now a national association of pregnancy massage therapists, numerous courses in prenatal massage, and a growing availability of such practitioners in many states. The negative effects of stress on health have become a widely recognized factor contributing to chronic health problems. Pregnant women are not immune to stress, and in fact, stress may be compounded by the physical discomforts associated with pregnancy, by the increased economic burden related to the responsibility of parenting, by shifting social and relationship roles, and by anxiety related to the experience of childbirth and parenting. The effects of maternal stress on the fetus are now recognized to translate into very real physical adverse outcomes[19] and increased levels of birth complications.[20] Stress is an established causal factor in postnatal depression, which can be severe and debilitating.

Several published studies point to the benefit of massage during pregnancy and labor for the reduction of anxiety, prenatal back pain, improvement of mood and sleep, and the reduction of complications of labor and postpartum, including a reduction in the rates of premature delivery.[21–23] Chang et al. conducted a randomized-controlled trial of massage during labor on 60 primiparous, low-risk mothers at a regional hospital in Taiwan. Eighty-seven percent of the women in the control group of 30 women reported reduction in pain and a sense of psychological support, with a reduction in anxiety in latent, active, and transitional stages of labor.

In another study,[21] 26 pregnant women were assigned to a massage therapy or a relaxation therapy group. The massage consisted of a 20-minute, twice-weekly massage given for 5 weeks. While both groups reported feeling less anxiety after the first session, and less after the last than after the first, only the massage therapy group reported a decrease in physical discomforts such as back pain and insomnia, and reported improvement in mood. Furthermore, only the massage therapy group showed a reduction in complications of labor and the postnatal period. In a previous study by Field et al.,[22] 28 women were recruited from prenatal classes and randomized to receive either massage during labor in addition to other support techniques such as breathing, or other support techniques alone. The women who received massage during labor had a significantly shorter hospital stay and less postpartum depression.

The general paucity of studies in this area is a reflection of the newness of prenatal massage as a discipline, and of the lack of attention from the medical community toward conducting studies in this area. Massage therapy may be used for the reduction of general stress and tension, mild general physical discomforts, reduction of stress on weight-bearing joints, reduction of tension, fatigue, and headaches, and possibly the reduction of hypertension.[15] Of course non-stress related etiological factors must be ruled out or addressed, as massage therapy is not a curative treatment for underlying disorders of pregnancy.

While there is little harm to be expected from the application of gentle massage therapy to pregnant women, certain precautions are advised by the National Association of Pregnancy Massage Therapists.[21] Table 32–2 outlines these contraindications and cautions.

▶ **TABLE 32-2** CONTRAINDICATIONS AND CAUTIONS FOR MASSAGE DURING PREGNANCY

General
Avoid the external application of essential oils during the first trimester with the exception of very mild and diluted oils such as lavender oil
High-risk pregnancies (do not proceed without written release of physician)
• Diabetic mother
• Cardiac disorders
• Chronic hypertension
• History of miscarriage
• Mothers younger than 20 years/older than 35 years of age
• Asthmatic mother
• Suspected Rh-negative mother or genetic problems
• Drug addiction or exposure
• Previous multiple births
Proceed with caution (physician's release advised)
• Incompetent cervix
• Complications caused by diethylstilbestrol
• Lung or liver disorder
• Severe anemia
• Convulsive disorder
• Abnormal fetal heartbeat
• Decrease or absence of fetal movement
• Intrauterine growth retardation
• Lupus erythematosus
• Poor lifestyle habits (drug abuse, poor nutrition, smoking, alcohol consumption)
• Low birth weight

Homeopathy

There are a number of common therapeutic applications of homeopathy during the childbearing cycle, including the prevention and treatment of miscarriage, anemia, cystitis, emotional instability, vaginitis, digestive complaints, pelvic pain, varicosities, abnormal bleeding, initiation of labor, failure to dilate, retained placenta, postpartum bleeding, and postnatal complications.[25–28] It is difficult, based upon literature review, to assess the efficacy of homeopathic treatments for such complaints. Table 32–3 summarizes several of the common homeopathic treatments for hemorrhoids.

In one review[29] of The Cochrane Pregnancy and Childbirth Group Trials Register, the Cochrane Controlled Trials Register, and bibliographies of related papers to determine the effects of homoeopathy for third-trimester cer-

vical maturation or induction of labor, randomized controlled trials comparing homeopathy used for third-trimester cervical ripening or labor induction with placebo/no treatment or other methods were reviewed. The reviewers concluded, based on the low quality of studies and insufficient information on such factors as methods of randomization, that there is insufficient evidence to recommend the use of caulophyllum, a popular "remedy" for homeopathic labor induction.

Conclusions regarding the efficacy of homeopathy for pregnancy-related problems are difficult to reach because of "methodological difficulties in comparing homeopathic and conventional medical intervention(s)" including lack of "specific research designs taking into account the different theoretical and practical approaches of the two disciplines,"[30] as well as generally inadequate numbers of sub-

▶ **TABLE 32-3** HOMEOPATHIC TREATMENTS FOR HEMORRHOIDS

	Homeopathic Treatment of Hemorrhoids: Sample of Homeopathic Assessment for Differentiation of Symptoms and Prescription		
	Arsenicum	**Nux-vomica**	**Pulsatilla**
Description of hemorrhoid	Blue/purple, bleeding	Burning, bleeding	Burning
External/internal	Internal	Internal, large, protruding in clusters of vesicles	Internal, hidden
Pain	Extreme	Extreme	Extreme
With	Debility	Itching, constipation, large, hard stool, backache	Continual itching and oozing
Worsened by	Advanced pregnancy	Advanced pregnancy	Advanced pregnancy; childbirth
Improved by	Warm-water baths	Cold-water baths	
Emotional behavior of patient	Restless, anxious, fear of being alone, wanted to be tended; difficult and demanding	Edgy, highly sensitive and irritable, impulsive, quarrelsome; irritable when questioned	Gentle, mild, yielding; clingy, desiring company and consolation
General attributes of patient	Very sensitive to cold; desires fresh air; tires suddenly	Very chilly, upset by smallest drafts	Chilly, dislikes stuffy rooms, no thirst

Adapted from Cummings B. Homeopathy for pregnancy and childbirth. In: Tiran D, Mack S, eds. Complementary Therapies for Pregnancy and Childbirth. *London: Bailliere Tindell; 1995:   .*

jects in most trials. However, it appears evident that for self-limiting and nonthreatening conditions there is no harm in attempting to use homeopathic preparations; for more severe conditions, as with other complementary therapies, the homeopath and primary practitioner should work in conjunction to assure that the patient is receiving adequate medical care.

Aromatherapy

Fragrance has been an important aspect of human evolution, with scent being a primal sense that carries associations, memories, and physical responses that resonate throughout the life of the human being. The history of spices, essential oils, perfumes, and their trade is rich, ancient, and extensive, with evidence of essential oil use ranging as far back in time as 4,500 BC in China and Egypt. The organic and oxygen based compounds in essential oils—terpenes, esters, aldehydes, phenols, ketones, and alcohols—have been recognized since the early nineteenth century; essential oils have been used as medicines in France, where much of the research on their activity and efficacy has been conducted.

As with other complementary therapies, aromatherapy has gained tremendously popularity in recent years.[31,32] Clinical aromatherapy, the use of specific essential oils for the prevention and treatment of health conditions, is increasingly being incorporated into the practices of naturopathic physicians, herbalists, midwives, nurses, and massage therapists, as well as becoming a discipline in its own right. In Europe, the Aromatherapy Organizations Council, an umbrella organization to ensure quality in aromatherapy training and practice, was established to promote a single body for professional aromatherapists.[33] While there is no formally recognized national certification in clinical aromatherapy in the United States, there is now a national certification examination offered through the National Association of Holistic Aromatherapists, and there are numerous clinical aromatherapy courses offered for certification, some of which are approved for continuing education for licensed health care providers.

Aromatherapy can be extremely beneficial to pregnant women. For example, relaxing scents can be added to a bath or diffuser to promote relaxation and sleep, or applied in diluted form as massage oils to ease aches and pains. Furthermore, the highly antiseptic nature of essential oils makes several of them, most notably lavender oil, traditionally valuable for the care of postcaesarean incisions, and for the treatment of perineal trauma from birth or episiotomy. However, a randomized clinical trial on the use of lavender oil for postnatal perineal comfort (n = 635), which compared pure lavender oil, synthetic lavender oil, and an inert substance as bath additives used daily for 10 days following normal childbirth, failed to show any statistically significant difference between the three groups on analysis of the total daily discomfort scores. The authors did note a nonsignificant decrease in mean discomfort scores on the third and fifth days in the lavender group, as compared to the two control groups. This is a time when the mother usually finds herself discharged home and perineal discomfort is high. As no side effects were found, the researchers concluded, that despite the lack of overall significant change in pain scores, "it seems that lavender oil may be a useful additional remedy to complement other forms of treatment helping postnatal mothers suffering from perineal discomfort."[34]

Because essential oils are extremely concentrated and potent substances with a wide range of chemical compounds and a real potential for toxicity, they should be used with a great deal of caution. Essential oils can cause negative reactions ranging from dermatitis to seizure, to hyper- and hypotension, and, in rare cases, even to death. Extreme care must therefore be taken to avoid excessive ingestion or other toxic exposure, particularly for pregnant women and newborns.

Essential oils that should be avoided during pregnancy can be divided into specific categories. Table 32–4 delineates these categories.[35] An exhaustive list of oils to be avoided is beyond the scope of this chapter; practitioners should consult an aromatherapy textbook before recommending oils not appearing on this list.

Conservative practitioners will avoid the use of the oils listed in Table 32–4 entirely during the first trimester, and use only 1–5% blends of essential oil to base oil with those herbs that appear in Table 32–4 but are considered safe for use externally after the first trimester. Base oils, also known as carrier oils, consist of nutritive oils that are completely safe for use. Most are food oils, such as almond oil, avocado oil, wheat germ oil, cocoa butter, and coconut oil.

Peppermint oil can be used in inhalation (a few drops of oil placed on a cotton ball and inserted into a vial, the vial to be open and the scent inhaled when there is nausea) for the treatment of NVP, but should be avoided internally. The volatile oil can cross the placental barrier and has an unknown effect on the developing fetal nervous system. Table 32–5 lists indications for other oils commonly used in pregnancy.

Herbal Medicine

If used with proper caution and taken in small amounts, herbs can provide relief for many minor pregnancy complaints; in expert hands, they can also be used for more complex pregnancy-related problems. However, herbs are also potent medicinal agents, and therefore great care and caution is advised for their use during pregnancy. Because the first trimester is a critical period of embryonic development and the effects of most herbs on the develop-

► **TABLE 32-4** ESSENTIAL OILS TO AVOID DURING PREGNANCY

Emmenagogues (oils that can initiate uterine bleeding/menses)			
Angelica	Basil*	Calamus	Camphor
Clary sage	Cypress	Jaborandi	Jasmine
Juniper	Lavender[‡]	Marjoram	Mugwort[†]
Mustard	Myrrh	Nightshade	Nutmeg
Pennyroyal	Peppermint[§]	Rose[‡]	Rosemary
Rue	Sage	Tansy	Thuja
Wormwood			
Toxic			
Bitter almond	Boldo	Clove	Horseradish
Mustard	Myrrh	Parsley	Oregano
Savin	Savory	Thyme	Wintergreen
Wormseed	Wormwood		
Abortifacients			
Mugwort	Pennyroyal	Rue	Sage
Tansy	Thuja	Wormwood	
Estrogenic			
Anise*	Fennel*		

*The use of herbs and spices for culinary purposes is not contraindicated; essential oils are highly concentrated substances, whereas food sources contain only small amounts of the essential oil.

[†]Chinese mugwort used for moxibustion in pregnancy is not considered contraindicated for use.

[‡]Considered safe for external use after the first trimester.

[§]Small amounts of these as herbs for use in tea, and as highly diluted essential oils used in diffusers or in baths, are not considered harmful.

ing fetus have not been well-documented, herbs should be avoided during this time.

While many herbal remedies are gentle and safe they are also pharmacologically active agents that should be administered with care. The following set of precautions can be used to ensure the safe use of botanical medicines during pregnancy:

• Natural is not synonymous with harmless or safe—many botanical medicines contain potent pharmacological substances.

• Many herbal constituents are capable of passing through the placenta and can therefore directly affect the fetus.

• Physiological and metabolic changes during pregnancy may influence the pharmacokinetics of the herbs.

• Preventive treatment and early intervention with herbs is safer and more effective than treating advanced problems, as dosage can typically be minimized and gentler herbs applied.

• Know each herb you are using by clearly

► **TABLE 32-5** ESSENTIAL OILS COMMONLY USED IN PREGNANCY

Essential Oil	Therapeutic Use
Lavender (*Lavandula officinalis*)	Antidepressant, antiseptic, relaxant, anxiolytic, carminative, antiviral, sedative, hypotensive, vulnerary for burns
Rose (*Rosa damscena*)	Antidepressant, antispasmodic, antiseptic, sedative, tonic
Tangerine (*Citrus reticulata*)	Antispasmodic, tonic, digestive, antispasmodic, antiseptic

understanding the side effects and the specific contraindications for the use of those herbs during pregnancy.

Table 32–6 provides a list of those herbs most commonly contraindicated for use during pregnancy. While there are a number of herbs on this list that may be used in small quantities for certain conditions, they should only be used under the supervision of a practitioner qualified in the use of herbs during pregnancy. Many naturopathic physicians, professional herbalists (for example, those registered with the American Herbalists Guild, Members of the National Institute of Medical Herbalists, and those certified in countries that have provisions for the legal practice of botanical medicine), and midwives specializing in the use of herbal medicines have specific training in this area. Certain herbs that are contraindicated by Western herbalists and Western scientific research for use during pregnancy are regularly used in other countries, such as dong quai *(Angelica sinensis)*, which is prescribed as a blood tonic for pregnant women in China. However, it is prudent to use such herbs cautiously if at

▶ **TABLE 32-6** HERBS CONTRAINDICATED IN PREGNANCY

Common Name	Botanical Name	Common Name	Botanical Name
Alder buckthorn	*Rhamnus frangula*	Juniper berries	*Juniperis communis*
Aloe	*Aloe vera*	Licorice	*Glycyrrhiza glabra*
Angelica	*Angelica archangelica*	Lily of the valley	*Convallaria magalis*
Arnica	*Arnica montana*	Lobelia*	*Lobelia inflata*
Autumn crocus	*Colchicum autumnale*	Male fern	*Dryopteris felix-mas*
Barberry	*Berberis vulgaris*	Mandrake	*Podophyllum peltatum*
Bethroot*	*Trillium* spp.	Mistletoe*	*Viscum album*
Black Cohosh*	*Cimicifuga racemosa*	Mugwort	*Artemesia vulgare*
Blessed thistle	*Carbenia benedicta*	Nutmeg (small	*Myristica officinalis*
Blood root	*Sanguinaria canadensis*	amounts fine)	
Blue Cohosh*	*Caulophyllum thalyctroides*	Osha	*Ligusticum porten*
Broom	*Sarpthamnus scoparius*	Parsley (small	*Carum petroselinum*
Butternut	*Juglans canadensis*	amounts fine	
Calamus	*Acorus calamus*	Pennyroyal	*Mentha pulegium*
Calendula	*Calendula officinalis*	Periwinkle	*Vinca* spp.
Cascara Sagrada	*Rhamnus purshiana*	Peruvian bark	*Cinchona* spp.
Coltsfoot	*Tussilago farfara*	Pleurisy root	*Aesclepius tuberosa*
Comfrey	*Symphytum officinale*	Poke root	*Phytolacca decondra*
Cotton root*	*Gossypium herbaceum*	Rue	*Ruta graveolens*
Cowslip	*Primula veris*	Rhubarb	*Rheum palmatum*
Damiana	*Turnera aphrodisiaca*	Sage	*Salvia officinalis*
Dong Quai	*Angelica sinensis*	Sarsaparilla	*Smilax officinale*
Ephedra	*Ephedra vulgaris*	Senna	*Cassia senna*
(Ma Huang)		Shepherd's purse*	*Capsella bursa-pastoris*
Feverfew	*Tanacetum parthenium*	Stillingia	*Stillingia sylvatica*
Ginseng*	*Panax quinquefolium*	Tansy	*Tanacetum vulgare*
Goldenseal*	*Hydrastis canadensis*	Thuja	*Thuja occidentalis*
Gotu kola	*Hydrocotyle asiatica*	Wormwood	*Artemesia absinthum*
Goat's rue	*Galega officinalis*	Yarrow	*Achillea millefolium*
Ipecac	*Ipecac ipechachuana*		

*Use these herbs with caution intrapartum. These herbs are generally contraindicated prior to the onset of labor.

all during pregnancy, and whenever possible to use them within traditional guidelines and formulae.

There are a few basic groups of herbs which are absolutely contraindicated during pregnancy. Herbs containing pyrrolizidine alkaloids can cause venoocclusive liver disease in fetuses when the herb is ingested regularly by pregnant women. Comfrey, coltsfoot, and borage all contain varying amounts of pyrrolizidine alkaloids. They should be avoided for internal use and should be used only topically for a short-course when there is no broken skin.

Herbs that have strong hormonal properties, as well as those that are known to promote menstruation (emmenagogues), are to be completely avoided; stimulating laxatives, as well as anthelmintics and vermifuges are contraindicated, as is the internal use of all essential oils. As noted in Table 32–6, certain herbs may be used with caution intrapartum, but are generally contraindicated prior to the onset of labor. For a more extensive list of herbs contraindicated in pregnancy, consult *The Botanical Safety Handbook.*[36]

Botanical medicines can be administered in a variety of forms. Internal routes of administration include teas, infusions, syrups, tinctures (alcohol and glycerol based), capsules, and enemas. External routes include oils, baths, compresses, peri-washes, and creams. Each of the internal forms offers specific advantages and disadvantages. For example, infusions are mild and effective, and therefore are a generally safe method of administration. Water is not as effective at extracting plant alkaloids, which are readily extracted when alcohol is used as a solvent. Thus water-based preparations are often milder and thereby safer. Water-based preparations also allow ease in evaporating off strong essential oils from teas that are considered safe for general use (chamomile, mints), but which do contain essential oil fractions. A clear disadvantage of water-based preparations is that the volume of tea one must consume for an effective dose may be prohibitive to the taste sensitivities of a pregnant woman. Decoctions are concentrated water-based preparations made by simmering or long-steeping of a larger quantity of herbs to water than is used for tea. They can be further simmered down to a concentrate to which a sweetener is added for flavor, thickening, and as a preservative, allowing tablespoon-sized doses rather than cup-sized doses of herbs to be administered.

Tinctures, which are hydroethanolic extractions, offer the advantage of being highly concentrated and are self-preserved, therefore allowing the patient to take them in small doses, and without the effort of preparation. Thus, they are easy to consume and convenient. However, because the water–alcohol combination is such an effective solvent, the medicines contain a full array of plant compounds, many of which may be undesirable for consumption during pregnancy. Additionally, some practitioners and some patients are uncomfortable with the use of alcohol during pregnancy, although the volume of alcohol per dose is typically very small (for example, in a 5-mL dose of a 40% alcohol tincture, the patient is receiving 2 mL of alcohol; even at 3 doses per day, this is 0.2 ounces of alcohol per day).

Capsules and pills, unless made from liquid extracts of freshly milled herb, are notoriously not fresh, and many herbalists consider them less than reliable medicines, preferring the use of water-based and alcohol-based extracts. Issues and challenges regarding herbal product quality and safety are of particular concern when prescribing herbs for pregnant women.

▶ SPECIFIC APPLICATIONS OF HERBS IN PREGNANCY

Some of the most common complaints and health concerns of pregnant women include NVP, miscarriage, urinary tract infections (UTIs), the use of herbs to induce labor, herbs for postnatal perineal discomfort, and the safety of herbs during lactation. These are addressed below.

Nausea and Vomiting of Pregnancy

NVP can be challenging to treat because it is difficult to find a single remedy that works consistently. Typically, women will find relief for a short duration only to find themselves nauseated by the remedy that helped in the first place. Most women are content to wait out the normal, mild to moderate first-trimester nausea without significant intervention as long as it does not interfere with their ability to function. Severe persistent nausea that is adversely affecting nutritional intake and hyperemesis gravidarum require further investigation for underlying causes and the use of more than just palliative therapies. However, even women with severe persistent nausea and hyperemesis will sometimes respond well to herbal therapies.

The best studied herb for NVP is ginger *(Zingiber officinale)*. In one double-blind, randomized crossover, placebo-controlled study, ginger was found to be significantly more effective than placebo for relieving the symptoms of morning sickness.[37] In a review of 10 randomized control trials reviewing the efficacy of ginger, vitamin B_6, hypnosis, and acupressure, evidence of benefit was found for each of these, with unequivocal benefit from ginger for the reduction of nausea, vomiting, and hyperemesis.[38] In a double-blind, placebo-controlled, randomized control trial using 1 tablespoon of commercially prepared ginger root syrup in 4–8 ounces of hot or cold water, the group receiving the ginger preparation experienced a significant reduction in severity and duration of symptoms (both nausea and vomiting), as compared to the placebo group.[39] The authors concluded that this dose, given at once or divided over the day, might be useful in the treatment of NVP in the first trimester. Numerous articles corroborate findings on the efficacy and safety of the use of ginger as an antinauseant and antiemetic in early pregnancy.[40–48]

While there are no reports of teratogenicity or mutagenicity from ginger found in the literature, some concern has arisen over its ability to inhibit platelet function and thromboxane synthetase.[19,50] Inhibition of testosterone binding to its receptor site has led to speculation that ginger could theoretically alter sex steroid-dependent differentiation of the fetal brain. While no mutagenic or teratogenic effects have been reported, the possibility of these or other idiosyncratic reactions cannot be entirely ruled out. Nonetheless, ginger is considered safe to use in small to moderate amounts for the reduction of nausea and vomiting of pregnancy. The dose should not exceed the quantity used in most of the clinical trials, 1 g/d. For best results, ginger is taken as a tea, syrup, or capsule.

Prevention and Treatment of Miscarriage

The causes of spontaneous abortion are often unknown. When there is threatened miscarriage as a consequence of insufficient progesterone levels, chastetree *(Vitex agnus-castus)* is sometimes used by midwives and herbalists[51–53] to prevent miscarriage. It may exert its effects via enhanced corpus luteal function. While researchers are still uncertain as to the exact mechanism of action of *Vitex*, it is suspected that it affects serum hormone levels and possibly has a regulatory effect on luteinizing hormone, follicle-stimulating hormone, and progesterone. Placebo-controlled studies for teratogenicity and mutagenicity were conducted in rats, and even when the animals were administered 74 times the dose typically consumed by humans, no toxicity or aberration in fetal development were seen. The dose is typically 5 mL BID-TID, 1:5 tincture.[53] It can be used alone or in conjunction with topical United States Pharmacopoeia (USP) progesterone when this is prescribed.

When there is threatened miscarriage with cramping, cramp bark *(Viburnum opulus)* or black haw *(Viburnum prunifolium)* can be used to arrest uterine spasm.[54,55] These plants, which can be used interchangeably, have a long history of use by North American indigenous tribes. Black haw was official in the United States Pharmacopoeia in 1882, its use as an antispasmodic having been popularized by the Eclectic physicians and the Shakers. Cramp bark is still included in the *British Herbal Pharmacopoeia*. In vitro studies demonstrate that constituents found in these related plants exert uterine smooth-muscle relaxant qualities. Low Dog[55] reports that in an in vitro study with an active glycoside, scopoletin, from black haw, there was demonstrable relaxation of both animal and human uteri. Other in vitro studies confirm similar clinical activity with several plants in the genus *Viburnum*, including the two mentioned here, which are the most commonly used medicinal species. Insufficient data on mutagenicity and teratogenicity are available, but a long historical record of use during pregnancy suggests safety. The dose is 2.5–5 mL q1–2h of 1:5 tincture until symptoms are relieved.[56]

Another herb with a long history of use for relieving spasms of the hollow organs is wild yam *(Dioscorea villosa)*. While this herb has developed the erroneous reputation for use as a progesterone supplement, wild yam, in fact, contains no progesterone, nor can it be converted by the body into progestogenic substances. This does not preclude its efficacy and reliability as a uterine antispasmodic, combining well both cramp bark and black haw. The typical dosage when taken alone is the same as for the tinctures of those herbs; in combination with either of the *Viburnum* herbs, it may be used as 30–50% of the formula.

Table 32–7 presents a typical formula that might be used for the prevention of miscarriage when there is known progesterone deficiency accompanied by cramping.

Urinary Tract Infections During Pregnancy

UTIs are common in pregnancy because of the physiologic displacement of the growing uterus

▶ **TABLE 32-7** HERBAL FORMULA FOR PREVENTION OF MISCARRIAGE

Vitex agnus-castus	50 mL (1:4)
Viburnum opulus	30 mL (1:4)
Dioscorea villosa	30 mL (1:4)
	Total 120 mL

Dose: 1 tsp BID-TID, or as needed up to 1 tsp q30m for 6 doses

onto the ureters and increased urinary stasis as a consequence of bladder compression. Repeated use of antibiotics is undesirable because of an increased likelihood of resistant UTIs and vaginal yeast infections; thus, alternative therapies for UTI that are safe and effective are important in the integrative approach to the pregnant patient. Numerous studies demonstrate the safety and efficacy of cranberry juice *(Vaccinium macrocarpon)* for the prevention of urinary tract infection.[57] Cranberry prevents the adherence of pathogenic *Escherichia coli* to the bladder wall and urinary tract lining, thus reducing infection. Daily intake of cranberry juice as a dietary beverage is advisable for women with a history of chronic UTI. For the treatment of acute UTI, a woman may consume up to 6 glasses of cranberry juice per day, although evidence of the efficacy of cranberry for treatment as opposed to prevention is still equivocal. Unremitting or worsening symptoms require medical attention. Cranberry juice and reconstituted cranberry concentrate are considered completely safe during pregnancy; however, avoid concentrated cranberry products, as these have not been evaluated for use during pregnancy.

Other herbs that are commonly employed by midwives and herbalists for the treatment of active urinary tract infections include echinacea *(Echinacea* spp.) and uva ursi *(Arctostaphylos uva-ursi)*. Echinacea has been conclusively demonstrated to be safe for mother and developing baby even when used throughout the duration of the pregnancy,[58] and should be used in large and frequent doses as part of an overall protocol for the treatment of UTI (5 mL

QID) to be effective. It is best when combined with cranberry juice. Although uva ursi is a highly effective urinary tract antiseptic, it has not been proven safe for and is generally contraindicated during pregnancy because of its arbutin content. The tea can be taken for a short duration (no more than 5 days) in small quantities (0.5 ounces of leaves per pint of boiling water, steeped for 1 hour; dose: up to 1.5 cups per day), and is generally combined with the gentle herb marshmallow root *(Althaea officinalis)*, a urinary demulcent that soothes inflammation in the urinary tract. Uva ursi should be avoided during the first trimester and is generally only used when gentler approaches, such as cranberry, are ineffective, when the infection is acute or recurrent, or when the mother prefers to avoid or cannot tolerate antibiotics. Conservative practitioners may prefer to avoid uva ursi during pregnancy.

Labor Induction

The use of herbs for labor stimulation is popular amongst pregnant women and midwives alike.[59] The pressure to give birth by a certain date to avoid being artificially induced is the primary incentive behind such use. However, the use of herbs to prepare women for labor begs the question of why one would use an herbal preparation to prepare the body for something it naturally knows how to do, and seems antithetical to the principles upon which herbal medicine philosophy is built—to trust the body's innate wisdom. The herbs most commonly used for labor induction are blue cohosh *(Caulophyllum thalictroides)* and black cohosh *(Actaea racemosa* syn. *Cimicifuga racemosa)*. The safety of blue cohosh prior to the onset of labor is highly questionable. This herb contains a number of potent alkaloids including methylcysteine and anagyrine, the latter being known to have an effect on cardiac muscle activity. At least one report published in 1998 in *Journal of Pediatrics* implicates the late pregnancy use of blue cohosh in the myocardial infarction of a neonate.[60] It is therefore prudent in general to avoid the use of herbs to stimulate labor, particularly those containing blue cohosh, and to only use labor-stimulating herbs at term of pregnancy under qualified supervision and with careful fetal monitoring. However, with careful monitoring of the uterus for intensity of contractions, along with diligent monitoring of the fetal heart rate, labor stimulation with herbs, when medically indicated, may be judiciously employed with perhaps greater safety and less intervention than other augmenting agents such as Pitocin (oxytocin) and misoprostol. Self-medication by patients is not recommended, and the expert guidance of an obstetrician or midwife trained in the use of botanical medicines is recommended.

Postpartum Perineal Discomfort and Healing

Astringent herbs such as witch hazel and white oak bark; vulnerary herbs such as calendula and comfrey; and antiseptic herbs such as sage and myrrh can be made into strong decoctions, which can be applied to the perineum via a peri-wash or sitz bath. These can accelerate the healing process from perineal tears and episiotomy, reduce swelling and bruising, and reduce pain and soreness. To prepare, use 7 g of each herb and steep in 2 L of water for 30 minutes. Strain and place in the peri-bottle or sitz bath. Use once or twice daily for up to 5 days postnatally. As mentioned earlier in this chapter, lavender also may reduce perineal pain associated with tearing and episiotomy; lavender blossoms may be added to the above preparation, or a dilute preparation of tinctures of lavender, calendula, witch hazel, and myrrh can be assembled and put into a spray bottle for ease of administration. This can be applied several times daily to promote healing and comfort. Table 32–8 outlines the formula.

▶ **TABLE 32–8** HERBAL FORMULA
FOR POSTPARTUM PERINEAL WASH

Witch hazel bark tincture	0.5 fl oz
Calendula tincture	0.5 fl oz
Lavender tincture	0.5 fl oz
Myrrh tincture	0.5 fl oz
	Total: 2 fl oz

Mix all tinctures and add 0.5 fl ounce of the
mix to a 2-cup spray bottle. Spray on
liberally as needed.

Herbs in Lactation

There are a number of herbs that should not
be consumed by lactating mothers during the
postnatal period because of possible harmful
effects on the newborn. A partial listing of these
appears in Table 32–9. For more information
on herbs contraindicated for breast-feeding
mothers, see *The Botanical Safety Handbook:*
"Class 2c . . . not to be used while nursing unless otherwise directed by an expert qualified
in the appropriate use of this substance."[36]

▶ **TABLE 32–9** HERBS TO AVOID
DURING LACTATION

Actaea racemosa syn. *Cimicifuga racemosa*
Alkanna tinctoria
Allium sativum
Aloe spp.
Artemisia absinthum
Borago officinalis
Dryopteris filix mas
Ephedra spp.
Eupatorium purpureum
Fucus vesiculosus
Glycyrrhiza spp.
Inula helenium
Lycopus spp.
Rhamnus spp.
Rheum spp.
Senna spp.
Stillingia sylvatica
Symphytum officinale
Tussilago farfara

REFERENCES

1. Mazzotta P, Magee L. Pharmacological and non-pharmacological management of nausea and vomiting of pregnancy (NVP); a systematic critical review of the literature on safety and effectiveness of treatment. 1998 (submitted for publication). Available at: http://www.nvp-volumes.org/p1_11.htm. Accessed: June 2003.

2. Upton R. TCM and gynecology. Unpublished presentation. Medicines from the Earth Conference, Asheville, NC; 2000.

3. Carlsson CP, Axemo P, Bodin A, Carstensen H, et al. Manual acupuncture reduces hyperemesis gravidarum. A placebo-controlled, randomized, single-blind, crossover study. *J Pain Symptom Manage.* 2000;20(4):273–279.

4. Norheim AJ, Pedersen EJ, Fonnebo V, Berge L. Acupressure treatment of morning sickness in pregnancy: a randomised, double-blind, placebo-controlled study. *Scand J Prim Health Care.* 2001;19(1):43–47.

5. Regutti A. "Pregnancy support with acupuncture and traditional Chinese medicine." *Infused: The Community Pharmacy Newsletter.* 2002;4(3):1–3.

6. Roscoe JA, Matteson SE. Acupressure and acustimulation bands for control of nausea review. *Am J Obstet Gynecol.* 2002; 185(5 suppl): S244–S247.

7. Stern RM, Jokerst MD, Muth ER, Hollis C. Acupressure relieves the symptoms of motion sickness and abnormal gastric activity. *Altern Ther Health Med.* 2001;7(4):91–94.

8. Slotnick RN. Safe, successful nausea suppression in early pregnancy with P-6 acustimulation. *J Reprod Med.* 2001;46(9):811–814.

9. Ho C-M, Hseu S-S, Tsai S-K, Lee T-Y. Effect of P-6 acupressure on prevention of nausea and vomiting after epidural morphine for post-cesarean section pain relief. *Acta Anaesthes Scand.* 1996; 40(3):372–375.

10. Hyodo M, Gega O. Use of acupuncture anesthesia for normal delivery. *Am J Chin Med.* 1977; 5(1) 63–69.

11. Wang DW, Jin YH. Present status of cesarean section under acupuncture anesthesia in China. *Fukushima J Med Sci.* 1989;35(2):45–52.

12. Cardini F, Weixin H. Moxibustion for correction of breech presentation: a randomized control trial. *JAMA.* 1998;280(18):1580–1584.

13. Packer-Tursman J. Alternative therapy struggles to bridge east-west divide. *Washington Post*. November 10, 2002. Available at: www.washingtonpost.com/wp-dyn/articles/A36744-2002Nov10html. Accessed.

14. Tremeau ML, Fontanie-Ravier R, Teurnier F, Demouzon J. Acupuncture for cervical maturation. *J Gynecol Obstet Biol Reprod*. 1992;21(4):375–380.

15. Tiran D, Mack S. *Complementary Therapies for Pregnancy and Childbirth*. London: Bailliere Tindall; 1995.

16. Duhnam C. *Mamatoto: A Celebration of Birth*. New York: Viking; 1992.

17. Chang MY, Wang SY, Chen CH. Effects of massage on pain and anxiety during labor: randomized-controlled trial in Taiwan. *J Adv Nurs*. 2002;38(1):68–73.

18. Romm A. *Natural Health After Birth*. Rochester, VT: Healing Arts Press; 2002.

19. Meek LR, Burda KM, Paster E. Effects of prenatal stress on development in mice: maturation and learning. *Physiol Behav*. 2000;71(5):543–549.

20. Hedegaard M. Lifestyle, work and stress, and pregnancy outcome. *Curr Opin Obstet Gynecol*. 1999;11(6):553–556.

21. Field T, Hernandez-Reif M, Hart S, et al. Pregnant women benefit from massage therapy. *J Psychosom Obstet Gynaecol*. 1999;20(1):31–38.

22. Field T, Hernandez-Reif M, Taylor S, et al. Labor pain is reduced by massage therapy. *J Psychosom Obstet Gynaecol*. 1977;18(4):286–291.

23. Keenan P. Benefits of massage therapy and the use of a doula during labor. *Altern Ther Health Med*. 2000;6(1):66–74.

24. National Association of Pregnancy Massage Therapists. Pregnancy contraindications. Available at: http://nampt.home.texas.net/napmtnews.html. Accessed   .

25. Katz T. The management of pregnancy and labour with homeopathics. *Complement Ther Nurs Midwifery*. 1995;1(6):159–164.

26. Moskowitz R. *Homeopathic Medicines For Pregnancy and Childbirth*. Berkeley, CA: North Atlantic Books; 1992.

27. Castro M. Homeopathy. A theoretical framework and clinical application. *J Nurse Midwifery*. 1999; 44(3):280–290.

28. Hochstrasser B, Mattman P. Mainstream medicine versus complementary medicine (homeopathic) intervention: a critical methodology study of pregnancy. *Forsch Komplementarmed*. 1999; 66(suppl 1):20–22.

29. Cummings B. Homeopathy for pregnancy and childbirth. In: Tiran D, Mack S, eds. *Complementary Therapies for Pregnancy and Childbirth*. London: Bailliere Tindall; 1995.

30. Hochstrasser B, Mattman P. Homeopathy and conventional medicine in the management of pregnancy and childbirth. *Schweiz Med Wochenschr Suppl*. 1994;62:28–35.

31. Wilkinson S, Aldridge J, Salmon I, et al. An evaluation of aromatherapy massage in palliative care. *Palliat Med*.1999;13(5):409–417.

32. Price S. Using essential oils in professional practice. *Complement Ther Nurs Midwifery*. 1998;4(5):144–147.

33. Baker S. Formation and development of the Aromatherapy Organisations Council. *Complement Ther Nurse Midwifery*. 1997;3(3):77–80.

34. Dale A, Cornwell S. The role of lavender oil in relieving perineal discomfort following childbirth: a blind randomized clinical trial. *J Adv Nurs*. 1994;19(1):89–96.

35. Balacs T. Safety in pregnancy. *Int J Aromather*. 1992;4(1):12–15.

36. McGuffin M, Hobbs C, Upton R, Goldberg A. *Botanical Safety Handbook*. Boca Raton, FL: CRC Press; 1997.

37. Jewell D, Young G. Treatments for nausea and vomiting in early pregnancy. In: Neilsen JP, Crowther CA, Hodnett ED, Hofmeyr GJ, Keirse MJNC, eds. Pregnancy and childbirth module of the Cochrane Database of Systematic Reviews [updated March 4, 1997]. *The Cochrane Collaboration*, Issue 2. Oxford, UK: Update Software; 1997.

38. Aikens M. Nausea and vomiting in pregnancy—ginger, vitamin C. *Obstet Gynecol*. 1998;91(1):149–155.

39. Keating A, Chez RA. Ginger syrup as an antiemetic in early pregnancy. *Altern Ther Health Med*. 2002;8(5):89–91.

40. Niebyl J, Goodwin T. Overview of nausea and vomiting of pregnancy with an emphasis on vitamins. *Am J Obstet Gynecol*. 2002;185(5 suppl): S253–S255.

41. Vutyavanich T, Kraisarin T, Ruangsri R. Ginger for nausea and vomiting in pregnancy: randomized, double-masked, placebo-controlled trial. *Obstet Gynecol*. 2002; 97(4):577–582.

42. Murphy P. Alternative therapies for nausea and vomiting of pregnancy. *Obstet Gynecol.* 1998; 91(1):149–155.

43. Fulder S, Tenne T. Ginger as an antinausea remedy in pregnancy: the issue of safety. *Herbal-Gram.* 1993;38:47–50.

44. Wilkinson J. What do we know about herbal morning sickness treatments? A literature survey. *Midwifery.* 2000;16:224–228.

45. Meltzer D. Complementary therapies for nausea and vomiting in early pregnancy. *Family Pract.* 2000;17:570–573.

46. Strong T. Alternative therapies of morning sickness. *Clin Obstet Gynecol.* 2001;144(4):653–660.

47. Backon J. Ginger in preventing nausea and vomiting of pregnancy: a caveat due to its thromboxane synthetase activity and effect on testosterone binding. *Eur J Obstet Gynecol Reprod Biol.* 1991;42:163–164.

48. Fischer-Rasmussen W, Kjaer SK, Dahl C, Asping U. Ginger treatment of hyperemesis gravidarum. *Eur J Obstet Gynecol Reprod Biol.* 1991;38:19–24.

49. Wilkinson J. What do we know about herbal morning sickness treatments? A literature survey. *Midwifery.* 2000;16:224–228.

50. Backon J. Ginger in preventing nausea and vomiting of pregnancy: a caveat due to its thromboxane synthetase activity and effect on testosterone binding. *Eur J Obstet Gynecol Reprod Biol.* 1991;42:163–164.

51. Upton R. Chaste tree fruit *(Vitex agnus-castus)*. In: *American Herbal Pharmacopoeia and Therapeutic Compendium.* Santa Cruz, CA: American Herbal Pharmacopoeia; 2001.

52. Romm A. Treatment of incomplete miscarriage with botanical therapies and continuing reproductive care. *J Am Herb Guild.* 2001;2(2): 16–17.

53. Romm A, Treasure J. American Herbalists Guild professional member botanical therapeutics survey: *Vitex agnus-castus. J Am Herb Guild.* 2001; 2(2):27–31.

54. Upton R. Cramp bark *(Viburnum prunifolium)*. In: *American Herbal Pharmacopoeia and Therapeutic Compendium.* Santa Cruz, CA: American Herbal Pharmacopoeia; 2001.

55. Low Dog T. *An Integrative Approach to Women's Health.* Albuquerque, NM: Integrative Medical Education Associates; 2001.

56. Romm A. *The Natural Pregnancy Book.* Freedom, CA: Crossing Press; 1997.

57. Upton R. Cranberry fruit *(Vaccinium macrocarpon)*. In: *American Herbal Pharmacopoeia and Therapeutic Compendium.* Santa Cruz, CA: American Herbal Pharmacopoeia; 2002.

58. Gall M, Sarkar M. Pregnancy outcome following gestational exposure to Echinacea. *Arch Intern Med.* 2000;160:3141–3143.

59. Allaire A, Moos M, Wells SR. Complementary and alternative medicine in pregnancy: a survey of North Carolina certified nurse-midwives. *Obstet Gynecol.* 2000;95(1):19–23.

60. Wright IM. Neonatal effects of maternal blue cohosh. *J Pediatr.* 1998;132(3):550–552.

CHAPTER 33

Integrative Approach to Common Conditions in Women's Health

ANDREA GIRMAN, ROBERTA LEE, BENJAMIN KLIGLER, SUSAN HADLEY, AND ELLEN TATTELMAN

▶ PREMENSTRUAL SYNDROME*

Pathophysiology

Many different etiologies have been proposed for the symptoms of premenstrual syndrome (PMS); none have been definitely established as a dominant cause. Possible influences include hormonal imbalance, specifically a low progesterone level during the luteal phase of the cycle; abnormal neurotransmitter response to ovarian signaling; disordered aldosterone function leading to sodium and water retention; abnormal hypothalamic–pituitary–adrenal axis function leading to deficient adrenal hormone secretion; nutritional deficiency including magnesium; pyridoxine; carbohydrate intolerance; and environmental factors, including stress.[1,2] Because no single etiology explains every case, many clinicians assume that this disorder is multifactorial in origin.

Prevalence

PMS is a condition of recurrent physical and psychological symptoms, occurring in a cyclic fashion during the 1–2-week period preceding a woman's menstrual period, significant enough to cause disruption in either family, personal, or occupational function.[3] In its most severe form, it affects roughly 2.5% of women of reproductive age[4]; in a more mild form, it is estimated to affect approximately 40% of women in this age group.[5] A variant of PMS that entails more severe psychological symptoms was recently described under the diagnosis of premenstrual dysphoric disorder (PMDD).

Conventional/Pharmacological Approaches

A wide range of pharmacological approaches have been used to treat the symptoms of PMS,

*Adapted with permission from Girman A, Lee R, Kligler B. Integrative approach to premenstrual syndrome. *Clin J Women's Health*. 2002;2(3):1–12.

including oral contraceptives and other hormonal supplementation, nonsteroidal antiinflammatories, bromocriptine, and diuretic agents. Most recently antidepressants, particularly the selective serotonin reuptake inhibitors, have become very popular in women for whom depression or mood instability is a major symptom. Although the use of conventional pharmacotherapeutic agents in the treatment of PMS and PMDD is an important component of the integrative approach, the applications of these agents are reviewed elsewhere,[6,7] and so are not discussed in detail in this chapter.

Integrative Treatment Approach

NUTRITIONAL APPROACHES
The information available on the use of nutritional approaches for PMS is compiled in Table 33–1.

Dietary Manipulation
Dietary manipulation is often used for PMS symptoms, although no food-based strategy has been properly evaluated to date. Based on findings by Abraham that women with PMS typically consume more dairy products, refined sugar, and high-sodium foods than do women without PMS,[8] many clinicians recommend reducing or eliminating these foods for women with severe symptoms. Limiting caffeine intake is often recommended as well, based on the findings in at least two studies associating in-

creased intake of caffeine-containing beverages with increased prevalence and severity of PMS symptoms.[9,10]

High estrogen levels are thought to be correlated with PMS symptoms in some women. Because diets higher in fat are believed to contribute to higher estrogen levels, and because high-fiber diets are thought to help reduce estrogen levels based on their effect on intestinal flora, another common approach in clinical practice is to recommend a relatively low-fat, high-fiber diet.[11] Although the rationale for all of these dietary approaches is appealing, and such a diet is health promoting for many people for other reasons, none of these dietary manipulation strategies has to date been adequately studied for efficacy in women with PMS.

Magnesium
Because low levels of red blood cell magnesium have been found in women experiencing PMS,[12] magnesium supplementation has been studied as adjunctive therapy in this condition. In a recent review published in the *Cochrane Library*, three small trials were included that compared magnesium and placebo. It was noted that the trials, although randomized with adequate methodological quality, were small, "with poor measurement and reporting outcomes."[13] One of the larger studies included data on the levels of prostaglandin $F_{2\alpha}$ ($PGF_{2\alpha}$). Women taking the magnesium therapy had substantially lower levels of $PGF_{2\alpha}$ in their menstrual blood than did those women on the

▶ **TABLE 33–1** SUMMARY OF EVIDENCE ON NUTRITIONAL APPROACHES FOR PMS

Supplement	Typical Dose	Efficacy	Level of Evidence
Magnesium	400–800 mg/d	Likely yes	Level B (small trials)
Vitamin B₆	50–100 mg/d	Likely yes	Level B (small trials, systematic review)
Calcium	1,200–1,600 mg/d	Yes	Level A (large trials, systematic review)
Caffeine cessation	N/A	Likely yes	Level B (small trials)
Dietary manipulation	N/A	Possible	Level C (expert opinion)

Level A = Large, high-quality, randomized, double-blind placebo-controlled trials; meta-analyses.
Level B = Lesser quality, randomized trials; retrospective studies, systematic reviews.
Level C = Expert opinion, case series, uncontrolled studies, consensus statements.

placebo ($p < .05$); these lower levels correlated with a decrease in pain by the participants.[11] In this study, 50 women were randomized and given the equivalent dose of 10 mval of magnesium aspartate or placebo for 6 months. Twenty-one of 25 women in the active treatment group reported improvement of their symptoms, with 4 reporting no therapeutic effects. A possible biological rationale for the effectiveness of magnesium is the inhibition of $PGF_{2\alpha}$ and the promotion of muscle relaxation and vasodilatation.[15,16] The overall conclusion in the Cochrane analysis was that magnesium was more effective than placebo for pain associated with PMS.[17] Furthermore, the need for additional medication was less in all the studies included. The limited evidence to date supports the use of magnesium in PMS, but more research is needed.

Vitamin B₆

Vitamin B_6, a water-soluble B vitamin, is another adjunctive dietary supplement used in treating PMS. The rationale for its use is for its positive effects on neurotransmitters—serotonin, norepinephrine, histamine, dopamine, and taurine.[18] A systematic review on the efficacy of vitamin B_6 on PMS done in 1999 included 9 published trials representing 940 patients with PMS, all of which were randomized, placebo-controlled, double-blinded studies.[19] Two studies included studied B_6 on mastalgia based on the frequency (60%) of women with PMS that report cyclical breast pain.[20] The odds ratio relative to placebo for overall improvement in PMS was 2.32 (95% confidence interval, 1.95–2.54). The odds ratio for improvement in depressive symptoms from four trials that included analyzing this aspect of PMS was 1.69 (1.39–2.06). The overall assessment of the review was that women with PMS are likely to benefit from B_6 supplementation at a dose of 50–100 mg/d, and may even have improvement of depressive symptoms. However, the conclusions, although positive, were limited, citing that there was "insufficient evidence of high quality to

give a confident recommendation for using vitamin B_6 in the treatment of premenstrual syndrome."

Pyridoxine has been given in clinical trials at doses ranging from 50 to 500 mg/d. It has been suggested that daily dosing not exceed 100 mg/d as it has been associated with reports of toxicity.[21] Furthermore, detailed animal studies indicate that nerve damage can occur before manifestation of the gross symptoms, such as ataxia and neuropathy.[22,23]

Calcium

Ovarian hormones influence calcium, magnesium, and vitamin D metabolism, and estrogen regulates calcium metabolism and intestinal calcium absorption, as well as parathyroid function and gene expression.[21] Several clinical trials have suggested that calcium supplementation can improve mood and somatic symptoms in PMS.[25]

A multicenter, randomized, placebo-controlled, double-blind study was done in 1998 with 720 women randomized to receive 1,200 mg of calcium carbonate or placebo for three menstrual cycles. These women were asked to report symptoms on a daily rating scale that had 17 core symptoms and 4 symptom factors (negative affect, water retention, food cravings, and pain).[26] By the third cycle of treatment, a reduction of 48% ($p < .001$) was found in symptoms in the treatment arm versus 30% in the placebo arm. Other trials have demonstrated similar modest but significant benefits, and a 1999 review on calcium as a treatment for PMS concluded that calcium 1,200–1,600 mg/d, unless contraindicated, "should be considered a sound treatment option for those who experience PMS."[27]

Recently, concerns have been raised regarding potential lead increases in those who take calcium supplements.[28] Ross published a study reporting on 4 of 7 natural products that had measurable lead content at 1 μg for 800 mg/d of calcium (calcium carbonate). However, the lead content was below the detection limit in two-thirds of the 22 products reported overall, and all of the products tested had a lead content less than both the 1993 Food and Drug Administration and the 1996 Food Chemicals Codex standards.[29] In a discussion section following the article, Heaney, an expert in calcium metabolism, pointed out that lead found in calcium supplements contributes only a small fraction of the total lead intake. Furthermore, it is stated that most of the lead is not absorbed and that calcium blocks lead absorption from other foods.[30] Therefore, it seems prudent to be mindful of the potential for lead contamination in some calcium carbonate products, but useful to continue recommending calcium as a supplement for improving PMS symptoms.

BOTANICAL MEDICINE

A number of the commonly used herbal medicines are discussed below. Table 33–2 summarizes information on botanicals.

Chastetree *(Vitex agnus-castus)* is commonly used for PMS. The Latin binomial means "chaste lamb" and refers to the reduction of sexual desire exhibited when one drinks a beverage prepared from the seeds of this plant.[31] The applicable part of the chastetree is the fruit. Active constituents in chasteberries are the essential oils, iridoid glycosides, and the flavonoids.[32] The mechanism of action relative to PMS is somewhat unclear. However, chastetree extracts at the lower dose of 120 mg/d diminish follicle-stimulating hormone release and increase luteinizing hormone, resulting in decreased estrogen, increased progesterone, and prolactin levels.[32,33] At higher doses of approximately 480 mg/d, prolactin levels seem to be inhibited.[34] Chastetree extracts also have multiple constituents that seem to have agonistic effects at dopamine receptors (D_2) when used at higher doses.[35]

Several clinical trials have been done using a proprietary chastetree extract (Agnolyt), which contains 9 g of a 1:5 tincture for each 100 g of aqueous-alcohol solution. In one large trial of 1,571 women with menstrual disturbances related to corpus luteum insufficiency, patients were treated for 135 days with 40 drops of Agnolyt. The response rate was around 90%, with both physicians and patients assessing the clinical outcome as being positive.[36] Adverse effects were reported at 1.9% (primarily malaise, gastrointestinal complaints, and nausea).

Another study done by Dittmar and Bohnert, involving 1,542 women with PMS, was done to monitor the effects of Agnolyt (40 drops). Thirty-three percent of the patients reported total relief of their symptoms, with an additional 57% reporting partial relief. Two percent of patients in this study reported adverse effects (nausea, allergy, diarrhea, weight gain, heartburn, hypermenorrhea, and gastric complaints). Seventeen patients stopped the study because of the side effects, while 562 patients continued to take the product after the monitoring period (4 months).[37]

▶ **TABLE 33–2** SUMMARY OF EVIDENCE ON BOTANICAL MEDICINES FOR PMS

Botanical	Typical Dose	Efficacy?	Level of Evidence
Chastetree (*Vitex*)	200 mg daily*	Likely yes	Level B (small or lesser-quality trials)
Evening primrose oil	2–3 g/d	Likely no	Level B (small trials)
Black cohosh	40 mg BID*	Possible	Level C (expert opinion)
St. John's wort	300 mg TID*	Possible	Level B (small trials)
Kava	100–300 mg/d*	Possible	Level C (expert opinion)
Ginkgo	80 mg BID*	Likely yes	Level B (small trials)

*Standardized extract.

Level A = Large, high-quality, randomized, double-blind placebo-controlled trials; meta-analyses.

Level B = Lesser quality, randomized trials; retrospective studies, systematic reviews.

Level C = Expert opinion, case series, uncontrolled studies, consensus statements.

A third randomized, double-blind, placebo-controlled study in 217 subjects with PMS taking chastetree (600 mg capsules three times a day) for 3 months showed only improvement in alleviating restlessness. There were no other differences noted for other PMS symptoms.[38] Finally, Schellenberg randomized 170 women with PMS to chastetree extract (20 mg) or placebo for three menstrual cycles. The reduction in symptoms was 52% versus 24% (active versus placebo, respectively) and considered statistically significant ($p < .001$).[39]

Vitex (Agnolyt capsule with approximately 3.5 mg of chastetree extract) was compared with vitamin B_6 (100 mg twice a day) in a 3-month randomized controlled study of 127 women with PMS. The chastetree and vitamin B_6 groups both had similar reductions in PMS scores; 77% in the chastetree and 66% in the vitamin B_6 groups showed improvements in PMS symptoms.[40]

No long-term randomized trials have been done comparing standard medical treatments (birth control pills or antidepressants) with chastetree. The German health authorities (Commission E) have approved the use of chastetree for irregularities of the menstrual cycle, PMS, and mastodynia.[32] Because of the potential effects on hormones it is recommended that the use of chastetree be avoided during pregnancy and during breast-feeding. Theoretically, chastetree might also interfere with medications that are dopamine antagonists.[32]

Evening primrose oil *(Oenothera biennis)* has been used for premenstrual syndrome in many patients, although it is used primarily for treatment of a variety of inflammatory disorders.[41] Some researchers have observed that women with PMS have impaired conversion of linoleic acid to gamma linolenic acid.[42] These two essential acids are important in the formation of one of the antiinflammatory prostaglandins, PGE1[43]; for this reason, evening primrose—a good source of both linoleic and gamma-linolenic acid—has been studied as a possible alternative treatment for PMS. Seven clinical trials have been done using evening primrose for PMS; only five clearly randomized their subjects. None of these trials found a beneficial effect for PMS; however, it was noted that the sample sizes in all might have been too small to detect a modest benefit.[44]

In one randomized trial, 27 women with PMS were randomized to four cycles of essential fatty acids or placebo with crossover after the fourth cycle. No differences were noted between either group, and the conclusion was that the essential fatty acids were ineffective for PMS.[45]

Another small, randomized, double-blind, placebo-controlled trial was done on 38 women with PMS. They received evening primrose or placebo for 3 months and were crossed over for another 3 months. An improvement was observed but considered not statistically significant. In addition, no "carryover" effect was observed. The conclusion was that "the improvement experienced by these women with moderate PMS was solely a placebo effect."[46] At this time, it does not appear that evening primrose will improve PMS.[47] If patients do choose to try this approach, the dose shown to be effective for other prostaglandin-related conditions is 2–3 g/d.[48]

Black cohosh *(Cimicifuga racemosa)* was first used medicinally by Native Americans who introduced it to European colonists.[49] It was introduced to Germany in the late nineteenth century and has been used in Germany since the late 1950s as an alternative to manage menopause.[50] The majority of studies looking at black cohosh have been in the treatment of menopausal symptoms. The mechanism of action remains somewhat unclear. Some clinical evidence suggests black cohosh suppresses luteinizing hormone secretion,[51] while another study shows no change in luteinizing hormone and follicle-stimulating hormone.[52] A number of studies using Remifemin, a proprietary extract of black cohosh, do show a benefit for various menopausal symptoms (hot flashes, profuse sweating, sleep disturbance, and depressive moods).[53] Because these symptoms often present as well in women with PMS, many clinicians have recommended the use of black cohosh in this population. Further clinical studies are needed to determine the efficacy of black cohosh in PMS. The recommended dose of black cohosh is 40–80 mg of a standardized extract twice daily, providing 4–8 mg of triterpene glycosides.[54]

Ginkgo *(Ginkgo biloba)* leaf extract comes from the oldest living tree species in the world.[55] Primarily known as a botanical useful for improving memory, ginkgo has also been evaluated as an extract that can improve PMS. Tamborini studied the effects of this botanical product in 165 women. Patients were randomized to placebo or a standardized extract (Egb761) for symptoms of PMS (congestion, breast tenderness, and mood) for two cycles. The results showed a statistically significant improvement in all symptoms, especially breast tenderness and fluid retention.[56] Ginkgo leaf extracts contain many active constituents including flavonoids and terpenoids. Ginkgo leaf flavonoids have antioxidant and free radical scavenging properties.[57] Ginkgo also inhibits platelet-activating factor[58] and has antiinflammatory effects.[59] Some constituents also can relax vascular smooth muscle.[60] Further study is needed to determine if there is a significant role for ginkgo in treatment of PMS.

Because ginkgo inhibits platelet-activating factor, its use in combination with medications that affect platelet aggregation could theoretically increase the risk of bleeding in some people. As ginkgo interacts with the cytochrome P450 enzymes in the liver, care should be taken in recommending ginkgo to patients with multiple medications that also effect these enzymes.[32] The dose used for PMS in clinical trials was 80 mg twice a day starting on the sixteenth day of the cycle and on through until the fifth day of menses.[58]

The use of serotonin reuptake inhibiting preparations for the mood symptoms of PMS and PMDD is well established.[61] With this in mind, St. John's wort *(Hypericum perforatum)* is often used as a botanical alternative for treating this aspect of PMS. A number of reviews have suggested that St. John's wort can be useful for mild depression[62] but not severe depression.[63] In a pilot study done in 2000 at the University of Exeter, 19 women with PMS were treated with St. John's wort 300 mg standardized to 0.3% hypericin. The results showed a reduction of 51% in PMS scores between baseline and the end of the trial with more than two-thirds demonstrating at least a 50% decrease in symptom severity.[64] The authors suggested that "there is scope for conducting a randomized, placebo-controlled, double-blind trial."

Those taking medications that increase photosensitivity should avoid the use of St. John's wort as this herb can induce photosensitivity if taken in large doses.[32] Patients taking protease inhibitors (for HIV), cyclosporine, or other medications that are metabolized by the P450 enzyme system should also avoid use of St. John's wort, as it has been shown to reduce serum levels of these medications and so potentially could interfere with their efficacy.[32] The dose recommended for mild depression in most clinical trials is hypericin 300 mg (standardized to 0.3% hypericin) three times a day.[32]

Kava *(Piper methysticum)*, a member of the pepper family used ceremonially to honor special events and esteemed guests in Oceania, has been investigated in Europe and the United States for its anxiolytic properties.[65] A recent review showed kava to be effective for mild anxiety.[66] A number of small trials have found improvement with the use of this herb in women suffering from menopause-related anxiety and neurovegetative symptoms.[67–69] No clinical studies have been done in women with PMS. The dose recommended in clinical trials is 100–300 mg daily of an extract standardized to 30% kava lactones.

Recent medical reports have warned of the use of kava and the development of hepatotoxicity. In Germany and Switzerland, brands concentrated to a 70% kava lactone concentration have been attributed as a possible cause for hepatotoxicity associated with kava use. Studies are underway at the Food and Drug

Administration to determine if hepatotoxicity is causally linked to kava use, as the case-by-case evaluation is not entirely convincing of this.[70] Currently, those who choose to use kava daily should work with a knowledgeable health care practitioner and monitor their liver function if use is for longer than 1 month. Those patients with liver problems, on multiple medications metabolized in the liver, or with heavy alcohol use should not take kava.[71] Furthermore, patients should be warned of the potential for sedation with this botanical and should avoid driving or using heavy machinery.[72]

Other botanicals used clinically for PMS but not well studied are cramp bark *(Viburnum opulus)*, dong quai root *(Angelica sinensis)*, blue cohosh *(Caulophyllum thalictroides)*, wild yam *(Dioscorea villosa)*, black haw *(Viburnum prunifolium)*, and pulsatilla *(Anemone pulsatilla)*.[73,74]

MIND–BODY APPROACHES

The evidence regarding most of the mind–body approaches for PMS is fairly limited. However, because most of these approaches are risk free, and because they include strategies traditionally accepted as important components of a healthy lifestyle (exercise, stress reduction, and relaxation), there is still a strong argument for their use in the treatment of PMS.

A randomized clinical trial of relaxation training in 46 women with PMS found that subjects assigned to the relaxation response group reported significantly greater reduction of mood symptoms as compared to controls assigned either charting of symptoms or reading over a 5-month period.[75]

Several small studies have investigated the effectiveness of cognitive therapy in alleviating negative symptoms in women with PMS. Blake et al. compared a group of women randomized to receive immediate weekly cognitive therapy to a group of controls allocated to a waiting list that kept a symptom diary over a 12-week period.[76] Results indicated that cognitive behavior therapy was significantly effective in relieving psychological and somatic symptoms, as well as impairment of functioning. Morse et al. found that women using cognitive behavior therapy with relaxation instructions had significantly reduced PMS symptoms as compared to women randomized to a nonactive control group during two menstrual cycles.[77] In a study by Kirkby, 37 women with severe premenstrual symptoms were nonrandomly assigned to cognitive-behavioral coping skills treatment, a nonspecific treatment, or a waiting-list group. The author found significant reductions in premenstrual symptoms in the coping skills group as compared to control subjects both at posttreatment and at a 9-month follow-up evaluation.[78] Christensen et al. randomized women to two different cognitive approaches, and found that both cognitive behavior therapy and information-focused therapy resulted in reduction of symptoms.[79] However, lack of a true placebo group makes these results difficult to interpret.

YOGA

A 10-month empirical study of 40 women with menstrual distress was undertaken to investigate the effectiveness of certain yogic practices in relieving negative symptoms.[80] Women assigned to the study group underwent yoga training (regular practice of specific yoga postures and transcendental meditation); the control group had no training. The authors found significantly lower scores on the subscales of the menstrual distress questionnaire for subjects in the yoga-trained group compared to the control group in both the premenstrual and menstrual periods.

AEROBIC EXERCISE

A number of studies have examined the role of aerobic exercise and evidence suggests this may be an effective therapy for PMS. One large survey of more than 1,800 women found that exercise was used by more than half of the women as a self-help measure for alleviating PMS symptoms.[81] Of those reporting exercise as a self-help measure, more than 80% found it helpful. Aganoff et al. also surveyed exercisers and nonexercisers to determine the effects of regular, moderate exercise on mood states and menstrual cycle symptoms. Regular exercisers obtained significantly lower scores on impaired concentration, negative affect, behavior change, and pain as compared to nonexercisers.[82]

Mood states and physical symptoms of 143 women (35 competitive sportswomen, two groups of exercisers [33 "high exercisers" and 36 "low exercisers"], and 39 sedentary women) were monitored for 5 days in each of the three phases of the menstrual cycle (mid-cycle, premenstrual, and menstrual) in another study.[83] "High exercisers" experienced a greater positive effect and the least negative effect; sedentary women experienced the least positive effect. Similarly, Prior et al. evaluated mood symptoms over a 6-month period in eight sedentary women who began to exercise and seven runners who began training for a marathon; six women who kept their activity level the same served as a control group. Both groups that increased activity were found to have a reduction in premenstrual mood symptoms, as compared to the control group.[84] The effects of aerobic and strength training exercise in a three-cycle randomized study of 23 healthy, premenopausal women were investigated.[85] The authors found that women participating in both groups had overall improvement in many premenstrual symptoms. However, the aerobic group showed improvement on more symptoms overall, especially premenstrual depression.

LIGHT THERAPY

It has been postulated that shifts in reproductive hormones throughout a woman's life may adversely affect neurotransmitter, neuroendocrine, and circadian systems.[86] It has also been hypothesized that the negative mood symptoms experienced in PMDD may be the result of a maladaptive response to light in the symptomatic luteal phase or to a disturbance in the circadian clock itself.[87] As a result of

these considerations, light therapy has been investigated as a possible therapeutic intervention in PMS.

A six-menstrual cycle randomized, double-blind, counter-balanced, crossover study of dim (500 lux red fluorescent light = placebo) versus bright-light therapy (10,000 lux cool-white fluorescent light = treatment) in 14 women with late luteal phase dysphoric disorder was undertaken by Lam et al.[88] The women completed two menstrual cycles of prospective baseline monitoring of premenstrual symptoms, followed by two cycles of each treatment; subjects were randomized to receive 30 min of evening light therapy using a light box at their homes. Results showed that the active bright white light condition significantly reduced depression and premenstrual tension scores during the symptomatic luteal phase, as compared to baseline, while the placebo dim red light condition did not.

Another 3-month crossover study evaluated the effects of bright (more than 2,500 lux) white morning, bright white evening, and placebo dim (less than 10 lux) red evening light administered daily for 1 week during the premenstrual phase of the menstrual cycle in 19 patients with late luteal phase dysphoric disorder and 11 healthy comparison subjects. The authors reported that depressive ratings were significantly reduced from baseline levels by all light treatments in the patients with late luteal phase dysphoric disorder.[89]

MANIPULATIVE MEDICINE APPROACHES

Twenty-four women with premenstrual dysphoric disorder were randomly assigned to receive either massage therapy or relaxation therapy.[90] The authors reported decreases in anxiety, depressed mood, and pain in subjects receiving massage (immediately following first and last massage), as compared to the control group.

Oleson et al. evaluated the effectiveness of reflexology therapy in alleviating symptoms in 35 women with PMS. Women receiving true reflexology demonstrated a significantly greater decrease in PMS symptoms compared to women receiving sham reflexology.[91]

A randomized, placebo-controlled, cross-over trial of chiropractic for treatment of PMS was done in 1999.[92] This study used a spring-loaded adjustment instrument as the placebo, included 25 subjects, and measured outcome using a standardized PMS questionnaire and daily symptom monitoring. Interestingly, although this study found an improvement over baseline in all groups in terms of symptom control, and a significant difference in scores between treatment and placebo in the group that had the active treatment first, there was no difference between treatment and placebo in the group that had the placebo treatment first. More study is obviously required to distinguish between the role of placebo adjustment and specific adjustment in the use of chiropractic for PMS.

HOMEOPATHY

A small but well-done study of individualized homeopathic prescription for PMS showed an improvement of at least 30% in symptoms in 90% of those receiving active treatment, as compared to 37.5% of those receiving placebo.[93] Additional larger studies are needed to determine if there is a significant role for homeopathy in treatment of this condition.

Conclusion

In the case of PMS, particularly given its multifactorial etiology and its tendency to present in different ways in different women, the integrative approach is well suited, and will provide benefit, for many patients. Although much of the clinical research is preliminary and/or inadequately controlled to this point, many of these therapies have an extremely wide margin of safety and so may have a role in treatment even as we wait for more substantial data to accumulate regarding efficacy.

▶ VAGINITIS

Pathophysiology

Vaginitis can be infectious, irritant, or atrophic. Normal vaginal secretions—the primary defense against vaginitis of all types—come from sebaceous, sweat, Bartholin, and Skene glands; vaginal walls; exfoliated cells of the cervix and vagina; mucus from the cervix; fluids from the endometrium and oviducts; as well as microorganisms and their metabolic products. There are at least six different aerobic bacteria in normal vaginal flora, which are also important in defense against vaginal infection. The most common microbe is hydrogen peroxide producing lactobacilli. Vaginal epithelial cells break down glycogen to monosaccharides, which can be converted by lactobacilli to lactic acid.[94] Healthy vaginal pH maintained by lactic acid is typically 4.

The most common forms of infectious vaginitis are bacterial or nonspecific vaginitis, candida, and trichomonas. Bacterial vaginitis results from an alteration in the normal vaginal flora with loss of lactobacilli and overgrowth of polymicrobial anaerobic bacteria with *Gardnerella* being the most prevalent.[95,96] Factors that influence bacterial survival include vaginal pH and the availability of glucose for metabolism. *Candida albicans* is a dimorphic fungus that exists as blastospores and mycelia. The blastospheres are responsible for transmission and asymptomatic colonization, and when they germinate, the resulting mycelia enhance colonization and facilitate tissue invasion.[97]

There is also speculation on the role of an extracellular toxin or enzyme in the pathogenesis of candidal vaginitis. In addition hypersensitivity may play a role. Uncomplicated candidal infections typically resolve quickly with either an integrative approach or conventional therapy. Complicated courses generally require an integrative approach.

Prevalence/Risk

Vaginitis is not a reportable disease. It is speculated that 40–50% of vaginal infections in women of child bearing age are caused by bacteria, and that 6 million cases in the United States annually are caused by trichomonas.[98] The remainder are most likely candidal. Increased risk of nonspecific vaginitis is seen with alkalinization of the vagina, as *Gardnerella* and trichomonas both survive in an alkaline environment. It is postulated that alkalinization of the vagina by frequent sexual intercourse over a short period of time (semen has a pH of 9),[99] use of douches, menstruation (alkaline blood), and predominance of progesterone favor overgrowth of pathogenic bacteria. Other influencing factors in favor of bacterial overgrowth and depression of normal flora include serious illness, pregnancy, prolonged use of steroids, immune dysfunction, depressed nutritional status, and antibiotics.

Candidal infections are most often self-diagnosed and self-treated. It is estimated that 75% of women experience one episode and 45% experience two or more episodes per year.

Predisposing factors include tight clothes, depressed immunity, antibiotic therapy, pregnancy, diabetes, allergies, and gastrointestinal (GI) candidiasis. GI candidiasis may have a role in recurrent vaginal candidiasis. One study showed that candida in the gut and vagina were linked; when no candida were found in the gut, none was found in the vagina.[100] Case reports link vaginitis to a candidal allergy; 70 selected patients with chronic candidal vaginitis were evaluated for allergy and 90% responded to allergy treatment, which included *Candida albicans* allergens in the hyposensitization injections.[101]

▶ Case Example 1: Vaginitis

E.P. is a 25-year-old female with a 4-day history of vaginal discharge and itching. She notes it is worse after intercourse with her partner. She has tried over-the-counter yeast treatments with no relief. She wonders if antibiotics are indicated at this time, but also wants to know what alternatives she may try first. Pelvic examination revealed a whitish-gray vaginal discharge with microscopy equivocal for clue cells. Several hyphae are seen on microscopy and no trichomonads are evident.

E.P. reports frequent vaginal infections over the past year, some of which have responded to over-the-counter yeast treatments and some of which have resolved with a period of abstention. She is interested both in treatment for this acute episode and in advice regarding a preventive approach for the future.

Conventional Treatment Approach

The choice of conventional treatment depends on the presumed etiology of the vaginitis. Antibiotics are the conventional treatment of choice for bacterial vaginitis. Metronidazole can be used orally or intravaginally. An alternative to metronidazole in the treatment of bacterial vaginitis is clindamycin orally or intravaginally. For trichomonas, metronidazole orally is thought to be 95% effective in single or multiple dosing options. The patient's sexual partner should be treated as well. Prolonged or recurrent antibiotic use can be a predisposing factor in the development of candidal vaginitis, and antibiotics may have gastrointestinal and other side effects.

Betadine has been used and recommended as a conventional treatment. Betadine has shown antimicrobial action against trichomonas and possibly other vaginal microbes, as well as demonstrable antimycotic activity. In a study of 74 women using a Betadine vaginal cleansing kit, 46 showed change on microscopy and all patients had improvement in symptomatology.[102] Betadine has no known side effects but should not be used if the patient has an iodine allergy.

Conventional therapies for candidal vaginitis include intravaginal agents butoconazole cream; clotrimazole cream and tablet; miconazole cream and suppository; and terconazole cream, suppository, or ointment. Oral agents are fluconazole, ketoconazole, and itraconazole. The intravaginal agents should not be used in a pregnancy before 12 weeks, and the oral forms are contraindicated in pregnancy. These agents are highly effective but side effects can include vaginal burning, irritation, headache, and gastrointestinal symptoms (especially for the oral forms). Betadine can be an effective treatment in candidal vaginitis and is safe in pregnancy.

Integrative Treatment Approach

The integrative medicine approach to vaginitis is to treat the underlying predisposing factors, restore balance to the system, and promote a return to healthy flora, as well as to combat or eradicate the offending organism. The goal of an integrative medicine provider in treating a vaginitis should be "to improve the vaginal immune system, support the systemic immune system, restore the proper balance of normal microflora in the vagina, restore the normal pH of the vagina, decrease the inflammation and irritation of the tissue itself, provide symptomatic relief, and, when necessary, also curb the population and overgrowth of the offending organism."[103]

NUTRITION/SUPPLEMENTS

The health of the entire body is important in the treatment of recurrent vaginitis as it is in dealing with any chronic or recurrent infectious process. Integrative medicine focuses on the importance of good nutrition and providing the body with the necessary fuel it needs while helping boost immune system function. Fresh whole foods are recommended. In addition, a diet low in refined sugars (simple carbohydrates), fat, processed foods (as these food have synthetic bonds which may actually tax the immune system) and alcohol is optimal. Most yogurt contains lactobacilli and can restore intestinal flora disrupted by antibiotics. Lactobacilli produce lactic acid to maintain acidic pH; interfere with pathogenic bacteria adherence to the vaginal wall and thus reduce colonization; and produce hydrogen peroxide, which prevents overgrowth of *Gardnerella* and other anaerobic bacteria. Lactobacillus may also act directly as an antibacterial agent against pathogenic bacteria, particularly *Gardnerella*.[104,105]

Supplements may also be indicated in the treatment of recurrent vaginitis, as immune dysfunction occurs with deficiencies in iron, zinc, and several vitamins. Vitamin E deficiency can depress a number of immune functions, including immune responses to antigens, lymphocytic proliferative responses to mitogens and antigens, delayed hypersensitivity reactions, and general host resistance.[106] Vitamin E can be used intravaginally once or twice daily for 7 or more days[107] in the treatment of vaginitis, as well as supplemented orally to support systemic immune function. It can also relieve external discomfort in the vaginal area when used topically. Caution should be taken with vitamin E as it can suppress the immune system in high doses; less than 800 IU/d is generally considered safe.

Vitamin A and beta-carotene also play an important role in maintaining healthy immune function.[108] Vitamin A can be toxic in large doses, and it is recommended that vitamin A and beta-carotene be used in supplements as mixed carotenoids.[109] Vitamin C helps improve connective tissue integrity and may reduce spread of infection. Zinc enhances epithelial growth and zinc deficiency has been associated with depressed immunity. In addition, zinc may have a direct antimicrobial action against trichomonas.[110]

BOTANICAL MEDICINES

Garlic *(Allium sativum)* is a potent antibacterial, antiviral, and antifungal. Allicin is the most active component in garlic. In numerous in vitro studies, garlic has demonstrated activity against gram-positive and gram-negative bacteria.[111] Garlic also has antimycotic properties: one study showed arrested lipid synthesis when a garlic extract was added to colonies of candida.[112] Another study, using an aqueous extract, demonstrated that garlic inhibits growth of candida by oxidizing thiol groups in the organism's essential proteins.[113]

Garlic can be used orally and intravaginally. No studies prove an absolute effective dose of garlic in the treatment of vaginitis, but recommendations from several sources include use of a "garlic suppository." The garlic suppository is a clove of skinned garlic in a small gauze inserted into the vagina. This can be used in the morning and taken out in evening (with addition of lactobacillus capsules in the evening),[114] or changed every 3–5 hours for 3–5 days,[115] or used overnight for 6 days.[116] Garlic can burn mucosal membranes so for topical use a small protective covering such as gauze is recommended. With oral use, it is recommended to add the garlic to food after the food is prepared so as to avoid the loss of volatile oils that can occur with heating or cooking.

Other botanicals used for the treatment of infectious vaginitis include goldenseal *(Hydrastis canadensis)* and Oregon grape root *(Berberis vulgaris)*. These herbs contain berberine, which has immune stimulating and antibacterial activity.[117] Berberine's mechanism of action is thought to be a result of its ability to inhibit microbial growth; in a study using group A streptococci, berberine was found to inhibit adherence of microbes to host cells.[118] Goldenseal has shown direct antimicrobial activity against several organisms, including *Trichomonas vaginalis*.[119] Tea tree oil *(Melaleuca alternifolia)* used topically demonstrates antibacterial, antifungal and monocyte activation properties.[120,121] One study has suggested that tea tree oil removes transient skin flora while suppressing but maintaining resident flora.

In the 1950s, intravaginal gentian violet was the treatment of choice for candidal vaginitis. As it is used externally, gentian violet can be messy and can stain clothing. Boric acid has also been used intravaginally in the treatment of candidal vaginitis. One study (n = 40) demonstrated fungistatic effects.[122] Another study comparing boric acid powder in gelatin capsules with nystatin capsules showed a cure rate of 92% at 7–10 days and 72% at 30 days for boric acid, and 64% at 7–10 days and 50% at 30 days for nystatin.[123] The study used boric acid 600 mg via vaginal insertion in gelatin capsules nightly for 2 weeks. This method is easy, less messy, and less expensive than gentian violet. Boric acid capsules can be used for recurrences.

MIND–BODY APPROACHES

Stress can play a major role in the development and recurrence of vaginitis. As discussed in detail in Chapter 3, stress has been related to depression of the immune system (making the vagina more susceptible to infection). Mind–body techniques potentially applicable in the approach to recurrent vaginitis include, but are not limited to, meditation, hypnosis, imagery, yoga, spirituality, and creative arts therapy. There is no specific research available on the impact of mind–body therapies on recurrent vaginitis.

▶ Case Example 1: Vaginitis Conclusions

Based on her history and physical exam, you conclude that E.P. most likely has recurrent candidal vaginitis. She may opt for conventional treatment of the current infection, either with topical or oral antifungal medication. In terms of prevention, the integrative approach should begin with recommendations for nutritional changes, vitamin supplements, and the addition of botanicals, as outlined below.

Nutritional strategies:

- Whole fresh foods with an emphasis on vitamin-rich fruits and vegetables and minimizing simple carbohydrates and simple sugars
- Vitamin E (D-alpha-tocopherol form) orally 400 IU/d a day and or intravaginally (using the oil from one to two 400-IU capsules); also external use of oil for symptomatic relief of the itching
- Mixed carotenoids 50,000 IU/d
- Zinc picolinate 10–15 mg/d
- Vitamin C 500 mg three times daily
- Lactobacillus 0.5 tsp twice daily

Botanicals: Recommend the patient start with one herb and may add another if symptoms only mildly improve or do not improve.

- Garlic—1 clove orally and 1 clove vaginally per day for 5 days
- Goldenseal tincture—20–60 drops every 2–4 hours or 2 capsules three to four times a day
- Tea tree oil—use topically for symptomatic relief

Other options:

- Betadine-soaked tampon if desired
- Boric acid—600-mg capsules intravaginally once daily
- Yoga, meditation, and/or acupuncture, to support the immune system and body as a whole
- No tight clothing, and keep the vaginal area dry
- Gentian violet—swab externally one to two times daily if desired

▶ FIBROIDS

Pathophysiology

Uterine fibroids, leiomyomas, and myomas are common, benign tumors of the smooth-muscle cells of the uterus. They can be submucosal, intramural, subserosal, or cervical, and are often multiple and of mixed type. Most women do not have symptoms from their fibroids and are unaware of them until they are noted on a routine pelvic examination. Symptoms that can occur include menorrhagia, pelvic pressure, or pain and complications with reproduction. Prolonged and heavy bleeding is more common with submucosal fibroids; irregular bleeding during the menstrual cycle can occur but should be evaluated with endometrial biopsy or dilatation and curettage to rule out endometrial disease. As the uterus grows, pelvic pressure or fullness in the abdomen, rectum, or lower back may occur. Anterior fibroids may cause urinary frequency and, occasionally, blockage of the ureter; posterior fibroids may cause constipation. Degeneration of a fibroid or torsion of a pedunculated fibroid can cause pelvic pain. Reproductive complications include infertility and, less frequently, pain, premature labor, or placental abruption if the fibroid is under the placenta.[124]

The pathophysiology of uterine fibroids is still unclear. There is a genetic predisposition to developing myomas.[125] However, the factors involved in their initiation and growth are not well understood. Uterine myomas are clearly hormone dependent, but the relationship between steroid hormones and local growth factors is complex. Estrogen had been considered the major culprit in fibroid growth, but evidence shows an important role for progesterone as well.[126] Both pregnancy and oral contraceptive use, with high concentrations of estrogen and progesterone, actually decrease the risk of fibroids; however, exposure to oral contraceptives between ages 13 and 16 years leads to an increased risk.[127] Timing may be important and some have suggested that unopposed estrogen plays a role in pathogenesis.[128] In rare cases (less than 1 in 1,000), the fibroid may develop into a malignant sarcoma, but karyotype discordance suggests that the pathogenesis of benign and malignant uterine tumors is different.[129]

Prevalence/Risk Factors

Uterine fibroids, usually becoming symptomatic when women are in their thirties or forties, are clinically present in 20–40% of women, but, in one study, meticulous pathological examinations of surgical specimens increased the prevalence to 77%.[130] Fibroids are the primary indication for 200,000–250,000 hysterectomies performed each year among premenopausal women. From 1988 to 1993, uterine leiomyomas accounted for 62% of hysterectomies among black women, 29% among white women, and 45% among women of other races.[131,132] Most symptoms from fibroids are relieved at menopause but may continue in those taking hormone replacement therapy.[133]

Women of African descent have a threefold greater frequency of uterine myomas and more severe disease for unknown reasons.[131,135] Positive associations have been shown between the risk of uterine fibroids and early menarche, nulliparity, and high body mass index, suggesting an association with increased exposure to ovarian hormones. Inverse associations were observed with oral contraceptive use and cigarette smoking.[136–139] Other nonhormonal factors including hypertension, pelvic inflammatory disease, intrauterine device use with infectious complications, and perineal talc use were also associated with increased risk.[140]

▶ Case Example 2: Fibroids

A.J. is a 40-year-old woman with a 16-week-size uterine fibroid diagnosed 1 year ago. The size has changed very little over the past year but the irregular bleeding and increased menstrual flow have worsened. She notices pelvic pressure and a small bulge in her lower abdomen. A.J. has a history of one pregnancy for which she chose to have a first-trimester abortion. She is not presently sexually active or in an ongoing relationship. She recently thought more about the earlier abortion and, although clearly not regretting the decision, she wonders whether she would ever like to have a child. She has been encouraged to try hormonal treatment or undergo myomectomy or hysterectomy, but is not interested in surgical or pharmacological interventions. A.J. is interested in any other options for symptom relief and possibly shrinking of the fibroids.

Conventional Treatment Approach

There is no need for treatment of uterine myomas unless they cause symptoms. The mainstay of treatment for symptomatic fibroids has been hysterectomy, often with oophorectomy, with most women reporting an improved quality of life.[111] However, the incidence of sexual dysfunction following this surgery can be as high as 45%.[112] For women wishing to keep their uterus or to have future children, myomectomy is available. However, the rate of new myomas and repeat surgery is high.[113,114] Abdominal myomectomy allows pregnancy after surgery, but there is a risk of uterine rupture after laparoscopic myomectomy.[115] Hysteroscopic myomectomy is an option for women with submucosal fibroids. Other surgical options include endometrial ablation and uterine artery embolization.

Hormonal treatments include androgenic steroids or gonadotropin-releasing hormone agonists. These agents cause amenorrhea and reduction in uterine size but are limited because of significant symptoms from the low estrogen state. Several new hormonal treatments are being studied including gonadotropin-releasing antagonists, progesterone antagonists, antiestrogen compounds, and selective estrogen receptor modulators.[116,117] Gene therapy may prove effective in the future.[118]

Integrative Treatment Approach

The integrative approach is predominantly based on traditional healing modalities and anecdotal experience with only a small number of clinical studies to date to substantiate the approach. One unifying principle is the reduction of estrogenic influence with resultant hormonal balance.

Another interesting approach looks at the symbolism of tumors in the reproductive organs. Northrup suggests that fibroids be considered a symptom a woman sends to herself in an unconscious effort to signal an emotional blockage. Fibroids emerge in an energetic pattern of stagnation of energy.[119]

A recent pilot study by Mehl-Madrona[150] looked at a combination of nonpharmacological and nonsurgical therapies for the treatment of women with fibroids. The study was designed to compare two approaches, integrative versus conventional, not to test the efficacy of a single modality. This approach addresses the possibility that one modality might fail to reach significance while several together—reflecting how integrative medicine is actually practiced—might reach a threshold of significance. In this study, 37 menstruating women between the ages of 24 and 45 years with palpable uterine fibroids were treated weekly for as long as 6 months. The treatment consisted of traditional Chinese medicine, including acupuncture, Chinese herbs, and nutritional therapy individualized to each patient; pelvic body work in the form of myofacial release and deep tissue massage; and guided imagery and self-hypnosis training. These women were compared to a matched sample of similar women using conventional treatment.

The fibroids either shrank or stopped growing in 22 patients in the treatment group, as compared to 3 in the comparison group, a statistically significant result. There was no statistically significant difference in the change in symptoms between the two groups. The women in the treatment group were significantly more satisfied with their care than were the women in the comparison group. The average cost for the treatment group was $3,800, significantly greater than the cost for the comparison patients, none of whom had surgery during the study.

This study showed that fibroid size and growth rate, as well as symptoms, could be affected by a combination of complementary therapies, although the cost of treatment was high. The patients in the treatment group actively sought complementary medicine, whereas the comparison group consisted of patients who had used the emergency department for any reason. What effect the role of this motivation had on the outcome is unclear. This study is the most comprehensive study of specific complementary therapies for fibroids to date but, as Mehl-Madrona[150] notes there is a need for further randomized, controlled trials with patients not specifically seeking complementary therapies to look at the individual and combined components of the treatment.

NUTRITIONAL APPROACHES— FOOD AND SUPPLEMENTS

A number of studies show an association between diet, estrogen levels, and breast and endometrial cancer, with red meat and pork associated with an increased cancer risk and vegetables and fruit demonstrating a protective effect.[151,152] A recent study shows a similar pattern when examining nutritional choices and the risk of myoma. Women with uterine fibroids report more frequent consumption of red meat and pork, and less frequent consumption of green vegetables, fruit, and fish.[153] Milk, eggs, butter, margarine, coffee, tea, and alcohol showed no association. Consumption of poultry was not evaluated. This study was done in Milan, Italy, where the use of hormone supplementation in the raising of poultry and cattle may be quite different than in the United States. Because of the extensive use of estrogens in the production of animal products in this country, the relationship between dairy, poultry, and egg consumption and uterine fibroid risk needs to be evaluated specifically in the United States.

If unopposed estrogen may increase the risk of myomas, then a diet that promotes high plasma estrogens may also increase this risk. In contrast, a diet rich in the phytoestrogens, lignans, and isoflavonoids, the precursors of which are found in soybean products, wholegrain cereals, seeds, and berries, may be protective. The lignans and isoflavonoids, which are weakly estrogenic, may compete with other endogenous estrogens and, therefore, influence sex-hormone production, metabolism, and biological activity.[154]

Obesity, especially truncal obesity, is associated with an increased risk of myomas.[155] A number of studies show that higher dietary intake of fat leads to higher plasma estrogen levels and lower fecal estrogen excretion.[156,157] Vegetarian women, with a higher fiber diet, have lower plasma and lower urinary estrogen levels along with higher fecal output and increased fecal excretion of estrogen.[158–160] Yet another study showed that plasma estrogen is positively associated with dietary fat and negatively associated with dietary fiber, and concluded that diet affects the route of excretion of estrogen by altering enterohepatic circulation and thus plasma estrogen levels.[161] Although food choices have been associated with the risk of fibroids, and although there is as described above a theoretical rationale for how these choices might impact this condition, there are no studies looking at a change in fibroid size, growth, or symptoms with a change in diet.

There are many recommendations about vitamin and mineral supplementation for fibroids. When foods rich in iron do not remedy the anemia caused by increased uterine bleeding, iron supplementation is indicated. Other recommendations include vitamins A, B complex, C, E, and K and magnesium, zinc, selenium, bioflavonoids, and essential fatty acids. The only study of any of these supplements is one using vitamin E 300 mg/d in the treatment of pregnancy complicated by fibroids. In the 25 women undergoing treatment, all pregnancies continued to term with no adverse effects in the mother or fetus.[162]

MIND–BODY APPROACHES

There are no studies using visualization or imagery, meditation, hypnosis, biofeedback, yoga, or relaxation training for treating fibroids. However, these therapies are often used and are anecdotally successful. Guided visual imagery and self-hypnosis training were part of the treatment protocol in Mehl-Madrona's study.[150] As mentioned previously, many physicians encourage women to work with the meaning of the fibroid in their lives and consider the possible source of energy "stuck" in the uterus. Relaxation breathing focusing on the pelvis and yoga are often recommended with imagery and journal writing focusing on releasing or even "birthing" the blocked energy or creativity to clarify areas for personal growth.[163–166]

ENVIRONMENTAL STRATEGIES
Regular exercise lowers circulating levels of estrogen and lowers the risk of myomas,[167,168] but there are no studies showing that an exercise program will reduce the symptoms in women with fibroids. Smoking cigarettes has an antiestrogen effect and lowers the risk of uterine fibroids.[169,170] Fibroids may be associated with heavy metal and pesticide contamination. One study showed increased cadmium excretion and elevated α-hexachlorocyclohexane concentrations in women with fibroids,[171,172] and an animal model demonstrated that organochlorine pesticides have estrogen effects on myometrial tissue.[173] Evaluation for these exposures should be considered.

BOTANICAL MEDICINES
There are many Western and Chinese herbs that traditionally have been used in the treatment of myomas. The Western herbs include chastetree berry *(Vitex agnus-castus),* black cohosh *(Cimicifuga vacemosa),* blue cohosh *(Caulophyllum thalictroides),* false unicorn root *(Chamaelirium luteum),* partridge berry *(Mitchella repens),* wild yam *(Dioscorea villosa),* cleavers *(Galium aparine),* yarrow *(Achillea millefolium),* and periwinkle *(Vinca major).* One combination from David Hoffman[166] that has been useful in clinical practice includes 2 parts blue cohosh, 2 parts periwinkle, 1 part chastetree berries, 1 part black cohosh, 1 part wild yam, and 1 part cleavers. This incorporates the actions of uterine tonic (blue and black cohosh), uterine astringent (periwinkle), alterative (cleavers, blue and black cohosh), antispasmodic (blue cohosh), and lymphatic (cleavers). Shepherd's purse *(Capsella bursa-pastoris),* bethroot *(Trillium pendulatum),* cotton root bark *(Gossypium),* and nettles *(Urtica dioica)* have been used to treat the heavy bleeding associated with fibroids. Warm castor oil packs over the lower abdomen also have a long history of use.

Although some of these herbs have been used cross-culturally,[174,175] and many show effects on hormonal balance in other studies,[176] there are no studies of the use of Western herbs to treat fibroids. Greater than 50% of estrogen metabolism and conjugation occurs in the liver, raising the possibility that herbs that improve liver function, such as milk thistle *(Silybum marianum),* may increase the excretion of estrogen and, therefore, lower the risk of, or even treat, uterine fibroids.[177,178] This has also not yet been studied.

Two studies have looked at traditional Chinese herbal remedies. Zhongli and Shurong[179] treated 223 premenopausal women with clinically apparent fibroids in an uncontrolled study. Treatment was individualized according to each patient's pattern of imbalance, using the principles of invigorating the blood and eliminating stasis, clearing heat and softening induration. The herbs were administered after menstruation. The authors reported a 72% reduction in menstrual blood flow for the 160 women complaining of menorrhagia. Forty-six percent of patients reported decrease in abdominal pain and leukorrhea. Backache improved in 59% of patients. Myomas disappeared in 13%, were markedly diminished in 29%, were slightly reduced in 19%, and were unchanged in 28% of cases. Overall, the treatment was effective in 92.4% of women.

Another study looked at the pharmacological effects of kuei-chih-fu-ling-wan (also known as keishi-bukuryo-gan or KBG in Japanese), a traditional Chinese herbal remedy combining 5 different roots, seeds, and barks, in 110 premenopausal women with uterine myomas. In this uncontrolled study, clinical symptoms of hypermenorrhea or dysmenorrhea were improved in 90% of the cases with shrinking of the fibroids in 60% of cases.[180]

TRADITIONAL SYSTEMS: ACUPUNCTURE, HOMEOPATHY, AND AYURVEDA

Acupuncture and acupressure, often to resolve a pattern of "blood stasis," have been traditionally used to treat uterine fibroids, although there are few studies to substantiate their effectiveness. Acupuncture was part of the treatment used in Mehl-Madrona's pilot study.[150] A recent review of esogetic colorpuncture therapy developed by German naturopath and acupuncturist Peter Mandel[181]—a therapy in which different colored light frequencies are placed on selected acupuncture points (determined by evaluating Kirlian photographs for energetic imbalances)—reported on 100 women 30–50 years old treated 30–60 times according to a particular esogetic colorpuncture therapy protocol. The study was not controlled or blinded. Fibroids disappeared in 33% and decreased in size in 45% of women. There was no change in 22% of cases, which included

12% who required surgery. All women reported an improvement, including less back or abdomen pain, sleeping better, feeling better emotionally, and the ability to be more physically active.

Another unblinded Chinese study compared women treated with acupuncture with those treated with Chinese and Western conventional medical treatments and found that acupuncture was more effective. The total effectiveness rate was 98% and cure rate was 73%.[182] A Russian study showed an electrical response correlation between acupuncture points and the presence and activity of uterine proliferation.[183]

Classical homeopathy has an extensive history of treatment of fibroids, but controlled studies have not been done as yet. Treatment of fibroids has also been traditional in Ayurveda and Tibetan medicine, through purifying the blood and improving liver detoxification, but again, there are no studies to substantiate its usage.

► Case Example 2: Fibroids Conclusions

A.J. began a low-fat, high-fiber diet with plenty of green vegetables, soy products, and whole grains. She substituted cold-water fish for red meat and poultry. She also began a regular aerobic exercise program. She did not have the resources to begin treatment with acupuncture, but she did start a combination of chastetree berry, black cohosh, blue cohosh, and milk thistle twice a day.

She started daily relaxation breathing with attention to the pelvic area and began to focus on the big question of whether she would like to have children at some point in her life. Within 2 months, her irregular, heavy bleeding and pelvic pressure ceased. She hopes the fibroid will begin to shrink as well as she continues these therapies.

REFERENCES

1. Reid R. Premenstrual syndrome. *N Engl J Med.* 1991;324:1208–1210.
2. Chrousos GP, Torpy DJ, Gold PW. Interactions between the hypothalamic–pituitary–adrenal axis and the female reproductive system: clinical implications. *Ann Intern Med.* 1998;129:229–240.
3. Reid R. Premenstrual syndrome. *N Engl J Med.* 1991;324:1208.
4. Mortola J. Premenstrual syndrome—pathophysiologic considerations. *N Engl J Med.* 1998;338:256–257.
5. Singh B, Berman B, Simpson R, Annechild A. Incidence of premenstrual syndrome and remedy usage: a national probability sample study. *Altern Ther Health Med.* 1998;4:75–79.
6. Johnson SR. Premenstrual syndrome therapy. *Clin Obstet Gynecol.* 1998;41(2):405–421.

7. Wyatt K, Dimmock P, Jones P, et al. Efficacy of progesterone and progestogens in management of premenstrual syndrome: systematic review. *BMJ.* 2001;323:776–780.

8. Abraham G. Nutritional factors in the etiology of the premenstrual tension syndrome. *J Reprod Med.* 1983;28:446–464.

9. Rossignol AM. Caffeine-containing beverages and premenstrual syndrome in young women. *Am J Public Health.* 1985;75(11):1335–1337.

10. Rossignol AM, Zhang JY, Chen YZ, Xiang Z. Tea and premenstrual syndrome in the People's Republic of China. *Am J Public Health.* 1989;79(1):67–69.

11. Low Dog T. Integrative treatments for premenstrual syndrome. *J Altern Ther Health Heal.* 2001;7(5):32–39.

12. Rosenstein DL, Elin RJ, Hosseini JM, et al. Magnesium measures across the menstrual cycle in premenstrual syndrome. *Biol Psychiatry.* 1994;35(8):557–561.

13. Proctor ML, Murphy PA. Herbal dietary therapies for primary and secondary dysmenorrhoea (Cochrane Review). In: *The Cochrane Library,* Issue 2, 2002. Oxford, UK: Update Software.

14. Seifert B, Wagler P, Dartsch S, Schmidt U, Nieder J. Magnesium-a new therapeutic alternative in primary dysmenorrhea. *Zentralblatt fur Gynakologie.* 1989;111(11):755–760.

15. Altura BM, Altura BT. New perspectives on the role of magnesium in the pathophysiology of the cardiovascular system. II. Experimental aspects. *Magnesium.* 1985;4(5–6):245–271.

16. Schindler R, Thoni H, Classen HG. The role of magnesium in the generation and therapy of benign muscle cramps. Combined in vivo/in vitro studies on rat phrenic nerve-diaphragm preparations. *Arneimittel Forschung.* 1998;48(2):161–166.

17. Proctor ML, Murphy PA. Herbal dietary therapies for primary and secondary dysmenorrhoea (Cochrane Review). In: *The Cochrane Library,* Issue 2, 2002. Oxford, UK: Update Software.

18. Ebadi M, Govitrapong P. Pyridoxal phosphate and neurotransmitters in the brain. In: Tryiates G, ed. *Vitamin B6: Metabolism and the Role in Growth.* Westport, CT: Food and Nutrition Press; 1980:223.

19. Wyatt K, Kimmock P, Jones PA, et al. Efficacy of vitamin B-6 in the treatment of premenstrual syndrome: systematic review. *BMJ.* 1999;318:1375–1381.

20. Blue J, Harman J. Mastalgia review: St Marks Breast Center. *NZ Med J.* 1998;111:34–37.

21. Cohen M, Bendich A. Safety of pyridoxine—a review of human and animal studies. *Toxicol Lett.* 1986;34:129–139.

22. Krinke G, Nalyor DC, Skorpil V. Pyridoxine megavitaminosis—an analysis of the early changes induced with massive doses of vitamin B6 in rat primary sensory neurons. *J Neuropathol Exp Neurol.* 1985;44:117–129.

23. Schaeppi U, Krinke G. Pyridoxine neuropathy: correlation of functional tests and neuropathology in beagle dogs treated with large doses of vitamin B6. *Agents Actions.* 1982;12:575–582.

24. Thys-Jacobs S. Micronutrients and the premenstrual syndrome: the case for calcium. *J Am Coll Nutr.* 2000;19(2): 220–227.

25. Thys-Jacobs S, Starkey P, Bernstein D, et al. Calcium carbonate and the premenstrual syndrome: effects on premenstrual and menstrual symptoms. Premenstrual Syndrome Study Group. *Am J Obstet Gynecol.* 1998;179(2):444–452.

26. Thys-Jacobs S, Starkey P, Bernstein D, et al. Calcium carbonate and the premenstrual syndrome: effects on premenstrual and menstrual symptoms. Premenstrual Syndrome Study Group. *Am J Obstet Gynecol.* 1998;179(2):444–452.

27. Ward MW, Holimon TD. Calcium treatment for premenstrual syndrome. *Ann Pharmacother.* 1999;33(12):1356–1358.

28. Bourgoin BP, Evans DR, Cornett JR, et al. Lead content in 70 brands of dietary calcium supplements. *Am J Public Health.* 1993;83:1155–1160.

29. US Food and Drug Administration. *Provisional Tolerable Exposure Levels for Lead* [memorandum]. Washington, DC: US Public Health Service, 1990.

30. Haney R. Lead in calcium supplements cause for alarm or celebration? *JAMA.* 2000;204(11):1432–1433.

31. Schultz V, Hansel R, Tyler V. *Rational Phytotherapy: A Physician's Guide to Herbal Medicine.* 3rd ed. Berlin: Springer; 1997:240.

32. Mills S, Bone K. *Principles and Practice of Phytotherapy.* London: Churchill Livingstone; 2000.

33. Natural Medicines Comprehensive Database. Available at: http://www.naturaldatabase.com. Accessed October 8, 2003.

34. Merz PG, Gorkow C, Schrodter A, et al. The effects of special *agnus-castus* extract (BP1095E1) on prolactin secretion in healthy male subjects.

Exp Clin Endocrinol Diabetes. 1996;104(6): 447–453.

35. Wutteke W. Dopaminergic action of extracts of *agnus-castus. Forschende Komplementarmedizen.* 1996;3(6):329–330.

36. Feldman HU, Albrecht M, Lamertz M, et al. The treatment of corpus luteum insufficiency and premenstrual syndrome. Experience in a multicenter study under clinical practice conditions. *Gynakol.* 1990;12:422–425.

37. Dittmar G, Bohnert K. Premenstrual syndrome: treatment with a phytopharmaceutical. *TW Gynakol.* 1992;5:60–68.

38. Turner S, Mills S. A double-blind clinical trial on a herbal remedy for premenstrual syndrome; a case study. *Complement Ther Med.* 1993;1:73–77.

39. Schellenberg R. Treatment for the premenstrual syndrome with *agnus-castus* fruit extract: prospective, randomized, placebo-controlled study. *BMJ.* 2001;322(7279):134–137.

40. Lauritzen C, Reuter H, Repges R. Treatment of premenstrual tension syndrome with *Vitex agnus-castus:* controlled double-blind study versus pyridoxine. *Phytomedicine.* 1997;4:183–189.

41. Kemper K. The Longwood Herbal Task Force. Available at: http://www.mcp.edu/herbal/default. htm. Accessed June 10, 2002.

42. Horrobin DF, Manku MS, Brush M, et al. Abnormalities in plasma essential fatty acid levels in women with premenstrual syndrome and nonmalignant breast disease. *J Nutr Med.* 1991;2: 259–264.

43. Koshidawa N, Tatsuma T, Furyya K, et al. Prostaglandins and premenstrual syndrome. *Prostaglandin Leukot Essent Fatty Acids.* 1992; 45:33–36.

44. Budeiri D, Li Wan Po A, Dornan JC. Is evening primrose oil of value in the treatment of premenstrual syndrome? *Control Clin Trials.* 1996; 17(1):60–68.

45. Collins A, Gerin A, Coleman G, et al. Essential fatty acids in the treatment of premenstrual syndrome. *Obstet Gynecol.* 1993;81(1):93–98.

46. Khoo SK, Munroe C, Battistutta D. Evening primrose and the treatment of premenstrual syndrome. *Med J Aust.* 1990;153(4):189–190.

47. Carter J, Verhoef MJ. Efficacy of self-help and alternative treatments of premenstrual syndrome. *Womens Health Issues.* 1994;4(3):130–137.

48. Evening primrose. Available at: http://www. naturaldatabase.com. Accessed June 23, 2002.

49. Foster S. Black cohosh *(Cimicifuga racemosa):* a literature review. *HerbalGram.* 1999;45:35–49.

50. Lieberman S. A review of the effectiveness of *Cimicifuga racemosa* (black cohosh) for the symptoms of menopause. *J Women's Health.* 1998;7(5);525–529.

51. Duker Em, Kopanski L, Jarry H, et al. Effects of extracts from *Cimicifuga racemosa* on gonadotropin release in menopausal women and ovariectomized rats. *Planta Med.* 1991;57(5); 420–424.

52. Jacobson JS, Troxel AB Evans J, et al. Randomized trial of black cohosh for the treatment of hot flashes among women with a history of breast cancer. *J Clin Oncol.* 2001;19(10):2739–2745.

53. Liske E. Therapeutic efficacy and safety of cimicifuga racemosa for gynecologic disorders. *Adv Ther.* 1998;15(1):45–53.

54. Black cohosh. Available at: http://www. naturaldatabase. com. Accessed June 23, 2002.

55. Ginkgo. Available at: http://www.naturaldatabase. com. Accessed June 23, 2002.

56. Tamborini A, Taurelle R. value of standardized ginkgo biloba extract (Egb 761) in the management of congestive symptoms of premenstrual syndrome. *Rev Fr Gynecol Obstet.* 1993;88(7–9): 447–457.

57. Liske E. Therapeutic efficacy and safety of cimicifuga racemosa for gynecologic disorders. *Adv Ther.* 1998;15(1):45–53.

58. Brautigam MR, Blommaert FA, Verleye G, et al. Treatment of age-related memory complaints with ginkgo biloba extract: a randomized, double-blind, placebo-controlled study. *Phytomedicine.* 1998;5(6);425–434.

59. Ranchon I, Gorrand JM, Cluzel J, et al. Functional protection of photoreceptors from light-induced damage by dimethyl urea and ginkgo biloba extract. *Invest Ophthalmol Vis Sci.* 1999;40(6); 1191–1199.

60. Paick J, Lee J. An experimental study of the effect of ginkgo biloba extract on the human and rabbit corpus cavernosum tissue. *J Urol.* 1996;156; 1876–1880.

61. Steiner M, Steinberg S, Stewart D, et al. Fluoxetine in the treatment of premenstrual dysphoria. Canadian fluoxetine/premenstrual dysphoria Collaborative Study Group. *N Engl J Med.* 1995;332: 1529–1534.

62. Williams JW, Mulrow CD, Chiquette E, et al. A systematic review of newer pharmacotherapies for depression in adults: Evidence report summary. *Ann Intern Med.* 2000;132:743–756.

63. Shelton RC, Keller MB, Gelenberg A, et al. Effectiveness of St. John's wort in major depression: A randomized placebo controlled trial. *JAMA.* 2001:285:1978–1986.

64. Stevinson C, Ernst E. A pilot study of hypericum perforatum for the treatment of premenstrual syndrome. *Br J Obstet Gynaecol.* 2000;107(7): 870–876.

65. Lebot V, Merlin M, Lindstrom L. *Kava: The Pacific Drug.* New Haven, CT: Yale University Press; 1992.

66. Pittler MH, Ernst E. Efficacy of kava extract for treating anxiety: systematic review and meta-analysis. *J Clin Pharmacol.* 2000;20(1):84–89.

67. Warnecke G. Psychosomatic dysfunctions in the female climacteric. Clinical effectiveness and tolerance of kava extract WS 1490. *Forschr Med.* 1991;109(4);119–122.

68. De Leo V, La Marca A, Lanzetta D, et al. Assessment of the association of Kava-kava extract and hormone replacement therapy in the treatment of postmenopausal anxiety. *Minerva Ginecol.* 2000;52:263–267.

69. De Leo, La Marca A, Morgante G, et al. Evaluation of combining kava extract with hormone replacement therapy in the treatment of postmenopausal anxiety. *Maturitas.* 2001;39(2): 185–188.

70. Blumenthal M. Expert analysis of case reports says there is insufficient evidence to make a causal connection. Available at: http://www. Herbalgram.org. Accessed April 8, 2002.

71. Packer-Tursman J. Anxiety over kava: FDA, others investigate reports of liver toxicity. *Washington Post.* January 22, 2002: F1.

72. Swensen JN. Man convicted of driving under the influence of Kava. *Deseret News.* August 5, 1996.

73. Low Dog T. Integrative treatments for premenstrual syndrome. *J Altern Ther Health Heal.* 2001; 7(5): 32–39.

74. Levitt A, Kohasu W, eds. *Premenstrual Syndrome. Complementary and Alternative Medicine Secrets.* Philadelphia: Hanley and Belfus; 2002.

75. Goodale IL, Domar AD, Benson H. Alleviation of premenstrual syndrome symptoms with the relaxation response. *Obstet Gynecol.* 1990;75: 649–655.

76. Blake F, Salkovskis P, Gath D, Day A, Garrod A. Cognitive therapy for premenstrual syndrome: a controlled trial. *J Psychosom Res.* 1998;45(4): 307–318.

77. Morse CA, Dennerstein L, Farrell E, Varnavides K. A comparison of hormone therapy, coping skills training, and relaxation for the relief of premenstrual syndrome. *Behav Med.* 1991;14: 469–489.

78. Kirkby RJ. Changes in premenstrual symptoms and irrational thinking following cognitive-behavioral coping skills training. *J Consult Clin Psychology.* 1994;62:1026–1032.

79. Christensen AP, Oei TP. The efficacy of cognitive behavior therapy in treating premenstrual dysphoric changes. *J Affect Disord.* 1995;33:57–63.

80. Sridevi K, Krishna Rao PV. Yoga practice and menstrual distress. *J Indian Acad Appl Psychology.* 1996;22(1–2):47–54.

81. Pullon SR, Reinken JA, Sparrow MJ. Treatment of premenstrual symptoms in Wellington women. *N Z Med J.* 1989;102(9862):72–74.

82. Aganoff JA, Boyle GJ. Aerobic exercise, mood states, and menstrual cycle symptoms. *J Psychosom Res.* 1994;38:183–192.

83. Choi PY, Salmon P. Symptom changes across the menstrual cycle in competitive sportswomen, exercisers and sedentary women. *Soc Sci Med.* 1995;41(6):769–777.

84. Prior JC, Vigna Y, Sciarretta D, Alojada N, Schulzer M. Conditioning exercise decreases premenstrual symptoms: a prospective controlled 6 month trial. *Fertil Steril.* 1987;47:402–408.

85. Steege JF, Blumenthal JA. The effects of aerobic exercise on premenstrual symptoms in middle-aged women: a preliminary study. *J Psychosom Res.* 1993;37:127–133.

86. Parry BL, Haynes P. Mood disorders and the reproductive cycle. *J Gend Specif Med.* 2000;3(5): 53–58.

87. Parry BL, Udell C, Elliott JA, et al. Blunted phase-shift responses to morning bright light in premenstrual dysphoric disorder. *J Biol Rhythms.* 1997;12(5):443–456.

88. Lam RW, Carter D, Misri S, Kuan AJ, Yatham LN, Zis AP. A controlled study of light therapy in women with late luteal phase dysphoric disorder. *Psychiatry Res.* 1999;86(3):185–192.

89. Parry BL, Mahan AM, Mostofi N, Klauber MR, Lew GS, Gillin JC. Light therapy of late luteal phase dysphoric disorder: an extended study. *Am J Psychiatry.* 1993;150(9):1417–1419.

90. Hernandez-Reif M, Martinez A, Field T, Quintero O, Hart S, Burman I. Premenstrual symptoms are relieved by massage therapy. *J Psychosom Obstet Gynaecol.* 2000;21:9–15.

91. Oleson T, Flocco W. Randomised controlled study of premenstrual symptoms treated with ear, hand, and foot reflexology. *Acta Obstet Gynecol Scand.* 1971;50:331–337.

92. Walsh MJ, Polus BI. A randomized, placebo-controlled clinical trial on the efficacy of chiropractic therapy on premenstrual syndrome. *J Manipulative Physiol Ther.* 1999;22:582–585.

93. Yakir M, Kreitler S, Brzezinski A, et al. Effects of homeopathic treatment in women with premenstrual syndrome: a pilot study. *Br Homeopathic J.* 2001;90:148–153.

94. Berek J, Adashi E, Hillard P. *Novak's Gynecology.* 12th ed. Baltimore, MD: Williams & Wilkins; 1988:430–431.

95. Spiegel C, Amsel R, Eschenbach D, et al. Anaerobic bacteria in nonspecific vaginitis. *N Engl J Med.* 1980;303:601–607.

96. Vontver L, Eschenbach D. The role of *Gardnerella vaginalis* in nonspecific vaginitis. *Clin Obstet Gynecol.* 1981;24:439–460.

97. Berek J, Adashi E, Hillard P. *Novak's Gynecology.* 12th ed. Baltimore, MD: Williams & Wilkins; 1988:432.

98. Thomason J, Gelbart S. *Trichomonas vaginalis. Obstet Gynecol.* 1989;74:536–541.

99. Northrup C. *Women's Bodies, Women's Wisdom.* New York: Bantam Books; 1994.

100. Miles MR, Olsen L, Rogers A, et al. Recurrent vaginal candidiasis—importance of an intestinal reservoir. *JAMA.* 1977;238:1836–1837.

101. Kudelko NM. Allergy in chronic monilial vaginitis. *Ann Allergy.* 1971;29:266–267.

102. Singha HSK. The use of a vaginal cleansing kit in non-specific vaginitis. *Practitioner.* 1979;223:403–404.

103. Hudson T. *Women's Encyclopedia of Natural Medicine.* Los Angeles: Keats; 1999:280.

104. Chan R, Bruce A, Reid G. Adherence of cervical, vaginal and distal urethral normal microbial flora to human uroepithelial cells and the inhibition of adherence of gram-negative uropathogens by competitive exclusion. *J Urol.* 1984;131:596–601.

105. Klebanoff S, Hiller S, Eschenbach D, Waltersdorph A. Control of the microbial flora of the vagina by H_2O_2 generating lactobacilli. *J Infect Dis.* 1991;164:94–100.

106. Beisel W, Edelman R, Nauss K, Suskin R. Single-nutrient effects on immunological functions—report of a workshop sponsored by the department of food and nutrition and its nutrition advisory group of the American Medical Association. *JAMA.* 1981;245(1):53–58.

107. Hudson T. *Women's Encyclopedia of Natural Medicine.* Los Angeles: Keats; 1999:281.

108. Sirisnha S, Daziy M, Moongkarndi P, et al. Impaired local immune response in vitamin A deficient rats. *Clin Exp Immunol.* 1980;40:127–135.

109. Pizzorno JE, Murray MT. *Textbook of Natural Medicine.* 2nd ed. New York: Churchill Livingstone; 1999.

110. Krieger J, Rein M. Zinc sensitivity of *Trichomonas vaginalis:* in vitro studies and clinical implications. *J Infect Dis.* 1982;146:341–345.

111. Cavallito C, Bailey J. Allicin, the antibacterial principle of *Allium sativum.* Isolation, physical properties and antibacterial action. *J Am Chem Soc.* 1944;66:1950–1951.

112. Adetumbi M, Javor G, Lau B. *Allium sativum* (garlic) inhibits lipid synthesis by *Candida albicans. Antimicrob Agents Chemother.* 1986;30(3):499–501.

113. Ghannaoum MA. Studies on the anticandidal mode of action of *Allium sativum* (garlic). *J Gen Microbiol.* 1988;134:2917–2924.

114. Gladstar R. *Herbal Healing for Women.* New York: Simon and Schuster; 1993:138–140.

115. Hudson T. *Women's Encyclopedia of Natural Medicine.* Los Angeles: Keats; 1999.

116. Soule D. *A Women's Book of Herbs—The Healing Power of Natural Remedies.* Toronto, Canada: Carol Publishing Group; 1998.

117. Hahn F, Ciak J. Berberine. *Antibiotics.* 1976; 3:577–588.

118. Murray M. *The Healing Power of Herbs.* Rocklin, CA: Prima Publishing; 1995:165.

119. Kaneda A, Torii M, Aikawa M. In vitro effects of berberine sulfate on the growth of *Entamoeba histolytica, Giardia lamblia,* and *Trichomonas vaginalis. Ann Trop Med Parasitol.* 1991;85:417–425.

120. Petry J, Hadley S. Medicinal herbs: answers and advice, part 1. *Hosp Pract.* 2001;36(7):59–60.

121. Pena E. Melaleuca alternifolia oil: its use for trichomonal vaginitis and other vaginal infections. *Obstet Gynecol.* 1962;19(6):793–795.

122. Swate T, Weed J. Boric acid treatment of vulvo-vaginal candidiasis. *Obstet Gynecol.* 1974;43(6): 893–895.

123. Van Slyke KK, Michel VP, Rein M. Treatment of vulvovaginal candidiasis with boric acid powder. *Am J Obstet Gynecol.* 1981;141(2):145–148.

124. Rice JP, Kay HH, Mahony BS. The clinical significance of uterine leiomyomas in pregnancy. *Am J Obstet Gynecol.* 1989;160:1212–1216.

125. Luoto R, Kaprio J, Rutanen, EM, et al. Heritability and risk factors of uterine fibroids—The Finnish twin cohort study. *Maturitas.* 2000;37: 15–26.

126. Rein MS. Advances in uterine leiomyoma research: the progesterone hypothesis. *Environ Health Perspect.* 2000;108(suppl 5):791–793.

127. Marshall LM, Spiegelman D, Goldman MB, et al. A prospective study of reproductive factors and oral contraceptive use in relation to the risk of uterine leiomyoma. *Fertil Steril.* 1998;70:432–439.

128. Ross RK, Pike MC, Bull D, et al. Risk factors for uterine fibroids: reduced risk associated with oral contraceptives. *Br Med J.* 1986;293:359–361.

129. Stewart E. Uterine fibroids. *Lancet.* 2001;357: 293–298.

130. Cramer SF, Patel A. The frequency of uterine leiomyomas. *Am J Clin Pathol.* 1990;94:435–438.

131. Farquhar CM, Steiner CA. Hysterectomy rates in the United States, 1990–1997. *Obstet Gynecol.* 2002;99:229–234.

132. Lepine LA, Hillis SD, Marchbanks PA, et al. Hysterectomy surveillance—United States, 1980–1993. *MMWR Surveill Summ.* 1997;46:1–15.

133. Sener AB, Seckin NC, Ozmen S, et al. The effects of hormone replacement therapy on uterine fibroids in postmenopausal women. *Fertil Steril.* 1996;65:354–357.

134. Kjerulff KH, Langenberg P, Seidman JD, et al. Uterine leiomyomas: racial differences in severity, symptoms and age at diagnosis. *J Reprod Med.* 1996;41:483–490.

135. Marshall LM, Spiegelman D, Barbieri RL, et al. Variation in the incidence of uterine leiomyoma among premenopausal women by age and race. *Obstet Gynecol.* 1997;90:967–973.

136. Parazzini F, La Vecchia C, Negri E, et al. Epidemiologic characteristics of women with uterine fibroids: a case-control study. *Obstet Gynecol.* 1988;72:853–857.

137. Faerstein E, Szklo M, Rosenshein N. Risk factors for uterine leiomyoma: a practice-based case-control study I. African-American heritage, reproductive history, body size, and smoking. *Am J Epidemiol.* 2001;153:1–10.

138. Chen C, Buck GM, Courey NG, et al. Risk factors for uterine fibroids among women undergoing tubal sterilization. *Am J Epidemiol.* 2001;153:20–26.

139. Parazzini F, Negri E, La Vecchia C, et al. Reproductive factors and risk of uterine fibroids. *Epidemiology.* 1996;7:440–442.

140. Faerstein E, Szklo M, Rosenshein NB. Risk factors for uterine leiomyoma: a practice-based case-control study II. Atherogenic risk factors and potential sources of uterine irritation. *Am J Epidemiol.* 2001;153:11–19.

141. Carlson KJ, Miller BA, Fowler FJ Jr. The Maine Women's Health Study: I. Outcomes of hysterectomy. *Obstet Gynecol.* 1994;83:556–565.

142. Zussman L, Zussman S, Sunley R, et al. Sexual response after hysterectomy-oophorectomy: recent studies and reconsideration of psychogenesis. *Am J Obstet Gynecol.* 1981;140:725–729.

143. Fedele L, Parazzini F, Luchini L, et al. Recurrence of fibroids after myomectomy: a transvaginal ultrasonographic study. *Hum Reprod.* 1995;10: 1795–1796.

144. Malone LJ. Myomectomy: recurrence after removal of solitary and multiple myomas. *Obstet Gynecol.* 1969;34:200–203.

145. Nezhat C. The "cons" of laparoscopic myomectomy in women who may reproduce in the future. *Int J Fertil Menopausal Stud.* 1996;41: 280–283.

146. Eldar-Geva T, Healy DL. Other medical management of uterine fibroids. *Baillieres Clin Obstet Gynaecol.* 1998;12:269–288.

147. Kettel LM, Murphy AA, Morales AJ, et al. Rapid regression of uterine leiomyomas in response to daily administration of gonadotropin-releasing hormone antagonist. *Fertil Steril.* 1993;60: 342–346.

148. Gross K, Morton C, Stewart E. Finding genes for uterine fibroids. *Obstet Gynecol.* 2000;95(suppl 1):S60.

149. Northrup C. *The Wisdom of Menopause: Creating Physical and Emotional Health and Healing During the Change.* New York: Bantam Books; 2001:19–20, 241–242.

150. Mehl-Madrona L. Complementary medicine treatment of uterine fibroids: a pilot study. *Altern Ther Health Med.* 2002;8:34–46.

151. Levi F, Franceschi S, Negri E, et al. Dietary

factors and the risk of endometrial cancer. *Cancer.* 1993;71:3575–3581.

152. Franceschi S, Favero A, La Vecchia C, et al. Influence of food groups and food diversity on breast cancer risk in Italy. *Int J Cancer.* 1995;63:785–789.

153. Chiaffarino F, Parazzini F, La Vecchia C, et al. Diet and uterine myomas. *Obstet Gynecol.* 1999; 94:395–398.

154. Adlercreutz H, Mazur W. Phytoestrogens and Western diseases. *Ann Med.* 1997;29:95–120.

155. Sato, F, Nishi M, Kudo R, et al. Body fat distribution and uterine leiomyomas. *J Epidemiol.* 1998; 8:176–180.

156. Goldin BR, Aldercreutz H, Gorbach SL, et al. The relationship between estrogen levels and diets of Caucasian American and Oriental immigrant women. *Am J Clin Nutr.* 1986;44:945–953.

157. Aldercreutz H, Gorbach SL, Goldin BR, et al. Estrogen metabolism and excretion in Oriental and Caucasian women. *J Natl Cancer Inst.* 1994;86: 1076–1082.

158. Armstrong BK, Brown, JB, Clarke HT, et al. Diet and reproductive hormones: a study of vegetarian and nonvegetarian postmenopausal women. *J Natl Cancer Inst.* 1981;67:761–767.

159. Goldin BR, Adlercreutz H, Dwyer JT, et al. Effect of diet on excretion of estrogens in pre- and postmenopausal women. *Cancer Res.* 1981;41: 3771–3773.

160. Goldin BR, Adlercreutz H, Gorbach SL, et al. Estrogen excretion patterns and plasma levels in vegetarian and omnivorous women. *N Engl J Med.* 1982;307:1542–1547.

161. Gorbach SL, Goldin BR. Diet and the excretion and enterohepatic cycling of estrogens. *Prev Med.* 1987;16:525–531.

162. Fruscella L, Ciaglia EM, Danti M, et al. Vitamin E in the treatment of pregnancy complicated by uterine myoma [abstract] [in Italian]. *Minerva Ginecol.* 1997;49:175–179.

163. Northrop C. *Women's Bodies, Women's Wisdom.* New York: Bantam Books; 1998:202–209.

164. Weed S. *Menopausal Years: The Wise Woman Way.* New York: Ash Tree Publishing; 1992:12–13.

165. Soule D. *The Woman's Book of Herbs: The Healing Power of Natural Remedies.* New York: Citadel Press; 1995:206.

166. Hoffman D. *Therapeutic Herbalism: A Correspondence Course in Phytotherapy.* c. 1986; 145–148, 173–174.

167. Stoll BA. Diet and exercise regimens to improve breast carcinoma prognosis. *Cancer.* 1996;78: 2465–2470.

168. Kaminski BT, Rzempoluch J. Evaluation of the influence of certain epidemiologic factors on development of uterine myomas [abstract]. *Wiad Lek.* 1993;46:592–596.

169. Baron JA, La Vecchia C, Levi F. The antiestrogenic effect of cigarette smoking in women. *Am J Obstet Gynecol.* 1990;162:502–514.

170. Parazzini F, Negri E, La Vecchia C, et al. Uterine myomas and smoking: results from an Italian study. *J Reprod Med.* 1996;41:316–320.

171. Gerhard I, Monga B, Waldbrenner A, et al. Heavy metals and fertility. *J Toxicol Environ Health.* 1998;54:593–611.

172. Gerhard I, Runnebaum B. The limits of hormone substitution in pollutant exposure and fertility disorders [abstract] [German]. *Zentralbl Gynakol.* 1992;114:593–602.

173. Hunter, DS, Hodges LC, Eagon PK, et al. Influence of exogenous estrogen receptor ligands uterine leiomyoma: evidence from an in vitro/in vivo animal model for uterine fibroids. *Environ Health Perspect.* 2000;108(suppl 5):829–834.

174. Hutchens A. *Indian Herbology of North America.* Ontario, Canada: MERCO; 1974.

175. Ososki A, Lohr P, Reiff M, et al. Ethnobotanical literature survey of medicinal plants in the Dominican Republic used for women's health conditions. *J Ethnopharmacol.* 2002;79:285–298.

176. Rotblatt M, Zimett I: *Evidence-Based Herbal Medicine.* Philadelphia: Hanley and Belfus; 2002: 98–101, 124–127, 283–286, 369–371.

177. Flora K, Hahn M, Rosen H, et al. Milk thistle *(Silybum marianum)* for the therapy of liver disease. *Am J Gastroenterol.* 1998;93:139–143.

178. Crocenzi FA, Sanchez Pozzi EJ, Pellegrino JM, et al. Beneficial effects of silymarin on estrogen-induced cholestasis in the rat: a study in vivo and in isolated hepatocyte couplets. *Hepatology.* 2001;34:329–339.

179. Zhongli S, Shurong Z. TCM treatment of uterine leiomyomas. Available at: http://library.ust.hsk/guides/tem/tem-ust.html. Accessed December 2002.

180. Sakamoto S, Yoshino H, Shirahata Y, et al. Pharmacotherapeutic effects of kuei-chih-fu-ling-wan (keishi-bukuryo-gan) on human uterinemyomas [abstract]. *Am J Chin Med.* 1992;20: 313–317.

181. Croke M, Bourne RD. A review of recent research studies on the efficacy of esogetic color-

puncture therapy—A wholistic acu-light system. *Am J Acupunct.* 1999;27:85–94.

182. Yan H, Wang J. The clinical study on hysteromyoma treated with acupuncture [abstract] [in Chinese]. *Zhen Ci Yan Jiu.* 1994;19:14–16.

183. Botwin MA, Sidorova IS, Zinevich AN, et al. Electric characteristics of acupuncture points in patients with benign and malignant uterine tumors [abstract] [in Russian]. *Akush Ginekol (Mosk).* 1989;4:27–30.

CHAPTER 34

Integrative Approach to Menopause

MONICA J. STOKES

The definition, scope of recognized symptoms, available drugs for, and goals of treatment of the menopausal period have all changed and expanded in recent years. Women have begun to question the conventional medical "wisdom" of the one-size-fits-all approach to what has been treated as a disease. In fact, the perimenopause is the normal transition period (of varying length in different women) from the years during which reproduction is possible, to the years when it is no longer (naturally) possible because of the final cessation of follicular development and ovulation leading to the ending of estrogen, inhibin, and progesterone production from the ovaries—the menopause. At this time there is a sustained reduction in circulating estrogens (estrone, rather than estradiol, becomes the predominant circulating estrogen) and sustained elevations of follicle-stimulating hormone (FSH) and luteinizing hormone (LH) that are no longer receiving the expected estrogen and inhibin feedback from the ovaries.

Symptoms of the perimenopause/menopause include vasomotor symptoms of hot flushing and night sweats; menstrual irregularities; vaginal dryness and related inflammation and atrophy; insomnia; a crawling feeling under the skin; palpitations; dyspareunia; irritability; mood instability; muscle and joint aches; poor concentration; fatigue; reduced libido; urethral inflammation and urinary incontinence; anxiety; and depression. The most common symptoms in the perimenopause are intermittent menstrual irregularity (heavier flow, lighter flow, shorter or longer cycle length or duration of bleeding), intermittent to extended periods of vasomotor symptoms, and vaginal dryness.

Menopause may occur naturally and gradually, or be induced with procedures that ablate or remove the ovaries (resulting in a sudden withdrawal of estrogen). Sudden menopause is usually associated with more severe symptomatology and more rapid bone loss than natural menopause. The clinical diagnosis of natural menopause is most conservatively defined retrospectively after 12 months of complete amenorrhea in the absence of other cause. During this 12-month period, intermittent ovulations are possible. This period of a woman's life is the most common time other than during adolescence for undesired pregnancy, therefore a reliable method for contraception is necessary. The rhythm method is no longer an option at this time in life. Barrier methods, sterilization (male or female), and low-dose contraceptives present the safest and most reliable methods. The latter has the added benefit of normalizing the timing and reducing the flow of menses and provides an even background hormone level that effectively controls symptomatology and helps maintain bone density during the transition years.

The details of the steroid physiology involved in the female reproductive system and of the physiologic changes that begin intermittently in the perimenopause and the ways in which these changes are influenced by other endocrine changes that occur with aging during the postmenopausal period are addressed elsewhere.[1,2]

There are estrogen receptors (ERs) present in most tissues (ER-alpha and ER-beta identified, so far); these are present in varying ratios of density in different tissues, and different substances may bind with different affinities to one receptor type over another. This diversity of receptor types is the basis for experimentation regarding the development of selective receptor modulators to achieve certain therapeutic goals while avoiding other, undesired actions. This is very loosely analogous to the evolution of beta-blocker therapies. In addition, there are actions that are "estrogen-like" produced by estrogen, phyto-estrogens (that also act weakly with a preference for ER-beta receptors) and a variety of other substances that may act through "nongenomic" mechanisms that do not involve receptor binding at all.[3] Over time, tissue receptors progressively experience changes associated with estrogen and progesterone deficiency resulting in a number of possible symptoms or signs. Of course, this is occurring concurrently with changes associated with aging.

Many women are now seeking more "natural" interventions for symptom control to improve the quality of the perimenopausal and the postmenopausal periods of their lives. They also want answers during this time of considerable uncertainty regarding the long-term risks and benefits of hormone replacement therapy.

This chapter focuses on lifestyle, nutrition, herbal interventions, hormones, and other management options for perimenopausal and the menopausal symptomatology, and reviews current evidence regarding hormones and how they may be related to selected chronic diseases and cancers. It is important to remember that any discussion of the perimenopause and early menopause must be linked to risk identification, prevention, and support of lifestyle modification (activity, nutrition, weight management, alcohol and drug use assessments, smoking cessation, sleep, social support, and spirituality) as needed to maximize health and minimize morbidity. Any discussion of the postmenopausal period of a woman's life is inextricably entwined with these and other issues surrounding healthy (optimal) aging.

Professional encouragement and education regarding these lifestyle and dietary issues before or during any discussion of pharmacologic intervention should now be the norm rather than the exception. In order to take advantage of their innate healing abilities, patients need to fully understand that these are modifiable risk factors, of which they may be in complete control, which will enhance their innate healing abilities.

▶ LABORATORY TESTING IN PERIMENOPAUSE

The issue of laboratory determination of the presence of the perimenopause is simple. Because of the wide fluctuations of estradiol[4] and follicle-stimulating hormone levels[5] during this period, a single measurement of either substance in the serum is unreliable for diagnosis. Two or three measurements of FSH over a period of several months may be helpful if they are consistently elevated well above the upper limits of normal and the patient remains amenorrheic during that time. However the diagnosis of the perimenopause may be made clinically without any laboratory confirmation with the emergence intermittently, and later more consistently, of the symptoms described above, after other causes for the symptoms have been ruled out by history or other testing.

Estrogen Testing

Historically, the gold standard for measuring estrogen levels was the 24-hour urine collection. This is quite cumbersome and expensive. Single-determination blood level represents only a spot measurement that may not always be clinically useful without other comparative measurements in the same individual. Salivary steroid hormone testing is being used more and more. The noninvasive nature of serial salivary testing makes it an attractive option for measuring hormone levels. These are typically enzyme-linked and direct radioimmunoassays. Unfortunately, most studies regarding salivary measurement of estrogens in women have been limited by small numbers of participants, drawn from regularly menstruating subjects, or measured in pregnancy when the hormones being measured circulate at much higher (more easily measured) levels. Most commercially available laboratory measurements are too inconsistent to be considered reliable for clinical use.

Selection of the proper assay for measuring steroid hormone levels during the course of therapy can be challenging. For example, during therapy with the transdermal administration of 17β-estradiol, salivary measurements are useless, but relatively direct measurements in the blood are accurate. Oral estrogen, as it is subjected to first-pass hepatic metabolism, is converted mostly to estrone and estrone sulfate. Despite this, the 12-hour postingestion measurement of estradiol, alone, is reflective of the dose actually prescribed.[6] Additionally, when dosing regimens are changed, retesting should be delayed for at least 4 weeks to ensure that a new metabolic steady state has been reached. If an FSH level, drawn during treatment with estrogen compounds of any type or any route, has been driven down into the reproductive age range, it indicates excessive estrogen dosing, which may place the patient at considerable iatrogenic risk.

Testosterone Testing

There are two reasons to measure testosterone levels in women: to monitor the dosage of testosterone supplementation and to diagnose hyperandrogenism. Testosterone in women circulates in considerably lower amounts in the blood (and consequently in the saliva), making measurements unreliable without very sensitive blood assays. Salivary tests for testosterone levels in women have not yet been validated. Most circulating testosterone is bound by sex hormone-binding globulin (SHBG) and is more loosely bound to albumin (making much of it easily bioavailable), and the unbound portion is immediately bioavailable. Growth hormone, glucocorticoids, androgens, and insulin decrease SHBG levels, whereas oral estrogen and thyroid hormone increase them (progestins appear to have a neutral influence). There appears to be poor correlation between blood and salivary levels and between salivary levels and clinical responses to testosterone administration in women.[7] The new "gold standard" for free testosterone measurement is equilibrium dialysis and ultracentrifugation-alpha, which is extremely labor intensive and requires strict temperature controls. Unfortunately, the very easy direct immunoassay measures only 20–60% of the actual levels. The free androgen (testosterone) index is calculated by dividing the total testosterone by the SHBG concentration and multiplying by 100, and correlates somewhat with the gold standard, but in situations with elevated SHBG and lower levels of testosterone (as often seen in women) the measurements may be falsely elevated.[8]

Testosterone is currently approved for use in women only in the current combination formulation with esterified estrogen or conjugated equine estrogen. Methyltestosterone (because it cannot be demethylated in the body) is not measurable for monitoring in the saliva or by any other testosterone assay. If supplemental androgens are to be used for an off-label indication in a female patient, it is best to choose a route that can be monitored by total testosterone levels in the serum, such as a transdermal gel, patch, or other individualized form compounded by a pharmacist. In addition the female patient should be educated regarding and closely monitored for signs and symptoms of androgen excess.

Progesterone Testing

Salivary progesterone measurements also are generally unreliable to monitor treatment, especially from transdermal administration.[9] Application of lower-dose progesterone cream does "show up" in salivary testing, but absorption is variable, and it is undetectable in urine or blood sampling done simultaneously.[10,11] Daily salivary measurements have been used successfully in studies evaluating potential luteal phase defects in (unsupplemented) reproductive age women.[12] On the other hand, salivary measurement of cortisol, dehydroepiandrosterone (DHEA) and growth hormone levels have shown reliable correlation with serum measurements and are becoming widely used for clinical diagnosis and monitoring of related conditions.

▶ THE PERIMENOPAUSE AS AN OPPORTUNITY FOR PREVENTIVE MEDICINE INTERVENTIONS AND PERSONAL GROWTH

The symptoms that bring a perimenopausal patient to the office present the physician with a golden opportunity to assess risk factors, perform early detection diagnostic studies, and to discuss and encourage health promotion and enhancement strategies. It also allows one to review the differential for the patient's symptoms to verify the absence of any medical problems that may have overlapping symptoms. It is best to refrain from overmedication for milder symptoms. Women are often fearful of conventional physicians' potentially dismissive or judgmental attitudes toward their symptoms or their use of unfamiliar treatments, so they may choose not to share potentially important information about these with their physicians. Openness to the patient's concerns and willingness to be a partner in her explorations of alternative or complementary interventions during this time will help educate the practitioner in areas that are now being actively researched, as well as enhance the patient's respect for the physician's opinions regarding other recommendations now and in the future.

Sleep

It is important not to underestimate the importance of the regular attainment of a good night's sleep. Insomnia causes or worsens many of the subjective symptoms of the perimenopause and menopause. Nighttime hot flushing is often the causative factor. In your evaluation, remember that alcohol, especially wine, will considerably worsen this occurrence. Consider the influence of other recreational, prescribed, or over-the-counter stimulant medications, and encourage the implementation of appropriate sleep hygiene habits.[13,14]

Estrogen supplementation has been shown to improve sleep and quality of life in menopausal women.[15] Warm beverages containing tryptophan taken near bedtime may be helpful, as are the caffeine-free teas of lemon balm and/or valerian root or chamomile. Valerian root capsules (*Valeriana officinalis* standardized to 0.8% valeric acid, 160–300 mg) taken 1 hour before bed are a relatively safe "next step" for short-term use. Acupuncture treatment is very helpful for this indication, as is hypnotherapy in selected patients. Pharmaceutical sleep agents should be reserved for very short-term use as a last resort because long-term continuous (or long-term intermittent) use may cause serious and/or chronic side effects.

Physical Exercise

The regular performance of physical activity is useful for the improvement of restful sleep and in the prevention and treatment of a variety of medical and psychological problems. There is no physical or psychological ailment not known to benefit from some amount of regular physical activity. The initiation or continuation (with modifications as necessary) of a physical activity program is an essential part of the successful transition through the perimenopause and of graceful aging in the menopause. For those who have never exercised or have completely stopped for some reason, it is important to emphasize that they begin with short durations and light intensity and advance very slowly to minimize the possibility of pain and injury. The subject should be revisited at each office visit so that the patient may be remotivated, have her progress validated, and encouraged to continue. Walking, increasing the pace over time, is a wonderful initial activity, and is effective for the reduction of cardiovascular disease risk in women.[16]

A recent report by Stampfer and colleagues, using the Nurses' Health Study cohort data, examined the question of primary prevention of coronary heart disease (the number one cause of mortality in American women) through diet and lifestyle.[17] They found it quite challenging to actually identify a group that could be categorized low risk in that population by currently defined standards of adherence to lifestyle guidelines involving diet, exercise, and abstinence from smoking. However, amongst the 3% of the pool of 84,129 women who did qualify, there was an extremely low associated risk of coronary heart disease. Sobngwi and colleagues have documented an evolution of development of obesity, hypertension, and diabetes as one developing nation's female population is transitioning from a predominantly rural community to an urban one with the associated reduction in physical activity.[18] Undoubtedly, with the trend toward Westernization of the developing world, the shift from traditional diets to more processed foods will further accelerate this worldwide trend toward earlier presentations of chronic disease.

Nutritional Recommendations

The problems with the standard American diet are discussed at length in Chapter 4. Addressing these problems in perimenopausal women is especially important with respect to the emerging associations between dietary intake, inflammation, and the development (and exacerbation of) chronic cardiovascular, neurodegenerative, and musculoskeletal diseases. It is clear that a poor diet will also exacerbate menopausal symptomatology. When you influence your female patients, you have the additional opportunity to influence the families for whom they shop and provide food.

Adherence to these recommendations will also help support optimal liver metabolism, improve elimination of excess estrogen from the circulation, enhance immune function, and help reduce levels of inflammatory markers. Despite the explosion of market supplements, whole foods should be recommended first to our patients. Supplements (with a few exceptions) should be used to supplement a healthy diet, not substitute for it.

The following 10 recommendations will maximize your patient's ability to sustain well-being through the perimenopause and after.

1. Drink at least 8–10 glasses of filtered water each day.
2. Choose whole, unprocessed, or minimally processed foods.
3. Because organic fruits and vegetables have been shown to retain the greatest amount of nutrients as compared to conventional and are exposed to fewer pesticides and

herbicides, choose organic products whenever possible.

4. Maximize fiber intake with whole grains, legumes, fruits, and vegetables.

5. Increase vegetable intake to 5–7 servings per day and fruits to 3–5 servings per day (consider purees and juicing)—the deeper and more varied the colors, the more nutrient dense the vegetables and fruits are.

6. Minimize intake of animal fats, refined sugar (sweets), and caffeine.

7. Eliminate or minimize alcohol intake; no more than one drink per day.

8. Eat cold-water fish or another omega-3 essential fatty acid source food 2–3 servings per week (or consider fish oil capsules).

9. Try using freshly ground flaxseed (contains an omega-3 fatty acid precursor) or flaxseed oil daily (1–2 tablespoons of ground or 1 of the oil).

10. Consider consuming 2–4 servings of soy foods per day.

The following supplements should also be considered:

- Multivitamin that contains 0.4–0.8 mg of folate and 400–800 IU of vitamin D per daily dose. If the following are not contained in the multivitamin, add at least calcium as noted below.
- Calcium 1,000 mg if perimenopausal, 1,500 if menopausal (avoid taking at same time with any acid suppressants; use citrate form if older than age 60 years). Take in divided doses for optimal absorption.
- Magnesium 300–600 mg/d (plus bone-supporting micronutrients such as boron, manganese, copper, and vitamin K found in the multivitamin and some calcium formulations).
- One B100 complex per day.

Consider, also, the following antioxidant regimen:

- Natural vitamin E with mixed tocopherols (400–800 IU/d)

- Vitamin C 200–500 mg once or twice per day
- Mixed carotenoids 10,000–20,000 IU/d (not just beta-carotene alone)
- Selenium 200 μg/d

To maximize digestive efficiency, it is also advisable to eat more frequent, smaller meals and to consider eating the largest meal at midday, reserving the lighter meal for the early evening; to eat slowly and eat no more (at any given meal) than enough to fill your stomach about 70% full or less (avoid eating to the point of discomfort); to avoid eating heavy foods after 7 PM; and to drink room temperature or warm fluids rather than ice-cold ones.

Botanical Medicines

Most herbs used for perimenopausal and menopausal symptoms have no known direct estrogen-receptor actions (except as noted). Despite this, several have been described in the traditional literature as effective for the treatment of menopausal symptoms. While most botanicals used for this purpose will elicit a response within 2 weeks, others take up to 12 weeks of continuous use for a full response to be realized. While most botanicals used in the traditional dosages and dosage-forms are very safe, patients must realize that natural does not mean safe at *any* dose. If a patient intends to use a formulation at greater than the recommended dose on the bottle, she will most safely do so in consultation with an herbalist or health care provider familiar with herbs and who has full awareness of the patient's medical history, current medical problems, risk profile, and current pharmaceutical medications.

There are several botanicals with long traditions of use for various menopausal symptoms. Some of these are supported to date by clinical trials, others only by anecdotal experience.

Evening primrose oil contains one of the most bioavailable forms of the essential fatty acid, gamma-linolenic acid. Evening primrose oil is very effective for treatment of cyclic mastalgia and is helpful in some women for the treatment of nighttime hot flushing. The dose is 500–1000 mg three to four times per day. To offset the production of pro-oxidants during metabolism of ≥4,000 mg/d, it is recommended that patients take vitamin E and selenium concurrently.

Mexican yams are used as a source of diosgenin, the precursor from which bioidentical hormones may be chemically modified into drugs that humans can assimilate. Mexican yam cream is sold to unsuspecting women claiming to have hormonal effects, but it has none at all. Wild yam extract has also been proven ineffective in a double-blind, placebo-controlled, crossover study.[19]

Red clover (Trifolium pratense) is a rich source of phytoestrogens, but no study has shown it to be more effective for hot flushing than placebo. It may have an effect of reducing bone resorption in pre- and perimenopausal women, but does not do so in postmenopausal subjects. Gut microorganisms produce dicoumarol during metabolism for absorption, but this is unlikely to have clinical significance. The dose is 500 mg, in tablet form, containing 40 mg of isoflavones. Skin eruptions may occur in sensitive individuals. The brand used most frequently in studies has been Promensil, a high-quality product. Larger trials to test the efficacy of red clover are in progress.

Licorice root (Glycyrrhiza glabra) has several actions, including antiinflammatory and immune-stimulating effects. It has been found to be estrogen antagonizing and progesterone sparing. It should be used with caution in patients with elevated blood pressure or cardiovascular disease because of its aldosterone effect. In others, it is safe for 4–5 weeks of use at a time in a dose of 250–500 mg of a solid, dry-powder extract (4:1) three times a day.

Dong quai (Angelica sinensis) root rhizome has been used as a uterine tonic and antispasmodic. Although it is touted as having estrogenic effects, those have not been proven with isolated use. It most often is used as a component of multiherb synergistic herbal preparations. There is a very small theoretical risk that the furanocoumarins in dong quai may enhance the action of anticoagulant medications. and may cause photosensitization in some individuals. The dose of the solid, dry extract is 1–2 g three times a day.

Chastetree berry (Vitex agnus-castus), considered a balancing herb for women, is very effective for the treatment of premenstrual symptoms and menstrual irregularities. As these tend to intensify in perimenopausal women this herb can be quite useful for this and for the treatment of mastalgia. Claims have been made that it may also be helpful for vasomotor symptoms. In premenopausal women, it is thought to work by a dopaminergic mechanism.[19] The mechanism of action in postmenopausal women is unknown. With continuous use, it may take 8–12 weeks for *Vitex* to achieve its full effect. The dose is a standardized hydroalcoholic extraction preparation containing 0.5% agnuside, 175–225 mg/d.

Ginseng (Panax ginseng) is considered in Chinese medicine to be a tonic and an adaptogen. Adrenocorticotrophic hormone is increased by ginseng, which enhances adrenal cortisol and DHEA production. This may be responsible for some of its antistress and antifatigue effects. It has an estrogen-like effect on the vagina and endometrium and there are several anecdotal reports of abnormal uterine bleeding and mastalgia with prolonged use of ginseng. Because of its high cost, it is important to find a high quality product from a reputable company. Otherwise, one may pay a high price for a highly substituted substance. The dosage range is 100–200 mg/d in 2–3 divided doses of a standardized product with at least 5–8% ginsenoside. Begin at low doses and increase gradually to measure your patient's response. Consider 3–8 weeks of cyclic use (with 3 weeks off). If bleeding occurs in a nonmenstruating woman taking ginseng, it should be investigated with transvaginal ultrasonography and/or endometrial sampling, unless she was very recently evaluated.

Ginkgo biloba has been subjected to a number of studies resulting in conflicting results regarding its memory-enhancing effects. There have been only infrequent reports of side effects such as headache, dizziness, palpitations, mild gastrointestinal complaints, and allergic skin eruptions in people beginning use with ginkgo; thus it is not unreasonable to trial it in a patient complaining of fogginess or forgetfulness. Ginkgo is a potent antioxidant and increases cerebral blood flow. It also may enhance the effectiveness of antidepressants.[20] Animal studies show that it increases the number of serotonin-binding sites in the brain. It may take up to 12 weeks of continuous use to determine whether ginkgo will work for your patient. The dose of a solid, dry extract (50:1), standardized to at least 24% ginkgo flavone glycosides and 3–7% terpene lactones, is 40–80 mg, three times per day.

St. John's wort (Hypericum perforatum) is comparable to fluoxetine for the short-term treatment of mild depression. It is not indicated for more severe depression. The dose is 300 mg three times a day of a preparation standardized to 0.3% hypericin or 10–15 mg three times per day for preparations standardized to 2–5% hyperforin. There are numerous herb–drug interactions described for St. John's wort as a consequence of its induction of cytochrome P450 enzyme systems and its additive effects with other antidepressant medications. It should be used with caution in patients taking other medications, and a patient's response or lack thereof should be monitored so that other interventions may be used as necessary.

Black cohosh (Cimicifuga racemosa) is the only solo-use botanical that has been shown in a number of well-designed clinical studies to be effective for vasomotor symptoms, sweating, headache, vertigo, palpitations, and sleep disturbances.[21] It influences neuroendocrine regulatory systems, but by a mechanism separate from that of estrogen. In vivo, black cohosh is not believed to bind to estrogen receptors[22] and appears not to exhibit any estrogenic effects despite its ability to reduce hot flash frequency.[23]

It is currently believed that black cohosh may be used safely for a trial of symptom control in women with a history of breast cancer. There is no known toxic dose of black cohosh. The dose of a nonstandardized solid, dry-powder extract (4:1) concentration is 250–600 mg three times a day; or of Remifemin, the brand used in most of the studies, 20–40 mg twice a day. The only adverse effect associated with black cohosh is headache. For those in whom this occurs, it appears that this is not dose-related. Mild gastric upset may also occur, but is unusual. It is currently recommended for only 6 months of continuous use, because there is no study data to prove it still safe and effective after that time frame. It is not known to be teratogenic or mutagenic, but use during pregnancy is not recommended except by those trained in its use during labor. Black cohosh should never be confused with blue cohosh, which has a completely different set of indications and several known adverse effects and contraindications.

Phytoestrogens and the Menopause

Phytoestrogens are plant compounds whose structures are dissimilar to estrogen (phenolic versus steroidal) but which are nevertheless able to conform to bind to estrogen receptors. They may also act as antiestrogens, which qualify them as adaptogens. Phytoestrogens have been found in in vitro studies to also have antioxidant, antiproliferative, antiangiogenic, and anticarcinogenic properties. Different phytoestrogens differ in the percentages of isoflavones, lignans, coumestans, and resorcylic acid lactones they contain. Isoflavones (followed, distantly, by lignans) have been the most extensively investigated. Isoflavones have the most potent estrogenic activity in comparison to other phytoestrogen components.[24] Both isoflavones and lignans are present in their source plants as precursors which are metabolized by gut bacteria into their respective mammalian forms that all bind reversibly to estrogen receptors. Lignans are found in highest concentrations in flaxseed but are also found in berries, whole grains, legumes, vegetables, and fruit. Isoflavones are found in highest concentrations in soybeans, legumes, chickpeas, red clover, sweet potatoes, green beans, carrots, and garlic.

Isoflavones bind preferentially to ER-beta receptors so they express their estrogenic activities in the central nervous system, blood vessels, bone, and skin without stimulating the uterus or the breast.[25] The major soy isoflavones are genistein and daidzein. These (and other phytoestrogens) are currently being studied extensively through a variety of avenues to determine the details of their possible health benefits. Studies suggest that soy isoflavones may be helpful for the treatment of vasomotor symptoms (conflicting results to date are probably due to poorly comparable study populations, products, dosages, scoring systems, and short study durations).[26] In most of these studies, the severity of hot flushes declined by 50–60% in both the treated and the placebo groups, so longer studies would have been helpful to detect some divergence with time. One recent, randomized, double-blind, placebo-controlled study using 100 mg of isoflavones daily for 4 months of treatment revealed a significant reduction in hot flush frequency and several other menopausal symptoms (the menopausal Kupperman index questionnaire was used); no change was noted in endometrial thickness as measured by transvaginal ultrasonography, and total and low-density lipoprotein cholesterol (LDL-C) levels decreased.[27]

The results are mixed for isoflavones' role in the prevention of bone loss.[28]

Generally, soy products' effect on plasma lipids reveals that there is an inverse dose-related reduction in total and LDL cholesterol, while high-density lipoprotein cholesterol (HDL-C) and triglyceride levels remain stable.[29] Soy appears to positively improve systemic vas-

cular compliance, as well. The epidemiological evidence regarding cancer development is as yet inconclusive in humans. But the fact that breast cancer incidence and mortality rates are so much lower in Asian countries where soy foods are consumed continues to drive studies to find out why.

Asian diets typically contain 100–200 mg of food-sourced isoflavones per day; this results in a heavy exposure to those beginning in utero and continuing through adulthood. It is possible that this exposure may confer certain advantages that reduce the likelihood of an untoward response and increase the likelihood of benefit when compared to those who begin exposure later in life. The source may also be of great importance; whole food is more complete and may carry with it protections that may be lost when isolated components are used as medicine. Safety data is being accrued. One notable study by the Baber group used varying doses (up to 85.5 mg/d) of a modified red clover isoflavone supplement to evaluate the effect of 6 months of daily exposure on the endometrium. Endometrial thickness did not change during the 6-month period and did not exceed 5 mm in any of the 50 study participants.[30]

At this time it is safest to recommend dietary isoflavone sources for your patients, as the safety of high-dose, isolated products is unknown. It is also probably prudent for now to advise your patients to eat soy foods daily, but avoid intake of greater than 100 mg/d of isolated soy isoflavones until these lingering issues are resolved.

► HORMONE REPLACEMENT THERAPY: SYNTHETIC, NATURAL, PLANT-SOURCED, AND "BIOIDENTICAL" HORMONES

There has been considerable confusion in both the medical and lay communities regarding what is "natural" and what is not. Synthetic medicines—compared to "natural"—are completely built from chemical components and generally have moieties that prevent them from being metabolized as quickly (and cleared as quickly) as they would be without them at the level of the gut, liver and in the circulation before they can reach their target tissues (e.g., ethinyl estradiol and diethylstilbestrol). There are plant-sourced hormones that have a moiety attached (such as an ester group) to inhibit rapid metabolism as well.

There are several other hormone delivery strategies for minimizing gut and hepatic metabolism. With matrix patch transdermal systems, gels, creams, and troches, the skin (or mucosa) must be traversed but the gut metabolism is initially bypassed, and the hepatic metabolism is delayed because the estrogen does not first have to go through the enterohepatic circulation before its first encounter with the target tissues. Micronized products (oral) are plant-sourced but avoid excessive metabolism in the gut, because of their small molecular size. This allows for absorption of more of the intended substance.

Premarin, currently the estrogen preparation most widely used for hormone replacement therapy, comes from a technically "natural" (but equine) source—pregnant mare's urine. However the conditions under which these animals are kept are a source of popular outcry. In addition, Premarin consists of more than 10 different estrogens that are bioconverted in the body and are obviously from a different mammalian species than our own.

Plant-sourced products are generally the ones considered natural by the general public. These products are "natural" in that they are derived from plant-based sources (e.g., wild yam, soy beans) but they must be chemically modified to be formulated into hormones absorbable and usable by the human body. The result (except with those with an attached moiety to slow breakdown, as mentioned above) is a product that is chemically indistinguishable from the hormones produced by the human body. The term "bioidentical" is now being used to describe this category of hormone-replacement preparations, and the current trend is to use more of this type of product.

Estriol is the weakest in potency of all of the plant-sourced estrogens currently in use. Based on animal studies showing antiproliferative effects on breast cancer in animals, claims have been made recently that, unlike some other forms of estrogen that may increase breast cancer risk and uterine cancer risk (if used unopposed by progesterone), estriol is "safe." These claims, however, are unsubstantiated; in the doses needed for symptom control, systemic estriol has been found to exert significant estrogenic effects on the endometrium, myometrium, and vagina.[31,32] If it is used systemically or in large vaginal doses, it should be treated as other estrogens, and must be opposed by progesterone in women with an intact uterus.

Bi-estrogen and tri-estrogen compounds (plant-sourced), usually supplied by a compounding pharmacy, typically contain estradiol 20% and estriol 80%, and estradiol 10%, estrone 10%, and estriol 80% respectively. Because the typical tri-estrogen preparation contains 12.5 μg of estradiol, the standard daily dose of 2 tablets twice daily would provide almost 0.05 mg of estradiol alone, which approaches a therapeutic dose. The components of these compounds are as quickly converted in the body as the bioidentical commercial pharmaceutical preparations. Few insurance companies cover the cost of these preparations, however, and there is no proof that they have any short- or long-term advantages for your patient. If your patient insists on them, you may be sure that they are relatively safe for symptom control, but the long-term benefits or risks are unclear at this time, and there are no studies in progress to evaluate them.

It is useful to be aware of selected substances that may cause changes in circulating estrogen levels in supplemented and/or unsupplemented patients to help guide the assessment of risks and expected responses to various doses of estrogen administered.

In postmenopausal women, alcohol[33,34] and grapefruit juice[35] ingestion delay the metabolic degradation of estrogen, transiently increasing plasma levels of bioavailable estrogen by three- to fivefold. Exogenous estrogen administered by either an oral or transdermal route is affected by alcohol, while grapefruit juice affects only orally administered estrogen levels. Substances that reduce sex hormone-binding globulin levels will also increase circulating bioavailable estrogen levels. These include growth hormone, glucocorticoids, androgens (including testosterone), and insulin. Substances that elevate SHBG include oral estrogen and thyroid hormone.

Tables 34–1 (estrogens), 34–2 (progesterones), and 34–3 (testosterones) summarize the major currently available hormone replacement preparations with the exception of progesterone-emitting intervention devices and the new lower dose Prempro.

Estrogen Replacement

Estrogen is best taken in the morning to avoid potential interactions with endogenous growth hormone release. The dosing of estrogen is most often adjusted by the clinical response of the patient. It is prudent to begin with the lowest effective dose to achieve your therapeutic goals. For example, 1 mg of micronized estradiol or 0.3 mg/d of conjugated equine estrogens (CEE) is effective for prevention of osteoporosis, but these doses may be ineffective if one of your goals is to treat vasomotor symptoms, especially in a younger, or surgically menopausal patient. If your patient is only presenting with vaginal symptoms unresponsive to nonhormonal moisturizers or lubricants such as Replens or Astroglide, you may want to use a product that will deliver estrogen to the local area only. If your patient's symptoms are more systemic in nature (which often include local lower genital symptoms) and they are not responding to the highest available single dosage forms (e.g., oral 1.25 mg CEE or 2 mg bioidentical), consider changing the route of administration (transdermal, vaginal-transmucosal, buccal) or type of formulation, or consider that they may be preferentially in need of progesterone. If these changes do not reduce the involved symptoms, consider the possibility that an unrelated disease process might be causing or complicating the clinical picture (e.g., thyroid, dermatologic, infectious, clinically significant psychological issues). Persistent iatrogenic hyperestrogenemia with the resultant risk exposure for your patient is inexcusable. Excessive dosing of estrogen must be avoided due to its association with estrogen-dependent neoplasia.

The current trend is to move away from CEE (Premarin) toward the plant-sourced bioidentical formulations for a variety of social and environmental reasons. Also, no one can be sure whether any of the adverse effects we associate with estrogen use may be a result of yet unknown mechanisms associated with some aspect of this particular equine-sourced formulation, and our literature has been dominated by studies done using only this preparation (without fair comparisons) for far too long. The historical lack of availability of reliable products and this skew in the scientific literature has resulted in Premarin's domination of our prescribing practices. It may not yet be necessary to switch patients from a regimen that they are comfortable with that includes it, but our patients must be made aware that other options are available to them should they wish to change formulations. Premarin should remain in our toolbox but should not be the only tool we reach for in every instance. There is no reason to initiate new patients on systemic estrogen therapy with a formulation containing equine estrogens when we now have better choices available to us. Table 34–1 summarizes the options currently available for estrogen replacement.

The choice of route of administration, which is beginning to favor transdermal over oral, should currently be based on your patient's history, risks, and personal preference given the ever-expanding evidence regarding benefits, risk, and specific bioinfluences of estrogens. For example, because oral estrogen is

► TABLE 34-1 ESTROGEN FORMULATIONS FOR MENOPAUSAL WOMEN

Chemical or Generic Name/Route	Commercial or Common Name	Dose Range (per day)	Notes
17-β-Estradiol Route:			Bioidentical to human estradiol Source: Plant—soy or wild yam
Oral tablets (micronized)	Estrace, estradiol USP	1–2 mg	1. Hepatic "first-pass effect"—increases HDL and triglycerides, clotting factors, sex hormone–binding globulin (SHBG) (as with all oral estrogens); reduces LDL 2. Peaking of serum levels within a few hours of administration, elimination within 24 hours 3. Micronized for rapid absorption but much metabolized in gastrointestinal tract before absorption, so sufficiently high doses must be used 4. Predominant metabolites reaching circulation are estrone and estrone sulfate
Transdermal patches	Climara, FemPatch Alora, Vivelle, Vivelle-Dot, Estraderm	0.025–0.1 mg delivered (25–100 µg)	1. Continuous release prevents peaking in serum 2. Recommended route for those at risk for thromboembolic disease or with hypertriglyceridemia (no "first pass") 3. Constant surface area of administration—consistent dosing 4. Adhesive may cause local skin irritation 5. Changed 2/wk (except Climara/FemPatch—once a week) 6. Press firmly on clean, dry, intact skin. Rotate application to abdomen, buttocks, lower back, lateral thorax, upper arm
Estradiol vaginal cream, ring	Estrace	0.01% cream with calibrated applicator 0.5, 1, 2, 3, or 4 mg	1. Local application and release reaching serum levels 25% of equivalent oral doses (higher if extreme atrophy) 2. Excellent for treatment of atrophic vaginal/vulvar/distal urinary symptoms
	Estring	7.5 µg release/day (2 mg per 90 days)	3. Creams capable of causing endometrial hyperplasia 4. Daily cream insertion until symptoms are reduced and then half or full dose 2–3× wk for maintenance 5. Estring—minimal absorption into circulation and minimal effect on endometrium
Estradiol vaginal tablet	Vagifem	25 µg tablet with single-use applicator	1. Minimal systemic absorption 2. 1 tablet inserted daily for 2 wk, then 1 tablet weekly for symptom control

800

Drug	Brand/Formulation	Doses	Comments
Estropipate	Ogen, Ortho-Est, estropipate USP	0.625, 1.25, 2.5 mg; 0.75, 1.5, 3 mg	1. Source: Plant 2. Begins bioidentical to human estrone 3. Sulfate makes formulation more soluble and protects the estrogen from rapid GI metabolism and extends time in circulation; piperazine further stabilizes 4. Vaginal cream also available (Ogen)
Esterified estrogens (oral)	Estratab, Menest	0.3 mg, 0.625 mg, 1.25 mg, 2.5 mg	1. Sources: Plant 2. Estrone sulfate (80%) and equilin sulfate (20%) 3. Approved only for symptoms, not prevention of end-organ sequelae of hypoestrogenism
Conjugated estrogens (oral)	Premarin—conjugated equine estrogens	0.3 mg, 0.625 mg, 0.9 mg, 1.25 mg, 2.5 mg	1. Source: Animal (horse)—PREgnant MAre urINe 2. Contains 10 different conjugated estrogens, including a bioidentical estrone and potent equine forms 3. Intravenous and intramuscular formulations and vaginal cream formulations available 4. The majority of studies regarding target tissue benefits have used Premarin
Synthetic (oral)	Cenestin—synthetic conjugated estrogen	0.625–1.25 mg	1. Source: Plant. Clinical data are lacking 2. Contains 9 of the 10 known conjugated estrogens found in Premarin 3. Currently approved only for vasomotor symptoms
Parenteral estrogens 1. Estradiol cypionate 2. Estradiol valerate 3. Estradiol pellets	1. Depo-Estradiol 2. Delestrogen 3. Estrapel	1. 1 mg/mL and 5 mg/mL 2. 10, 20, and 40 mg/mL 3. 25 mg pellet implant	1, 2. Administered every 3–6 weeks 3. 1–4 pellets (implanted subcutaneously with trocar in lower abdomen or gluteal region) every 6 months 4. All pellets have a cumulative effect with persistent blood levels up to 2 years after the last insertion. Monitor blood estradiol levels to remain below 100 pg/mL. 5. Mostly used in extended-care elderly patients.

Continued

▶ TABLE 34-1 ESTROGEN FORMULATIONS FOR MENOPAUSAL WOMEN (Continued)

Chemical or Generic Name/Route	Commercial or Common Name	Dose Range (per day)	Notes
Combination formulations (oral) (estrogen/progestin)			Combinations of above with synthetic progestins
17 β-estradiol + norethindrone acetate (NETA)	Activella	1 mg 17 β-estradiol + 0.5 mg NETA	
17 β-estradiol + norgestimate (NGM)	Ortho-Prefest	1 μg 17 β-estradiol + 90 μg NGM	Estradiol on days 1–3 then estradiol + norgestimate on days 4–6. The pattern is repeated continuously
Ethinyl estradiol + NETA	Femhrt	5 mg ethinyl estradiol + 1 mg NETA	Ethinyl estradiol is an extremely potent synthetic estrogen that greatly increases SHGB levels, but is not bound by SHGB; may not be the best choice for postmenopausal hormone supplementation
Conjugated equine estrogens (CEE) + medroxyprogesterone acetate	Prempro vs Premphase	Continuous 2.5 mg MPA vs cyclic, sequential 5 mg MPA with 0.625 CEE (continuously) in each	Equine estrogens
Transdermal combination Preparation of norethindrone and estradiol (E²)	CombiPatch	0.05 mg E2 + 0.14 mg NETA/ day or 0.05 mg E2 + 0.25 mg NETA/day	The first approved of a series of combination patches in the pipeline for FDA approval

Compounded estrogen combinations (Oral or troches)	Triestrogen 80% estriol 10% estrone 10% estradiol	1.25–5.0 mg/d
	Biestrogen 80–90% estriol 10–20% estradiol	1.25–5.0 mg/d

1. No objective evidence to support long-term target tissue effects as yet
2. Usual dose range provides therapeutic dose of estradiol

Estriol USP (compound oral dose, troches, or vaginal cream)	Compounded	2–5 mg/d—oral micronized Other compounded to specification

1. Weak estrogenic effect—requires higher dosing
2. In therapeutic doses, can cause endometrial hyperplasia
3. Studies in progress to evaluate potential protective effect against breast cancer in humans
4. Predominant estrogen during pregnancy (fetoplacental metabolism)

Compounding pharmacists Estrogens and other steroids	Can produce a wide variety of dosage forms in multiple vehicles for administration (troches, creams, ointments, gels, capsules, injectables)	Wide range— recommend communication with local or mail order pharmacy's compounding pharmacist

When using formulations and routes without clear evidence of serum level ranges with particular doses, be sure to verify with testing that the patient is getting enough but not too much estrogen, progesterone, or androgen

803

Chemical or Generic Name/Route	Commercial or Common Name	Dose Range (per day)	Notes
Micronized progesterone (oral capsules)	Prometrium	100 mg/capsule Cyclic: 200–300 mg/d (BID or single daily QHS administration 13–14 days per month)	1. Bio-identical; plant source 2. Produces 5 α- and 5 β-pregnenolone via gut metabolism—potential CNS-sedating effect 3. Fewer adverse effects than synthetic progestins (less thrombotic risk) 4. Adequately opposes estrogen effect on the endometrium 5. Micronized form increases GI absorption and reduces less from "first-pass" hepatic metabolism
		Continuous: 100–200 mg/day (BID or single daily QHS administration)	
Norethindrone acetate (oral)	Aygestin	5 mg	Synthetic—resists metabolism
Medroxy-progesterone acetate (oral)	Provera Cycrin Amen, Curretab	2.5, 5, 10 mg 5, 10 mg 10 mg	Synthetic—resists metabolism
Micronized progesterone in oil (oral capsules)	Compounded	50–300 mg/d	1. Plant source 2. Reaches higher peak serum levels at similar mg doses than Prometrium 3. First-pass effect from oral administration
Micronized progesterone in troche	Compounded	50-mg/d average dose	1. Troches dissolve between cheek and gum 2. No first-pass effect—lower doses can be used

Progesterone cream	Many manufacturers (e.g., Pro-Gest); prescription, over-the-counter, and compounded sources	20–40 mg/d	1. Choose commercial preparations that contain approx 500 mg/oz (at this concentration = ⅛–¼ tsp/d) 2. Compounded preparations may be of higher concentrations and come with a calibrated dosing applicator 3. Check baseline levels and repeat 3 months after therapy begins (baseline <0.3 ng/mL; should increase to 3–4 ng/mL with proper use) 4. Any product that contains mineral oil prevents skin absorption even if it contains adequate amounts of progesterone 5. Improperly stabilized products deteriorate over time as they are repeatedly exposed to the air 6. Rotate application sites: upper chest, breast, inner arms, and thighs 7. Vaginal application—may use lower doses for symptom control 8. No first-pass effect
Micronized progesterone bioadhesive vaginal gel	Crinone 4% and 8%	4% (45 mg) in pre-filled applicators per vagina QOD at bedtime for 12 days (6 doses) every 3 months	1. Progesterone suspended in a polycarbophil gel which adheres to vaginal mucosa—sustained release of hormone over time 2. Provides a significant local protective effect from estrogen's influence on the endometrium. Expect withdrawal bleeding flow commensurate with degree of estrogen priming and number of months between applications 3. Not yet approved by FDA for this indication
Progesterone in oil (injectable)	Progesterone in oil	IM administration 100 mg q 2–3 months	1. Discomfort of injection 2. Most commonly used to induce a withdrawal bleed in an estrogen-primed endometrium

Note: In women with a uterus receiving supplemental estrogen, use of progesterone for endometrial production is necessary.

▶ **TABLE 34–3** TESTOSTERONE SOURCES FOR USE IN WOMEN*

Chemical or Generic Name/Route	Commercial or Common Name	Dose Range (per day)	Notes
17 β-hydroxy-androst-4-ene-3-one	Testosterone USP—used for compounding	Route dependent; 1–5 mg/d	Source: Plant **General notes regarding testosterone use (any form) in women:** 1. The long-term effects of supplemental testosterone exposure in women are unknown 2. The potential adverse effects are dose and duration of exposure dependent and include virilization (principally acne, hirsutism, and clitoromegaly), liver dysfunction, clotting factor suppression, and hypoglycemic effect. Increased low-density lipoprotein and decreased high-density lipoprotein, triglycerides, and total cholesterol 3. When used in women, close monitoring of response and for appearance of adverse effects is strongly recommended 1. Source: Synthetic derivative 2. Most effective in women with surgical or ablative menopause (libido, energy level, mood, sense of well-being) 3. Results mixed in non-oophorectomized women; may benefit selected women. 4. Hirsutism seen in 15–36% of patients with long-term use 5. Combination forms approved for use in women 6. Oral—subject to (hepatic) first-pass effect 7. FDA approved for use in women
Oral estrogen/ testosterone combinations			
Esterified estrogen (EstE) +	Estratest	1.25 mg EstE +	
Methyltestos-terone (MT)	Estratest HS (half-strength)	2.5 mg MT/d 0.625 mg EstE + 1.25 mg MT/d	
Conjugated equine estrogen (CEE) +	Premarin with methyltestos-terone	1. 0.625 mg CEE + 5 mg MT/d	
Methyltestos-terone (MT)		2. 1.25 mg CEE + 10 mg MT	
Methyltestos-terone USP (oral tablet)	Android, tested	10 mg	1. FDA approved for use only in men 2. Subject to first-pass effect

Formulation	Product	Dose	Notes
Micronized testosterone in oil (oral capsules)	Compounded	2.5–5 mg	Subject to first-pass effect
Micronized testosterone in troches	Compounded	1 mg, 2.5 mg, 5 mg	1. Troches dissolved between cheek and gum 2. No first-pass effect
Micronized testosterone in cream	Compounded	1. 2% Cream in jar 2. 2 mg/g—¼ teaspoon equals 1 g of cream	1. For libido, apply 2% cream "sparingly" (i.e., small amount on tip of finger) to perivaginal region and/or clitoris; titrate for effect 2. If more precise dosing is required for other desired effects, choose the precisely compounded formulation
Transdermal patches (testosterone) (USP)	1. Androderm 2. Testoderm TTS transdermal system	Testosterone delivery/day: 1. 2.5 mg or 5 mg 2. 5 mg	1. FDA-approved use for men only 2. Daily application 3. Rotate application to back, upper buttock, and upper arm
Parenteral Testosterones			
Testosterone cypionate Testosterone enanthate	Virilon I.M. Depo-Testosterone Delatestryl	200 mg/mL 100 and 200 mg/mL 200 mg/mL	FDA-approved for men only
Testosterone pellet implants	Testopel	75 mg	1. FDA-approved for men only 2. Usually used in conjunction with estrogen pellet placement in long-term care elderly patients 3. Trocar subcutaneous application 4. High supraphysiologic levels will occur initially

*The injectable forms, patches, and higher dose tablets are FDA approved only for use in men and for treatment of selected late-stage breast cancer in women. They are included here for completeness, with the realization that off-label short-term treatment situations may arise.

known to mildly elevate triglyceride levels, it should not be used in women who are known to have high triglycerides. Oral estrogen may necessitate an increase in thyroid hormone replacement dosage, while transdermal estrogen usually will not. This highlights the importance of reviewing pertinent baseline laboratory studies during the initial evaluation of perimenopausal and menopausal women before initiating treatments, and at 1–2 yearly intervals thereafter in order to tailor each patient's regimen accordingly.

Selective Estrogen-Receptor Modulators

For some patients, one of the selective estrogen receptor modulators will be the most appropriate choice of hormonal therapy. A recent review by Riggs and Hartmann described the mechanisms of action and application to clinical practice of currently available selective estrogen receptor modulators.[36] Different selective estrogen receptor modulators exert selective agonist or antagonist effects on different estrogen target tissues. Tamoxifen, raloxifene, and recently approved toremifene are being tested to determine the long-range risks and benefits. For example, raloxifene, developed originally to treat osteoporosis, increases bone density at all scanning sites but, with regard to the clinical end points, it only reduces vertebral fracture incidence, with no change in incidence at the hip or other sites, and it is unclear why. Raloxifene is also associated with worsening of vasomotor symptoms and vaginal atrophy in some women, appears to have neutral effects on the endometrium and the breast, and affects lipids similarly to estrogen, but does not increase triglyceride levels. The long-term effect on the incidence of cardiovascular events in low-risk women is not yet known. Selective receptor modulators for various types of steroid hormones are likely to evolve into a major role in the prevention and treatment of problems associated with the menopause in the years to come.

Progesterone Replacement

Progesterone has a more relaxed dosing range than estrogen, because there are no disease processes yet proven to be progesterone-induced or dependent. As long as the goals of administration are met (symptom relief and/or endometrial protection) and the patient has no problems with fatigue or somnolence dosing is quite flexible. The latter problem most often occurs with oral, synthetic preparations. With rare exception, no woman with a uterus should be using (other than vaginal ring, vaginal tablet, or intermittent cream form) systemic estrogen without it being opposed with progesterone to prevent estrogen-induced endometrial neoplasia. If taken orally as a separate pill, it is best taken in the late evening, as it might cause slight somnolence in some women. Progesterone is usually given continuously/daily in a 2.5 or 5 mg dose for medroxyprogesterone acetate (MPA) and 200–300 mg/d for micronized progesterone (Prometrium). The latter form is associated with less blunting of the beneficial lipid effects of estrogen. MPA is available in combination with CEE as Prempro and Premphase. Other synthetic progesterones, norethindrone and norgestimate, have become available in combination oral formulations with 17β-estradiol as Activella and Ortho-Prefest, respectively. These may be better choices for women who have prolonged (heavier) bleeding on other continuous regimens because these progestins may be associated with less breakthrough bleeding during the early months of the continuous regimen. This regimen is usually associated with some intermittent spotting and bleeding for the first 6–12 months of administration, at which time most women become amenorrheic. If your patient on continuous therapy has more than spotty bleeding after the first 6 months or so, and she is not missing pills, an evaluation with an endo-metrial biopsy should be considered to rule out endometrial neoplasia. In addition, if there is any bleeding after 12 months, an evaluation should be undertaken. The alternative to continuous therapy is to use 5–10 mg of MPA for days 1 through 14–16 of each month, but this will result in some degree of monthly withdrawal bleeding indefinitely in most women.

For vaginal dryness, a more localized application of a progesterone gel or cream formulation may be as helpful as estrogen cream. Transdermal progesterone cream (400–600 mg/oz concentration, ⅛ to ¼ teaspoon or 20–40 mg/d, rotated site application) administration may be quite helpful for the treatment of vasomotor symptoms as well, but has not yet been proven adequate for prevention of bone loss,[37] despite the anecdotal claims. Transdermal or intravaginal administration of the above cream is inadequate for endometrial protection.[38,39] Crinone, a sustained-release progesterone in a bioadhesive gel for intravaginal application, may be used intermittently every 2–4 months for those who do not tolerate other forms of progesterone but who require endometrial protection. Crinone establishes a local (regional) protective effect opposing estrogen's endometrial stimulatory action. It may induce withdrawal bleeding, after each use, in those on estrogen supplementation. Although it is not yet FDA approved for this indication, it remains a valuable option for selected reliable, adherent patients who you can follow closely. The insertion of a levonorgestrel-secreting intrauterine device (synthetic progesterone, trade name Mirena, recently FDA approved for this indication) may also be an option in selected women who require endometrial protection. Currently in the research stages are selective progesterone receptor modulators that are likely to have a role in postmenopausal hormone replacement therapy and treatment of endometriosis. Optimally, their effect will be more targeted and they will be able to avoid the adverse effects of synthetic progestins such as bloating, breast tenderness, and irregular bleeding associated with continuous use.

Testosterone Replacement

In women, testosterone is often used to treat reduced libido and has incidentally been noted to improve a patient's sense of well being and some cognitive skills. It is also associated with the prevention of bone loss. The only testosterone formulations FDA approved for use in women at this time are oral dosage forms of a low (1.25 mg or 2.5 mg) dose of methyl-testosterone dose found commercially in combination with an esterified estrogen (Estratest, or Estratest HS). This particular form is most effective for improving libido in younger women who have experienced abrupt surgical menopause. Larger doses of testosterone are approved for treatment in women with advanced breast cancer, when the goal of treatment is also ablation of ovarian function. Testosterone dosing (beyond the approved doses), in women especially, must be closely monitored because of the seriousness of potential adverse effects, including alteration in lipid levels, especially HDL-C; glucose levels in diabetics; prothrombin time measurements in anticoagulated patients; hepatic function derangements; and, of course, virilization (duration of administration and dose-dependent effect), including voice deepening, acne, and hirsutism. Because biotransformation of exogenously administered DHEA (given for deficiency states) results in significant increases in serum androstenedione, testosterone, and dihydrotestosterone, it confers the same risk profile as other androgens and should be monitored closely as well. When DHEA is deficient, as in some patients with systemic lupus erythematosus, the transmucosal is the most reliable route of administration.

In the past, few commercial dosing options were available. A much greater number of different hormonal preparations are now available and more are currently in the FDA approval pipeline, which will allow greater flexibility in dosing and application routes. In the meantime, for those who request or require them, compounding pharmacists are happy to work with clinicians to tailor dosages more specifically for oral, transmucosal, and transdermal administration of estrogens, progesterone, testosterone, or DHEA as needed.

► RISKS AND BENEFITS OF HORMONE REPLACEMENT THERAPY

The historic paucity of attention and research focused on women's health has recently evolved into a hotbed of efforts to accumulate new data from long-followed cohorts and to perform and publish studies to determine whether, when, and which pharmacologic interventions should be offered to "treat" or prevent disease in perimenopausal and menopausal women. Current thought regarding hormones and cancer and hormones and chronic disease is selectively reviewed below in "HRT and Cancer."

A serious limitation in the vast majority of studies of the effects of hormones is that only the standard preparations of CEE, some other synthetic estrogens, and synthetic progestational agents (usually MPA) have been used. None of the larger trials have used plant-sourced bioidentical estrogens or progesterones (or other routes of administration), so we are still left wondering if the same conclusions would be true for those preparations. There is an increasing number of small, usually short-term studies that are beginning to shed light on the beneficial effects of alternate preparations and routes of administration that may help guide us regarding selections for individual patient profiles. Newer drugs are also entering the market to target specific problems. Furthermore, certain older drugs have been found to have side benefits that treat some of the issues previously treated preferentially with hormone supplementation therapy. An example of this is the recent discovery that statins may improve bone mineral density, reduce inflammatory markers, improve endothelial function, and contribute to plaque stabilization, as well as reducing cholesterol levels and blocking the oral estrogen effect on triglyceride elevation.[40]

The sweeping generalizations originally drawn from observational epidemiologic studies such as the Nurse's Health Study[41] and the Lipid Research Clinics Program[42] regarding hormone supplementation therapy and the prevention of chronic disease (including, especially, heart disease[43]) are being more rigorously questioned with the performance of more prospective clinical trials. Some of the larger of these randomized intervention trials include the Women's Health Initiative (WHI);[44] the Heart and Estrogen/Progestin Replacement Study (HERS)[45]; the Women's Angiographic Vitamin and Estrogen (WAVE) Trial;[46] HERS II, the open-label design, extended follow-up of the HERS participants;[47] the Postmenopausal Hormone Replacement Against Atherosclerosis (PHOREA) study[48]; and the Postmenopausal Estrogen/Progestin Interventions (PEPI) Trial.[49,50] In addition, various longitudinal studies on aging have become valuable sources of information about the potential benefits and risks of postmenopausal hormone supplementation. Study end points secondary to the primary questions these studies were originally designed to address have been generously reported to support or negate long-held beliefs about the potential benefits or risks of hormone supplementation therapy.

In the past few years, conclusions from some of these studies have received uncritical and usually unbalanced media exposure. This has made patients wary and has made it difficult for providers of women's health to counsel patients regarding perimenopausal or menopausal hormonal treatments. In addition, the above studies (with the exception of the PEPI Trial that found that micronized bioidentical progesterone had less of a blunting of the beneficial lipid effects from estrogen and beneficial effects on carbohydrate metabolism) used only the historically "standard" oral preparations noted above (CEE and MPA), thereby limiting each study's generalizability to bioidentical, transdermal, or transmucosal preparations of estrogen and progesterone.

For many years, unopposed oral estrogen (CEE) was given to every woman who presented with bothersome symptoms of apparent estrogen deficiency (vasomotor symptoms, vaginal dryness, decreased libido, or mood "problems"). It has become clear that the perimenopause is more often characterized by wide fluctuations in estrogen and FSH levels.[51] More often than not, a woman will be hyperestrogenic during this period of her life. Therefore, while an estrogen prescription might help lessen symptoms by preventing the nadirs of these endogenous fluctuations, it may also encourage the development of situations associated with estrogen excess, including dysfunctional uterine bleeding, endometrial hyperplasia, endometrial cancer, and possibly an increased risk of breast cancer. The problem of unopposed estrogen with the development of endometrial cancer in women with a uterus can be avoided (reduced to the rate of those on no estrogen supplementation at all) with the addition of a progesterone to the regimen. Progestins (synthetic or bioidentical) stabilize the endometrium when given in a dose that the local endometrium "sees" as adequate to control its proliferation. For this use progestins appear to be equally effective given in a low dose continuously or cyclically.

Until recently, the above situation appeared to be all there was to be concerned about. Women's symptoms were controlled, osteoporosis was usually avoided, and women were relatively "safe." The only other associated "significant" risks were increased gallbladder and thrombotic disease. Contraindications to hormone replacement therapy (HRT) included previous history of thrombotic disease, serious or currently active liver disease, undiagnosed genitourinary bleeding, suspected pregnancy, breast cancer (now a relative contraindication), and the suspicion of other estrogen-dependent cancers. Not only was hormone supplementation therapy considered relatively safe, but in the last 10–25 years there have been numerous study reports of the coincidental prevention or successful treatment of a number of other debilitating chronic diseases, including cardiovascular disease; hyperlipidemia; mild early Alzheimer disease; osteoarthritis; periodontal disease and tooth loss; age-related macular degeneration; memory deficits; cognitive decline; symptoms of treated Parkinson's disease; type 2 diabetes and insulin resistance; colon cancer; hemorrhagic stroke and migraine headaches; and, of course, osteopenia and osteoporosis.

More recent studies cast doubt on some of the claims of benefit for HRT. To adequately counsel patients, many more answers are needed. The answers regarding hormone use are not likely to be simple and easily generalizable as they have seemed in the past. Individualization of hormones and other treatments will be necessary and close follow-up will likely be the norm in order to ensure that our patients benefit from the best evidence available as it relates to estrogen, progesterone, and other pharmacologic therapies.

HRT and Cancer

Breast Cancer

The early belief that menopausal use of estrogen did not cause or increase the likelihood of cancers other than endometrial was apparently founded on a number of negative studies in the literature especially with regard to breast cancer.[52–55] However, more recent studies, other retrospective data source derivations, and the continued observation of ongoing cohorts (e.g., Nurses Health Study, the Breast Cancer Demonstration Project) suggest a slightly increased breast cancer risk in current and past users (especially over 10 years of use) of supplemental estrogen and an even higher risk with estrogen/progestin (combination therapy).[56,57] The questions of risk are now felt to be most likely related to duration of use, current use versus past use, estrogen-only versus an estrogen/progestin regimen, and family history.

Most recently, the combination regimen arm of the Women's Health Initiative trial[58] (16,608 arm enrollees) was prematurely discontinued (at 5.2 years of the originally planned 8.5 years) because of the finding of an unexpected increase in the incidence of invasive breast cancer, strokes, cardiovascular events, and thromboembolic events. The increased venous thrombosis and pulmonary embolus risk was concentrated in the first 2 years of use. While the absolute numbers involved were very small for all of these end points, the hazard risk was 1.26 for invasive breast cancer (i.e., a 26% increase over the rate noted with placebo). The estrogen-only arm of the study has been allowed to continue.

The Women's Health Initiative trial was designed to be a pure primary prevention trial enrolling women from 40 clinical centers across the country. Unfortunately, the study excluded women currently experiencing a significant number of hot flushes. This excluded a large number of women, especially those in the early years of the menopausal period. Furthermore, as with many studies before it, it considered only one hormonal formulation of estrogen (CEE) and one of progestin (medroxy-progesterone acetate), one set of dosages, and only the oral route of administration was used. In addition, other confounding factors have not yet been explained fully. It is possible that body weight or body mass index with the "standard" doses used in the study may have affected outcomes. Alcohol use has been linked to an increased risk of breast cancer, and the effect may be enhanced in association with hormone replacement therapy.[59] Generalization to other doses, bioidentical formulations, or other routes of administration can only be made without direct supportive data regarding the potential risks and benefits. A final dilemma

is that the natural history of the growth of breast cancer indicates that these foci of breast cancer may have been present but yet undetectable prior to the onset of the study. Thus the question remains unanswered whether postmenopausal hormone therapy initiates the development of new breast cancers, or serves as a promoter for already established neoplastic foci.

This picture is further complicated by the consistent observation that women who use (and have used) menopausal hormone supplementation are diagnosed at earlier stages, develop better differentiated tumors, have less metastatic disease (more localized), and significantly lower mortality rates than do women who have not used estrogen or estrogen/progestin supplementation therapy.[60] While this finding was originally thought only to be a result of detection/surveillance bias, it is possible that other mechanisms may be at work that accelerate the growth of a preexisting malignant locus. In addition, this increase in relative risk has consistently been found to expire 5 years after discontinuation of hormone therapy.

This apparent positive effect on outcomes of HRT for women with breast cancer has progressed to the point that it is no longer taboo to discuss the possibility of using hormone therapy in women previously treated for breast cancer for symptom control and as a tool to factor into disease prevention strategies. As yet, there are no large, randomized controlled trials and only a few small nonrandomized studies regarding this subject. The first controlled study on hormone therapy in women with breast cancer was published by Eden and colleagues,[61] in 1995, showing a significantly lower risk of breast cancer recurrence and mortality from all causes as compared to nonusers (the average duration of use after diagnosis and treatment for breast cancer was 1.5 years). The conclusion drawn from this was that at least short-term usage of combined hormone therapy was safe, and possibly protective against recurrence (the relative risk of recurrence in users was 0.4). These findings been confirmed by Durna and colleagues[62] and expanded by Verheul et al. to show that estrogen-only and combination therapy also appear not to effect responsiveness to breast cancer therapies.[63]

HRT and Epithelial Ovarian Cancer

Ovarian cancer is diagnosed most commonly in the advanced stages of the disease and has a very low survival rate despite numerous heroic efforts to find appropriate treatments. With the lowering of age of first menses in girls and the reduction in the number of pregnancies per woman that has been occurring over the last 100 years, the incidence of ovarian cancer may continue to increase in the future. The strategy of transvaginal ultrasonography combined with serum CA125 measurements for screening is plagued by false positives and is not cost-effective in a low-risk population. Serial transvaginal ultrasonography and CA125 used together in a high-risk population have a better yield, but not all ovarian cancers produce CA125 and a very small aggressive tumor may metastasize early, so false negatives remain an issue. Prophylactic bilateral oophorectomy performed in women at high risk reduces, but does not eliminate, the risk of ovarian cancer, as peritoneal carcinomas may still occur.[64,65] Currently, anything that can be even loosely associated with a reduced incidence of this disease is certainly worth much closer investigation.

Ovarian cancer has not historically been linked to menopausal hormone therapy use. In fact, 5 or more years of pharmacologic dosing of estrogen and synthetic progestins in oral contraceptives has been found to be chemoprotective against the ever-development of epithelial ovarian cancer with a relative risk reduction of 50%.[66,67] This finding has been extrapolated to include women with a positive family history of ovarian cancer as an accepted risk-reduction strategy.

There is little doubt that the postmenopausal ovary is quite a different entity from the ovary during the reproductive years, and the history of the number of lifetime ovulations seems to affect a woman's lifetime risk of ovarian cancer. We are unsure in how many other ways it differs and what to do about it. If oral contraceptives are so "good" for the prevention of the scourge of ovarian cancer (possibly through the reduction of the number of lifetime ovulations), how could the considerably lower dosing with menopausal hormone supplementation cause harm? There is no randomized trial data to help us evaluate any relationship between menopausal estrogen and combination therapy and ovarian cancer. There have been no positive secondary end points regarding the issue from any large epidemiologic study as yet. One population-based, case-controlled study revealed no association between epithelial ovarian cancer and any use of combination hormone replacement (categorized by CEE and non-CEE preparations with or without the progestin).[68] There was a reduced risk in those without a uterus who had used an estrogen, unopposed, of any type. There has been one meta-analysis[69] and two prospective cohort studies that showed an increased risk of epithelial ovarian cancer with 10 and more years of estrogen-only use (relative risk of 1.27–1.8).[70,71] Estrogen/ progestin therapy (combined) was not associated with an increased risk of developing the disease.

HRT, Colorectal Cancer, and Endometrial Cancer

The same WHI data set that revealed the aforementioned findings for breast cancer (that prompted the early discontinuation of the estrogen/progestin arm of the study) also revealed reduced risks of colorectal cancer with a hazard risk of 0.63, and endometrial cancer with a hazard risk of 0.83, as compared to placebo. The reduction in colorectal cancer is consistent with the results from a large number of case-controlled studies. The reduction in endometrial cancer with the use of opposing progestin in women with a uterus supports information proven and accepted over the last 30 years.

HRT and Other Chronic Diseases

Fracture Risk

The Women's Health Initiative trial data for the prematurely discontinued combination hormone therapy study arm (5.2 years) is the first randomized trial data to show not only an increased bone mineral density, but also a measurable change in the morbid end point clinicians and patients are most concerned about: reduced fracture risk at both the hip and the spine (hazard risk 0.66 for each site). The details of estrogen, progesterone, and other medical therapies for prevention and treatment of osteopenia and osteoporosis are discussed in detail in Chapter 24. It was recently noted, however, that there are women who are nonresponders with respect to the degree of the antiresorptive effect of estrogen on their bones. It is, therefore, unwise to assume that every woman receiving estrogen supplementation will automatically be protected against osteoporosis.

Alzheimer's Disease

Women are three times more likely to develop Alzheimer's disease than men of the same age. There has been much speculation regarding the effect of estrogen on the aging brain. There are many mechanisms by which estrogen is capable of protecting the central nervous system: it protects against local oxidation, resulting in neuronal cytotoxicity;[72] reduces the concentration in the serum of amyloid P[73] (a glycoprotein seen in neurofibrillary tangles in Alzheimer's disease); increases neuronal growth and synapses, especially dendritic spine density;[74] and increases cerebral and cerebellar blood flow in postmenopausal women.[75] Progesterone does not exert these actions.

Earlier, small studies that showed that estrogen replacement enhanced memory skills in postmenopausal women were plagued by small sample sizes and self-selection biases. More recent studies have failed to show an impact of estrogen on the course of already established Alzheimer's disease. This is probably due to the presence of changes in the brain for prolonged periods prior to phenotypic expression of the disease. More recently, efforts have turned to examination of, and have begun to reveal the benefit of, estrogen for the prevention and delay of onset of some of the debilitating effects of Alzheimer disease.[76,77] Here also, results are somewhat conflicting.

The Rancho Bernardo retirement community prospective cohort study did not support a cognitive function benefit of postmenopausal estrogen, and the number of subjects was too small to infer any effect on the development of Alzheimer disease.[81] Other smaller studies suggested a considerable benefit with up to a 60% reduction of the risk of Alzheimer disease and related dementia in estrogen users with the benefit increasing with greater dosage and duration of use.[82,83] Similar findings were noted in the prospective cohorts of the Italian Longitudinal Study of Aging[84] and the Baltimore Longitudinal Study of Aging.[85] Most recently, the prospective cohort Cache County Study set out to examine the relationship between hormone replacement therapy and the risk of dementia among 1,357 men and 1,889 women (mean age: 74.5 years) in a single county in Utah.[86] In the follow-up done 3 years after the initial interview (in which a history of women's previous and current use of HRT was assessed), 2.7% of the men and 4.7% of the women had developed Alzheimer disease. The risk varied with increasing duration of use, so that a woman's gender-specific increase in risk disappeared entirely after 10 years of treatment (predominantly former estrogen use). The adjusted hazard risks were 0.41 for users as compared to never-users, and 0.77 as compared to men. There was no effect with current use unless the "former use" threshold level had been met.

DHEA is also being considered in this preventative context,[78,79] as are nonsteroidal anti-inflammatory drugs and antioxidant vitamin E, especially that from food sources.[80]

Carbohydrate Metabolism and the Development of Type 2 Diabetes Mellitus

Type 2 diabetes and obesity in women has become epidemic in this country over the last 20 years. More processed and fast foods have contributed to these problems, as has the reduction in activity levels beginning in childhood. While true prevention with improved food choices and regular exercise should be our first emphasis with our patients, hormone replacement may have a role in prevention and treatment of impaired glucose metabolism in menopausal women.

Pharmacologic doses of the synthetic ethinyl estradiol found in oral contraceptives decrease insulin sensitivity in normal women.[87] Additionally, different progestins reduce insulin clearance to varying degrees. In prospective studies of postmenopausal women with type 2 diabetes, estrogen supplementation has improved all glucose metabolic parameters, including lipoprotein profile, insulin resistance, and measurements of androgenicity.[88,89] Estrogen replacement, especially with natural bioidentical estrogens may also counteract the age-related changes of glucose metabolism.[90-92] Most studies show that standard doses of progestins do not appear to significantly blunt these positive effects, but the least-worsening effect has been noted with bioidentical micronized progesterone. Several smaller, shorter trials compared oral versus transdermal routes of estrogen administration and found either no difference or a slight enhancement of the beneficial influence on glucose levels.[93] One 60-day study on healthy postmenopausal women found that transdermal estradiol, alone, improved insulin sensitivity, but the effect was considerably blunted with the addition of a 10-mg synthetic progestin (MPA) dose given cyclically.[94]

The largest randomized trial to consider glucose metabolism before the Heart and Estrogen/Progestin Replacement Study was the PEPI trial, which evaluated a younger group of postmenopausal women without heart disease. While the initial reports found a general worsening of 2-hour postchallenge glucose levels in study participants in the hormone replacement arm, later analysis revealed decreasing fasting glucose levels over time in women who actually adhered to the hormone replacement regimen.[95]

Diabetes is a major contributor to the development of heart disease. It is considered the equivalent of a previous myocardial infarction in newer global risk assessment models.[96] The HERS randomized, placebo-controlled, double-blind trial, published in the *Annals of Internal Medicine* in 2002, evaluated the effect of hormone therapy on fasting glucose level and incident diabetes involving 2,763 (naturally) postmenopausal women with coronary heart disease who were followed for 4.1 years. It concluded that in women with coronary heart disease, hormone therapy (CEE and MPA, daily versus placebo) reduced the incidence of diabetes by 35%.[97]

Heart Disease

Heart disease is the number one cause of death of women in the United States. The mortality rate exceeds the mortality from all cancer types combined and exceeds the number of breast cancer deaths per year by 10-fold.[98] Women tend to experience the first manifestations of heart disease 10–15 years later, and have worse outcomes after cardiac events, than men. Unfortunately, there is inconsistent knowledge of and adherence to primary prevention measures that might avert or lessen the phenotypic expression of coronary heart disease. These measures include weight management/reduction; regular physical activity; nutrition education and follow-up; supplement use; stress reduction education; encouragement of social involvement (prevent isolation); smoking cessation; low-dose aspirin; and assertive treatment of hypertension and hyperlipidemia as needed *during* the time these interventions are being implemented and evaluated for efficacy, or if they are unsuccessful for any reason.

The topic of hormones and heart disease has been studied extensively in the last several years. The earlier reports from ongoing observational trials (including the Nurses Health Study[99] with 48,470 enrollees) consistently supported the benefit of postmenopausal estrogen therapy for the reduction of cardiovascular risk, reporting risk reductions of 40–50% for cardiovascular events and deaths. The women at highest risk or who had already had an event, seemed to enjoy the greatest benefits. After all, estrogen was known to exert beneficial influences on a number of factors known to affect the development and severity of cardiovascular disease, and the decline of estrogen levels at the menopause seemed temporally related to the rise in the female incidence of heart disease. Estrogen exerts (at least) several effects[100]: it reduces low-density lipoprotein cholesterol levels, as well as lipoprotein a and homocysteine levels; increases the beneficial high-density lipoprotein cholesterol levels; increases nitric oxide, vasodilator prostaglandin levels, and fibrinolytic activity; augments antiplatelet aggregation factors; exerts a number of favorable direct and indirect vascular effects; reduces endothelin (vasoconstrictor) levels; improves endothelial function; has calcium channel-blocking and local antioxidant actions; and exerts positive effects on glucose metabolism and insulin resistance. On the negative side, the positive effect of estrogens on lipoprotein levels is blunted by synthetic progestins. The PEPI trial[101,102] was the first large trial to show that micronized, oral progesterone (Prometrium) had less of an antagonistic effect on estrogen's beneficial lipid effects. Oral estrogens, but not alternate route formulations (e.g., transdermal), increase triglyceride levels (known to be an independent risk factor for heart disease in women) and increase the inflammatory marker C-reactive protein.[103]

Studies of selective estrogen receptor modulators such as raloxifene (typically used for the treatment of osteoporosis) reveal that they have similar, but less potent, effects on lipoproteins and vascular reactivity as estrogens, while not elevating C-reactive protein levels as does estrogen.[104] However, the long-term effects on cardiovascular end points of selective estrogen receptor modulators are as yet unknown. Analysis of the MORE (Multiple Outcomes of Raloxifene Evaluation) trial showed a reduction in cardiac events only in high-risk women.[105] Currently available selective estrogen receptor modulators share estrogen's ability to increase thromboembolic events, while differing in that they worsen vasomotor symptoms. The ongoing Raloxifene Use for The Heart (RUTH) trial is sure to be the first of many studies to examine the cardiovascular outcomes question.

Follow-up reports from the 20 years of follow-up in the Nurses' Health Study were published by Grodstein et al. in 2000 and 2001. They first noted that when all cardiovascular risk factors were considered, the risk for major *primary* coronary events was lower among current, even short-term, hormone users as compared to never-users (CEE 0.3 or 0.625 dose-associated with relative risk of 0.61).[106] In 2001, Grodstein et al. reported that the risk for *recurrent* major coronary events in the same population increased among short-term users with previous coronary disease, but decreased with longer-term use as compared to never-users with coronary heart disease.[107]

The first randomized prospective trial to challenge these assumptions that hormone supplementation therapy was "good" for the heart was the 1998 report from the HERS,[108] a secondary prevention trial that studied more than 3,000 postmenopausal women, younger than age 80 years, each with a uterus and known coronary heart disease for 4.1 years. The women were not taking hormones immediately prior to the study. They received either placebo or continuous CEE and MPA (estrogen/progesterone [E/P]). This study showed that, overall, there was no reduction in cardiovascular events during the study period and that there was actually an unexpected increase in number of events during the first year. There was no effect on stroke incidence.[109] Surprisingly, there was a threefold increase in the rates of deep venous thrombosis and pulmonary embolus as compared to rates reported in most previous studies.

Significant controversy followed the release of the HERS results. It was soon supported by yet more randomized trials (and several smaller trials). The Estrogen Replacement and Angiography (ERA) trial[110] enrolled 309 women with known coronary heart disease who had a greater than 30% obstruction of at least one coronary artery. They were given estrogen, E/P combination, or placebo. Follow-up angiography done 3 years later revealed no difference between any of the groups regarding new lesion development, lumen diameter, or clinical events. The Postmenopausal Hormone Replacement Against Atherosclerosis was the next large prospective trial enrolling 321 healthy women randomized to placebo or E/P therapy. The marker chosen for subclinical atherosclerosis was carotid intimal thickening. There was no difference in progression between the two groups over the study period.[111] The WAVE trial also concluded that hormone therapy was actually harmful, but in the result section of the publication the author's stated that once diabetes and diabetes-related variables were adjusted for, the increase in risk was no longer significant.[112]

In 2001, based on all of these compelling trial results and new information drawn from previously collected data, the American Heart Association published recommendations that hormone supplementation therapy should be discontinued if a cardiovascular event occurs in a patient using it, and that it not be prescribed for the secondary prevention of heart disease.[113]

As a consequence of the controversy, the HERS participants were followed for another 31 months to see if a cardiac benefit would emerge in this population with preexisting disease (HERS II). Still, no significant difference was found in the number of cardiac events or mortality in the E/P group as compared to placebo.[111] In July 2002, soon after the HERS II report was released, the WHI trial,[115] the multicenter study with 27,348 pre-

sumed healthy total enrollees, prematurely discontinued the E/P (CEE/MPA) arm that included 16,608 participants (noted previously) because of the unexpected increased occurrence over placebo in the number of cases of invasive breast cancer (26%), coronary heart disease events (29%), stroke (41%), and pulmonary embolic events (50%). Incidentally, the risk for fractures of the hip and spine as well as colorectal cancer were reduced by nearly 35% for each. The estrogen-only arm (CEE) is being allowed to continue until 2005.

Again, it is unfortunate that all of these trials leave the question open whether any difference in risk and benefit profiles would have been found with transdermal estradiol or other forms of oral estrogens and progestins.

Thyroid Dysfunction, Hormones, the Heart, and Mortality

With the progression now to the extremely sensitive fourth generation thyroid-stimulating hormone (TSH) assays, the effect of subclinical thyroid dysfunction has entered the picture as a silent contributor to heart disease including impaired left ventricular diastolic function at rest, systolic dysfunction on effort, and increased risk for atherosclerosis and infarction.[116] Another recent study report revealed an increase in all-cause mortality (particularly caused by circulatory and cardiovascular diseases) in a cohort (60 years old, not on thyroid or antithyroid medication) followed for up to 11 years that had just one low serum TSH measurement at the beginning of the study.[117]

It is important to screen perimenopausal and menopausal women for thyroid dysfunction because of the gender prevalence of dysfunction. Many of the symptoms overlap between the two states and the prevalence of thyroid dysfunction increases with age. An expanded diagnostic panel to include antithyroid peroxidase antibodies may be necessary in symptomatic (and possibly in the asymptomatic, as well) patients that have a high-normal TSH and a normal or low-normal free T_1 level. Previously held tenets regarding the goals of replacement in light of the serious potential morbidity caused by subclinical disease in older patients, may require replacement dosages be increased in order to push the T_4 level into the upper portion of the reference range and push TSH level into the lower portion of the reference range for treated patients who still do not feel well after the usual replacement dosage brings the TSH and the T_4 into the midranges for your reference laboratory.[118]

Oral estrogen therapy will most likely prompt the need for a dosage change (increase of up to 45%) of thyroid medication because of the estrogen-induced increase to the thyroid-binding globulin synthesis by the liver. Transdermal estrogen preparations will not require such modification. The TSH level is not thought to be directly affected by estrogen by any route or by these binding protein changes. Estrogen and progesterone may also exert direct effects on thyroid cell function,[119] but the full scope of their role in the hypothalamic–pituitary–thyroid axis remains unclear.[120]

HRT and Immune Competence

Several small studies show that estrogen therapy increases levels of several immune factors in postmenopausal women. In one study, the greatest increases were found in interleukin-2 and gamma-interferon levels.[121] In another case-controlled study, combination hormone replacement therapy appeared to reverse the immune alterations (negative) associated with normal aging.[122] The degree of these changes may be route dependent.

Oral contraceptives may cause deficiencies of the antioxidant vitamin E in reproductive-age women, but postmenopausal hormone supplementation appears to have no effect on vitamin E status.[123]

HRT and Weight Gain

Many women believe that hormone supplementation during the menopause causes sustained weight gain. Becoming menopausal, whether surgically or naturally, is associated with some weight gain because the basal metabolic rate tends to decline, but food intake patterns and activity levels usually do not. What does seem to be the case, however, is that the distribution of the weight gain is in an android pattern in hormone users (pear shaped) and more gynecoid pattern (apple shaped) in nonhormone users.[124] In addition, the weight gain that may occur early after the initiation of replacement is often lost after the first 5 months of treatment when the body adjusts to the altered growth hormone secretory response and reaches a new homeostatic state.[125] The perimenopause and early menopause is a time for a woman to reevaluate her lifestyle habits and food choices and to develop a regular activity routine that positively maximizes her body and mind's responses to the changes that will occur in the last half to third of her life span. Even for women who feel that they are already "doing enough," adjustments may be required.

▶ OTHER TREATMENT OPTIONS FOR CONTROL OF MENOPAUSAL SYMPTOMS

The first line of treatment for alleviation of vasomotor symptoms is behavioral. This may include dressing in layers, lightening make-up product use, carrying a hand-held fan, relaxation exercises, imagery, carrying an extra shirt to change into if necessary and avoiding spicy foods, very hot drinks, and alcohol, as well as anything that is identified with a worsening of vasomotor symptoms. This may be all many women need, and should certainly be attempted before trying medications or other more time- and money-consuming interventions.

Given the current situation surrounding the uncertainties of hormone supplementation therapy, it makes more sense than ever to try other means not potentially associated with major adverse effects to help your patient with menopausal symptom relief. There are other ancient traditional systems of healing and effective techniques that overtly rely more on energy and the mind–body continuum than conventional medicine with its reliance on drugs. Given the potential risks, drugs may be reserved for short-term use or for those women who do not benefit from less-invasive interventions.

Ayurvedic medicine, traditional Chinese medicine, and/or acupuncture are very effective for balancing and treatment of menopausal symptoms. While studies have not yet proven the efficacy of homeopathy for this indication, there is significant anecdotal evidence that homeopathic remedies prescribed by a trained practitioner may be very helpful for the alleviation of symptoms.

Social support and a sense of community are invaluable during this time when a woman may suffer from a myriad of symptoms unfamiliar to her. This is also a time to consider connecting with something larger than herself; meditation, breathing techniques, and prayer, as well as simple relaxation[126] and stress management techniques,[127] can all provide a healthier perspective on the challenges of menopause. Guided imagery and medical hypnotherapy are helpful, with and without concurrent cognitive behavior therapy, for treatment of hot flushes, mood changes, irritability, and sleep disturbance symptoms. These techniques can empower the patient by helping her reframe the situation, change internalized negative beliefs, and "reconstruct and recreate" herself. Halas has outlined the details of this process with specific respect to menopause.[128]

Where behavioral change, Bach flower remedies, mind–body techniques, and traditional medicine approaches do not result in symptom relief, medications can be very useful. As noted previously, progesterone cream may be very effective, as are estrogen and progesterone replacement via other routes.

Megestrol acetate, a synthetic progestin (20–80 mg/d in two divided doses) and cloni-dine (0.05–0.1 mg orally once or twice a day, or a 0.1-mg patch that is replaced weekly), each titrated to clinical response, may be helpful for severe vasomotor symptoms. Selective serotonin reuptake inhibitors (such as venlafaxine, paroxetine, fluoxetine) and anti-seizure medications (such as gabapentin) have been trialed and found modestly effective for the treatment of vasomotor symptoms. Because of their potential adverse side-effect profile (short- and long-term) these medications should be reserved as last resort trial medications in women for whom other interventions are ineffective or contraindicated. If they are used, consider using them for the shortest time possible to achieve your therapeutic goals.

▶ CONCLUSION AND FUTURE DIRECTIONS

The debate regarding optimal management of menopause continues. It makes the greatest sense to educate the population beginning early in life regarding optimal activity, nutrition, and sleep habits and reducing our use of and exposure to environmental toxins of all sorts, and to encourage everyone to perform some form of regular stress management on a daily basis and to actively work to maintain our sense of interconnectedness with each other and everything around us.

In the near future there will be considerable advances in receptor selectivity studies so that we may more specifically treat what needs to be treated in menopause more safely with the least perturbation to the rest of our bodies. Eventually we will have tests to predict who is most likely to benefit from a particular intervention, and of those, who is most likely to suffer an adverse effect of that intervention, and within what time frames these might occur. A recent article by Herrington and colleagues discusses variants in a gene encoding estrogen receptor alpha that might enhance the effects of hormone replacement therapy on levels of high-density lipoproteins and other outcomes related to estrogen treatment in postmenopausal women.[129] Tribble et al. have suggested a gene mutation that might increase the risk of myocardial infarction in women with hypertension who receive hormone supplementation therapy.[130] This field of pharmacogenetics is likely to help guide our discussions with our patients in the future.

Our hope is that, unlike the current environment of uncertainty in which we practice and advise patients, the future will provide more answers than questions.

REFERENCES

1. Eskin B, ed. *Menopause: Comprehensive Management*. 4th ed. Pearl River, New York: 2000: 3–19.

2. Speroff L, Glass R, Kase N, eds. *Clinical Gynecologic Endocrinology and Infertility*. 6th ed. Baltimore, MD: Lippincott, Williams and Wilkins; 1999.

3. Revelli A, Massobrio M, Tesarik J. Nongenomic actions of steroid hormones in reproductive tissues. *Endocr Rev*. 1998;19:3–17.

4. Santoro N, Brown JR, Adel T, et al. Characterization of reproductive hormonal dynamics in the perimenopause. *J Clin Endocrinol Metab*. 1996; 81:1435–1501.

5. Stellato R, Crawford S, McKlinky S, Longcope C. Can follicle-stimulating hormone be used to define menopausal status? *Endocr Pract*. 1998;4: 137–141.

6. Natchigall L, Raju U, Banerjee S. Serum estradiol profiles in postmenopausal women undergoing three common estrogen replacement therapies: association with sex hormone-binding globulin, estradiol and estrone levels. *Menopause*. 2000;7: 243–250.

7. Shirtcliff EA, Granger DA, Likos A. Gender differences in the validity of testosterone measured in saliva by immunoassay. *Horm Behav*. 2002; 41(1):62–69.

8. Speroff L. Measuring testosterone. *OBGYN Clin Alert*. 2003;19(11):86–87.

9. Lewis JG, McGill H, Patton VM, Elder PA. Cau-

tion on the use of saliva measurement to monitor absorption of progesterone from transdermal creams in postmenopausal women. *Maturitas*. 2002;41(1):1–6.

10. O'Leary P, Feddema P, Chan K, et al. Salivary, but not serum or urinary levels of progesterone are elevated after topical application of progesterone cream to pre- and postmenopausal women. *Clin Endocrinol*. 2000;53(5):615–620.

11. Wren BG, McFarland K, Edwards L, et al. Effect of sequential transdermal progesterone on endometrium, bleeding pattern, plasma progesterone and salivary progesterone levels in postmenopausal women. *Climacteric*. 2000;3(3): 155–160.

12. Ishikawa M, Sengoku K, Tamate K, et al. The clinical usefulness of salivary progesterone measurement for the evaluation of corpus luteum function. *Gynecol Obstet Invest*. 2002;53(1):32–37.

13. Siegal DL. Habits worth changing. In: Doress P, Siegal D, Brown P, eds. *Ourselves Growing Older: Women Aging With Knowledge and Power*. New York: Touchstone Books; 1994:33–34.

14. Weil A. Getting a good night's sleep. *Self Healing Newsletter*. September 1998:1, 6.

15. Polo-Kantola P, Erkkola R, Irjala K, et al. Effect of short-term transdermal estrogen replacement therapy on sleep: a randomized, double-blind cross-over trial in postmenopausal women. *Fertil Steril*. 1999;71:873–890.

16. Manson JE, Greenland P, LaCroix A, et al. Walking compared to vigorous exercise for the prevention of cardiovascular events in women. *N Engl J Med*. 2002;347:719–725.

17. Stampfer M, Hu F, Manson J, et al. Primary prevention of coronary heart disease in women through diet and lifestyle. *N Engl J Med*. 2000; 343:16–22.

18. Sobngwi E, Mbanya JC, Unwin NC, et al. Physical activity and its relationship obesity, hypertension and diabetes in urban and rural Cameroon. *Int J Obes Relat Metab Disord*. 2002; 26:1009–1016.

19. Murray M. *The Healing Power of Herbs*. 2nd ed. ND Prima Health. Rocklin, CA; 1995:35.

20. Lieberman SA. A review of the effectiveness of *Cimicifuga racemosa* for the symptoms of menopause. *J Womens Health*. 1998;7:525–529.

21. Liske E. Therapeutic efficacy and safety of *Cimicifuga racemosa* for gynecologic disorders. *Adv Ther*. 1998;15:45–53.

22. Liske E, Hanggi W, Henneicke-von Zepelin HH, et al. Physiological investigation of a unique extract of black cohosh: a 6-month clinical study demonstrates no systemic estrogen effect. *J Womens Health Gend Based Med.* 2002;11:163–174.

23. Jones KP. Menopause and cognitive function: estrogens and alternative therapies. *Clin Obstet Gynecol.* 2000;41:198–208.

24. Kuiper GG, Carsson B, Grandien K, et al. Comparison of the ligand binding specificity and transcript tissue distribution of estrogen receptors alpha and beta. *Endocrinology.* 1997;138:863–870.

25. Kronenberg G, Fugh-Berman A. Complementary and alternative medicine for menopausal symptoms: a review of randomized, controlled trials. *Ann Intern Med.* 2002;137:805–813.

26. Han KK, Soares JM, Haidar MA, et al. Benefits of soy isoflavone therapeutic regimen on menopausal symptoms. *Obstet Gynecol.* 2002;99: 389–394.

27. Ewies AA. Phytoestrogens in the management of menopause: up-to-date. *Obstet Gynecol Surv.* 2002;57:306–315.

28. Baber R, Clifton-Bligh P, Fulcher G, et al. The effect of an isoflavone dietary supplement (p-081) on serum lipids, forearm bone density and endometrial thickness in postmenopausal women. Proceedings of the 10th annual meeting of the North American Menopause Society; September 23–25, 1999; New York.

29. Crouse JR 3rd, Morgan T, Terry JG, et al. A randomized trial comparing the affect of casein with that of soy protein containing varying amounts of isoflavones on plasma concentrations of lipids and lipoproteins. *Arch Intern Med.* 1999;159: 2070–2076.

30. Murray M, Pizzorno J. *Encyclopedia of Natural Medicine.* Revised 2nd ed. Rocklin, CA: ND Prima Health; 1998:348.

31. Grandberg S, Ylostald P, Wikland M, Karlsson B. Endometrial sonographic findings in women with and without hormonal replacement therapy suffering from postmenopausal bleeding. *Maturitas.* 1997;27:35–40.

32. van Haaften M, Donker G, Sie-Go D, et al. Biochemical and histological effects of vaginal estriol and estradiol applications on the endometrium, myometrium and vagina of postmenopausal women. *Gynecol Endocrinol.* 1997; 1:175–185.

33. Ginsberg ES, Mello NK, Mendelson JG, et al. Effects of alcohol ingestion on estrogens in postmenopausal women. *JAMA.* 1996;276:1747–1751.

34. Ginsberg ES, Walsh BW, Shea BF, Gao X, et al. The effects of ethanol on the clearance of estradiol in postmenopausal women. *Fertil Steril.* 1995;63:1227–1230.

35. Schubert W, Cullberg G, Edgar B, Hedner T. Inhibition of 17-beta estradiol metabolism by grapefruit juice in ovariectomized women. *Maturitas.* 1995;20:155–163.

36. Riggs BL, Hartmann LC. Selective estrogen-receptor modulators. Mechanisms of action and application to clinical practice. *N Engl J Med.* 2003;248:618–629.

37. Leonetti H, Longo S, Anasti J. Transdermal progesterone cream for vasomotor symptoms and postmenopausal bone loss. *Obstet Gynecol.* 1999; 94:225–228.

38. Wren BG, McFarland K, Edwards L. Micronised transdermal progesterone and endometrial response [letter]. *Lancet.* 1999;354:1447–1448.

39. Cooper A, Spencer C, Whitehead MI, et al. Systemic absorption of progesterone from progesterone cream in postmenopausal women [letter]. *Lancet.* 1998;351:1255–56.

40. Herrington DM, Potvin Klein K. Statins, hormones and women: benefits and drawbacks for osteoporosis. *Curr Atheroscler Rep.* 2001;3:35–42.

41. Stampfer MJ, Colditz GA, Willett WC, et al. Postmenopausal estrogen therapy and cardiovascular disease. Ten-year follow-up from the Nurses' Health Study. *N Engl J Med.* 1991;325:756–762.

42. Bush T, Barrett-Conner E, Cowan L, et al. Cardiovascular mortality and noncontraceptive use of estrogen in women: results from the Lipid Research Clinics Program follow-up study. *Circulation.* 1987;75:1102–1109.

43. American Heart Association. *2002 Heart and Stroke Statistical Update.* Dallas, TX: American Heart Association; 2002.

44. Rossouw JE, Anderson GL, Prentice RL, et al. Risks and benefits of estrogen plus progestin in healthy postmenopausal women: principal results from the Women's Health Initiative randomized controlled trial. *JAMA.* 2002;288: 321–333.

45. Hulley S, Grady D, Bush T, et al. Randomized trial of estrogen plus progestin for secondary prevention of coronary heart disease in postmenopausal women. Heart and Estrogen/Progestin Replacement Study (HERS) research group. *JAMA.* 1998;280:605–613.

46. Waters DD, Alderman EL, Hsia J, et al. Effects of hormone replacement therapy and antioxidant supplements on coronary atherosclerosis in postmenopausal women: a randomized controlled trial. *JAMA*. 2002;288:2432–2440.

47. Grady D, Herrington D, Bittner V, et al. Cardiovascular disease outcomes during 6.8 years of hormone therapy: Heart and Estrogen/Progestin Replacement Study follow-up (HERS II). *JAMA*. 2002;288:49–57.

48. Angerer P, Stork S, Kothny W, et al. Effect of oral postmenopausal hormone replacement on the progressive of atherosclerosis: a randomized controlled trial. *Arterioscler Thromb Vasc Biol*. 2001;104:499–503.

49. The Writing Group for the PEPI Trial. Effects of estrogen/progestin regimen on heart disease risk factors in postmenopausal women. The Postmenopausal Estrogen/Progestin Interventions (PEPI) trial. *JAMA*. 1995;273:199–208.

50. Barrett-Conner E, Slone S, Greendale G, et al. The Postmenopausal Estrogen/Progestin Interventions study: primary outcomes in adherent women. *Maturitas*. 1997;27:261–274.

51. Stellato R, Crawford S, McKlinky S, Longcope C. Can follicle-stimulating hormone be used to define menopausal status? *Endocr Pract*. 1998;4:137–141.

52. Newcomb PA, Longnecker MP, Storer BE, et al. Long-term hormone replacement therapy and risk of breast cancer in postmenopausal women. *Am J Epidemiol*. 1995;142:788–795.

53. Moorman PG, Kuwahara H, Mullican RC, Newman B. Menopausal hormones and breast cancer in a biracial population. *Am J Public Health*. 2000;90(6):966–997.

54. Schairer C, Lubin J, Troisi R, et al. Menopausal estrogen and estrogen-progestin replacement therapy and breast cancer risk. *JAMA*. 2000;283:485–491.

55. Collaborative Group on Hormonal Factors in Breast Cancer. Breast cancer and hormone replacement therapy: collaborative meta-analysis of data from 51 epidemiologic studies of 52,505 women with breast cancer and 108,411 women without breast cancer. *Lancet*. 1997;350:1046–1059.

56. Colditz GA, Rosner B. Cumulative risk of breast cancer to age 70 years according to risk factor status: data from the Nurses' Health Study. *Am J Epidemiol*. 2000;152(10):950–964.

57. Rossouw JE, Anderson GL, Prentice RL, et al. Risks and benefits of estrogen plus progestin in healthy postmenopausal women: principal results from the Women's Health Initiative randomized controlled trial. *JAMA*. 2002;288:321–333.

58. Rodriguez C, Calle EE, Patel AV, et al. Effect of body mass on the association between estrogen replacement therapy and mortality among elderly US women. *Am J Epidemiol*. 2001;153(2):145–152.

59. Chen W, Colditz G, Rosner B, et al. Use of postmenopausal hormones, alcohol and risk of invasive breast cancer. *Ann Intern Med*. 2002;137:798–804.

60. Willis DB, Calle EE, Miracle-McMahill HL, Heath CW Jr. Estrogen replacement therapy and the risk of fatal breast cancer in a prospective cohort of postmenopausal women in the United States. *Cancer Causes Control*. 1996;7:449–457.

61. Eden JA. Should women who have breast cancer take hormone replacement therapy? *Maturitas*. 1995;22(2):69–70.

62. Durna EM, Wren BG, Heller GZ. Hormone replacement therapy after diagnosis of breast cancer: cancer recurrence and mortality. *Med J Aust*. 2002;177(7):340–344.

63. Verheul HA, Coelingh-Bennicnk HJ, Kenemans P, et al. Effects of estrogens and hormone replacement therapy on breast cancer risk and on efficacy of breast cancer therapies. *Maturitas*. 2000;36(1):1–17.

64. Piver MS, Jishi ME, Tsukada Y, Nava G. Primary peritoneal carcinoma after prophylactic oophorectomy in women with a family history of ovarian cancer: a report of the Gilda Radner Familial Cancer Registry. *Cancer*. 1993;71:2751–2755.

65. Tobacman JK, Greene MH, Tucker MA, et al. Intra-abdominal carcinomatosis after prophylactic oophorectomy in ovarian cancer-prone families. *Lancet*. 1982;2:795–797.

66. Franceschi S, Parazzini F, Negri E, et al. Pooled analysis of three European case-control studies of epithelial ovarian cancer: III. Reproductive factors and risk of epithelial ovarian cancer. *Int J Cancer*. 1991;49:57–60.

67. Negri E, Franceschi S, Tzonou A, et al. Pooled analysis of three European case-control studies of epithelial ovarian cancer: I. Reproductive factors and risk of epithelial ovarian cancer. *Int J Cancer*. 1991;49:50–66.

68. Sit AS, Modugno F, Weissfeld JL, et al. Hormone replacement therapy formulations and risk of epithelial ovarian cancer. *Gynecol Oncol.* 2002;86:118–123.

69. Garg PP, Kerlikowske K, Subak L, et al. Hormone replacement and the risk of epithelial ovarian carcinoma: a meta-analysis. *Obstet Gynecol.* 1998;92:472–479.

70. Rodriguez C, Patel AV, Calle EE, et al. Estrogen replacement therapy and ovarian cancer mortality in a large prospective study of US women. *JAMA.* 2001;285:1460–1465.

71. Lacey JV, Mink PJ, Lubin JH, et al. Menopausal hormone replacement therapy and risk of ovarian cancer. *JAMA.* 2002;288:334–341.

72. Behl C, Skutella T, Lezoualc'h F, et al. Neuroprotection against oxidative stress by estrogens: structure-activity relationship. *Mol Pharmacol.* 1997;51:535–541.

73. Hashimoto S, Katou M, Dong Y, et al. Effects of hormone replacement therapy on serum amyloid P component in postmenopausal women. *Maturitas.* 1997;26:113–119.

74. Woolley CS, Weiland NG, McEwen BS, et al. Estradiol increases the sensitivity of hippocampal CA1 pyramidal cells to NMDA receptor-mediated synaptic input: correlation with dendritic spine density. *J Neuroscience.* 1997;17:1848–1859.

75. Ohkura T, Teshima Y, Isse K, et al. Estrogen increases cerebral and cerebellar blood flows in postmenopausal women. *Menopause.* 1995;2:13–18.

76. Brinton RD. Estrogen replacement therapy and Alzheimer's disease. *Menopausal Med.* 1997;1:5–8.

77. Tang-Ming X, Jacobs D, Stern Y, et al. Effects of oestrogen during the menopause on risk and age at onset of Alzheimer's disease. *Lancet.* 1996;348:429–432.

78. Robel P, Baulieo EM. Dehydroepiandrosterone (DHEA) is a neuroactive neurosteroid: DHEA and aging. *Ann N Y Acad Sci.* 1995;774:82–110.

79. Sunderland T, Merril CR, Harrington MG, et al. Reduced plasma dehydroepiandrosterone concentrations in Alzheimer's disease [letter]. *Lancet.* 1989;341:570.

80. Morris MC, Evans DA, Bienias JL, et al. Dietary intake of antioxidant nutrients and risk of Alzheimer disease in a biracial community. *JAMA.* 2002;287:3230–3237.

81. Barrett-Conner E, Kritz-Silverstein D. Estrogen replacement therapy and cognitive function in older women. *JAMA.* 1993;269:2637–2641.

82. Paganini-Hill A Henderson VW. Estrogen replacement therapy and risk of Alzheimer's disease. *Arch Intern Med.* 1996;156:2213–2217.

83. Henderson VW. The epidemiology of estrogen replacement therapy and Alzheimer's disease. *Neurology.* 1997;48(suppl 7):S27–S35.

84. Baldereschi M, DiCarlo A, Lepore V. Estrogen replacement therapy and Alzheimer's disease in the Italian Longitudinal Study on Aging. *Neurology.* 998;50:996–1002.

85. Kawas C Resnick S, Morrison A, et al. A prospective study of estrogen replacement therapy and the risk of Alzheimer's disease. *Neurology.* 1997;48:1517–1521.

86. Zandi PP, Carlson MC, Plassman BL, et al. Hormone replacement therapy and incidence of Alzheimer's disease in older women: the Cache County study. *JAMA.* 2002;288:2123–2129.

87. Kojima T, Lindheim SR, Duffy DM. Insulin sensitivity is decreased in normal women by doses in ethinyl estradiol oral contraceptives. *Am J Obstet Gynecol.* 1993;169(6):1540–1542.

88. Andersson B, Mattsson L, Hahn L. Estrogen replacement therapy decreases androgenicity and improves glucose homeostasis and plasma lipids in postmenopausal women with noninsulin-dependent diabetes mellitus. *J Clin Endocrinol Metab.* 1997;82:638–643.

89. Brusaard HE, Gevers Leuven JA, Frolich M, et al. Short-term oestrogen replacement therapy improves insulin resistance, lipids and fibrinolysis in postmenopausal women with noninsulin-dependent diabetes mellitus. *Diabetologia.* 1997;40:843–849.

90. Nabushi AA, Folsom AR, White A, et al. Association of hormone replacement therapy with various cardiovascular risk factors in postmenopausal women. *N Engl J Med.* 1993;328:1069–1075.

91. Gaspard UJ, Gottal JM, van den Brule FA. Postmenopausal changes of lipid and glucose metabolism: a review of their main aspects. *Maturitas.* 1995;21:171–178.

92. Barrett-Conner E, Slone S, Greendale G, et al. The Postmenopausal Estrogen/Progestin Interventions study: primary outcomes in adherent women. *Maturitas.* 1997;27:261–274.

93. Karjalainen A, Paassilta M, Heikkinen J, et al. Effects of peroral and transdermal oestrogen

therapy on glucose and insulin metabolism. *Clin Endocrinol (Oxf)*. 2001;54:165–173.

94. Lindheim SR, Duffy DM, Kojima T, et al. The route of administration influences the effect of estrogen and insulin sensitivity in postmenopausal women. *Fertil Steril*. 1994;62: 1176–1180.

95. Espland MA, Hogan PE, Fineberg SE, et al. Effect of postmenopausal hormone therapy on glucose and insulin concentrations. PEPI investigators, Postmenopausal Estrogen/Progestin Interventions. *Diabetes Care*. 1998;21:1589–1595.

96. Executive Summary of the National Cholesterol Education Program Expert Panel (NCEP) on detection, evaluation and treatment of high blood cholesterol in adults (Adult Treatment Panel III). *JAMA*. 2001;285:2486–2497.

97. Kanaya A, Herrington D, Vittinghoff E, et al. Glycemic effects of postmenopausal hormone therapy: the Heart and Estrogen-progestin Replacement Study. A randomized, double-blind, placebo-controlled trial. *Ann Intern Med*. 2003; 138:1–9.

98. American Heart Association. 2002 Heart and Stroke Statistical Update. Dallas, TX: American Heart Association; 2002.

99. Stampfer MJ, Colditz GA, Willett WC, et al. Postmenopausal estrogen therapy and cardiovascular disease: Ten year follow-up from the Nurses' Health Study. *N Engl J Med*. 1991;325:756–762.

100. Mendelsohn ME, Karas RH. The protective effects of estrogen on the cardiovascular system. *N Engl J Med*. 1999;340:1801–1811.

101. The Writing Group for the PEPI Trial. Effects of estrogen/progestin regimens on heart disease risk factors in postmenopausal women. The Postmenopausal Estrogen/Progestin Interventions (PEPI) trial. *JAMA*. 1995;273:199–208.

102. Barrett-Conner E, Slone S, Greendale G, et al. The Postmenopausal Estrogen/Progestin Intervention Study: primary outcomes in adherent women. *Maturitas*. 1997;27:261–274.

103. Pradham AD, Manson JE, Rossouw JE, et al. Inflammatory biomarkers, hormone replacement therapy, and incident coronary heart disease: prospective analysis from the Women's Health Initiative observational study. *JAMA*. 2002;288: 980–987.

104. Walsh BW, Paul S, Wild RA, et al. The effects of hormone replacement therapy and raloxifene in C-reactive protein and homocysteine in healthy postmenopausal women: a randomized, controlled trial. *J Clin Endocrinol Metab*. 2000;85: 214–218.

105. Barrett-Conner E, Grady D, et al. Raloxifene and cardiovascular events in osteoporotic menopausal women. *JAMA*. 2002;287:847–856.

106. Grodstein F, Manson JE, Colditz GA, et al. A prospective, observational study of hormone therapy and primary prevention of cardiovascular disease. *Ann Intern Med*. 2000;133 (12): 933–941.

107. Grodstein F, Manson JE, Stampfer MJ. Postmenopausal hormone use and secondary prevention of coronary events in the Nurses' Health Study, a prospective observational study. *Ann Intern Med*. 2001;135 (1):1–8.

108. Hulley S, Grady D, Bush T, et al. Randomized trial of estrogen plus progestin for secondary prevention of coronary heart disease in postmenopausal women. Heart and Estrogen/Progestin Replacement Study (HERS) research group. *JAMA*. 1998; 280:605–613.

109. Simon JA, Hsia J, Cauley JA, et al. Postmenopausal hormone therapy and risk of stroke: The Heart and Estrogen/Progestin Replacement Study (HERS). *Circulation*. 2001;103:638–642.

110. Herrington D, Reboussin D, Brosnihan B, et al. Effects of estrogen replacement on the progression of coronary artery atherosclerosis: a randomized, controlled trial. *Arterioscler Thromb Vasc Biol*. 2001;21:262–268.

111. Angerer P, Stork S, Kothny W, et al. Effect of oral postmenopausal hormone replacement on the progression of atherosclerosis: a randomized, controlled trial. *Arterioscler Thromb Vasc Biol*. 2001;104:499–503.

112. Waters DD, Alderman L, Hsia J, et al. Effects of hormone replacement therapy and antioxidant supplements on coronary arteriosclerosis in postmenopausal women: a randomized controlled trial. *JAMA*. 2002;288:2432–2444.

113. Mosca L, Collins P, Herrington DM, et al. Hormone therapy and cardiovascular disease: a statement for healthcare professionals from the American Heart Association. *Circulation*. 2001;102: 499–503.

114. Grady D, Herrington D, Bittner V, et al. Cardiovascular disease outcomes during 6.8 years of hormone therapy: Heart and Estrogen/Progestin Replacement Study follow-up (HERS II). *JAMA*. 2002;288:49–57.

115. Rossouw JE, Anderson GL, Prentice RL, et al.

Risks and benefits of estrogen plus progestin in healthy postmenopausal women: principal results from the Women's Health Initiative randomized controlled trial. *JAMA.* 2002;288: 321–333.

116. Biondi B, Palmieri E, Lombardi G, et al. Effects of subclinical thyroid dysfunction on the heart. *Ann Intern Med.* 2002;137:904–914.

117. Parle JV, Maisonneuve P, Sheppard MC, et al. Prediction of all-cause mortality and cardiovascular mortality in elderly people from one low thyrotropin result: a 10-year cohort study. *Lancet.* 2001;358:861–865.

118. Toft A, Beckett G. Thyroid-function tests and hypothyroidism [editorial]. *BMJ.* 2003;326:295–296.

119. Onitsuka T. Sex hormones in papillary carcinoma of the thyroid gland and pleomorphic adenoma of parotid gland. *Acta Otolaryngol.* 1994; 114:218–222.

120. Adlersberg M, Burrow G. Focus on primary care: thyroid function and dysfunction in women. *Obstet Gynecol Surv.* 2002;57(supple 3):S1–S7.

121. Alder MA, Lobo R. Estrogen replacement therapy alters immune competence in postmenopausal women. Abstracts of oral and poster presentation: abstract 34. The Pacific Coast Fertility Society; Birmingham, AL; April 1995; American Society for Reproductive Medicine.

122. Porter VR, Greendale GA, Schocken M. Immune effects of hormone replacement in postmenopausal women. *Exp Gerontol.* 2001;36(2): 311–326.

123. Wen Y, Doyle MC, Harrison RF, Feely J. The effect of hormone replacement therapy on vitamin E status in postmenopausal women. *Am J Epidemiol.* 1996;144:612–644.

124. Reubinoff BE, Wurtman J, Rojansky N, et al. Effects of hormone replacement therapy on weight, body composition, fat distribution and food intake in early postmenopausal women: a prospective study. *Fertil Steril.* 1995;64:963–968.

125. Hartmann BW, Kirchengasts, Albrecht E, et al. Altered growth hormone secretion in women gaining weight during hormone replacement therapy. *Maturitas.* 1996;276:1747–1751.

126. Irvin JH, Domar AD, Clark C, et al. The effects of relaxation response training on menopausal symptoms. *J Psychosom Obstet Gynaecol.* 1996;17: 202–207.

127. Wijma K, Melin A, Nedstrand E, Hammar M. Treatment of menopausal symptoms with applied relaxation: a pilot study. *J Behav Ther Exp Psychiatry.* 1997;28:251–261.

128. Halas M. Hypnosis for the many faces of menopause: enhancing normal development and treating trauma-related disruptions. In: Hornyak L, Green J, eds. *Healing from Within.* Washington, DC: American Psychological Association; 2002.

129. Herrington DM, Howard TD, Hawkins GA, et al. Estrogen-receptor polymorphisms and effects of estrogen replacement on high-density lipoprotein cholesterol in women with coronary disease. *N Engl J Med.* 2002;346:967–974.

130. Tribble DL, Krauss RM. HDL and coronary artery disease. *Adv Intern Med.* 1993;38:1–29.

CHAPTER 35

Integrative Approach
to Geriatrics

LEWIS MEHL-MADRONA, ROBERT SCHILLER, AND KENNETH MERCER

Geriatrics presents unique opportunities for integrated care. Unlike the other fields of medicine, geriatrics has few diseases not shared with the other branches of medicine. Even the difficulties found among extended care patients are not unique to geriatrics. Patients with spinal injuries share the bowel and bladder difficulties of immobilization. Teenagers with anorexia can experience osteoporosis, although it is more common among the elderly. All ages can be visually or hearing impaired. All ages can experience dementia, delirium, and confusion. Geriatric patients (generally defined as those over age 65) do share the tendency for more than one organ system to be impaired, complicating their care over the younger person with only one compromised system. Because of the synergy in organ system breakdown, the need for discussion of integration of care and synergy of healing is warranted. The art of geriatrics is to use the least toxic and simplest interventions to protect and promote health; this is also the essence of integrative medicine.

Geriatrics requires complete assessments. Quality of life for the aged includes mental, physical, familial, social, and spiritual elements, all of which must be integrated. Geriatric assessment must examine the nutritional life of the aged; their supplements and herbal intake; medication intake; interactions among herbs, drugs, and supplements; movement and exercise; social restrictions; presence or absence of community; family conflict, resources, and relationships; spiritual beliefs and resources; relationship strain; cognitive impairment; functional independence; abilities to carry out activities of daily life; and issues regarding purpose and meaning. The geriatric practitioner must be truly integrated—treating body, mind, family, and spirit.

Aging has changed in modern times. Descriptions by early European explorers of aging in Native America paint a picture of a better nourished, more vigorous, more respected elder than today.[1] These early descriptions portray a role for the elder that was full of meaning and purpose—essential to longevity and well-being.[2] The challenge of geriatrics is more than the reduction of symptoms and the prevention of disease. It must include the restoration of meaning, purpose, and dignity to aging, a task shared by psychiatry, but not by many of the other conventional medical specialties. This challenge can only be met by revisioning the practice of medicine through the eyes of complex systems theory in which the whole equals more than the sum of its parts.[3] Through this lens, aging is a complex psychobiosocial and spiritual process that is inextricably linked to every other aspect of society and culture. Accomplishing this task requires a change in the assumptions by which conventional medicine is now practiced.[4]

One of the few remaining contemporary examples of indigenous cultures' treatment of aging comes from the hunter-gatherer societies of the Inglalik people of Alaska, representing a material culture in which the elderly were deeply honored, integral members of the society. The Inglalik strongly promoted and supported cooperation and mutual dependence among men and women, young and old. Their primary foods and sources of materials for artifacts were wild species. Manufacturing involved hand labor and individual skills applied to locally available raw materials. Little differentiation existed in social roles by age or sex.[5] Meaning and purpose was not denied to the elderly through forced retirement. Rather, elders were venerated for their knowledge of habitats, weather patterns, and memory of recent and remote events. One might, in such a setting, anticipate fewer "diseases of meaning," for example, cancer, heart disease, and depression. Skeletal remains largely confirm the absence of modern degenerative diseases among these people. The context and the larger community system affects the health of the individual.

Integrative geriatrics, therefore, is the treatment of systems—humans, families, and communities—with multiple modalities and levels of entry, including nutritional, energetic, physical, psychological, molecular, familial, community, and spiritual. Its goal is to reduce suffering and to promote well-being among the elderly by whatever means possible while limiting side effects. If movement therapies, for example, decrease falls, we can better prevent the morbidity related to osteoporosis. Thus the ideal approach is a prevention-oriented practice that includes a balanced life with proper nutrition, exercise, movement, meditation, self-exploration, and spiritual practice.

Integrative geriatrics is also concerned with the process of care, specifically addressing the relationship and the language between the provider and the patient. For example, how does the doctor understand a specific patient's experience of aging, and make recommendations consistent with that patient's beliefs? How do patient expectations affect outcome? How does the culture within which treatment occurs encourage or discourage a therapeutic response? Because of the many potential organ system weaknesses incipient to geriatrics and the existence of other specialists for each of these organ systems, geriatrics must necessarily concern itself with the health and healing of the person and family rather than any narrow focus on a specific disease in a particular organ. It must focus on restoring health more than treating disease, compatible with the World Health Organization's definition of health as "a state of complete physical, mental, and social well-being and not merely the absence of disease or infirmity."[6] Multidisciplinary, special-care geriatric teams[7] and end-of-life programs to optimize quality of life in hospice care represent conventional medical attempts to be integrative and to maintain health more than just treat disease.[8]

As we did in the discussion of integrative psychiatry (see Chap. 28), we can draw parallels from indigenous cultures and from traditional systems of healing, for our further understanding of integrative geriatrics. Cherokee medicine, as discussed earlier, for example, included seven major categories of healing, each reflecting a separate, but interactive, and therefore synergistic, level of intervention. Depending on the severity of an illness, anywhere from one to all seven of these levels might be addressed as part of the treatment plan. An understanding of humans as existing within larger systems including family and community, and of the potential for synergy between different levels of healing are intrinsic to this approach.

Traditional Chinese medicine operates within similar principles. Chinese treatments seek balance, harmony, and proper energy flow throughout the person. Systemic patterns of dysfunction are diagnosed, leading to person-centered treatment more than disease-specific treatment. Cherokee medicine seeks to restore balance and harmony through correcting imbalances in relationships among all the above-mentioned levels. This correction is termed restoring "right relationship." Other indigenous healing systems (Ayurvedic and African, for example) and homeopathy share this focus on systemwide diagnosis and treatment, falling outside of any conventional biomedical framework.[9,10]

Homeopathy, in particular, is well suited for the elderly, because it has virtually no side effects. The constitutional remedies, in particular, are similar conceptually to what psychology has termed temperaments, or Jungian analysts call archetypes. The principles which govern selection of constitutional remedies in homeopathy are discussed in depth in Chapter 12 and will not be reviewed here. In one case example from the author's (LMM) practice the homeopathic remedy natrum muriaticum (nat mur) was prescribed to an elderly patient who was failing to thrive. No specific medical diagnosis stood out as the single cause of his ennui, although multiple organ systems were operating at reduced efficiency. Suppressed grief was evident in his story, along with a general tendency to avoid emotion. Although everyone around him felt sadness as he discussed his wife's lingering illness and death, he was unaware of feeling any sadness at all. (The keynote—the homeopathic archetype which corresponds to the remedy—for prescribing nat mur is suppressed emotion.) We found that he had a tendency toward addictions: excess drinking at one time in his life, coupled with tobacco addictions, and even television addictions. As is common with what homeopaths call "nat mur constitution," he had a rebellious streak, manifesting in the past as war protests and a certain unconventionality in his lifestyle and dress. In selecting his constitutional remedy, we were only pe-

ripherally interested in the specific organ system manifestations of his condition—his arthritis, the status of his kidneys, his level of dementia, how much he was wheezing—although all of these were important in his overall geriatric assessment. By treating him from the whole-person perspective of homeopathy, giving him nat mur improved all of these areas of function progressively and helped him maintain a higher level of health than he had previously demonstrated. Chinese medicine and Ayurvedic medicine are similarly holistic in their approach to the elderly patient, and could have easily been substituted for homeopathy in this case.

Chinese, Native American, Ayurvedic, and other indigenous systems of healing share with integrative geriatrics the idea that a given disease may manifest spiritually as well physically.[11,12] This view holds that the most effective interventions must address the spiritual disturbance as a source for the physical manifestation.[13] Integrative geriatrics proposes that the origins of disease are multifactorial more than hierarchical, and include genetic, physical, emotional, psychological, environmental, socioeconomic, *and* spiritual contributions. This does not necessarily emphasize spirituality as root cause. Integrative geriatrics assumes that the individual has the potential for healing at the spiritual level, even when physical curing does not take place.[14,15] This differs from conventional geriatrics, which has largely confined itself to the primary domain of the physical manifestations of disease.

Synergy

Synergy between therapeutic interventions and between the different "levels of healing" plays a critical role in integrative geriatrics. For example, a home-based intervention for depression by a psychogeriatric team provided more benefit than what was found for medication alone.[16] The team provided an individualized package of care optimized for each client, focused upon problem-solving psychotherapy, development of social support, and community intervention. Fifty-eight percent of the intervention group recovered as compared with only 25% of the control group. Even after controlling for possible confounders in logistic regression analysis, patients of the geriatric team were nine times more likely to recover than were patients receiving only medication alone. The odds of recovering with medication alone was only 0.3. Critical human elements of what the geriatric team did, above and beyond its use of medications, contributed to patient improvement, emphasizing the importance of the human aspect of care.

▶ FALLS AND FALL PREVENTION

We have chosen falls and fall prevention as an area of geriatrics not discussed elsewhere in this book, and exemplifying the multi-focused, integrative nature of geriatrics.

Functional independence is a hallmark of successful aging. Elderly individuals with compromised physical function are limited in their ability to participate fully in society.[17] Falls among the elderly contribute to reduced function, impaired mobility, injury, extensive hospital stays, premature nursing home admission, and even death, related in part to the greater fragility of bones among the elderly (osteoporosis and osteopenia).[18–21] Falls can be considered signs of more complex processes that represent "symptoms and signs of disordered functions in a disordered environment."[22]

Nearly one-third of elderly individuals older than age 65 years fall each year,[23–26] and of those who reach age 80 years, approximately 50% will fall in a given year and half again will do so repeatedly.[27] Falls cause most of the deaths from unintentional injury among geriatric populations, with at least 10% suffering serious injuries.[28] One percent of falls cause hip fractures, and 90% of hip fractures are a result of falls.[29] Considering that approximately 280,000 hip fractures occur annually in the United States among those older than age 65 years, the associated morbidity, complications, and costs are substantial.[30] Falls may be responsible for up to 6% of all medical costs for this population.[31]

Loss of confidence in the performance of daily activities is a logical consequence of falls, especially for those who repeatedly fall.[32] Fear of falling may precipitate a vicious cycle of isolation, further restriction of activity, and increased risk of falls and fractures because of instability.[33,34] Falls represent significant predictors for admission to long-term care facilities[35] with an even greater incidence of falls there than in the community.[36]

Risk Factors for Falls

Falls result from multiple, interacting factors with the risk increasing proportionately to the number of factors. Risk factors include living alone and having inadequate resources for food and necessities; safety hazards in the home (e.g., loose rugs, defects in the floor, slippery surfaces, poor lighting, extension cords); outdoor safety hazards (e.g., cracked sidewalks, animals, curbs, inclement weather); ill-fitting footwear; and risk-taking behavior, such as not using assistive devices for ambulation.[37] Intervening in these areas can prevent falls.

Other risk factors for falls include physical changes in eyes, ears, feet, muscles, and joints; medical conditions (heart failure, postural hypotension, arrhythmias, neurologic disorders, dementia, incontinence, arthritis); acute illness; medication use (sedatives, hypnotics, antihypertensives), including multiple interacting medications; alcohol consumption; and functional parameters related to muscle strength, gait, balance, mobility, and flexibility.[38] In an examination of risk factors in a community-based elderly population, of the 423 falls deemed to be a result of causes within the person, only 88 were ascribed to a single factor.[39] Correcting these risk factors also prevents falls. When individuals with a history of falls are compared to those with no falls, significant differences are found on measures of balance, leg strength, heel width, and flexibility.[40,41]

Cognitive Impairment and Fall

Fall prevention requires careful assessment of cognitive function and impairment. Assessment of cognitive impairment requires taking a thorough history of the patient's functional status over time.[42,43] We inquire about the patient's independence in functioning and how this has changed over time. Is the patient driving? Is the patient preparing meals? Is the patient able to pay bills? Can the patient take responsibility for appointments and for managing supplements and medications? How has the patient's level of activity changed? Have the declines been gradual or acute? Were there any antecedent events (medical, social, or familial)? For example, family conflict worsens congestive heart failure, presumably through the increased release of catecholamines. Family members need to be included in assessments, because the patient may be unaware of his or her decline.

Clinical assessments, such as the Folstein Mini-Mental Status Examination,[44] are helpful, although they may not detect early dementia[45] or impairment in executive functioning (planning, organizing, judging).[46] A quick assessment of functioning should include the SCOPED for safety procedure, in which the patient is checked for *spend* (Are finances being handled appropriately?), *cook* (Does the patient leave the stove on or water running?), *operate a car* (ask about driving accidents and incidents; consider driving evaluation), *pills* (Can the patient follow health care instructions for medications, supplements, and other forms of self-care?), *everyday activities* (safety in ambulating, dressing, toileting, and bathing), and *decisions* (competence in decision making and exercise of judgment).[47,48]

Delirium leads to falls, and the most common causes of delirium are metabolic encephalopathies and drug intoxications.[49] Delirium can be mild, and can wax and wane. At its worst point, falls are more likely. At its best point, the patient appears entirely normal, even to family. One of the greatest services of integrative medicine for the elderly is the replacement of delirium-producing medications with gentler herbs and vitamins that produce sufficient clinical effect for symptom relief. The most common medications that precede both delirium and falls include narcotics, sedative-hypnotics, and anticholinergics.[50]

Elsewhere in this volume (see Chapter 26) a number of nonnarcotic therapies for pain relief have been described, including hypnosis, biofeedback, neurofeedback, meditation, Qigong, acupuncture, St. John's wort, and Reiki. The use of integrative principles and therapies to reduce pain and narcotic consumption also prevents falls and fosters functional independence. Sedative-hypnotics are commonly used for anxiety. In Chap. 28 on psychiatric disorders, a number of procedures and supplements are proposed to reduce anxiety, and therefore the consumption of medications, thereby preventing falls. Anticholinergics are commonly used for symptom relief, especially of digestive symptoms, where integrative medicine also offers hope (see Chap. 21). Sleeping medications often have anticholinergic properties; these can be avoided with valerian, melatonin, and biofeedback offering help with sleeplessness (see Chapter 28). Other common delirium-producing drugs that can be replaced by gentler alternatives include cimetidine (aloe vera gel, slippery elm), steroids (omega-3 fatty acids, glucosamine-chondroitin-methylsulfonylmethane, other fatty acids), nonsteroidal antiinflammatory drugs (glucosamine; beta-glucan), salicylates *(Ginkgo biloba)*, and antispasmodics (food allergy elimination, digestive enzymes).

Important metabolic causes of delirium and of falling include abnormal thyroid function, electrolyte imbalance, dehydration, hyperglycemia, hypoglycemia, hypoxia, acute blood loss, and end-stage organ failure.[51] By attending to adequate nutrition and appropriate supplementation of minerals and vitamins, the integrative approach can help prevent these metabolic disturbances as well, particularly given the high prevalence of poor nutrition in the elderly.

Blood Pressure and Falls

Falls are often related to blood pressure changes. Sudden falls in blood pressure can lead to orthostatic hypotension, a common precursor of passing out and falling. Arteriosclerosis makes arteries more rigid and less able to readily adjust to changing conditions that require changes in blood pressure as manifested in tension of the arterial wall. Besides the conventional treatment for stroke prevention in the face of small vessel disease (antiplatelet therapies, including aspirin, ticlopidine, clopidogrel, and dipyridamole), reduction of blood pressure is important for stroke prevention. Medications used to reduce blood pressure can contribute to falls. Applying integrative strategies to control hypertension with reduced dosages of these medications can reduce the incidence of postural hypotension and other complications, also reducing falls.

Falls can also occur from transient ischemic attacks, for which conventional medicine has few preventive therapies other than the antiplatelet inhibitors. The integrative approach can add to transient ischemic attack prevention. *Gingko biloba* may prevent cerebral ischemia and transient ischemic attacks.[52,53] Qigong, which emphasizes tranquil mind, relaxed body, and smooth breathing, lowers blood pressure along with its other benefits of increased social interaction and of building self-confidence.[54] Comprehensive stress management programs, including biofeedback and home blood pressure monitoring, can help reduce the need for medication.[55] A machine that trains a person to breathe slowly and regularly is effective in reducing blood pressure[56]; breathing slowly for just 10 minutes daily with this device, in conjunction with music, significantly lowers blood pressure.[57]

Sleep Disorders and Falls

Lack of sleep has more profound consequences among geriatric populations. Insomnia predisposes to confusion and to unmasking incipient dementia. Sleeplessness lowers the threshold for expression of delirium and dementia, and increases coordination difficulties and disorientation, both of which predispose directly to falls. A number of integrative therapies can help to improve sleep, and thereby reduce falls. Valerian and kava kava both produce decreased sleep onset time and promote deeper sleep.[58] German chamomile, lavender, hops, lemon balm, and passion flower are reputed to be mild sedatives, but need further experimental confirmation.[59] Two hundred two outpatients, aged 18 to 73 years and diagnosed with nonorganic insomnia were treated in a multicenter, double-blind, randomized parallel group comparison with either valerian extract LI 156 (Sedonium) 600 mg/d or oxazepam 10 mg/d taken for 6 weeks. Mean duration of insomnia was 3.5 months at baseline. Valerian was equivalent to oxazepam.[60]

In another study, the hypnotic effect and safety of *Valeriana edulis* standardized extract 450 mg was evaluated in patients with insomnia in a double-blind, crossover, placebo-controlled study. Polysomnographic (PSG) recordings were performed to analyze the quantity and architecture of sleep; morning sleepiness, memory quotient, and side effects were also evaluated. The experimental procedures were conducted on four consecutive nights of 8 hours each. Twenty patients were admitted to the sleep unit. Based on the PSG results, *V. edulis* reduced the number of awakening episodes while both treatments, *V. edulis* and control (including *V. officinalis*, a control), increased the rapid eye movement (REM) sleep. This last parameter was better improved by *V. officinalis* extract. Other PSG data did not achieve outstanding statistical differences, but the clinical tendency with both treatments was to increase the sleep efficiency index. The *Valeriana* extracts produced beneficial effects on sleep architecture because they diminished the time of stages 1 and 2 in non-REM sleep while they increased delta sleep. Validated clinical tests showed that both species of *Valeriana* reduced morning sleepiness, and did not affect anterograde memory. In only three cases were slight side effects observed, one a result of the experimental extract.[61] Biofeedback and mindfulness-based stress-reduction practices have also been successfully used for insomnia.[62]

Impaired Vision and Falls

Impaired vision is often a significant contributor to falls. Impairment can arise from glaucoma, macular degeneration, and cataracts, among other causes. Fall prevention through integrative therapies for visual maintenance and improvement can be very effective.

Higher intake of carotenoids, including lutein and zeaxanthin (found in dark-green, leafy vegetables such as spinach and collard greens) may reduce progression of macular degeneration.[63] Increased intake of fruits and vegetables contributes to a reduction in macular degeneration progression as well,[64] as do combinations of antioxidants, including selenium 600 mg, vitamin E 1.2 g, vitamin B_6 80 mg, vitamin B_2 15 mg, and vitamin C 2 g daily, all taken over a 5 month period.[65] In another study of macular degeneration and antioxidants, a daily dose of vitamin C (500 mg), vitamin E (400 IU), beta-carotene (9 mg), and selenium (250 µg) halted or improved the degenerative changes in 60% of subjects tested.[66] Clearly there is a role for antioxidant supplementation in treatment and prevention of macular degeneration, although the exact dose needed remains unclear.

Vitamins C[67] and E[68] may be helpful in patients with cataracts. Multivitamins did not further reduce the risk in one study,[69] but did in another.[70] As for glaucoma, supplementation with cod liver oil decreased mean intraocular pressure in patients with this condition.[71] Mag-

nesium supplementation (122 mg BID as Magnesiocard granules) also slowed progression.[72,73] Zinc may also have a role in treatment of glaucoma.[74]

Osteoporosis and Falls

Falls are significant because of osteoporosis, which renders bones brittle and more likely to break from small injuries. Prevention of osteoporosis—discussed in detail in Chapter 24—reduces the direct damage caused by falls, but may also stop falls by providing a restored sense of strength, vitality, and confidence.

In addition to ensuring adequate intake of calcium and vitamin D, and encouraging adequate weight-bearing exercise, a number of other nutritional measures may be helpful in treatment of osteoporosis. Reduction of grain intake, which can interfere with calcium absorption in some patients, can be helpful,[75,76] as can reducing the amount of sodium in the diet.[77] Increasing magnesium is critical to bone health,[78,79] as is supplementing vitamin D.[80] Diagnosing and treating celiac disease, which increases intestinal losses of fat-soluble minerals and vitamins, especially calcium and vitamin D, is helpful.[81] Avoiding nicotine[82–84] is important, as is avoiding phosphoric acid, as found in soft drinks.[85,86] Calcium supplementation, as well as the importance of trace minerals and other micronutrients such as boron, strontium, and vitamin K, is discussed in detail in Chapter 24.

Osteoarthritis and Falls

Arthritis of all kinds affects joint mobility and the ability to balance and move. Restoration of joint function and stability can help prevent falls. Current therapies for osteoarthritis include the use of orthoses, physical therapy, treatment of depression, patient education,[87] monthly telephone calls from lay personnel,[88] and drugs given systemically or intraarticularly.

Drugs for osteoarthritis are classified as either symptomatic or structure-modulating, based on their mechanism of action.[89] Symptomatic drugs include analgesics and nonsteroidal antiinflammatory drugs (NSAIDs), which have a fast onset and short duration of action, and slow-acting drugs, whose lasting beneficial effects on pain and function require several months to develop and can persist for some time after treatment discontinuation.[90,91] Slow-acting drugs may help to reduce the need for analgesics and NSAIDs, which are commonly responsible for adverse effects. A number of nutritional interventions may possibly serve this function safely in elderly patients with osteoarthritis.

Avocado/Soybean Unsaponifiables

Fatty acids, including avocado/soybean unsaponifiable (ASU) mixture, may be active in osteoarthritis. In vitro, ASU inhibited interleukin-1 and stimulated collagen production in articular chondrocyte cultures.[92] The deleterious effects of interleukin-1 on human synovial cells were partly prevented, and those on articular chondrocytes from rabbits were abolished.[93] Another in vitro effect was inhibition of interleukin-1β–induced stimulation of the production of stromelysin, interleukins 6 and 8, prostaglandin E_2, and collagenase.[94] In vivo, ASU prevented the occurrence of joint lesions in a rabbit postcontusive model of osteoarthritis.[95] An open study in patients with knee or hip osteoarthritis showed a good safety profile and suggested symptomatic efficacy after 2 months.[96] In a 6-month, randomized, double-blind, placebo-controlled study, significant improvements in conventional symptomatic efficacy criteria were found in the ASU group after 2 months and persisted 2 months after treatment discontinuation.[97]

Niacinamide

Seventy-two patients with osteoarthritis were treated with niacinamide 500 mg six times daily for 12 weeks or with a placebo in double-blind fashion. In the niacinamide group, global arthritis impact improved 29% ($p < .05$), joint mobility increased significantly, sedimentation rate fell 22% ($p < .005$), and NSAID intake was reduced 13% ($p = .01$), compared to no changes in the placebo group.[98]

S-Adenosyl Methionine

S-adenosyl methionine (SAMe) has been used on more than 22,000 osteoarthritis patients.[99] In one double-blind trial, SAMe (1,200 mg/d) was as effective as naproxen in 676 patients with osteoarthritis of the hips and knees.[100] The onset of action is slower than that of NSAIDs, and the benefits persisted longer than NSAIDs when they were stopped. SAMe also improves depression, which is another contributor to falling.

Vitamin D

In a study of 516 subjects, those consuming 400 IU/d of vitamin D were two- to fourfold less likely to have serious osteoarthritis knee disease than were those consuming less than 170 IU/d.[101] From 1983 to 1985, 516 subjects were seen; they were rechecked in 1992–1993 as part of the Framingham study follow-up. The relative risk for progression of osteoarthritis in the lower tertile versus the upper tertile for vitamin D intake was 4.0 ($p = .009$), and for serum vitamin D levels at baseline, 2.9 ($p = .05$). In those with disease at baseline, the relative risk for loss of cartilage by comparison radiographs in the lowest tertile compared to the highest was 2.3 (95% confidence interval [CI], 0.9–5.5), and for osteophyte growth it was 3.1 (95% CI, 1.3–7.5).

Movement Therapies for Reduction of Risk Factors

A multiple-risk-factor intervention strategy among elderly individuals in the community, which involved exercise programs, behavioral training, medication adjustments, and environmental changes, demonstrated significant risk factor reduction when compared with a control group that did not receive the intervention.[102] The risk of falling decreased by 11% in the intervention group, which was significant. The greatest and most significant differences between the two groups lay among those subjects with impairments in balance or transfer skills. In a study assessing the contributions of resistance (or strength), balance, and gait training to a reduction in fall risk factors in a population of community elderly individuals, subjects were randomly assigned to a strength and balance/gait group or a strength and relaxation training control group. The authors measured strength, static balance, and dynamic balance, finding that the addition of balance training was responsible for a significant improvement in balance-related tasks among intervention group participants.[103]

Tai Chi

Conventional means for preventing falls focus primarily on muscle strengthening, balance improvement, and enhancement of lower extremity flexibility. Tai chi is a low-intensity movement exercise of Oriental origin, practiced in China for centuries, and recently transposed to Western society. Tai chi, which is also discussed in Chapter 11, is short for tai chi chuan a traditional Chinese exercise developed centuries ago as a martial arts form to ward off foreign invaders.[104,105] In China, persons of all ages have practiced tai chi since then, especially elderly individuals, as an art form, religious ritual, relaxation technique, exercise, and form of self-defense.[106] During the past century, tai chi has been promoted in China and, more recently in the West, for the improvement and maintenance of health, as well as the treatment of chronic illness.[107]

Traditional Chinese geriatrics—in which tai chi practice plays an important role—focuses on the preventive elements of the human–nature and the mind–body relationships.[108] Harmony between man and nature requires a coordination of one's daily activities with the seasons and with one's circadian rhythm. Integration of the mind and body demands moderation in

physical and emotional activities and the practice of moderate exercise.[109] In particular, exercises like tai chi, which encompass both mental and physical elements, facilitate a peaceful and serene mind during the performance of gentle and flexible movements. Its movements are thought to stimulate the flow of chi (vital energy, or life-giving force) through the body's energy meridians. Restoring balance and vitality to the energy body (as manifested in the meridians) can slowly but surely restore balance and vitality to the physical body, sometimes curing illness.[110] Tai chi is sometimes called "moving meditation" because a goal is to banish extraneous thoughts and to focus upon relaxation, balance, and harmony.[111] The process of tai chi is an embodiment of an integrated mind–body approach to healing.

Chinese studies report that tai chi practitioners experience less osteoporosis and spinal deformity, better spinal flexibility, greater vital capacity, lower resting blood pressure, and better cardiovascular response to exercise than do nonpractitioners.[112,113] Long-time practitioners (more than 6 years) age 50–64 years had significantly higher maximum oxygen consumption, O_2 pulse, and work rate responses to maximal exercise testing than did sedentary controls.[114] Similar results were found in an older age group (66–80 years),[115] and in another group of people ranging in age from 58–70 years.[116] Among postmyocardial infarction males ranging in age from 39–80 years, tai chi resulted in decreases in systolic and diastolic blood pressures.[117] Resting blood pressure, both systolic and diastolic, fell significantly in two studies of healthy, elderly people,[118,119] but nonsignificantly in a third study.[120]

A cross-sectional study comparing long-time elderly tai chi practitioners with elderly sedentary individuals showed significantly higher trunk flexibility among the tai chi group.[121] A year-long tai chi program for older adults resulted in significant improvements in thoracolumbar flexibility as compared to controls.[122] Joint flexibility in the knees and shoulders improved significantly after only a 12-week program compared to a control group.[123] Trunk and hamstring flexibility and total body flexibility was significantly better among long-time elderly male practitioners of tai chi than for a sedentary control group,[124] but a 10-week program of a Westernized version of tai chi did not have an effect on naive subjects.[125]

Tai chi has been useful in rheumatoid arthritis and osteoarthritis to improve general arthritis symptoms, reduce pain, decrease joint swelling, and increase joint mobility.[126,127] Range of Motion Dance, a program based on tai chi principles, increased joint flexibility among individuals with chronic conditions that limit movement. In another study, tai chi subjects performed significantly better on single-leg standing tasks with eyes closed in comparison to nonpractitioners.[128] Tai chi practitioners of 2–35 years experience showed significantly better balance results than did a control group of active elderly individuals under more complicated conditions of visual, vestibular, and proprioceptive disturbances.[129]

Tai chi training substantially reduced the rate of falls by 47.5% after 4 months follow-up with conventional therapies having no effect.[130] Tai chi also resulted in significantly decreased fear of falling (when compared with controls), as well as a reduction in blood pressure and an increased sense of being able to do all that one would like to do. Tai chi was also associated with less fear of falling, though postural stability improved less than with conventional therapies.[131]

Among a small group of community-dwelling elderly persons, when flexibility training and balance exercises in a control group were compared to a combination of resistance training, walking, flexibility training, and balance exercises (including tai chi movements), the treatment group showed a 17% improvement (only trending toward significance) in a measure of balance at posttest, as compared to no appreciable change by the control group.[132] A different study of 24 months duration recruited participants from within two long-term

care facilities who were able to ambulate, and randomized them to one of three groups: resistance/endurance plus basic enhanced programming, tai chi plus basic enhanced programming, and a control group consisting of basic enhanced programming alone.[133] Participants were equally satisfied with the two exercise regimens without statistically significant differences in fall outcome measures among the three groups. Overall adherence was low (approximately 40%) and many participants were at least mildly cognitively impaired (although initially screened for ability to follow simple directions), which may have affected their ability to fully participate in tai chi.

Both balance training and overall exercise were significant for fall reduction (incidence ratios 0.83 and 0.90, respectively) in a multicenter trial, with resistance, endurance, and flexibility training showing trends toward less falls. One site of this large study (the Frailty and Injuries: Cooperative Studies on Intervention Techniques trials) used tai chi as a form of dynamic balance training with pronounced effects on fall outcome parameters.[134]

Spirituality and Falls

Today we see a virtual explosion of interest in examining the implications of spirituality for health in medicine, nursing, psychology, and other disciplines, with a growing impetus to integrate spirituality into conventional conceptions of the person.[135] The occurrence of spiritual experiences is associated with psychological and physical well-being.[136–143] As a consequence, spirituality has been gaining recognition, even within conventional medicine, as a legitimate and important aspect of human functioning, related reliably to health and well-being, even though the mechanism behind that relationship cannot be readily explained.[144,145] Ample evidence supports an association of psychological functioning with measures of religious commitment.[146] Religious behavior (for example, church attendance) is a highly reliable predictor of health and well-being.[117] Analytic literature surveys and meta-analyses of some or all of the more than 1,100 relevant studies suggest that spirituality and associated constructs/phenomena like religiousness, spiritual beliefs, and practices, are positively related to health and longevity.[118,119] Spirituality appears to be robustly associated with lower levels of substance abuse, depression, and suicide, with improved treatment outcomes and higher levels of life satisfaction and general well-being.[150] Meaning and purpose in life are central to many extant models and measures of spirituality,[151–153] and have been proposed as one of the main mechanisms through which spirituality affects health and well-being.

Boredom and boredom proneness are negatively associated with perceived meaning and purpose in life[151–158] and self-actualization.[159] Among retired persons, boredom was associated with ill health.[160] Transforming boredom is therefore a potential means to improve geriatric health. One of the means for this transformation is through volunteerism. Spiritual development and spiritual practice derived activities (e.g., feeding the homeless) provide important avenues for the transformation of boredom. The research has yet to be done to explore the relationship between boredom and falls, but we suspect that the relationship exists. Boredom arises in the absence of purpose and meaning and self-actualization. Therefore, geriatrics must cultivate these traits.

Recovery from Hip Fracture

When falls do occur and fractures result, improving their rate of healing is paramount. Patients with femoral neck fractures randomized

---

▶ Case Example: Integrative Geriatrics

How might integrative geriatrics work in practice? Consider Ms. Howard, an elderly diabetic patient. First, we consider her diabetes. Could she exercise more? The integrative approach, acknowledging the barriers to exercise in her age group, might recommend an "exercise buddy." Exercise buddies are very effective for encouraging each other. Group exercise programs facilitate social interaction and also bolster the motivation of individual patients. Tai chi and Qigong might be considered as exercise strategies that add meditation and energy healing to movement practices. Reducing grains and sugars in the diet improves diabetic control. Supplements such as fenugreek may improve carbohydrate metabolism. Higher dose antioxidants prevent diabetic complications, including retinopathy, nephropathy, and neuropathy. A dementia assessment for Ms. Howard reveals mild impairment. *Ginkgo biloba* is often helpful in early dementia, along with vitamin E in higher dosages (2,000 IU daily). Naturalistic behavior therapy can be used to shape behavior through natural environmental consequences. One possible cause of dementia is medication. We ask what medications can be reduced or eliminated. For example, the use of an antihistamine for sleep, common among the elderly, can often add to daytime confusion. Ms. Howard is on high-dose NSAIDs. We know that these drugs, even the newer versions like Vioxx, are potentially associated with risk of ulcer. Replacing NSAIDs with glucosamine/chondroitin, which is effective for joint pain, may allow safer control of her arthritis pain. Movement therapies may also be helpful for the various musculoskeletal disorders, as well as to reduce her risk of falls.

to receiving a daily comprehensive vitamin and mineral supplement achieved a favorable outcome 56% of the time, as compared to 13% for those patients who were not supplemented ($p < 0.05$).[161] The death and complication rate in the supplemented group was 44% versus 87% in the control group. Length of hospital stay was 24 days versus 40 days in the control group ($p < .02$). Six-month all-cause mortality was 24% among those supplemented, and 37% among control patients. Another study supplemented elderly patients with femoral neck fractures with protein, calcium, vitamin A, and vitamin D resulting in 79% favorable outcomes compared to 36% without protein, and a lower percentage without any supplementation.[162] Mean hospital stay was 69 days for protein supplementation and 102 days without.

▶ CONCLUSION

As the aging population increases, living longer and more active lives, the challenges in their medical care become more complex. Surgery and medications are used more aggressively in the elderly, as people have more active lives in their late seventies and eighties. However, the goals of care in geriatrics require a balance between optimizing the quality of life and minimizing the disabilities often associated with treatments. The approach of integrative geriatrics can assist the practitioner in achieving this balance with its wide range of therapeutic choices and its emphasis on emotional well-being and spirituality. The practitioner can educate the older patient about prioritizing choices in nutrition, herbs, homeopathy, and movement therapy, collaboratively developing a plan for starting with the more appealing or accessible treatments. Coping with a culture that currently fails to value the wisdom of its older citizens is another crucial role for the practitioner. Assisting these patients to engage in personally meaningful social activities will be of enormous value in minimizing boredom, isolation, and depression. The discussion of spirituality between the patient and the practitioner may be the most important intervention, and it elevates the quality of the relationship between them. The spiritual practice may vary considerably from traditional religious practice to a more individual meditation. However, assisting our patients in making the connections between their health and their spirit as they confront their mortality may be our greatest gift.

REFERENCES

1. Mehl-Madrona L. Native American medicine: herbal pharmacology, therapies, and elder care. In: Selin H, ed. *Medicine Across Cultures: The History of Non-Western Medicine*. Lancaster, UK: Kluwer; 2003:253–270.
2. Cunningham AJ, Edmonds CVI, Jenkins GP. A randomized controlled trial of the effects of group psychological therapy on survival in women with metastatic breast cancer. *Psychooncology*. 1998;7: 508–517.
3. Bell IR, Caspi O, Schwartz GER, et al. Integrative medicine and systemic outcomes research: issues in the emergence of a new model for primary health care. *Arch Intern Med*. 2002;162: 133–140.
4. Zollman C, Vickers A. What is complementary medicine? *BMJ*. 1999;319:693–696.
5. Mehl-Madrona L. Native American medicine: herbal pharmacology, therapies, and elder care. In: Selin H, ed. *Medicine Across Cultures: The History of Non-Western Medicine*. Lancaster, UK: Kluwer; 2003:253–270.
6. World Health Organization. *About WHO: Definition of health*. Available at: http://www.who.int/aboutwho/en/definition.html. Accessed October 9, 2001.
7. Burns R, Nichols LO, Martindale-Adams J, Graney MJ. Interdisciplinary geriatric primary care evaluation and management: two-year outcomes. *J Am Geriatr Soc*. 2000;48:8–13.
8. Bretscher M, Rummans T, Sloan J. Quality of life in hospice patients: a pilot study. *Psychosomatics*. 1999;40:309–313.
9. Ernst E, White A, eds. *Acupuncture: A Scientific Appraisal*. Oxford, England: Butterworth Heinemann; 1998.
10. Ernst E, White AR. Acupuncture for back pain. *Arch Intern Med*. 1998;158:2235–2241.

11. Jonas WB, Levin JS. *Essentials of Complementary and Alternative Medicine.* Philadelphia: Lippincott, Williams, & Wilkins, 1999.

12. Fulder S. *The Handbook of Alternative and Complementary Medicine.* 3rd ed. Oxford, England: Oxford University Press, 1996.

13. Bell IR, Caspi O, Schwartz GER, et al. Integrative medicine and systemic outcomes research: issues in the emergence of a new model for primary health care. *Arch Intern Med.* 2002;162:133–140.

14. Maizes V, Caspi O. The principles and challenges of integrative medicine. *West J Med.* 1999;171: 148–149.

15. Gaudet TW. Integrative medicine. *Integr Med.* 1998;1:67–73.

16. Banerjee S, Shamash K, Macdonald AJ, Mann AH. Randomised controlled trial of effect of intervention by psychogeriatric team on depression in frail elderly people at home. *BMJ.* 1996;313(7064):1058–1061.

17. Mercer KA. Use of tai chi in the elderly as a means for improvement in physical performance and fall prevention. Master's Integrative Project, MPH—Aging Track; 2002. Available from the co-author.

18. Tinetti ME, Williams CS. Falls, injuries due to falls, and the risk of admission to a nursing home. *N Engl J Med.* 1997;337:1279–1284.

19. Rubenstein LZ, Powers CM, MacLean CH. Quality indicators for the management and prevention of falls and mobility problems in vulnerable elders. *Ann Intern Med.* 2001;135:686–693.

20. Rubenstein LZ. Patient education forums. Falls and balance problems. The Foundation for Health in Aging. 2001. Available at: http://www.healthinaging.org/pef/falls_balance.html. Accessed June 16, 2002.

21. Sattin RW. Falls among older persons: a public health perspective. *Annu Rev Public Health.* 1992;13:489–508.

22. Sattin RW. Falls among older persons: a public health perspective. *Annu Rev Public Health.* 1992;13:489–508.

23. Tinetti ME, Speechley M, Ginter SF. Risk factors of falls among elderly persons living in the community. *N Engl J Med.* 1988;319:1701–1707.

24. McElhinney J, Koval KJ, Zuckerman JD. Falls and the elderly. *Arch Am Acad Orthop Surg.* 1998; 2:60–65.

25. Nickens H. Intrinsic factors in falling among the elderly. *Arch Intern Med.* 1985;145:1089–1093.

26. Tinetti ME, Baker DI, McAvay G, et al. A multifactorial intervention to reduce the risk of falling among elderly people living in the community. *N Engl J Med.* 1994;331:821–827.

27. Tinetti ME, Speechley M, Ginter SF. Risk factors of falls among elderly persons living in the community. *N Engl J Med.* 1988;319:1701–1707.

28. Province MA, Hadley EC, Hornbrook MC. The effects of exercise on falls in elderly patients. A preplanned meta-analysis of the FICSIT trials. *JAMA.* 1995;273:1341–1347.

29. McElhinney J, Koval KJ, Zuckerman JD. Falls and the elderly. *Arch Am Acad Orthop Surg.* 1998;2: 60–65.

30. Verfaillie DF, Nichols JF, Turkel E, Hovell MF. Effects of resistance, balance, and gait training on reduction of risk factors leading to falls in elders. *J Aging Phys Act.* 1997;5:213–218.

31. Rubenstein LZ. Patient education forums. Falls and balance problems. The Foundation for Health in Aging. 2001. Available at: http://www.health inaging.org/pef/falls_balance.html. Accessed June 16, 2002.

32. Alexander NB, Edelberg HK. Assessing mobility and preventing falls in older patients. *Patient Care.* 2002;36:18–29.

33. Campbell AJ, Borrie MJ, Spears GF. risk factors for falls in a community-based prospective study of people 70 years and older. *J Gerontol Med Sci.* 1989;44:M112–M117.

34. Petrells RJ. Exercise for older patients with chronic disease. *Physician Sports Med.* 1999;27: 79–104.

35. Tinetti ME, Williams CS. Falls, injuries due to falls, and the risk of admission to a nursing home. *N Engl J Med.* 1997;337:1279–1284.

36. Rubenstein LZ. Patient education forums. Falls and balance problems. The Foundation for Health in Aging. 2001. Available at: http://www.healthinaging.org/pef/falls_balance.html. Accessed June 16, 2002.

37. Norwalk MP, Predergast JM, Bayles CM, D'Amico FJ, Colvin GC. A randomized trial of exercise programs among older individuals living in two long-term care facilities: The Falls FREE Program. *J Am Geriatr Soc.* 2001;49:859–865.

38. Norwalk MP, Predergast JM, Bayles CM, D'Amico FJ, Colvin GC. A randomized trial of exercise programs among older individuals living in two long-term care facilities: The Falls FREE Program. *J Am Geriatr Soc.* 2001;49:859–865.

39. Campbell AJ, Borrie MJ, Spears GF. Risk factors for falls in a community-based prospective study of people 70 years and older. *J Gerontol Med Sci.* 1989;44:M112–M117.

40. Gehlsen GM, Whaley MH. Falls in the elderly: part II, balance, strength, and flexibility. *Arch Phys Med Rehabil.* 1990;71:739–741.

41. Gehlsen GM, Whaley MH. Falls in the elderly: part I, gait. *Arch Phys Med Rehabil.* 1990;71:735–738.

42. Fleming KC, Evans JC, Weber DC, Chutka DS. Practical functional assessment of elderly persons: A primary care approach. *Mayo Clin Proc.* 1995;70:890–910.

43. Chan D, Brennan NJ. Delirium: making the diagnosis, improving the prognosis. *Geriatrics.* 1999;54(3):28–42.

44. Folstein MF, Folstein SE, McHugh PR. Mini-mental state: A practical method of grading cognitive state of patients for the clinicians. *J Psychiatr Res.* 1975;12:189–198.

45. Galasko D, Klauber MR, Hofstetter CR. The mini-mental state examination in the early diagnosis of Alzheimer's disease. *Arch Neurol.* 1990;47: 49–52.

46. Royal D, Cordes J, Polk M. Clox: an executive clock drawing task. *J Neurol Neurosurg Psychiatry.* 1998;64:588–594.

47. Beck J, Freedman M, Warshaw G. Geriatric assessment: focus on function. *Patient Care.* 1994; Feb:12–37.

48. Dohrenwend A, Kusz H, Eckleberry J, Stucky K. Evaluating cognitive impairment in the primary care setting. *Clin Geriatr.* 2003;11(2):21–36.

49. Victor M, Ropper A. The acquired metabolic disorders of the nervous system. In: Victor M, Ropper A, Adams R, eds. *Principles of Neurology.* 7th ed. New York: McGraw-Hill; 2001:1175–1204.

50. Ranjan A. Recognizing delirium in the hospitalized elderly. *FPR/MWR.* 2001;May (special issue):11–18.

51. Dohrenwend A, Kusz H, Eckleberry J, Stucky K. Evaluating cognitive impairment in the primary care setting. *Clin Geriatr.* 2003;11(2):21–36.

52. Calapai G, Crupi A, Firenzuoli F, et al. Neuroprotective effects of ginkgo biloba extract in brain ischemia are mediated by inhibition of nitric oxide synthesis. *Life Sci.* 2000;67(22):2673–2683.

53. Clark WM, Rinker LG, Lessov NS, Lowery SL, Cipolla MJ. Efficacy of antioxidant therapies in transient focal ischemia in mice. *Stroke.* 2001; 32(4):1000–1004.

54. Mayer M. Qigong and hypertension: a critique of research. *J Altern Complement Med.* 1999;5(4): 371–382.

55. Stein F. Occupational stress, relaxation therapies, exercise and biofeedback. *Work.* 2001;17(3): 235–245.

56. Schein MH, Gavish B, Herz M, et al. Treating hypertension with a device that slows and regularises breathing: a randomised, double-blind controlled study. *J Hum Hypertens.* 2001;15(4): 271–278.

57. Grossman E, Grossman A, Schein MH, Zimlichman R, Gavish B. Breathing-control lowers blood pressure. *J Hum Hypertens.* 2001;15(4):263–269.

58. Lewis Mehl-Madrona. Integrative approach to psychiatry. In: Kligler B, Lee R. *Integrative Medicine.* New York: McGraw-Hill; 2004.

59. Gyllenhaal C, Merritt SL, Peterson SD, Block KI, Gochenour T. Efficacy and safety of herbal stimulants and sedatives in sleep disorders. *Sleep Med Rev.* 2000;4(3):229–251.

60. Lewis Mehl-Madrona. Integrative approach to psychiatry. In: Kligler B, Lee R. *Integrative Medicine.* New York: McGraw-Hill; 2004.

61. Herrera-Arellano A, Luna-Villegas G, Cuevas-Uriostegui ML, et al. Polysomnographic evaluation of the hypnotic effect of *Valeriana edulis* standardized extract in patients suffering from insomnia. *Planta Med.* 2001;67(8):695–699.

62. Futterman AD, Shapiro D. A review of biofeedback for mental disorders. *Hosp Community Psychiatry.* 1986;37(1):27–33.

63. Seddon JM, Ajani UA, Sperduto RD, et al. Dietary carotenoids, vitamins A, C, and E, and advanced age-related macular degeneration. Eye Disease Case-Control Study Group. *JAMA.* 1994;272(18): 1413–1420.

64. Goldberg J, Flowerdew G, Smith E, Brody JA, Tso MO. *Am J Epidemiol.* 1988;128(4):700–710.

65. Sommerburg O, Keunen JE, Bird AC, van Kuijk FJ. Fruits and vegetables that are sources for lutein and zeaxanthin: the macular pigment in human eyes. *Br J Ophthalmol.* 1998;82(8):907–910.

66. Christen WG, Ajani UA, Glynn RJ, et al. Prospective cohort study of antioxidant vitamin supplement use and the risk of age-related maculopathy. *Am J Epidemiol.* 1999;149(5):476–484.

67. Valero MP, Fletcher AE, De Stavola BL, Vioque J, Alepuz VC. Vitamin C is associated with reduced risk of cataract in a Mediterranean population. *J Nutr.* 2002;132(6):1299–1306.

68. Gale CR, Hall NE, Phillips DI, Martyn CN. Plasma antioxidant vitamins and carotenoids and age-related cataract. *Ophthalmology.* 2001;108(11): 1992–1998.

69. Kuzniarz M, Mitchell P, Cumming RG, Flood VM. Use of vitamin supplements and cataract: the Blue Mountains Eye Study. *Am J Ophthamol.* 2001;132(1):19–26.

70. Chasan-Taber L, Willett WC, Seddon JM, et al. A prospective study of vitamin supplement intake and cataract extraction among U.S. women. *Epidemiology.* 1999;10(6):679–684.

71. Arnarsson A, Jonasson F, Sasaki H, et al. Risk factors for nuclear lens opacification: the Reykjavik Eye Study. *Dev Ophthalmol.* 2002;35:12–20.

72. Gaspar AZ, Gasser P, Flammer J. The influence of magnesium on visual field and peripheral vasospasm in glaucoma. *Ophthalmologica.* 1995; 209(1):11–13.

73. Johnson S. The multifaceted and widespread pathology of magnesium deficiency. *Med Hypotheses.* 2001;56(2):163–170.

74. Akyol N, Deger O, Keha EE, Kilic S. Aqueous humour and serum zinc and copper concentrations of patients with glaucoma and cataract. *Br J Ophthalmol.* 1990;74(11):661–662.

75. Lindeberg S. Available at: http://maelstrom. stjohns.edu/CGI/wa.exe?A2=ind9706&L= paleodiet&P=850. Accessed January 8, 2003.

76. Cordain L. Cereal grains: humanity's double-edged sword. *World Rev Nutr Diet.* 1999;84:19–73.

77. Lau EM, et al. Nutrition and osteoporosis. *Curr Opin Rheumatol.* 1998;10(4):368–372.

78. Rude RK. Magnesium deficiency: possible role in osteoporosis associated with gluten-sensitive enteropathy. *Osteoporos Int.* 1996;6(6):453–461.

79. Varo P. Mineral element balance and coronary heart disease. *Int J Vit Nutr Res.* 1974;44:267–273.

80. van der Wielen RP. Serum vitamin D concentrations among elderly people in Europe. *Lancet.* 1995;346(8969):207–210.

81. Green P. Unmasking celiac disease. Presented at American Celiac Society Conference; November, 1996.

82. Laroche M. Osteocalcin and smoking. *Rev Rhum Ed Fr.* 1994;61(6):433–436.

83. Broulik PD. The effect of chronic nicotine administration on bone mineral content in mice. *Horm Metab Res.* 1993;25(4):219–221.

84. Ernst E. Smoking, a cause of back trouble? *Br J Rheumatol.* 1993;32(3):239–242.

85. Meinig G. Available at: http://members.aol. com/ppnf/articles/softdrk.html. Accessed January 31, 2003.

86. Lukert BP. Influence of nutritional factors on calcium-regulating hormones and bone loss. *Calcif Tissue Int.* 1987;40(3):119–125.

87. Weinberger M, William MT, Booher P, Katz BP. Can the provision of information to patients with osteoarthritis improve functional status? *Arthritis Rheum.* 1989;32:1577–1583.

88. René J, Weinberger M, Mazzuca SA, Brandt KD, Katzz BP. Reduction of joint pain in patients with knee osteoarthritis who have received monthly telephone calls from lay personnel and whose medical treatment regimens have remained stable. *Arthritis Rheum.* 1992;35:511–515.

89. Altman R, Brandt K, Hockberg M, et al. Design and conduct of clinical trials in patients with osteoarthritis: recommendations from a task force of the Osteoarthritis Research Society. Results of a workshop. *Osteoarthritis Cartilage.* 1996;4:217–243.

90. Lequesne M. Symptomatic slow-acting drugs in osteoarthritis: a novel therapeutic concept? *Rev Rhum [Engl Ed].* 1994;61:69–73.

91. Lequesne M, Maheu E. Traitements anti-arthrosiques. In: Bardin T, Kuntz D, eds. *Thérapeutique Rhumatologique.* Paris: Flammarion-Médecine-Sciences; 1995:95–104.

92. Mauviel A, Aireaux M, Hartmann DJ, Galera P, Loyau G, Pujol JP. Effets des insaponifiables d'avocat et de soja (PIAS) sur la production de collagène par des cultures de synoviocytes, chondrocytes articulaires et fibroblastes dermiques. *Rev Rhum Mal Ostéoartic.* 1989;56:207–211.

93. Mauviel A, Loyau G, Pujol JP. Effet des insaponifiables d'avocat/soja (Piascledine) sur l'activité collagénolytique de cultures de synoviocytes rheumatödes humaines et de chondrocytes articulaires de lapin traités par l'interleukine 1. *Rev Rhum Mal Ostéoartic.* 1991;58: 241–5.

94. Henrotin Y, Labasse A, Zheng SX. Effects of three avocado/soybean unsaponifiable mixtures on human articular chondrocytes metabolism [abstract]. *Arthritis Rheum.* 1996;39:S227.

95. Mazières B, Tempesta C, Tiechard M, Vaguier G. Pathologic and biochemical effects of a lipidic avocado and soya extract on an experimental post-contusive model of OA [abstract]. *Osteoarthritis Cartilage.* 1993;1:46.

96. Maheu E. Les insaponifiables d'avocat-soja dans le traitement de la gonarthrose et de la coxarthrose. *Synoviale.* 1992;9:31–38.

97. Maheu E, Mazières B, Valat JP, et al. Symptomatic efficacy of avocado/soya unsaponifiables the treatment of osteoarthritis of the knee and hip. *Arthritis Rheum.* 1998;41.

98. Jonas WB, Rapoza CP, Blair WF. The effect of niacinamide on osteoarthritis: a pilot study. *Inflamm Res.* 1996;45(7):330–334.

99. di Padova C. S-adenosylmethionine in the treatment of osteoarthritis. Review of the clinical studies. *Am J Med.* 1987;20;83(5A):60–65.

100. Caruso I, Pietrogrande V. Italian double-blind multicenter study comparing S-adenosylmethionine, naproxen, and placebo in the treatment of degenerative joint disease. *Am J Med.* 1987;20; 83(5A):66–71.

101. McAlindon TE, Felson DT, Zhang Y, et al. Relation of dietary intake and serum levels of vitamin D to progression of osteoarthritis of the knee among participants in the Framingham Study. *Ann Intern Med.* 1996;125(5):353–359.

102. Tinetti ME, Baker DI, McAvay G, et al. A multifactorial intervention to reduce the risk of falling among elderly people living in the community. *N Engl J Med.* 1994;331:821–827.

103. Verfaillie DF, Nichols JF, Turkel E, Hovell MF. Effects of resistance, balance, and gait training on reduction of risk factors leading to falls in elders. *J Aging Phys Act.* 1997;5:213–218

104. Wolf SL, Coogler C, Xu T. Exploring the basis for tai chi chuan as a therapeutic exercise approach. *Arch Phys Med Rehabil.* 1997;78:886–892.

105. Kessenich CR. Tai chi as a method of fall Prevention in the elderly. *Orthop Nurs.* 1998;17: 27–29.

106. Chen K-M, Snyder M, Krichbaum K. Clinical use of tai chi in elderly populations. *Geriatr Nurs.* 2001;22:198–200.

107. Sun WY, Dosch M, Gilmore GD, Pemberton W, Scarseth T. Effects of a tai chi chuan program on Hmong American older adults. *Educ Gerontol.* 1996;22:161–167.

108. Da-hong Z. Preventive geriatrics: an overview from traditional Chinese medicine. *Am J Chin Med.* 1982;10:32–39.

109. Da-hong Z. Preventive geriatrics: an overview from traditional Chinese medicine. *Am J Chin Med.* 1982;10:32–39.

110. Wolf SL, Coogler C, Xu T. Exploring the basis for tai chi chuan as a therapeutic exercise approach. *Arch Phys Med Rehabil.* 1997;78:886–892

111. Koh TC. Tai chi and ankylosing spondylitis—a personal experience. *Am J Chin Med.* 1982;10: 59–61.

112. Farrell SJ, Ross ADM, Sehgal KV. Eastern movement therapies. *Phys Med Rehabil Clin N Am.* 1999;10:617–629.

113. Wolf SL, Barnhart HX, Ellison GL. The effect of tai chi quan and computerized balance training on postural stability in older subjects. *Phys Ther.* 1997;77:371–381.

114. Lai J-S, Wong M-K, Lan C, Chong C-K, Lien I-N. Cardiorespiratory responses of tai chi chuan practitioners and sedentary subjects during cycle ergometry. *J Formos Med Assoc.* 1993;92:894–899.

115. Lan C, Lai J-S, Wong M-K, Yu M-L. Cardiorespiratory function, flexibility, and body composition among geriatric tai chi chuan practitioners. *Arch Phys Med Rehabil.* 1996;77:612–616.

116. Lan C, Lai J-S, Chen S-Y, Wong M-K. 12-Month tai chi training in the elderly: its effect on health fitness. *Med Sci Sports Exerc.* 1997;63:345–351.

117. Channer KS, Barrow D, Barrow R, Osbourne M, Ives G. Changes in haemodynamic parameters following tai chi chuan and aerobic exercise in patients recovering from acute myocardial infarction. *Postgrad Med J.* 1996;72:349–351.

118. Schaller KJ. Tai chi chuan. An exercise option for older adults. *J Gerontol Nurs.* 1996;22:12–17.

119. Sun WY, Dosch M, Gilmore GD, Pemberton W, Scarseth T. Effects of a tai chi chuan program on Hmong American older adults. *Educ Gerontol.* 1996;22:161–167.

120. Channer KS, Barrow D, Barrow R, Osborne M, Ives G. Changes in haemodynamic parameters following Tai Chi Chuan and aerobic exercise in patients recovering from acute myocardial infarction. *Postgrad Med J.* 1996;72(848):349–351.

121. Lan C, Lai J-S, Wong M-K, Yu M-L. Cardiorespiratory function, flexibility, and body composition among geriatric tai chi chuan practitioners. *Arch Phys Med Rehabil.* 1996;77:612–616.

122. Lan C, Lai J-S, Chen S-Y, Wong M-K. 12-Month tai chi training in the elderly: its effect on health fitness. *Med Sci Sports Exerc.* 1997;63:345–351.

123. Sun WY, Dosch M, Gilmore GD, Pemberton W, Scarseth T. Effects of a tai chi chuan program on Hmong American older adults. *Educ Gerontol.* 1996;22:161–167.

124. Hong, Y, Li JX, Robinson PD. Balance control, flexibility and cardiorespiratory fitness among older tai chi practitioners. *Br J Sports Med.* 2000; 34:29–34.

125. Schaller KJ. Tai chi chuan. An exercise option for older adults. *J Gerontol Nurs.* 1996;22:12–17.

126. Kirsteins AE, Dietz F, Hwang SM. Evaluating the safety and potential use of a weight-bearing exercise. Tai-Chi Chuan, for rheumatoid arthritis patients. *Am J Phys Med Rehabil.* 1991;70(3): 136–141.

127. Hartman CA, Manos TM, Winter C, et al. Effects of t'ai chi training on function and quality of life indicators in older adults with osteoarthritis. *J Am Geriatr Soc.* 2000;48:1553–1559.

128. Hong Y, Li JX, Robinson PD. Balance control, flexibility and cardiorespiratory fitness among older tai chi practitioners. *Br J Sports Med.* 2000; 34:29–34.

129. Wong AM, Lin Y-C, Chou S-W, Tang F-T, Wong P-Y. Coordination exercise and postural stability in elderly people: effect of tai chi chuan. *Arch Phys Med Rehabil.* 2001;82:608–612.

130. Wolf SL, Barnhart HX, Kutner NG, et al. Reducing frailty and falls in older persons: an investigation of tai chi and computerized balance training. *J Am Geriatr Soc.* 1996;44:489–497.

131. Wolf SL, Barnhart HX, Ellison GL. The effect of tai chi quan and computerized balance training on postural stability in older subjects. *Phys Ther.* 1997;77:371–381.

132. Judge JO, Lindsey C, Underwood M, Winsemius D. Balance improvements in older women: effects of exercise training. *Phys Ther.* 1993;73: 254–265.

133. Norwalk MP, Predergast JM, Bayles CM, D'Amico FJ, Colvin GC. A randomized trial of exercise programs among older individuals living in two long-term care facilities: The Falls FREE Program. *J Am Geriatr Soc.* 2001;49:859–865.

134. Wolf SL, Kutner NG, Green RC, McNeely E. The Atlanta FICSIT study: two exercise interventions to reduce frailty in elders. *J Am Geriatr Soc.* 1993;41:329–332.

135. MacDonald DA, Holland D. Examination of the psychometric properties of the temperament and character inventory self-transcendence dimension. *Personality Individual Diff.* 2002;32: 1013–1027.

136. Hay D, Morisy A. Reports of ecstatic, paranormal, or religious experience in Great Britain and the United States—a comparison of trends. *J Sci Study Religion.* 1978;17(3):255–268.

137. Hood RW, Hall JR, Watson PJ, Biderman M. Personality correlates of the report of mystical experience. *Psychol Rep.* 1979;44(3):804–806.

138. Hood RW. Eliciting mystical states of consciousness with semi-structured nature experiences. *J Sci Study Religion.* 1977;16(2):155–163.

139. Hood RW. Differential triggering of mystical experience as a function of self-actualization. *Rev Religious Res.* 1977;18(3):264–270.

140. Hood RW. Psychological strength and the report of intense religious experience. *J Sci Study Religion.* 1974;13(1):65–71.

141. Maslow A. *Toward a Psychology of Being.* New York: Van Nostrand; 1962.

142. Murphy M. *The Future of the Body: Explorations into the Further Evolution of Human Nature.* Los Angeles, CA: Tarcher Perigee; 1992.

143. Maslow A. *Religions, Values, and Peak Experiences.* New York: Viking; 1970.

144. Gartner J. Religious commitment, mental health, and prosocial behavior: a review of the empirical literature. In: Shafranske EP, ed. *Religion and the Clinical Practice of Psychology.* Washington, DC: American Psychological Association; 1996:187–214.

145. George LK, Larson DB, Koenig HG, McCullough ME. Spirituality and health: what we know, what we need to know. *J Soc Clin Psychol.* 2000;19(1): 102–116.

146. George LK, Larson DB, Koenig HG, McCullough ME. Spirituality and health: what we know, what we need to know. *J Soc Clin Psychol.* 2000; 19(1): 102–116.

147. Gartner J. Religious commitment, mental health, and prosocial behavior: a review of the empirical literature. In: Shafranske EP, ed. *Religion and the Clinical Practice of Psychology.* Washington, DC: American Psychological Association; 1996:187–214.

148. Koenig HG. *Handbook of Religion and Mental Health.* San Diego, CA: Academic Press; 1998.

149. Koenig HG. Correspondence. *Lancet.* 1999; 353:1804.

150. Gartner J. Religious commitment, mental health, and prosocial behavior: a review of the empirical literature. In: Shafranske EP, ed. *Religion and the Clinical Practice of Psychology.* Washington, DC: American Psychological Association; 1996:187–214.

151. Ellison CW. Spiritual well-being: conceptualization and measurement. *J Psychol Theol.* 1983; 11(4):330–340.

152. Howden JW. *Development and psychometric characteristics of the Spirituality Assessment Scale* [dissertation]. Houston, TX: Texas Women's University; 1992.

153. Elkins DN, Hedstrom LJ, Hughes LL, Leaf JA, Saunders C. Toward phenomenological spirituality: definition, description, and measurement. *J Hum Psychology.* 1988;28(4):5–18.

154. Weinstein L, Xie X, Cleanthous CC. Purpose in life, boredom, and volunteerism in a group of retirees. *Psychol Rep.* 1995;76(2):482.

155. Wink P, Donahue K. The relation between two types of narcissism and boredom. *J Res Personality.* 1997;31(1):136–140.

156. Tolor A, Siegel MC. Boredom proneness and political activism. *Psychol Rep.* 1989;65(1):235–240.

157. Drob SL, Bernard HS. The bored patient: a developmental/existential perspective. *Psychother Patient.* 1987;3(3–4):63–73.

158. Barghill RW. The study of life boredom. *J Phenomenol Psychology.* 2000;31(2):188–219.

159. McLeod CR, Vodanovich SJ. The relationship between self-actualization and boredom proneness. *J Soc Behav Personality.* 1991;6(5):137–146.

160. Weinstein L, Xie X, Cleanthous CC. Purpose in life, boredom, and volunteerism in a group of retirees. *Psychol Rep.* 1995;76(2):482.

161. Bonjour JP, Schurch MA, Rizzoli R. Nutritional aspects of hip fractures. *Bone.* 1996;18(3 suppl): 139S–144S

162. Delmi M, Rapin CH, Bengoa JM, et al. Dietary supplementation in elderly patients with fractured neck of the femur. *Lancet.* 1990;335(8696): 1013–1016.

PART V

Legal and Ethical Issues

CHAPTER 36

Legal and Ethical Issues in Integrative Medicine

ALAN DUMOFF

As physicians explore the legitimate role that many complementary and alternative medical (CAM) approaches can play in their practice, a number of legal questions should arise. Because CAM therapies are by definition nonstandard therapies, the potential for malpractice liability, medical board discipline, fraud and abuse investigations by insurers, and violations of drug and device regulation, to name the most serious concerns, require special care. Appropriate CAM practices can be safely practiced, particularly given the steady increase in acceptance of CAM as evidenced by increased funding for research through the National Center for Complementary and Alternative Medicine at the National Institutes of Health (NIH); increased medical school participation, including the founding of the Consortium of Academic Health Centers for Integrative Medicine; more accepting guidelines for CAM practice by the Federation of State Medical Boards; and a favorable White House Commission Report on Complementary and Alternative Medicine Policy. However, safe practice does require thoughtful investigation and awareness of a wide array of legal considerations.

Physicians often feel vulnerable and frustrated, with some cause, when issues of legal liability and risk management are raised. In some ways physicians have greater legal rights to practice as they see fit than members of any other profession, given their relatively broad scope of practice and the respect generally afforded a physician's independent judgment. This can be small consolation, however, given the extensive oversight and legal exposure to which medical practice is subjected. Physicians exploring the integration of CAM services into their practice should take advantage of assistance in crafting legally acceptable methods of practice prior to adoption.

Some integrative therapies can only be offered by physicians; these range from treating chronic fatigue syndrome with prescription thyroid supplementation, even in the face of normal thyroid-stimulating hormone and T_4 values, to more clearly experimental treatments such as autologous vaccines for cancer. Other integrative approaches—such as acupuncture and manipulative therapies—are practiced both by physicians and by credentialed and licensed nonphysician professionals. Some bodies of knowledge, such as homeopathy, do not have recognized national credentialing bodies and can only be practiced by physicians, or in some states, by acupuncturists, naturopaths, or a few other professions, if at all. Yet other developing sciences, such as nutritional and botanical medicines, are represented by a wide array of professions and professional bodies, yet can be a central part of integrative practice.

In some states, however, medical boards have taken internal policy positions that some or all CAM therapies pose a patient risk, and physicians need to be aware of state policies. Where integrative physicians employ experimental therapies, the burden of delivering non-standard care may be the greatest with respect to liabilities and regulatory oversight. Where physicians bring therapies to bear that do not have national credentialing in place, such as homeopathy, such practice can be risky, particularly in states that have not chosen to license such care through any practitioner. The practice of distinct CAM disciplines, such as acupuncture, not barred by a physician's state medical board is generally less troublesome, and more often revolves around issues of qualification to practice.

Integrative programs present particularly complex challenges. The extent to which there may be legal or regulatory difficulties depends not only on the nature of the practitioners and services offered, but also on the type of program, the setting, and the business structure. Requirements for credentialing, hidden kickbacks for referrals, and laboratory regulation are but some of the matters that may need to be addressed. Whatever the situation, physicians can take steps to reduce their risk.

▶ UNDERSTANDING AND MANAGING MALPRACTICE LIABILITY

For many physicians, the legal risk that springs to mind when considering unusual therapeutic approaches is the risk of malpractice claims. Because CAM methods are by definition "non-standard" therapies, a distressed patient would have an easier task demonstrating that the physician violated accepted standards of care in their treatment. Where a breach in standard

of care can be shown to cause a patient's injury, a physician will be found liable in malpractice.

While malpractice suits are occasionally brought against physicians for integrative therapies, in practice, this has not been a significant area of risk. Disciplinary actions from medical boards, FDA actions for unapproved therapies, and other complex regulatory issues have been the primary concern for integrative physicians. Even so, physicians should have a full understanding of how to manage malpractice risks, both for its own sake and because these same steps will help defer these regulatory risks as well.

While a defense attorney will be concerned about the nonstandard nature of the care, this risk is offset to a significant degree when patients choose CAM treatment with an understanding of the nonstandard nature of the care. Particularly where informed consent forms are properly used, the patient's agreement to use a CAM therapy assumes at least the known risks of such care. This was clearly tested in the matter of Emanuel Revici, MD, whose finding of liability for providing alternative cancer treatment was overturned by the court of appeals because the patient, who signed an informed consent form setting forth potential adverse reactions, assumed the listed risks of the treatment.[1]

Rather than the availability of legal defenses, however, the relatively low levels of malpractice claims may primarily be a result of the quality of the doctor-patient relationship in the "holistic," patient-centered approaches that are a hallmark of integrative practice. Studies show that physicians who draw the most suits are those seen by their patients as distant and arrogant.[2,3] In contrast, a hallmark of complementary settings is a time-intensive approach in which physicians spend time listening, exploring options, educating about illness and lifestyle, and discussing these novel treatments. Patients are generally not disposed to bring suit against physicians they believe are working with them to offer the best possible solutions. This highlights that good communication is not only a vital clinical skill, but also a necessary risk management strategy.

Malpractice Risk

Where physician use of CAM leads to a suit, the most likely claims are that a serious medical condition was missed, resulting in harm, or that there was a mismatch between the diagnosis and the proffered treatment. With regard to diagnosis, physicians need to keep their conventional diagnostic skills sharp and follow patients with a conventional eye, even when pursuing a strictly alternative course of treatment. Good documentation of diagnostic impressions and the use of conventional testing in addition to any CAM methods of diagnosis are essential. Where the treatment is unusual, especially for serious conditions such as cancer or diabetes, the medical record should show a rational basis for the choice and the consideration that was given to conventional treatments. The record should also note any potential interactions between a complementary therapy and concurrent pharmaceutical or other conventional therapies. A patient presenting with borderline high blood pressure, for example, could receive nutritional counseling, herbal recommendations, stress management, acupuncture or other nonstandard interventions, offered either instead of or in conjunction with antihypertensive medication. Before prescribing magnesium or olive leaf *(Olea europaea)*, for example, interactions with any antihypertensive medications need to be assessed. If antihypertensive medication is reduced or discontinued because of CAM interventions, then the patient needs to be aware of the risks and closely followed. And were an integrative physician to consider such a change in a patient being followed by a cardiologist, consultation, and perhaps provision of supporting literature, would be vital.

A threshold issue in analyzing malpractice risk is whether the physician is using an innovative medical practice or incorporating a therapy from a discipline recognized as a separate body of knowledge. Where a physician brings tools from recognized professions to bear, such as mind–body interventions, training in these approaches is of central importance. Where innovative medical practices are used, such as using rapid magnesium infusions in emergency room treatment of tachycardia, or intravenous vitamin and mineral therapies for infectious disease, it is important to assess and document the literature supporting the therapy.

One suggested approach is that physicians evaluate potential malpractice liability issues by classifying whether the evidence reported in the literature for the therapy (1) supports both safety and efficacy; (2) supports safety, but with little evidence of efficacy; (3) supports efficacy, but with little evidence of safety; or (4) indicates either serious risk or inefficacy.[1]

Under this rubric, physicians evaluate their exposure based upon the current state of the literature and inform patients of the status of the evidence. Because peer-reviewed medical literature tends to limit publication to treatments within accepted mechanisms of action, a wide net may need to be cast for studies of innovative methods. Physicians should weigh the status of this evidence against the risks and benefits of recognized therapies and document the basis for their recommendation. Where a physician is performing a CAM modality within the scope of their practice that is also recognized as a separate profession, such as acupuncture, the acceptance of the profession should overcome concerns about the "nonstandard" nature of the care and, in the event of patient harm, the question would be whether the physician standards for acupuncture practice were violated.

Risks of Collaborative Practice

An issue critical to the development of integrative health care involves the liabilities physicians have referring to or working directly with acupuncturists, chiropractors, massage therapists, mind–body professionals, and other practitioners in collaborative practice settings. Physicians can be subject to liability for negligent referral, which occurs where the CAM approach referred to is inappropriate or where the physician knew or should have known of competency problems with the practitioner.[5–8] Physicians should have confidence in, and know the credentials of, any health care practitioner to whom they refer a patient. These suits are rare and physicians should simply approach collaborative opportunities by becoming educated and comfortable with a community of CAM professionals.

An area of potential liability in conventional medicine is the failure to refer to a needed specialist. As CAM becomes more well entrenched, we may see suits for failure to refer for appropriate CAM services. Another area that may develop are suits against physicians who countermand the orders of licensed colleagues, an experience that is not unusual. Physicians with no training in nutrition have been known, for example, to order patients to cease taking supplementation recommended by a nutritionist.

In collaborative, multidisciplinary settings in which integrative physicians and nonphysician CAM practitioners work in team practice, physicians assume a primary role in health care services virtually by default. This is partly a result of the physician's wide scope of practice, unlike the limited, specific scopes of practice granted to the licensed CAM professions. In practice, physicians often function as a medical director in integrative settings. As a result, physicians' imagined deep pockets are a likely target in suits where the alleged harm was caused by a CAM practitioner within an integrated practice setting. The clinical and legal realities of shared practice serve to both increase and decrease risk; in some senses these practices are safer even while there is increased potential exposure.

Physician liability for harm is increased in integrative practices to the extent that the therapies themselves pose a risk, and physicians can be liable for harm caused by another either directly or vicariously. Direct liability arises when the physician performs an overt act that contributes to the harm, such as directly supervising the negligent treatment.[5] Another direct liability arises from negligent hiring or credentialing, in which due diligence obligations are not met and the physician, clinic, or hospital retaining the CAM practitioner did not discover or heed adverse information, such as peer-review or health board sanctions.[6,7] Vicarious liability occurs were the physician is in control of a practitioner who causes harm, a matter very clear when there is a supervisory relationship. The issue of control also can attach when the public reasonably believes that the physician or health entity is in a position to control the quality of care. Some integrative practices, for example, use a "medical mall" concept in which independent practitioners rent space in a single clinic, acting individually but appearing to the public as one entity working under a common name. The perception that it is a single entity will likely trump the business reality of independent professionals, so that liability will be shared. The public will often assume that a physician in such a practice is the medical director, bringing liability to the physician's doorstep.

As a result, physicians in collaborative settings may be well-advised to engage in a supervisory role that minimizes the risks of harm, rather than attempt to avoid any appearance of association that will likely prove unsuccessful. Shared practice can also reduce some risks. Team interaction offers a cross-check on diagnosis and treatment, making a missed diagnosis or poor treatment planning less likely. For CAM practitioners, legal risks can occur for exceeding their scope of practice. Multidisciplinary team practice reduces this risk because of the combined scopes of practice of the available practitioners.

Malpractice Experience

Actuarial data tracking suits against physicians for integrative practice is very difficult to find, not only because it is not tracked, but because it is difficult to assess whether a suit arises because of CAM practice. If a physician misses a cancer diagnosis, for example, would their use of CAM diagnostics for unrelated matters be material to the suit? While suits alleging difficulties with CAM services are known to happen, experience does not suggest that they are significant in number.

While the potential for shared liability with CAM practitioners in integrative settings is real, the risk of malpractice exposure is tempered by the comparatively low levels of risk historically experienced by CAM practitioners. That CAM practitioners' exposure is significantly less than physicians' should be no surprise, given that physicians take responsibility for the most seriously ill and their armamentarium includes invasive surgical techniques and medications with potentially serious side effects, while even the most aggressive of the alternative techniques, such as spinal manipulation and acupuncture needling, are less invasive and relatively free of ill effects.

While it is not uncommon for physicians to remark upon the dangers of chiropractic, even the most significant risk of harm—the risk of stroke resulting from a cervical adjustment—is between 2 per 1 million and 1 per 4–5 million adjustments.[9] The actual claims experience for chiropractors is about 2.7 claims per 100, compared to about 8.9 claims per 100 for primary care physicians. The financial risks are not on the same order of magnitude, however. The average paid claims per 100 policyholders is $66,150 for chiropractors versus $45.5 million for physicians. Other CAM practitioners' claim experience is even lower; massage therapists' rate, for example, is about 0.2 claims per 100, totaling less than a $1,000 paid claim per 100 policyholders.[10]

In some cases, low rates of adverse events are partly a result of standards adopted within CAM professions. The primary concern when exposed to acupuncture needling, for example, is the risk of infection from a contaminated needle. The standard of care is the use of the "clean needle technique" developed by the National Commission for the Certification of Acupuncturists and Oriental Medicine (NCCAOM) in cooperation with the Centers for Disease Control. This technique combines a sterile swipe with the use of a sterilized, disposable needle. This standard of care virtually eliminates risk of infection, and the AMA has acknowledged that acupuncture results in ". . . remarkably few serious complications. . . ."[11] While there are currently more than 14,000 practicing acupuncturists in the United States, there are only a handful of reported cases in which allegations of malpractice have been made. These allegations are primarily a result of pneumothorax; a needle breaking off in the skin; fainting during treatment; or to pain or injury from an inaccurate deep insertion. Adverse events have been reported at an average of one event every 5 years for a full-time acupuncturist.[12]

Risk Management

A first, easily overlooked risk management requirement is the notification of one's malpractice carrier of any unusual additions to one's practice. Where nonstandard therapies are adopted without notice and a claim is filed, the carrier may refuse coverage because of a material misrepresentation of the nature of the practice. If the carrier balks at covering the practice, and the physician is willing to go without coverage with regard to practices that are reasonably safe but merely unknown to the carrier, it may be possible to negotiate an exception that would allow the core coverage to continue. For many of the CAM professions malpractice coverage is now available through their professional associations.

Where nonstandard therapies are applied, it is important to document that the patient has given informed consent. Well-developed, detailed informed consent forms are very helpful in limiting liability where they educate the patient about their condition, the potential risks and benefits of the proposed therapy, and the conventional medical alternatives to the CAM treatment. The form should be very explicit that the treatment is not accepted by the medical community and may be considered not medically necessary and therefore noncovered by the patient's insurer. If the treatment uses a substance or device that is not approved by the FDA, or is experimental, these facts need to be clearly stated. Some states have specific requirements for informed consent. In Florida, for example, to have protection against discipline for using CAM approaches requires that informed consent forms describe the practitioner's training for the particular therapy.[13]

Integrative physicians can play a number of roles in their patients' health care, and it is important to be clear with the patient about the nature of that role. While an integrative approach counsels taking a whole view of the patient no matter what role is played, an integrative physician can nonetheless function as a primary care physician, a specialist within the physician's medical specialty, or as a specialist in the use of appropriate CAM services for a patient being followed by conventional physicians. Where a physician is not functioning as the primary care physician, but is acting as a specialist, it is vital that the form include a statement that the physician is not the patient's primary care physician and that the patient identify their primary care physician to ensure that the specialist does not assume these much larger legal obligations.

When working with CAM practitioners, basic concepts of credentialing and quality assurance need to be put in place. Within innovative medical practice, credentialing is as yet underdeveloped, but there are some standards such as training and certification as discussed below. Physicians should work with practitioners that maintain the highest and best state and private credentialing in the physician's area. An acupuncturist, for example, might be required to maintain NCCAOM diplomate status, and if herbs are used in the practice, required to possess NCCAOM or other relevant certification, or at least evidence of training.[14]

It is worth noting that physicians offering a holistic orientation seem to attract their share of troubled patients who are either disorganized or who carry resentment from previous medical management. An essential risk management strategy is having trained office staff defuse and manage patients who present with complex, often psychosomatic, issues. In addition to the protection provided by positive human relationships, studies suggest that patients are reluctant to discuss their CAM use with their primary care physician. This certainly makes coordinating care difficult, and even physicians not practicing integrative medicine need to create an atmosphere in which physician and patient both feel comfortable discussing the pros and cons of all therapies undertaken or being considered.

► HEALTH OCCUPATION BOARDS: REGULATORY REACTIONS TO CAM

Most physicians responsibly integrating CAM methods into their practice never face difficulty with their state medical boards, especially when simply incorporating a specific discipline such as acupuncture. Usually all that is required in these instances is to determine the state regulatory requirement. Some states allow acupuncture practice by any physician, some simply require registration prior to practice, while others have minimal training requirements such as the 200-hour postdoctoral training course that is the national standard.[16] Other activities may require registration, such as a creating a dispensary to supply compounded or other pharmaceuticals onsite.

Medical Board Disciplinary Responses to Physician CAM Practice

While most physicians practice without incident, some state medical boards have been quite active in disciplining physicians they find

▶ Case Example: Herbal Medicines in the Hospital

When the parents of a child admitted at Children's Hospital in Detroit, Michigan, wanted to continue providing him melatonin, valerian root, and algae while hospitalized, the hospital decided that it needed to review its policy regarding inpatient self-prescribing of herbs.

The Pharmacy and Therapeutics Committee reviewed the matter, and while initially favoring patient choice, the health system's lawyers counseled that the hospital would be liable for reasonably foreseeable problems such as lack of effectiveness, worsening of the underlying medical condition, and potential interactions with conventional therapies and tests. Counsel advised the hospital that informed consent that discloses information about the effectiveness and potential risks associated with alternative therapies would not relieve the health system of liability, given that all potential risks are unknown.[15]

This is an extreme position; it is unlikely that the hospital would be held to assume liability for all unknown risks of herbs patients self-prescribe. This presumes courts would adopt an entirely unreasonable burden on the hospital to protect the patients from their own behavior. It is important, however, that physicians avail themselves of developing databases that note adverse herb–drug interactions.

engaging in practices they consider suspect. Physicians have been disciplined for practicing a wide variety of CAM care, such as alternative cancer therapies,[17] homeopathy,[18] ethylenediaminetetraacetic acid IV chelation therapy,[19] or referring patients for dental mercury amalgam removal to resolve systemic health complaints.[20] These disciplinary actions have been viewed as either legitimate efforts to maintain standards or as anticompetitive, reactionary responses to the growth of CAM practices. To be fair, the truth probably spans this spectrum, and approaches vary from state to state. There has been sufficient concern about board motives that 14 state legislatures have enacted laws designed to minimize the ability of their own boards to discipline physicians for using CAM.[21,22] The impact of these laws has been modest, at best, as boards can target physicians for common errors in documentation or billing. These laws are narrowly drafted, so boards can bring charges for practices that do not meet the particular protections defined in the statute, such as for therapies the practitioner cannot show are effective.

State standards for practice brought to any investigation are not matters of clear record but rather of interpretation by board membership of a diffuse body of thought that includes medical school curricula, peer-reviewed publication, learned society opinion, and federal regulatory views. There are considerable variations in judgment about innovative and alternative treatments, such that some boards generally accept responsible practice, some fault physicians for practicing a nonstandard modality, and other boards accept integrative practice in principle but rest charges on a lack of informed consent or the inadequacy of documentation pertaining to medical evaluation and CAM treatment decisions. The best stance is to consistently practice good, well-documented care no matter what its source. Strident advocacy of CAM methods can suggest to regulators that use is a matter of fervor rather than reason. Materials and behavior of practitioners should suggest a balanced and reasoned approach to controversial issues, one that informs patients about the pros and cons of CAM and conventional treatments and works with patients to make reasonable decisions.

Federation of State Medical Board CAM Guidelines: 2002 Developments

State boards taking strident positions against CAM practice have historically been encouraged by the Federation of State Medical Boards, Inc. (FSMB), a private national body offering nonbinding policy guidance to their member state boards. Until recently, FSMB's guidelines have been sharply critical of alternative medicine. The original FSMB assessment of CAM was conducted by their Special Committee on Health Care Fraud. As recently as 1999, the committee was called the Special Committee on Questionable and Deceptive Health Care Practices, a name that was finally transformed in 2002 into the Special Committee for the Study of Unconventional Health Care Practices. The FSMB originally defined CAM by rejecting the term, saying that it had "not been utilized by the committee due to a lack of consensus among both practitioners and the public as to [its] meaning." Instead, the "committee has chosen to use the term 'questionable health care practices' to include those treatments, . . . conventional or unconventional, which may be unsafe and thereby considered a risk to the public's health, safety, and welfare and/or which may be worthless and thereby likely to deceive or defraud the public."[23] While not overtly equating CAM and "questionable health care practices," the implication was not lost, and these pejorative descriptions of CAM have been at the heart of many state board disciplinary actions.

Against this background, the Model Guidelines adopted in 2002[24] by the FSMB are a striking turn of events. While some of these policies, if adopted by state boards, could continue to create disciplinary problems for CAM physicians, the Guidelines reflect how far CAM acceptance has come in the past decade. The Model Guidelines include protective language similar to that adopted by many states that "a licensed physician shall not be found guilty of unprofessional conduct for failure to practice medicine in an acceptable manner solely on the basis of utilizing CAM." The Guidelines now acknowledge that ". . . standards [of medicine] allow a wide degree of latitude in physicians' exercise of their professional judgment and do not preclude the use of any methods that are reasonably likely to benefit patients without undue risk." In addition to recognizing physicians' right to use their judgment without being constrained by established doctrine, the Guidelines recognize that "patients have a right to seek any kind of care for their health problems."

Despite this more accepting posture, physicians should be aware that each state board has to decide if it will adopt this new language, and some boards will likely continue to target practices of concern. Even in states with express statutory protection, charges can be brought for problems such as poor medical documentation or upcoding visits without making the CAM target of the action apparent. Drafting protective language that allows medical boards to discipline truly fraudulent practices while protecting against actions targeting legitimate integrative practices is difficult, as is the threshold question of whether a therapy is legitimate.

Creating a Level Playing Field
This underlying issue of legitimacy pervades virtually any legal assessment of CAM regulation. A frequently expressed concern is the difficulty achieving a fair and even-handed assessment of safety and effectiveness. Many CAM proponents argue that established medicine

holds CAM to a higher standard than it applies to its own efforts; the majority of conventional therapies have not been subjected to randomized controlled trials. Many experts in the integrative medicine field believe that randomized, single-agent research methodologies often are ill suited for multiagent, system-based therapies. This message was at least partially heard by the FSMB, whose Model Guidelines now expressly call for a "level playing field." Whether parity of evaluation can be achieved in practice is an open question. Even the description in the Guidelines, urging a level playing field through "the application of medical science to any clinical approach," in practice may be a call to use the very methods that arguably skew evaluation toward conventional thinking where outcome or multifactorial testing methodologies may be more appropriate.

This difficulty in crafting a level playing field frequently arises when weighing risks and benefits. The Guidelines would create potential disciplinary action where a treatment "may be potentially harmful," yet most therapies carry some risk, and, to be fair, conventional treatments are often laden with risk. The "appropriate" use of pharmaceuticals is estimated to fatally injure 106,000 US patients per year, with significant injuries estimated in excess of 2 million hospital patients annually,[25,26] while another 88,000 die from hospital-acquired infections.[27] As noted previously, the adverse effects of most CAM therapies that have been tracked are of a much smaller magnitude, although physicians should stay vigilant with regard to herb–drug interactions, the potential toxicity of novel treatments, and other potential risks. Conventional therapies are maintained in spite of these risks because of proven or presumed benefits, a calculation not applied to CAM in the FSMB formulation.

Cautions within the FSMB Guidelines

The Model Guidelines also provide that physicians may make referrals to CAM practitioners. This is an improvement over historical animosity to such referrals, most notably prohibi-

tions against referral to chiropractors that resulted in that profession's successful antitrust suit against the AMA in *Wilk v. AMA*.[28] The Guidelines limit acceptable referrals to licensed practitioners, an understandably cautious step. The Guidelines also create ongoing responsibility for the work of any CAM practitioner to which a physician refers a patient. This could result in regulatory exposure for a misadventure by a licensed nutritionist, for example, even where there is no supervision or fault on the part of the referring physician. No board would place such an ongoing legal obligation upon a referral to a medical specialist, and whether a state board can place such an obligation on a physician will be subject to challenge should it occur.

Finally, another area integrative physicians need to note are guidelines that would effectively ban physician sales of supplements. For many integrative/CAM clinics, supplement sales form a significant portion of a practice's revenues.[29] This has been a disputed area since a similar policy was adopted by the AMA Ethics Committee in 1998,[30] a position that has been followed by some state boards.[31] The stated reason for this policy is that a physician with a self-interest in a product will be influenced to inappropriately recommend these products. A level playing field is not apparent here, as dermatologists sell skin creams and orthopedic surgeons sell splints and braces, and all physicians are inundated by detail staff urging them to prescribe their pharmacological solutions. Yet physicians who wish to provide high-quality vitamins are required under this policy to send their patients to their local health food store, catalogues, or the Internet—resources not without self-interest in terms of product recommendations.

Keeping Good Medical Records

The first and last place a medical board or a plaintiff's attorney will look is the patient's medical record. Careful documentation of a conventional work-up is a critical part of any record. Even where the focus is upon an alternative method of care, a review of the chart by a conventional physician should show that sound evaluation and reasoning lay underneath any CAM methods that may also be used.

Even if using unusual diagnostic methods or complementary therapies, physicians should make sure that their documentation reflects a proper conventional medical evaluation and that the basis for any deviation from expected, standard care is documented in the chart. If working directly with CAM practitioners, physicians should recognize that most CAM practitioners have not been trained in charting. When establishing close collaboration with CAM practitioners, it is important to educate them in SOAP (subjective, objective, assessment, plan) notes and in legal charting requirements. Practitioners should cross-train each other in their clinical language. Notes should be kept in the chart when integrative staff meets as a team in order to show the level of care and supervision.

Ethical Challenge: Evaluating Poor Treatment Choices in Cancer Care

When reviewing the appropriateness of the therapeutic tools physicians have available, the ethical dilemmas physicians face in the CAM or conventional arena are not so different. While the institutional view of standards provides legal weight to conventional methods, the ethical obligation to grapple with the value of therapies remains the same. Treatments for cancer provide an unfortunate case-in-point.

While chemotherapeutic agents are widely used as the best hope in many situations, numerous authors and studies have questioned the value of using these toxic methods of treatment for some cancers, raising issues about the efficacy, side effects, methods of research, and biased interpretation of data.[32,33] Studies reveal that oncologists would not, in fact, subject themselves to some of the treatments they provide their patients.[34] Chemotherapy, in many situations where it offers little hope, is too often driven by a fear of litigation if standard efforts are not offered, even when it is clear that

the debilitating effects of the drugs far outweigh any benefit.

Where integrative physicians use innovative treatment methods that have little evidence of safety and effectiveness, similar questions arise. Some integrative physicians feel that providing alternatives to chemotherapy is, in many situations, an ethical obligation even if the evidence for the alternative is sparse. A malpractice action asks whether a physician met the standard of care, so that where a course of action is accepted by the community of physicians as a reasonable one despite weak evidence, it is legally defensible as standard care despite the weak state of the evidence. But when a physician acts outside of these professional standards, the burden of directly demonstrating scientific evidence is much greater. A physician comparing a poor track record for a conventional treatment with a poorly tested but more promising integrative treatment thus faces a dilemma with regard to legal risk; the law and ethical obligations may be at odds in some of these situations.

One ethical thread of key importance is the use of informed consent forms. Integrative physicians must take great care in ensuring that patients understand the alternative, experimental nature of the care. Ethical and legally safe practice in any setting, but particularly in an integrative setting, requires that patients understand the potential risks and benefits, that a therapy may not be accepted by the medical community, the FDA, or other significant decision makers in the medical community, and the nature of other methods that might be available instead of the proposed therapy.

► FDA REGULATION: SUPPLEMENTS, DEVICES, AND DRUGS

Most CAM therapeutics are regulated by the FDA. Experimental pharmaceuticals, medical devices, biologics, as well as botanicals, herbs, and other dietary supplements are all subject to regulations that can be especially difficult to apply to the fast-moving, innovative arena of CAM therapies. Given natural conflicts between the interests of manufacturers and advocates of these therapies, on the one hand, and conservative regulatory interests on the other, claims as to legal status need to be carefully evaluated when adopting new therapies.

This review of nonstandard therapies must include an understanding of a complex web of FDA regulations and policies. Recommending over-the-counter remedies such as vitamins, minerals, botanical products, or homeopathics directly to patients is legally acceptable under food and drug law, although physicians should be aware of the boundaries regarding health claims for public consumption. More esoteric therapies, such as experimental drugs, unusual, off-label uses of approved drugs, compounding of specialty products, and intravenous injections of vitamins and minerals require legal review.

Many innovative therapies rapidly go to market, in contrast to the lengthy drug approval process, so treatment choices include a myriad of products offered as dietary supplements, including herbal remedies, and even unapproved, experimental drug products. Integrative physicians may be offered the use of experimental drugs claimed to be under an investigational auspice such as approval from an Institutional Review Board (IRB). Against this already complex backdrop of issues, integrative physicians are frequently approached by patients with requests that push the boundaries of other FDA policies, such as requests for assistance importing drugs that are not approved in the United States under personal use exemptions. These situations are all manageable, but do require awareness on the part of a physician.

Unapproved Use of Pharmaceuticals

Generally, physicians may prescribe an approved drug for a use other than that listed as an indication, the so called "off-label" use.

While there may be malpractice liability for such use, it is nonetheless routinely done in conventional settings as new uses are discovered through clinical experience. While there have been disputes about the extent to which manufacturers can advertise off-label uses,[35] once a drug is made available to a physician, he or she may prescribe it according to the dictates of their clinical judgment because the FDA does not have jurisdiction to interfere with the practice of medicine, and, as a general rule, seeks not to interfere with the independent judgment of physicians.

In the CAM arena, however, the FDA has taken enforcement actions against physicians for their use of therapies such as therapeutic doses of vitamins. Although these actions have been rare, they remain troubling for physicians committed to these therapies. State medical boards, as well, may decide that certain off-label uses are off limits, as some boards have done with the off-label use of human growth hormone.[36] Regulatory agencies are particularly watchful where they believe there is a high potential for exploitation, such as exists with HIV or cancer patients. A number of unapproved drugs and devices are sold by manufacturers under approved IRBs, many of which are not based in medical institutions but are independent panels. These can be acceptable, but in some cases are merely ploys to circumvent premarketing approval requirements; physicians should examine the legal status of IRB approvals carefully. Numerous medical devices on the market also may not have FDA approval, although manufacturers have been known to inaccurately represent the status of their products. A review of the requirements for an IRB should be done to assure legitimacy and then performed only with patients who meet the clinical protocol.

A special case worth noting are homeopathic remedies, which are mentioned in the Food, Drug, and Cosmetic Act.[37] There is a common misperception that the FDA is prohibited from regulating homeopathic remedies under this provision, but it is more accurate to say that the FDA has chosen as a matter of policy to leave this arena unregulated. With regard to FDA policy, physicians can prescribe homeopathic remedies without concern.

Alternative Cancer Products

There are a wide variety of pharmaceutical entities that are not approved for use that are offered by some CAM physicians. These more often appear in cancer treatment than other areas, and include various immunoaugmentive treatments such as Livingstons' autologous vaccines, Lawrence Burton's Immuno-Augmentive Therapy, or Coley's Toxins, or herbally derived products such as Carnivora (Dionaea muscipula) or the infamous Hoxsey cure.[38] Even if such therapies are not of interest, or their unproven nature exceeds a physician's level of acceptable risk, patients may seek information and possibly referral to physicians who provide such therapies. An informed understanding on the part of the physician about the legal risks of providing and of referring to these therapies is critical.

One case that drew a great deal of legal attention was that of antineoplastins developed by Stansilaw Burzynski. A battle over this innovative and highly controversial cancer treatment erupted in the struggle between Dr. Burzynski, the FDA, and the Texas Medical Board. Dr. Burzynski developed his approach while at Baylor College of Medicine in the late 1970s, isolating certain peptides in human urine that appear to act as biochemical switches that "turn off" cancer genes. After years of conflict over Dr. Burzynski's use of antineoplastins, the United States tried unsuccessfully to prosecute Dr. Burzynski on criminal charges, including mail and insurance fraud, and using unapproved drugs in interstate commerce. Federal prosecutors had to convene four grand juries before they were finally able to obtain charges against the doctor and tried him twice because the first jury could not reach a verdict. After the second jury refused to convict on 74 of 75 charges, Dr. Burzynski was convicted on one count of contempt of court for defying a court order not to ship antineoplastins in interstate commerce. A consent agreement was reached that expanded clinical trials but limited use to approved clinical subjects and prohibited any advertising.

Many aspects of the Burzynski case highlight the political complexities of CAM policy. While the FDA's enforcement branch pursued a prison sentence for Dr. Burzynski, other branches in the FDA were working with him to develop investigational new drug clinical trials. The trials were developed in the face of an increasing consensus in the medical community that his clinical results indicated anticancer activity, based in part on a site visit by National Cancer Institute (NCI) scientists 4 years before criminal charges were brought; an internal FDA memo concluded that the "human brain tumor responses are real."[39] Earlier animal testing done by the NCI in 1983 had used the P338 mouse leukemia tumor model, which showed no activity. Dr. Burzynski's attorney, Rick Jaffe, points out that antineoplastins have never been offered to treat leukemia, which is quite a different disease than the tumors targeted by antineoplastins, and that such tests are designed to fail rather than to provide a true test of this work.[40] This has been a frequent criticism of testing by established medical institutions of CAM therapies, such as the laetrile cancer trials at the Memorial Sloan-Kettering Cancer Center.[41,42]

Innovative cancer treatments remain a rich arena, in which the lines between CAM practice and developments within conventional medicine are often blurred. As biomedical views slowly accept immunoaugmentive approaches, therapies such as interferon, which had roots in Lawrence Burton's immunoaugmentive therapy, have moved more into the mainstream.[43]

Dietary Supplements: Herbs, Botanicals, Vitamins, and Minerals

Herbs and botanical products are a core modality in many traditions, including traditional Chinese medicine, Tibetan medicine, and Ayurvedic medicine, as well as many Western traditions. Practitioners using a metabolic nutritional approach use therapeutic doses of vitamins and minerals to treat a wide variety of conditions, many of which show poor responsiveness to conventional treatments, such as autism, chronic fatigue syndrome, and chronic infections. Physicians may recommend supplement products for treatment of disease in the privacy of the treatment room, but claims made by manufacturers are more limited under a regulatory approach reached after a long history of struggles and compromise between Congress and the FDA about health claims for dietary products.

Supplement policy has undergone a contentious evolution over the past four decades. FDA efforts to protect consumers by restricting access based on conservative scientific assessments of potentially unfounded claims have been repeatedly counterbalanced by congressional recognition that consumers want access to supplement information and products. The FDA has proposed that vitamins and minerals bear warning labels stating that there is an abundant supply of vitamins and minerals in the food supply, that potencies exceeding 150% of the recommended daily allowance be regulated as drugs, and that supplement manufacturers not be allowed to make any health claim. The only restriction that has survived congressional review, albeit after significant modification, is the limitation on health claims.[44] The principal legal distinction that turns a product into a drug is the claim; a mushroom marketed to cure infectious disease is no longer a food, but is now a drug. While a few specific claims have been reviewed by the FDA and approved, such as the connection between sodium and hypertension,[45] dietary fat and cancer,[46] dietary saturated fat and cholesterol and risk of coronary heart disease,[47] and fiber-containing grain products, fruits, and vegetables and cancer,[48] manufacturers are generally prohibited from health claims that a product can be used "to diagnose, cure, mitigate, treat, or prevent disease."[49] Under the compromise worked out in the Dietary Supplement Health and Education Act of 1994 (DSHEA),[50] manufacturers may explain the impact a product has on the structure or function of the body. An example of this distinction is that calcium cannot be marketed to "prevent or relieve osteoporosis," or even to implicitly treat osteoporosis with a claim that a calcium product "prevents bone fragility in postmenopausal women," but a label may state that the product "helps build healthy bones."[51]

A casual perusal of the Internet or the local health food store makes it clear that thousands of products are marketed in violation of this prohibition against implied health claims. The FDA simply does not have the resources to police this enormous marketplace. It is therefore important to recognize that, while there is a significant body of research supporting a more expansive and vital role for supplementation in practice, the claims advanced by manufacturers may have little basis and need to be evaluated on a case-by-case basis independently. Physicians who market supplements either directly or as part of their practice also must take heed of these restrictions, as statements made to the general public are subject to FDA jurisdiction. Integrative settings that offer supplements for sale should review the claims they make in their promotional literature.

Nonconventional Medical Devices

Medical devices are regulated by the FDA. As with drugs, a device becomes subject to regulation as a medical device where a health claim is made. Due diligence requires evaluation of the FDA regulatory stance on unconventional devices, including careful examination of claims made by manufacturers.

Numerous devices are based on mechanisms that are implausible, at best, from a Western biomedical perspective. One widely used device, originally developed by Dr. Voll of Germany in the 1920s, is known as Electroacupuncture According to Voll, and used for electrodermal screening or meridian health analysis. This tests the galvanic skin resistance along the acupuncture meridians for specific disease responses. The test claims to sense energetic precursors or subtle etiologies to disease, including sensitivities to food or environmental triggers. The FDA has approved galvanic skin responses as evidence of anxiety, but this expansive use is more troubling and is based on an energetic view that is not sensible from a Western physiologic perspective.

Restrictions on Nonconventional Diagnostic Laboratory Devices

There are other federal regulatory authorities that can have an impact on the use of diagnostic devices. Certification for laboratory testing under the Clinical Laboratory Improvement Act (CLIA)[52] is focused on ensuring that laboratory personnel are proficient and have equipment capable of providing accurate results. CLIA requires that tests of any complexity be demonstrated and certified as valid. A number of laboratories and manufacturers offer nonstandard tests and devices used by some integrative physicians. Many of these are CLIA approved, but this should be confirmed. Some tests have been rejected by CLIA given differences in orientation. In a mark of growing changes in regulation of CAM, the General Counsel's office wrote a memo raising questions about the CLIA approach to CAM.[53]

► LEGAL ISSUES IN COLLABORATIVE PRACTICE WITH NONPHYSICIAN CAM PRACTITIONERS

Collaborative practice between physicians and nonphysician CAM practitioners is a key component of integrative practice. Medical training should familiarize all physicians in the relative safety and efficacy of CAM practices and in how to work in consultation and referral with CAM practitioners. Medical training cannot, nor should it, attempt to provide comprehensive

training in CAM disciplines such as acupuncture, herbal medicine, and naturopathy. Other CAM practices, such as bodywork and massage, healing touch, or aromatherapy only make economic sense when delivered by these CAM practitioners. Across this entire spectrum of practitioners, the cross-training and fertilization generated within team practice is an enriching experience for staff and promotes quality patient care.

Whether referring, supervising, or partnering with nonphysician CAM practitioners, there are legal concerns that must be taken into account. Some are more obvious, such as the care that should be taken when considering incorporating practitioners who have certificates in "holistic medicine" from unaccredited institutions. These practitioners often perform nutritional or herbal counseling, massage, colonic irrigation, iridology, and a host of other services. Even though there is no state license or other authorization for such practice, these practitioners are infrequently prosecuted even though they work on their own. Practitioners with legitimate training may be able, under some circumstances, to reasonably collaborate with physicians, although legally safe practice requires proper due diligence and supervision and should be limited to those with legitimate training.

Scope of Practice Considerations

Setting up collaborative efforts requires a comparison of intended practices with allowed practices under these acts and planning for methods, such as delegated responsibilities, to deliver care outside the scope of practice. Practicing outside these designated scopes of practice is one of the primary legal risks faced by nonphysician CAM practitioners, and can result in administrative discipline, malpractice liability, and, in some cases, even direct civil or criminal liability for the practice of medicine without a license.[6,8]

Many CAM professions have achieved state boards of their own. In various states, there are boards for acupuncture, chiropractic, homeopathy, massage, naturopathy, and midwifery. Other professions, such as nursing with a strong interest in holistic approaches, and psychology with an interest in mind–body approaches, are valuable resources in integrative settings that should not be overlooked. Some states offer considerable freedom for CAM practitioners. The Nevada Homeopathic Board, for example, allows the state's licensed homeopaths to engage in a number of therapies, including herbal, vitamin, and nutritional treatments, and trigger point and thought field therapy.[54] In Washington state, naturopathic physicians function as primary care practitioners.[55] Other boards and their enabling statutes may be fairly restrictive, such as states in which chiropractors cannot give nutritional advice or acupuncturists cannot prescribe traditional Chinese herbs.

Because many CAM disciplines are a quilt of overlapping fields, conflicts in scope of practice can arise. In some states that license massage therapists, a reflexology therapist or movement reeducation therapist may be required to have a license. Unfortunately, many of these practitioners may not meet state licensing criteria. Other practitioners trained in bodywork have resisted massage licensure even though the scopes of practice are equivalent. In some states, chiropractors can practice acupuncture, although not in others. National associations are often knowledgeable about other practitioners' use of methods. The NCCAOM, for example, tracks which states allow chiropractors to perform acupuncture.[56]

Delegated and Supervised Duties

Delegating duties can, when properly executed, expand the limited scope of practice of CAM practitioners in collaborative settings. Medical supervision of CAM practitioners can provide a legal basis for some CAM services and reduce the risk of negligent actions by staff. Depending on the state scope of practice, a licensed nutritionist, for example, may more reasonably offer nutritional interventions for disease, rather than simply advice about diet under medical supervision. Given the lack of training most physicians receive in nutrition, such teams provide an effective clinical and legal collaboration. Most states have fairly liberal rules regarding physicians' ability to delegate duties, even to unlicensed medical assistants that they train and for which they take responsibility.[57] This generally requires that a physician have first seen the patient during the course of treatment, train and supervise the practitioner, review and sign notes for services rendered, and take legal responsibility for the care.

Nutritional Advice

Many CAM practitioners focus on nutrition as a key aspect of health. Providing nutritional education that is grounded in research should not present legal difficulty, and general counseling about wellness should also present little concern. Applying nutritional advice to specific signs and symptoms or diagnoses of disease, however, requires a scope of practice allowing such a discussion. Acupuncturists, chiropractors, massage therapists, naturopaths in unregulated states, unlicensed nutritional consultants, as well as self-styled "holistic practitioners" and others may have education in nutrition and dispense advice that can go beyond lay discussion or exceed a licensed scope of practice. Chiropractors have frequently found themselves in difficulty for giving nutritional advice. Even in states where practice acts expressly allow chiropractors to give dietary advice, courts have held that they cannot make a suggestion that their patients take a dietary supplement, a suggestion that a layperson could make.[58,59] The preceding discussion of the DSHEA has application here, as one useful approach is to adhere to the "structure–function" restriction according to the preceding guidelines when discussing food or dietary supplements, which serves to make the conversation more clearly educational and lessens, if not removes, the intent to prescribe for a particular illness.

Issues Affecting Business and Program Structure

When designing collaborative practice, there are restrictions on financial arrangements that could have the appearance of affecting practitioners' judgments about referrals. Of greatest concern are federal and state prohibitions against receiving kickbacks in exchange for referrals and the Stark prohibition against referring to laboratories or other entities for services in which a practitioner has an ownership interest. While Stark[60] is limited to physicians referring to specific, designated services in which the physician has ownership, the antikickback statute[61] is broad and can be violated by any person as it is not limited to physicians. These complex regulations present considerable ambiguity; therefore any but the most straightforward situations should be reviewed for conflicts with these provisions.

These issues are prevalent in integrative settings because independent contractors are often used, or affiliations entered with other groups, which introduces a separate entity into the picture. In some health systems, a separate entity is created to isolate legal risk or to create a separate business structure for billing noncovered services apart from participating provider agreements. Because kickback and Stark problems arise when multiple entities are working together, these arrangements can give rise to violations.

When multiple entities contract together and base remuneration on the volume of referrals or on production, they are likely in violation of these laws. Because the law is so broad, numerous safe harbors have been developed that, although they do not have to be met for conduct to be legal, give safe ground for practices useful in integrative settings, such as group practice, arrangements for space rental, and for personal and management services contracts. When CAM practitioners are retained as independent contractors who make a percentage of what they earn, the patients should belong to the practice, and the practitioner reimbursed on a production basis, which is acceptable. If the patients are those of the practitioners, then the practice is being reimbursed by the practitioner based on the volume of referrals the practitioner receives from the practice.

Under the Stark self-referral prohibition, a physician may not refer for certain designated services to another entity in which the physician has an ownership interest. This was originally a narrow prohibition barring referrals of Medicare patients to clinical laboratories owned in part by the physician, but has been expanded into one of the more arcane federal regulations. Sharing patients in an effort to establish integrative methods needs to be reviewed for these issues.[62]

▶ BILLING AND REIMBURSEMENT ISSUES

Payment Sources for CAM Services

Payment for CAM services comes from a wide array of sources, although third-party coverage for most services is still the exception rather than the rule. Much of the current boom in CAM development exploded after research published in the early 1990s by David Eisenberg, who found that more money is spent out-of-pocket by patients on CAM visits than on primary care visits.[63] Out-of-pocket payment remains the principal source of payment.[64]

Direct reimbursement for CAM care has significantly increased over the past decade. Acupuncture, chiropractic, nutrition, massage, mind–body programs, and other CAM care are being covered by some plans. Covered benefits are often quite narrow; acupuncture, for example, can be used in some plans only as an alternative to anesthesia, or for specific disorders such as chronic pain or musculoskeletal conditions. Similarly, biofeedback and hypnotherapy may be limited to conditions such as migraine or stress-related conditions. Coverage for CAM can vary widely by state. Some plans may offer a CAM benefit, but only in specific states. Some plans have developed products specific to the CAM marketplace. American Health Specialty Plans, the largest of such specialized companies, offers benefit packages with a wide array of CAM benefits.

The key obstacle to continuing development of CAM benefits is a lack of an actuarial base allowing for proper pricing of insurance products. Several attempts have been made, including a paper by Millman and Robertson, (San Francisco), "Considerations in the Design and Pricing of an Alternative Medicine Benefit," a document that offers some perspective for hospitals negotiating with insurance plans as well as those developing these products.

A number of other vehicles exist for CAM reimbursement, such as carve-outs, riders, or unlisted coverage for services only offered if a primary care physician or specialist indicates something is medically necessary. One of the most common CAM "benefits" is an affinity or discount access network, which does not provide reimbursement; instead it provides access to a "panel" of practitioners who offer a prenegotiated, discounted rate. Self-insured employers are among the strongest CAM participants, as they are not beholden to medical directors but have immediate self-interest in cost-effective outcomes.

Obtaining Reimbursement: Issues that Arise During Contracting

While participating provider agreements in CAM networks are not yet common, there are some contracting possibilities. Chiropractic networks are expanding into broader CAM offerings. Following a disease management approach, some hospitals are creating programs that offer predesigned protocols for particular patient populations. Wellness programs are receiving considerable marketing interest. As CAM network contracting becomes more avail-

able, negotiations about price, risk sharing, and the definitions of services to be offered are all central considerations.

Integrative physicians should be aware that their conventional contracts can bind them into only providing medically necessary care at contract rates to beneficiaries in any setting. Where physicians enter into agreements in their personal capacity, it becomes more difficult later to see patients for CAM services without being held to these provider agreements. Physicians may wish to create separate practice structures, one for conventional contracts and another for fee-for-service CAM services. Leaving open an option to create separate entities with separate tax IDs for this purpose can be an important business strategy for establishing integrative centers.

Increasing Reimbursement: "Incident to" Billing

Where physicians and CAM practitioners work together in integrated settings, an important method of obtaining or increasing levels of reimbursement is an arrangement in which CAM practitioners work and bill under the physician. The physician works with these practitioners as a type of "physician extender." This method, which can be done in both outpatient and inpatient settings, frames the services as delivered "incident to" the physician's management of the patient, allowing for reimbursement at physician, rather than the extenders' rates.[65] The increased reimbursement is intended to offset the physician's time in supervision.

Historically, this has involved services such as nurse-administered injections or other technical components provided incident to the office visit with the physician. The payment was simply made for the physician office visit, with the fee for the nursing service built in, or bundled, in that payment. As physician extenders such as nurse practitioners and physician assistants came on the scene, adding a "professional" component as well, the physician was allowed to bill as if the physician performed these services, even though they were provided by the extender. Many CAM practitioners can properly be billed in this fashion, as long as specific requirements for such billing are met.

Fraud and Abuse Issues

Given the intensive levels of regulatory oversight of physician treatment decisions, it is not surprising that integrative services require special care about how practices are billed to avoid charges of fraud or abuse. One pervasive issue is whether differences in the philosophy of medicine and the resulting disparity in diagnostic and treatment methods lead to a therapy being considered medically unnecessary. Repetitive billing for services seen as medically unnecessary can draw an investigation into fraudulent or abusive practices.

One way that insurers track medical necessity is by checking the match between the Physicians' Current Procedural Terminology Procedures (CPT) codes[66] and International Classification of Diseases (ICD) codes.[67] Insurers run checks to see if the procedure is acceptable for the patient's diagnosis; a mismatch suggests that the procedure may be unnecessary. Where a nutritional intravenous code (90780) appears for treatment of chronic fatigue, for example, an insurer may balk at payment and questions could be raised.

Another auditing method used is to track the number of visits per year for repetitive treatments. Perhaps one of the most common red flags for insurers are excessive office visits, particularly when submitted as detailed or comprehensive, suggesting that the physician is upcoding visits. This creates difficulty for holistic physicians whose approach requires a review of numerous systems and who spend a considerable time educating patients. A patient's insurer may well find this a signal that claims are being submitted for unnecessary services. This issue can be complicated when using CAM

practitioners. The number of expected visits for musculoskeletal problems, for example, may be based upon experience with physical therapy. A neuromuscular therapist may require a different frequency or number of visits. Lack of experience with these CAM practitioners can cause misunderstanding with an insurer.

Medicare Reimbursement Policies Affecting Integrative Practice

Medicare has a number of specific restrictions on billing, some of which are troubling for integrative physicians. Billing for multiple services the same date of service, for example, can trigger denials. This issue can appear quite readily in integrative practices, as it is not uncommon for a patient to see a physician for evaluation and then be referred to an acupuncturist, massage therapist, or other practitioner for treatment. Generally, billing Medicare an Evaluation and Management (E/M) code and a procedure code the same day can only be done where the purpose of the E/M visit is distinct from the purpose of the procedure and the E/M and the procedure are both medically necessary. Unfortunately, Medicare patients desiring coverage may need to return for services on a later day.

One common problem is submitting claims to Medicare for clearly noncovered services, such as acupuncture services (97780). Acupuncture or other clearly noncovered CAM services are only billed to Medicare if the patient asks for submission in order to obtain a denial for coverage by the patient's secondary insurance company. Such a bill should be clearly marked that it is submitted for a denial, otherwise it may be considered fraud. Physicians should consult their malpractice carrier about how this should be done. Physicians have been held liable for fraud charges even when they specifically request their patients in writing not to submit because they believe the service to be noncovered.[70]

Medicare Opt-Out/ Private Contracts

Physicians whose focus is integrative care and who find most of their services are not covered may be well advised to opt-out of the Medicare program. This allows the physician to privately contract with Medicare beneficiaries for out-of-pocket payments that will not be reimbursed by Medicare. Physicians are then no longer limited by the Medicare fee schedule, and no longer responsible for Medicare's fraud and abuse provisions.

Since January of 1998, physicians have been able to opt-out of the Medicare program for a 2-year interval.[68] The patient agrees not to submit claims to Medicare but instead to pay the physician's fees directly. If a physician has responsibilities other than working in an outpatient integrative clinic, this should be done with great care. This is not a case-by-case election depending upon the patient or the setting, but applies to all patients seen in any setting except for those seen in an emergency. To opt-out, the physician must submit an affidavit to Medicare and have each Medicare-eligible patient sign a contract explaining the situation, including an agreement not to submit claims and acknowledging that they are responsible for payment.

Procedural Coding: Proper Use of CPT Codes

The primary language used for submitting claims for payment to any third-party payer are CPT codes, primarily authored by the American Medical Association (AMA). These codes must be used to accurately depict the procedures and services provided. Not surprisingly, CAM procedure codes are very limited; the AMA identifies only 8 codes of its more than 8,000 CPT codes for CAM practices. In addition, codes for E/M visits, physical therapy, counseling, and others may be used in some circumstances. But applying codes designed for conventional care to alternative methods can be risky, and the potentially ill-fitting nature of the codes requires careful review.

The most troublesome and common example are E/M codes, which were developed in light of a medical view of health care decision making and contain standards requiring documentation of medical complexity, morbidity, and organ–system assessments that do not correspond closely with integrative thinking. Coding holistic or CAM practices can be especially problematic, as a practice orientation requires spending more time with patients in pursuit of a more "whole" view. A searching differential diagnosis requires an understanding of symptoms across a wide spectrum of health systems. As a result, the face-to-face time spent by integrative physicians is often equivalent to the 40–60 minutes implied by a level 5 comprehensive office visit. But comprehensive visits can only be coded with patients who exhibit problems of moderate or high severity and can only be charged for established patients when significant treatment milestones or changes in symptom presentation occur. Integrative physicians need to be aware that they may not be able to justify higher levels of visit by conventional standards. With advance notice to patients, physicians may be able to bill a lower, appropriate E/M code, but charge an additional, noncovered fee for consultation time.

One issue that caused a great deal of concern in the aftermath of the expansive fraud and abuse provisions passed as part of the Health Insurance Portability and Accountability

Act (HIPAA)[69] was the erroneous belief that physicians could not bill for an office visit where some alternative modalities are discussed. The concern was based on a fear that using an E/M code would imply that the visit was strictly a conventional visit when it was not. While a visit that is primarily CAM related may raise such a concern, a physician can certainly discuss a range of conventional and alternative therapies within a billable visit. If a psychiatrist reviewing treatment options for depression considers St. John's wort as well as Prozac (fluoxetine), consideration of the herbal remedy does not convert the entire visit to an unbillable conversation. If, however, an MD homeopath conducts an entire visit for the sole purpose of suggesting homeopathic remedies, and biomedical treatments are never a consideration, an E/M coding would misrepresent the visit, given that few insurers would ever consider homeopathic remedies to be medically necessary, and Medicare will not cover self-administered medications in any event. Coding entirely CAM, presumably noncovered visits, should be done in a way in which the super-bill makes it clear that the visit is for homeopathic or other integrative service.

Another issue that causes confusion are codes that can refer to either covered or non-covered services. Vitamin B_{12} injections are covered with documented B_{12} deficiency, but can be used by integrative physicians for fatigue, viral conditions, and other uses that generally will not be reimbursed. Where a code can describe either covered or noncovered services, physicians should use the code with a modifier that makes it clear that the practitioner does not believe the service is covered. Physicians are also obligated for Medicare patients, and well-advised for other patients, to have the patient sign an "anticipated beneficiary notice" that informs the patient that the claim will not be paid.

Nonphysician CAM practitioners who have a scope of practice that involves clinical judgment may use E/M codes. Practitioners can also use codes within their scope of practice

unless the descriptive materials limit their use to physicians. Some of the codes for maternity care and delivery, for example (59000–59899), may be used by licensed midwives. The difference in scope of practice, however, limits which codes can be used. A midwife could use code 59400, "routine obstetric care including antepartum care, vaginal delivery and postpartum care,"[1] but could not use 59510, the code for cesarean delivery, as this is clearly outside a midwife's scope of practice. Similarly, a massage therapist can use 97124, "massage, including effleurage, pétrissage and/or tapotement (stroking, compression, percussion)," in the physical medicine section, but should be very cautious about using 97110, "therapeutic procedure . . . to develop . . . range of motion and flexibility," given that range of motion is generally within the scope of practice of physical therapists and not of massage therapists.

Pending Developments: A Unique Code Set for CAM Practice

A lack of CPT codes has been an impediment to reimbursement. A number of companies, most prominently ABC codes (Alternative Billing Concepts developed by Alternative Link, Inc.), are proposing literally thousands of codes for CAM procedures and supplies for federal approval. These codes are designed to be used on insurance claims by integrative physicians as well as acupuncturists, chiropractors, naturopaths, homeopaths, massage therapists, nurses, and other practitioners. Insurers presume that the lack of a code implies a lack of medical necessity, so that code development could portend additional coverage,[71] and thus additional interest on the part of patients in these approaches. At the very least, additional codes would make it easier to track outcomes from CAM treatments and make the actuarial decisions that would make changes in reimbursement policy more likely.

These new code sets are being reviewed by the National Committee for Vital and Health

Statistics and by the Healthcare Financing Administration's Common Procedure Coding System Committee, within the Department for Health and Human Services, for designation in electronic claims filing. While the AMA continues to believe there is no real gap in their code set, and maintains that the existence of only eight CAM CPT codes reflects a lack of need rather than any resistance on its part,[72] this view is becoming a minority one. The National Committee for Vital and Health Statistics has recognized that there is a gap in codes.[73]

► CREDENTIALING AND QUALITY ASSURANCE ISSUES

While there have been extensive efforts to develop credentialing programs for integrative physicians and CAM practitioners, the availability of recognized credentials is very uneven. The emerging field of practice by integrative physicians has made some progress, but clearly established ways to credential and privilege practice are only slowly evolving.

Credentialing the CAM Physician

An area in great need of continued development are credentialing programs that provide some assurance of competence in CAM techniques. Some of this is a result of the large number of specific modalities that can be included within the rubric of "integrative physician," drawing from a wide range of practices such as herbal medicine, homeopathy, mind–body approaches, and manipulative therapies, as well as many others. There are numerous specific emerging specialties and organizations that have their own training programs, such as training and certifications in antiaging medicine, the American Holistic Medical Association, the American Association for Medical Acupuncture, and the American College for the Advancement of Medicine for ethylenediaminetetraacetic acid IV chelation practice.

Some efforts at establishing broader certifications, such as by the American Board of Holistic Medicine, are slowly developing.

Hospital committees expanding their offerings must make difficult privileging decisions about what specific therapies they will allow. Some therapies have recognized standards and professional organizations, such as the 200-hour certification in acupuncture of the American Academy of Medical Acupuncture, which meets the recommended policy that has been adopted by many state medical boards. Others, such as homeopathy, are the subject of wide-ranging differences in education and approach and have no recognized certification programs. Documentation in these areas is currently limited to continuing medical education and training programs of varying credibility, membership, and participation in professional societies, and mentoring by senior physicians in these fields.

Whether physicians should be granted privileges in areas short on documentation rests in part on the risk presented by the modality and how it will be practiced. Homeopathy practiced as a complement to conventional care poses virtually no risk, but as a replacement for conventional care can present significant risk. Privileging can be done in a way that limits the nature of a practice to minimize its potential for harm or to control the range of services offered, such as limiting chiropractors to spinal manipulation.

Some conventional specialty boards have a greater share of members with CAM interests, such as the American Board of Pain Medicine, which is helping to develop the North American Society of Acupuncture and Alternative Medicine. There have also been attempts to create private associations to develop integrative medicine as a board specialty, although this has proven very difficult. Integrative medicine is still at the early stages and the standards of what are considered appropriate vary considerably. Additional professional and educational development is needed before providers and patients can have assurances of CAM medical competence.

Credentialing the Nonphysician Practitioner

While physicians occupy a central seat in the health care system, other practitioners have extensive training in CAM. The diverse community of CAM practitioners includes professions that are long established and with well-developed credentialing mechanisms, such as acupuncture and chiropractic, to emerging professions that are still at the threshold of establishing a professional infrastructure, such as herbal medicine. Credentialed naturopathic physicians, for example, have high-quality, 4-year postgraduate training with a great deal of crossover with medical training but a focus on natural remedies, such as homeopathics and herbs, as their frontline healing modalities. As medical practitioners supplement their training, collaborative work with practitioners who have focused on CAM as their core training is one way to further efforts at integration.

Whether bringing CAM practitioners into a hospital or other large health organization, or as part-time contractors into an integrative group practice, attention should be paid to issues of credentialing and quality assurance. When the profession itself is considered to be "complementary" or "alternative," a provider's task must begin with an evaluation of the profession itself before determining what standards to apply to its practitioners. There has been a tremendous infusion of credentials among the diverse CAM professions; some of these credentials document an independently verified education and national examination process as well-designed as medical mechanisms, while others are self-recognized correspondence programs or offered by small clinics as a sideline.

The profession of acupuncture, for example, has recognized bodies that credential and discipline members and accredit its schools. The NCCAOM, established in 1984, developed and administers the national certification examination to acupuncturists qualified by training or experience. Of the 33 jurisdictions that license acupuncturists, 27 rely in whole or in part on the NCCAOM examination. This examination process includes a written examination and a practical examination of point location skills and of clean needle technique. Successful applicants may represent that they are a NCCAOM Diplomate. Of the more than 14,000 non-MD acupuncturists, about 10,000 have achieved this credential. The NCCAOM and its examination are recognized by the National Commission of Certifying Agencies, and provides a forum for disciplinary review of any complaints that are filed. The NCCAOM has also developed an examination in Chinese herbology and Oriental bodywork. Some of the states that do not license acupuncturists allow acupuncture to be practiced in some circumstances under medical supervision. Acupuncture may be performed by medical physicians in most of the remaining states.

► CONSUMER ISSUES: THE HEALTH FREEDOM MOVEMENT

CAM advocates have raised the issue of access to practice as an issue of freedom of patient choice. This has been sought in federal and state legislatures, as well as brought before the courts in a variety of postures with limited success.

Legislative Efforts

At the federal level, the American Association for Health Freedom[74] has been steadily moving toward congressional adoption of the Access to Medical Treatment Act. This bill would allow state-licensed practitioners to use treatments within their scope of practice even though the FDA has not approved them for use, as long as there is reasonable evidence of safety and efficacy, patients are informed of the treatment's status, and a national data bank of adverse reactions is created. At the state level, the most significant development has been the limitations upon board disciplinary actions against physicians for practicing CAM, which exist in Alaska, Colorado, Florida, Georgia, Louisiana, Massachusetts, Nevada, New York, North Carolina, Ohio, Oklahoma, Oregon, Texas, and Washington state. Creative approaches include the Complementary and Alternative Health Freedom of Access law[75] passed in Minnesota, with similar laws passed in California and Rhode Island, allows health practitioners to practice without licensure, relying on full disclosure of training and registration to allow handling of complaints instead. The results of this experiment, begun in 2000, are still not clear.[76]

Judicial Reactions to Arguments for a Right to Access the Care of One's Choice

Efforts to obtain judicial recognition of a common law right to access the health care of one's choice have largely been unsuccessful. Given decisions asserting rights in reproductive freedom at the beginning of life and to seek or reject heroic medical efforts at the end of life,[77] the rejection of a right to manage major life events during the interim appears at odds with these cases.

The issue of a patient's right to receive cancer treatment reached the United States Supreme Court in *United States v. Rutherford.*[78] The 10th Circuit Court of Appeals had ruled that FDA requirements that a drug has to be demonstrated safe and effective had no reasonable application to patients without hope of recovery. That court ordered the FDA to allow laetrile to be available for administration by physicians to terminally ill patients. The Supreme Court reversed and held that terminally ill patients had no rights to obtain laetrile without FDA approval.[79,80] This decision came in the midst of a significant public battle over the use of laetrile in the 1970s; 17 states had legalized the use of laetrile for cancer treatment, with 14 other states rejecting such legislation, by the time this case reached the Supreme Court in 1979.

The plaintiffs argued that their rights grew out of their terminal status, which removed them from ordinary considerations about safety or effectiveness. In rejecting this argument, the Supreme Court referred to a history of "purportedly simple and painless cures for cancer, including liniments of turpentine, mustard, oil, eggs, and ammonia; peat moss; arrangements of colored flood lamps; pastes made from glycerin and limburger cheese; mineral tablets; and 'Fountain of Youth' mixtures of spices, oil, and suet . . ." and found that terminal patients also require regulatory protection, particularly given their vulnerability to fraudulent cures.

Citing an often-heard concern, the Court accepted the argument that if an individual suffering a potentially fatal disease rejects conventional therapy in favor of a drug with no demonstrable curative properties, the consequences can be irreversible. That a terminally ill patient by definition faces no real possibility of reversal was not accepted by the Supreme Court, as "[e]ven critically ill individuals may have unexpected remissions and may respond to conventional treatment. . . . A patient can be said to be terminal only after he dies." Critically, the essential right to make medical choices grounded in a constitutional right of privacy and self-determination were not raised in *Rutherford.*

In forecasting whether the Court may ever recognize a right to patient autonomy and choice, a careful reading of *Roe v. Wade*[81] and its progeny, which established privacy rights for contraceptive choices, offers some surprising guidance. The language in these cases suggest that the Supreme Court was not as impressed with the right of a woman to have an abortion as it was distressed at the idea that the state would have the right to impose upon the medical judgment of the physician. This reaction by the Court is consistent with the great deference with which courts have treated the judgments of medical physicians in virtually all areas of the law. This deference has been a significant source of the difficulty faced by CAM providers, as the courts turn to the very profession whose professional bodies have opposed CAM approaches for guidance in how these matters should be addressed. With this background, it may be less surprising that a right to choose treatment not approved by professional medicine was not found.

Privacy Rights and the Ninth Amendment

When privacy rights have been argued, courts have almost universally rejected this argument as well. The issue has been raised about various therapies[82] such as nutritional and herbal treatments for cancer.[83] The one remarkable exception to this trend is *Andrews v. Ballard*,[84] in which a Texas court found a statute restricting acupuncture to the hands of medical physicians unconstitutional, finding that the right to privacy includes the right to access the health care of one's choice. Much of the court's reasoning was based upon those cases in which patients have been found to have a right to accept or decline treatment; the court saw the choice of the type of treatment to be a logical consequence of these holdings. Unfortunately, courts have generally declined to follow *Andrews*.[85,86]

Another effort to gain a judicial recognition of medical freedom lay in the Ninth Amendment to the United States Constitution, which provides that "The enumeration in the Constitution of certain rights shall not be construed to deny or disparage others retained by the people."

The argument is that the right to seek the health care of one's choosing is a fundamental constitutional right "retained by the people." Courts have unequivocally ruled that the argument for medical freedom based upon the Ninth Amendment has no legal merit.[87] The only rights courts have found within the meaning of the amendment are those in the "'traditions and [collective] conscience of our people' . . . ranked as fundamental."[88] While those seeking alternatives to Western care would certainly rank such freedom as fundamental, the

courts have disagreed. These are consistent with definitive case law that allows states the greatest possible latitude when regulating the public health and safety.

Some holistic practitioners place a statement about the patient's rights under the Ninth Amendment in their consent forms; the problem with these forms is that all they accomplish is to document awareness of practice outside the law and need of a constitutional protection that is absent.

► THE ROLE OF EXPERIENCE IN CLINICAL AND LEGAL JUDGMENTS

It is widely recognized that the adoption of CAM approaches follows experience more than publication. When physicians and others turn to CAM approaches out of need, or experience the wellness advantages of modalities such as massage or nutritional modification, it is their experience, more than peer-reviewed studies, that brings them to participation. This affects legal results as well, as the law is also based upon deference to prevailing scientific views of what practices are sensible as much as what is "proven."

While randomized trials are seen as the gold standard for scientific validation, the decisions of regulators, prosecutors, courts, and scientists is to some extent based upon their view of the mechanisms of action. The real test may be whether a therapy fits within our world view. If one cannot conceive of how the treatment could work, evidence of efficacy may meet insurmountable obstacles of disbelief. Claims that do not fit preconceptions become extraordinary claims. Conventional medicine therefore tends to place higher expectations of proof on CAM, following the old maxim of the skeptic that "extraordinary claims require extraordinary proof." Over time, many claims that were once "extraordinary" are now recognized, as the level of evidence finally overcomes this skepticism.

The converse of this maxim is that therapies that fall within the expected paradigm are often uncritically accepted. As a result, therapies accepted by established medicine have frequently been the subject of headlines in which well-accepted, presumably evidence-based practices may in fact be no better than placebo or potentially dangerous, such as hormone replacement therapy[89,90] or arthroscopic knee surgery for osteoarthritis.[91] While continuing research may suggest a role for these therapies, the presumption of safety and effectiveness is more questionable than belief in them originally allowed. Yet, together, these few treatments affect the majority of patients in the United States and billions of dollars in medical spending.[21]

Perceptions, more than uncertain realities, create standards of care. As more physicians experience the value in legitimate CAM approaches for themselves, not only does quality of care improve for patients, but the legal atmosphere for physicians improves as well. Both continuing research and scientific validation on the one hand, and greater acceptance of therapies successfully practiced for centuries (in some cases for millennia), on the other hand, are critical for continuing legal safety as well as professional development.

► CONCLUSION

Practicing integrative therapies does take some special attention to risk and regulatory concerns. While many CAM therapies can be practiced in legal safety, an aspect of the nonstandard nature of some therapies is that they can exist in a legal "gray" zone, a limbo in which it may be hard to give complete assurance that no agency or patient will take exception. Physicians who believe such therapies can be useful to their patients in these cases must make decisions about how risk-adverse they are. Understanding the basic legal precepts about proper practice will greatly reduce one's exposure to legal risks, whether simply incorpo-

rating basic therapies such as vitamin therapies or acupuncture, or exploring more radical approaches such as experimental cancer drugs.

A legal maxim worth noting is that the law is 10 years behind the culture. This appears to be true here, as legal changes more accepting of CAM, such as portended by the White House Commission or the FSMB guidelines, are now arriving. Physicians in the near future should anticipate a continuing trend toward greater acceptance and less risk. Much of this development is circular; as more and more physicians accept responsible integrative practice, the courts and agencies will become more accepting as well.

REFERENCES

1. *Boyle v. Revici,* 961 F.2d 1060 (2d Cir. 1992); *Schneider v. Revici, M.D., and Institute of Applied Biology, Inc.,* 817 F.2d 987; 1987 U.S. App. LEXIS 5725; 22 Fed. R. Evid. Serv. (Callaghan) 1493.
2. Adamson TE, Bunch WH, Baldwin DC Jr, et al. The virtuous orthopaedist has fewer malpractice suits. *Clin Orthop.* 2000;(378):104–109.
3. Pfifferling JH. Ounces of malpractice prevention. *Physician Exec.* 1994;20(2):36–38.
4. Cohen MH, Eisenberg DM. Potential physician malpractice liability associated with complementary and integrative medical therapies. *Ann Intern Med.* 2002;136(8):596–603.
5. Dumoff A. Malpractice liability of alternative/complementary health care providers: a view from the trenches. *Altern Complement Ther.* 1995; 1(4):248–253, 1(5):333–334.
6. Dumoff A. Including alternative providers in managed care—managing the malpractice risk (parts I & II). *Med Interface.* 1995;8(5):95–97, 1995;8(6):127–128.
7. Cohen MH. *Beyond Complementary Medicine: Legal and Ethical Perspectives on Health Care and Human Evolution.* Ann Arbor, MI: University of Michigan Press; 2000.
8. Cohen MH. *Complementary and Alternative Medicine: Legal Boundaries and Regulatory Perspectives.* Baltimore, MD: Johns Hopkins University Press; 1998.
9. Lauretti WJ. The comparative safety of chiropractic. In: Redwood D, ed. *Current Controversies in Chiropractic.* New York: Churchill Livingstone; 1997.

10. Studdert DM, Eisenberg DM, Miller FH, et al. Medical malpractice implications of alternative medicine. *JAMA.* 1998;280(18):1610–1615.

11. AMA. House of Delegates of the American Medical Association, Resolution 55. December; 1974.

12. Norheim AJ, Fonnebo V. Acupuncture adverse effects are more than occasional case reports: results from questionnaires among 1135 randomly selected doctors, and 197 acupuncturists. *Complement Ther Med.* 1996;4:8–13.

13. Florida Statutes Ann., § 456.41 (2001).

14. ANCCAOM Brochure. Available at: http://www.nccaom.org/. Accessed November 24, 2002.

15. Walker PC. Evolution of a policy disallowing the use of alternative therapies in a health system. *Am J Health Syst Pharm.* 2000;57(21):1984–1990.

16. Available at: http://www.medicalacupuncture.org/aama_marf/aama.html. Accessed November 24, 2002.

17. In the Matter of Glenn Warner, M.D. Washington State Medical Quality Assurance Board, License revoked 7/14/95. https://fortress.wa.gov/doh/hpqa1/Application/Credential_Search/profile.asp. Accessed 9/5/03.

18. *Guess v. Bd. of Medical Examiners,* 967 F.2d 998 (4th Cir. 1992).

19. In the Matter of Binyamin Rothstein, D.O. Maryland Board of Physicians Case No: 94-0718; 1997.

20. Connick N. Before the State Board of Dental Examiners, State Board of Colorado. Case No. 95-04. In the matter of the disciplinary proceedings regarding the license to practice dentistry in the State of Colorado of Hal A. Huggins, D.D.S., License No. 3057. Feb 29, 1996.

21. Dumoff A. Protecting ACM physicians from undeserved discipline: legislative efforts in Maryland. *Altern Complement Ther.* 2002; 8(2):120–126.

22. The text of these laws can be found at http://www.healthlobby.com (accessed October 14, 2002) the web site of Monica Miller, the lobbyist instrumental in some of these state efforts. The states with legislation include Alaska, Colorado, Florida, Georgia, Louisiana, Massachusetts, Nevada, New York, North Carolina, Ohio, Oklahoma, Oregon, Texas, and Washington state.

23. Federation Services. Special Committee on Questionable and Deceptive Health Care Practices, a report to the Federation of State Medical Boards' governing body, April 1997. This report is available at: http://www.fsmb.org. Accessed 1/5/03.

24. The Model Guidelines are available at: http://www.fsmb.org. Accessed 1/5/03.

25. Lazarou J, Pomeranz B, Corey PN. Incidence of adverse drug reactions in hospitalized patients: a meta-analysis of prospective studies. *JAMA.* 1998;279:1200–1205.

26. Kohn L, Corrigan J, Donaldson M, eds. *To Err is Human: Building a Safer Health System.* Washington, DC: National Academy Press; 1999.

27. Centers for Disease Control and Prevention. Fourth Decennial International Conference on Nosocomial and Healthcare-Associated Infections. *MMWR Morb Mortal Wkly Rep.* 2000; 49(7):138.

28. *Wilk v. American Medical Association,* 895 F.2d 352 (7th Cir. 1990) (finding the AMA violated antitrust laws by banning its members from referring to chiropractors.)

29. Weeks J. Natural product sales: life saver for CAM networks. *Integr Bus Altern Med.* 1999; 4(5):6.

30. AMA. Council on Ethical and Judicial Affairs, H-385.972 *Capitation Method Of Payment* (Sub. Res. 87, I-90).

31. Dumoff A. Medical board prohibitions against physician supplements sales: a critical review. *Altern Complement Ther.* 2000;6(4):226–236.

32. Bross ID. Is toxicity really necessary? II. Sources and analysis of data. *Cancer.* 1996;19:1785–1795.

33. Moss RW. *Questioning Chemotherapy.* New York: Equinox; 1995.

34. Moore MJ, Tannock IJ. How expert physicians would wish to be treated if they developed genitourinary cancer [abstract no. 455]. *Proc ASCO.* 1988;7:118.

35. *Washington Legal Foundation v. FDA,* 340 U.S. App. D.C. 108; 202 F.3d 331 (D.C. Cir. 2000).

36. See, for example, K.A.R. § 100–28a-8 (Kansas Administrative Regulations).

37. 21 U.S.C. § 321(g)(1).

38. Diamond WJ, Cowden WL, Goldberg G. *The Alternative Medicine Definitive Guide to Cancer.* Tiburton, CA: Future Medicine Publishing; 1997.

39. Friedman M. Internal FDA memo from later acting FDA commissioner, October 31, 1991.

40. Jaffe R. FDA abuse and retaliation: Dr. Stanislaw Burzynski. *Townsend Letter for Doctors.* 1995.

41. Moss RW. *The Cancer Syndrome.* New York: Grove Press; 1980.

42. Moss RW. *The Cancer Industry: Unraveling the Politics.* New York: Paragon House; 1989.

43. Kennedy R. Immune therapies for cancer. Available at: http://www.medical-library.net/sites/framer.html?/sites/_immune_therapies_for_cancer.html. Accessed November 24, 2002.

44. Dumoff A. Defining "disease:" the latest struggle for turf in dietary supplement regulation. *Altern Complement Ther.* 2000;6(2):95–104.

45. 21 C.F.R. § 101.74.

46. 21 C.F.R. § 101.73.

47. 21 C.F.R. § 101.75.

48. 21 C.F.R. § 101.76.

49. Dietary Supplement Health and Education Act of 1994, codified at 21 U.S.C. §§ 321, 331, 342, 343, 343-2, 350, 350b; 42 U.S.C. §§ 281, 287c-11.

50. 21 U.S.C. § 343(r)(6).

51. Federal Register: 65;4:999–1050 January 6, 2000.

52. Office of Inspector General, Department of Health and Human Services, CLIA Regulation of Unestablished Laboratory Tests, July 2001 (OEI-05-00-00250). The regulations governing CLIA are found at 42 C.F.R. 493 *et seq.*

53. Available at: http://oig.hhs.gov/oei/reports/oei-05-00-00250.pdf. Accessed November 24, 2002.

54. Nev. Rev. Stat. § 630A.020 *et seq.*

55. Rev. Code Wash. § 43.70.470 (2003).

56. Available at: http://acupuncture.com/StateLaws/StateLaws.htm. Accessed November 22, 2002.

57. MD Code Health Occ. § 14-306.

58. *Foster v. Board of Chiropractic Examiners.* 359 S.E.2d 877 (Ga. 1987).

59. *In re Stockwell.* 622 P.2d 910, 914 (Wash. 1981).

60. 42 U.S.C. § 42-1395nn and 42 CFR § 411.350.

61. 42 U.S.C. § 42-1320a-7b(b) and 42 CFR 1001.952.

62. Dumoff A. Regulating professional relationships: kickback and self-referral restrictions on collaborative practice. *Altern Complement Ther.* 2000; 6(1):41–46.

63. Eisenberg DM, Kessler RC, Foster C, et al. Unconventional medicine in the United States. *N Engl J Med.2* 1993;328:246, 251.

64. Eisenberg DM, Davis RB, Ettner SL, et al. Trends in alternative medicine use in the United States, 1990–1997: results of a follow-up national survey. *JAMA.* 1998; 280(18):1569–1575.

65. Center for Medicare Services. *Medicare Carrier Manual.* § 2050. Available at www.cms.gov.

66. *Physician's Current Procedural Terminology CPT—2002.* Denver: AMA Press; 2002.

67. *International Classification of Diseases: 9th Revision; Clinical Modification.* Denver: AMA Press; 2003.

68. 42 C.F.R. § 405.420.

69. Health Insurance Accountability and Portability Act of 1996, Pub. L. No. 104–191 (Aug. 21, 1996) (HIPAA), 18 U.S.C. § 1035 (false statements regarding health care); 18 U.S.C. § 1347 (criminal health care fraud); and the two primary Medicare proscriptions, 42 U.S.C. § 1395nn (physician self-referral proscription) and 42 U.S.C. § 1320a–1327b(b) (antikickback proscriptions); and 31 U.S.C. § 3729–3733 (civil false claims act).

70. See, for example, *HHS v. Virginia Livingston, M.D.,* United States District Court in the District of Columbia Case No. 89–2281-OG, which discusses the administrative record in this case.

71. Information is available at: http://www.alternativelink.com. Accessed September 8, 2003.

72. Statement of Michael Beebe, Director of CPT Editorial and Information Services, American Medical Association. Hearing before the National Committee on Vital and Health Statistics, Subcommittee on Standards and Security, May 30, 2002.

73. National Committee on Vital and Health Statistics, Subcommittee on Standards and Security [transcript]. April 10, 2002. Available at:http://www.ncvhs.hhs.gov/020410tr.htm#discussion. Accessed June 6, 2002.

74. Available at: at http://www.apma.net/. Accessed September 8, 2003.

75. Minn. Stat. § 146A.01 *et seq.*

76. See http://www.minnesotanaturalhealth.org/billtext.htm.

77. See, for example, *Matter of Quinlan.* 348 A.2d 801 (N.J. Super. Ct. Div. 1975), *modified.* 355 A.2d 647 (N.J. 1976); *In re Boyd.* 403 A.2d 744 (D.C. 1979).

78. *Rutherford v. United States.* 442 U.S. 544, 99 S. Ct. 2470, 61 L. Ed. 2d 68 (1979).

79. Food, Drug, and Cosmetic Act, 21 USCS § 355.

80. 21 USCS § 321(p)(1).

81. 410 US 113 (1973).

82. *Majebe v. North Carolina Bd. of Medical Examiners.* 416 S.E.2d 404, 407 (N.C.Ct.App. 1992) (finding no privacy right to practice unconventional medical approach, such as acupuncture).

83. *People v. Privitera.* 591 P.2d 919 (Cal. 1979) (there is no right of privacy that requires the state allow access to laetrile).

84. *Andrew v. Ballard.* 498 F. Supp. 1038 (S.D. Tex. 1980).

85. See, for example, *Majebe v. North Carolina Board*

of Medical Examiners, 416 S.E.2d 404 (N.C. Ct. App. 1992) (MD physician had no privacy right to practice acupuncture).

86. There have been some other cases supporting such a right. See, for example, *Rogers v. State Board of Medical Examiners,* 371 So.2d 1037 (Fla. Dist. Ct. App. 1979).

87. *US v. Vital Health Products,* 786 F. Supp. 761, 777–778 (E.D. Wisc. 1992), *aff'd* 985 F.2d 563 (1993).

88. *Griswold v. Connecticut,* 381 U.S. 479, 493 (1965).

89. Rossouw JE. Risks and benefits of estrogen plus progestin in healthy postmenopausal women: principal results from the Women's Health Initiative Randomized Controlled Trial. *JAMA.* 2002; 288:321–333.

90. White E. Hormone replacement therapy in relation to breast cancer. *JAMA.* 2002;287: 734–741.

91. Moseley JB, O'Malley K, Peterson NJ. A controlled trial of arthroscopic surgery for osteoarthritis of the knee. *N Engl J Med.* 2002;347: 81–88, 132–133.

PART VI

Selected Cases in
Integrative Medicine

CHAPTER 37

Selected Cases in Integrative Medicine

MaryBeth Augustine, Karen Erickson, Benjamin Kligler,
Roberta Lee, Suzanne Little, Arya Nielsen,
Aurora Ocampo, Edward Shalts, and Lauren Vigna

In this chapter, we use three cases studies from the Continuum/Beth Israel Center for Health and Healing to illustrate some of the possibilities inherent in the integrative approach to health and illness. The first is a case of recurrent otitis and respiratory infection in a young child; the second is that of a middle-aged woman with fatigue and recurrent inflammatory symptoms; and the third is an older woman with cardiovascular disease, anxiety, and chronic pain. In each of these cases, the patient was seen at the Center by a multidisciplinary team, each of whom made a distinct and important contribution to the person's treatment. Our hope is that these cases will illustrate how the diverse voices of the various healing arts that comprise the integrative health care team can come together in a given case to offer an approach to treatment much more powerful than that which any of the disciplines can provide on their own.

Of course, the manner in which these cases were handled by our team represents only one of the many ways in which these patients' problems could have been effectively treated. Because we view the patient and/or the family as the primary decision maker on the health care team, our choices for therapies and approaches in these cases were guided in large measure by the patients' previous experience, personal preferences, and intuition, as well as by our clinical experience and knowledge of the evidence. Different people presenting with these same sets of problems could very well have been treated in dramatically different ways in each of these scenarios, and still with potential benefit.

▶ Case Example 1: Jared C.

Description

Jared first came to our practice as a newborn in February 2000. He is the first child in his family, and the product of a normal, uncomplicated full-term pregnancy. His birth was unremarkable as was his initial newborn period.

Family history is remarkable for asthma in his father, as well as childhood eczema. Jared was breast-fed for the first 4 months of life and his growth and development during his first year were normal. He was vaccinated according to a modified schedule as per his parents wishes, receiving diphtheria, tetanus toxoids and acellular pertussis (DTaP) and *Haemophilus influenzae* type b (HIB) immunizations at 2, 4, and 6 months but deferring polio and hepatitis B vaccinations to the second year. Jared started in day care at 4 months of age, 3 days per week.

At 7 months of age, Jared developed a cough and fever; this was treated conservatively in our office and seemed to resolve. At 8 months of age he again developed cough and fever, this time with rapid respiratory rate. On our advice by phone the parents had him seen at a local emergency room, where he was diagnosed with bronchiolitis, treated with nebulizers, and released, on albuterol syrup. His fever continued; when seen in our office 2 days later for follow-up he had a right otitis media. This was treated conservatively and his fever resolved. However, 1 week later he again developed a worsening cough, with his parents reporting that he "was having a hard time catching his breath." In the office, at that point, he had expiratory wheezing bilaterally and looked fairly ill; the right tympanic membrane at this point was dull and still slightly red with persistent effusion. Our impression at this point was reactive airway disease, possibly asthma, with a persistent middle ear effusion. He was treated with albuterol syrup and referred for craniosacral therapy at this point. Based on his mother's wish to treat as actively as possible, he was also given Zithromax for the otitis. The next day his mother called to report discharge from the ear, from a ruptured tympanic membrane, with rapid resolution of his fever and discomfort.

One month later (now 10 months of age) Jared presented again with fever and otitis. Because of the perforation on the previous episode, we opted to treat more aggressively and gave Cefzil. This episode resolved quickly. One month later he was seen again in the emergency room for respiratory distress accompanied by fever. He was started on oral steroids.

Integrative Primary Care Physician Perspective: Benjamin Kligler

At this point, we were seeing a pattern of both repeated episodes of otitis and repeated episodes of respiratory distress, probably asthmatic in nature. Based on conversations with the parents and previous experience in our practice with similar cases, we recommended a more aggressively proactive prevention-oriented approach to these two conditions consisting of a combination of nutritional manipulation, frequent chiropractic/craniosacral treatment to assist both with pulmonary function and with eustachian tube drainage, and homeopathic treatment to address what appeared to be an underlying constitutional vulnerability in these areas. We recommended a change from a milk-based formula to a soy-based formula, as well as avoidance of other dairy-containing products. Elimination of dairy, and at times other food groups, including wheat, soy, and citrus, can be helpful in certain children with recurrent upper respiratory illness.

The conventional approach to the child with recurrent otitis relies mainly on repeated courses of antibiotics, followed by suppressive antibiotics if needed, and then, ultimately, by myringotomy, especially if there is evidence of hearing loss and/or language delay. Although these approaches can be helpful for certain cases, they do have drawbacks, and should be applied only in cases where more conservative natural approaches have been unsuccessful. The repeated use of antibiotics, for example, has potential consequences both for the individual patient—in whom it can disturb the intestinal flora repeatedly, potentially leading to recurrent diarrhea and to an increased susceptibility to food sensitivities as a consequence of intestinal dysbiosis—and for the public health—in that antibiotic-resistant microbes that are now widely prevalent are thought to have emerged in part in response to the overuse of antibiotics in treating childhood otitis and respiratory infection.

The integrative approach seeks to address the recurrent ear and respiratory problems by addressing the underlying causes: nutritional inputs predisposing to systemic inflammatory response; structural problems in eustachian tube drainage and lung function potentially addressed by manipulative approaches; and predisposing constitutional or energetic factors potentially addressed by homeopathy.

Homeopathic Perspective: Edward Shalts

Jared struck me as a very personable, beautiful child. I felt immediately closely connected with him. And he immediately connected with me. I invited him to sit on my lap and he did. He was a nice, smiley little boy. Extroverted, open, with an abundance of energy, Jared could not stay still in my office. He started walking early. He did not speak yet, but was very easy to communicate with.

This first impression played a very important role in the selection of the homeopathic remedy. As in any type of healing practice, the data obtained from direct observation is very important for a homeopath. I also knew that he developed ear and upper respiratory infections early in his life. Jared had a history of serious diaper rashes that tended to be located more in the genital area. His father had a history of kidney stones. I learned that he had a lot of energy at night. Calming him down before sleep was a bit of a task. His skin was somewhat oily. I learned that his favorite position in sleep was on his abdomen, and that earlier in life he used to sleep in genupectoral position.

In such a young person, much of the information a homeopath uses is not necessarily readily available. Consequently, the choice of homeopathic remedy for an infant or a toddler requires very close observation and an intensive knowledge of homeopathic pharmacology. A homeopath has to be able to pay very close attention to even small details of the person's behavior and family history. In many cases, previous experience of successfully prescribing to similar individuals (although not necessarily for the same nosological problem) can be of tremendous help. For me, the combination of extreme extroversion, history of intense perineal rash, family history of kidney problems, early onset of upper respiratory problems and otitis, oily skin and genupectoral position in sleep pointed to the homeopathic remedy Medorrhinum. One dose of Medorrhinum 200c caused a very significant improvement in Jared's condition. It had to be repeated only once or twice in a course of a year.

I have to say that this course of treatment is more the norm than the exception in general homeopathic practice. Medorrhinum is the remedy very frequently indicated for children with chronic respiratory problems and asthma. Herscu provides one of the best clinical descriptions of this remedy available to date.[1] As in any other medical discipline, however, generalizations are often inaccurate, and prescribing specific homeopathic remedies for serious chronic conditions requires years of education and expertise.

Medorrhinum belongs to the class of Nosodes. Nosodes are homeopathic preparations of various secretions. Medorrhinum is a nosode of gonorrhea. It is a sterile lysate. The basic preparation from which the remedy is diluted and potentized corresponds to 0.01 mL of secretion per mL of distilled water, This dilution is frozen at $-20°C$ ($-4°F$) and then thawed at room temperature; this procedure is done four times successively. The lysate obtained is filtered through a sterilizing membrane, then distributed in 10-mL fractions in sterile containers. These fractions are freeze-dried for preservation. The freeze-dried product of each container is dissolved in 100 mL of sterile distilled water. This final solution is filtered through a sterilizing membrane. It is used as the starting point for preparation of homeopathic dilutions. (From the *Homeopathic Pharmacopeia of the United States*, 1988.)

Chiropractic Perspective: Karen Erickson

The clinical research shows that chiropractic is an effective technique for reducing the frequency and severity of recurrent otitis media in children. This has certainly been my experience in treating Jared and other infants and children at the Center. Chiropractic care and cranial sacral therapy works by helping to drain the eustachian tubes, thereby reducing the opportunity for infection to develop. In young children, the eustachian tubes are still horizontal and can more easily occlude, allowing the middle ear to fill with fluid. With cranial development and growth, the eustachian tubes become more vertical, allowing them to more easily drain. This makes them less susceptible to infection. Additionally, in Jared's case, gentle lymphatic massage was used to help drain the cervical chain lymph nodes. This technique was taught to the parents so they could support his care between visits. As with any child under my care, I did a full spinal evaluation. Although no serious abnormalities were found I did notice restrictions in the cervical spine.

The philosophy of chiropractic care is to restore the normal relationship between the structure and function of the body, which, in part, is modulated by the nervous system. Through the proper alignment and function of the upper cervical spine and cranium, we are able to assist the natural healing capabilities of the body to prevent recurrent otitis media. Treatment of the sinus reflexes is often an important component of care in these cases, as sinus congestion is often a concomitant condition with otitis. Reflex points over the maxillary and frontal sinuses are gently pressed or tapped to facilitate drainage. Often, a postnasal drip cough is heard during or after the treatment, as fluid drains down the back of the throat. This usually only lasts a short time, perhaps no more than an hour, and is a sign that drainage is occurring. In very rare cases, we may see a child with a particularly chronic history who develops a fever after this drainage. It is as if we are releasing pathogens that have been confined to the eustachian tube and sinuses back into the system at large and the child's immune system reacts with a fever. Usually this is mild and short-lived. In our Center, there is a close collaboration between the patient's family, the physician, and myself. This type of communication is essential in monitoring a child's progress.

Occasionally, essential oils containing eucalyptus, lavender, lemon, and wintergreen among others are used to help improve lymphatic circulation and reduce the inflammation of otitis and the surrounding musculoskeletal imbalances. However, we do not add essential oils when homeopathic remedies are being used as some essential oils might interfere with the effect of the homeopathic remedies.

Jared was treated a total of 6 times over a 3-month period. This is a typical treatment plan for chiropractic care in a case like this. Parents should monitor their child for factors that might make the recurrence of otitis more likely, such as colds or flu, swollen cervical lymph nodes, excessive stress, falls, injury to the neck or spine, or poor diet. At these times, an additional chiropractic evaluation and treatment might be warranted.

Follow-up

Jared did very well following the combination of homeopathic and chiropractic treatment. During his next upper respiratory illness at age 12 months, he ran a high fever as he had previously but did not develop any wheezing or other respiratory distress. At that time, he also had a left serous otitis media, which resolved over the following month. At 20 months he developed a right otitis media, which was treated with mullein-garlic drops for pain control, but without antibiotics. Parents were encouraged to resume the craniosacral therapy at this point which they had stopped several months earlier. One month later he again developed high fever and was seen at an emergency room and diagnosed with acute otitis and treated with amoxicillin. Because the pattern of the previous winter seemed to be repeating itself, we recommended a repeat visit with the homeopath. Chiropractic therapy was also continued. Again, he responded well and over the following 6 months had no further episodes of otitis and no respiratory difficulties despite at least two upper respiratory infections.

Jared has now moved out of the area but we recently heard from his parents that he has been healthy and will be turning 5 years old next summer.

► Case Example 2: Hannah T.

Description

Hannah is a 47-year-old woman who first came to our practice 2 years ago. She came primarily with the complaint of fatigue, reporting that over the 2 years prior to her first visit she had persistent tiredness, much more than she felt could be blamed on having a young son. She had been diagnosed by her previous physician as having "subclinical hypothyroidism"—symptoms of hypothyroidism despite normal function as measured on laboratory testing—and started on a low dose of Armour thyroid (15 mg). Her fatigue symptoms had responded somewhat to this treatment but she remained unsatisfied with how tired she felt upon awakening in the morning.

Hannah had a medical history significant for tonsillectomy as a child, hospitalization for pneumonia at age 15 years, and mild childhood asthma. She was frequently on courses of antibiotics during her early years for these recurrent upper respiratory problems. She also had several months of severe abdominal pain in her early twenties for which she eventually underwent laparoscopy with no clear diagnosis. This pain gradually resolved and has not recurred.

In addition to her complaint of fatigue, Hannah also reported frequently recurrent vaginal yeast infections over the past 2 years. She has one sexual partner, her husband, and is confident that he is monogamous. She has generally treated these yeast infections with over-the-counter antifungals, and has taken an oral antifungal on two occasions. Her most recent episode of vaginitis was last month. Hannah reports that her menstrual periods have become shorter in duration and lighter over the past year. They remain regular, occurring every 28 days; however she believes she is perimenopausal. Her mother entered menopause at age 46 years. This is a somewhat saddening experience for her because until recently she was considering having a second child and she now feels this would no longer be possible.

Hannah also complains of recurrent facial rash, which has been diagnosed in the past as rosacea. She has been prescribed both topical and oral antibiotics for this condition but has resisted taking them for fear of worsening her vaginal infections. She reports that she feels the skin condition is worse during periods of higher stress.

She describes her mood as "down," but does report enjoying the company of her husband and son. She is a potter, and has enjoyed this work in the past, but reports difficulty finding time to do this over the past year. She has produced pottery professionally in the past, but is not doing so now. Hannah describes her marriage as "stable and supportive," and does take pleasure in caring for her son as a full-time mother. Her son is now 4 years of age and healthy, except for mild eczema. Hannah reports no problems with sleep. She does report that her libido is fairly low, but states that this has been the case for several years and that

it has not posed a problem in her marriage. She began seeing a psychotherapist 1 year ago and has found this somewhat helpful; she plans to continue with this therapy, which she describes as "insight-oriented therapy."

Hannah describes her diet as "basically good," reporting that she tries to eat at least two servings of fruits and vegetables daily, tries to eat fish or chicken as the main sources of animal protein, and avoids snack foods and processed foods as much as possible. She has always been slim, and remains so currently; she reports a stable weight over the past 2 years.

Mind–Body Medicine Perspective: Suzanne Little

This is one of those challenging presentations where nothing is acutely wrong, but many things are at least somewhat wrong. Hannah just feels poorly all over, her symptoms recur and never fully resolve, and this is frustrating to her because the clinical findings are nebulous. The working diagnosis—fatigue—is one of exclusion, and most of the interventions she has tried have missed the mark.

What is warranted at this point is a health prescription to boost her entire system—a mind–body tune-up. Hannah is functioning at a low, lethargic level, so it is not surprising that her mood is also muted; I wonder if she is not actually downplaying her emotions. What seems to be missing is vitality, a feeling of joy and hope about life. I get the sense that her sadness is about loss and yearning—a sense of being personally unfulfilled. She seems to lack a quality of "generativity," which Erik Erikson thought gave purpose and meaning in midlife. This is a woman who mourns that she cannot have another child because she is fated for premature menopause like her mother; she's an artist who is not making art; and a wife who doesn't feel sexually aroused. And her lack of expressiveness is consistent with functional somatic disorders, where the focus is on what is external, concrete, and "fixable."

The tendency, as a provider, is to offer a patient like this a long list of recommendations—try this, change that, do this, take that—but this runs the risk of making her feel more helpless and ineffectual. She is not managing her response to stress very well. So, a good therapeutic place to begin is to confront the sadness and helplessness—but constructively. First, one could ask, is there a core belief that supports the idea that *she can't get well*? Core beliefs are a kind of structure around which symptoms take root. The thought could be, "I am too tired to help myself," or "I need someone stronger than myself to rely on," or "It's easier to avoid difficulties than to face them." If she can identify an operating belief, she can also disprove it. We can help in that process by giving her a graded task she can succeed at—such as increasing physical activity over time—because it is intrinsically motivating to effect tangible change. Second, we can frame physical activity as a way to "wake up" her spirit. We can use whatever she responds to—breathing, visualization, biofeedback, physical exercise—to increase body aliveness. It's easy to overlook how we can lose touch with our bodies, go into a kind of passive, sensory numbness, where fatigue or sadness becomes a natural state, and a kind of tacit alienation results, in which one feels physically disengaged. This poses a challenge for mind–body work; it erodes self-compassion, breeds demoralization, and chips away at feeling competent or authorized to take care of oneself.

All the symptoms she initially talked about—rosacea, allergies, vaginitis—seem to be related, and suggest something is going on with the whole person that is much larger than any single or simple condition. I think there is a picture emerging here of a lot of things "flaring up." To me, the idea of inflammation is interesting because it suggests heat, a generative force, gone awry, like an electrical charge that cannot find a ground and simply fizzles out. So, inflammation, a nonspecific body defense, can be seen as an intense reaction with no place to go. I have learned from Arya Nielsen that from an East Asian medicine perspective, reactivity to exogenous agents always has an endogenous basis, and I agree. There's a lot of emphasis on this woman's external problems, but why aren't they being addressed on an internal level? We have to ask ourselves what is being defended against? And why is that defense failing? Her behavior, in contrast to her physical symptoms, seems to be one of *underreactivity*. So we have this intriguing juxtaposition where the body is breaking out, the skin gets raw and rashy, there's vaginal overgrowth, she is basically on immune overdrive, and yet, subjectively, she is physically and emotionally depleted, lacks libido, and feels resigned to her circumstances. It's as if she doesn't protest enough, perhaps because her body is doing it for her.

I want to address the point of dealing with inflammation as an expression of psychic reactivity. If you consider the problem of misplaced heat or energy psychically, it can be construed, perhaps, as bound up anger that eventually peters out and becomes fatigue. As providers we often unwittingly take on the suppressed feelings, and then get irritated without knowing why. I think this accounts in part for the subtle pressure to *do* something, or to get the *patient* to do something, which is a way of getting rid of the discomfort. The thyroid gland, site of the fifth Chakra, is the organ of speech, but I think it is fair to say she is not giving voice to what is bothering her. Of course, it is not as simple as encouraging her to say what's on her mind; it's a matter of helping her become more conscious, more awake. A spiritually based therapy could help her reengage with what inspires her most deeply; it could fire up her artistic passions and give her a healthier, more creative channel for energy and expression.

Treatment of "Subclinical" Hypothyroidism: Benjamin Kligler

Hannah's case from the physician perspective is quite complex—an intersection between possible thyroid dysfunction, perimenopause, depression, and functional fatigue. I focus here on the use of thyroid hormone in this situation.

The treatment of hypothyroid symptoms in the context of normal laboratory indicators of thyroid function has been called, somewhat incorrectly, treatment of "subclinical" hypothyroidism. In fact the presence of symptoms makes "subclinical" not the correct label, and this condition, which has not been accepted to date by conventional endocrinology as a legitimate indication for thyroid hormone therapy, might be more appropriately named "laboratory-euthyroid hypothyroid state." The fact is many patients do present with fatigue, constipation, dry skin, and other potentially thyroid-related symptoms, requesting treatment with low-dose thyroid replacement. The rationale proposed for this treatment is that in some cases, current laboratory testing is not accurate enough to detect dysfunction either in conversion of T_4 to T_3 or in the more subtle dimensions of thyroid-related intracellular signaling systems.

In our experience, this approach can be helpful in some patients and so long as thyroid function is maintained within the normal laboratory range it does not seem to pose any risks. Low axillary temperature is

sometimes used as a marker for this condition, but functional markers—that is, target symptoms—are often more useful in determining whether the therapy is effective. We typically start at a low dose of a T_3/T_4 preparation (Armour or Thyrolar, for example) and titrate to symptoms while monitoring laboratory values to keep thyroid function tests within normal range. In Hannah's case, she came to us already on a dose of Armour thyroid, which she felt had led to some improvement in her symptoms but, as is often the case in these complex, multidetermined clinical situations, not as great an improvement as she had hoped for. Her thyroid function tests were within normal range, so we opted, at her request, to continue her current dose of Armour (15 mg) for whatever benefit it was bringing her.

Functional Medicine Perspective: Roberta Lee

Fatigue is a challenging condition with many possible etiologies. Its description as a medical complaint reflects a loss of optimal function that forces the diligent practitioner to consider a wide range of possible medical causes involving multiple systems which may contribute to this functional imbalance. Facing this particular problem through the framework of a reductionistic "lens" brings with it the assumption that the array of tests available to the clinician will be enough to highlight exactly where the imbalance lies. Following this line of reasoning, one assumes that the basic pathophysiology will be revealed, a plausible explanation for the patient's symptoms will be evident, and a treatment plan subsequently obvious to the practitioner. However, as we know, clinical medicine can often defy this assumption and this case represents one of those instances.

One of the reasons in this case for Hannah's fatigue, as in many cases of fatigue, may be that Hannah's condition represents a synergistic malfunction rather than a dysfunction in a single system. A second reason for the challenging nature of the diagnosis in this case may be that our reductionistic model might be ignoring certain pathophysiologic systems that provide information that explain the malfunction. Looking at the intestinal "terrain" may be one of the key systems that has been ignored in her previous medical assessments.

The functional medicine model of gut dysbiosis suggests that the predominant organisms that live in the gut serve to either augment the digestion of needed nutrients for the host (the patient) or to create potentially toxic substances, which can contribute to a subtle shift in physiologic function as a negative effect. This dysfunction is mediated through an increase in permeability of the intestinal wall to very small particles that "leak" through the intestine. In severe gut dysbiosis, the villi of the small intestine become flattened and unhealthy. The end result of this process is the loss of efficient absorptive capacity to transport some nutrients while simultaneously letting in others which may be undesirable. Conditions that create this intestinal imbalance include the repeated use of antibiotics without adequate replenishment of the "good" organisms. This particular patient does have such a history, having been repeatedly given antibiotics to treat recurrent upper respiratory problems. The consequence of this "leaky gut syndrome" is the presentation of small antigen particles to the macrophages in the liver and the gut-activated lymphatic system; this can cause an upregulation of inflammatory cytokine production, leading, in turn, to increased systemic inflammation. The possible clinical manifestations of this process in Hannah's case include the recurrence of her facial rash with worsening during periods of stress. The influence of stress

as a contributor to systemic inflammation has been well-documented in the psychoneuroimmunology literature. Fatigue can also be a manifestation of systemically upregulated inflammatory processes; thus gut dysbiosis could very well be contributing to Hannah's primary complaint.

Further adding to the complexity of this case is Hannah's age and family history, which suggest an early transition into menopause. She is having normal but subtle signs of transition into a state where estrogen levels, although cycling, may be lessening. Estrogen is excreted in the urine and bile after being conjugated in the liver.[2] If the gut milieu is dysbiotic, the predominant "bad" gut flora can uncleave the conjugated excretory estrogen products, allowing reabsorption back into the body. This has been described as the enterohepatic recirculation of estrogen and its metabolites. At any given time, depending on the influences of cortisol, nutrition, and oxidative stress, one can see alterations in the predominance in the circulation of the different forms of estrogen. At times of higher concentrations of 16α-hydroxyestrone and 4-hydroxyestrone (toxic estrogen metabolites), a patient may experience more perimenopausal symptoms than when 2-hydroxyestrone (a more favorable estrogen metabolite) predominates. The end result of all the above may partially account for Hannah's increasing moodiness, a propensity for vaginal dryness interpreted as "vaginal infections," and a drop in libido.

The role of the adrenal glands as a secondary reservoir of estrogen also becomes critical in menopause: as ovarian production of estrogen decreases, the adrenals become a more primary source of estrogen. In addition, as the pathways of sex steroid synthesis shift in menopause, the synthesis of progesterone, which is derived from cholesterol and pregnenolone, may be altered as well, resulting in progesterone levels either too low or too high relative to the concentrations of estrogen. With added stress there may be further drains on estrogen production as catecholamine releases from the adrenals increase.

The strategy for treating gut dysbiosis in this particular patient to help correct or rebalance these subtle physiologic shifts was to add daily supplements of acidophilus, green tea extracts, glutamine (restores the intestinal villi), and alternating fish oil and flax seed meal (to increase both lignans and omega-3 fatty acids). In addition, we recommended increasing indole-3-carbinol-containing foods in the diet (e.g., broccoli), and reducing the consumption of high-glycemic-index foods, which can also up-regulate inflammation through their influence on insulin metabolism. It is important to note that this nutritional approach can be somewhat slow to take effect, often requiring a minimum of 2 months to show an impact on clinical markers.

East Asian Medicine Perspective: Arya Nielsen

There is not a thyroid per se in East Asian medicine. The functions attributed to thyroid in the West are the province of several traditional East Asian organs and channels, so each hypothyroid patient has a unique organ/channel configuration. In Hannah's case, the thyroid was the branch, not the root of her problem. Treating her hypothyroidism, whether subclinical or frank, may not represent a comprehensive or effective intervention.

In treating Hannah, I thought her history of repeated use of broad-spectrum antibiotic therapy without restorative measures was significant. Antibiotics are considered "cold" medicines that can injure the stomach and spleen, interfering with digestion and absorption. She was presenting to us noticeably underweight with signs of blood deficiency and errant heat. Her pale complexion with pale tongue and slight menses corroborated her blood deficiency. The errant heat manifested as damp heat and stasis in the lower burner in the form of chronic fungal leukorrhea and constipation, and heat in the stomach and lung channels congesting at the face in the form of acne.

I like how Suzanne Little put it by saying her "generativity" was lacking. The aphorism in East Asian medicine that applies to Hannah is "earth feeds all"; in clinical terms, this means that digestion is central to well-being. If the earth element is not working, the blood becomes deficient and heat congests, with ensuing fatigue, depression, acne, constipation, and potentially subclinical hypothyroidism. If the digestion is good, then vitality and tissues are maintained and the ability to generate in the world is sustained.

The intervention I used with Hannah had to resolve the errant heat in the short-term and nourish the blood and vitalize in the long-term. I placed a lot of emphasis on restoring the digestion as the root treatment. I used acupuncture, herbs, diet, and other recommendations, reinforcing also the functional medicine approach of restoring gut ecology. It was also very important to eliminate coffee. The use of caffeine fatigues people who are already tired. Coffee, even decaffeinated, depletes the Qi and can create errant heat in the form of flushing.

Hannah had also been eating a large amount of bread. Whereas some people cannot eat bread because they are allergic to wheat, gluten, or yeast, others do not do well with it because they do not break it down completely. The physical nature of incomplete digestion of bread is cloying, leading to constipation. This seemed to be true for Hannah. As we eliminated bread, of course we also virtually eliminated gluten, and Hannah responded well. In many patients, there is a relationship between gluten sensitivity and failing thyroid, and this may explain part of the benefit Hannah experienced.

As it was her acne cleared, the vaginitis resolved, and her bowels became regular, so many of the subclinical thyroid signs resolved. She began to try for a second child, reflecting a change in the "generativity," of her earth element. At this point, she also decided to discontinue the thyroid medication. She has periods of relapse, but never to the extent of original severity. She feels better and is happy about that, but also expresses appreciation for knowing more about what helps her be well. I think where it stands now for Hannah is finding "what is asking to be born of her."

The Physical Exam and Somatic Rapport

LITTLE: What do you think is the importance of the physical exam in the integrative approach to the patient? Does one find a significant physical finding very often? Do patients expect an exam? Do patients generally get anxious if you don't do an exam?

KLIGLER: Some patients definitely do. But there is currently one school of thought in medicine that states that because the physical exam is not an evidence-based procedure, it does not add any benefit to the annual screening visit, and so it should be de-emphasized in favor of lifestyle counseling and other interventions more proven to be beneficial. This group believes that we should limit the "physical exam" to blood pressure checks and Papanicolaou smears, as these are the only interventions that have actually been shown to make a difference. But patients don't necessarily agree with this approach.

NIELSEN: I would think the physical exam is important in helping develop a somatic rapport. In East Asian medicine, you consciously engage in a somatic rapport as well as a cognitive discourse. Somatic rapport starts with noticing how the patient walks in the door, and continues through the visit as part of every element that assesses the patient. And the point is not necessarily just to get information, like heart rate and breath sounds as in the case of a medical exam. There is a shared physical journey that is reassuring, healing even. It goes deeper than the cognitive exchange alone.

KLIGLER: Well, I'm not saying there's no value to the physical exam in certain clinical settings; I'm talking about solely in the context of the initial screening.

NIELSEN: I agree, and it also probably matters what the patient brings in terms of issues whether you can or need to do a physical exam at first meeting. It's unfortunate that the more technological medicine gets in terms of diagnosis, the less touching of a person takes place. I am not suggesting that any touch would build rapport, but that the skills of assessment through palpation are valuable because it's where the patient lives. In that body.

LITTLE: It is very interesting, because for the physician, the stethoscope enables you to "hear" them. Patients want to be listened to, and this can be another tool, even if symbolic at times, to facilitate that listening. Also, frequently, a patient comes in thinking, "No matter what I say, you already know things that I don't know about myself, so I want you to hear me, on a very deep level, because there may be things that you know and I don't know."

KLIGLER: The physical exam does mean a lot to people, and I don't think that meaning is adequately captured in the evidence-based analyses of screening techniques.

NIELSEN: The real question is are you doing what you are doing only to find or rule out something—signs of severe disease or life-threatening illness. An integrative practitioner is involved in something more. We are looking to be effective in short-term, yes, but also to establish a long-term relationship of somatic trust with the patient and the patient's family.

KLIGLER: And the long-term goal is to promote wellness. This is much more difficult to measure in terms of evidence-based analysis. But one could argue that if that's really the goal, then what we should institutionalize in the initial visit would be some other sort of physical contact, and it doesn't have to be the physical exam. It could be part of the way we make contact with the person physically; the exam may, in fact, be an old-fashioned way to do that.

VIGNA: A handshake seems too formal and a hug too personal. . . .

NIELSEN: Yes, it's finding what you are comfortable with to open and close a session.

KLIGLER: It does come back to the dilemma of how important is determining evidence-based practice, as opposed to art? And that's a lot of what this discussion is about: the art of medicine, the art of the doctor–patient relationship.

NIELSEN: The critical question, again, is what evidence exactly are we looking for to demonstrate that a given intervention is or is not worthwhile? Presence or absence of disease? What about the value of a good therapeutic relationship that also teaches a person how to be present, how to be well, and ensures ongoing collaboration?

KLIGLER: Evidence of a good therapeutic relationship that then has positive outcomes in the long-term is not what most people are talking about with evidence-based medicine. They are talking much more about the question of whether listening to the patient's lungs does or does not increase my probability of detecting lung cancer. The fact is, however, that both streams of thought are legitimate—we need both evidence-based medicine to inform our care, and a firm connection to the art and intuition of medicine. The challenge currently is that there is a giant juggernaut of evidence-based medicine, to a degree to which the art of medicine and the intangible, unprovable dimensions of healing relationship are not being adequately emphasized.

► **Case Example 3: Mary S.**

Mary is a 69-year-old woman who initially came to our practice in January 2002. She was 6 months postcoronary artery bypass surgery and came to us looking for help with an integrative approach to promoting cardiovascular health and minimizing her risk of further coronary artery disease progression. Fortunately, she had no history of myocardial infarction prior to her surgery; her coronary artery disease was diagnosed during a work-up for new-onset angina, and she went to surgery rather than angioplasty because of significant left main coronary artery stenosis.

Prior history was significant for a long history of hypertension, intermittently controlled with medications; however, because she had experienced side effects from multiple antihypertensives, there were a number of extended periods over the 15 years since her diagnosis of hypertension during which her blood pressure was not well-controlled. She also had a history of hyperlipidemia, for which she was at her initial visit taking Lipitor. Mary had a distant history of smoking, having stopped 10 years prior to her surgery, no history of diabetes, and no significant family history of heart disease.

Her other major presenting problem was left hip pain with sciatica, as well as ongoing pain at the site of her cardiac surgery scar. At the time she was taking Tylenol with codeine intermittently for this pain, and recently had been requiring this almost daily; physical therapy had not been helpful, and she did not tolerate nonsteroidal antiinflammatory drugs because of gastrointestinal upset. The hip pain was constant, although typically worse when she was stationary for a long period of time, and at times radiated down the posterior left leg.

Medical history was otherwise significant for Hashimoto's thyroiditis, diagnosed 30 years earlier and stable on thyroid replacement medication.

Mary is widowed, with two grown sons and three grandchildren. One son is in the New York area with no children; the other is in California. In the past year, she had been unable to travel to visit her grandchildren because of her back pain and she views this as a major loss. Mary is a retired school administrator and enjoys reading. She does have a network of friends, although three of her close friends have been ill over the past year and she has not been able to see them very often.

Mary's physical examination was remarkable for blood pressure of 140/80, a systolic murmur, and mild peripheral edema. Mary's mood was upbeat, although she did report a fair amount of loneliness in recent months as a consequence of her growing disability from her back pain. She also reported an ongoing sadness since the events of 9/11 with occasional bouts of significant anxiety, in which she was particularly focused on the safety of her children and grandchildren. This did not tend to occur prior to 9/11. She also reported feeling more tired than she would like to. Her cardiologist did not feel that this was cardiac in origin as her ejection fraction and left ventricular function were normal.

Mary was followed by a cardiologist in whom she has great confidence. Recently, however, he had been urging her to add a fourth antihypertensive medication and she was reluctant based on her experience of adverse effects from multiple medications in the past. He was aware of her visit to the Center for Health and Healing and was supportive of her wish to pursue other approaches to blood pressure and lipid control as long as these were done cautiously and he was kept informed.

Medications at the time of her initial presentation were atenolol, Zestril, Dyazide, Lipitor, enteric-coated baby aspirin, Synthroid, and Tylenol with codeine. She takes a multivitamin. She reported that she tries to keep to a "low-fat" diet in general.

Laboratory tests on initial evaluation were all normal, with total cholesterol 162, low-density lipoprotein 102, high-density lipoprotein 43, thyroid function in normal range, and homocysteine 7.2.

Integrative Physician Perspective, Initial Evaluation: Roberta Lee

Integrative medicine seeks to understand the whole person, addressing the mind, body, and spirit. In order to explore this perspective with Mary, I began my 90-minute visit by asking her, "What brings you here today?" She replied that in the past 6 months she had a significant event happen—coronary bypass surgery—and she was experiencing difficulty with fatigue. This fatigue was especially severe when she went to cardiac rehabilitation. Her coach was encouraging her to push herself physically to improve cardiovascular resilience, but she was anxious about pushing too hard.

Mary brought all of her medical records from her internist and cardiologist for me to review. She volunteered that she had recently had a "great report" from her cardiologist, and was told that she had normal left ventricular function and ejection fraction; but this knowledge did not seem to comfort her. When I asked her why, she volunteered that prior to her surgery she had been following her primary care physician's recommendations for hypertension, hyperlipidemia, and hypothyroidism, but the surgery made her feel like a failure. Furthermore, she felt "isolated and trapped" by her fatigue: she was afraid that every time she had shortness of breath it represented another anginal episode. She was afraid to travel, she missed her grandchildren, and noted that she felt isolated. She felt like much of her focus these days was attending to all the doctor visits and was especially alarmed at her cardiologist's suggestion that she add another medication to control her hypertension. With each medication that was added, she felt less in control of her health.

When I asked Mary if she had anything in her life that she enjoyed, she remarked upon her inability to concentrate on reading. Her closest friends had been ill and this added increasing tension within, as she wanted to spend time with them but could not because of her medical conditions. Furthermore, she was not sleeping well. Her primary care physician had offered her a medication to help her sleep through the night (Ambien), but she decided that she would approach this using a more integrative approach. I asked her, based on past experiences, if she could recall how anxiety usually manifested itself. She replied that under pressured circumstances she would sleep more, but that she did not feel rested after sleep. For a number of years when she slept excessively she would have more aches and pains, with the discomfort usually focused in her lower back. However, with her recent anxiety she would also awaken in the middle of the night. Her first thoughts on these awakenings were always to notice whether she was experiencing any difficulty with chest pressure or palpitations.

Mary revealed that once she had seen a TV show explaining progressive relaxation and simple breathing techniques and found it intriguing. She was interested in exploring this. I taught her a simple breathing exercise in the first visit. I asked her to sit comfortably in the chair, focus on her breath, breathing in to a count of four through her nostrils, holding her breath to a count of seven, and exhaling through her mouth to a count of eight with her tongue on the roof of her mouth (this is a breathing technique that I learned from the Program in Integrative Medicine). Her instructions were to practice this breathing twice a day, four breaths in the morning and four in the evening. She felt this was too much for her. I asked her if there was something else she found relaxing. She remarked how much she enjoyed walking, but never seemed to have enough time to do this. We decided that rather than implementing the breathing exercises twice a day, she would walk for 20 minutes in the morning and before retiring she would sit comfortably and practice her breathing exercise before going to sleep. I suggested that the most important aspect of these exercises were really to make them part of a daily routine.

I screened for signs of depression, asking about suicidal ideation, but Mary denied any plans for action or feelings of significant despair. We acknowledged that she could be mildly depressed with anxiety present, especially in view of her recent slide downward after 9/11. A recommendation to consider psychological counseling was made during this first visit.

We moved on to exploring her diet. She recently had stopped adding salt to her food, but admitted that she did not actually understand the relationship between sodium and hypertension. We explored the need to begin reading labels for sodium. I began to explain the relationship of cholesterol and coronary artery disease to omega-3 fatty acids, *trans*-fatty acids, and saturated fat. I suggested specific protein sources that represented sources containing less saturated fat (fish, lean chicken, and soy). We discussed the need to have five to seven servings of fruits and vegetables in her daily diet. She expressed a wish to learn more about nutrition, so I suggested that she might benefit from nutritional consultation.

We reviewed her medications and with the exception of her antihypertension medication she had been on most of her medications for more than a year. She did not take any supplements. The statin family of hypolipidemic medications have been reported to deplete coenzyme Q10 stores in the body, so I suggested that she begin by taking 200 mg/d of this supplement. In addition, I also suggested that she take 2 tablespoons of flax seed meal a day to increase fiber and omega-3 content. Garlic supplements are mildly hypolipidemic, and I recommended she add this at a dose of 1,000 mg/d (standardized to contain 6–10 mg alliin or 2–5 mg of allicin). In addition, I suggested that she take a daily multivita-

min containing the following vitamins and micronutrients for their possible role in preventing progression of heart disease: vitamin C (500 mg), vitamin E (mixed tocopherols and tocotrienols 800 IU), selenium (200 μg), folic acid (400 μg), vitamin B_{12} (500 μg), vitamin B_6 (50 mg), and mixed beta carotenes (25,000 IU). For prevention of osteoporosis, I also recommended adding calcium citrate 1,500 mg and magnesium gluconate 400 mg.

Mary raised the question of what alternatives were available for treatment of pain if she did not want to take a nonsteroidal antiinflammatory medication. I suggested either glucosamine sulfate (500 mg TID) with chondroitin sulfate (400 mg TID) or a combination of turmeric *(Curcuma longa)*, ginger *(Zingiber officinale)*, and boswellia *(Boswellia serrata)* in a blended product; these are botanical medicines with antiinflammatory activity.

Mary's exercise routine to this point had been guided by her cardiac rehabilitation team. I explained that deconditioning can occur with inactivity, and encouraged her to continue her rehabilitation. We explored the need to add stretches to her exercise regimen; balance is an aspect of physical health that is overlooked. We agreed that yoga even once a week might provide an enjoyable way to bring this dimension to her health. I suggested that physical activities like swimming and pool walking can be incorporated in substitution for the yoga.

We agreed to meet in 8 weeks. A long-range goal from Mary's perspective was to eventually reduce her antihypertensive medications. At the close of the visit, we prioritized the interventions in accordance with what seemed most important and potentially meaningful to her. Anxiety seemed to be a big obstacle and along with it her inability to relax. I therefore recommended a series of visits with Aurora Ocampo, our clinic mind–body specialist. In addition, as Mary had a desire to learn more about the applications of nutrition to her cardiovascular/hypertensive history, we agreed on a nutritional consult as part of the treatment plan. For pain relief—and a different perspective on her overall health—I also recommended acupuncture. To prevent "overmedicalizing" Mary's treatment, we agreed to reevaluate each of these interventions and the treatment plan as a whole after 2 months.

Mind–Body/Energy Medicine Perspective: Aurora Ocampo

In collaboration with the patient and the physician, I chose to use the following approaches to help manage the hypertension and anxiety of this patient: biofeedback, guided imagery, Reiki, and essential oil therapy. I believed that biofeedback would work particularly well as a relaxation training strategy for this patient. This technique is particularly effective in eliciting the vasodilatation response that can help control blood pressure. Mary was extremely motivated to make it work. Adding to this motivation was the fact that she had experienced significant side effects from her multiple antihypertensive drugs and her blood pressure remained uncontrolled.

Biofeedback training is virtually the opposite of any drug treatment; rather than relying on an external input (the medication) to lower blood pressure, it teaches the patient to use their internal resources for the same purpose. It allows the patients to remain totally in control, responsible, and empowered to work it out for themselves. It is a useful tool that allows them to learn self-regulation. This can be particularly effective in a patient such as Mary for whom anxiety is a significant contributor to hypertension. I learned on my first visit with her that her blood pressure control had become much

worse after 9/11 as a consequence of her increased anxiety. This confirmed my belief that, especially given her high motivation level, biofeedback would be an effective approach.

I also used imagery, Reiki, and essential oil therapy to complement biofeedback. My experience with these modalities with other patients has been that these additional techniques can greatly enhance the relaxation-oriented management of anxiety and hypertension.

The goal of the treatment that Mary and I agreed to during our first visit was the recognition and minimizing of the stress and anxiety in her everyday life through the learning and home practice of relaxation skills, which can also reduce the blood pressure.

During the first session we discussed the rationale of the treatment, what the feedback equipment does, how it is used, and the immediate temperature training goals. We also discussed how the mind and the body work together and how through imagination (imagery) she could easily affect the temperature of her hands. The average person cannot tell the temperature of their hands within 4–5 degrees; the sensitivity of the temperature feedback machine, however, can detect and feedback to the patient subtle changes in the activity of the sympathetic nervous system as reflected in hand temperature change. This feedback signal can be used to teach the patient how to consciously control a process (vasodilatation) that is normally not controlled by the conscious mind. Because vasodilatation leads to decreased blood pressure, this approach is extremely useful in treatment of hypertension.

The peripheral vascular system, which controls surface body temperature, does not have significant parasympathetic innervation. The smooth muscles of the blood vessel walls that control vasoconstriction are almost completely regulated by the level of sympathetic nervous system input. Because of this, blood flow in the hands and other peripheral areas is easily affected by stress. Because it responds so readily to changes in stress level, hand temperature is a particularly effective feedback measure.

In the first biofeedback training session, the thermistor was attached to the index finger of the dominant hand. I then gave instruction on breathing technique and a 15-minute autogenic session with heaviness, warmth, and inner quietness phrases. The initial hand temperature (26.1°C [79°F]) was recorded; the temperature was recorded again at the beginning of each phrase. At the end of the autogenic session, the patient shared the thoughts and emotions she felt during the session. At the conclusion of the first session, the temperature unit was turned toward the patient and we reviewed the current temperature and the recorded temperatures during the session in the context of her inner experience of relaxation. Her hand temperature ranged from 33.9°C (93°F) to 35.6°C (96.1°F). Her blood pressure was lowered to 140/70 from 160/88 at the start of the session. This was a very successful first experience, and I encouraged Mary to go forward with her home practice as instructed and to return to me in 1 week to continue with the training. She was instructed to use the "script" of autogenic phrases that were used during her session with me as part of the home practice.

During the second session, a review of the home practice experience revealed that Mary was practicing the techniques throughout the day as instructed. Her blood pressure following this second session was lowered to 130/70; the hand temperature during this session was maintained between 32.2°C (90°F) and 35°C (95°F). Reiki and essential oil therapy were also used during this session to further enhance the treatment. These techniques often allow the patient to achieve an even deeper state of relaxation during the session.

After 2 weeks of home training, the patient was instructed to discontinue the use of the autogenic phrases (the script) and to replace them with her own personal visualization relating to the temperature control. She chose the image of lying on a sunny, warm beach. The transition from scripted phrases to a more personal image allows the patient to realize that the use of set phrases or listening to a recorded tape is unnecessary to initiate a desirable physiological behavior. I strongly recommended to Mary that regular home practice with relaxation, warmth, and breathing exercises be done until the newly developing skill at handling stress "becomes a way of life." This can often take several months.

At the third and final session several weeks later, the patient determined that she had the self-mastery of the techniques that she needed to continue to apply this approach to her everyday stressful life. Mary shared with me descriptions of several incidents of acute stressful situations and how she was able to cope with these using her practice of breathing, imagery, and hand warming. I encouraged her to continue her practice and to come back as needed for refresher sessions.

East Asian Medicine Perspective: Arya Nielsen

Mary and I decided it was best for us to focus on several unresolved problem areas that were significant to her but not addressed by her cardiologist beyond ruling out disease. These problems were the pain in her chest from the surgery itself, the scar that had healed with a disturbing keloid that pulled and was sore, her general anxiety, and her hip pain. Her hip pain and sciatica were preventing her from participating fully in cardiac rehabilitation. The anxiety she identified was both in relation to the 9/11 disaster that she had witnessed and to her surgery. She was still in the process of learning how to interpret sensation in her changed body and her changed world.

Because Mary was already taking a few medications and a number of supplements prescribed by Dr. Lee, I opted to forego herbs, even though there are options in the East Asian pharmacopeia specific to cardiac and hypertensive cases. We relied on acupuncture and gua sha to resolve the sciatica right away so she could comfortably begin exercising.

Mary experienced anxiety reduction during acupuncture treatment for her heart and chest, and this worked synergistically with the skills she was learning with Aurora Ocampo to reduce anxiety on her own. After the first 2 months of weekly treatments, her chest pain resolved completely, and she could exercise without dyspnea. As her condition improved, she began to question the need for some of her medications, feeling her blood pressure was too low. She addressed those questions to her physician who adjusted her medication.

Each time I treated Mary, I also used acupuncture to reduce the keloid scar. Our first sessions eliminated the pulling pain she suffered, breaking the adhesion of the scar tissue from deeper fascia so the skin at her chest could move. Over time, the keloid cord has become softer and smaller in width and height.

The East Asian medicine perspective is that even a necessary corrective surgery still represents a trauma with all the attending forms of stasis and altering of channel pathways. The very definition of pain in East Asian medicine is that something is "stuck." In Mary's case, acupuncture and gua sha were used together to resolve the blood stasis that had resulted from her surgery and to restore proper channel function. Blood stasis at the chest is felt as oppression and heaviness. In this sense, anxiety is not considered a mind state alone. Removing the blood stasis clears the sensation of chest oppression resolving anxiety associated with it.

Mary is now doing very well in cardiac rehabilitation and is able to push herself physically; this has also greatly improved her stamina and health status, while enabling her to lose some weight. She sustained a slight shoulder injury that is common with people returning to exercise programs, and this was also easily treated.

Nutritional Medicine: Mary Beth Augustine

My primary goal on my initial visit with this patient was to develop a nutritional plan that would help her with her hypertension. I have used the DASH (dietary approach to stopping hypertension) diet extensively in this setting, and found it extremely effective in the motivated patient. I was very impressed with Mary's motivation level, and felt she was ready to make some significant changes in her diet. Her body mass index was 34 on this initial visit, which concerned me, given her history of coronary disease, but I opted not to focus on weight control in our visit as I believed this was not her top priority. I have also found that in certain patients the DASH diet leads naturally to weight loss, without a need to identify weight control as a specific goal.

After taking the initial diet history, I made the following initial recommendations to Mary:

1. 1 or more pieces of fruit at breakfast every day; minimize fruit juices and concentrate on whole fruits to help with fiber intake

2. 1 cup of cooked or raw vegetables at both lunch and dinner every day
3. 1 leafy green salad daily
4. 1 yellow-orange-red colored fruit or vegetable daily
5. 1 citrus fruit daily
6. Cruciferous vegetables every other day
7. 1 oz nuts every other day

In addition, I recommended that she eat fish at least once a week and ideally as often as four times per week; fish intake and omega-3 essential fatty acid intake are effective in reducing risk of adverse cardiac events. Sardines, canned tuna, herring, and anchovies are all good options because they do not contain high levels of mercury. I also recommended a specific dish—Tuscany tuna salad, which contains tuna, white beans, olive oil, olives, vinegar, walnuts, and canned tuna. The Mediterranean diet, in which many of these ingredients play a major part, also lowers cardiac risk. Garlic and onions are also important components in this diet, and I recommended liberal consumption of these for Mary.

We also discussed the possible use of hawthorne berry extract and of herbal teas and/or supplements for lipid-lowering effects, but we chose to focus on the dietary measures outlined above for this first visit and held these herbal options in reserve for possible use in the future. We also discussed weight management as a goal for future visits, as Mary's body mass index did put her in a high-risk category for cardiovascular disease.

On our follow-up visit 6 weeks later, I was pleased to find that Mary was doing quite well with the DASH diet, and that her blood pressure control appeared to be improving. At this point, she and I decided to add weight loss as a second goal in hopes of increasing the impact of her diet on her hypertension. I also made a set of additional recommendations aimed at enhancing cardiovascular health. Our plan at this second visit was as follows:

1. Continue with the DASH diet.
2. Decrease/limit wheat intake; Mary reported a heavy emphasis on wheat-containing foods in her diet and moving toward a more low-glycemic-index/higher-protein diet seemed the best approach to weight control for her. I suggested substituting lentil pastas for wheat pastas, taking more brown rice as a carbohydrate source in moderate amounts, and trying other grains such as quinoa and spelt.
3. Decrease simple sugars overall, especially sorbet, which she was eating almost daily at this point.
4. Increase her emphasis on allium family vegetables, including leeks, shallots, onions, and garlic to take advantage of their potential lipid-lowering effects.
5. Increase red-purple-blue fruits and vegetables, including cabbage, radishes, eggplant, grapes, and berries, as sources of cardioprotective flavonoids.
6. Drink 1 cup daily of a "cardioprotective" tea containing hawthorne, green tea, raspberry leaf, blueberry, and elderberry, again as a good source of flavonoids.

Integrative Physician Follow-up: Roberta Lee

Mary was seen 8 weeks after our initial visit for follow-up. She reported that she was sleeping more soundly, especially after she initiated a daily relaxation exercise and breathing exercises that Aurora Ocampo and I had taught her. Her acupuncture sessions reduce her chest pain, dyspnea, and sciatica, so Mary could resume cardiac rehabilitation. She continued her cardiac rehabilitation and now reported improved exercise tolerance. She felt "less scared."

She now had somewhat improved blood pressure readings, mostly because her anxiety was reduced, but still clearly had hypertension. At this visit, Mary spoke of her need to look at this anxiety in greater depth and now has made a commitment to undergo cognitive therapy.

Because one of her major initial goals was to reduce her medication intake, and because she had shown significant improvement in her blood pressure control, we decided to eliminate one of her hypertensive medications. This was done with the caveat that she report daily blood pressure readings on a weekly basis. Parameters for unacceptably high readings were set in case she rebounded, at which point she would resume the removed medication and notify me of the change. We agreed on regular follow-up visits at intervals of 6–8 weeks. Mary has continued to do well on this combination of therapeutic approaches and we anticipate being able to reduce her antihypertensive medications further as she continues to progress.

REFERENCES

1. Herscu P. *The Homeopathic Treatment of Children.* Berkeley, CA: North Atlantic Books; 1991:91–138.

2. Speroff L, Glass R, Kase N. *Clinical Gynecologic Endocrinology and Infertility.* 6th ed. Philadelphia: Lippincott Williams & Wilkins; 1999.

Index

Page numbers followed by *f* indicate figures, by *t* indicate tables.

intended use of, 119
intestinal permeability and, 469
intestinal system motility and, 461
Latin names of, 112
literature sources on safety and drug interactions, 127–28t
misbranding, 123–24
pharmacologic actions of, 110
pharmacologic drugs vs., 108, 111–12
poisonous plants, 107
preparations, 112, 114
in prescription drugs, 108, 109t
production techniques, 114–15
product labels, 112, 113f
quality control, 115, 117, 124
restricted for children, 130t
safety classifications for, 121t
safety standards and regulation, 110–11, 119–30
secondary active constituents, 111
self-regulatory safety labeling initiatives, 121–23
standardization issues, 111
as substitutes for pharmacologic drugs, 112
toxic medicinal plants, 119, 121–22, 123, 130t
whole-plant products, 111
Hernandez-Reif, M., 595
heroic medicine, 5–6, 108
herpes simplex 6, 515
Herrington, D. M., 819–20
Herscu, 880
HERS study, 816–17
high-efficiency particulate air (LHEPA) filtration, 614
hip arthroplasty, 169
hip fractures
falls and, 830
osteoporosis and, 295, 551–52
recovery from, 837
hip pain, 889, 894
hippocampal atrophy, 508
Hippocrates, 107, 153, 271
Hippocratic medicine, 184
dietetics, 72
Hippocratic Oath, 3
hippotherapy, 524
histamine, 243
Hitayu (public health), 222
hives. See urticaria, chronic
hoarseness, 568–69
hobby activities, 287t
Hochu-ekki-to, 638
Hofer, M. A., 43, 56
Hoffer, Abram, 653
Hoffman, David, 779
holding therapy, 730–31
holistic medicine, 5, 9

Ayurvedic medicine, 219
botanical medicine use in, 112
defined, 10
scientific study design and, 20–21
home birth, 697–99
Homeopathic Educational Services, 329
homeopathic immunotherapy, 614
Homeopathic Pharmacopeia of the United States, 258
homeopathic proving model, 20
Homeopathic Trust, 329
homeopathy, 255–69
for acute conditions, 261–69
acute vs. chronic conditions in, 261–63
for adenotonsillar disease, 581
for allergic conjunctivitis, 380
for asthma, 614
for atopic dermatitis, 720–21
case example, 879–80
centesimal dilutions, 258
certification, 261
for chronic fatigue syndrome, 423
"classical" vs. homeopathic polypharmacy, 262
clinical research, 261
concentrations in, 256
databases, 314
decimal dilutions, 258
defined, 255
for diabetes mellitus, 444
differential therapeutics in, 255
dilutions, 257–59
dose size, 257–59
efficacy of, 269
environmental sensitivity and, 389
for fibroids, 780
for fibromyalgia syndrome, 677
geriatrics and, 829
homeopathic evaluation, 259–60
for obstructive sleep apnea, 582
for otitis media, 574–75
for pain relief, 598
pregnancy and, 750–51
for premenstrual syndrome, 771
principle of similars, 255–56
principles of, 255–59
promptness of response in, 263
provings, 256–57
remedy choice in, 263
for schizophrenia, 655
for sinusitis, 579
skepticism of, 255, 269
theory of signatures, 255
training, 260
for vertigo, 586
websites, 324t, 329
Homeopathy Medicine Research Group, European Commission, 260

homeostasis, 39, 41, 43–44
home water filtration products, 346–47
HomInform, 314
homocysteine, 408, 506–7, 632
HONCode (Health on the Net Foundation), 323
honeysuckle (Lonicera japonica), 581
hopelessness, 31, 79
hormonal treatments, for fibroids, 777
hormone replacement therapy (HRT)
alternatives, 818–19
Alzheimer's disease and, 814
breast cancer and, 811–13
carbohydrate metabolism and, 815
colorectal cancer and, 813
contraindications, 811
delivery strategies, 798
diabetes mellitus and, 815
endometrial cancer and, 813
epithelial ovarian cancer and, 813
fracture risk and, 814
heart disease and, 815–17
hormone sources, 797–98
immune competence and, 818
osteoporosis and, 558–59
plant-sourced products, 798
risks and benefits of, 810–18
thyroid dysfunction and, 817–18
types of, 797–810
weight gain and, 818
hormones, in meat and dairy food, 558
horseradish, 579
Horvath, Karoly S., 729, 730
hospital privileges, for acupuncturists, 207
hostility. See also anger
health effects, 29–30
intestinal system motility and, 461
H_1-receptor antagonists, 374, 375
bridroga (heart disease), 236–37
britsbula (ischemic heart disease), 237
Huang qin, 426
Hughes, S., 713
human body, Ayurvedic structural and functional units, 226
human growth hormone, 554
human herpes virus, 418
human leukocyte antigen (HLA)-B27, 459
human vibrational matrix, 50
Hume, David, 5
humors, 3, 5
in East Asian medicine, 190
Greco-Roman tradition and, 72
"hunter-gatherer" diet, 139–40

CPSIA information can be obtained at www.ICGtesting.com
Printed in the USA
BVOW04*1450060815

411843BV00009B/167/P